AF778623

Essentials of Blood Product Management in Anesthesia Practice

Corey S. Scher • Alan David Kaye • Henry Liu
Seth Perelman • Sarah Leavitt
Editors

Essentials of Blood Product Management in Anesthesia Practice

Springer

Editors
Corey S. Scher
NYU-Grossman School of Medicine
Department of Anesthesiology
New York, NY
USA

Henry Liu
Department of Anesthesiology and Perioperative Medicine
Milton S. Hershey Medical Center
Penn State College of Medicine
Hershey, PA
USA

Sarah Leavitt
NYU-Grossman School of Medicine
Department of Anesthesiology
New York, NY
USA

Alan David Kaye
Departments of Anesthesiology and Pharmacology
Toxicology, and Neurosciences
Louisiana State University School of Medicine-Shreveport
Shreveport, LA
USA

Seth Perelman
NYU Grossman School of Medicine
Department of Anesthesiology
Perioperative Care and Pain Medicine
New York, NY
USA

ISBN 978-3-030-59294-3 ISBN 978-3-030-59295-0 (eBook)
https://doi.org/10.1007/978-3-030-59295-0

© Springer Nature Switzerland AG 2021
This work is subject to copyright. All rights are reserved by the Publisher, whether the whole or part of the material is concerned, specifically the rights of translation, reprinting, reuse of illustrations, recitation, broadcasting, reproduction on microfilms or in any other physical way, and transmission or information storage and retrieval, electronic adaptation, computer software, or by similar or dissimilar methodology now known or hereafter developed.
The use of general descriptive names, registered names, trademarks, service marks, etc. in this publication does not imply, even in the absence of a specific statement, that such names are exempt from the relevant protective laws and regulations and therefore free for general use.
The publisher, the authors and the editors are safe to assume that the advice and information in this book are believed to be true and accurate at the date of publication. Neither the publisher nor the authors or the editors give a warranty, expressed or implied, with respect to the material contained herein or for any errors or omissions that may have been made. The publisher remains neutral with regard to jurisdictional claims in published maps and institutional affiliations.

This Springer imprint is published by the registered company Springer Nature Switzerland AG
The registered company address is: Gewerbestrasse 11, 6330 Cham, Switzerland

Foreword

Blood and blood products have been experimented with and employed to treat clinical disease processes since the early 1600s. Today the indications for the therapeutic use of blood and blood products have expanded significantly. Recent outcome studies have found a wide range of beneficial indications for the use of blood or blood components. Today, in clinics and hospitals worldwide, the patient's own blood is harvested, and components are reinjected strategically to reduce inflammation and promote healing for a wide variety of clinical conditions.

The use and ordering of blood products based on clinical disease processes or procedural necessity can be a complex issue fraught with economic, physiologic, and religious matters. Knowledge of disease processes, patient risk factors, and modern-day testing specificity creates an ever-expanding knowledge base for the practicing clinician. A thorough understanding of standard practice involving appropriate testing, selection, and screening of donors, storage of blood products, compatibility testing, storage of donations, and clinical use indications are all requirements for today's practitioner.

Regarding blood needs and blood supply, the American Red Cross states that someone needs blood in the United States every two seconds, and less than 38% of the population has the ability or is eligible to donate blood or platelets. It is critical for those having surgery, receiving cancer treatment, experiencing a chronic illness, or someone involved in a traumatic injury that an intact blood supply exists. In the United States alone, nearly 21 million blood components are transfused yearly.

This book was created under the leadership of Corey S. Scher, MD, Henry Liu, MD, Seth Perelman, MD, and Alan David Kaye, MD, PhD all of whom are my long-time esteemed colleagues and friends. Together they have worked tirelessly to recruit experts from diverse medical fields and professional disciplines to share their expertise and knowledge in the following chapters. Students and professional practitioners alike will be able to utilize the material in this book both in their medical practice and for continued education. It is my honor to introduce Essentials of Blood Products and my hope that the reader will take deep satisfaction in their efforts to create a timeless volume of information that will continue our shared commitment to the Hippocratic Oath: "To treat the ill to the best of one's ability, to preserve a patient's privacy, to teach the secrets of **medicine** to the next generation, and so on."

Charles Fox, MD
President and CEO, Ochsner-LSU Health Shreveport
Professor and Chairman
Departments of Anesthesiology and Pharmacology,
Toxicology, and Neurosciences
Louisiana State University School of Medicine-Shreveport
Shreveport, LA, USA

Contents

Contributors

Alaa Abd-Elsayed, MD, MPH Department of Anesthesiology, University of Wisconsin School of Medicine and Public Health, Madison, WI, USA

Caroline Raasch Alquist, MD, PhD, D(ABHI) Transplantation Immunology Division, Hoxworth Blood Center, University of Cincinnati, Cincinnati, OH, USA

Ariunzaya Amgalan, BS Georgetown University School of Medicine, Washington, DC, USA

Prathima Anandi, MD Department of Anesthesiology, LSU Health Shreveport, Shreveport, LA, USA

Erica Ash, MD NYU Langone Medical Center, Department of Anesthesiology, Perioperative Care, and Pain Medicine, New York, NY, USA

Douglas R. Bacon, MD, MD Department of Anesthesiology, University of Mississippi Medical Center, Jackson, MI, USA

Philip G. Boysen II, MD, MBA, FACP, FCCP, FCCM Department of Anesthesiology, University of Mississippi Critical Care Organization, University of Mississippi Medical Center, Jackson, MS, USA

Jason M. Buehler, MD University of Tennessee at Knoxville Medical Center, Department of Anesthesiology, Knoxville, TN, USA

John C. Cargile, MD Texas A&M University – College of Medicine, Bryan, TX, USA

Baylor Scott and White Medical Center – Temple, Department of Anesthesiology, Temple, TX, USA

Samuel Carlson, BS Medical College of Wisconsin, Department of Anesthesiology, Wauwatosa, WI, USA

Joseph Cassis, MD University of Kentucky, Department of Anesthesiology, Lexington, KY, USA

Pierre Alex Casthely, MD NYU Langone Medical Center, NYU Department of Anesthesiology, Perioperative Care, & Pain Medicine, New York, NY, USA

Destiny F. Chau, MD Division of Anesthesiology, Children's Hospital of the King's Daughters, Department of Pediatric Anesthesiology, Norfolk, VA, USA

Luis Chabla-Penafiel, MD NYU Langone, Department of Anesthesiology, Perioperative Care, and Pain Medicine, Brooklyn, NY, USA

Karina Charipova, MD Georgetown School of Medicine, Washington, DC, USA

Lin Chen, MD, PhD Department of Anesthesiology, Hubei Women & Children's Hospital, Wuhan, Hubei, China

Chrissy Cherenfant, MD NYU Langone Health, NYU Langone Orthopedic Hospital, Department of Anesthesiology, Perioperative Medicine, and Pain Medicine, New York, NY, USA

Samuel Chijioke Onyewu, MBCHB Virginia Commonwealth University Health System, Department of Anesthesiology, Richmond, VA, USA

Hyung Sun Choi, MD Department of Anesthesiology, Montefiore Medical Center, Bronx, NY, USA

Alice Tolbert Coombs, MD, MPA, FCCP Virginia Commonwealth University Health System, Department of Anesthesiology, Richmond, VA, USA

Daniel E. Core, MS LSU Health Shreveport, Shreveport, LA, USA

Elyse M. Cornett, PhD LSU Health Shreveport, Department of Anesthesiology, Shreveport, LA, USA

Jayanth Dasika, MD University of Florida–Jacksonville, Department of Anesthesiology, Jacksonville, FL, USA

Joseph Dean, BS Virginia Commonwealth University School of Medicine, Richmond, VA, USA

Mario DeAngelis, MD Department of Anesthesiology, Methodist Division, Thomas Jefferson University Hospital, Philadelphia, PA, USA

Keith P. Delaune, MS4 Department of Anesthesiology, LSU Health Shreveport, Shreveport, LA, USA

Yi Deng, MD Baylor College of Medicine, Department of Anesthesiology, Houston, TX, USA

Hermandeep Dhami, MD New York University, Anesthesiology, New York, NY, USA

Monica M. DiLorenzo, MD The Mount Sinai Hospital, Department of Anesthesiology, Perioperative, and Pain Medicine, New York, NY, USA

Dallas L. Domangue Department of Anesthesiology, LSUHSC New Orleans, New Orleans, LA, USA

Abigail P. Erwin, BS, MD Candidate Department of Anesthesiology, LSUHSC New Orleans, New Orleans, LA, USA

Joshua M. Etienne, BS, MD Candidate Department of Anesthesiology, LSUHSC New Orleans, New Orleans, LA, USA

Lisa Farmer, MD Department of Anesthesiology, The University of Texas Medical Branch at Galveston, Galveston, TX, USA

Justin B. Feit, MD NYU Langone Health, NYU School of Medicine, Department of Anesthesiology, Perioperative Care, and Pain Medicine, New York, NY, USA

Mitchell C. Fuller, BS Froedtert Hospital, Medical College of Wisconsin, Milwaukee, WI, USA

Robert Gaiser, MD University of Kentucky, Department of Anesthesiology, Lexington, KY, USA

Meera Gangadharan, MD University of Texas Medical Branch, Department of Anesthesiology, Galveston, TX, USA

Andrew Jesse Garcia, PharmD George Washington University School of Medicine and Health Sciences, Department of Anesthesia, LSU Health Sciences Center, Washington, DC, USA

Michael Godbold, MD University of Tennessee Medical Center – Knoxville, Department of Anesthesiology, Knoxville, TN, USA

Eric Gomez, MD Department of Anesthesiology, Thomas Jefferson University Hospital, Philadelphia, PA, USA

Amanda L. Granier, BS, MD Candidate Department of Anesthesiology, LSUHSC New Orleans, New Orleans, LA, USA

Kyle Gress, BS Georgetown School of Medicine, Washington, DC, USA

Ryan T. Gualtier, MD Department of Anesthesiology Perioperative Care and Pain Medicine, NYU Langone, Department of Anesthesiology, New York, NY, USA

Erik M. Helander, MD Department of Anesthesiology, LSUHSC New Orleans, New Orleans, LA, USA

Louise Helander, MBBS University of Colorado, ClinImmune Labs, Denver, CO, USA

Amie L. Hoefnagel, MD Department of Anesthesiology, Jacksonville, FL, USA

Christopher Hoffman, DO Department of Anesthesiology, Thomas Jefferson University Hospital, Philadelphia, PA, USA

Hannah J. Hsieh, MD NYU Langone Health, Department of Anesthesiology, Perioperative Care and Pain Medicine, New York, NY, USA

Albert Hsu, MD University of Florida – Jacksonville, Department of Anesthesiology, Jacksonville, FL, USA

Liang Huang, MD, PhD Department of Anesthesiology, New York University Langone School of Medicine, New York, NY, USA

Jose C. Humanez, MD University of Florida – Jacksonville, Department of Anesthesiology, Jacksonville, FL, USA

Larry R. Hutson Jr., MD Texas A&M University – College of Medicine, Bryan, TX, USA

Baylor Scott and White Medical Center – Temple, Department of Anesthesiology, Temple, TX, USA

Mary Im, MD Department of Anesthesiology, Lewis Katz School of Medicine Temple University, Temple University Hospital, Philadelphia, PA, USA

Usama Iqbal, MD Department of Anesthesiology, NYU Langone School of Medicine, New York, NY, USA

George M. Jeha, BS Department of Anesthesiology, LSUHSC New Orleans, New Orleans, LA, USA

Yang Jiang, MD University of California Los Angeles School of Medicine, Department of Hematology and Oncology, Los Angeles, CA, USA

Robert Jungerwirth, MD NYU Langone Health, Department of Anesthesiology, Perioperative Care, and Pain Medicine, New York, NY, USA

Jennifer Kaiser, BS Medical College of Wisconsin, Department of Anesthesiology, Wauwatosa, WI, USA

Jay Karri, MD, MPH Baylor College of Medicine, Department of Physical Medicine and Rehabilitation, Houston, TX, USA

Daniel Katz, MD Icahn School of Medicine at Mount Sinai, Department of Anesthesiology, New York, NY, USA

Philip J. Katzman, MD University of Rochester Medical Center, Department of Pathology and Laboratory Medicine, Rochester, NY, USA

Alan David Kaye, MD, PhD Departments of Anesthesiology and Pharmacology, Toxicology, and Neurosciences, Louisiana State University School of Medicine-Shreveport, Shreveport, LA, USA

LSU Health Shreveport School of Medicine, New Orleans, LA, USA

Tulane School of Medicine, New Orleans, LA, USA

Samir Kendale, MD NYU Langone Health, Department of Anesthesiology, Perioperative Care & Pain Medicine, New York, NY, USA

Norma J. Klein, MD University of California Medical Center Davis (UCDMC), University of California, Davis, Department of Anesthesiology & Pain Medicine, Sacramento, CA, USA

Cody Koress, BS LSU Health Sciences Center, Department of Anesthesiology, New Orleans, LA, USA

Brandan Kovacs, MD New York University School of Medicine, Department of Anesthesiology, Perioperative Care, and Pain Medicine, NYU Langone Medical Center, New York, NY, USA

Fatoumata Kromah, MD, FASA Virginia Commonwealth University Health System, Department of Anesthesiology, Richmond, VA, USA

Dustin Latimer, MS Department of Anesthesiology, LSU Health Shreveport, Shreveport, LA, USA

Sarah Leavitt, MD NYU-Grossman School of Medicine, Department of Anesthesiology, New York, NY, USA

Mingqiang Li, MD, PhD Xiangyang Central Hospital, Department of Anesthesiology, Xiangyang, Hubei, China

Na Li, MD, PhD Hubei Women & Children's Hospital, Department of Anesthesiology, Wuhan, Hubei, China

Craig J. Lilie, MD Baylor Scott and White Medical Center – Temple, Department of Anesthesiology, Temple, TX, USA

Henry Liu, MD, MS, FASA Department of Anesthesiology and Perioperative Medicine, Milton S. Hershey Medical Center, Penn State College of Medicine, Hershey, PA, USA

Alaina Lofaso, MSIV LSU Health Shreveport, Shreveport, LA, USA

Sanjana A. Malviya, MD, MBA Baylor College of Medicine, Department of Anesthesiology, Houston, TX, USA

Deepinder S. Mann, MD Department of Anesthesiology, The University of Texas Medical Branch at Galveston, Galveston, TX, USA

Haig Mannasian, MD Thomas Jefferson University Hospital, Department of Anesthesiology, Philadelphia, PA, USA

Kristen Mathias, MD University of Chicago, Department of Internal Medicine, Chicago, IL, USA

David Matson, DO Reading Hospital/Tower Health, Department of Anesthesiology, West Reading, PA, USA

Patrick O. McConville, MD, FASA The University of Tennessee Medical Center, Department of Anesthesiology, Knoxville, TN, USA

David C. McEnerney, DO University of Florida – Jacksonville, Department of Anesthesiology, Jacksonville, FL, USA

Patrick D. McFarland, MD, MBA – candidate Department of Anesthesiology, University of Tennessee Graduate School of Medicine, Knoxville, TN, USA

Shairko Missouri, MBChB, MD NYU-Grossman School of Medicine, Department of Anesthesiology, New York, NY, USA

Paul D. Mongan, MD University of Florida – Jacksonville, Department of Anesthesiology, Jacksonville, FL, USA

Jose V. Montoya-Gacharna, MD NYU Langone Medical Center, Department of Anesthesiology, New York, NY, USA

Blake A. Moore, MD Section on Cardiothoracic Anesthesia, University of Tennessee Graduate School of Medicine, Knoxville, TN, USA

Phillip Morris, MD Baylor Scott and White Medical Center – Temple, Department of Anesthesiology, Temple, TX, USA

Chris Murphy, MD Department of Anesthesiology, University of Mississippi Medical Center, Jackson, MS, USA

Nikita Nayyar, MD New York University Langone School of Medicine, Department of Anesthesiology, New York, NY, USA

Melissa Nikolaidis, MD Baylor College of Medicine, Department of Anesthesiology, Houston, TX, USA

Matthew B. Novitch, MD University of Washington Medical Center, Department of Anesthesiology, Seattle, WA, USA

Matthew E. Nungesser, BS, MD Candidate Department of Anesthesiology, LSUHSC-New Orleans, New Orleans, LA, USA

Chikezie N. Okeagu, MD Department of Anesthesiology, LSU School of Medicine, New Orleans, LA, USA

Natalia Okon, BS Department of Anesthesiology, Medical College of Wisconsin, Milwaukee, WI, USA

Oladapo Oshikoya, MD University of Florida College of Medicine – Jacksonville, Department of Anesthesiology, Jacksonville, FL, USA

Anne Lee Parsiola, MS Department of Anesthesiology, LSU Health Shreveport, Shreveport, LA, USA

Atish Patel, MD Vanderbilt University Medical Center, Department of Anesthesiology, Nashville, TN, USA

Divya Patel, MD NYU-Grossman School of Medicine, Department of Anesthesiology, New York, NY, USA

Shukan Patel, MS Department of Anesthesiology, LSU Health Sciences Center, New Orleans, LA, USA

Seth Perelman, MD, FASA NYU Grossman School of Medicine, Department of Anesthesiology, Perioperative Care and Pain Medicine, New York, NY, USA

Alex D. Pham, MD Department of Anesthesiology, LSUHSC New Orleans, New Orleans, LA, USA

Amit Prabhakar, MD, MS Emory University School of Medicine, Department of Anesthesiology, Atlanta, GA, USA

Aaron N. Primm, MD NYU Langone Health, Department of Anesthesiology, Perioperative Care and Pain Medicine, New York, NY, USA

Donald S. Prough, MD Department of Anesthesiology, The University of Texas Medical Branch at Galveston, Galveston, TX, USA

Jordan S. Renschler, BS, MD Candidate Department of Anesthesiology, LSUHSC New Orleans, New Orleans, LA, USA

Christa L. Riley, MD VCU Health, Department of Anesthesiology, Richmond, VA, USA

Pamela R. Roberts, MD, FCCM, FCCP Department of Anesthesiology, University of Oklahoma College of Medicine, Oklahoma City, OK, USA

Diana Romano, MD The Icahn School of Medicine at Mount Sinai Hospital, Department of Anesthesiology, Perioperative and Pain Management, New York, NY, USA

Renira Rugnath, BS University of Mississippi Medical Center, School of Medicine, Jackson, MS, USA

Jaime Sanders, MD Drexel University College of Medicine, West Reading, PA, USA

J. Arthur Saus, MD Department of Anesthesiology, LSU Health Shreveport, Shreveport, LA, USA

John E. Scheinuk, BS, MD Candidate Department of Anesthesiology, LSUHSC New Orleans, New Orleans, LA, USA

Corey S. Scher, MD NYU-Grossman School of Medicine, Department of Anesthesiology, New York, NY, USA

Anitha Shelvan, MBBS, DNB Department of Anesthesiology, Lahey Hospital & Medical Center, Burlington, MA, USA

Saurin J. Shah, MD University of Florida – Jacksonville, Department of Anesthesiology, Jacksonville, FL, USA

Michelle M. Sheth, MD UMMC, Department of Anesthesiology, Jackson, MS, USA

Harish Siddaiah, MD Department of Anesthesiology, LSU Health Shreveport, Shreveport, LA, USA

Lauren Smajdor, MD University of Florida, Department of Anesthesiology, Gainesville, FL, USA

Natalie Smith, MD The Icahn School of Medicine at Mount Sinai, Department of Anesthesia, Perioperative, and Pain Medicine, New York, NY, USA

Allyson L. Spence, PhD Department of Pharmaceutical Science, Regis University, Denver, CO, USA

Bruce D. Spiess, MD, FAHA University of Florida Health, Gainesville, FL, USA

Garrett D. Starling, MD Texas A&M University – College of Medicine, Bryan, TX, USA

Baylor Scott and White Medical Center – Temple, Department of Anesthesiology, Temple, TX, USA

Lu Sun, PhD LSU Health Shreveport, Department of Anesthesiology, Shreveport, LA, USA

Rayhan Tariq, MD Thomas Jefferson University Hospital, Department of Anesthesiology, Philadelphia, PA, USA

Shruthima Thangada, MD NYU Langone Health, Department of Anesthesiology, Perioperative Care, & Pain Medicine, New York, NY, USA

Jacob Tiegs, MD NYU Langone Medical Center, Department of Anesthesiology, New York, NY, USA

J. Clint Tippett, MD Baylor Scott and White Medical Center – Temple, Department of Anesthesiology, Temple, TX, USA

Anuragh Trikha, MD NYU Langone Health, Department of Anesthesiology, New York, NY, USA

Uchenna Umeh, MD, FASA NYU Langone Health, NYU Langone Orthopedic Hospital, Department of Anesthesiology, Perioperative Care and Pain Medicine, New York, NY, USA

Ivan Urits, MD Beth Israel Deaconess Medical Center Harvard Medical School, Boston, MA, USA

Arnaldo Vera-Arroyo, MD Department of Anesthesiology and Perioperative Medicine, University of Miami Miller School of Medicine, Miami, FL, USA

Division of Anesthesiology, Bruce W. Carter VA Medical Center, Miami, FL, USA

Christine T. Vo, MD University of Oklahoma College of Medicine, Department of Anesthesiology, Oklahoma City, OK, USA

Michael P. K. Webb, BHK, MSc, MBChB Middlemore Hospital, Department of Anaesthesia and Pain Medicine, Auckland, New Zealand

Marie-Christine Wright, MD, JD, MSc Tulane University School of Medicine, New Orleans, LA, USA

Hao Wu, MD NYU Medical Center, Department of Anesthesiology, New York, NY, USA

Hong Yan, MD Department of Anesthesiology, Wuhan Central Hospital, Wuhan, Hubei, China

Longqiu Yang, MD, PhD Huangshi Central Hospital, Department of Anesthesiology, Huangshi, Hubei, China

Colleen B. Yen, MD The Mount Sinai Hospital, Department of Anesthesiology, Perioperative and Pain Medicine, New York, NY, USA

Richard A. Zack-Guasp, MD Department of Anesthesiology and Perioperative Medicine, University of Miami Miller School of Medicine, Miami, FL, USA

Division of Anesthesiology, Bruce W. Carter VA Medical Center, Miami, FL, USA

Jeron Zerillo, MD The Mount Sinai Hospital, Department of Anesthesiology, Perioperative and Pain Medicine, New York, NY, USA

Jianli Zhao, MD Thomas Jefferson University Hospital, Department of Pathology, Philadelphia, PA, USA

The History of Blood Transfusion and Blood Management

1

Philip G. Boysen II and Douglas R. Bacon

Introduction

Blood was mystery rather than science for thousands of years. Blood, and its function, was surrounded by religious beliefs, rituals, social customs, and human experiences. That blood was a "life force" was obvious. One had only to observe that when blood was drained from humans and animals, weakness and death followed as a result. In every language, blood is used as a symbol for family relationships; being "related by blood" refers to the concept of family ancestry or descent, as opposed to related by marriage. We emphasize bloodlines when we speak of "royal blood," or assert that "blood is thicker than water."

Perhaps the most emphatic statement on the power of blood is made by William Shakespeare in his famous history play, Henry V. King Henry is exhorting his outnumbered, undernourished, fatigued, and diseased soldiers to engage the French forces. He exclaims:

> And Crispin Crispian shall ne'er go by,
> From this day to the ending of the world,
> But we in it shall be remembered-
> We few, we happy few, we **band of brothers,**
> For he today that sheds his blood with me
> Shall be my brother; be he ne'er so vile,
> This day shall gentle his condition;
> And gentlemen in England now-a-bed
> Shall curse themselves they were not here,
> And hold their manhoods cheap whilst any speaks
> That fought with us on Saint Crispin's Day!

The absent historical fact in the play is that the English were trapped. Their retreat to Calais, the embarking point to return to England was blocked by the French. Their position was desperate. But the English had perfected the long bow, with spear-like arrows, allowing the English army to launch a hail of projectiles in rhythm to cut down the French before they were able to engage the battle line. The point is made that spilling blood in desperate battle brings the soldiers as close together as any family tie. For centuries humans really knew nothing about blood, how and where it was made in the body, the actual composition of blood, and its purpose. Accepting it as a life force led to the conclusion that drinking blood or rubbing it on the body would make one stronger. The stronger the animal or human from whence the blood came, the greater the effect. Spectators would rush the field of battle to drink the blood of wounded and slain gladiators to assimilate their courage and strength.

Notable cultural exceptions to the ingestion of blood are found in religious texts. In the Old Testament, Jewish dietary laws forbid consuming blood in even the smallest quantity (Leviticus 17:13). Blood must be purged from meat by salting and soaking in water. However, the next statement (Leviticus 17:14) reasserts the life force of blood: "because the life of every animal in in its blood." Similarly, consumption of food that is contaminated with blood is contrary to Islamic dietary law. "Forbidden to you are dead meat, blood, the flesh of swine, and that on which hath been invoked the name of other than Allah." (Qur'an sura Al-Maida 5:3).

The Legacy of Hippocrates

The teachings of Hippocrates were viable for 2000 years and the basis of Western medicine [1]. His basic theory identified four "humors" operating in the body: health and wellness depended on these four humors operating in balance, a conceptual humoral homeostasis. The four humors were blood, phlegm, yellow bile, and black bile. Hippocrates proposed that no single one of these humors were more important than the other. Well into the Renaissance period, the language of

P. G. Boysen II (✉)
Department of Anesthesiology, University of Mississippi Critical Care Organization, University of Mississippi Medical Center, Jackson, MS, USA
e-mail: pboysen@umc.edu

D. R. Bacon
Department of Anesthesiology, University of Mississippi Medical Center, Jackson, MI, USA

© Springer Nature Switzerland AG 2021
A. D. Kaye, S. Leavitt (eds.), *Essentials of Blood Product Management in Anesthesia Practice*,
https://doi.org/10.1007/978-3-030-59295-0_1

humoral theory, *sanguine, phlegmatic, melancholic, and choleric,* indicated which of these humors were out of balance, and the resulting personality and demeanor.

- Sanguine: cheerfully optimistic, hopeful, confident, even arrogant
- Phlegmatic: calm, or even an apathetic temperament
- Melancholic: gloomy, dejected, depressive personality
- Choleric: irritable, easily angered, and unpredictable

Given the physical state associated with the humors, early physicians concluded that the major function of blood was to control one's mental state. Therefore, it followed that "bad blood" could be addressed by bleeding the patient to let the offending humor out of the body.

The ancient Greeks had a limited knowledge of anatomy. Advancing the science of anatomy and physiology would be in direct contradiction to the theory of Hippocrates. However, the legacy of Hippocrates is a positive one. He proposed a holistic view of medicine and the expectation that a physician should be selfless in the care of patients and hold to the highest ethical and moral standard.

Antiquity and the Concept of Transfusion

In antiquity, the first "transfusionist" was Medea, a character in the epic poem by Ovid [2]. She is the protagonist in Metamorphosis, Book VII. Medea is enjoined by her husband Jason to rejuvenate his aging and failing father, Aeson. At first, he begs her to transfer some of his own life-years to his father, a plan which she rejects as offensive to the gods. Her plan is to drain the blood from Aeson and replace it with a secret potion. The ingredients are many and secret:

> Meanwhile the strong potion in the bronze pot is boiling and leaping, and frothing white with swollen foam… and wherever the froth bubbled over from the hot pot and fell upon ground the earth grew green and flowers and grass sprang up. When she saw this Media unsheathed her knife and cut the old man's throat; then letting the blood run out, filled his veins with her brew… his beard and hair lost their hoary gray and became black again; his leanness vanished, away went the pallor and look of neglect, deep wrinkles were filled out with new flesh, his limbs had the strength of youth.

Medea is described as moving round the "blazing altar" while dipping many cleft sticks in the dark pools of blood, to which she added a long list of additional ingredients including animal organs and parts.

When the daughters of King Pelias heard of this achievement, they begged Media to similarly rejuvenate their father. Media used this art and sorcery as a method for murder. She scolded the daughters.

> Why do you hesitate now, you laggards? Come now, draw your swords and let out his blood that I may fill his veins with young blood again!

The daughters set upon the father, their king, stabbing him repeatedly, but when the time came for the rejuvenation, Medea was nowhere to be found, and the two daughters realized they had murdered their father.

The Discovery of the Circulation

The physiology of blood and circulation was hampered by slow discovery of human anatomy, and incorrect assumptions. The first known treatise on circulation is found in the Ebers Papyrus, a book of medical knowledge written in the sixteenth century B.C. [2]. Although mainly concentrating on remedies and "prescriptions" of the day, it asserts the connection of arteries to veins, but believed the circulatory system carried air and not blood. Air entrained from the atmosphere was thought to enter both the lungs and the heart.

The circulation of vital fluids in the body was described in the *Sushruta Samhita,* sixth century B.C., describing the arteries as channels [3]. Sushruta also understood the valves of the heart had something to do with directional flow of vital fluids, but did not offer complete understanding of how that function was achieved. The concept of arteries, veins, and blood therein was misunderstood due to lack of anatomical study and cadaveric dissection. After death, the veins' arteries appear empty, and the assumption was made that in life arteries and veins carried air. Three specific errors, all proposed by Aristotle, and physicians of his time, led to three misconceptions:

1. Aristotle opined the arteries carried air not blood.
2. Veins carried blood to the extremities, not from them.
3. The interventricular septum separated right ventricle from left, but the septum had pores or perforations.

Greek physician Herophilus is the first true anatomist, and has been dubbed the "father of anatomy" [4]. As a young man, he emigrated to Alexandria, the most progressive city in the world during the reign of the Ptolemaic Pharaohs [5]. The city collected books as well as scholars of all sorts. With the death of Alexander the Great in 325 B.C., the leadership void was filled by one of his general who took the name Ptolemy, and his dynasty was in power from 305 B.C. to 30 B.C. During that time, all the Pharaohs took the name Ptolemy, and all the Ptolemaic queens regnant became Cleopatra, Arsinoe, or Berenice. Cleopatra VII was the last ruler of the dynasty when Romans captured the city in 30 B.C. During this period of academic enlightenment, Herophilus practiced dissection for an estimated 30–40 years. At some point, he was accused of vivisection of prisoners, but this was probably a false accusation. He still believed that the vascular system carried air not blood, and would have corrected that error in thinking had he been performing vivisection. With the passing of the Ptolemaic dynasty, cadaveric dissection was abandoned for the next 1800 years, restarting in the middle of the sixteenth century.

The Greek physician Galen corrected the first error in thinking in the second century A.D. He established the fact that arterial blood was a brighter red color than the darker hue of venous blood. He established two separate functions for arterial versus venous blood, different and unrelated [6]. Venous blood, responsible for growth and energy, was created from chyle in the liver. Arterial blood was created in the heart, and its function was to carry air. Blood flowed from the arterial and venous system to the periphery and all organs, there to be dissipated and not returned. Thus, the heart was not a pump, there was no venous return of blood to the heart, and the interventricular septum had pores to allow venous blood to pass from the left ventricle to the right ventricle.

The false assumption of pores in the ventricular septum of the heart was corrected by the Arabic physician Ibn al-Nafis in 1242 [7]. His manuscript was discovered in 1924 in the Prussian State Library in Berlin. In that document, he states:

> …the blood from the right chamber of the heart must arrive at the left chamber, but there is no direct pathway between them. The thick septum of the heart is not perforated and does not have visible pores as some people have thought or invisible pores as Galen thought. The blood from the right chamber must flow through the vena arteriosa (pulmonary artery) to the lungs, spread through its substances, be mingled there with air, passed through arteria venosa (pulmonary vein) to reach the left chamber of the heart, and there form the vital spirit…

So, the assumed perforation in the ventricle of the heart did not exist and blood went through the pulmonary circulation and parenchyma, and returned to the left side of the heart (Fig. 1.1). Ibn al-Nafis and his work were largely unknown for three centuries in Europe. It was again described in 1552 in Spain, and in 1558 in Italy. During that same time, Andrea Cesalpino coined the term "circulation," postulating that the arteries and veins were connected by a thin vascular network [8].

Finally, the English physician William Harvey put it all together [9]. In 1628, he published Exercitatio Anatomica de Motu Cordis et Sanguinis in Animalibus. The *magnus opus*, a book of 100 pages, was widely read and rapidly influenced thinking. He described the true function of the cardiac and venous valves, and asserted that the arterial pulsation is only due to blood. He did not mention the capillary system, the network connecting arteries and veins, and elucidated by Marcello Malpighi [10].

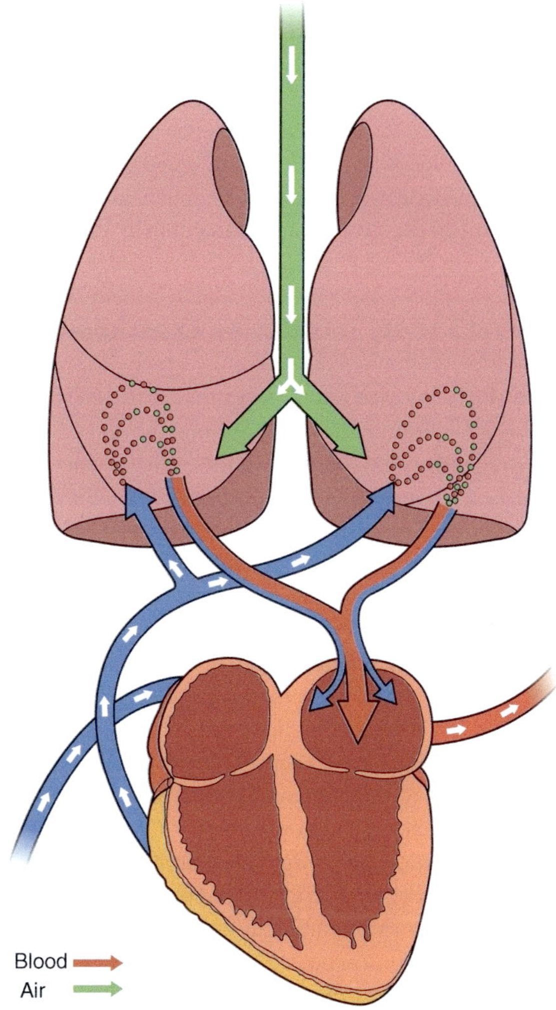

Fig. 1.1 A representation of the pulmonary circulation as described in his writings c. 1236 A.D. [11]

The Cellular Elements of Blood

The microscope became available in the mid-seventeenth century, a Dutch biologist reported its use to study amphibian blood in 1658, and with this instrument gave the first report describing the red blood cell [12]. Unaware of this report by Jan Swammerdam, the Dutch physician Anton von Leeuwenhoek made a second report 16 years later, in 1674 [13].

Nearly 200 years later, the first microscopic description of the platelet was published in the journal *Archiv fur mikroskopische Anatomie.* The journal was founded by the German anatomist Max Schultze 1865, and he published his work in the first issue of his own journal. In his investigation, he describes another component of blood which he dubbed "spherules," later known as platelets. Further he noted these spherules often occurred in clumps and seemed to collect fibrous material [14].

Giulio Bizzozero developed a microscopic technique to examine red blood cells passing in single file in an amphibian web using a live animal. He confirmed the description Schultze made of platelets and also confirmed their role in coagulation at a site of injury [15].

The work of Paul Ehrlich, German physician, was a giant leap forward for hematology. He developed dyes to stain blood smeared on a glass plate. With his dyes he not only garnered information on the red blood cell, but described the white blood cell, clearly showing the difference between lymphocytes and granulocytes [16]. He was awarded the Nobel Prize for these investigations. Finally, and much later, Dr. Max Perutz described the structure of hemoglobin in 1959 [17].

The Royal Society Transfusion Experiments

The Royal Society was founded in London in 1661, obtaining a Royal Charter in 1662 [18]. Among the early founders and participants were Thomas Willis, Christopher Wren, Richard Lower, Robert Hooke, Robert Boyle, Sir William Petty, Thomas Sydenham, and Samuel Pepys. Although other Europeans (Italian, French, and English) wrote about transfusion as a concept, the first documented transfusion belongs to Christopher Wren who employed an animal bladder and two quills to establish a circulatory connection. The knighted Sir Christopher Wren is better known for his contributions to astronomy and architecture. Wren's experiments were later described by Robert Boyle when he published "The Usefulness of Experimental Philosophy" in 1663 [19].

Another member of the Royal Society, Cornish physician Dr. Richard Lower, made a significant contribution of transfusion science in February in the year 1665 [20]. He described the first animal to animal transfusion using a bled dog and transfusing blood from another dog. The first dog was bled to the point of being in extremis, then revived by blood transfusion. He described his work in his book "Tractatus de Corde" published in 1669, his work previously having been read to the Royal Society by Robert Boyle [21].

Lower published the first description of direct transfusion from donor artery to recipient vein after he was unsuccessful in transfusing from vein to vein. This blood transfer failed due to clotting before it could be completed. Of further significance is his ability to use transfusion to replace blood lost for whatever reason, in an era when blood transfusion was viewed as therapy for mental disorders.

Nevertheless, when Lower pushed his technique even further to achieve transfusion from animal to man, he selected a mental patient for the procedure. Arthur Coga, a 32 year-old man, was suffering from anxiety and depression, apparently without benefit from any therapy (including presumably blood-letting). Lower enlisted Dr. Edmund King, a well-known surgeon, to establish the connection from the carotid artery of a sheep to one of Coga's arms. The operation was a success, but the patient showed minimal or no improvement in his mental state. A second transfusion was scheduled but never took place.

A young French physician, Dr. Jean Baptiste Denys, in the employ of King Louis XIV, read of Lower's experiments. He had been experimenting with animal to animal transfusion with the cooperation with his own surgical associate, Dr. Paul Emmerz. He was asked to treat a 15-year old boy who had been suffering with fever for months, again with no improvement after being bled multiple times. In this procedure, the boy was transfused 9 ounce of sheep blood, having been first bled by that same amount. Except for feeling local heat in his arm, the patient tolerated the transfusion but again with little apparent benefit. Denys is credited with performing the first animal to man transfusion in 1667 [22].

Denys continued to expand his transfusion practice using sheep's blood so as not to transmit vices or passions from one human to another. He eventually became aware of the erratic behavior of Antoine Mauroy following a display of public nudity causing his wife to seek Denys in hopes of a cure by transfusion. Denys could not resist this challenge and transfused a small amount of calf blood to Mr. Mauroy, noting no apparent complication or benefit. Within two days, Mauroy transfused the man again resulting in what is now a classic description of a transfusion reaction including hematuria. Denys mistakenly mistook hemoglobinuria as proof of release of "black choler" and a positive sign that his brain would be favorably changed.

However, several months later, Mauroy was irrational and violent, and he was subjected to another transfusion. It was never performed as adequate blood flow could not be established. Mauroy died the following evening. The medical community persuaded the widow to file charges against Drs. Denys and Emmerz. Many physicians of the day still refused to believe Harvey's demonstration of blood circulation; also, the practice of the day continued to bleed patients to remove bad humors in the body. Denys filed his own lawsuit against the widow and had his day in court. He was acquitted when it was discovered that the man had died of arsenic poisoning and the widow confessed!

With his macabre ending came a serious and unfortunate outcome. The Faculty of Medicine of Paris issued a decree that transfusion could not be performed without the permission of a member of the Faculty, which would never be forthcoming. Then in 1678, the French Parliament decreed that transfusion henceforth would be a criminal act. A year later the Royal Society in London followed suit, and wanted nothing to do with the public outcry against the procedure. For the next 150 years, the practice of transfusion was prohibited by law in France and England.

James Blundell and Obstetricians Revive Transfusion Medicine

James Blundell was the first to transfuse human blood (1818) and has been referred to as the father of modern blood transfusion [23]. He was motivated to save women from fatal hemorrhage during childbirth. He also developed a science of transfusion while reawakening interest in the technique. He had first repeated the experiments of Lower by transfusing exsanguinated dogs. He established that transfusing blood from another dog to the exsanguinated dog was not accomplished without complications, and decided to investigate human to human transfusion. He was the first investigator to wonder about availability of a suitable donor (in this case a dog) to accomplish an emergency transfusion [23].

Blundell was aware of the work of one of his contemporaries, John Henry Leacock who asserted that transfusion is life-saving in the face of acute blood loss, such as the bleeding parturient or wounded soldiers, rather than transfusing for mental disorders.

Blundell had a mechanical mind, and in 1824, published a book introducing a device he called an "impellor" consisting of a funnel to collect donor blood, a surrounding water bath to keep the blood warm, and tubing to push the blood into the patient. A subsequent invention, known as the "Gravitator" provided enhanced blood delivery [24]. An illustration published in 1829 shows a standing donor watching his blood flow into the Gravitator (Fig. 1.2).

In his reports, Blundell noted that some patients reported fever, backache, headache, and passed dark urine, presumably due to transfusion with ABO-incompatible blood.

The Legacy of Karl Landsteiner

Karl Landsteiner (Fig. 1.3) investigated the problem of blood incompatibility, working along the same scientific observations started by Blundell. When he began his work the issue of blood incompatibility was recognized between species, but not within any given species. Landois published a manuscript, "Die Transfusion des Blutes" in 1875 demonstrating that mixing blood from one animal with the blood of another species caused coagulation and lysis

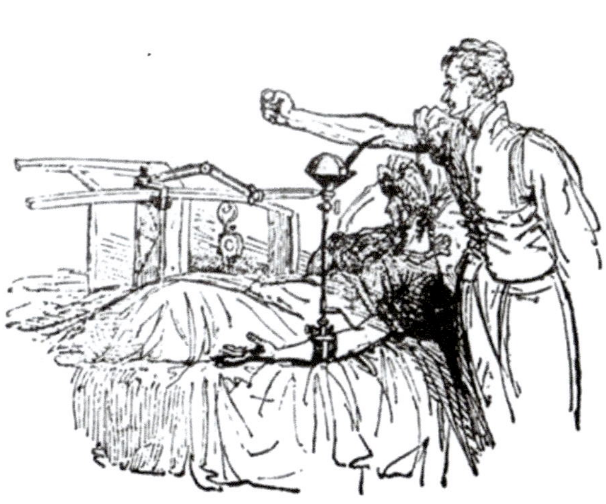

Fig. 1.2 Blood transfusion with the Gravitator, shown in *Lancet* (1828)

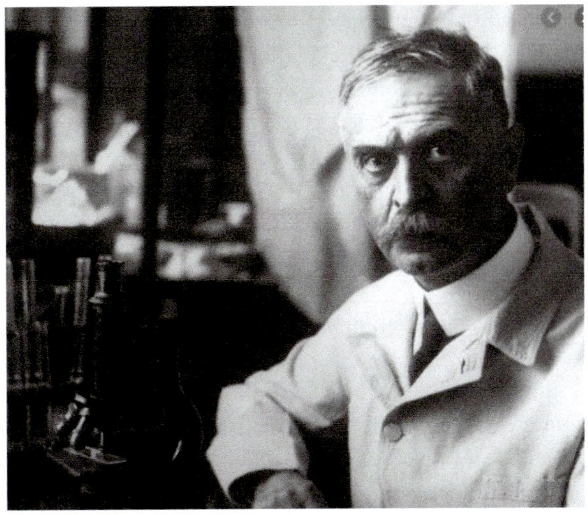

Fig. 1.3 Karl Landsteiner

within minutes [25]. Then 25 years later, Landsteiner did similar experiments limited to human blood. He described his results when mixing red blood cells and serum in 22 subjects. He made two important observations, the first being that clumping of the mixed blood was observed in some specimens but not in others (the blood mixed was "compatible"), and secondly that this was an immunologic phenomenon. He was able to identify three blood groups, A, B, and C [26]. The following year two of his students studied 4.155 patients who had no agglutinins in their own serum, but all three of the previously discovered blood types (group AB). Further they noted that isoagglutinins were present in healthy people and not associated with a disease state [25]. Written in German, Landsteiner's work was not put into common practice until the 1920s. He received the Nobel Prize for his work in 1930 [27].

In that interim, other groups were duplicating his findings unknowingly. Moss described four groups also by naming them in reverse order: IV, III, II, I [28]. It took a meeting of the Congress of the International Society of Blood Transfusion in 1937 to adopt the ABO terminology. Genetic aspects of blood formation and blood inheritance were under investigation since the 1920s racial distribution of blood groups was documented during World War II in Germany [29]. Blood discrimination followed as blood group A was determined to be of Aryan descent, and blood group was a marker for Jewish and Slavic descent. Similarly, in the United States, blood was segregated according to donor by the American Red Cross. Blood from black donors was not acceptable for pooled plasma from which albumin was derived. Such laws were in place in the United States until the late 1960s. In fact, in the 1950s, a law was passed in Louisiana charging physicians with a misdemeanor if blood from a black donor was transfused into a Caucasian without explicit and informed consent. The law remained in effect until it was repealed in 1983 [30].

Another of Landsteiner's students, Philip Levine began work with him in the Rockefeller Institute in 1925. Levine published a case report of a couple, both with blood group O, experienced a bleeding episode after the husband's blood was transfused into the wife. The ensuing post-transfusion hemolysis was investigated by incubating the husband's blood with the wife's blood, which resulted in immediate agglutination. Levine then incubated the woman's blood with 140 compatible samples of ABO blood. Agglutination was observed in 80 samples, thus demonstrating the presence of what came to be known as Rhesus antibodies [31]. The antibodies were so named due to previous work that Levine had performed with Landsteiner that had similar results and did involve Rhesus monkeys. Sir Ronald Fisher, a Cambridge geneticist, established the complexity of the Rh antibody describing several alleles, which he named C and c, D and d, E and e.

In the ensuing years, researchers discovered many new antigens in blood. Coombs developed the anti globulin test to identify new antigenic systems often named for the first patient who had those new antibodies [32]. Further progress was made when Morton and Pickles discovered that enzymes such as trypsin could be incubated with blood to enhance antigenic expression [33]. Coombs identified the Kell antigens in a case of hemolytic disease of the newborn that could not be explained by the Rh antibody. Joseph Duffy (Fy) was a hemophiliac who received multiple transfusion and carried the gene. Mrs. Kidd (Jk) delivered a son, her fifth child, who had hemolytic disease of the newborn. An antibody in her blood agglutinated the blood of 146/189 donors [34].

The Search for an Anticoagulant

Further limiting transfusion medicine was the vexing problem of blood coagulation, which resulted in the requirement of fresh blood for transfusion and donor and recipient in the same place and at the same time. An early approach to this problem was the arterio-venous anastomosis first described in 1913 by the French surgeon Alexis Carrel, a donor radial artery to recipient vein graft. Once again, the immediacy and emergency of the situation involved a mother who had delivered a baby with erythroblastosis fetalis. Carrel was rewarded the Nobel Prize in Medicine for his work [35]. However, the technique has definite limitations. Donor and recipient must be immediately present for the procedure. It is not possible to know how much blood is being transfused, or even to estimate the volume. The blood vessels of donor and recipient could not be used a second time.

A second technique was simply to defibrinate the blood by collecting it into a reservoir and stir with a device to promote clotting, lift out the clot, and use the remaining fluid for transfusion. Prevost and Dumas used defibrillated blood to resuscitate animals that had been exsanguinated and reported their results in 1821 [36]. They also reported severe febrile reactions after the transfusion. What was needed was a third option, i.e., find a stable non toxic anticoagulated environment so that blood could be collected and stored for a prolonged period of time.

The British obstetrician Braxton-Hicks tested a phosphate of soda as an anticoagulant, but it proved to be a toxic medium [37]. Richard Lewinsohn experimented with sodium citrate at a concentration of 1%, noting that some laboratories used it as an anticoagulant for specimens not collected for transfusion as the solution was also toxic. Lewinsohn continued his work, exploring the theory that a lower concentration of citrate might provide anticoagulation without ensuing toxicity [38]. Finally, in 1915, he published his results using 0.2% citrated solution with good anticoagulant effect and no toxicity even if 2500 cc of blood was transfused [38]. But the blood still had to be stored for only a short time. Adding dextrose to stored blood extended red cell survival to two weeks; acid-citrate-dextrose (ACD) improved red blood survival without effect of acid–base milieu in the recipient [39]. Citrate-phosphate-dextrose (CPD) extended red blood cell survival to 28 days [40, 41].

The ability to store blood in a non toxic solution and the ability to prevent coagulation were major achievements in the transition to blood management. Prior to that the blood service concentrated on enlisting donors who had been processed and examined, and able to respond to the need for blood donation in short notice. The first blood service was established in 1921 by Percy Oliver, a civil servant working with the British Red Cross [42]. Establishing a list of prospective donors was a slow process, but the need was evident in post-war England. There were few homes with phones, so the donors were summoned by police and escorted to the facility. The blood donor service expanded throughout the UK in spite of resistance by some physicians to use anticoagulants, and the challenge of having to perform a surgical procedure to access the vascular anatomy. There were still deaths resulting from ABO incompatibility since blood typing was not widely available. The process of enlisting a panel of donors, in essence a "walking blood bank" continues to exist in the American military, and has recently been activated by US Navy physician and corpsmen in a desert post [43]. Eventually, the term "blood bank" meant a physical space, not a living person. Dr. John Lundy at the Mayo Clinic initiated blood banking in 1935 [44]. In 1937, Bernard Fantus opened a blood bank at the Hektoen Institute of Cook County Hospital in Chicago, storing refrigerated blood in bottles for 10 days prior to infusion [45]. Whether blood is collected at the site of transfusion, or collected and stored for later use, a panel of donors is still a requisite.

The shortage of blood donors in Russia in the 1930s demanded a different approach and the result was the collection of cadaveric blood [46, 47]. The premise was that rapid access to a trauma patient, and drainage of blood from a dead donor from the inferior vena cava would result in an adequate amount of blood for transfusion. Shamov reported transfusion of blood from trauma patients and patients who died from cardiac arrest in 2500 recipients with only seven deaths. In the United States, Dr. Jack Kevorkian (who later became famous for his work in physician-assisted suicide) reported similar results [48]. Other physicians collected and transfused placental blood, which was plentiful, but more likely to be infected prior to transfusion [49]. The establishment of blood banks supplanted the use of these and other techniques [50].

Fractionated Blood Products

The fact that blood contains cellular elements and platelets was well established. It wasn't until 1940 that Professor Edwin Cohn, a physical chemist at Harvard Medical School, began to methodically search for other "fractions" in blood and plasma. His technique involved repeatedly exposing blood to ethyl alcohol. With each iteration of the experiment, he varied salt content, temperature, and pH [51]. The isolated fraction I contained mostly fibrinogen, fractions II and III were mainly globulins, and fraction V was albumin. The albumin-rich factor V was reported to restore circulation in accident victims with "circulatory collapse." On December 7, 1941 – the date of the Japanese attack on Pearl Harbor, albumin was immediately deployed to the base and infused into 84 victims, mainly burn injuries with reported improvement enhancing survival. Albumin was introduced into clinical medicine with no randomized clinical trials as would be required today [52].

Immunoglobulins in fractions II and III were employed to provide prevention infectious diseases including measles and Rh hemolytic syndrome [52]. The anti-Rh(D) given by IM injection in male volunteers coated Rh erythrocytes that had been previously injected. Subsequently a combined study between the United States and UK found efficacy in the protection of Rh-negative parturients [53].

Fractionation of blood and treatment of hemophilia is a crowning achievement in modern medicine. Before such treatment became available, young boys died prior to adolescence [54]. Inbreeding of Royal families of Europe who carried the gene for hemophilia saw their line die out due to the disease. Up until the 1950s, bovine and porcine plasma were used to treat hemophiliacs since both were rich in the missing factor, or factor VIII [55]. Severe allergic reactions were noted with repeated exposure stimulating further research [56].

Dr. Judith Graham Poole of Stanford University discovered cryoprecipitate in 1965 noting much greater clotting activity than plasma [57]. Stored in a refrigerator, it could be thawed and administered by a physician [58].

Dr. Kenneth Merle Brinkhous of the University of North Carolina at Chapel Hill discovered the factor VIII deficiency which was responsible for hemophilia in 1935. He later described von Willebrand's disease [59]. Another form of hemophilia, deficiency of clotting factor IX was discovered in 1952 [60].

Blood Management in the Modern Era

It took centuries to develop the concept and practicality of human blood transfusion as a means of treating anemia and blood loss rather than transfusing to treat mental disorders. Safe collection of blood, and storage for prolonged periods, prevention of coagulation, and the fractionation of non-cellular components led to the ability to "manage" the product and extend the ability to treat more patients with a targeted approach to therapy. Subsequent acquisition of knowledge during the past 50 years has been impressive.

- 1967: Rh immune globulin was released as a commercial product
- 1969: Platelet storage at room temperature was reported
- 1970: Blood was collected only from volunteer donors
- 1972: Apheresis is introduced to extract donor platelets, returning the rest of blood
- 1981: Gay Related Immune Deficiency Syndrome (GRID) reported
- 1983: GRID, now AIDS virus isolated at Pasteur Institute in France
- 1985: ELISA test applied to blood donors to detect AIS virus
- 1987: Indirect screening for hepatitis B introduced
- 1990: Testing for Non A–Non B (now hepatitis C) introduced
- 1992: Donor blood now direct testing for HIV-1 and HIV-2 virus
- 1996: Testing for HIVp24 antigen introduced

In addition to addressing hepatitis A, B, C and AIDS, the technology is introduced to screen for and diagnose malaria, toxoplasmosis gondii, and cytomegalovirus. The search for a technique to perform "blood less" surgery has been partially achieved by autologous transfusion, a technology that retrieves the patient's own blood during the surgical procedure, processes it through a "cell saver" to be reinfused into the patient prior to the end of the procedure [61, 62].

The Future of Blood Management

Implementation of blood management has been made possible due to recent advances. The triggers for transfusion have been re-examined and are based on individual patient physiology rather than absolute rules. Rapid assessment of clot formation and fibrinolysis is available using thromboelastography leading to precise replacement of red blood cells, platelets, and blood products. The search for substitutes for hemoglobin and platelets continues. Genetic approaches have been under evaluation such as experiments with transgenic livestock and cultivation of stem cells to grow cellular components of blood. The Joint Commission offers certification in blood management as a means of maximizing the benefit of the resources collected from volunteer blood donors. The search for a hemoglobin substitute continues. The need for blood and blood products, however, will continue for decades to come [63].

References

1. Lloyd GF. Hippocratic writings. London: Penguin Classics; 1978.
2. Kay AB. Eber papyrus. The book of medical knowledge of the 26th century B.C. Egyptians. Arch Hist Filoz Med. 2014;64:5–14.
3. Champaneria MC, Workman AD, Gupta SC. Sushruta: father of plastic surgery. Ann Plastic Surg. 2011;73:2–7.
4. Keynes G. Tercentenary of blood transfusion. Brit Med J. 1967;1v:410–1.
5. Hunt C. The Ptolemies: dynastic Egypt from Alexander to Cleopatra, the last Pharaoh's of Egypt were Greek. 2019. https://www.thoughtco.com/rulers-of-the-ptolemies-172247.
6. Aird WC. Discovery of the cardiovascular system: from Galen to William Harvey. J Thromb Haemost. 2011;73:2–7.
7. West JB. Ibn el-Nafis, the pulmonary circulation and the Islamic Golden Age. J Appl Physiol. 2008;105:1877–80.
8. https://en.wikipedia.org/wiki/Andrea_Cesalpino.
9. Ribatti D. William Harvey and the discovery of the circulation of the blood. J Angiogen Res. 2009;1:3.
10. Forrester JM. Malpighi's De Polypo Cordis: an annotated translation. Med Hist. 1995;39:477–92.
11. Blundell J. Observation on transfusion of blood by Dr. Blundell with a description of his gravitator. Lancet. 1828;ii:321–4.
12. Cole F. Jan Swammerdam (1637-1680). Nature. 1937;131:218–20.
13. Lane L. The unseen world: reflections on Leeuwenhoek. Philos Trans R Soc B. 2015;370:1.
14. Schultze M. Ein heizbarer objectissch und seine verwendung bei untersuchengen des blutes. Archiv fur Microskopische Anatomie. 1865;1:1–42.
15. Brewer DB. Max Schultze, G Bizzero and the discovery of the platelet. Brit J Haemotol. 2001;133:251–8.
16. Kay AB. Paul Ehrlich and the early history of granulocytes. Microbiol Spectr. 2016;4:1128–32.
17. Steensma DP, Shampo MA, Kyle RA. Max Perutz and the discovery of hemoglobin. Mayo Clin Proc. 2015;90:e89.
18. www.royalsociety.org.
19. Barry FB, Parker HS. Dir Christopher Wren: complete philosopher. JAMA. 1962;181:117–20.
20. Fastag E. Richard Lower: the origins of blood transfusion. J Emerg Med. 2013;44:1146–50.
21. Lower R. Tractatus de Corde: De Motu & Colore Sanguinis. Schaumburg: The Wood Library Museum of Anesthesiology; 1669.
22. Myhre BA. The first recorded blood transfusions. Transfusion. 1990;30:358–62.
23. Dzik S. James Blundell, obstetrical hemorrhage, and the origins of transfusion medicine. Transfus Med Rev. 2018;32:205–12.
24. Jones HW, Mackmul G. The influence of James Blundell on the development of blood transfusion. Bri Med J. 1928;iv:410–1.
25. Landois L. Transfusion des Blutes. 1875. F Vogel, Leipzig. Transfusion available www.wellcomelibrary.org.
26. Landsteiner K. On agglutination of normal human blood. Wiener Klinische Wochenschrift. 1901;14:1132–4. Translation in Transfusion. (1961). Transfusion 1, 5–8.
27. Levine F. A review of Landsteiner's contribution to human blood groups. Transfusion. 1961;I:45–53.
28. Moss WL. Studies in isoagglutinins and isohemolysins. Johns Hopkins Med J. 1910;21:63–9.
29. Hirszfeld L, Hirszfeld H. Serological differences between the blood of different races. The result of researches on the Macedonian front. Lancet. 1919;ii:675–9.
30. Marcus F. Louisiana repeals black blood laws. New York Times Archives, July 26, 1983, Section A, Page 10.
31. Levine P, Stetson R. An unusual case of intragroup agglutination. J Am Med Assoc. 1939;113:126–7.
32. Coombs R, Mourant A, Race RR. In-vivo isosensitization of red cells in babies with haemolytic disease. Lancet. 1946;I:264–6.
33. Morton J, Pickles MM. Use of trypsin in the detection of incomplete anti-Rh antibodies. Nature. 1947;159:7780790.
34. Coombs R, Mourant A, Race R. A new test or the detection of weak and "incomplete" Rh agglutinins. Pathology. 1945;26:255–66.
35. Cutbush M, Mollison P, Parkin D. A new human blood group system. Nature. 1950;165:188–9.
36. Clarke TW. The birth of transfusion. J Hist Med. 1949;4:337–8.
37. Hicks J. On transfusion and a new mode of management. Brit Med. 1868;J2:151.
38. Lewinsohn R. Blood transfusion by the citrate method. Surg Gyn Obstet. 1915;21:37–47.
39. Rous P, Turner JR. Preservation of living red blood cell corpuscles in-vitro II. The transfusion of kept cells. J Exp Med. 1916;231:219.
40. Loutit J, Mollison P. Advantages of disodium-citrate-glucose mixture as a preservative. Brit M J. 1943;ii:744.
41. Gibson J, Gregory C, Britton L. Citrate-phosphate-dextrose solution for preservation of human blood. Transfusion. 1961;I:280–7.
42. Gunson H, Dodsworth H. Toward a National Blood Transfusion Service in England and Wales. Transfus Med. 1966;6:4–16.
43. Scott C. The Sand Docs. The story of a Navy Forward Surgical Team in Afghanistan. 2010. Sanddocs.blogspot.com/2010/11/walking-blood-bank.html.
44. Ellis TA, Narr BJ, Bacon DR. Developing a specialty: 3 contributions of John Lundy to the specialty of anesthesiology. J Clin Anesth. 2004;16:226–9.
45. Fantus B. The therapy of the Cook County Hospital. JAMA. 1937;109:128–31.
46. Cohn E, Strong L, Hughes W, Mulford D, Ashworth J, Melin M, Taylor H. Preparation and properties of serum and plasma proteins. IV. A system for the separation into fractions of the proteins and lipoprotein components of biological tissue and fluids. J Am Chem Soc. 1946;68:459–75.
47. Tarssov MM. Cadaveric blood transfusions. Ann NY Acad Sci. 1960;87:512.
48. Shamov RE. The transfusion of stored cadaver blood. Lancet. 1937;8:306–9.
49. Kevorkian J, Marra JJ. Transfusion of human corpse blood with additives. Transfusion. 1964;4:112–7.

50. Goodall JR, Anderson PO, Altemas GT, McPhaill FG. An inexhaustible source of blood for transfusion and its transfusion. Surg Gyn Obstet. 1938;66:176–8.
51. Boland CR, Craig NS, Jacobs AL. Collection and transfusion of preserved blood. Lancet. 1939;I:388–9.
52. Ordman CW, Jennings CG, Janeway CA. Chemical, clinical, and immunological studies on the products of human plasma fractionation. XII. The use concentrated normal serum gamma globulin (human serum immune globulin) in the prevention and attenuation of measles. J Clin Investig. 1944;23:541–55.
53. Combined Study from Centres in England and Baltimore. Prevention of Rh haemolytic disease; results of the clinical trial. Brit Med J. 1966;ii:k907–13.
54. Larsson SA. Life expectancy of Swedish hemophiliacs 1831-1980. Brit J Haemotol. 1985;59:593–602.
55. Kekwick RA, Wolf P. A concentrate of anti-haemophilic factor in blood and its use in 6 patients. Lancet. 1957;I:647–50.
56. Biggs R, Bidwell E, Handley DA, McFarlane RG, Trueta J, Elliot-Smth A, Dike GW, Ash BJ. The preparation of an assay of a Christmas factor (factor IX) concentrate and its use in the treatment of patients. Brit J Haemotol. 1961;7:349–64.
57. Poole JG, Hershgold EJ, Pappenhagen AR. High potency anti-haemophilic factor concentrate prepared rom cryoglobulin precipitate. Nature. 1964;203:312.
58. Poole JG, Shannon AE. Production of high potency of anti-hemophilic globulin in a closed bag system. N Engl Med. 1965;273:1443–4.
59. Shulman NR, Cowan DH, Libre EL, Watkins SP, Marder VJ. Physiologic basis for therapy of classic hemophilia (factor VIII deficiency and related disorders: combined clinical staff conference at the National Institutes of health). Ann Int Med. 1967;67:856–82.
60. Brinkhous KM, Hedner U, Carris JB, Dinness JB, Read MS. Wddwxt of recombinant factor VIIa on the hemostatic defect in dogs with Hemophilia A, hemophilia B and von Willebrand's disease. Proc Natl Acad Sci U S A. 1986;86:1382–6.
61. Lubori HK, Paleyanda RK, Velander WH, Drohan WN. Blood proteins from transgenic animal bioreactors. Transfus Med Rev. 1996;10:131–43.
62. Grant RC. Autotransfusion. Am J Surg. 1921;74:253–4.
63. Ovid metamorphosis, Books 1-8: translated by Frank Justus Miller; 1977. Cambridge: Loeb Classic Library, Harvard University Press.

Modern Blood Banking

2

Louise Helander and Caroline Raasch Alquist

Abbreviations

AABB	formerly the American Association of Blood Banks
AIDS	Acquired Immunodeficiency Syndrome
C:T ratio	Crossmatch-to-transfusion (C:T) ratios
CJD	Creutzfeldt–Jakob disease
DAT	Direct antiglobulin test
EDTA	Ethylenediaminetetraacetic acid
FDA	Food and Drug Administration
FNHTR	Febrile non hemolytic transfusion reaction
HDFN	Hemolytic disease of the fetus and newborn
HLA	Human leukocyte antigens
HPA	Human platelet alloantigens
HTR	Hemolytic transfusion reaction
MHC	Major Histocompatibility Complex
NAIT	Neonatal alloimmune thrombocytopenia
PRT	Pathogen reduction technologies
RBC	Red blood cell
RhD	D antigen of Rh blood group
TA-GVHD	Transfusion-associated graft-versus-host disease
TRALI	Transfusion-related acute lung injury

The ABO and Rh Blood System

The ABO antigens are recognized as the most clinically significant blood group system. Two antigens, A and B, determine ABO typing. The presence or absence of these two antigens create the four common blood group phenotypes: A, B, AB, and O. These antigens are found on red blood cell membranes, lymphocytes, platelets, vascular endothelium, and a wide variety of other tissues. In predisposed type A, B, or AB individuals, antigens are secreted in body fluids, with the exception of cerebrospinal fluid [1]. Those with group O blood type produce a nonfunctional enzyme, which is responsible for the constitutive absence of A and B antigens. ABO phenotypes vary with race and ethnicity (Table 2.1).

Inversely correlated to the expression of A and B antigens, are the expression of anti-A and anti-B antibodies (Table 2.2). Group A, B, and AB individuals express predominantly IgM antibodies. These antibodies are said to be "naturally occurring" because they do not require exposure to a reciprocal antigen for formation. For example, a group A

Table 2.1 ABO & RH phenotypes by race (%)

–	O	A	B	AB	D Pos	D Neg
White	45	40	11	4	83	17
Black	50	40	11	4	93	7
Hispanic	56.5	31	10	2.5	93	7
Asian	40	28	25	7	98	2
Donors	47	37	12	4	85	15

Adapted from Garretty et al. [5]
Decimals have been rounded to the nearest whole number

Table 2.2 ABO antigens and antibodies

Antigens on RBCs[a]			Antibodies in plasma/serum[b]		
A	B	D	Anti-A	Anti-B	Interpretation
0	0	0	+	+	O Neg
+	0	+	0	+	A Pos
0	+	0	+	0	B Neg
+	+	+	0	0	AB Pos

[a]Forward/Front type: Patient RBCs with reagent antisera containing antigen antibodies
[b]Reverse/Back type: Patient serum with reagent RBCs with known antigens added

L. Helander (✉)
University of Colorado, ClinImmune Labs, Denver, CO, USA
e-mail: Louise.helander@cuanschutz.edu

C. R. Alquist
Transplantation Immunology Division, Hoxworth Blood Center, University of Cincinnati, Cincinnati, OH, USA
e-mail: Raaschce@ucmail.uc.edu

© Springer Nature Switzerland AG 2021
A. D. Kaye, S. Leavitt (eds.), *Essentials of Blood Product Management in Anesthesia Practice*,
https://doi.org/10.1007/978-3-030-59295-0_2

individuals will produce anti-B antibodies in their serum as early as three months of age [2]. It is hypothesized that these naturally occurring antibodies are formed in response to environmental and gastrointestinal flora that form structures similar to the ABO antigens and elicit an immune response [2]. The anti-A and anti-B antibodies can agglutinate or cause red cell clumping at room temperature (20–24 °C) and can activate the complement cascade at 37 °C, causing red cell hemolysis.

In contrast, group O individuals express predominantly IgG anti-A and anti-B antibodies. Similar to IgM antibodies, these are capable of activating complement and causing hemolysis. Additionally, group O individuals possess IgG anti-A,B. This unique antibody is believed to react with a common region on the A and B antigens of A, B, or AB individuals, leading to hemolysis [2]. Unlike IgM antibodies, IgG immunoglobulins can cross the placenta and are responsible for the higher rates of hemolytic disease of the fetus and newborn (HDFN) seen in group O pregnant women (see Chapter 23).

The Rh antigens are the second most significant group after the ABO blood system. Originally discovered in 1939 [1], the Rh group is composed of 61 different antigens. Of these, D, C, c, E, and e are known as the primary antigens. Rh genes are closely linked and inherited as a group on chromosome 1. This system is considered to be the most immunogenic of all the minor blood group antigens, with the D-antigen (RhD) being the most immunogenic and clinically significant of the group [3, 4]. "Rh-positive" and "Rh-negative" terminology is generally accepted as denoting the RhD antigen status of a patient. Using "RhD-positive" or "RhD-negative" terminology when referring to a RBC unit is more accurate.

Unlike ABO antibodies, anti-RhD antibodies require exposure to D-antigen for formation. They are predominantly IgG antibodies which can bind and agglutinate red blood cells, leading to extravascular hemolysis. RhD antibodies do not typically activate complement. As with the ABO system, phenotype frequency varies by race and ethnicity. Overall, roughly 85% of individuals are classified as RhD-antigen positive [1, 5].

ABO group and RhD testing of donated blood is performed after collection. Additionally, the ABO group and RhD-negative status of all products containing red cells (RBCs, whole blood, and granulocytes) must be confirmed by the receiving hospital prior to use [2]. Testing consists of typing for antigens attached to the red blood cell membrane with antigen-specific reagent (forward type), as well as screening for suspended antibodies in serum or plasma with antigen-positive test cells (reverse type).

Similarly, prior to routine transfusion, a patient's ABO and RhD type must be confirmed with forward and reverse typing. ABO type in this setting must be confirmed by two determinations prior to transfusion. A second determination can consist of comparison to previous records, testing a second patient sample, or retesting of the same sample if the patient's identity was verified with a validated process to reduce misidentification [6]. This check helps ensure that donor RBCs will be compatible with the recipient's plasma to minimize the risk of life-threatening hemolysis.

Table 2.3 Compatible recipients and donor units

Recipient ABO/Rh type	Compatible RBC units	Compatible platelet units	Compatible plasma units[a]
O -	O –	Platelets are not ABO or Rh matched	O, A, B, AB
A +	O +, A +		A, AB
B +	O –, B –		B, AB
AB +	O +, A +, B +, AB +		AB

Adapted from Technical Manual, Nineteenth Edition
[a]Plasma does not need to be Rh matched

A RBC unit is compatible if the ABO and Rh antibodies in the recipient's serum will not react with antigens on the donor's cells. For example, a group A recipient with anti-B antibodies in their serum would likely be compatible with a group A donor (same type) or with a group O donor whose red blood cells lack A and B antigens to be acted on by the anti-B antibodies. Group O red cells and platelets lack ABO surface antigens and are referred to as universal donor cells. Conversely, group O plasma containing IgG anti-A,B and IgM anti-A and -B is not compatible with Group A or B recipients. Group AB individuals lack ABO antibodies in their serum, making AB plasma products compatible with any blood group recipient. Group AB individuals can receive RBC-containing products from any ABO blood group (Table 2.3). Please note that these examples only hold true in the absence of recipient alloimmunization, further discussed below.

In the absence of a confirmed patient ABO typing during emergent situations, group O RBCs can be safely used. The RhD antigen status of products selected for emergent transfusion may vary by patient type. Similarly, either group AB or A plasma products may be issued for transfusion in emergency settings with unknown recipient ABO and RhD typing. These two notable exceptions to historic blood bank dogma are discussed below in the Inventory Management section.

Other Blood Antigen Systems

Beyond ABO groups and the Rh system, over 350 additional RBC antigens have been identified [7]. Only some are considered clinically significant and capable of causing hemolysis, HDFN, and reduced RBC survival [8]. Clinically insignificant RBC antigens have little to no clinical consequences when transfused to alloimmunized recipients. Red cell antibodies are typically IgG and are regularly screened for in standard patient antibody screen testing [6, 7, 9]. This testing uses recipient serum or plasma and watches for agglutination with screening red blood cells of known antigen type. If a screening cell agglutinates with the recipient serum or plasma, additional work up is warranted to identify the specific antibody/antibodies. If clinically significant antibodies are identified, the patient will need to receive crossmatch-compatible red blood cells that lack the corresponding antigen [6].

The Human Leukocyte Antigen System

The human leukocyte antigen (HLA) system is encoded by a group of closely linked genes located on chromosome 6 in a region known as the major histocompatibility complex (MHC). HLA antigens have an essential immune function in the binding and presentation of antigens for T cell recognition [10]. Because we develop tolerance to our own HLA type, our immune system can identify non self cells within the body by their foreign HLA antigens [10]. For the purposes of transfusion medicine, Class I and Class II are significant for transfusion management.

Class I antigens are found on the surface of all nucleated cells in the body, including platelets, the products of nucleated megakaryocytes. Immature nucleated RBCs also express HLA antigens. These are generally lost in maturation with the exception of Bennett-Goodspeed (Bg) antigens, Class I HLA antigens retained on mature red cell membranes [11]. Class II antigens are found on antigen-presenting cells, including B-lymphocytes, monocytes, macrophages, dendritic cells, and activated T-lymphocytes. Class I and II HLA antigens and antibodies are of particular importance when selecting appropriate platelet and plasma donor units.

Platelets carry Class I HLA antigens, in addition to ABO antigens and human platelet alloantigens (HPA). They do not express Rh or Class II HLA antigens. Given a short shelf life of 5–7 days and commonly limited inventory (see Chapter 3: Component Therapy), platelet units may be transfused without matching for ABO, HLA, or HPA status. ABO, HLA, or HPA-incompatible units may be associated with a lower platelet number increases following transfusion, but this has not been shown to have a measurable impact on clinical bleeding [12]. As an exception to this rule, if a patient demonstrates significant platelet transfusion refractoriness on two occasions and non immune mechanisms (e.g., fever, hypersplenism, or sepsis) are ruled out, HLA and HPA antibodies must be considered [13]. HLA antigens are the most common cause of immune-mediated refractoriness [13]. Consulting with the Transfusion Medicine Service or blood bank can help clarify the need for additional HLA antibody testing and subsequent HLA-matched product requests in select individuals.

HLA antigens are also implicated in transfusion reactions. Plasma products are a suspension of proteins, immunoglobulins, coagulation factors, and a multitude of other dissolved substances necessary for cellular metabolism. HLA antibodies may be included in this suspension, which can result in HLA antibody-mediated transfusion reactions. Transfusion of plasma-containing products, which may harbor HLA antibody, have the potential to cause transfusion-related acute lung injury (TRALI). Leukocytes with HLA Class I and II antigens are commonly found in cellular blood products, which have the potential to cause HLA-mediated febrile non hemolytic transfusion reaction (FNHTR), rare hemolytic transfusion reactions (HTR), potentially fatal transfusion-associated graft versus host disease (TA-GVHD), as well as TRALI [14, 15]. All transfusion reactions are described in greater detail in Chapter 12: Complications of Blood Transfusions.

In the event of a transfusion reaction, the transfusion must be stopped immediately and a workup is required [14]. The initial work up steps include checking all clerical work for errors, retyping the patient ABO, visually assessing for plasma discoloration indicative of hemolysis, and performing a direct antiglobulin test (DAT) [14]. The DAT can help distinguish immune from non immune-mediated hemolysis causes and is also used in HDFN and autoimmune hemolytic anemia workups. The DAT can determine if an individual's RBCs are coated with immunoglobulin and/or complement. An appropriate specimen must be received in an ethylenediaminetetraacetic acid (EDTA) tube, to chelate calcium from the sample and stop the in-vitro fixation of complement, which could cause a false-positive result. Unfortunately, there are many causes of a false-positive DAT (infections, high serum immunoglobulins, antiphospholipid syndrome, medications), and up to 15% of hospitalized patients with no signs of hemolysis will have a positive test [16]. A positive DAT is therefore not diagnostic of hemolytic anemia, but must be examined in the context of the patient's diagnoses, medication history, pregnancy status, and transfusion history. If the work up rules out hemolysis, other etiologies must be investigated to classify the transfusion reaction [15].

Alloimmunization

An alloantibody is an antibody produced to an antigen that an individual lacks [8]. Alloimmunization (alloantibody formation) is a known complication of transfusion and transplant therapy. Alloantibodies to cellular antigens can also be formed naturally during pregnancy and can put subsequent pregnancies at risk (see Chapter 23). Studies have demonstrated that the risk of alloimmunization is dependent on a number of factors including the number of red cell containing units administered, the health of the recipient, and recipient genetic factors [17, 18]. Once an alloantibody has been generated, recipients may be at risk for future platelet refractoriness and transfusion reactions, described above.

Historically, the formation of an anti-D alloantibody has been considered the most concerning. D-antigens are highly immunogenic and anti-D antibodies can cause severe and potentially fatal hemolytic reactions. In the 1970s, it was demonstrated that 80% of healthy male volunteers formed an anti-D antibody when exposed to small doses of Rh-positive red blood cells [19]. The majority of hospitalized patients receiving red blood cell transfusions, however, are not "healthy." Subsequent studies have demonstrated a much lower rate of alloimmunization, ranging 20–30% in non-immunosuppressed individuals and massively transfused recipients [20, 21]. Alloimmunization rates of less than 10% were identified in immunosuppressed patients, including those with hematologic malignancies, acquired immunodeficiency syndrome (AIDS), or on immunosuppressive therapy [17, 22]. Decreased rates of alloantibody formation may be secondary to dampened responses to foreign antigens encountered in these states [9, 23].

Platelets differ from RBCs in that they express HPA antigens, in addition to ABO and Class I HLA antigens. Exposure to foreign HLA and HPA antigens can lead to the generation of HLA and HPA antibodies. Class I HLA antigens are the most immunogenic platelet antigens. Of acute myelogenous leukemia patients transfused with platelets, 45% formed HLA antibodies [9]. Conversely, only 8% of recipients demonstrated HPA antibodies following platelet transfusions [9]. Both types of antibodies can cause rapid clearance of transfused platelets, decreasing or eliminating their therapeutic benefit. Some of these platelet antibodies are capable of crossing the placenta, leading to neonatal alloimmune thrombocytopenia (NAIT). Platelet units may also contain variably small quantities of suspended RBCs. Rarely, passively transfused RhD-positive RBCs can cause anti-D antibody formation in RhD-negative individuals at a rate of less than 4% [24].

Chronically transfused patients pose a unique and difficult challenge to a transfusion service when considering alloimmunization risk. Treatment of patients with both benign and malignant hematologic diagnoses may require frequent red blood cell or platelet transfusions, but repeated exposure to foreign red cell and platelet antigens may result in the formation of multiple red cell, HLA, and/or HPA alloantibodies. Beyond the aforementioned complications of alloimmunization, finding compatible units for these patients may be difficult, leading to transfusion delays [9]. In these cases, providers must be aware that anywhere from hours to weeks may be required to obtain compatible RBC or platelet units. In some instances, nationwide donor searches are required.

Inventory Management

Since 2010, the National Blood Collection and Utilization Survey has noted a decrease in both blood donations and usage [25]. Modern blood banking practice has evolved to do more with less, challenging historical concepts of unit selection.

RBC Considerations

As our knowledge of alloimmunization and associated transfusion reactions has increased, demand for the least immunogenic blood products has increased. Universal RBC donor units were once identified as group O, RhD-negative (O-negative), but demands for this product have begun to outstrip availability [26]. In emergent situations requiring massive transfusion or large volume hemorrhage where the patient's blood type is unknown, O-negative product is the preferred standard for initial resuscitation to reduce the risk of RhD-alloimmunization and likelihood of an anti-RhD hemolytic transfusion reaction. Additionally, O-negative RBCs are almost exclusively used in neonates secondary to typing, sampling, and name challenges; those with significant alloimmunization; and in patients undergoing bone marrow transplant [26, 27]. Donor centers actively recruit group O donors, but D-negative individuals make up only 15% of the Caucasian and 8% of the Black populations [1]. In 2014, only 8.2% of American blood donors were O-negative [28]. These numbers highlight the scarcity and finite availability of O-negative RBC units.

To balance high demands with decreasing supply, blood conservation strategies and blood management programs are being instituted across the United States. Blood management programs are recommended by many professional societies and improve transfusion practices via evidence-based guidelines [29, 30]. Implemented programs may include written policies and procedures to prevent unnecessary transfusions via restrictive RBC transfusion recommendations (hemoglobin of <7.0 g/dL), lab-guided emergency transfusion protocols, or single unit orders with required interim RBC counts in the absence of a life-threatening bleed [24, 26, 31]. These strategies have been shown to reduce product use by 40%, while reducing patient morbidity and mortality [31, 32].

Strategies specific to conservation of O-negative units include transfusing this resource only to proven O-negative patients, using patient-specific criteria to switch from O-negative to O-positive product, adhering to restrictive transfusion thresholds, and limiting blood unit wastage [20, 24, 26, 27] (Table 2.4). Inventory management is crucial for all patient types. Even in neonatal centers, where O-negative product is almost exclusively used, aliquots of the same RBC

Table 2.4 Transfusion threshold recommendations [52–54]

Product	Indication	Recommendation to transfuse
Packed red blood cell units[a]	Hospitalized, hemodynamically stable adult	<7 g/dL
	Orthopedic surgery Cardiac surgery Preexisting cardiovascular disease	<8 g/dL
Platelet units[b]	Hospitalized, hemodynamically stable adult	<10 x 10^9 cells/L
	Elective central venous catheter placement	<20 x 10^9 cells/L
	Diagnostic lumbar puncture or major elective nonneuroaxial surgery	<50 x 10^9 cells/L
Plasma (FFP) products	Trauma patients requiring massive transfusion	Suggested to give (no specific recommendations made)

[a]These recommendations do not apply to those with acute coronary syndromes or transfusion-dependent anemia

[b]No official recommendations have been made regarding transfusion thresholds for those with intracranial hemorrhage

unit can be used for multiple neonates. Additionally, during large trauma or emergent situations where ABO and RhD type are unavailable, many centers have protocolized the use of O-positive RBCs in men and women beyond childbearing age [26]. Delayed hemolytic reactions due to RhD-alloimmunization in these populations are extremely rare and pose limited risk to the patient [24, 26]. This approach reserves RhD-negative product for known RhD-negative individuals and young women of childbearing age without a known type, who would be at risk for potentially fatal HDFN during pregnancy if alloimmunized.

Individual patient factors can also be considered when allocating O-negative units. Even with young females, hospital policies may advocate for switching to O-positive products during large volume resuscitations given local inventory and the patient's likelihood of survival [24]. Additionally, intensive care units have been identified as a location where switching to O-positive RBCs may be beneficial in times of product shortage. These patients are less likely to be chronically transfused and may have shorter life spans, making RhD-alloimmunization less significant [26].

Platelet Considerations

Various inventory management strategies have been implemented to address platelet product shortages. Bacterial contamination in platelets is a significant concern due to their room temperature storage (see Chapter 3). Accordingly, platelet shelf life was restricted to five days until 2016, when the US Food and Drug Administration (FDA) provided guidance on improving platelet safety while extending apheresis platelet shelf life to seven days with the use of approved storage containers, pathogen reduction technologies (PRT), and appropriate bacterial detection protocols (see Pathogen Reduction Technologies section below) [33]. These new guidelines have led to improved platelet availability and decreased outdating wastage [34].

Efforts to encourage responsible transfusion practices have also helped with shortages. Platelet transfusion thresholds are generally well established and have resulted in decreased use over time, though variation exists between centers [35, 36]. Platelet doses necessary to maintain hemostasis are controversial. Prophylactic administration of low-dose platelets ($1.1x10^{11}$–$4.4x10^{11}$) had no effect on bleeding incidence when compared to more standard doses [37]. Based on this evidence, medical directors may routinely split apheresis-derived platelet units in certain clinical situations to better ration platelet inventory.

Plasma Considerations

Plasma products present a unique challenge to inventory management. The universal plasma donor is group AB, representing only 4% of the population [5]. Especially in the Level 1 Trauma Center setting, having immediately available thawed plasma for emergent resuscitation is a necessity. While AB plasma would be the optimal choice, many centers now provide group A plasma for initial resuscitation efforts secondary to inventory limitations. Despite the concern for potential acute hemolytic transfusion reactions between A plasma and non compatible B recipients, no increased mortality or ABO-related acute hemolytic transfusion reactions have been reported with this change [38]. These outcomes are partially attributed to 85% of the population being compatible (either group O or A recipients) [5]. Additionally, recipients of massive transfusions are likely receiving high volumes of group O RBCs, which would not be affected by the transfused group A plasma anti-B antibodies [38, 39]. Furthermore, anti-B antibodies may be neutralized by secreted antigens in incompatible group B individuals [38]. Group A plasma is a safe alternative to group AB plasma during initial massive resuscitation while preserving group AB plasma inventory for other deserving patients in the hospital [9, 14, 23, 39].

Ordering Practices

Surgical service blood ordering practices are critical to inventory management in the hospital-based setting. Orders including:

- **Type and Hold**: Recipient ABO and RhD determined without antibody testing.
- **Type and Screen**: Recipient ABO, RhD, and antibody identification performed. No crossmatch performed on specific units, but compatible blood is available in most situations.
- **Type and Crossmatch**: Recipient ABO, RhD, and antibody identification performed. Units are removed from inventory and crossmatched to the recipient for compatibility.

A type and crossmatch order results in units being removed from inventory and assigned to a specific patient. These units are therefore unavailable in an emergency or for another patient. Over ordering of crossmatched products can result in inventory shortages and outdating of products that go unused. To mitigate these issues, crossmatch-to-transfusion (C:T) ratios are monitored, and a ratio > 2.0 suggests excessive ordering of crossmatched blood [6]. Strategies to reduce this waste include policies for preferential ordering of type and screens and the development of a hospital-specific Maximum Surgical Blood Order Schedule for common procedures that sets the number of units to be designated based on the intervention.

By combining their knowledge of hospital usage patterns, component outdating, and distance from their supplier, each transfusion services must determine their blood supply needs. Inventory levels must meet routine daily needs, while maintaining enough product for emergency-related transfusion requirements [6]. In particular, maintaining an adequate supply of O-negative RBCs (universal donor) for emergency procedures and rapidly expiring platelets levels remain daily challenges. Specialty products (e.g., cytomegalovirus negative, HLA-matched platelets) and modified products (e.g., leukoreduced, irradiated) requirements also need to be considered in terms of demand and supplier availability for delivery.

Serologic Versus Computer Crossmatch

Crossmatching is required on any product containing ≥2 mL of RBCs [6]. Serologic crossmatch has traditionally been used to demonstrate ABO compatibility between a recipient and donor product unit. Following ABO and Rh determination, an antibody screen is completed on the intended recipient. A potentially compatible unit is then selected for transfusion by the blood bank staff. The recipient's plasma is mixed with a red blood cell suspension made from donor unit. This mixture can then be examined for evidence of red blood cell clumping, indicating incompatibility.

Alternatively, an electronic records review or "computer crossmatch" can be used for the selection and verification of ABO-compatible RBC or whole blood products if the intended recipient has no current or historical clinically significant antibodies [40]. If computer crossmatching is used, the system must be validated on-site to select only ABO-compatible products, recognize required donor and recipient data, verify correct data entry, and be capable of identifying and alerting the user to discrepancies between the unit label and confirmatory testing, as well as between donor and recipient ABO and Rh types [40]. Additionally, electronic crossmatching is not permitted if ABO typing discrepancies are present [41].

Advantages of the electronic crossmatch use include decreased sample volume requirements, decreased workload for the transfusion service, and improved blood inventory management [6].

Emerging Infections

Beyond inventory concerns, modern transfusion medicine practice is also focused on the management of infectious disease risk. Transfusion-transmitted infections were described by the AABB in 2009 as "agents that pose a real or theoretical threat to transfusion safety, but for which existing effective interventions are lacking" [42]. Currently, the most dangerous emerging infections are those that have asymptomatic infectious phases, making donor screening difficult [43]. Difficult screening strategies equate with increasing the risk of transmission. The emergence of new pathogens is unpredictable, but mathematical modeling predicts a new transfusion-transmissible infection will emerge every five years [44]. Commonly considered infections in transfusion medicine are described below.

Arboviruses

Mosquitoes transmit the majority of medically significant arboviruses. Symptomatology can range from asymptomatic to severely debilitating disease to lethal. These viruses are frequently initially asymptomatic, making donor screening difficult to impossible in the early stages of disease. Transfusion-transmission has been documented for multiple arboviruses including Dengue and Zika virus, both recognized as emerging infection risks to the blood supply [43]. Unlike the majority of arboviruses that are unable to develop sufficient viremia within human hosts, these viruses maintain their viremia allowing for mosquito infection and continued spread in urban locations [45].

Dengue virus usually produces a self-limiting flu-like illness that rarely develops into life-threatening hemorrhagic fever. It can be transmitted by mosquitoes, blood transfusion, or solid organ transplant. There is currently no vaccine or treatment for infection, but symptomatology is usually asymptomatic to mild, and has not been demonstrated to be significantly different from non infected controls [42, 44].

Currently, donated blood products are not screened for Dengue in the United States [46] nor most other developed countries due to the general mildness of disease. This may change over the coming decades as mosquito grounds expand and cases become more prevalent.

Like Dengue, Zika virus infection initially begins with an asymptomatic viremia that usually results in a mild flu-like illness. Infection can result in a Guillian Barre-like syndrome or can cause miscarriage or congenital defects of pregnancy [42, 47]. Transmission may occur via mosquito, sexual contact, and blood transfusion. The FDA currently requires nucleic acid amplification testing (NAT) or the use of pathogen-reduced products in an attempt to limit the transmission risk [46].

Babesia Species

Babesiosis is a tick-borne protozoan illness endemic to the Northeastern and Midwestern United States [42]. Clinical manifestations range from asymptomatic to potentially fatal severe hemolytic disease. The most common species identified in the United States is *Babesia microti*. All known *Babesia* species can be transmitted through tick bite and red blood cell transfusion. The FDA recommends selective testing of blood donations for *Babesia* parasites in endemic regions. RNA NAT donor screening assays are currently available for testing, but only identify a limited number of *Babesia* species, including *B. microti* [42, 46].

Creutzfeldt–Jakob Disease (CJD)

CJD is a fatal neurodegenerative spongiform encephalitis resulting from abnormally folded proteins (prions). The majority of cases are due to sporadic mutations, with genetic and iatrogenic causes making up the remainder (6–16% of cases combined) [48]. Transmission has been identified in certain forms of transplant including corneal and human dura mater grafts, from the use of previously contaminated neurosurgical equipment or the use of human pituitary growth factor [7]. There have been no identified cases of CJD transfusion-transmission, but the risk remains theoretical [46]. Since 2000, the FDA has recommended permanent donor deferral based on risk factor screening for CJD as there are no commercially available tests or treatments [42, 48].

Pathogen Reduction Technology (PRT)

The FDA recommends PRT to aid in the reduction of infectious risk of some blood products. Blood donor screening and testing reduce the risk of transfusion-transmitted infections, but cannot address all asymptomatic yet viremic infection windows or screen for the disease in the absence of a developed test. It is also logistically and fiscally unrealistic to screen every donor unit for every known infectious risk [49]. PRT, however, reduces the need for extensive testing by eliminating bacteria and certain virus reproduction.

PRT uses a photochemical compound that is excited by light to cause nucleic acid cross-linking [50]. This cross-linking results in the inability of a pathogen to replicate. *Babesia microti,* Dengue, Zika virus, and other arboviruses are effectively inactivated using PRT, significantly decreasing their transmission risk [44, 50]. This treatment is also effective in reducing the transmission risk of other known bacteria, viruses, and protozoa [44]. Additionally, the technology disables leukocyte proliferation, reducing the need for irradiation while still decreasing the risk of TA-GVHD [51]. This technology may allow for the discontinuation of some currently required infectious disease testing in the future, helping to offset the costs associated with pathogen reduction.

PRT is approved for use on plasma and platelet products in the United States. Technologies for red blood cells and whole blood unit pathogen reduction are currently in trials. PRT has been especially beneficial in reducing transmission risk in platelet products. Due to platelet storage conditions (20–24 °C with continuous agitation for 5–7 days (see Chapter 3), bacterial proliferation is a known hazard. Transfusion services are currently required to have methods to detect or inactivate bacteria for these reasons [6]. As an alternative, the FDA allows the use of PRT.

PRT does have its limitations. Prion diseases are not affected by nucleic acid cross-linking and PRT is not as effective at inactivating non-enveloped viruses [50]. PRT platelets have lower corrected count increments following transfusion, more frequent transfusion failures and platelet refractoriness, and more platelet transfusions required per patient with shorter transfusion time intervals in between. There were no differences found in significant bleeding or adverse outcomes however when comparing PRT to non-PRT platelets [46].

Conclusion

Blood banking and transfusion medicine is a complex and evolving discipline. Familiarity with red blood cell and human leukocyte antigen (HLA) systems is essential to understand the impact of alloimmunization in clinical settings. Transfusion practices have adapted in an era of limited inventory. Blood donation campaigns have begun to target the younger generations, in an attempt to reinvigorate donors and protect long-term supplies, but an era of conservation and limited availability may be the new norm of modern blood banking. Clinicians who transfuse must be aware of modern transfusion topics to include evidence-based transfusion guidelines, shelf-life limitations, the use of O-positive red blood cells and thawed group A plasma in emergency transfusions, platelet product splitting, the effect of ordering practices on product availability, and the potential impact of emerging infections and PRT on transfusion risk. As always, your clinical pathology and transfusion medicine colleagues remain an available resource in this changing field.

References

1. Reid ME, Lomas-Francis C, Olsson ML. The blood group antigen facts book. Boston: Academic Press; 2012.
2. Westman JS, Olsson ML. ABO and other carbohydrate blood group systems. Technical manual. 19th ed. Bethesda: AABB; 2017. p. 265–75.
3. Avent ND, Reid ME. The Rh blood group system: a review. Blood. 2000;95(2):375–87.
4. Denomme GA, Westhoff CM. The Rh system. Technical manual. 19th ed. Bethesda: AABB; 2017. p. 295–9.
5. Garratty G, Glynn SA, McEntire R. Retrovirus epidemiology donor study. ABO and Rh (D) phenotype frequencies of different racial/ ethnic groups in the United States. Transfusion. 2004;44(5):703–6.
6. Harm SK, Dunbar NM. Transfusion-service-related activities: pretransfusion testing and storage, monitoring, processing, distribution and inventory management of blood components. Technical manual. 19th ed. Bethesda: AABB; 2017. p. 457–84.
7. Storry JR. Other blood group systems and antigens. Technical manual. 19th ed. Bethesda: AABB; 2017. p. 319–45.
8. Hamilton JR, Bailey DJ. Identification of antibodies to red cell antigens. Technical manual. 19th ed. Bethesda: AABB; 2017. p. 349–66.
9. Zimring JC, Welniak L, Semple JW, Ness PM, Slichter SJ, Spitalnik SL. NHLBI Alloimmunization working group. Current problems and future directions of transfusion-induced alloimmunization: summary of an NHLBI working group. Transfusion. 2011;51(2):435–41.
10. Petersdorf EW. HLA. In: Wingard JR, Gastineau DA, Leather HL, Snyder EL, Szczerpiorkowski ZM, editors. Hematopoietic stem cell transplantation: a handbook for clinicians. 2nd ed. AABB: Bethesda; 2015.
11. Eisenbrey AB, Kopko PMRA. The HLA system. Technical manual. 19th ed. Bethesda: AABB; 2017. p. 435–56.
12. Triulzi DJ, Assmann SF, Strauss RG, Ness PM, Hess JR, Kaufman RM, Granger S, Slichter SJ. The impact of platelet transfusion characteristics on posttransfusion platelet increments and clinical bleeding in patients with hypoproliferative thrombocytopenia. Blood. 2012;119(23):5553–62.
13. Vassallo RR, Curtis BR. Platelet and granulocyte antigens and antibodies. Technical manual. 19th ed. Bethesda: AABB; 2017. p. 413–9.
14. Harmening D. Modern blood banking and transfusion practices, 6th ed. Philadelphia: F.A. Davis Company; 2012.
15. U.S. Centers for Disease Control and Prevention. The National Healthcare Safety Network (NHSN) manual: Biovigilance Component v2.4. Atlanta: Division of Healthcare Quality Promotion, National Center for Emerging and Zoonotic Infectious Diseases. Available at: http://www.cdc.gov/nhsn/PDFs/Biovigilance/BV-HV-protocol-current.pdf. Accessed [8/24/19].
16. Parker V, Tormey CA. The direct antiglobulin test: indications, interpretation, and pitfalls. Arch Pathol Lab Med. 2017;141(2):305–10.
17. Meyer E, Uhl L. A case for stocking OD+ red blood cells in emergency room trauma bays. Transfusion. 2015;55(4):791–5.
18. Zalpuri S, Evers D, Zwaginga JJ, Schonewille H, de Vooght KM, le Cessie S, van der Bom JG. Immunosuppressants and alloimmunization against red blood cell transfusions. Transfusion. 2014;54(8):1981–7.
19. Gunson HH, Stratton F, Cooper DG, Rawlinson VI. Primary immunization of Rh-negative volunteers. Br Med J. 1970;1(5696):593–5.
20. Gonzalez-Porras JR, Graciani IF, Perez-Simon JA, Martin-Sanchez J, Encinas C, Conde MP, Nieto MJ, Corral M. Prospective evaluation of a transfusion policy of D+ red blood cells into D− patients. Transfusion. 2008;48(7):1318–24.
21. Yazer MH, Triulzi DJ. Detection of anti-D in D–recipients transfused with D+ red blood cells. Transfusion. 2007;47(12):2197–201.
22. Dutton RP, Shih D, Edelman BB, Hess J, Scalea TM. Safety of uncrossmatched type-O red cells for resuscitation from hemorrhagic shock. J Trauma Acute Care Surg. 2005;59(6):1445–9.
23. Frohn C, Dümbgen L, Brand JM, Görg S, Luhm J, Kirchner H. Probability of anti-D development in D− patients receiving D+ RBCs. Transfusion. 2003;43(7):893–8.
24. Callum JL, Waters JH, Shaz BH, Sloan SR, Murphy MF. The AABB recommendations for the choosing wisely campaign of the American Board of Internal Medicine. Transfusion. 2014;54(9):2344–52.
25. Ellingson KD, Sapiano MR, Haass KA, Savinkina AA, Baker ML, Chung KW, Henry RA, Berger JJ, Kuehnert MJ, Basavaraju SV. Continued decline in blood collection and transfusion in the United States–2015. Transfusion. 2017;57:1588–98.
26. Dunbar NM, Yazer MH, OPTIMUS Study Investigators on behalf of the Biomedical Excellence for Safer Transfusion (BEST) Collaborative. O–product transfusion, inventory management, and utilization during shortage: the OPTIMUS study. Transfusion. 2018;58(6):1348–55.
27. Zeller MP, Barty R, Aandahl A, Apelseth TO, Callum J, Dunbar NM, Elahie A, Garritsen H, Hancock H, Kutner JM, Manukian B. An international investigation into O red blood cell unit administration in hospitals: the GRoup O Utilization Patterns (GROUP) study. Transfusion. 2017;57(10):2329–37.
28. Sapiano MR, Savinkina AA, Ellingson KD, Haass KA, Baker ML, Henry RA, Berger JJ, Kuehnert MJ, Basavaraju SV. Supplemental findings from the National Blood Collection and Utilization Surveys, 2013 and 2015. Transfusion. 2017;57:1599.
29. Meybohm P, Richards T, Isbister J, Hofmann A, Shander A, Goodnough LT, Muñoz M, Gombotz H, Weber CF, Choorapoikayil S, Spahn DR. Patient blood management bundles to facilitate implementation. Transfus Med Rev. 2017;31(1):62–71.
30. Patient Blood Management [Internet]. AABB [cited 2019 Aug 27]. Available from http://www.aabb.org/pbm/Pages/default.aspx. Accessed [8/24/19].
31. Nunnes GR, Moore EE, Stettler GR, Moore HB, Ghasabyan A, Cohen M, Huebner BR, Silliman CC, Banerjee A, Sauaia A. Empiric transfusion strategies during life-threatening hemorrhage. Surgery. 2018;164(2):306–11.
32. Salpeter SR, Buckley JS, Chatterjee S. Impact of more restrictive blood transfusion strategies on clinical outcomes: a meta-analysis and systematic review. Am J Med. 2014;127(2):124–31.
33. Food and Drug Administration. Draft guidance for industry: bacterial risk control strategies for blood collection establishments and transfusion services to enhance the safety and availability of platelets for transfusion. Silver Spring: CBER Office of Communication, Outreach, and Development; 2016. Available at: https://www.fda.gov/downloads/BiologicsBloodVaccines/GuidanceComplianceRegulatoryInformation/Guidances/Blood/UCM425952.pdf. Accessed [8/24/19].
34. Harm SK, Szczepiorkowski ZM, Dunbar NM. Routine use of day 6 and day 7 platelets with rapid testing: two hospitals assess impact 1 year after implementation. Transfusion. 2018;58(4):938–42.

35. Kaufman RM, Shehata N. Hemotherapy decisions and their outcomes. Technical manual. 19th ed. Bethesda: AABB; 2017. p. 511–8.
36. Rebulla P, Finazzi G, Marangoni F, Avvisati G, Gugliotta L, Tognoni G, Barbui T, Mandelli F, Sirchia G. The threshold for prophylactic platelet transfusions in adults with acute myeloid leukemia. N Engl J Med. 1997;337(26):1870–5.
37. Slichter SJ, Kaufman RM, Assmann SF, McCullough J, Triulzi DJ, Strauss RG, Gernsheimer TB, Ness PM, Brecher ME, Josephson CD, Konkle BA. Dose of prophylactic platelet transfusions and prevention of hemorrhage. N Engl J Med. 2010;362(7):600–13.
38. Dunbar NM, Yazer MH, Biomedical Excellence for Safer Transfusion (BEST) Collaborative and the STAT Study Investigators, Carey PM, Christie JD, Fadeyi EA, Fontaine MJ, George MR, Harm SK, Hess JR, Karp JK. Safety of the use of group A plasma in trauma: the STAT study. Transfusion. 2017;57(8):1879–1884.
39. Dunbar NM, Yazer MH. Biomedical Excellence for Safer Transfusion Collaborative. A possible new paradigm? A survey-based assessment of the use of thawed group A plasma for trauma resuscitation in the United States. Transfusion. 2016;56(1):125–9.
40. American Association of Blood Banks. Committee on Standards. Standards for blood banks and transfusion services. Bethesda: AABB; 2018.
41. Food and Drug Administration Guidance for Industry: "Computer Crossmatch" (computerized analysis of the compatibility between the donor's cell type and the recipient's serum or plasma type). Rockville: Food and Drug Administration; 2011.
42. Busch MP, Bloch EM, Kleinman S. Prevention of transfusion-transmitted infections. Blood. 2019;133(17):1854–64.
43. Petersen LR, Busch MP. Transfusion-transmitted arboviruses. Vox Sang. 2010;98(4):495–503.
44. Schlenke P. Pathogen inactivation technologies for cellular blood components: an update. Transfus Med Hemother. 2014;41(4):309–25.
45. Marano G, Pupella S, Vaglio S, Liumbruno GM, Grazzini G. Zika virus and the never-ending story of emerging pathogens and transfusion medicine. Blood Transfus. 2016;14(2):95.
46. Cohn CS, Allen ES, Cushing MM, Dunbar NM, Friedman DF, Goel R, Heddle N, Hopkins CK, Klapper E, Perumbeti A, Ramsey G. Critical developments of 2018: a review of the literature from selected topics in transfusion. A committee report from the AABB's Clinical Transfusion Medicine Committee. Transfusion. 2019;59:2733.
47. Fryk JJ, Marks DC, Hobson-Peters J, Watterson D, Hall RA, Young PR, Reichenberg S, Tolksdorf F, Sumian C, Gravemann U, Seltsam A. Reduction of Zika virus infectivity in platelet concentrates after treatment with ultraviolet C light and in plasma after treatment with methylene blue and visible light. Transfusion. 2017;57(11):2677–82.
48. Crowder LA, Schonberger LB, Dodd RY, Steele WR. Creutzfeldt–Jakob disease lookback study: 21 years of surveillance for transfusion transmission risk. Transfusion. 2017;57(8):1875–8.
49. Stramer SL, Glael SA. Infectious disease screening. Technical manual. 19th ed. Bethesda: AABB; 2017. p. 193–5.
50. Magron A, Laugier J, Provost P, Boilard E. Pathogen reduction technologies: the pros and cons for platelet transfusion. Platelets. 2018;29(1):2–8.
51. Kleinman S, Reed W, Stassinopoulous A. A patient-oriented risk-benefit analysis of pathogen-inactivation blood components: application to apheresis platelets in the United States. Transfusion. 2013;53(7):1603–18.
52. Carson JL, Guyatt G, Heddle NM, Grossman BJ, Cohn CS, Fung MK, Gernsheimer T, Holcomb JB, Kaplan LJ, Katz LM, Peterson N. Clinical practice guidelines from the AABB: red blood cell transfusion thresholds and storage. JAMA. 2016;316(19):2025–35.
53. Kaufman RM, Djulbegovic B, Gernsheimer T, Kleinman S, Tinmouth AT, Capocelli KE, Cipolle MD, Cohn CS, Fung MK, Grossman BJ, Mintz PD. Platelet transfusion: a clinical practice guideline from the AABB. Ann Intern Med. 2015;162(3):205–13.
54. Roback JD, Caldwell S, Carson J, Davenport R, Drew MJ, Eder A, Fung M, Hamilton M, Hess JR, Luban N, Perkins JG. Evidence-based practice guidelines for plasma transfusion. Transfusion. 2010;50(6):1227–39.

Blood Component Therapy

3

Christine T. Vo and Pamela R. Roberts

Introduction

In the United States, the US Food and Drug Administration (FDA) Center for Biologics Evaluation and Research sets the standards regarding collection of blood components and whole blood. All entities that collect, prepare, store, process, or distribute blood products must be registered with the FDA and inspected by them at defined intervals. Many institutions that collect or prepare blood products also get accreditation by the American Association of Blood Banks (AABB) since this organization sets standards that help maintain quality and safety of blood banking and transfusion practices. Other parts of the world have similar entities.

Combat history and related medical care during the last century contributed much of what we know about treatment of trauma and principles of resuscitation and contributed to blood banking technology. From the 1940s through 1960s, the military program mostly used whole blood. But following the Vietnam War, interest grew in the civilian medical arena to conserve blood and focus on treating specific component deficiencies resulting in the predominance of component therapy in the 1970s–1990s [1–3]. Component therapy allowed longer storage times and lower rates of infection. By the mid-2000s, persistent coagulopathy was recognized as contributing to deaths from severe trauma. [4] In 2012, Pidcoke and colleagues published a large retrospective cohort study of patients injured in Operation Iraqi Freedom and Operation Enduring Freedom and reported that use of a 1:1:1 ratio of red blood cells (RBCs), platelets, and fresh frozen plasma conveyed a significant survival benefit as opposed to transfusion of then traditional large volumes of packed RBCs [5]. Over the last decade, clinical studies of improved outcomes with whole blood for hemorrhaging patients led to renewed interest in utilizing whole blood for transfusion of critically injured trauma patients or those with severe hemorrhaging. Massive transfusion strategies are covered elsewhere in this book. This chapter will focus on specifics of blood components derived from blood donation.

PRBCs

Provision of packed red blood cells (PRBCs) or red blood cell (RBC) units relies on donation of blood from volunteers. These donors first undergo screening of their medical history which specifically addresses risk factors for infectious diseases or other complications. For example, women that have been pregnant should be screened as they may have developed HLA antibodies and therefore convey a risk of a recipient developing transfusion associated acute lung injury (TRALI). Then, all donated blood undergoes laboratory testing for specific infectious organisms and viruses. Details of all elements of screening and laboratory testing are beyond the scope of this chapter, but have led to significant reduction of transmission of disease via blood transfusion. However, the risk of new emerging infections is a constant potential threat to our blood supply, as was seen most recently with Zika virus and West Nile virus.

Most commonly a unit of whole blood with a volume of 500–600 mL is donated and undergoes routine centrifugation to separate it into components including RBCs, platelets, and plasma. Alternatively, RBC units can be obtained via apheresis; in the United States, about 20% of RBC units are collected via apheresis [6]. For apheresis, a donor with an adequate hematocrit is connected to an apheresis machine which separates other constituents from the RBCs and returns the other cellular and plasma constituents to the donor. Typically, this type of apheresis will yield two units of

C. T. Vo
University of Oklahoma College of Medicine, Department of Anesthesiology, Oklahoma City, OK, USA
e-mail: christine-vo@ouhsc.edu

P. R. Roberts (✉)
Department of Anesthesiology, University of Oklahoma College of Medicine, Oklahoma City, OK, USA
e-mail: pamela-roberts@ouhsc.edu

© Springer Nature Switzerland AG 2021
A. D. Kaye, S. Leavitt (eds.), *Essentials of Blood Product Management in Anesthesia Practice*,
https://doi.org/10.1007/978-3-030-59295-0_3

RBCs. However, some apheresis systems can collect a single unit of RBCs along with a unit of platelets and/or plasma. The number of RBCs in an RBC unit from donated whole blood will vary based on the donor's hemoglobin level. In contrast, apheresis units are collected in a manner that provides more standardized numbers of RBCs per unit. Both types of RBC units provide sufficient RBCs for transfusion.

In the early 1960s, bags made of polyvinyl chloride became available for storage of blood products, permitting separation of collected products into components in a sterile, closed environment. The plasticizer used in bags for RBC storage is di-2-ethylhexylphthalate (DEHP) and it is key to preservation of the integrity of the RBC membrane during prolonged storage. It is believed that small amounts of DEHP leak into the stored unit but no deleterious effects of DEHP have been found from transfused RBCs in patients. That said, concerns of potential exposure to DEHP from other medical devices are extended to RBC recipients and in particular neonates who may be vulnerable to related adverse effects of DEHP or toxic metabolites. Due to these concerns, efforts are underway to develop an alternative plasticizer that is also capable of stabilizing red cell membrane integrity [7].

Preservation of blood requires an anticoagulant-preservative (A-P) solution. It was a major breakthrough in the 1940s when acid citrate dextrose was developed as the first A-P solution allowing storage for up to 21 days. Since then, other A-P solutions were developed: citrate phosphate dextrose (CPD) with 21-day storage, CDP-adenine with 35-day storage, and current generation additive solutions with 42-day storage. There are several additive formulations used in the United States from different manufacturers denoted as AS-1, AS-3, and AS-5. A solution similar to AS-1 is used in Europe and it is saline, adenine, glucose, mannitol (SAGM). These additive solutions maintain the pH and other essential parameters for RBC shelf life [6]. This has resulted in less loss of RBC units due to being outdated. Less additive is used than the volume of plasma that was removed resulting in a higher hematocrit and lower volume than in the original unit of whole blood. See Table 3.1 for expected volumes and hematocrits of RBCs obtained from the methods described. Whole blood is collected into an anticoagulant solution and the additive preservative solution is added to the RBC units through an integral bag system soon after collection and component preparation. Apheresis-derived RBCs undergo similar procedures depending on the apheresis device.

Table 3.1 Practical differences of RBCs from current common methodologies

Type of storage or additive	Final volume (mL)	Hematocrit (%)
CPD-adenine (CPD-A1)	225–350	65–80
AS formulations	300–400	55–65
Apheresis-derived	175–200	55–60

Table 3.2 Populations that should receive leukocyte-reduced blood components [8]

History of a previous febrile nonhemolytic transfusion reaction
Undergoing cardiac surgery [9]
Recipients or potential recipients of solid organ or hematopoietic cell transplants [10]
Acute leukemias and probably other malignancies
Chronically transfused
CMV seronegative at risk patients if they are not given seronegative components

Leukocytes are naturally collected along with other cellular elements during blood donation. A unit of whole blood or packed RBCs has about 2–5 billion leukocytes and these are believed to convey risk of adverse effects such as human leukocyte antigen (HLA) alloimmunization, febrile nonhemolytic reactions, transmission of cytomegalovirus (CMV) or intracellular organisms, and potentially other immunologic and inflammatory mediated events. Leukocyte depletion or reduction refers to the process of filtering the blood to remove leukocytes and can be done before storage or at the time of transfusion. Leukoreduction prior to storage is preferred since it results in removal of more leukocytes as well as better quality control and standardization of the process. Such processes decrease the leukocyte load by approximately 99.9%, thereby significantly decreasing adverse events. Leukoreduction decreases the hemoglobin concentration by up to 15%. Some clinical populations are at higher risk of leukocyte-related adverse reactions, so it is recommended that they receive leukocyte-reduced blood components when transfused [8] (See Table 3.2). Currently, universal leukoreduction is a standard practice in many developed countries. In the United States, more than 80% of institutions provide universally leukoreduced RBCs with an estimated 85% of these using pre-storage leukoreduction processes [6]. When ordering transfusions, one needs to be familiar with local processes such as leukoreduction so that ordering for at-risk patients is clinically appropriate. If RBC units are not universally leukoreduced, this should be specifically requested for selected patients. In general, pre-storage leukoreduction is preferable to bedside leukoreduction; bedside leukoreduction is preferable to transfusion of non-leukoreduced RBC units. Of note, leukoreduction techniques do not prevent transfusion-associated graft versus host disease (TAGVHD) since even a small number of cells can contribute to this disorder. Susceptible patients should receive irradiated blood to prevent graft versus host disease.

Irradiation of RBC units prior to transfusion is sufficient to inactivate lymphocytes that can attack recipient cells in immunologically impaired individuals resulting in TAGVHD. All hematopoietic cells as well as other tissues can be targets of TAGVHD. Bone marrow aplasia as well as other fatal complications can occur from

Table 3.3 Populations that should receive irradiated blood components [11]

Premature neonates and recipients of intrauterine or neonatal exchange transfusion
Recipients of autologous or allogeneic hematopoietic stem cell transplants
Individuals with any stage of Hodgkin lymphoma
Individuals receiving treatment with potent immune-suppressing therapies (e.g., some monoclonal antibodies, antithymocyte globulin); may include those with hematologic malignancies and non-Hodgkin lymphoma
Individuals at risk for partial HLA-matching with the donor due to directed donations, HLA-matched products, or genetically homogenous populations

Table 3.4 Populations that should receive CMV-negative blood components if they are not CMV-positive

Low birth weight neonates
Pregnant women
HIV-infected individuals
Recipients of solid organ transplants
Recipients of hematopoietic stem cell transplants

TAGVHD. Randomized trials have not been performed to establish which patients must be given irradiated blood and recommendations are based on observational evidence and attempts to predict the degree of immunosuppression of populations. Table 3.3 lists patient populations for which irradiated components are recommended; some of these are lifelong needs while others may be time-limited [11]. In the United States, each hospital typically develops its own policy regarding which patient populations should be given irradiated products [12]. Society guidelines should be consulted for specific recommendations.

Cytomegalovirus (CMV) seronegative components have tested negative for the presence of CMV using antibody testing. Enough units are typically tested for CMV so that an adequate supply of CMV-negative units is available to be administered to individuals at risk of clinically serious CMV infection (See Table 3.4). In the general adult population, at least 40% have been exposed to CMV; however, exposure varies geographically. Individuals that are immunocompetent generally do not need CMV-negative blood as they can mount their own immune responses. However, immunocompromised individuals that are CMV-negative can develop serious CMV infections if given a unit of CMV-positive blood. Conversely, if they are already CMV-positive, they can likely receive CMV-positive units [6]. Of note, leukoreduction is considered to be of equivalent safety to administering CMV-negative components for individuals at risk of severe CMV infections and may be an alternative to transfusion of seronegative units.

RBC units must be stored at controlled refrigeration temperatures of 1–6 °C to preserve viability and prevent bacterial growth. During transport between facilities such as from a blood collection facility to a hospital, temperatures of 1–10 °C must be sustained. Similarly, during transport from a blood bank to a patient care area for transfusion, these same transport temperatures must be maintained. Changes to RBCs during storage include depletion of ATP, membrane changes, oxidative damage to lipids and proteins, leakage of potassium, and loss of the ability to change shape for flow in the microvasculature.

In the United States, RBCs can be stored up to 42 days; average storage of RBC units is estimated to be between 15–19 days [6]. Numerous randomized clinical trials have evaluated whether longer storage times result in more recipient morbidity or not. These have demonstrated similar outcomes from transfusion of fresh compared to longer or standard issue RBCs. These include the ARIPI trial (Age of Red Blood Cells in Premature Infants), the TOTAL trial in children (Tissue Oxygenation by Transfusion in Severe Anemia with Lactic Acidosis), the RECESS trial in cardiac surgery patients (Red Cell Storage Duration Study), and the TRANSFUSE trial (Standard Issue Transfusion versus Fresher Red-Cell Use in Intensive Care) [13–16]. Additionally, a meta-analysis by Alexander et al. also confirmed lack of clinical benefit of use of RBC units with shorter storage times [17].

RBC units can be frozen in 40% glycerol and are approved by the United States FDA and AABB to be stored at -80 °C for up to ten years. The major reasons for freezing RBC units is to maintain a supply of very rare blood group phenotypes (e.g., Bombay phenotype) or for those who have developed numerous alloantibodies directed against common RBC blood group antigens [18]. A randomized trial of 57 trauma patients comparing refrigerated RBC units to frozen then deglycerolized RBC units did not demonstrate significant differences in effects on hematocrit, thromboelastography parameters, or clinical outcomes [19]. However, preparing RBCs for freezing, thawing, then removing the glycerol is time consuming and thus delays transfusion as well as increases the costs, so is not utilized unless necessary.

Administration of RBC units should start with informed consent except in emergency situations where consent cannot be immediately obtained. Care must be taken to assure the intended unit is given to the intended recipient to prevent transfusion reactions (e.g., acute hemolytic transfusion reactions due to ABO mismatch). Data do not support routine pre medication with acetaminophen or antihistamines for prevention of allergic transfusion or febrile nonhemolytic reactions. The unit should be visually inspected for any abnormalities. RBC units must be transfused through a 170–260 micron filter to remove clots or aggregates of cellular components. Patients at risk of hypothermia or those with autoimmune cold-induced hemolysis can receive blood warmed to near body temperature but no higher than 40 °C as heat can cause hemolysis.

As a general rule, fluids containing calcium should not be administered through the same tubing concurrently with RBCs as the calcium may chelate the citrate and thus overcome the anticoagulant effect of citrate and clotting may occur in the tubing. Compatible fluids for concurrent transfusion include 0.9% sodium chloride, plasma, and albumin. Generally, use of Ringer's lactate is prohibited as it contains calcium, although some have advocated it for emergency trauma cases due to immediate needs of therapy [6]. The safety of this practice has not been verified and we recommend the safety of avoiding Ringer's lactate in this circumstance. Dextrose containing intravenous fluids should not be administered through the same tubing concurrently as the dextrose can be taken up rapidly by the RBCs which will then uptake water and then lyse. When transfusing via a multi-lumen central line, other meds may be administered simultaneously via other lumens. When concurrently administered with RBC units, it can be challenging to distinguish potential adverse effects of medications versus transfusion reactions. If the same lumen is to be used for medications before or after a transfusion, the lumen should be flushed with normal saline both before and after a medication.

RBC units should be given at rates that are efficient but that do not increase risk of volume overload. Typically, a rate of 1–2 mL/min over the first 15 minutes followed by a faster rate as tolerated is adequate. One RBC unit should be transfused over no more than 4 hours. For patients at higher risk of circulatory overload, slower rates using partial units may be indicated to avoid complications. Concomitant diuretics may be helpful in preventing circulatory overload in some patients.

Indications for RBC unit transfusions include symptomatic anemias and acute blood loss. Physiologic triggers include shock with marginal hemoglobin levels, orthostatic hypotension, and evidence of end-organ damage from inadequate tissue oxygenation to maintain vital organ function. For example, symptomatic anemia may manifest as dyspnea or fatigue with exercise. Anemia itself warrants investigation into its cause, so appropriate diagnostic studies and treatment can be administered. Historically, RBC transfusion was guided by a "10/30 rule" which aimed to maintain a hemoglobin of 10 g/dL and a hematocrit of 30%. Along with this goal, it was a historic standard practice to transfuse two or more RBC units per transfusion [20]. Over the last 20 years, clinical concerns of risks of transfusions led to recognition of the need to establish indications that provide greater benefit than risk to patients receiving RBC unit transfusions. Multiple randomized trials in varied populations demonstrated either noninferiority or superiority of restrictive transfusion strategies (aimed for hemoglobin levels of 7–8 g/dL) versus more liberal ones [21]. The Choosing Wisely Campaign started in the United States in 2012 and now includes participating clinical groups from over 20 countries on five continents. Single unit transfusions followed by reassessment and treating iron deficiency anemia with iron instead of transfusion in patients that are hemodynamically stable are both strategies promoted in the Choosing Wisely recommendations from the American Society of Hematology, the AABB, and the Canadian Society for Transfusion Medicine [22]. Further, it is recommended that a restrictive threshold of 7–8 g/dL hemoglobin be used for most hospitalized stable patients without evidence of inadequate tissue oxygenation. For patients with pre existing cardiovascular disease, they note that evidence supports a threshold of 8 g/dL. The recommendations also make the point that a decision to transfuse should include assessment of symptoms as well as hemoglobin level.

An international consensus statement recommends that anesthesia providers take a lead role with pre operative assessment using strategies aimed at reducing need for peri operative transfusions starting with assessment and treatment of pre operative anemia. They even recommend delay of major non urgent surgery to allow diagnosis and treatment of anemia and iron deficiency [23]. A recent meta-analysis by Chong et al. compared studies using restrictive vs liberal transfusion strategies for critically ill vs surgical patients [24]. These authors reported that restrictive strategies led to better outcomes which included reduced risk of stroke, transfusion reactions, packed RBC exposure, hospital length of stay, and 30-day mortality in critically ill patients. For surgical patients, the restrictive compared to a liberal strategy was associated with an opposite direction effect on mortality which was reported as a potentially increased risk or no difference between strategies. Both populations were exposed to lower RBC units with restrictive strategies. Caution should be taken at over extrapolation of this meta-analysis as future studies are required to target specific goals for different perioperative stages of care as well as varied surgical populations.

Improved donor questionnaires and sophisticated laboratory screenings for infectious diseases has significantly reduced infectious complications of transfusions. Noninfectious serious complications of blood transfusions are now more common than infectious ones [25]. Transfusion reactions include febrile, hemolytic, septic, allergic, urticarial, and anaphylactic reactions. Other complications such as mistransfusion, TRALI, transfusion-associated circulatory overload (TACO), TAGVHD, alloimmunization, iron overload, and metabolic derangements to name a few. Complications of RBC transfusions are covered in detail elsewhere in this book. Some strategies to reduce complications are obvious such as avoiding unnecessary transfusions and others employ use of electronic systems to help assure patient identification and appropriate blood matching to the patient [26]. Appropriate use of RBC units and attention to details of administration are vital to provide safe delivery of this vital resource to patients.

Fresh Frozen Plasma

Fresh Frozen Plasma (FFP) is obtained from whole blood or apheresis donations using a centrifugal process. Citrate-containing anticoagulants and preservatives are added to whole blood prior to separation into its components to increase its shelf life and reduce biochemical changes. Blood separates into its components via centrifugation, with plasma precipitating to the top, leukocytes and platelets to the middle, and RBCs to the bottom. Essentially, platelet-rich plasma is expressed after the first centrifugation step. It is further separated into plasma and platelet concentrates with a second, higher speed centrifugation. Within eight hours of collection, plasma is immediately frozen to −18 °C or colder and stored for up to one year. FFP can be further processed to produce cryoprecipitate [27]. When plasma is frozen greater than 8 hours from collection, but less than 24 hours, this is termed plasma frozen within 24 hours of phlebotomy (PF24). The clinical efficacy of clotting factors in PF24 are similar to FFP except for a mild decrease in the labile clotting factors VIII and protein C when thawed [28]. To prevent contamination, FFP is thawed at 33 °C and 37 °C in a vacuum-sealed overwrap bag. Once thawed, FFP should be transfused within four hours as long as maintained in temperatures at approximately 22 ± 2 °C. If transfusion is not going to be immediate, thawed FFP may be stored up to a maximum of 120 hours at 4 ± 2 °C [29].

Often, when clinicians order FFP, there is not a clear designation of the "type" of plasma being released from the blood bank. In fact, most plasma that is transfused is PF24 and not actually FFP. Studies have shown that integrity of most clotting factors are maintained in PF24. However, the clinician should keep in mind that factor VIII is 15–20% lower in thawed PF24 compared to FFP but factors V, VII, and VIII decrease over time in thawed plasma [28, 30]. The drop in factor VIII can be greater than 50%, and the drop in factor V and VII can be by approximately 20% activity by day 5 [31]. FFP can also be processed with solvent detergents or methylene blue to reduce pathogen contamination. But doing so results in loss of clotting factors and natural anticoagulants [32].

FFP contains the following: all coagulation factors except platelets, factors II, V, VII, VIII, IX, X, XI. FFP contains fibrinogen (400–900 mg/unit), albumin, protein C, protein S, antithrombin, tissue factor pathway inhibitor, and vWF [33]. A standard dose of 10–20 mL FFP/kg (4–6 units FFP in adults) will raise factor levels by approximately 20%. An increase of approximately 10% of several factors is enough to effect hemostasis. When accounting for fibrinogen levels of at least 75–100 mg/dL with no other inhibiting agent such as heparin, increasing coagulation factors to 25–30% of normal is enough to obtain hemostasis. Infusing approximately one-fourth to one-third of the patient's total plasma volume, or 10–15 mL/kg, should achieve this effect [34].

Table 3.5 Transfusion reactions and associated signs and symptoms

Reaction	Signs and symptoms
Acute hemolytic transfusion reaction	Jaundice, hemoglobinuria, hypotension, disseminated intravascular coagulation, feeling of impending doom, fever, and chills
Allergy	Urticaria, hives, flushing
Anaphylaxis	Dyspnea, wheezing, coughing, nausea/vomiting, hypotension, loss of consciousness, cardiopulmonary collapse
TACO	Acute dyspnea, hypoxia, pulmonary edema, possible elevated systolic pressure, enlarged heart, increased BNP, significant response to diuretic
TRALI	Sudden dyspnea, pulmonary edema, hypoxemia, bilateral pulmonary infiltrates, occurs within 6 hours of transfusion

Fresh frozen plasma (FFP) is often used to treat conditions in which a quantitative or qualitative deficit in coagulation factors is present. This includes disseminated intravascular coagulation, severe liver disease, and massive bleeding/trauma. It can also be used in the reversal of vitamin K deficiency and warfarin-induced coagulopathy if sufficient time for vitamin K repletion is not an option. This could be due to urgent surgery in which massive blood loss is anticipated, trauma or hemodynamic instability. FFP may be indicated in rare coagulation disorders when a specific factor concentrate or recombinant product is not readily available.

Transfusion of any blood product is not without risks. ABO compatibility must be considered due to the presence of alloantibodies in plasma. Failure to screen for ABO compatibility could result in an acute hemolytic transfusion reaction. Other reactions include allergy, anaphylaxis, TACO, and TRALI [35]. Common symptoms of transfusion reactions are shown in Table 3.5. TRALI is now the leading cause of transfusion associated mortality in the United States, with FFP the most frequently implicated blood product [36]. Occurrence of infection is low but not zero. Processes to reduce these risks include nucleic acid testing, donor-retested plasma, or pathogen-inactivated/reduced plasma.

Platelets

Platelets can be obtained from whole blood donations by two different methods. Platelet-rich plasma is preferred in the United States whereas the buffy coat method is primarily utilized in Europe. To generate platelet-rich plasma, whole blood undergoes a low-speed centrifugation or "soft" spin that separates the RBCs from the platelet-rich plasma. The platelet-rich plasma then undergoes a higher centrifugation or "hard" spin to separate platelets from plasma. In the buffy coat method, whole blood is subjected to high-speed centrifugation to separate red blood cells, plasma, and a buffy coat that contains mostly platelets with a small amount of RBCs and leukocytes. Buffy coats from 4–6 whole blood donations are then added to a unit of plasma from one donation. After that, a low-speed centrifugation yields platelet-rich plasma which is then removed for potential transfusion. Platelets are obtained from whole blood or apheresis in a similar fashion to FFP. Each donation of approximately 500 mL of whole blood is collected in a citrate preservative solution within 8 hours of donation. From 500 mL of whole blood, approximately $5–7 \times 10^{10}$ platelets are extracted as a volume of about 50 mL in 50–70 mL of plasma for a total volume of about 100–120 mL. The plasma helps maintain the pH greater than or equal to 6.2.

A single unit of platelets from one unit of whole blood is not enough to raise platelet counts to hemostatic levels in clinical practice. Typically, 4–6 units are pooled from multiple donors to provide adequate platelet counts for clinical purposes. Alternatively, apheresis uses specialized equipment that selectively removes plasma and platelets from a single donor and returns RBCs and leukocytes to the donor. This allows extraction of approximately 200 mL of platelets suspended in about 200 mL of plasma from one donor. A unit of pooled platelets or one unit of apheresis platelets is expected to raise the platelet count by approximately 30,000–50,000/microL in a 70 kg adult. In an infant, administration of 10–15 mL platelets/kg should increase the platelet count by 50,000–100,000/microL.

Platelets are stored at room temperature (20–24 °C) with continuous gentle agitation to extend their clinical lifespan. Platelets that are cooled to 4 °C have shown poor survival due to an irreversible clustering of alpha subunits of glycoprotein Ib on the platelet surface. Chilled platelets undergo rapid clearance by phagocytosis from the circulation when transfused. Once collected, platelets must be transfused within five days of collection. Once platelets are processed via pooling or washing, it must be transfused within four hours. A standard 170–260 micron filter should be used to transfuse platelets since a smaller filter could remove platelets from the transfusion. Caution should be taken to avoid infusing platelets through extreme heat (i.e., temperature greater than 43 °C) due to the risk of altering cytoskeletal membrane components and impairing aggregation [37]. There is not much data available to recommend for or against infusion through standard OR warming devices.

Platelet transfusion is indicated when platelet dysfunction exists or in the presence of significant thrombocytopenia. When a patient with thrombocytopenia is actively bleeding, transfusion to maintain platelet counts above 50,000/microL is recommended for most circumstances. Recommended platelet counts for safe performance of common perioperative procedures are shown in Table 3.6. Platelets may also be transfused prophylactically in preparation for invasive procedures. Platelet transfusion is contraindicated for both thrombotic thrombocytopenic purpura and heparin-induced thrombocytopenia due to risk of further thrombosis and associated morbidity [38].

Table 3.6 Recommended platelet counts for common perioperative procedures

Type of procedure	Pre-procedure platelet count goal/microL
Major surgery and/or actively bleeding	50,000 [39]
Neurosurgery, ocular, and cardiopulmonary bypass	100,000 [39]
Central line placement	20,000 [40]
Epidural placement	80,000 [41]

Platelet transfusions have risks for complications. Bacterial contamination is highest with platelet transfusions compared to other blood components due to storage conditions. The rate of bacterial contamination of platelets is approximately1:2000 as compared to RBC units at 1:30,000 [42]. Because platelets contain plasma, the risks are similar between components with regards to TRALI, TACO, allergic and anaphylactic reactions. Post transfusion purpura is unique to transfusion of platelets or platelet containing products. Lingering leukocytes may cause febrile non hemolytic transfusion reactions, alloimmunization, and TAGVHD [43]. Although ABO compatibility does not apply to platelets, consideration should be given to RhD-negative women of childbearing age due to the risk for development of alloimmunization to RBC antigens that are potentially present in platelet units. If ABO compatibility cannot be attained due to scarcity of resources, then Rho(D) immune globulin should be given after transfusion [44].

Cryoprecipitate

Cryoprecipitate contains specific products from fresh frozen plasma. These include fibrinogen, factor VIII, factor XIII, von Willebrand factor, and fibronectin. Each unit of cryoprecipitate is expected to raise fibrinogen concentration by 7–10 mg/dL. Cryoprecipitate is typically pooled to include either five or ten units. Normal fibrinogen levels range from 150 to 400 mg/dL. The minimum level of fibrinogen to maintain hemostasis is 100 mg/dL. Although the recommended goal is higher at 150–200 mg/dL for individuals with significant risks of bleeding, such as intracerebral hemorrhage [45].

Cryoprecipitate is prepared by thawing FFP at 4 °C to precipitate out the higher molecular weight proteins, called cryoproteins. The thawed and cooled FFP is then separated by centrifugal forces and after removal of the supernatant the cryoprecipitate is stored with a small volume of plasma at –20 °C [46]. One unit (~10–20 ml) of cryoprecipitate is produced from one unit of FFP (~250 ml). Cryoprecipitate can be stored for up to 12 months. It should be noted that cryoprecipitate cannot be derived from PF24 due to the decreased availability of labile clotting factors in PF24 as compared to FFP. In particular, factor VIII is mild to moderately reduced in PF24. If transfusion is indicated, cryoprecipitate takes approximately 10–30 minutes to thaw. And once a unit has been thawed, it must be transfused within six hours. If pooled with other units, it must be transfused within four hours.

Administration of cryoprecipitate is indicated when a deficiency in specific clotting factors VIII, XIII, vWF, or fibrinogen exists. It is commonly used for acquired hypofibrinogenemia states instead of inherited deficiencies due to the availability and safety of commercial fibrinogen concentrates, recombinant or plasma-derived factor concentrates [47]. Currently, the use of fibrinogen concentrates is limited to inherited disorders in the United States. Factor VIII and von Willebrand's factor are now produced as purified recombinant concentrates making cryoprecipitate dedicated to the treatment of hypo- or dysfibrogenemia, It was once thought of as a "last resort" to treat a trauma-induced coagulopathy but now is deployed as the desired first component to treat trauma resuscitative coagulopathy, especially in scenarios where whole blood is not utilized for massive transfusions. Fibrinogen levels are commonly low upon arrival to the trauma emergency room. Cryoprecipitate is a part of many massive transfusion protocols. Cryoprecipitate may also be used in patients with liver disease, disseminated intravascular coagulation, and uremic bleeding. The decision to replace fibrinogen with cryoprecipitate, fibrinogen concentrate, or FFP is based on clinical judgment and availability.

Risks associated with cryoprecipitate include potential pathogen transmission since viral inactivation can result in a significant decrease in available fibrinogen. ABO compatibility must be considered since it is suspended in plasma. The risks are similar to those with plasma, although likely lower depending on rate and volume infused. The process of thawing can be a problematic rate-limiting step, especially when massive bleeding necessitates expedient availability of blood components [46].

References

1. Cap AP, Beckett A, Benov A, Borgman M, Chen J, Corley JB, et al. Whole blood transfusion. Mil Med. 2018;183(suppl_2):44–51.
2. Miller RD. Massive blood transfusions: the impact of Vietnam military data on modern civilian transfusion medicine. Anesthesiology. 2009;110(6):1412–6.
3. Neel SH, United States. Department of the Army. Medical support of the U.S. Army in Vietnam, 1965–1970. Washington, D.C.: Dept. of the Army; for sale by Supt. of Docs.; 1973.
4. Brohi K, Cohen MJ, Ganter MT, Matthay MA, Mackersie RC, Pittet JF. Acute traumatic coagulopathy: initiated by hypoperfusion: modulated through the protein C pathway? Ann Surg. 2007;245(5):812–8.
5. Pidcoke HF, Aden JK, Mora AG, Borgman MA, Spinella PC, Dubick MA, et al. Ten-year analysis of transfusion in operation Iraqi freedom and operation enduring freedom: increased plasma and platelet use correlates with improved survival. J Trauma Acute Care Surg. 2012;73(6 Suppl 5):S445–52.
6. Kleinman S. Practical aspects of red blood cell transfusion in adults: storage, processing, modifications, and infusion. Silvergleid AJ ed. Waltham, MA. UpToDate Inc. https://uptodate.com Accessed October 26, 2020.
7. Almizraq RJ, Acker JP. Closing in on DEHP-free red blood cell concentrate containers. Transfusion. 2018;58(5):1089–92.
8. Ratko TA, Cummings JP, Oberman HA, Crookston KP, DeChristopher PJ, Eastlund DT, et al. Evidence-based recommendations for the use of WBC-reduced cellular blood components. Transfusion. 2001;41(10):1310–9.
9. Fung MK, Rao N, Rice J, Ridenour M, Mook W, Triulzi DJ. Leukoreduction in the setting of open heart surgery: a prospective cohort-controlled study. Transfusion. 2004;44(1):30–5.
10. Bynum JP, Zachary A, Ness PM, Luo X, Bagnasco S, King KE, et al. Transfusion of leukoreduced blood products and risk of antibody-mediated rejection of renal allografts. Transfusion. 2018;58(8):1951–7.
11. Treleaven J, Gennery A, Marsh J, Norfolk D, Page L, Parker A, et al. Guidelines on the use of irradiated blood components prepared by the British Committee for Standards in Haematology blood transfusion task force. Br J Haematol. 2011;152(1):35–51.
12. King KE, Ness PM. How do we prevent transfusion-associated graft-versus-host disease in children? Transfusion. 2011;51(5):916–20.
13. Fergusson DA, Hebert P, Hogan DL, LeBel L, Rouvinez-Bouali N, Smyth JA, et al. Effect of fresh red blood cell transfusions on clinical outcomes in premature, very low-birth-weight infants: the ARIPI randomized trial. JAMA. 2012;308(14):1443–51.
14. Dhabangi A, Ainomugisha B, Cserti-Gazdewich C, Ddungu H, Kyeyune D, Musisi E, et al. Effect of transfusion of red blood cells with longer vs shorter storage duration on elevated blood lactate levels in children with severe anemia: the TOTAL randomized clinical trial. JAMA. 2015;314(23):2514–23.
15. Steiner ME, Ness PM, Assmann SF, Triulzi DJ, Sloan SR, Delaney M, et al. Effects of red-cell storage duration on patients undergoing cardiac surgery. N Engl J Med. 2015;372(15):1419–29.
16. Cooper DJ, McQuilten ZK, Nichol A, Ady B, Aubron C, Bailey M, et al. Age of red cells for transfusion and outcomes in critically ill adults. N Engl J Med. 2017;377(19):1858–67.
17. Alexander PE, Barty R, Fei Y, Vandvik PO, Pai M, Siemieniuk RA, et al. Transfusion of fresher vs older red blood cells in hospitalized patients: a systematic review and meta-analysis. Blood. 2016;127(4):400–10.
18. Lecak J, Scott K, Young C, Hannon J, Acker JP. Evaluation of red blood cells stored at −80 degrees C in excess of 10 years. Transfusion. 2004;44(9):1306–13.
19. Fabricant L, Kiraly L, Wiles C, Differding J, Underwood S, Deloughery T, et al. Cryopreserved deglycerolized blood is safe and achieves superior tissue oxygenation compared with refrigerated red blood cells: a prospective randomized pilot study. J Trauma Acute Care Surg. 2013;74(2):371–6; discussion 6–7.
20. Hebert PC, Fergusson DA, Stather D, McIntyre L, Martin C, Doucette S, et al. Revisiting transfusion practices in critically ill patients. Crit Care Med. 2005;33(1):7–12; discussion 232-2.
21. Shih AW, Liu A, Elsharawi R, Crowther MA, Cook RJ, Heddle NM. Systematic reviews of guidelines and studies for single versus multiple unit transfusion strategies. Transfusion. 2018;58(12):2841–60.

22. Circular of Information Regarding Transfusions from the Choosing Wisely Campaign. American Association of Blood Banks, 2014. Available at http://www.aabb.org/pbm/Documents/Choosing-Wisely-Five-Things-Physicians-and-Patients-Should-Question.pdf. Accessed October 26, 2020.
23. Munoz M, Acheson AG, Auerbach M, Besser M, Habler O, Kehlet H, et al. International consensus statement on the peri-operative management of anaemia and iron deficiency. Anaesthesia. 2017;72(2):233–47.
24. Chong MA, Krishnan R, Cheng D, Martin J. Should transfusion trigger thresholds differ for critical care versus perioperative patients? A meta-analysis of randomized trials. Crit Care Med. 2018;46(2):252–63.
25. Hendrickson JE, Hillyer CD. Noninfectious serious hazards of transfusion. Anesth Analg. 2009;108(3):759–69.
26. Vamvakas EC, Blajchman MA. Blood still kills: six strategies to further reduce allogeneic blood transfusion-related mortality. Transfus Med Rev. 2010;24(2):77–124.
27. Rudmann SV. Textbook of blood banking and transfusion medicine. 2nd ed. Philadelphia: Elsevier/Saunders; 2005.
28. Scott E, Puca K, Heraly J, Gottschall J, Friedman K. Evaluation and comparison of coagulation factor activity in fresh-frozen plasma and 24-hour plasma at thaw and after 120 hours of 1 to 6 degrees C storage. Transfusion. 2009;49(8):1584–91.
29. Fresh Frozen Plasma Leucocyte Depleted. Guidelines for the blood transfusion services. 8th ed: Joint United Kingdom: The Stationary Office; 2013.
30. Smith JF, Ness PM, Moroff G, Luban NL. Retention of coagulation factors in plasma frozen after extended holding at 1-6 degrees C. Vox Sang. 2000;78(1):28–30.
31. Shehata N, Blajchman M, Heddle N. Coagulation factors in FFP and cryosupernatant. Transfus Med. 2001;11:391–401.
32. MacLennan S, Williamson LM. Risks of fresh frozen plasma and platelets. J Trauma. 2006;60(6 Suppl):S46–50.
33. Khawar H, Kelley W, Guzman N. Fresh frozen plasma (FFP). Treasure Islands: StatPearls; 2019.
34. O'Shaughnessy DF, Atterbury C, Bolton Maggs P, Murphy M, Thomas D, Yates S, et al. Guidelines for the use of fresh-frozen plasma, cryoprecipitate and cryosupernatant. Br J Haematol. 2004;126(1):11–28.
35. Dean L, National Center for Biotechnology Information (U.S.). Blood groups and red cell antigens. Bethesda: NCBI; 2005.
36. Pandey S, Vyas GN. Adverse effects of plasma transfusion. Transfusion. 2012;52(Suppl 1):65S–79S.
37. Jhang JS, Spitalnik SL. Glycosylation and cold platelet storage. Curr Hematol Rep. 2005;4(6):483–7.
38. Rao GH, Smith CM 2nd, Escolar G, White JG. Influence of heat on platelet biochemistry, structure, and function. J Lab Clin Med. 1993;122(4):455–64.
39. Haematology BCfSi, Force BTT. Guidelines for the use of platelet transfusions. Br J Haematol. 2003;122(1):10–23.
40. Kumar A, Mhaskar R, Grossman BJ, Kaufman RM, Tobian AA, Kleinman S, et al. Platelet transfusion: a systematic review of the clinical evidence. Transfusion. 2015;55(5):1116–27. quiz 5
41. Zeidler K, Arn K, Senn O, Schanz U, Stussi G. Optimal preprocedural platelet transfusion threshold for central venous catheter insertions in patients with thrombocytopenia. Transfusion. 2011;51(11):2269–76.
42. Van Veen JJ, Nokes TJ, Makris M. The risk of spinal haematoma following neuraxial anaesthesia or lumbar puncture in thrombocytopenic individuals. Br J Haematol. 2010;148(1):15–25.
43. Centers for Disease C, Prevention. Fatal bacterial infections associated with platelet transfusions – United States, 2004. MMWR Morb Mortal Wkly Rep. 2005;54(7):168–70.
44. Goldfinger D, McGinniss MH. Rh-incompatible platelet transfusions – risks and consequences of sensitizing immunosuppressed patients. N Engl J Med. 1971;284(17):942–4.
45. Schochl H, Maegele M, Solomon C, Gorlinger K, Voelckel W. Early and individualized goal-directed therapy for trauma-induced coagulopathy. Scand J Trauma Resusc Emerg Med. 2012;20:15.
46. Franchini M, Lippi G. Fibrinogen replacement therapy: a critical review of the literature. Blood Transfus. 2012;10(1):23–7.
47. Yang L, Stanworth S, Baglin T. Cryoprecipitate: an outmoded treatment? Transfus Med. 2012;22(5):315–20.

The Coagulation System and Blood Clot Stability

4

Nikita Nayyar, Haig Mannasian, Longqiu Yang, and Henry Liu

Introduction

Hemorrhage is a very common complication in perioperative settings and other invasive procedures. This complication can be caused by various factors, usually by surgical technical difficulties and coagulation abnormalities [1, 2]. Reduction of surgery-related blood loss will be addressed in other chapters in this book. Here we will discuss normal coagulation system, coagulation regulations, and clot stability. The coagulation system is a series of enzymatic reactions that plays an important role in hemostasis and normal human life. Coagulation cascade is a very dynamic process that involves multiple enzymes that propagate to the clot formation [2]. A delicate balance between the coagulation system and the fibrinolytic system is critical in order to maintain a normal blood circulation. Hemostasis is to stop bleeding after an injury. It is categorized as primary hemostasis and secondary hemostasis [3, 4]. In primary hemostasis, the blood vessel contracts and platelets adhere to the site of injury. In a series of integrative reactions, the platelets form a temporary hemostatic plug that prevents extravasation from the site of injury. The final step is secondary hemostasis [5]. In secondary hemostasis, the coagulation system is activated and a series of enzymatic reactions and a cascade of factor activations take place to form fibrin which subsequently reinforces the primary platelet plug [6].

Blood maintains its fluidity in the vascular system and its ability to clot when a blood vessel is damaged by various etiologies. In 1905, Morawitz described the classic theory of blood coagulation (Fig. 4.1), in which he first described the conversion of prothrombin to thrombin and then the conversion of fibrinogen to fibrin, utilizing thromboplastin and calcium ions [7]. More intricacies and details of the coagulation cascade were discovered via clinical observations and experimental studies in subsequent decades. It was unveiled that there was an abnormality in the blood of patients with hemophilia that leads to the prolongation of clotting time in 1936. Both in vivo and in vitro investigations led to the discovery of Factor VIII deficiency [8]. Furthermore, heparin and antithrombin were discovered after multiple experiments looking into the coagulation of blood with enzymes derived from the livers of dogs [9]. Each of the new factors that were discovered were given their own name by different researchers which led to enormous confusion regarding the interplay between various factors and their roles in coagulation cascade. An international committee for the nomenclature of blood coagulation factors was established in 1954 with a goal of creating common terminology for the known clotting factors at that time [10]. With the discovery of procoagulants also came the discovery of anticoagulants. The role of Protein C in anticoagulation was also discovered after significantly lower Protein C levels were found in a family with many members prone to thrombosis as opposed to normal Protein C levels in those without coagulation issues [11]. After the discovery of Protein C deficiencies, laboratory tests were developed and revealed that deficiencies in Protein S also lead to procoagulant tendencies [6, 12].

As our understanding of clotting factors deepened, adjustments to the classic theory were made and the role of the coagulation factors was more specifically defined.

N. Nayyar
New York University Langone School of Medicine, Department of Anesthesiology, New York, NY, USA

H. Mannasian
Thomas Jefferson University Hospital, Department of Anesthesiology, Philadelphia, PA, USA

L. Yang
Huangshi Central Hospital, Department of Anesthesiology, Huangshi, Hubei, China

H. Liu (✉)
Department of Anesthesiology and Perioperative Medicine, Milton S. Hershey Medical Center, Penn State College of Medicine, Hershey, PA, USA

© Springer Nature Switzerland AG 2021
C. S. Scher et al. (eds.), *Essentials of Blood Product Management in Anesthesia Practice*,
https://doi.org/10.1007/978-3-030-59295-0_4

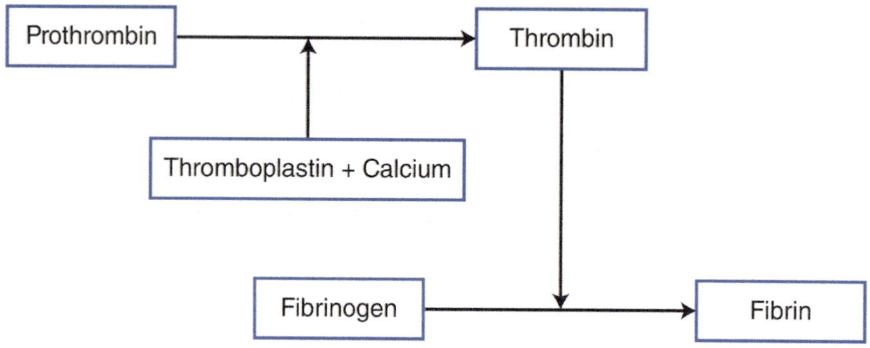

Fig. 4.1 The classic theory of blood coagulation by Morawitz (1905) [7]

Table 4.1 Coagulation factors and their functions [15]

Factor number	Coagulation actor name	Biological function	Plasma concentration (mg/L)	Plasma $T_{1/2}$ (h)
I	Fibrinogen	Clot formation	3000	90
II	Prothrombin	Activates I, V, VII, VIII, protein C, platelet	100	65
III	Tissue factor	Cofactor of VIIa		
IV	Calcium	Facilitates factor binding to phospholipids		
V	Labile factor/Proacclerin	Cofactor of X-prothrombinase complex	10	15
VI	Unassigned			
VII	Stable factor/Proconvertin	Activates IX, X	0.5	5
VIII	Antihemophilic factor A	Cofactor of IX-tenase complex	0.1	10
IX	Antihemophilic factor B/Christmas factor	Activates X: forms tenase complex with factor VIII	5	25
X	Stuart-power factor	Prothrombinase complex with factor V, activates II	10	40
XI	Plasma thromboplastin antecedent	Activates IX	5	45
XII	Hageman factor	Activates factor XI, VII, Prekallikrein		
XIII	Fibrin-stabilizing factor	Cross-link fibrin	30	200
XIV	Prekallikrein(F Fletcher)	Serine protease zymogen		35
XV	HMWK- (F Fitzgerald)	Cofactor		150
XVI	vWF	Binds to VIII, mediates platelet adhesion	10 ug/ml	12
XVII	Antithrombin III	Inhibits IIa, Xa, other proteases	0.15–0.2 mg/ml	72
XVIII	Heparin cofactor II	Inhibits IIa		60
XIX	Protein C	Inactivates Va, VIIIa		0.4
XX	Protein S	Cofactor for activated protein C		

The waterfall hypothesis, which was developed in 1964 by Davie and Rantoff, provided a detailed schematic for the interactions of the factors leading to clot formation and is the basis of coagulation cascade today [13]. As the roles of the various factors began to be better defined, the waterfall hypothesis has also been continually modified [6].

The coagulation cascade can be broken down into two pathways, the intrinsic pathway and the extrinsic pathway. The intrinsic pathway, so named because all of the components in the cascade are found in plasma, it is triggered when plasma comes into contact with an artificial surface, such as a glass test tube. The extrinsic pathway requires blood to come into contact with an extrinsic molecule, tissue factor, which then triggers the clotting cascade [3]. Both pathways are explained in greater depth in subsequent sections.

Coagulation Factors and Their Functions

Most of the coagulation factors are zymogens which are inert precursors of enzymes. Zymogens are activated by limited proteolysis which results in active serine proteases with low inherent enzymatic activity. When these active proteases bind specific protein cofactors, the activity of the proteases increases significantly. The cofactors of the clotting cascade also circulate in the plasma as inert procofactors, which must be converted to active cofactors via proteolysis. So, both the enzymes and cofactors of the coagulation cascade require an activation process prior to exerting their biological effects. Once these enzymes and cofactors become active, they are appended with a lower case 'a' [14]. Table 4.1 lists all the coagulation factors currently known and their physiological functions (Table 4.1) [15].

Thromboplastin (TF) is a glycosylated integral membrane protein and it is unique because it does not require activation. It functions as a receptor (for involved in inflammation, apoptosis, cell migration) and also as a cofactor for Factor VII/VIIa [3, 14]. It is expressed in many extravascular tissues as in the brain, heart, lungs, and kidneys. Furthermore, it can also be expressed on vascular endothelium in response to inflammatory stimulation, lipopolysaccharides in sepsis, adhesion molecules, and inflammatory cytokines. TF expression has also been found on some cancer tissues [14]. Factor VII/VIIa, Factor VII is synthesized in the liver. Factor VII contains a gamma-carboxyglutamic acid-rich (GLA) domain which allows calcium-dependent binding of Factor VII to membranes containing negatively charged phospholipids. Factor VII circulates in both active VIIa and inactive VII form in the blood. VIIa is not susceptible to most plasma protease inhibitors and has a half-life of 2 hours. Factor VII can be activated by IXa, Xa, XIIa, thrombin, plasmin, and TF:VIIa complex [3, 14]. TF:VIIa Complex can activate Factors IX and X, and it can be inhibited by Tissue Factor pathway inhibitor XII/XIIa (thrombin).

Thrombin is produced in the liver and is activated by kallikrein, plasmin, Factor XIIa. XII/XIIa activates Protein C, so thrombin can be both procoagulant and anticoagulant. PK/Kallikrein is produced in the liver and activated by XIIa. High-molecular-weight kininogen (HK) is synthesized in liver but also contained in granulocytes, platelets, and endothelial cells. HK binds to cell surface in a zinc-dependent manner. HK activates Factor XII to XIIa.

Normal Coagulation Cascade

Intrinsic pathway depends on the activation by a negatively changed surface and involves coagulation Factors XII, XI, IX, VIII, and V. The extrinsic pathway depends on the activation by TF and tissue factor (Factor III) and Factor VII. Both pathways converge on a common pathway to activate Factor X, which leads to the conversion of prothrombin (Factor II) to thrombin (IIa). This subsequently converts fibrinogen to form fibrin. The Partial thromboplastin time (PTT) can be used to assess the intrinsic pathway and the Prothrombin time (PT) can be used to assess the function of the extrinsic pathway. The three stages of coagulation are initiation, amplification, and propagation [2, 16], (Fig. 4.2).

The initiation phase begins with the exposure of TF to the blood by damage to or activation by the endothelium. TF then forms a complex with Factor VIIa on the surface of the cell membrane and activates the zymogens Factors IX and X. Activated Factor X then generates Factor IIa (thrombin). Tissue Factor pathway inhibitor neutralizes Factor Xa and TF:VIIa complexes. The duration of the initiation phase is

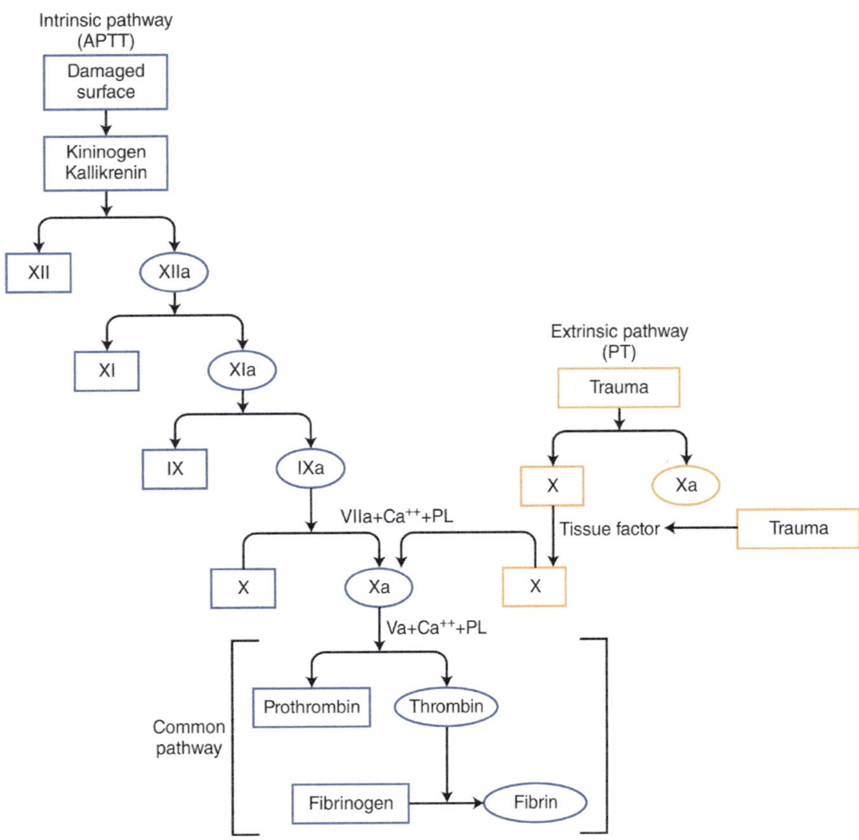

Fig. 4.2 Coagulation pathways [2, 14]

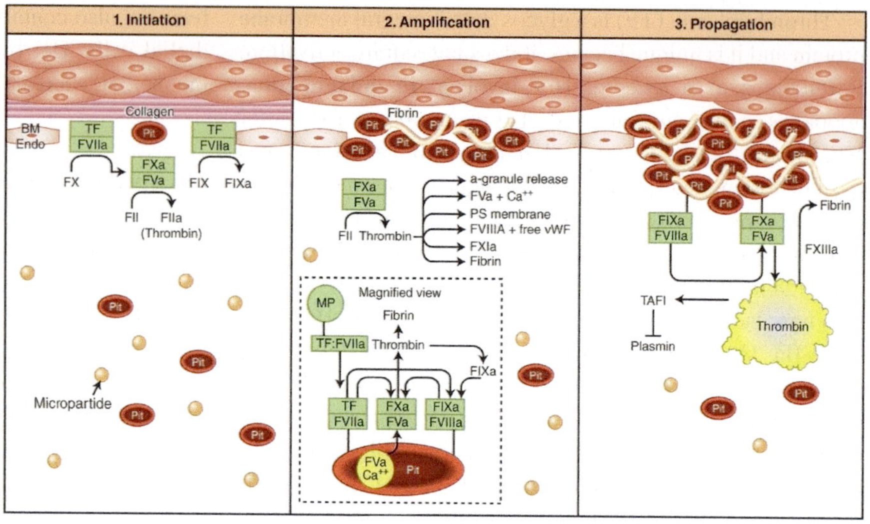

Fig. 4.3 Stages of coagulation [2, 14]

dependent on the balance between the concentration of TF:VIIa and tissue Factor pathway inhibitor [2, 17], (Fig. 4.3).

In the amplification phase, Factor IXa and Factor VIIa form an intrinsic Factor tenase complex (FIXa:FVIIa) in the presence of calcium. This process greatly enhances the production of Factor Xa which significantly accelerates thrombin production. The prothrombinase complex (FXa:FVa) is also increased by its proximity to the tenase complex and the presence of calcium, resulting in more thrombin production. A positive feedback loop forms between the tenase and prothombinase complexes to generate substantial quantity of thrombin to stabilize the newly formed clot [2, 17]. Thrombin also interacts with platelets via platelet receptor GPIb which allows interaction of other platelet components and activates GPIIb/IIIa receptor, further promoting platelet aggregation. Thrombin also increases Factor VIIIa by releasing it from vWF:VIII complex and also activates Factor XI to XIa. Subsequently, Factor XIa adheres to platelets and causes activation of the intrinsic pathway. The platelets in the hemostatic plug are stimulated by both collagen and thrombin and then generate more thrombin by further activating tenase and prothombinase complexes. The main result of the amplification phase is to generate as much thrombin as possible [2, 4, 14, 18], (Fig. 4.3).

The propagation phase is the final step in stabilizing the clot. It involved the recruitment of all components, tenase complex, platelets, prothrombinase complexes, calcium to the phospholipid surface. Then platelets are activated by thrombin and the "thrombin burst" leads to the accelerated formation of fibrin from fibrinogen. These fibrin monomers form fibrin layers. Thrombin also activates Factor XIII to Factor XIIIa which then covalently crosslinks the fibrin strands to form a more stable fibrin network. Thrombin also activates thrombin-activatable fibrinolysis inhibitor which protects the clot from plasmin fibrinolysis [2, 4, 14, 18], (Figs. 4.3 and 4.4).

The intrinsic or contact pathway is generally activated by Factor XII. Contact of plasma with an artificial surface leads to activation of Factor XII to XIIa. Factor XIIa then activates Factor XI to XIa. Factor XIa activates Factor IX to IXa and it allows for the formation of tenase complexes with VIIIa. This then activates Factor X to Factor Xa. The generation of Factor Xa leads to the common pathway of thrombin generation and blood clot stabilization. The intrinsic pathway also produces bradykinin when kallikrein cleaves HK. Subsequently, bradykinin binds to its receptors and results in vasodilation, increased vascular permeability, pain, and neutrophil activation [14, 18], (Fig. 4.2).

Regulation of Coagulation

The coagulation cascade is regulated at every step in order to maintain a balance between procoagulation and anticoagulation. The most important regulation mechanisms are multiple zymogens and cofactors requiring activation prior to exerting their effects. Tissue factor pathway inhibitor (TFPI) neutralizes Factor Xa and it inhibits the TF:VIIa complex. TFPI is primarily produced by the endothelium and it can also be found on platelets. When heparin is administered, the endothelial form of TFPI is released [2, 14]. In mice whose TFPI have been knocked out, these mice do not survive, indicating that lack of TFPI is incompatible with life [19]. Endothelial cells secrete heparan sulfate which activates antithrombin. This antithrombin heparan complex can inhibit multiple coagulation enzymes [2, 14]. When Protein C is activated by thrombin, Protein C inhibits the procoagulant functions of Factors VIIIa and Va. Protein C is vitamin K dependent. Protein S further supports the activity of protein C in inactivating Factors

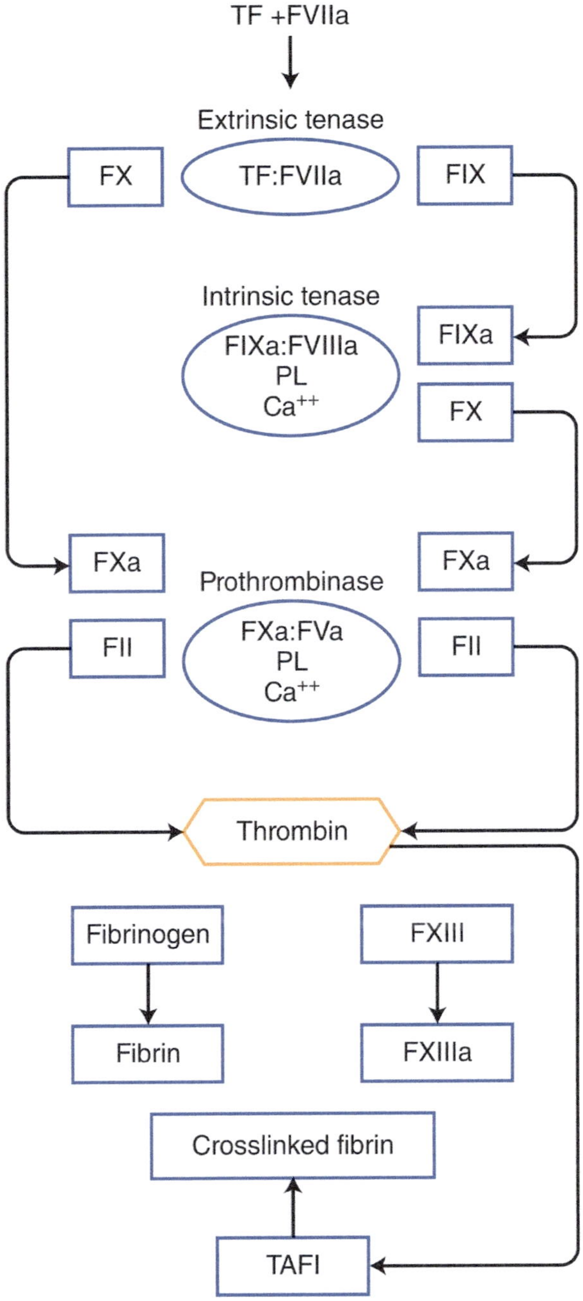

Fig. 4.4 Regulation of coagulation cascade [2, 14]

VIIIa and Va. Deficiencies of both protein C and S will clinically present significant prothrombotic conditions [19].

Mechanisms of Clot Stability and Fibrinolysis

Precise regulation of clot stability is of paramount importance, as an insubstantial or excessively robust clot can lead to hemorrhage or thrombosis, respectively. The fundamental principle of clot stability is that it is a balance between clot formation and fibrinolysis. This balance can be skewed in either direction by a multitude of factors, including those molecular, metabolic, mechanical, and pharmacologic in nature. Furthermore, the processes of coagulation and fibrinolysis occur simultaneously in many clinical scenarios. It is necessary to first mitigate the inherent complexity of this topic by providing a global roadmap for how coagulation and fibrinolysis interrelate to afford hemostasis. We will then point to specific factors in this framework that influence clot stability, and fibrinolysis and its role in disease process. After the blood coagulation cascade is initiated and subsequently thrombin is activated, which then catalyzes the formation of fibrin from its parent zymogen, fibrinogen. Fibrin creates a hemostatic milieu in the blood vessels due to its low solubility in the blood. The fibrin peptides are then cross-linked at lysine residues by the action of Factor XIIIa in the process known as "polymerization". Simultaneously, leukocytes, erythrocytes, and platelets assimilate into the fibrin cross-link network to enhance the structural integrity of the clots [20–22]. Once the injured tissue has healed, then the process of fibrinolysis begins to take effect. The core of fibrinolysis process is the enzyme plasmin, which is converted from plasminogen via tissue plasminogen activator (tPA) or urokinase-type plasminogen activator (uPA) on the surface of the fibrin clot, and one of its main functions is to "dissolve" the fibrin clot through its serine protease activity [23, 24]. However, a fibrinolytic cross-talk mechanism may potentially bypass the requirement for their molecular coassembly on the same surface, plasmin can be formed by uPA [25].

Factors Affecting Clot Stability

The stability of a clot is dependent on the structural integrity with which it was formed, as well as external factors. Fibrin fiber diameter and the specific geometry of the fibrin network are the main determinants of clot stability [21]. Even the local blood flow rate in the vessel affects how fibrin networks are oriented as the thrombus forms [26]. Higher concentrations of thrombin also seem to have an impact on the quality of the fibrin structure [21]. Understandably, if the newly formed clot is loose and fragile to begin with, then it is more susceptible to fibrinolysis. Fibrinogen polymorphisms can also impact fibrin clot architecture and create a prothrombotic or antithrombotic state [27]. The biological environment in which the clot forms can also affect the various reactions involved in forming and stabilizing a clot, including local calcium concentration, pH, and platelet count [21, 26].

Fibrinolysis: Regulation and Its Role in Disease Process

As above mentioned, plasmin is the primary molecular factor in fibrinolysis, and it is activated from plasminogen by either tPA or uPA. The function of endothelial cells and monocytes that produce tPA and uPA, respectively have significant impact on the rate of fibrinolysis. Plasminogen activator inhibitor-1 (PAI1) is an important serine protease inhibitor ("serpin") that protects against excessive fibrinolysis by inhibiting tPA and uPA and ultimately limiting their half-lives. Serpins are present in the blood in excess concentrations to ensure that tPA and uPA are rapidly neutralized [28]. There is also thrombin-activated fibrinolysis inhibitor (TAFI), which is a nonserpin and is activated by thrombin as the name suggests [29]. TAFI serves as just one of the many molecular links between coagulation and fibrinolysis, illustrating the inter relatedness of the two processes.

Clinical applications of fibrinolysis in perioperative period are vast. The fibrinolytic system itself is usually subject to perturbations from the level of organ system functions (e.g., organ failure) to that of genetic polymorphisms (e.g., fibrinogen). These "acquired" disorders of fibrinolysis can be categorized into hyperfibrinolysis and hypofibrinolysis. Examples of acquired hyperfibrinolysis include disseminated intravascular coagulation, coagulation factor deficiency secondary to chronic liver disease, and nephrotic syndrome [30, 31]. Examples of acquired hypofibrinolysis include multiple myeloma, antiphospholipid syndrome, and diabetes [30]. There are also pharmaceutical means of intentionally altering fibrinolysis to achieve a desirable clinical outcome, such as administering tPA in the setting of early ischemic stroke and tranexamic acid to prevent excessive bleeding in surgical procedures and in patients with hemophilia.

Summary

Normal coagulation is a very dynamic process involving a series of enzymatic reactions. Activation of either intrinsic pathway or extrinsic pathway will lead to fibrin production and clot formation. Coagulation has three stages (initiation, amplification, and propagation). A delicate balance between clot formation and fibrinolysis, which often occurs simultaneously, is critical to normal blood circulation and hemostasis. Coagulation system is regulated by ways of multiple zymogens and cofactors all requiring activation prior to exerting their effects. And the clot stability is also regulated by numerous factors. The many steps in coagulation and fibrinolysis pathways also offer targets for pharmacological interventions.

References

1. Levi M, Sivapalaratnam S. Coagulation and anticoagulation in the intraoperative setting. Transfus Apher Sci. 2019. pii: S1473-0502(19)30106-5. https://doi.org/10.1016/j.transci.2019.06.013. PMID: 31307835.
2. Adams RL, Bird RJ. Coagulation cascade and therapeutics update: relevance to nephrology. Part 1: overview of coagulation, thrombophilias and history of anticoagulants. Nephrology. 2009;14(5):462–70. https://doi.org/10.1111/j.1440-1797.2009.01128.x. PMID: 19674315.
3. Boon GD. An overview of hemostasis. Toxicol Pathol. 1993;21(2):170–9. https://doi.org/10.1177/019262339302100209. Sage Publications. Thousands Oaks, CA.
4. Bombeli T, Spahn DR. Updates in perioperative coagulation: physiology and management of thromboembolism and haemorrhage. Br J Anaesth. 2004;93(2):275–87.
5. Bhagavan N. Medical biochemistry. San Diego: Harcourt/Academic Press; 2006. p. 839–872i.
6. Saito H, Matsushita T, Kojima T. Historical perspective and future direction of coagulation research. J Thromb Haemost. 2011;9:352–63.
7. Morawitz P. Die chemie der blutgerinnung. Ergebnisse der Physiologie. 1905;4(1):307–422. (translated text was: Beck EA. The chemistry of blood coagulation: a summary by Paul Morawitz (1905). Thrombosis and haemostasis. 1977 Jan;37(01):376–9.)
8. Patek AJ, Stetson RP. Hemophilia. I. the abnormal coagulation of the blood and its relation to the blood platelets. J Clin Invest. 1936;15(5):531–42.
9. Howell WH, Holt E. Two new factors in blood coagulation—heparin and pro-antithrombin. Am J Physiol-Legacy Content. 1918;47(3):328–41.
10. Wright HP. Blood coagulation. Br Med J. 1955;2(4932):184. PMC1980349.
11. Griffin JH, Evatt BR, Zimmerman TS, Kleiss AJ, Wideman C. Deficiency of protein C in congenital thrombotic disease. J Clin Invest. 1981;68(5):1370–3.
12. Nixon RR, Cooper MR, Esmon CT. Familial protein S deficiency is associated with recurrent thrombosis. J Clin Invest. 1984;74(6):2082–8.
13. Davie EW, Ratnoff OD. Waterfall sequence for intrinsic blood clotting. Science. 1964;145(3638):1310–2.
14. Smith SA, Travers RJ, Morrissey JH. How it all starts: initiation of the clotting cascade. Crit Rev Biochem Mol Biol. 2015;50(4):326–36.
15. https://www.researchgate.net/figure/Nomenclature-of-the-coagulation-proteins-clotting-factors_tbl1_270005500. Accessed 18 Aug 2019.
16. Palta S, Saroa R, Palta A. Overview of the coagulation system. Indian J Anaesth. 2014;58(5):515.
17. Hoffman M, Pawlinski R. Hemostasis: old system, new players, new directions. Thromb Res. 2014;133:S1–2.
18. O'Donnell JS, O'Sullivan JM, Preston RJ. Advances in understanding the molecular mechanisms that maintain normal haemostasis. Br J Haematol. 2019;186(1):24–36.
19. Dahlbäck B. Blood coagulation and its regulation by anticoagulant pathways: genetic pathogenesis of bleeding and thrombotic diseases. J Intern Med. 2005;257(3):209–23.
20. Furie B. Pathogenesis of thrombosis. ASH Education Program Book. 2009;2009(1):255–8. PMID: 20008207.
21. Wolberg AS, Pieters M. Fibrinogen and fibrin: an illustrated review. Blood Rev. 2007;21(3):131–42. Res Pract Thromb Haemost. 2019 Apr;3(2):161–72. https://doi.org/10.1002/rth2.12191. PMCID: PMC6462751.

22. Aleman MM, Walton BL, Byrnes JR, Wolberg AS. Fibrinogen and red blood cells in venous thrombosis. Thromb Res. 2014;133:S38–40. https://doi.org/10.1016/j.thromres.2014.03.017. PMID: 24759140.
23. Chapin JC, Hajjar KA. Fibrinolysis and the control of blood coagulation. Blood Rev. 2015;29(1):17–24. https://doi.org/10.1016/j.blre.2014.09.003. PMCID: PMC4314363.
24. Hajjar KA. The molecular basis of fibrinolysis. In: Hematology of infancy and childhood, vol. 2; 1998. p. 1557–73.
25. Dejouvencel T, Doeuvre L, Lacroix R, Plawinski L, Dignat-George F, Lijnen HR, et al. Fibrinolytic cross-talk: a new mechanism for plasmin formation. Blood. 2010;115(10):2048–56. https://doi.org/10.1182/blood-2009-06-228817. PMCID: PMC2896557.
26. Gersh KC, Edmondson KE, Weisel JW. Flow rate and fibrin fiber alignment. J Thromb Haemost. 2010;8(12):2826–8. PMCID: PMC3071618.
27. Cooper AV, Standeven KF, Ariëns RA. Fibrinogen gamma-chain splice variant γ' alters fibrin formation and structure. Blood. 2003;102(2):535–40. https://doi.org/10.1182/blood-2002-10-3150. PMID: 12663453.
28. Travis J, Salvesen GS. Human plasma proteinase inhibitors. Annu Rev Biochem. 1983;52(1):655–709. https://doi.org/10.1146/annurev.bi.52.070183.003255. PMID: 6193754.
29. Broze GJ, Higuchi DA. Coagulation-dependent inhibition of fibrinolysis: role of carboxypeptidase-U and the premature lysis of clots from hemophilic plasma. Blood. 1996;88(10):3815–23. PMID: 8916945.
30. Cesarman-Maus G, Ríos-Luna NP, Deora AB, Huang B, Villa R, del Carmen CM, Alarcón-Segovia D, Sánchez-Guerrero J, Hajjar KA. Autoantibodies against the fibrinolytic receptor, annexin 2, in antiphospholipid syndrome. Blood. 2006;107(11):4375–82.
31. Cucuianu M, Knauer O, Roman S. α2-Antiplasmin, plasminogen activator inhibitor (PAI) and dilute blood clot lysis time in selected disease states. Thromb Haemost. 1991;66(05):586–91.

Fibrinolysis, Antifibrinolytic Agents, and Perioperative Considerations

5

Aaron N. Primm

Abbreviations

A2AP	Alpha-2-antiplasmin
ACT	Activated clotting time
APTT	Activated partial thromboplastin time
ATC	Acute traumatic coagulopathy
BART	Blood conservation using antifibrinolytics in a randomized trial
CABG	Coronary artery bypass graft
CPB	Cardiopulmonary bypass
CRASH	Clinical randomization of an antifibrinolytic in significant hemorrhage
EACA	Epsilon-aminocaproic acid
FDA	Food and drug administration
GABA/A	Gamma-aminobutyric acid type A
INR	International normalized ratio
IV	Intravenous
LY30	Lysis measurement 30 minutes
MATTERs	Military application of tranexamic acid in trauma emergency resuscitation study
PAI-1	Plasminogen activator inhibitor-1
PAI-2	Plasminogen activator inhibitor-2
PATCH	Prehospital antifibrinolytics for traumatic coagulopathy and hemorrhage
PPH	Postpartum hemorrhage
RCT	Randomized control trial
ROTEM	Rotational thromboelastometry
SAH	Subarachnoid hemorrhage
TAFI	Thrombin-activated fibrinolysis inhibitor
TBI	Traumatic brain injury
TEG	Thromboelastography
THA	Total hip arthroplasty
TKA	Total knee arthroplasty
tPA	Tissue plasminogen activator
TXA	Tranexamic acid
ULTRA	Ultra-early tranexamic acid after subarachnoid hemorrhage
uPA	Urokinase plasminogen activator
WHO	World health organization

A. N. Primm (✉)
NYU Langone Health, Department of Anesthesiology, Perioperative Care and Pain Medicine, New York, NY, USA
e-mail: aaron.primm@nyulangone.org

Introduction

Fibrinolysis is a process that works to limit clot formation and is tightly controlled by cofactors, receptors, and inhibitors. Its actions are integrally counterbalanced by the coagulation process, maintaining physiologic homeostasis and protecting against excessive clot formation or hemorrhage. When plasmin or plasminogen is produced in excess quantities through, for example, trauma and surgery, multiple inflammatory responses can be generated, leading to coagulopathy and unwanted pathophysiology. To combat these unwanted events, clinicians have employed antifibrinolytic agents to reduce surgical blood loss, allogenic blood transfusion, and other potential adverse outcomes. Of the antifibrinolytic agents, tranexamic acid has been the most widely studied and utilized and will be the focus going forward. This chapter will review fibrinolysis and its measurement, antifibrinolytic agents, and the role of tranexamic acid in the most studied perioperative settings.

Fibrinolysis and Molecular Regulation

Fibrinolysis is an integral component of hemostasis that acts to regulate fibrin formation. Generally, hemostasis is the process of maintaining the integrity of the vascular system after damage [1]. Vessel wall injury and extravasation of blood from the circulation will trigger multiple processes to begin the repair. To do this, expressed tissue factor and circulating platelets combine to achieve vascular hemostasis and thrombin is generated through the coagulation cascade

© Springer Nature Switzerland AG 2021
C. S. Scher et al. (eds.), *Essentials of Blood Product Management in Anesthesia Practice*,
https://doi.org/10.1007/978-3-030-59295-0_5

[2]. More specifically, after endothelial cell disruption, platelets are activated when they come in contact with subendothelial matrix proteins such as collagen, fibronectin, and von Willebrand factor [3]. This activation exposes anionic phospholipids, which attract procoagulant proteins to the cell surface. A sequential series of enzymatic cleavage events lead to thrombin activation from its zymogen prothrombin [4, 5]. Thrombin will catalyze the conversion of soluble fibrinogen to insoluble fibrin, and hence achieves hemostasis [4]. Fibrin will be cross-linked through Factor XIIIa, a transglutaminase, as more platelets, red blood cells, and white blood cells are incorporated for greater clot stability to resist fibrinolysis [6].

As the clot forms, the fibrinolytic system is activated to counterbalance the coagulation response at the site of injury, as well as throughout the body. Plasmin is formed on the surface of the fibrin clot, or cell surfaces, from plasminogen [7]. Plasmin is the primary fibrinolysin that is activated by two primary serine proteases, tissue plasminogen activator (tPA) and urokinase (uPA) (Fig. 5.1) [4]. Endothelial cells synthesize and release tPA, while uPA is made in macrophages, monocytes, and urinary epithelium. Both are cleared by the liver [8]. Plasminogen also exhibits positive feedback on its activation because plasmin increases activator activity by converting single-chain tPA and uPA to their two-chain counterparts [4]. In response to vascular injury, tPA and uPA are released in high concentrations, although they exist in plasma at a low, "surveillance," concentration [9].

Plasmin is the key enzyme of fibrinolysis, acting to cleave fibrin and release fibrin degradation products. This action is facilitated by sites in the plasminogen molecule that can bind fibrin's lysine residues [10]. However, plasmin can also be involved in multiple enzymatic pathways leading to worsening coagulopathy, bleeding, and inflammation [10]. Plasmin, especially when bound to the surface of macrophages, is critical in monocyte activation and inflammation. Activated plasmin conveys chemotaxis and actin polymerization in monocytes leading to cytokine release [11]. Also, plasmin can be generated from inflammation secondary to bacterial infection and exposure to lipopolysaccharide, which can contribute to disseminated intravascular coagulation and sepsis [12]. By whatever means, these actions can occur when plasmin is present in concentrations that exceed its physiologic inhibitors and is the basis for the use of antifibrinolytic therapy [10, 13]. Bursts of free plasmin lead to degradation of coagulation factors like fibrinogen and factors V and VII. Additionally, the cleavage of glycoprotein Ib and IIb/IIIa receptors on platelets through fibrinolysis will hinder platelet adhesion and aggregation [14]. By all of these processes, plasmin can bring on a serious pathophysiologic state that will lead to poor clinical outcomes if left unchecked.

Molecular inhibitors are vitally important in fibrinolysis to control any surplus of plasmin or plasminogen activator. Serine protease inhibitors form covalent complexes with circulating plasmin and plasminogen activators, neutralizing their effects [15]. The most important serine protease inhibi-

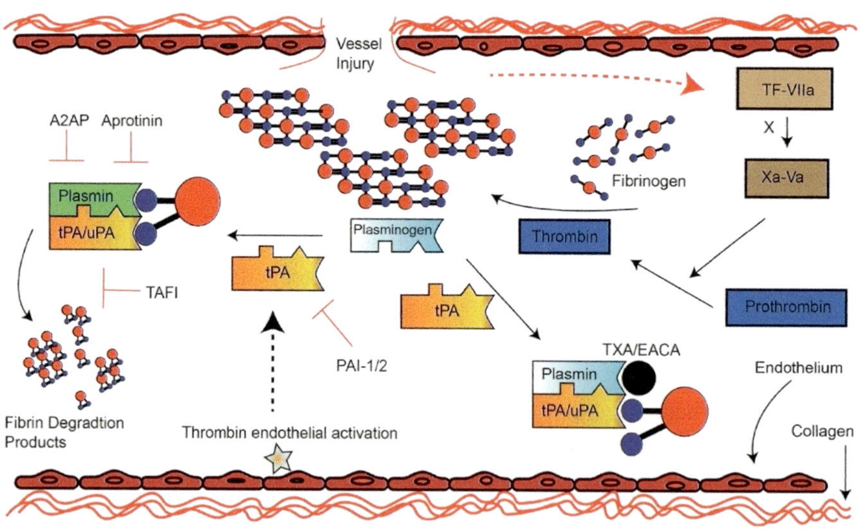

Fig. 5.1 Schematic of hemostasis and fibrinolysis with inhibitors. After vessel wall injury (red dashed arrow), expressed tissue factor (TF) binds with factor VIIA, leading to the generation of thrombin and hemostasis. Thrombin will catalyze the conversion of soluble fibrinogen into an organized fibrin meshwork that will lead to clot formation. Thrombin also stimulates release of tissue plasminogen activator (tPA) from the endothelium (black dashed arrow) that will form a complex with plasminogen on the surface of fibrin to release active plasmin. Plasmin formation can also be achieved with urokinase plasminogen activator (uPA), which is released from macrophages, monocytes, and urinary epithelium. Plasmin will cleave fibrin to soluble fibrin degradation products. Tranexamic acid (TXA) and epsilon-aminocaproic acid (EACA) inhibit fibrinolysis intravascularly by competitive inhibition on plasminogen's lysine-binding site. This prevents plasmin release and allows for a stable fibrin clot. Aprotinin reversible inhibits free plasmin. Fibrinolysis is inhibited by plasminogen activator inhibitors (PAI-1 and PAI 2), alpha-2-antiplasmin (A2AP), and thrombin-activated fibrinolysis inhibitor (TAFI)

tors are plasminogen activator inhibitor-1 (PAI-1), plasminogen activator inhibitor-2 (PAI-2), and α2-antiplasmin (A2AP). A2AP acts to irreversibly inactivate plasmin by a suicide inhibition mechanism [15]. However, when plasmin is bound to fibrin, it is protected from this inhibition and can allow fibrinolysis [16]. PAI-1 and PAI-2 inhibit both tPA and uPA. However, PA-2 is only present in appreciable quantities during pregnancy [17]. C1-esterase inhibitor, α2-macroglobulin, and other aspects of the contact pathway of the coagulation cascade also represent less prominent non-serpin plasmin inhibitors.

Thrombin-activated fibrinolysis inhibitor (TAFI) is activated by thrombomodulin-associated thrombin. It is a carboxypeptidase that removes C-terminal lysine and arginine residues on fibrin. By doing so, it can decrease the number of available plasminogen-binding sites and help stabilize clots [18]. TAFI may play a key role in regulating the interplay between inflammation and coagulation [18, 19].

Measuring Fibrinolysis

The development of methods to assess fibrinolytic activity has lagged behind the progress seen in coagulation testing, which is standardized for routine high-throughput screening [20]. Fibrinolysis, in normal blood and conditions, may take hours or days to develop and limits its clinical applications [21]. Coagulation reactions (international normalized ratio (INR) and activated partial thromboplastin time (APTT), for example) can take only seconds to minutes to run. To facilitate the assessment of fibrinolysis, one must add plasminogen activators or remove inhibitors. However, this will limit the applicability to an in vivo scenario [20]. No "gold standard" assay exists to assess fibrinolytic activity, and the various methods available can be grouped according to a sample from whole blood, plasma, or euglobulin fraction of plasma [22].

Whole blood preparations are useful in that they can represent truly "global" activity, as the cellular components of blood have a significant impact on coagulation and fibrinolysis [22]. These samples are often used perioperatively by point-of-care testing. However, this approach is limited by assay standardization, storage issues, the absence of endothelium, and the inability to use the sample in other types of assays [22]. The most studied perioperative tool to measure fibrinolysis is thromboelastography. This test is performed with a thromboelastograph (TEG) or rotation thromboelastometery (ROTEM) by measuring viscoelastic changes in whole blood over time with the addition of different activators like tissue factor and kaolin [22]. Thromboelastography can assess coagulation parameters but can also be modified to reflect any endogenous fibrinolytic activity. In ROTEM, maximal lysis reflects the percent decrease of maximal amplitude over time. Small decreases can be due to tapering of the clot, allowing additional rotation of the sample [10, 22]. Maximal lysis of greater than 15% could indicate hyperfibrinolysis, whereas greater than 3% is an important benchmark to initiate antifibrinolytic therapy in trauma [23, 24].

TEG and ROTEM are the most frequently utilized tools to assess fibrinolysis in trauma patients and have become increasingly popular [25]. However, there is controversy regarding the need to assess fibrinolysis in these patients given the frequent use of pre-emptive antifibrinolytic therapy [10, 26]. Studies have suggested that they lack sensitivity to detect small changes in fibrinolytic activation, and there is questionable evidence to suggest that they would be helpful to guide antifibrinolytic therapy [10, 26].

Plasma turbidity methods rely on the measurement of changes in optical density after the initiation of coagulation. Fibrin formation and lysis are reflected by the optical density [18]. A common method utilized to measure fibrinolytic and coagulation activity is overall hemostasis potential. The assay relies on spectrophotometer readings in two sets of wells containing platelet-free plasma mixed with phosphatidylserine-containing phospholipids, calcium chloride, and tissue factor [22]. The other sample of wells has the addition of tPA. The readout will give an overall hemostasis potential and overall coagulation potential, allowing calculation of the overall fibrinolysis potential. Clot lysis time, the time from 50% of maximal clotting to 50% lysis, can also be obtained [27]. The overall fibrinolysis potential and clot lysis time can give insight for determining pro hemorrhagic and pro thrombotic states.

Lastly, the euglobulin fraction of plasma has been known for its strong fibrinolytic activity. It has greatly reduced amounts of PAI-1 with preserved levels of plasminogen activators when compared to untreated platelet free plasma [28]. This rebalanced plasminogen activator: PA-1 ratio allows the measurement of intrinsic fibrinolytic activity without exogenous activators [22]. The classic test is the euglobulin clot lysis time, which is a visual recording of the time it takes the euglobulin fraction to completely lyse [22].

Antifibrinolytic Agents

By the 1950s, the amino acid lysine was known to inhibit the activation of plasminogen in vitro, but the effect was too weak to be clinically relevant. In efforts to reduce maternal deaths from postpartum hemorrhage, investigations in 1953 by a Japanese team showed several mercapto- and aminocarbonic acids had antiplasminic effect [29]. During this work, they showed that epsilon-aminocaproic acid (EACA) was a strong inhibitor of plasminogen. EACA had been used clinically before this time, but the antiplasminic effect was not potent enough and required large doses. In 1962 a more potent compound was found: 4-amino-methyl-cyclohexane-carbonic acid [30]. The compound contains two stereoisomers of which the trans-form was discovered to be antifibrinolytic (trans-4-aminomethylcyclohexanecarboxylic acid). This substance is now known as tranexamic acid (TXA) [31, 32]. EACA and TXA are synthetic lysine analogs that inhibit fibrinolysis by attaching to the lysine-binding site of the plasmin(ogen) molecule and displacing plasminogen from fibrin. TXA was found to be about 6–10 times more potent than EACA while also better tolerated [29]. Of countries that incorporate TXA into clinical practice, the United States has most strongly adapted the use of EACA, likely related to costs and early availability [10].

Aprotinin is another antifibrinolytic which acts as a broad-spectrum protease inhibitor. First isolated in cow parotid glands in 1930, its first clinical use was in treating of hyperfibrinolytic conditions, notably pancreatitis [33]. In the early 1980s, the Kirkland group in Alabama began using aprotinin in an attempt to attenuate the inflammatory response after protamine administration. The surgical field was found to be unusually dry after cardiopulmonary bypass (CPB), which led to a trial-and-error approach to developing aprotinin protocols and the further study of its interaction with the fibrinolytic system [34]. By 1993, aprotinin was approved by the FDA for use in coronary artery bypass grafting (CABG). Widespread use of aprotinin to reduce perioperative blood loss and transfusions also became popular in major orthopedic and hepatic surgery.

Other potential antifibrinolytic agents, not approved for clinical use, include nafamostat, MDCO-2010, and textilinins from *Pseudonaja textilis* [10]. The three clinically used agents will be reviewed as follows.

Tranexamic Acid

TXA is a synthetic lysine analog with a molecular weight of 157 Da that reversibly and competitively blocks the lysine-binding site on plasminogen, hence inhibiting fibrinolysis. Plasminogen is believed to have 4–5 low-affinity binding sites and one high-affinity binding site. TXA acts on the high-affinity binding site [35, 36].

The pharmacokinetics will vary based on the route of administration and overall renal function. TXA is produced under several brand names (see Table 5.1) and can be admin-

Table 5.1 Antifibrinolytic agents

Drug	Tranexamic acid	Epsilon-aminocaproic acid	Aprotinin
Composition	Synthetic lysine analog	Synthetic lysine analog	Naturally occurring polypeptide, isolated from bovine lung tissue
Molecular weight	157 Da	131 Da	6512 Da
Mechanism of action	Antifibrinolytic Inhibits conversion of plasminogen to plasmin through reversible, competitive blockade of plasminogen's lysine-binding site	Antifibrinolytic Inhibits conversion of plasminogen to plasmin through reversible, competitive blockade of plasminogen's lysine-binding site	Serine protease inhibitor Reversible inhibition of free plasmin, trypsin, chymotrypsin, kallikrein Inhibition of fibrinolysis, Factor XIIa-mediated kallikrein activation, thrombin-induced platelet activation Possible anti-inflammatory effects
Elimination	Renal	Renal	Proteolysis, renal
Terminal elimination half-life	3 h	2 h	10 h
Select adverse effects	Possible thrombosis Seizures	Possible thrombosis	Possible thrombosis Renal dysfunction
Prescription products (North America)	Cyklokapron (IV, oral) Erfa-tranexamic (IV) Lysteda (oral)	Amicar (IV, oral)	Trasylol (IV)
Market approval	USA Canada Europe	USA Canada	Complete removal from market in 2008 Reintroduced in Canada in 2011 and Europe in 2012 Select availability in United Kingdom, the Netherlands, Sweden, Canada Still suspended in the USA

Abbreviations: *IV* intravenous

istered intravenous (IV), intramuscular, oral, and topical. IV administration of a 10 mg/kg bolus gives a plasma concentration of 10 mg/L [37]. Additionally, the half-life is about 80 min with 30% renal elimination within the first hour, 55% by 3 h, and 90% by 24 h [38]. Oral TXA doses of 10–15 mg/kg give a peak plasma concentration within 3 h [38]. In an in vitro tissue study, it has been shown that 100 mg/L of TXA will reduce fibrinolytic activity by 98–100% [39]. TXA has little plasma-protein binding with minimal metabolism [36]. It passes through the placenta and equilibrates with fetal blood levels, with no adverse effects on the fetus. TXA is present in breast milk but at a concentration 100 times less than found in maternal blood, and does not have any effects on breast-fed babies [37, 40].

IV dosing can range from 0.5 to 25 g based on patient and clinical conditions and must be adjusted for renal insufficiency [10]. In earlier work, Nillson et al. describes a dose of 10 mg/kg IV, 3–4 times hourly, in the treatment of systemic fibrinolysis with massive bleeding [37]. In a landmark study of TXA, the Clinical Randomization of an Antifibrinolytic in Significant Hemorrhage (CRASH-2) trial analyzed a group with major bleeding after severe trauma to receive a loading dose of 1 g IV followed by an infusion of 1 g over 8 h [41]. In pediatric (less than 12-years-old) trauma, an expert consensus would dose TXA in a similar matter as adults at 15 mg/kg (maximum 1 g) followed by an infusion of 2 mg/kg/h for at least 8 h until bleeding stops [42].

For the treatment of heavy menstrual bleeding, the U.S. Food and Drug Administration (FDA) recommends oral TXA (Lysteda; Ferring-Parsippany, New Jersey) 1.3 g, three times daily for up to five days [43]. Several other European agencies have similar protocols for oral TXA. Oral TXA formulation should be given 2 h before any indicated surgical procedure.

Side effects are uncommon, and TXA has had a strong safety record. Mild nausea and diarrhea have been observed in a high-dose trial of TXA, but improve with a diminished dose [44]. Macroscopic hematuria from the upper renal tract is often considered a contraindication to TXA due to the risk of clot burden and ureteral obstruction. There are reports of acute renal cortical necrosis with oliguria and renal failure caused by TXA [29]. Patients on estrogens that have additional risk factors for thrombosis should take caution; however, evidence is lacking. Absolute contraindications include hypersensitivity, active thromboembolic disease, and fibrinolytic conditions with consumption coagulopathy.

Epsilon-Aminocaproic Acid

EACA is a synthetic, highly water-soluble crystal with a molecular weight of 131Da that acts as a lysine analog. Both EACA and TXA act to block the conversion of plasminogen to plasmin resulting in the inhibition of fibrinolysis. Its volume of distribution is about 30 L with IV dosing, and max serum concentrations are reached in 10 min [45]. The drug eventually distributes throughout both intravascular and extravascular compartments while penetrating blood and tissues [46]. Total body clearance is 169 ml/min, and terminal half-life is about 2 h [47–49].

Studies evaluating IV EACA of 10 g or 100 mg/kg in humans produced an initial concentration of about 1.5 g/L that decreased to 35 mg/L within 3–4 h, with 80–100% eliminated by urine filtration [10]. Patients with renal failure have markedly decreased total body clearance, and only 25% can be removed via hemodialysis [50]. EACA undergoes rapid excretion in the urine and thus needs to be administered as an IV infusion to achieve therapeutic levels. Studies have identified that an EACA concentration of about 130 mcg/mL is required to inhibit systemic fibrinolytic activity. These studies recommend a dose of 0.1 g/kg bodyweight every 3–4 h or an initial loading dose of 10 g to be followed by a continuous infusion of 1 g/h [47–49]. EACA likely crosses the blood-brain barrier, but it is unclear whether it crosses the placenta or distributes in breast milk [46].

EACA is predominantly administered IV, with some case reports describing topical use [51, 52]. There are no standard guidelines for EACA dosing, and many dosing protocols have been developed for perioperative use. Like TXA, EACA has been studied most extensively in cardiac surgery. EACA protocols have shown reduced chest tube drainage following cardiac surgery, making EACA a preferred drug in many institutions in the United States [46].

Most safety concerns of EACA are based on the potential for promoting a prothrombotic state through action on the fibrinolytic pathway. Reports of adverse events are from isolated case reports or low-powered studies. To date, no trial has been able to show a significant difference in thrombotic events when compared to TXA or aprotinin [46]. Caution should always be taken when considering the mechanism of the drug and any pre-existing patient coagulopathies. Overall, EACA is well tolerated.

Aprotinin

Aprotinin is a naturally occurring 58 amino acid polypeptide, with a molecular weight of 6512 Da, isolated from bovine lung but currently manufactured by recombinant technology. It is a serine protease inhibitor with its antifibrinolytic effect via direct noncompetitive inhibition of plasmin. The structure is similar to tissue factor pathway inhibitor, and its dosing is calculated in kallikrein-inhibiting units [10]. Aprotinin may falsely elevate or prolong partial thromboplastin time and celite-activated clotting time (ACT) measurements. Therefore these should not be used to monitor heparin anticoagulation during surgery. If ACT monitoring is necessary after aprotinin administration, a minimal ACT of 750 s or kaolin-ACT of 480 s is recommended by the European Society of Anesthesiology task force [33].

Due to its nonspecific nature, aprotinin is also an inhibitor of trypsin, chymotrypsin, platelet protease-activated receptor-1, and kallikrein. The inhibition of protease-activated receptor-1 is a possible mechanism for stroke reduction during cardiac surgery after aprotinin administration [10]. Additionally, aprotinin inactivates free plasmin but does not greatly affect bound plasmin. Aprotinin is renally excreted with a plasma half-life of 150 min and an elimination half-life of 5–10 h after lysosomal enzyme metabolization [53].

In the mid-2000s, concerning reports regarding the safety of aprotinin were widely published, which suggested multiple adverse events and increase in 5-year mortality [46]. By 2006, the FDA added renal dysfunction, stroke, graft occlusion, and anaphylaxis to aprotinin's list of safety issues [33]. Further research in 2007 gave conflicting evidence surrounding aprotinin's safety but only cast doubt on the drug.

In 2008, the Blood Conservation Using Antifibrinolytics in a Randomized Trial (BART) was published [54]. This blinded, randomized controlled trial (RCT) compared aprotinin, TXA, and EACA in patients undergoing high-risk cardiac surgery. The trial was stopped by the safety committee in October 2007 due to nonsignificant increased mortality associated with aprotinin. Results from BART, previous studies, and the FDA warning led to the withdrawal of aprotinin from the United States in late 2007 and from Canada and Europe in 2008. Subsequent criticism and reanalysis of the data eventually convinced Health Canada in 2011 to allow aprotinin for patients undergoing isolated CABG. The European Medicines Agency also lifted its suspension in the European Union in 2012 but enforced the establishment of a European registry for aprotinin use [55]. Aprotinin is currently available in the United Kingdom, the Netherlands, Sweden, and Canada.

Perioperative Considerations

Cardiac Surgery

Cardiac surgery is the most studied area in the fibrinolytic literature. TXA became key in antifibrinolytic therapy after its comparative safety was shown in the BART trial, and has been extensively examined in cardiac surgery, CPB, or off-pump [54]. TXA has been consistently shown to be efficacious in reducing blood loss and transfusion requirements during cardiac surgery. The Society of Thoracic Surgeons and the Society of Cardiovascular Anesthesiologists blood conservation guidelines strongly (class IA) recommend the use of TXA or EACA in cardiac surgery [56].

There is no optimal dose of TXA, and large variations in dosing recommendations have been cited. In a prospective, double-blinded dosing study on CPB by Horrow et al. [57], 148 patients were given placebo, while five groups received TXA IV with a loading dose before incision (2.5–40 mg/kg) and followed by infusion of one-tenth the loading dose for 12 h. A major finding was a significant reduction in chest tube drainage from the patients who received a 10 mg/kg loading with additional maintenance dose (now referred to as the "Horrow low dose" regimen). However, TXA did not change transfusion requirements. Increasing the dosage (20 and 40 mg/kg bolus) did not provide additional reductions in bleeding. Fiechtner et al. [58] showed that a bolus 10 mg/kg dose followed by an infusion of 1 mg/kg/h gave a TXA concentration sufficient to inhibit fibrinolytic activity in vitro. Dowd et al. [59] calculated a bolus of 30 mg/kg TXA IV, followed by 16 mg/kg/h for 6 h, and 2 mg/kg added to the pump prime would get a 100% inhibition of fibrinolytic activity. Using this regimen, Sharma et al. [60] found that the mean plasma TXA concentration was consistently higher than the previously suggested threshold.

After FDA withdrawal of aprotinin in 2007 and the implementation of TXA during cardiac surgery, there were increased reports of postoperative generalized convulsive seizures in the absence of new ischemic lesions on brain imaging [10]. In retrospective analysis, it was found that patients were receiving doses of 100 mg/kg followed by 20–50 mg/kg/h with a total dose up to 259 mg/kg during surgery [61]. Given concern for seizure activity at these high doses, lower dose guideline modifications were made with 30 mg/kg loading followed by 15 mg/kg/h plus 2 mg/kg in the CPB priming solution. It was recommended not to exceed a maximum TXA total dose of 100 mg/kg in patients over 50 years old who underwent CPB open-heart procedures [62].

A recent, large RCT that gives the strongest evidence of the benefits of TXA in cardiac surgery is from Myles et al. [63]. The administration of a single initial bolus of 50 or 100 mg/kg of TXA was associated with a decreased incidence of transfusion of RBCs and other blood products and a reduction of redo surgery for major hemorrhage for tamponade. The incidence of seizures was 0.7% with TXA-treated patients compared to 0.1% of patients given placebo.

TXA has also been specifically studied for use in off-pump CABG, with several studies showing a reduction in perioperative bleeding when compared to placebo without increased thrombotic complications [46].

Tranexamic Acid and the Risk of Seizures

Seizures are a major concern with the use of TXA as they have been an associated complication with cardiac surgery. A recent meta-analysis of 28 RCTs of TXA administration, in patients undergoing CABG, found an increase in the incidence of postoperative seizures with a relative risk of 6.67 [64]. The mechanism for the increased risk of seizures is unknown but may involve the competitive antagonism of TXA on hippocampal gamma-aminobutyric acid type A (GABA/A) and the glycine receptor [65]. TXA, GABA, and glycine have similar molecular structures. The proconvulsant properties of TXA are likely via direct effects on the central nervous system, as the application of TXA in experimental animal models will cause systemic, as well as intracranial, hypertension, and seizures [66]. Case reports have found that maximal TXA concentrations from the cerebral spinal fluid occurred after the termination of drug infusion [65]. EACA has not been known to cause seizure activity, although there is inadequate data.

The incidence of seizures associated with TXA is likely dose-related, particularly with doses greater than 50 mg/kg [67]. Studies have shown that predictors of seizure activity include: open chamber cardiac surgery, advanced age, female sex, redo surgery, ascending aortic disease, deep hypothermic circulatory arrest, cross-clamp time, chronic renal dysfunction, and TXA [68–71]. It has been speculated that cerebral emboli causing local blood-brain barrier disturbances leading to seizure activity could be an alternate or contributory mechanism for these findings. In other scenarios, such as TXA loading in menstrual or traumatic bleeding, seizure activity is much less significant [10, 72].

Although shown to occur, the significance of seizures associated with cardiac surgery and TXA is not known. A Japanese database of pediatric cardiac surgeries showed a significant increase in the incidence of seizures (1.6% versus 0.2%) in patients who received TXA but no difference in outcomes [73]. In contrast, Myles et al. [63] showed an increased incidence of stroke and death associated with TXA. Overall, it is unclear if TXA is the direct cause of stroke after cardiac surgery or if it only enables other mechanisms to exert their effects on the central nervous system.

Trauma, the Role of Fibrinolysis, and Traumatic Brain Injury

Trauma and traumatic bleeding is a leading cause of death and disability worldwide, with an estimated 400,000 deaths every year [74]. The past decade has seen the growing popularity of utilizing antifibrinolytic agents in traumatic bleeding after the CRASH-2 and Military Application of Tranexamic Acid in Trauma Emergency Resuscitation Study (MATTERs) trials [41, 75]. Based on findings in these landmark studies, TXA was added to the World Health Organization's list of essential medicines.

The CRASH-2 trial was a randomized trial to evaluate the effects of TXA in 20,211 adult trauma subjects who experienced or were at risk of significant bleeding. Subjects were randomized within 8 h of injury to 1 g IV over 10 min followed by a 1 g infusion over 8 h, or matching placebo. The primary outcome was 28-day in-hospital mortality. All-cause mortality was 14.5% in the treatment group and 16% in the placebo group (RR 0.91, 95% CI 0.85–0.97, P = 0.0035). Additionally, there was a reduction in risk of death due to bleeding of 4.9% vs. 5.7% (RR 0.85, 95% CI 0.76–0.96, P = 0.0077). Other cardiothoracic and thromboembolic events were similar between the groups. There was no significant difference in the number of transfusions or need for surgery. Post hoc analysis of the 35% of patients that died from bleeding suggested that the benefit of TXA was greatest when injected within the first hour after injury. However, treatment that was started 3 h after injury paradoxically increased the risk of death from bleeding.

CRASH-2 was the first trial to demonstrate a mortality benefit using TXA in trauma, however, the results were controversial considering these results were not obtained in the setting of an advanced trauma network [76]. There were concerns about subjects being treated in facilities with limited resources, no protocols for identifying thromboembolic events, and no insight into the mechanism of TXA's protective effect. More trials are being conducted to give answers to these lingering questions, including the Pre hospital Antifibrinolytics for Traumatic Coagulopathy and Hemorrhage (PATCH) trial [77].

The MATTERs trial was a retrospective observational study designed to evaluate TXA in combat injury and to assess the effects of its administration on total blood product use, thromboembolic complications, and mortality. In the patient group treated with TXA, there was an unadjusted in-hospital mortality of 17.4% vs. 23.9% in the nonTXA-treated group, as well as an independent association of TXA-treated patients with greater survival and less coagulopathy. Conflicting with the CRASH-2 study, MATTERs reported an associated increased risk of thromboembolic events in TXA subjects, however with further analysis, no association was found. Future studies will aim to clarify these findings.

The concept of acute traumatic coagulopathy (ATC) began to emerge in the literature after theorizing that another form of coagulopathy exists in patients, unrelated to fluid and blood product administration, related to tissue injury and bleeding [78]. During the response to traumatic injury, there arises a primary coagulopathy that has been associated with increased activated protein C. Shock and tissue injury results in a large tPA release from intracellular endothelial stores. A resultant sympathetic surge and "endotheliopathy" with glycocalyx damage further exacerbate coagulopathy and stimulate hyperfibrinolysis [79]. Additionally, the response is characterized by dysfibrinogenemia, endothelial dysfunction, and thrombocytopathia [80]. Hyperfibrinolysis has been identified as a significant contributor to mortality in adult trauma patients [76]. Although data suggests an important role of hyperfibrinolysis as a pathological cause of bleeding, there can be individual variability in fibrinolysis.

With this in mind several investigators have raised caution to the practice of giving TXA, or other antifibrinolytics, to all trauma patients due to the concern of fibrinolytic shutdown, or reduced fibrinolytic activity [81]. Giving TXA to these patients may cause unwanted thrombotic effects. In one study, Moore et al. [81] describe three fibrinolytic phenotypes: hyperfibrinolysis, physiologic, and shutdown. Using a TEG databank from trauma subjects presenting to the emergency department over three years, they grouped subjects by lysis measurement 30 min after maximum amplitude (LY30, percent). The most common phenotype was fibrinolysis shutdown (46%), while hyperfibrinolysis (18%) independently increased risk of mortality (OR 3.3, 95% CI 2.4–4.6, $P < 0.0001$). Acute blood loss was the leading cause of death in the hyperfibrinolysis group, while multiple organ failure was most common in fibrinolysis shutdown. Possible mechanisms to explain these results have been put forward, but none have been proven in vivo [82]. There is ongoing debate concerning the relevance of fibrinolytic shutdown.

Traumatic brain injury (TBI) is a leading cause of death after trauma and commonly presents with coagulopathy. Coagulopathy is a poor prognostic indicator for patients with TBI and is associated with hemorrhagic injury and high mortality [83]. Hyperfibrinolysis is also present in these patients with a mechanism likely similar to patients that present with other traumas. What is known is that patients with TBI will have increased release of tissue factor in the circulation from injured brain tissue, temporal changes in tPA and uPA, and depletion of antiplasmin [84]. Evidence of the efficacy of antifibrinolytics on TBI is lacking, but several trials are attempting to address this issue. CRASH-3: tranexamic acid for the treatment of significant traumatic brain injury, is estimated to be completed in 2020 [85].

Orthopedics

Antifibrinolytics have been studied extensively in orthopedic surgery, particularly in the most common procedures like total knee arthroplasty (TKA) and total hip arthroplasty (THA). During TKA, blood loss can be significant and under estimated, averaging between 762 and 1789 mL in the absence of TXA [86]. In a recent study, 25% of patients required red blood cell transfusion with a median of 2.2 units [87]. The total blood loss in THA averages 1600 mL, depending on surgical technique. About 30% of patients receive at least one blood transfusion with a median of 2.2 units [87].

Overall, TXA is efficacious in reducing perioperative blood loss and transfusion requirements over a range of procedures. Intraoperative dosing of TXA for joint arthroplasty varies greatly. Many centers administer 10–15 mg/kg TXA prior to the release of the tourniquet, or prior to skin incision for THA, followed by 1 or more repeat 10–15 mg/kg boluses 3–8 h later. A 2015 meta-analysis of 2720 TKA and THA procedures found that TXA significantly reduced blood loss and transfusion requirements [88]. For both TKA and THA, the number of patients receiving at least one unit of packed red blood cells were decreased in the TXA group compared to the control group. These results have been supported in several studies involving TKA and THA patients [89, 90]. Having established the efficacy of TXA in major joint surgeries, Xu et al. [91] conducted a systemic review and meta-analysis of 211 publications to investigate the safety of different routes of TXA, with a secondary aim to identify the safest and most efficacious route of TXA. Studies were examined with drug administration via: IV, intra-articular, topical, oral, and their combinations. TXA via IV and topical had the lowest risk ratio (RR = 0.11, 95% CI 0.03–0.41) with all routes showing significantly lower transfusion rates compared to placebo.

Spine surgery has also been studied in single and multi-level procedures. A 2015 meta-analysis with a total of 644 patients concluded that TXA reduced intraoperative blood loss by 219 mL (95% CI −116 mL to −322 mL, $P < 0.05$) [92]. They did not find an associated increased incidence of pulmonary embolism, deep venous thrombosis, or myocardial infarction. A more recent review and meta-analysis of TXA looking at blood loss and blood transfusion in multi-level spine surgery showed a decrease in blood loss and transfusion compared to controls, as well as a higher hemoglobin value post-surgery [93]. The RCTs in the analysis reviewed several different dosing regimens with many following 10–15 mg/kg TXA loading dose IV with an infusion of 1–2 mg/kg/h [93]. Recent studies show promising results utilizing high-dose TXA with a 50 mg/kg loading dose IV followed by an infusion of 5 mg/kg/h. Current literature and future studies in orthopedic surgery focus on the role of TXA in intertrochanteric fractures, total shoulder replacement, pediatrics, and topical TXA application.

Liver Surgery and Transplantation

Patients undergoing hepatic surgery face a unique challenge due to potential alterations in hemostatic function leading to coagulopathy and excess bleeding. Hemostatic function is determined by a complex relationship between vascular endothelium, platelets, coagulation, and fibrinolytic activity [94]. Patients with compromised liver function often have derangement in hemostasis and can develop a primary hyperfibrinolysis from the inflammation and trauma of surgery. Hyperfibrinolysis is particularly common during liver transplantation [95]. Early reports of hyperfibrinolysis during transplant, diagnosed by thromboelastography, spurred the use of antifibrinolytics for treatment until reports gave concern over increases in venous thromboembolism and mortality [10]. During hepatic transplantation, tPA levels increase during the anhepatic phase due to vascular trauma and reduced clearance. This perturbation is usually corrected after hepatic reperfusion, as PAI-1 is released and tPA is cleared.

RCTs have shown that TXA reduces blood loss and transfusion requirements during orthotopic liver transplantation (OLT) by 30–40% compared to placebo [96]. Subsequently, most liver transplant centers have developed protocols that determine when TXA and other antifibrinolytics are appropriate during transplantation. TXA use is not universal due to lingering concerns about safety and thromboembolic complications. Large-scale safety data exist for aprotinin but are lacking for TXA, particularly in subgroups that are low risk for blood loss or high risk for thromboembolic complications. Additionally, there has been great change in surgical and anesthetic technique for OLT over the last 15 years that may change blood management practices.

A propensity score matched study by Badenoch *et al.* [96] looked to describe the clinical use of TXA and to appraise effectiveness and safety. Data was collected from 1799 liver transplant patients and retrospectively analyzed using propensity matching to account for thrombotic risk and transfusion confounders. In matched pairs, patients exposed to TXA received less red blood cell and fresh frozen plasma transfusions. No difference in thromboembolic events were found between matched groups. They concluded that TXA is effective in modern clinical practice. However, the magnitude of effectiveness was reduced when compared to previous studies, possibly accounting for the improvements in modern practice.

The efficacy of TXA in hepatic resection is less studied. Resection is the optimal treatment for primary metastatic liver malignancies, benign liver tumors, and some biliary disease [94]. Like OLT, bleeding is a regular obstacle in hepatic resections and would seem amenable to antifibrinolytic therapy. A prospective, randomized trial in 2006 found that TXA lowered blood loss and operative times in hepatic tumor resections [97]. In a 2016 prospective cohort study, 18 patients undergoing major hepatic resection were sequentially assigned to one of three cohorts: control, TXA dose I (1 g bolus followed by 1 g infusion over 8 h), and TXA dose II (1 g bolus followed by 10 mg/kg/h until the end of surgery) [94]. Blood samples were collected for TEG, coagulation components, and TXA concentration. They concluded that there was no thromboelastographic evidence of hyperfibrinolysis in these major liver resections and that TXA did not influence a change in systemic fibrinolysis. Further research is warranted in this area.

Obstetrics

Postpartum hemorrhage (PPH) is an obstetric emergency and the leading cause of maternal death worldwide. At delivery, PAI-2 synthesis stops and tPA is rapidly increased, causing hyperfibrinogenemia to levels of 500–600 mg/dL [29]. Based on previous work, World Health Organization (WHO) guidelines recommend TXA in PPH if uterotonics fail to stop bleeding, or if bleeding is thought to be from trauma [98]. However, the efficacy of TXA in this scenario is uncertain, and a 2016 analysis of 26 RCTs was inconclusive due to poor study design and serious flaws [99]. Many of the studies used a 1 g IV dose of TXA before incision for cesarean section, or 1 g IV after vaginal delivery.

A recent, large trial published in 2017 was able to add to our understanding of TXA in PPH [100]. The study aimed to analyze the effects of TXA on death and hysterectomy in woman with PPH. Woman aged 16 years and older from 193 hospitals in 21 countries were recruited after being diagnosed with PPH after vaginal birth or caesarean section. Subjects were assigned to either 1 g IV TXA or matching placebo, but if bleeding persisted or restarted within 24 h of the first dose, a second 1 g dose or placebo could be given. The composite primary endpoint was death from all-causes or hysterectomy within 42 days of giving birth. They found that death due to bleeding was significantly reduced in women given TXA, especially when given within 3 h of birth where deaths were reduced by nearly one-third. There were no significant differences in other causes of death between groups. Hysterectomy was not reduced with TXA, although it did substantially reduce the number of laparotomies to control bleeding. The composite primary endpoint of all-cause mortality or hysterectomy was not reduced with TXA.

Subarachnoid Hemorrhage

When a patient suffers a subarachnoid hemorrhage (SAH), rebleeding is a significant cause of morbidity and mortality. Currently, the rate of rebleeding has decreased to about 15% due to more sophisticated endovascular and surgical techniques early in the hospital course. The highest risk of rebleed is during the first 24 h after SAH, peaking in the first 6 h. After rebleed, approximately 60% of patients will die, and another 30% will remain dependent for activities of daily living [101].

The literature supports considering a short-course use of TXA to prevent rebleeding after SAH, with studies reporting a reduction in rebleeding by 35–40% [46, 102, 103]. However, these studies emphasized that outcomes were diminished by cerebral ischemia. A 2017 systematic review to assess the evidence for the role of TXA in the treatment of SAH and subdural hemorrhage found that TXA significantly reduced rebleeding in SAH patients and trended toward reducing mortality, but did not improve Glasgow Outcome Scale scores [104].

Initiated in 2013, the ultra-early tranexamic acid after subarachnoid hemorrhage (ULTRA) trial will aim to determine whether ultra-early and short-term administration of TXA (1 g bolus as soon as possible after randomization followed by 1 g over 8 h infusion to maximum of 24 h), in addition to standard SAH management will lead to better functional outcome scores at six months [105]. The TXA dose used in this trial will be lower than in previous studies in an effort to prevent delayed cerebral ischemia.

Pediatrics

Antifibrinolytic drugs, particularly TXA, are effective when used in both adult and pediatric surgical patients. Prospective RCTs in children undergoing cardiac surgery, spinal fusion, and craniosynostosis repair have shown that IV TXA is effective in reducing blood loss and transfusions [106]. Although without significant evidence, TXA has been used clinically in major pediatric plastic and maxillary procedures, organ transplantation, trauma, and major abdominal surgeries. Additionally, the WHO, American Society of Anesthesiologists, European Society of Anesthesiology, and Australian National Blood Authority have comprehensive blood management guidelines that suggest prophylactic TXA administration.

Pharmacokinetic studies over the past 10 years have elucidated TXA dosing regimens for children. These regimens are mostly based on the assumption that plasma TXA concentrations should target between 20 and 100 mcg/mL. However, these assumptions are based on in vitro models of fibrinolysis inhibition, and further studies are needed to validate this concept in vivo [106].

Topical Tranexamic Acid

Given the potential benefits of decreased risk of adverse events compared to systemic TXA, there is increased interest in utilizing the topical form of TXA [107]. When applied topically, the plasma concentration of TXA is 90% less than when administered IV [36]. However, local tissue drug concentrations from the topical application may also increase the risk of adverse events. A previous Cochrane review, covering a wide range of procedures, concluded that locally applied TXA might reduce bleeding and transfusions, but had concerns about the lack of safety data [108].

A recent systematic review and meta-analysis were conducted to evaluate the efficacy and safety of topically administered TXA [107]. A total of 67 studies were included, the majority of which evaluated orthopedic procedures. Administration of topical TXA, compared to placebo, significantly reduced the odds of receiving a blood transfusion (OR 0.28, 95% CI 0.20–0.38; $P < 0.001$) and significantly reduced mean blood loss. When compared to IV administration, there was no difference in transfusion requirements or blood loss. There was also no difference in the odds of developing a venous thromboembolic complication between topical TXA and control groups, or the topical and IV groups. No major differences were found between topical and systemic TXA concerning safety and efficacy. However, most of the included trials were not powered sufficiently to detect these differences. Besides orthopedic surgery, comparisons between systemic and topical TXA warrant further exploration.

Conclusions

The antifibrinolytic agents, particularly TXA, have been studied widely in a variety of perioperative settings. Most concerns about potential thromboembolic events using the antifibrinolytics have not been seen in the literature, although many studies are underpowered to detect them. The efficacy of aprotinin has been shown in cardiac surgery, but early safety concerns shelved its use in the United States. The reintroduction of aprotinin in Europe, along with a large safety registry, will be closely examined. The three described antifibrinolytics had shown reduced blood loss and transfusion rates in cardiac surgery, but concern over seizure activity in patients treated with TXA remain. Seizures in cardiac surgery are likely related to higher dosages, and it will be important to investigate the real impact on outcomes. CRASH-2 was a landmark trial showing reduced mortality in patients treated early with TXA after traumatic injury. The controversy surrounding measuring fibrinolytic shutdown and its impact on therapy is an area requiring further work. Several on-going trials will further enlighten the use of TXA in trauma, including CRASH-3 for traumatic brain injuries. Orthopedic surgery has established the benefits of perioperative TXA administration and continues to investigate alternate routes of administration to improve safety. Liver transplant has clear reductions in blood loss with antifibrinolytic treatment, although the magnitude of such reductions may be explained by improved surgical and blood management practices. There is no clear evidence for improved outcomes with TXA administration after SAH, and the results of the ULTRA trial are highly anticipated. Death due to bleeding is significantly reduced in women given TXA during PPH, particularly within the first 3 h. Like adults, antifibrinolytic therapy is effective in pediatric surgery, but optimum dosages are still under investigation.

References

1. Furie B, Furie BC. Mechanisms of thrombus formation. N Engl J Med. 2008;359:938–49.
2. Sim D, Flaumenhaft R, Furie B, Furie B. Interactions of platelets, blood-borne tissue factor, and fibrin during arteriolar thrombus formation in vivo. Microcirculation. 2005;12:301–11.
3. Broos K, Feys HB, De Meyer SF, Vanhoorelbeke K, Deckmyn H. Platelets at work in primary hemostasis. Blood Rev. 2011;25:155–67.
4. Chapin JC, Hajjar KA. Fibrinolysis and the control of blood coagulation. Blood Rev. 2015;29:17–24.
5. de Witt SM, Verdoold R, Cosemans JMEM, Heemskerk JWM. Insights into platelet-based control of coagulation. Thromb Res. 2014;133(Suppl 2):S139–48.
6. Bagoly Z, Koncz Z, Hársfalvi J, Muszbek L. Factor XIII, clot structure, thrombosis. Thromb Res. 2012;129:382–7.
7. Michalets E, Harris L. Antifibrinolytics. Cardiovascular Thrombus [Internet]. Elsevier; 2018 [cited 2019 Apr 29]. p. 615–49. Available from: https://linkinghub.elsevier.com/retrieve/pii/B9780128126158000442.
8. Bu G, Warshawsky I, Schwartz AL. Cellular receptors for the plasminogen activators. Blood. 1994;83:3427–36.
9. Foley J. Plasmin(ogen) at the nexus of fibrinolysis, inflammation, and complement. Semin Thromb Hemost. 2017;43:135–42.
10. Levy JH, Koster A, Quinones QJ, Milling TJ, Key NS. Antifibrinolytic therapy and perioperative considerations. Anesthesiology. 2018;128:657–70.
11. Gong Y, Hart E, Shchurin A, Hoover-Plow J. Inflammatory macrophage migration requires MMP-9 activation by plasminogen in mice. J Clin Invest. 2008;118:3012–24.
12. Syrovets T, Simmet T. Novel aspects and new roles for the serine protease plasmin. Cell Mol Life Sci. 2004;61:873–85.
13. Longstaff C, Kolev K. Basic mechanisms and regulation of fibrinolysis. J Thromb Haemost. 2015;13 Suppl 1:S98–105.
14. Ouimet H, Francis S, Loscalzo J. Structural changes in platelet glycoprotein IIb/IIIa by plasmin: determinants and functional consequences. Blood. 1994;83(2):404–14.
15. Travis J, Salvesen GS. Human plasma proteinase inhibitors. Annu Rev Biochem. 1983;52:655–709.
16. Schneider M, Nesheim M. A study of the protection of plasmin from antiplasmin inhibition within an intact fibrin clot during the course of clot lysis. J Biol Chem. 2004;279:13333–9.
17. Sprengers ED, Kluft C. Plasminogen activator inhibitors. Blood. 1987;69:381–7.
18. Broze GJ, Higuchi DA. Coagulation-dependent inhibition of fibrinolysis: role of carboxypeptidase-U and the premature lysis of clots from hemophilic plasma. Blood. 1996;88:3815–23.
19. Bajzar L, Jain N, Wang P, Walker JB. Thrombin activatable fibrinolysis inhibitor: not just an inhibitor of fibrinolysis. Crit Care Med. 2004;32:S320–4.
20. Longstaff C. Measuring fibrinolysis: from research to routine diagnostic assays. J Thromb Haemost. 2018;16:652–62.
21. Fearnley GR, Lackner R. The fibrinolytic activity of normal blood. Br J Haematol. 1955;1:189–98.
22. Ilich A, Bokarev I, Key NS. Global assays of fibrinolysis. Int J Lab Hematol. 2017;39:441–7.
23. Ives C, Inaba K, Branco BC, Okoye O, Schochl H, Talving P, et al. Hyperfibrinolysis elicited via thromboelastography predicts mortality in trauma. J Am Coll Surg. 2012;215:496–502.
24. Schöchl H, Frietsch T, Pavelka M, Jámbor C. Hyperfibrinolysis after major trauma: differential diagnosis of lysis patterns and prognostic value of thrombelastometry. J Trauma. 2009;67:125–31.
25. Theusinger OM, Levy JH. Point of care devices for assessing bleeding and coagulation in the trauma patient. Anesthesiol Clin. 2013;31:55–65.
26. Chapman MP, Moore EE, Ramos CR, Ghasabyan A, Harr JN, Chin TL, et al. Fibrinolysis greater than 3% is the critical value for initiation of antifibrinolytic therapy. J Trauma Acute Care Surg. 2013;75:961–7; discussion 967.
27. He S, Bremme K, Blombäck M. A laboratory method for determination of overall haemostatic potential in plasma. I. Method design and preliminary results. Thromb Res. 1999;96:145–56.
28. Urano T, Nishikawa T, Nagai N, Takada Y, Takada A. Amounts of tPA and PAI-1 in the euglobulin fraction obtained at different pH: their relation to the euglobulin clot lysis time. Thromb Res. 1997;88:75–80.
29. Tengborn L, Blombäck M, Berntorp E. Tranexamic acid – an old drug still going strong and making a revival. Thromb Res. 2015;135:231–42.
30. Okamoto S, Okamoto U. Amino-methyl-cyclohexane-carboxylic acid: amcha. Keio J Med. 1962;11:105–15.
31. Okamoto S, Sato S, Takada Y, Okamoto U. An active stereo-isomer (trans-form) of amcha and its antifibrinolytic (anti-plasminic) action in vitro and in vivo. Keio J Med. 1964;13:177–85.
32. Melander B, Gliniecki G, Granstrand B, Hanshoff G. Biochemistry and toxicology of amikapron; the antifibrinolytically active isomer of AMCHA. (A comparative study with epsilon-aminocaproic acid). Acta Pharmacol Toxicol (Copenh). 1965;22:340–52.
33. European Society of Anaesthesiology task force reports on place of aprotinin in clinical anaesthesia. Aprotinin: is it time to reconsider? Eur J Anaesthesiol. 2015;32:591–5.
34. Westaby S. Aprotinin: twenty-five years of claim and counterclaim. J Thorac Cardiovasc Surg. 2008;135:487–91.
35. Hoylaerts M, Lijnen HR, Collen D. Studies on the mechanism of the antifibrinolytic action of tranexamic acid. Biochim Biophys Acta Gen Subj. 1981;673:75–85.
36. McCormack PL. Tranexamic acid: a review of its use in the treatment of hyperfibrinolysis. Drugs. 2012;72:585–617.
37. Nilsson IM. Clinical pharmacology of aminocaproic and tranexamic acids. J Clin Pathol. 1980;33:41–7.
38. Eriksson O, Kjellman H, Pilbrant Å, Schannong M. Pharmacokinetics of tranexamic acid after intravenous administration to normal volunteers. Eur J Clin Pharmacol. 1974;7:375–80.
39. Andersson L, Nilsoon IM, Colleen S, Granstrand JB, Melander B. Role of urokinase and tissue activator in sustaining bleeding and the management thereof with EACA and AMCA. Ann N Y Acad Sci. 1968;146:642–56.
40. Gilad O, Merlob P, Stahl B, Klinger G. Outcome following tranexamic acid exposure during breastfeeding. Breastfeed Med. 2014;9:407–10.
41. CRASH-2 trial collaborators, Shakur H, Roberts I, Bautista R, Caballero J, Coats T, et al. Effects of tranexamic acid on death, vascular occlusive events, and blood transfusion in trauma patients with significant haemorrhage (CRASH-2): a randomised, placebo-controlled trial. Lancet. 2010;376:23–32.
42. Beno S, Ackery AD, Callum J, Rizoli S. Tranexamic acid in pediatric trauma: why not? Crit Care. 2014;18:313.

43. Drug Approval Package: Lysteda (tranexamic acid) NDA #022430 [Internet]. [cited 2019 Jul 7]. Available from: https://www.accessdata.fda.gov/drugsatfda_docs/nda/2009/022430_lysteda_toc.cfm
44. Preston JT, Cameron IT, Adams EJ, Smith SK. Comparative study of tranexamic acid and norethisterone in the treatment of ovulatory menorrhagia. Br J Obstet Gynaecol. 1995;102:401–6.
45. Amicar (Aminocaproic Acid): side effects, interactions, warning, dosage & uses [Internet]. RxList. [cited 2019 Jul 9]. Available from: https://www.rxlist.com/amicar-drug.htm.
46. Gerstein NS, Brierley JK, Windsor J, Panikkath PV, Ram H, Gelfenbeyn KM, et al. Antifibrinolytic agents in cardiac and noncardiac surgery: a comprehensive overview and update. J Cardiothorac Vasc Anesth. 2017;31:2183–205.
47. Nilsson IM, Andersson L, Björkman SE. Epsilon-aminocaproic acid (E-ACA) as a therapeutic agent based on 5 year's clinical experience. Acta Med Scand Suppl. 1966;448:1–46.
48. Nilsson IM, Sjoerdsma A, Waldenstrom J. Antifibrinolytic activity and metabolism of 6-aminocaproic acid in man. Lancet. 1960;1:1322–6.
49. Mcnicol GP, Douglas AS. Epsilon-aminocaproic acid and other inhibitors of fibrinolysis. Br Med Bull. 1964;20:233–9.
50. Fish SS, Pancorbo S, Berkseth R. Pharmacokinetics of epsilon-aminocaproic acid during peritoneal dialysis. J Neurosurg. 1981;54:736–9.
51. Sucher MG, Giordani M, Figoni A, Nedopil AJ. Peri-operative blood loss after total hip arthroplasty can be significantly reduced with topical application of epsilon-aminocaproic acid. Int Orthop. 2016;40:2019–23.
52. Gurian DB, Meneghini A, de Abreu LC, Murad N, de Matos LL, Pires AC, et al. A randomized trial of the topical effect of antifibrinolytic epsilon aminocaproic acid on coronary artery bypass surgery without cardiopulmonary bypass. Clin Appl Thromb Hemost. 2014;20:615–20.
53. Koster A, Faraoni D, Levy JH. Antifibrinolytic therapy for cardiac surgery: an update. Anesthesiology. 2015;123:214–21.
54. Fergusson DA, Hébert PC, Mazer CD, Fremes S, MacAdams C, Murkin JM, et al. A comparison of aprotinin and lysine analogues in high-risk cardiac surgery. N Engl J Med. 2008;358:2319–31.
55. McMullan V, Alston RP. Aprotinin and cardiac surgery: a sorry tale of evidence misused. Br J Anaesth. 2013;110(5):675–8.
56. Ferraris VA, Brown JR, Despotis GJ, Hammon JW, Reece TB, Saha SP, et al. 2011 update to the Society of Thoracic Surgeons and the Society of Cardiovascular Anesthesiologists blood conservation clinical practice guidelines. Ann Thorac Surg. 2011;91:944–82.
57. Horrow JC, Van Riper DF, Strong MD, Grunewald KE, Parmet JL. The dose-response relationship of tranexamic acid. Anesthesiology. 1995;82:383–92.
58. Fiechtner BK, Nuttall GA, Johnson ME, Dong Y, Sujirattanawimol N, Oliver WC, et al. Plasma tranexamic acid concentrations during cardiopulmonary bypass. Anesth Analg. 2001;92:1131–6.
59. Dowd NP, Karski JM, Cheng DC, Carroll JA, Lin Y, James RL, et al. Pharmacokinetics of tranexamic acid during cardiopulmonary bypass. Anesthesiology. 2002;97:390–9.
60. Sharma V, Fan J, Jerath A, Pang KS, Bojko B, Pawliszyn J, et al. Pharmacokinetics of tranexamic acid in patients undergoing cardiac surgery with use of cardiopulmonary bypass*: Pharmacokinetics of tranexamic acid in cardiac surgery. Anaesthesia. 2012;67:1242–50.
61. Murkin JM, Falter F, Granton J, Young B, Burt C, Chu M. High-dose tranexamic acid is associated with nonischemic clinical seizures in cardiac surgical patients. Anesth Analg. 2010;110:350–3.
62. Menkis AH, Martin J, Cheng DCH, Fitzgerald DC, Freedman JJ, Gao C, et al. Drug, devices, technologies, and techniques for blood management in minimally invasive and conventional cardiothoracic surgery a consensus statement from the International Society for Minimally Invasive Cardiothoracic Surgery (ISMICS) 2011. Innovations. 2012;7:229–41.
63. Myles PS, Smith JA, Forbes A, Silbert B, Jayarajah M, Painter T, et al. Tranexamic acid in patients undergoing coronary-artery surgery. N Engl J Med. 2017;376:136–48.
64. Zhang Y, Bai Y, Chen M, Zhou Y, Yu X, Zhou H, et al. The safety and efficiency of intravenous administration of tranexamic acid in coronary artery bypass grafting (CABG): a meta-analysis of 28 randomized controlled trials. BMC Anesthesiol. 2019;19:104.
65. Lecker I, Wang D-S, Romaschin AD, Peterson M, Mazer CD, Orser BA. Tranexamic acid concentrations associated with human seizures inhibit glycine receptors. J Clin Invest. 2012;122:4654–66.
66. Gupta S, Bhiwal A, Sharma K. Tranexamic acid: beware of anaesthetic misadventures. J Obstet Anaesth Crit Care. 2018;8:1.
67. Hessel EA. What's new in cardiopulmonary bypass. J Cardiothorac Vasc Anesth. 2019;33:2296–326.
68. Sharma V, Katznelson R, Jerath A, Garrido-Olivares L, Carroll J, Rao V, et al. The association between tranexamic acid and convulsive seizures after cardiac surgery: a multivariate analysis in 11, 529 patients. Anaesthesia. 2014;69:124–30.
69. Couture P, Lebon J-S, Laliberté É, Desjardins G, Chamberland M-È, Ayoub C, et al. Low-dose versus high-dose tranexamic acid reduces the risk of nonischemic seizures after cardiac surgery with cardiopulmonary bypass. J Cardiothorac Vasc Anesth. 2017;31:1611–7.
70. Lin Z, Xiaoyi Z. Tranexamic acid-associated seizures: a meta-analysis. Seizure. 2016;36:70–3.
71. Takagi H, Ando T, Umemoto T, All-Literature Investigation of Cardiovascular Evidence (ALICE) group. Seizures associated with tranexamic acid for cardiac surgery: a meta-analysis of randomized and non-randomized studies. J Cardiovasc Surg (Torino). 2017;58:633–41.
72. Koster A, Levy JH. Understanding potential drug side effects: can we translate molecular mechanisms to clinical applications? Anesthesiology. 2017;127:6–8.
73. Maeda T, Sasabuchi Y, Matsui H, Ohnishi Y, Miyata S, Yasunaga H. Safety of tranexamic acid in pediatric cardiac surgery: a Nationwide Database Study. J Cardiothorac Vasc Anesth. 2017;31:549–53.
74. Ker K, Kiriya J, Perel P, Edwards P, Shakur H, Roberts I. Avoidable mortality from giving tranexamic acid to bleeding trauma patients: an estimation based on WHO mortality data, a systematic literature review and data from the CRASH-2 trial. BMC Emerg Med. 2012;12:3.
75. Morrison JJ. Military Application of Tranexamic Acid in Trauma Emergency Resuscitation (MATTERs) Study. Arch Surg. 2012;147:113.
76. Ramirez RJ, Spinella PC, Bochicchio GV. Tranexamic acid update in trauma. Crit Care Clin. 2017;33:85–99.
77. Pre-hospital anti-fibrinolytics for traumatic coagulopathy and haemorrhage (The PATCH Study) - Full Text View - ClinicalTrials.gov [Internet]. [cited 2019 Jul 16]. Available from: https://clinicaltrials.gov/ct2/show/NCT02187120.
78. Brohi K, Singh J, Heron M, Coats T. Acute traumatic coagulopathy. J Trauma. 2003;54:1127–30.
79. Ostrowski SR, Henriksen HH, Stensballe J, Gybel-Brask M, Cardenas JC, Baer LA, et al. Sympathoadrenal activation and endotheliopathy are drivers of hypocoagulability and hyperfibrinolysis in trauma: a prospective observational study of 404 severely injured patients. J Trauma Acute Care Surg. 2017;82:293–301.
80. Davenport RA, Brohi K. Cause of trauma-induced coagulopathy. Curr Opin Anaesthesiol. 2016;29:212–9.
81. Moore HB, Moore EE, Liras IN, Gonzalez E, Harvin JA, Holcomb JB, et al. Acute fibrinolysis shutdown after injury occurs fre-

quently and increases mortality: a multicenter evaluation of 2,540 severely injured patients. J Am Coll Surg. 2016;222:347–55.

82. Moore EE, Moore HB, Gonzalez E, Sauaia A, Banerjee A, Silliman CC. Rationale for the selective administration of tranexamic acid to inhibit fibrinolysis in the severely injured patient: rationale for the selective administration of TXA. Transfusion. 2016;56:S110–4.
83. Yuan Q, Sun Y-R, Wu X, Yu J, Li Z-Q, Du Z-Y, et al. Coagulopathy in traumatic brain injury and its correlation with progressive hemorrhagic injury: a systematic review and meta-analysis. J Neurotrauma. 2016;33:1279–91.
84. Gall LS, Davenport RA. Fibrinolysis and antifibrinolytic treatment in the trauma patient. Curr Opin Anaesthesiol. 2018;31:227–33.
85. Dewan Y, Komolafe EO, Mejía-Mantilla JH, Perel P, Roberts I, Shakur H, et al. CRASH-3 - tranexamic acid for the treatment of significant traumatic brain injury: study protocol for an international randomized, double-blind, placebo-controlled trial. Trials. 2012;13:87.
86. Alshryda S, Sarda P, Sukeik M, Nargol A, Blenkinsopp J, Mason JM. Tranexamic acid in total knee replacement: a systematic review and meta-analysis. J Bone Joint Surg Br. 2011;93:1577–85.
87. Gombotz H, Rehak PH, Shander A, Hofmann A. The second Austrian benchmark study for blood use in elective surgery: results and practice change. Transfusion. 2014;54:2646–57.
88. Wei Z, Liu M. The effectiveness and safety of tranexamic acid in total hip or knee arthroplasty: a meta-analysis of 2720 cases: the effectiveness and safety of tranexamic acid in total hip or knee arthroplasty. Transfus Med. 2015;25:151–62.
89. Yu X, Li W, Xu P, Liu J, Qiu Y, Zhu Y. Safety and efficacy of tranexamic acid in total knee arthroplasty. Med Sci Monit. 2015;21:3095–103.
90. Farrow LS, Smith TO, Ashcroft GP, Myint PK. A systematic review of tranexamic acid in hip fracture surgery: tranexamic acid in hip fracture surgery. Br J Clin Pharmacol. 2016;82:1458–70.
91. Xu S, Chen JY, Zheng Q, Lo NN, Chia S-L, Tay KJD, et al. The safest and most efficacious route of tranexamic acid administration in total joint arthroplasty: a systematic review and network meta-analysis. Thromb Res. 2019;176:61–6.
92. Cheriyan T, Maier SP, Bianco K, Slobodyanyuk K, Rattenni RN, Lafage V, et al. Efficacy of tranexamic acid on surgical bleeding in spine surgery: a meta-analysis. Spine J. 2015;15:752–61.
93. Zhang Y, Liu H, He F, Chen A, Yang H, Pi B. Does tranexamic acid improve bleeding, transfusion, and hemoglobin level in patients undergoing multilevel spine surgery? a systematic review and meta-analysis. World Neurosurg. 2019;127:289–301.
94. Karanicolas PJ, Lin Y, Tarshis J, Law CHL, Coburn NG, Hallet J, et al. Major liver resection, systemic fibrinolytic activity, and the impact of tranexamic acid. HPB. 2016;18:991–9.
95. Roullet S, Pillot J, Freyburger G, Biais M, Quinart A, Rault A, et al. Rotation thromboelastometry detects thrombocytopenia and hypofibrinogenaemia during orthotopic liver transplantation. Br J Anaesth. 2010;104:422–8.
96. Badenoch A, Sharma A, Gower S, Selzner M, Srinivas C, Wąsowicz M, et al. The effectiveness and safety of tranexamic acid in orthotopic liver transplantation clinical practice: a propensity score-matched cohort study. Transplantation. 2017;101:1658–65.
97. Wu C-C, Ho W-M, Cheng S-B, Yeh D-C, Wen M-C, Liu T-J, et al. Perioperative parenteral tranexamic acid in liver tumor resection: a prospective randomized trial toward a "blood transfusion"-free hepatectomy. Ann Surg. 2006;243:173–80.
98. World Health Organization. WHO recommendations for the prevention and treatment of postpartum haemorrhage. Geneva: World Health Organization; 2012.
99. Ker K, Shakur H, Roberts I. Does tranexamic acid prevent postpartum haemorrhage? A systematic review of randomised controlled trials. BJOG. 2016;123:1745–52.
100. Shakur H, Roberts I, Fawole B, Chaudhri R, El-Sheikh M, Akintan A, et al. Effect of early tranexamic acid administration on mortality, hysterectomy, and other morbidities in women with postpartum haemorrhage (WOMAN): an international, randomised, double-blind, placebo-controlled trial. Lancet. 2017;389:2105–16.
101. Fleming JB, Hoh BL, Simon SD, Welch BG, Mericle RA, Fargen KM, et al. Rebleeding risk after treatment of ruptured intracranial aneurysms. J Neurosurg. 2011;114:1778–84.
102. Roos Y, Rinkel G, Vermeulen M, Algra A, van Gijn J. Antifibrinolytic therapy for aneurysmal subarachnoid hemorrhage: a major update of a cochrane review. Stroke. 2003;34:2308–9.
103. Baharoglu MI, Germans MR, Rinkel GJ, Algra A, Vermeulen M, van Gijn J, et al. Antifibrinolytic therapy for aneurysmal subarachnoid haemorrhage. Cochrane Stroke Group, editor. Cochrane Database Syst Rev [Internet]. 2013 [cited 2019 Jul 27]; Available from: http://doi.wiley.com/10.1002/14651858.CD001245.pub2.
104. Anker-Møller T, Troldborg A, Sunde N, Hvas A-M. Evidence for the use of tranexamic acid in subarachnoid and subdural hemorrhage: a systematic review. Semin Thromb Hemost. 2017;43:750–8.
105. Germans MR, Post R, Coert BA, Rinkel GJE, Vandertop WP, Verbaan D. Ultra-early tranexamic acid after subarachnoid hemorrhage (ULTRA): study protocol for a randomized controlled trial. Trials. 2013;14:143.
106. Goobie SM, Faraoni D. Tranexamic acid and perioperative bleeding in children: what do we still need to know? Curr Opin Anaesthesiol. 2019;32:343–52.
107. Montroy J, Hutton B, Moodley P, Fergusson NA, Cheng W, Tinmouth A, et al. The efficacy and safety of topical tranexamic acid: a systematic review and meta-analysis. Transfus Med Rev. 2018;32:165–78.
108. Ker K, Beecher D, Roberts I. Topical application of tranexamic acid for the reduction of bleeding. Cochrane Database Syst Rev. 2013;(7):CD010562.

Hypercoagulation and Thrombotic Disorders

6

Saurin J. Shah, Jayanth Dasika, and David C. McEnerney

Introduction

Hypercoagulable states, sometimes referred to as thrombophilias or thrombotic disorders, are clinical conditions whereby individuals are predisposed to arterial and/or venous thromboembolisms [1]. Clinical manifestations of thrombotic disorders can range from the asymptomatic to lethal; the causes of these manifestations may be complicated and multifactorial. Research over the last several decades has aided in identifying many of the risk factors associated with hypercoagulable states and has helped streamline chronic management of predisposed individuals. Acute management of these individuals, such as during surgery, poses a unique set of challenges for the anesthesia care team.

Individuals with hypercoagulable states are considered high risk for thromboembolic phenomenon in the perioperative setting [2]. The occurrence of venous thromboembolism (VTE) in the non-surgical population is 1–2 out of 1000; this frequency increases anywhere from 10 to 25 out of 1000 depending on the surgical procedure [3]. In addition, the administration of blood products, which may occur more frequently during surgery, may increase VTE occurrence two fold to threefold when compared to bloodless surgery [4]. Special consideration and management need to be given to surgical patients that may receive blood products in the setting of preexisting risk factor(s) for thrombotic disease.

Hypercoagulable States

Hypercoagulable states have been described since 1856 when Rudolph Virchow described a triad of conditions that promoted coagulation in the circulatory system [1]. The majority of these states can be classified into two groups: primary (congenital) and secondary (acquired); there are some conditions of mixed etiology that may fall into both categories or are of unknown etiology.

Primary (Congenital) Hypercoagulable States

Primary hypercoagulable states are due to either (1) a defect/deficiency of an antithrombotic protein or (2) an abnormally increased level of a prothrombotic clotting factor. The most common conditions are listed in Table 6.1.

Antithrombin Deficiency

Antithrombin is a natural anticoagulant that inhibits thrombin (factor IIa), factor Xa, and other serine proteases in the coagulation cascade. Inherited antithrombin deficiency is estimated to occur in 1 in 2000–3000 individuals. It is an autosomal dominant disease with variable penetrance; laboratory evidence does not necessarily lead to the development of VTE or require maintenance anticoagulant therapy. Type I Deficiency is the most severe and usually is the result of a quantitative deficit of Antithrombin; Type IIb deficiency is less severe and usually the result of a qualitative defect

Table 6.1 Primary hypercoagulable states (thrombophilias)

1. Decreased antithrombotic proteins
(a) Antithrombin deficiency
(b) Protein C deficiency
(c) Protein S deficiency
2. Increased prothrombotic proteins
(a) Factor V Leiden (activated protein C resistance)
(b) Prothrombin gene mutation G20210A
(c) Increased levels of factors VII, XI, IX, VIII, von Willebrand factor

S. J. Shah (✉) · J. Dasika · D. C. McEnerney
University of Florida – Jacksonville, Department of Anesthesiology, Jacksonville, FL, USA
e-mail: saurin.shah@jax.ufl.edu

© Springer Nature Switzerland AG 2021
C. S. Scher et al. (eds.), *Essentials of Blood Product Management in Anesthesia Practice*,
https://doi.org/10.1007/978-3-030-59295-0_6

within the structure of the Antithrombin protein. Other disease states may indirectly lower the concentration of antithrombin; however, this is usually associated with abnormalities in other factors, thus making it more difficult to evaluate and manage these acquired deficiencies [1, 5].

Perioperative management of these patients can vary based on the complexity of the procedure, anticipated blood loss, and preexisting comorbid situations. As noted, the risk of deep vein thrombosis (DVT) can be as high as 3% in the general surgical population; the risk may be higher in patients predisposed to VTE secondary to a thrombophilia such as Antithrombin Deficiency. Preoperative and postoperative prophylaxis with unfractionated (UFH) or low-molecular-weight heparin (LMWH) or Antithrombin concentrates may be absolutely indicated in this patient population except in trauma or non-trauma cases with significant anticipated blood loss – although the exclusion in the latter group is still under debate. Intraoperative management is usually routine and uneventful except in the setting of blood transfusions, most notably red blood cell (RBC) transfusions. Blood transfusions may impair the balance between coagulation factors and the inflammatory cascade triggering a hypercoagulable state. While the exact mechanisms are unknown, it is clear that there is a dose response effect between the number of RBCs transfused and the risk of a VTE [6]. In the setting of a known thrombophilia, such as Antithrombin Deficiency, this can be problematic and potentially lethal. Consideration should be given to blood sparing techniques when possible as blood transfusions are not without risks. In patients that require blood transfusions, the use of Antithrombin concentrates may be given to minimize the risk of a VTE.

Protein C and S Deficiency

Protein C deficiency causes impaired deactivation of Factors V_a and VIII_a, leading to increased production of thrombin and fibrin. Inherited deficiency is estimated at about 1 per 200–500 in the general population and up to 15–30 per same number in patients with VTE. It is an autosomal dominant disease with variable penetrance and, like Antithrombin, may be divided into two general forms. Type I deficiency is characterized by a quantitative reduction in Protein C with a proportionate reduction in functional activity; type II deficiencies are due to a qualitative abnormality in Protein C with a variable reduction in functional activity. Protein C deficiency may also be acquired in certain disease states such as liver disease, disseminated intravascular coagulation (DIC), and sepsis [1, 5].

Protein S deficiency causes decreased activity of activated Protein C, thus leading to increased production of thrombin and fibrin. Protein S and protein C work in concert as a natural anticoagulant system; Protein S serves as the binding protein for activated Protein C to form an anticoagulant complex on cell surfaces. Congenital Protein S deficiency (mild) is estimated to occur in 1 per 500 individuals; severe deficiency is rare, prevalence is unknown, and is associated with a myriad of life-threatening symptoms from birth. It is an autosomal dominant disease caused by a mutation in the PROS1 gene. It has variable penetrance and may be divided into type I-III based on how the PROS1 gene mutation affects Protein S. Type I disease is characterized by a quantitative defect in both total and free Protein S, whereas type II is characterized by a qualitative defect with normal levels; type III has normal total levels, but low free protein levels. Types I and III are the most common and have similar symptomology. Acquired Protein S deficiency can occur to a lesser extent with liver disease, vitamin K deficiency, and pregnancy [1, 5, 7].

Perioperative management of these patients is based on the severity of the disease, complexity of the procedure, and comorbid diseases. The occurrence of VTE in protein C- and/or S-deficient patients is considered to be less than that of patients with Antithrombin Deficiency; however, the combination of surgery and a preexisting protein C and/or S deficiency is believed to increase one's risks of perioperative VTE above the 3% occurrence rate of otherwise healthy surgical patients. The mainstay of preoperative treatment is UFH or LMWH to reduce this increased risk [7]. In patients at higher risk – decreased ambulation, other comorbid disease states, anticipated RBC transfusion – prophylactic administration of protein C concentrates and/or fresh-frozen plasma (no protein S concentrate exists) may be given to further reduce the risk of VTE [2].

Factor V Leiden (Activated Protein C Resistance)

Factor V is a protein of the coagulation system that once activated works in conjunction with activated Factor X to convert prothrombin to thrombin. Factor V Leiden (FVL) is caused by a point mutation in the gene that renders the protein resistant to activated Protein C resulting in decreased breakdown of thrombin and an increased risk of VTE [1].

Heterozygous FVL is very common in individuals of Caucasian descent. It is present in about 5% of healthy individuals and up to 40–50% in individuals presenting with or for evaluation of VTE. The homozygous form is rare, but carries a 10-fold increase in the risk of thrombosis. Most FVL patients are asymptomatic and usually require another "hit" or predisposing factor to present with a VTE [5].

Surgery and/or blood transfusions may be the other "hit" to increase the occurrence of VTE. Standard perioperative VTE prophylaxis should be followed in these patients;

special considerations should be given to those patients with a previous history of VTE. No specific guidelines or recommendations currently exist for blood transfusions in the setting of FVL. As noted, most patients are asymptomatic even in the setting of blood product administration. In fact, current studies suggest a beneficial link between FVL and reduced blood loss in cardiovascular surgery. Those same studies have raised concerns about antifibrinolytic therapy and the increased potential for thrombosis in FVL patients.

FVL may also occur in pregnancy. Whether as a primary or secondary (acquired) condition, FVL is found in 20–45% of women with pregnancy-associated VTE. Homozygous patients carry the highest risk of VTE during pregnancy when compared to heterozygous patients; the risk of thrombosis during pregnancy is almost 50% greater in FVL patients as compared to non-FVL patients [1]. Prophylactic anticoagulation is usually not recommended in patients with no previous history of VTE; anticoagulation is recommended in the setting of pregnancy, FVL, and previous VTE [3]. All patients should be counseled about the risks and benefits of these therapies during pregnancy. Additionally, high-risk patients should consider a 4- to 6- week course of anticoagulation during the postpartum period. No current recommendations exist for FVL, pregnancy, and blood product administration.

Table 6.2 Relative risk – first episode of VTE – Inherited States

Risk factor	Relative risk
Factor V Leiden	
Homozygous	25
Heterozygous	5
Antithrombin deficiency	5
Protein C deficiency	3
Protein S deficiency	2
Hyperhomocysteinemia	2

Table 6.3 Secondary hypercoagulable states (thrombophilias)

1. **Deficiency of coagulation inhibitors**
(a) Malignancy
(b) Surgery
(c) Immobilization
2. **Increased prothrombotic proteins**
(a) Trauma
(b) Pregnancy
(c) Medications (OCP/HRT)
(d) Antiphospholipid Syndrome

Hyperhomocysteinemia

Homocysteine is an intermediary amino acid formed by the metabolism of methionine. Congenital alterations in this pathway, as well as acquired deficiencies in various vitamins and certain disease states, can produce elevated levels of homocysteine in the blood. Hyperhomocysteinemia may predispose individuals to arterial and venous thrombosis [5].

The incidence of hyperhomocysteinemia has been reported to be as high as 10%; however, the cause is multifactorial and varies greatly across different ethnicities and geographic regions. Homocysteinemia is suspected to cause endothelial dysfunction and promote an imbalance between procoagulant and antithrombotic activity; decreases in protein C activation, endothelial resistance to thrombosis, and nitric oxide may play a key role in this thrombotic disorder [8].

Perioperative management usually consists of standard DVT prophylaxis – LMWH and placement of pneumatic lower extremity compression devices. In the patient with elevated homocysteine levels, administration of pyridoxine, methylcobalamin, and folic acid may help to reduce homocysteine levels and the risk of a thrombotic event. Maintenance of euvolemia and avoidance of nitrous oxide are also recommended for these patients. As noted, blood product administration carries its own risk of thrombosis; any treatment that lowers homocysteine levels should be considered for procedures where blood product administration is anticipated.

Other Primary Hypercoagulable States

A number of other congenital thrombophilia exists such as Prothrombin Gene Variant, increased levels of specific coagulation factors (VII, XI, IX, and vWF) and tissue plasminogen activator deficiency [7]. Many of these other hypercoagulable states have a much lower occurrence rate (<2–3% incidence across all populations). Thus, studies and recommendations are limited regarding management of these disease states during surgery and in the setting of blood product administration. As always, treatment should be patient specific (Table 6.2).

Secondary (Acquired) Hypercoagulable States

Secondary hypercoagulable states encompass a variety of conditions that may predispose individuals to thrombotic events. The pathophysiology of these states is usually complex, multifactorial, and poorly understood. Most individuals with acquired hypercoagulable states are at risk for both arterial and venous thrombosis due to suspected abnormalities in all parts of Virchow's triad of thrombogenesis (Table 6.3).

Pregnancy/Puerperium

Pregnancy and puerperium are well-recognized and well-studied hypercoagulable states. The risk of VTE during pregnancy/puerperium is six to eight times greater than in non-pregnant women; however, VTEs are still only seen in approximately 1% of pregnancies [1, 5]. The increased risk is present for 8–10 weeks postpartum and can present with life-threatening symptoms to both the mother and fetus [9].

The pathophysiology of hypercoagulability during pregnancy and the postpartum period involves a number of anatomical, physiological, and biochemical changes that may predispose an individual to thrombotic events. There is an increased concentration of various factors within the coagulation cascade, increased platelet count, and decreased fibrinolysis [10, 11]. This imbalance within the coagulation cascade coupled with stasis from a gravid uterus on lower extremity venous return increases one's thrombogenic potential [12–14].

Concomitant genetic risk (primary), older age, previous VTE, higher parity, and preeclampsia are independent risk factors that may further increase one's predisposition for a thrombotic event [1, 5, 15].

Diagnosis and management of VTEs in pregnancy can be challenging. Overlapping signs and symptoms as well as limited radiologic and laboratory testing can complicate timely diagnosis of a VTE. Previous history or high suspicion of current VTE is to be treated with anticoagulation for up to 8 weeks postpartum [16, 17]. LMWH or UFH are the mainstays of therapy as they do not cross the uteroplacental barrier and allow for timely discontinuation for neuraxial anesthesia administration [18]. Warfarin is reserved for high-risk cases due to its teratogenic effects and potential for fetal bleeding. Blood product administration should be judicious with reasonably high transfusion triggers, reserving administration for the most high-risk patients (placenta accreta, severe anemia, DIC, etc.) [19–21].

Oral Contraceptives and Hormone Replacement Therapy

The administration of estrogen is associated with a two fold to six fold increase in the incidence of VTE in individuals with no other predisposing thrombotic factors [22–24]. Use of oral contraceptive pills (OCP)/hormone replacement therapy (HRT) is associated with increased levels of Factor VII and decreased activity of protein S and thrombomodulin [25]. Smoking, obesity, Polycystic Ovary Syndrome, older age, and immobilization, as well as a primary hypercoagulable disease, may significantly increase the risk of VTE in the setting of OCP/HRT [26].

Table 6.4 Relative risk – first episode of VTE – acquired states

Risk factor	Relative risk
Pregnancy	4
Recent postpartum	14
OCP/HRT	3
Antiphospholipid antibody	9
Immobilization	10
Surgery	6

Data from Liem and Deloughery, Seminars in Vasc Surg 2008

Individuals who are considered high risk for VTE or have previously had a VTE should be candidates for anticoagulation while on OCP/HRT [27, 28]. Prophylaxis with either LMWH or UFH is recommended and the mainstay of treatment. Blood product administration should be clinically indicated with reasonable triggers as no additional therapies exist to reduce the incidence of VTE from blood transfusions in the setting of OCP/HRT (Table 6.4).

Antiphospholipid Syndrome

Antiphospholipid Syndrome (APS) is a thrombotic disorder mainly associated with auto antibodies toward plasma proteins on the surface of phospholipids [5, 29]. Two main subsets of auto antibodies exist in APS – anticardiolipin and lupus anticoagulant associated with lupus erythematosus [7, 30]. There are secondary states that may be acquired in the setting of infections, drugs, or collagen vascular diseases. Regardless of the etiology, venous or arterial thromboembolic phenomenon may occur in up to one-third of individuals with APS [31].

Thrombosis often occurs at unusual sites and may present with a myriad of symptoms such as skin necrosis – livedo reticularis, acute renal failure, cerebrovascular pathology (strokes, ocular disturbances, etc.), or recurrent miscarriages [32]. APS is the most common cause of initial thrombosis in pregnancy when compared to other thrombophilias. Currently, no recommendations exist for anticoagulation in APS individuals with no history of thromboembolic phenomenon [33]. Individuals with other risk factors or previous VTE should be placed on long-term anticoagulation therapy; patients with "high" APS antibody titers should also consider long-term therapy even in the absence of VTE [34, 35]. The mainstay of long-term therapy is warfarin with goal INRs of 2–3; LMWH may be used in patients with allergies to warfarin [32, 36].

No current recommendations exist for blood product administration either. Individuals with APS may have a concomitant quantitative thrombocytopenia. Blood product administration should be based on reasonable transfusion triggers and the needs of the individuals.

Other Secondary Hypercoagulable States

Thromboembolic phenomenon may occur in individuals with gastrointestinal disorders such as inflammatory bowel disease and Behcet's disease. Intestinal inflammation, which may occur cyclically in these disease states, may activate the coagulation system and increase the risk of thrombosis [5].

Nephrotic Syndrome may lead to an acquired Antithrombin III deficiency through the excess excretion of protein. Myeloproliferative disorders can create a myriad of acquired thrombotic disorders [37, 38].

Hemolytic diseases or diseases with abnormal RBCs, such as sickle cell disease, may lead to alterations in the surface of RBCs that promote increased thrombin formation.

Summary

Hypercoagulable states, or thrombophilias, are disease states that predispose individuals to thrombotic phenomenon; these disease states are either congenital or acquired and may present with no symptoms or be life-threatening. The occurrence of thromboembolic events is usually complex and multifactorial; laboratory testing and treatment will vary based on the severity of the disease and concomitant co morbidities. The administration of blood products increases the incidence of thrombotic events. While specific recommendations do not exist for blood transfusions in many of these disease states, caution and judicious practices should be used to minimize any risks for VTE in predisposed individuals.

References

1. Kojima T, Saito H. Hypercoagulable states. In: Tanaka K, Davie EW, Ikeda Y, Iwanaga S, Saito H, Sueishi K, editors. Recent advances in thrombosis and hemostasis 2008. Tokyo: Springer; 2008.
2. Martlew VJ. Peri-operative management of patients with coagulation disorders. Br J Anaesth. 2000;85(3):446–55.
3. Schafer A, Levine MN, Konkle BA, Kearon C. Thrombotic disorders: diagnosis and treatment. Am Soc Hematol Educ Prog. 2003:520–39.
4. Lin SY, Chang YL, Yeh HC, Lin CL, Kao CH. Blood transfusion and risk of venous thromboembolism: a population-based cohort study. Thromb Haemost. 2020;120(1):156–67.
5. Schafer AI. Hypercoagulable state: cardiovascular medicine. London: Springer; 2007.
6. Goel R, Patel EU, Cushing MM, et al. Association of perioperative red blood cell transfusions with venous thromboembolism in a north American registry. JAMA Surg. 2018;153(9):826–33. https://doi.org/10.1001/jamasurg.2018.1565.
7. Thomas RH. Hypercoagulability syndromes. Arch Intern Med. 2001;161(20):2433–9.
8. Aggarwal S, Verma S, Singh B, Kumar M. Hyperhomocysteinemia: anesthetic concerns. Saudi J Anaesth. 2014;8(1):143–4.
9. Greer IA. Thrombosis in pregnancy: maternal and fetal issues. Lancet. 1999;353:1258–65.
10. Bremme KA. Haemostatic changes in pregnancy. Best Pract Res Clin Haematol. 2003;16:153.
11. Cerneca F, Ricci G, Simeone R, et al. Coagulation and fibrinolysis changes in normal pregnancy. Increased levels of procoagulants and reduced levels of inhibitors during pregnancy induce a hypercoagulable state, combined with a reactive fibrinolysis. Eur J Obstet Gynecol Reprod Biol. 1997;73:31.
12. Chan WS, Spencer FA, Ginsberg JS. Anatomic distribution of deep vein thrombosis in pregnancy. CMAJ. 2010;182:657.
13. Heit JA, Kobbervig CE, James AH, et al. Trends in the incidence of venous thromboembolism during pregnancy or postpartum: a 30-year population-based study. Ann Intern Med. 2005;143:697.
14. Polak JF, Wilkinson DL. Ultrasonographic diagnosis of symptomatic deep venous thrombosis in pregnancy. Am J Obstet Gynecol. 1991;165:625.
15. Egan K, Kevane B, Ní Áinle F. Elevated venous thromboembolism risk in preeclampsia: molecular mechanisms and clinical impact. Biochem Soc Trans. 2015;43(4):696–701.
16. Bates SM, Greer IA, Middeldorp S, et al. VTE, thrombophilia, antithrombotic therapy, and pregnancy: antithrombotic therapy and prevention of thrombosis, 9th ed: American College of Chest Physicians Evidence-Based Clinical Practice Guidelines. Chest. 2012;141:691.
17. Greer IA, Nelson-Piercy C. Low-molecular-weight heparins for thromboprophylaxis and treatment of venous thromboembolism in pregnancy: a systematic review of safety and efficacy. Blood. 2005;106:401.
18. Forestier F, Daffos F, Capella-Pavlovsky M. Low molecular weight heparin (PK 10169) does not cross the placenta during the second trimester of pregnancy study by direct fetal blood sampling under ultrasound. Thromb Res. 1984;34:557.
19. Kline JA, Williams GW, Hernandez-Nino J. D-dimer concentrations in normal pregnancy: new diagnostic thresholds are needed. Clin Chem. 2005;51:825.
20. Sood SL, James AH, Ragni MV, et al. A prospective study of von Willebrand factor levels and bleeding in pregnant women with type 1 von Willebrand disease. Haemophilia. 2016;22:e562.
21. Simpson EL, Lawrenson RA, Nightingale AL, Farmer RD. Venous thromboembolism in pregnancy and the puerperium: incidence and additional risk factors from a London perinatal database. BJOG. 2001;108:56.
22. Stegeman BH, de Bastos M, Rosendaal FR, et al. Different combined oral contraceptives and the risk of venous thrombosis: systematic review and network meta-analysis. BMJ. 2013;347:f5298.
23. Gomes MPV, Deitcher SR. Risk of venous thromboembolic disease associated with hormonal contraceptives and hormone replacement therapy. Arch Intern Med. 2004;164:1965–76.
24. Heinemann LA, Dinger JC. Range of published estimates of venous thromboembolism incidence in young women. Contraception. 2007;75:328.
25. Rosendaal FR, Vessey M, Rumley A, et al. Hormonal replacement therapy, prothrombotic mutations and the risk of venous thrombosis. Br J Haematol. 2002;116:851.
26. Cushman M, Kuller LH, Prentice R, et al. Estrogen plus progestin and risk of venous thrombosis. JAMA. 2004;292:1573.
27. Marjoribanks J, Farquhar C, Roberts H, et al. Long-term hormone therapy for perimenopausal and postmenopausal women. Cochrane Database Syst Rev. 2017;1:CD004143.
28. Gris JC, Bouvier S, Molinari N, et al. Comparative incidence of a first thrombotic event in purely obstetric antiphospholipid syndrome with pregnancy loss: the NOH-APS observational study. Blood. 2012;119:2624.
29. Finazzi G, Brancaccio U, Moia M, et al. Natural history and risk factors for thrombosis in 360 patients with antiphospholipid anti-

bodies: a four year prospective study from the Italian registry. Am J Med. 1996;100:477–80.

30. Moll S, Ortel TL. Monitoring warfarin therapy in patients with lupus anticoagulants. Ann Intern Med. 1997;127:177.
31. Barbhaiya M, Erkan D. Primary thrombosis prophylaxis in antiphospholipid antibody-positive patients: where do we stand? Curr Rheumatol Rep. 2011;13:59.
32. Levine SR, Brey RL, Tilley BC, et al. Antiphospholipid antibodies and subsequent thrombo-occlusive events in patients with ischemic stroke. JAMA. 2004;291:576.
33. Erkan D, Cervera R, Asherson RA. Catastrophic antiphospholipid syndrome: where do we stand? Arthritis Rheum. 2003;48:3320–7.
34. Crowther MA, Ginsberg JS, Julian J, et al. A comparison of two intensities of warfarin for the prevention of recurrent thrombosis in patients with the antiphospholipid antibody syndrome. N Engl J Med. 2003;349:1133.
35. Kasthuri RS, Roubey RA. Warfarin and the antiphospholipid syndrome: does one size fit all? Arthritis Rheum. 2007;57:1346.
36. Dentali F, Manfredi E, Crowther M, Ageno W. Long-duration therapy with low molecular weight heparin in patients with antiphospholipid antibody syndrome resistant to warfarin therapy. J Thromb Haemost. 2005;3:2121.
37. van Genderen PJ, Mulder PG, Waleboer M, et al. Prevention and treatment of thrombotic complications in essential thrombocythaemia: efficacy and safety of aspirin. Br J Haematol. 1997;97:179.
38. Passamonti F, Malabarba L, Orlandi E, et al. Polycythemia vera in young patients: a study on the long-term risk of thrombosis, myelofibrosis and leukemia. Haematologica. 2003;88:13.

Diseases or Conditions of Platelet Disorders

7

George M. Jeha, Alex D. Pham, Ivan Urits, Lu Sun, Dallas L. Domangue, Karina Charipova, Kyle Gress, Elyse M. Cornett, and Alan David Kaye

Introduction

Platelets are small, anucleate cells circulating in the blood at concentrations of approximately 150,000–400,000/μL. They form from projections known as proplatelets off megakaryocytes in the bone marrow. Thrombopoietin is important in the process of megakaryopoiesis and stimulation of other stems cells in the bone marrow [1, 2]. The typical lifespan of a platelet is 10 days before they are removed from circulation by the spleen [3]. Platelets primarily function in hemostasis. Platelets contain alpha granules and dense granules, which play major roles in coagulation. The alpha granules contain larger proteins (e.g., von Willebrand factor) while the dense granules contain small non-protein particles (e.g., ADP) [3]. Platelets are involved in inflammation and atherosclerosis related to their production of inflammatory mediators (e.g., thromboxanes) and aid in cancer progression by impeding the immune system. They may even be involved in the progression of Alzheimer's dementia given their ability to carry amyloid precursor protein. Platelet dysfunction has been noted in various other systemic diseases such as diabetes mellitus, liver disease, and renal disease, which can all lead to plasma membrane alterations that affect their function [4].

There are various inherited and acquired disorders associated with platelets. Inherited platelet disorders are typically rare compared to the acquired platelet disorders (with the exception of inherited versus acquired vWF disease) [1]. The inherited platelet disorders have increased in prevalence in part due to routine blood counts but are still often misdiagnosed as an acquired platelet disorder or are simply not classified, making accurate measurements of prevalence difficult [2]. These disorders can cause alterations in platelet number (quantitative) or function (qualitative). The qualitative changes involve impairment in platelet adhesion, activation, secretion, or aggregation. The quantitative changes can predispose to thrombosis or bleeding depending on the presence of thrombocytosis or thrombocytopenia, respectively. The bleeding from platelet disorders usually involves mucocutaneous bleeding, epistaxis, petechiae, and postsurgical bleeding. This contrasts with the larger and deeper bleeds associated with hemophilia [1, 3]. Given that several genes involved with inherited platelet disorders (e.g., WAS, MYH-9, GP2B) are also utilized by other cell lines, multisystem disease is common with platelet disorders [2, 3].

Related to the systemic involvement of platelets in hemostasis and the effects of other diseases on them, platelet disorders are an important consideration for afflicted patients. Up to 25% of the population has thrombocytopenia, which can cause mild bleeding at platelet concentrations lower than 100,000/μL [1]. Screening tools in the form of questionnaires have been utilized to screen for platelet disorders without significant success, deferring to the patient's ability to recount a history of bleeding and multisystem involvement as the primary screening modality [1, 3]. When an inherited disorder is suspected, flow cytometry is commonly implemented, taking advantage of the fact that platelets do not contain DNA [4]. Various other tests are used to assess platelet function (e.g., Aggregation tests) [3]. Many different

G. M. Jeha · A. D. Pham · D. L. Domangue
Department of Anesthesiology, LSUHSC New Orleans, New Orleans, LA, USA

I. Urits
Beth Israel Deaconess Medical Center Harvard Medical School, Boston, MA, USA

L. Sun · E. M. Cornett (✉)
LSU Health Shreveport, Department of Anesthesiology, Shreveport, LA, USA
e-mail: ecorne@lsuhsc.edu

K. Charipova · K. Gress
Georgetown School of Medicine, Washington, DC, USA

A. D. Kaye
Departments of Anesthesiology and Pharmacology, Toxicology, and Neurosciences, Louisiana State University School of Medicine-Shreveport, Shreveport, LA, USA

LSU Health Shreveport School of Medicine, New Orleans, LA, USA

Tulane School of Medicine, New Orleans, LA, USA

© Springer Nature Switzerland AG 2021

A. D. Kaye, S. Leavitt (eds.), *Essentials of Blood Product Management in Anesthesia Practice*,
https://doi.org/10.1007/978-3-030-59295-0_7

drugs, foods, and supplements are known to affect platelet function (e.g., aspirin). Patients with platelet disorders must therefore be identified and educated on their bleeding risk and advised to avoid compounds which could increase their risk. The role of platelets should be carefully considered by the physician when evaluating patients. This chapter focuses on summarizing platelet disorders, as well as their diagnosis, management, and perioperative considerations, for the clinical anesthesiologist.

Types of Disorders

Platelets play an important role in hemostasis, initiation of blood coagulation, and wound healing [4–7]. Disorders of platelet function, whether inherited or acquired, can range in clinical expression from asymptomatic to mild bruising, mild mucocutaneous bleeding, and even acute life-threatening bleeding [7–9]. Patients with platelet counts less than 150×10^3 per μL 10 but greater than 50×10^3 per μL may be clinically asymptomatic. As platelet count continues to decline, patients may experience petechiae, purpura, and ecchymoses. Severely low platelet counts can lead to bleeding with minimal trauma and eventually spontaneous bleeding [9, 10].

Platelet disorders encompass a vast spectrum of disease, varying from syndromes with abnormally decreased platelet numbers (thrombocytopenia), abnormally increased platelet numbers (thrombocythemia or thrombocytosis), or abnormal platelet function [6].

Thrombocytopenia

Thrombocytopenia is a commonly encountered clinical entity with a multitude of potential etiologies, making diagnosis challenging [11–13]. Potential causes include decreased platelet production in the bone marrow, increased platelet destruction or consumption in the periphery, enhanced splenic sequestration, and hemodilution [14, 15].

Consumptive thrombocytopenic disorders involve increased consumption of platelets in the periphery, such as that which occurs in disseminated intravascular coagulation (DIC), septicemia, and thrombotic microangiopathies such as thrombotic thrombocytopenic purpura and hemolytic-uremic syndrome [15–17]. Platelet destruction often refers to the clearance of platelets via platelet-reactive antibodies, alloantibodies, or drug-dependent antibodies [15, 18, 19].

Several medications have the potential to lead to thrombocytopenia by either inducing destruction of platelets via antibody-mediated processes or inhibiting production of platelets in the bone marrow. Drugs with known potential for causing drug-induced thrombocytopenia include beta-lactam antibiotics such as penicillins and cephalosporins, vancomycin, phenytoin, piperacillin, trimethoprim-sulfamethoxazole, sulfonamides, rifampin, quinine, quinidine, carbamazepine, abciximab, eptifibatide, and tirofiban; drugs with the potential for dose-dependent bone marrow suppression include valproic acid, linezolid, daptomycin, and gold compounds [20–29].

Heparin-induced thrombocytopenia (HIT) is a life-threatening condition related to heparin exposure caused by antibodies recognizing complexes of platelet factor 4 and heparin. These antibodies also activate platelets and lead to arterial and venous thrombosis which can be fatal in up to 20% of untreated cases [30, 31].

Acquired causes of decreased bone marrow platelet production include malignancies, chemical agents, or infectious agents [14]. Thrombocytopenia is a common finding in patients with solid tumors and may be related to several factors such as tumor infiltration of the bone marrow and spleen, chronic DIC, microangiopathy, alterations in cytokine profiles, and the use of chemotherapeutic agents [32, 33]. In patients with leukemias, impaired hematopoiesis, abnormalities in hematopoietic cell morphology, and infiltration of bone marrow can lead to thrombocytopenia [34]. Chronic myeloid leukemia may be the cause of thrombocytopenia when neutrophilia is also present and infectious etiologies have been excluded [10]. Significant elevations in white blood cell counts accompanying thrombocytopenia may suggest the presence of lymphoid malignancy [35].

If thrombocytopenia is present in the context of neutrophilia, an infectious process should be considered [10]. Several infectious agents are associated with thrombocytopenia, with the most common mechanisms being immune-mediated destruction, bone marrow suppression, and consumption. Some viruses may influence platelet and megakaryocyte function and induce the generation of antiplatelet antibodies [36]. Infection with viruses such as Epstein-Barr, mumps, rubella, parvovirus, varicella, and hepatitis C virus may lead to thrombocytopenia.

Thrombocytopenia has also been reported after Zika virus infection [37]. Since thrombopoietin is produced in the liver, any viral infection leading to severe hepatitis may potentially cause thrombocytopenia [38, 39]. In thrombocytopenia related to chronic hepatitis C infection, bone marrow inhibition, hypersplenism, and auto-immunogenicity are also contributory factors [38, 40].

Mild platelet dysfunction has been associated with consumption of several food products and supplements including onion, cumin, turmeric, curcumin, clove, garlic, fish oil, and vitamin E, with possible etiologies related to decreased synthesis of thromboxane A2, decreased metabolism of arachidonic acid, and inhibition of fibrinogen binding to platelets [41–43].

Thrombocythemia and Thrombocytosis

Thrombocytosis, often defined as a platelet count greater than 450 × 10^9/L, has numerous potential causes which can generally be organized as spurious, reactive, or clonal in nature [44–46]. Reactive etiologies are the most common, comprising up to 97% of cases of thrombocytopenia [47, 48]. Patients with thrombocytosis may be at risk of both thrombotic complications and paradoxical bleeding [46, 49, 50].

A major branchpoint in the diagnostic evaluation of thrombocytosis involves determining whether a reactive or clonal process is taking place [46]. Common causes of reactive thrombocytosis include infection, tissue damage, chronic inflammatory disorders, iron deficiency anemia, and malignancy [46–48, 51].

After excluding reactive thrombocytosis, a clonal etiology should be investigated. The most common clonal causes of thrombocytosis are essential thrombocythemia, CML, polycythemia vera, and primary myelofibrosis [46].

Spurious thrombocytosis occurs when non-platelet structures in peripheral blood, such as cryoglobulin crystals, cell fragments, or bacteria, are counted as platelets by automated blood counters. This can be avoided by evaluation of a peripheral blood smear [46].

Inherited Platelet Disorders

Compared to acquired causes, inherited causes of platelet disorders are less frequent but often portend a higher tendency for bleeding [52, 53]. Although rare, these inherited platelet disorders have contributed greatly to our understanding of platelet function and hemostasis.

Inherited platelet disorders may affect the number of platelets or impair normal platelet functions such as adhesion, receptor functionality, secretion, enzymatic activity, or signaling pathways [2, 54–57]. Inherited thrombocytopathies are often organized into disorders of platelet adhesion, aggregation, and secretion, [2].

Oftentimes, the platelet phenotype can be of significance when evaluating differential diagnosis of thrombocytopenia. For example, Wiskott-Aldrich syndrome and X-linked thrombocytopenia may both lead to small platelet size [2, 58, 59]. Alternatively, abnormally large platelets may be seen in disorders such as velocardiofacial syndrome, Mediterranean macrothrombocytopenia, platelet-type von Willebrand disease, May-Hegglin anomaly, Fechtner syndrome, Sebastian syndrome, or Epstein syndrome [2, 58, 60–64].

Bernard-Soulier syndrome and platelet-type von Willebrand disease are examples of disorders of platelet adhesion. Bernard-Soulier syndrome is an autosomal recessive bleeding syndrome involving defects of the platelet glycoproteins Ib, IX, and V, which form a complex to aid in the adherence of platelets to the vascular endothelium via binding of von Willebrand Factor (vWF) [65, 66]. The syndrome is characterized by bleeding tendency, abnormally large platelets, and thrombocytopenia [53, 66]. Homozygous mutations typically manifest after birth with purpura, epistaxis, or gingival bleeding [53]. Bleeding tendencies have been reported in heterozygous individuals, but these patients more often remain asymptomatic [67, 68]. Platelet-type von Willebrand disease is a rare autosomal dominant disorder characterized by increased affinity for glycoprotein Ib for vWF, leading to abnormal enhanced binding of vWF by platelets [69–71]. Consequently, complexes of platelets bound to high-molecular-weight multimers of vWF are removed from circulation, leading to thrombocytopenia and decreased levels of vWF multimers [72]. Platelet-type von Willebrand disease and type 2B von Willebrand disease are very similar in clinical and laboratory findings, and diagnosis can be made using genetic analysis [70, 72]. The former disorder requires treatment with platelet transfusions, while the latter requires administration of exogenous vWF [71]. Due to misdiagnosis, the prevalence of platelet-type von Willebrand disease is likely underestimated [72–74].

Glanzmann's thrombasthenia is a classic disorder affecting platelet aggregation. This is an autosomal recessive syndrome affecting the quantity or quality of the $\alpha_{IIb}\beta_3$ integrin (glycoprotein IIb/IIIa) present on platelets, which is involved in platelet aggregation at the site of vessel injury [75]. The syndrome is characterized by a lack of platelet aggregation and commonly manifests at birth with bleeding symptoms such as purpura, epistaxis, and gingival bleeding [75]. Glanzmann thrombasthenia should be suspected when mucosal bleeding is accompanied by lack of platelet aggregation in the presence of normal platelet count and size; the diagnosis may be confirmed via flow cytometry [53].

Inherited disorders involving the number, contents, storage, or release of platelet granules belong to a heterogeneous group of disorders called storage pool disease (SPD). Alpha-SPD, or the gray platelet syndrome, is a deficiency involving alpha granules and their contents. Delta-SPDs involve abnormalities in the dense bodies, causing a deficiency of adenosine diphosphate, adenosine triphosphate, and serotonin [8, 76, 77]. The most commonly known delta-SPDs include Hermansky-Pudlak syndrome, Chediak-Higashi syndrome, and the Quebec platelet syndrome [8, 53, 78, 79].

Disorders of platelet membrane receptors affecting platelet extension and aggregation are a growing area of research [8]. Examples include defects in the P2Y12 receptor, which is necessary for adenosine diphosphate-induced platelet aggregation, defects in the glycoprotein VI platelet collagen receptor, thromboxane A2 receptor, and the epinephrine receptor [8, 80, 81].

Several inherited platelet disorders involve abnormalities in platelet enzymes required for normal platelet function. Some examples include deficiencies in thromboxane A2 synthase, cytosolic phospholipase A2, cyclooxygenase-1, prostaglandin H synthetase 1, lipoxygenase, glycogen-6 synthetase, and enzymes involved in the metabolism of adenosine triphosphate [56, 57].

Diagnosis

Diagnosis of platelet disorders can be challenging. First, it is important to determine whether the patient has a bleeding disorder. Bleeding history is often highly subjective. For example, patients with hereditary bleeding disorders may have not experienced bleeding challenges, while patients without bleeding disorders may exaggerate their symptoms [82, 83]. Occasionally, it is difficult to discern profuse bleeding from bleeding in the upper normal range. Secondly, manifestation of bleeding disorders may be complicated by patients' pathophysiological conditions and medication use. Patients without bleeding disorders are still predisposed to bleeding in medical conditions such as cancer, alcohol use disorder, liver disease, kidney disease, connective tissue disorders, and hypothyroidism. Medications including but not limited to NSAID, aspirin, glucocorticoid, antibiotics, and SSRI also increase the risk of bleeding. Thirdly, when a bleeding disorder is suspected, it is crucial to determine which component of blood clot formation has been impacted. Platelet dysfunction needs to be differentiated from coagulopathy to insure efficacious treatment [84].

In the initial evaluation, physicians should obtain detailed personal bleeding and family history. These include the reason for the visit, prior bleeding events, history of bruising or iron deficiency, outcome of bleeding challenges, bleeding episodes severe enough for surgical intervention, and menstrual and pregnancy history in female patients [85]. Frequent mucosal bleeding is a sign of bleeding disorder. Excessive menstrual bleeding should raise suspicion because of the high prevalence of bleeding disorders (10–30%) in this population of women [85–89]. In contrast, if a patient did not require transfusion during past hemorrhagic trauma, major surgical procedures, or dental extraction, they are unlikely to have a bleeding disorder. Many institutions employ a standardized bleeding assessment tool (BAT) to evaluate the likelihood of bleeding disorders. BAT generates a bleeding score based on answers to questions about the frequency and severity of epistaxis, cutaneous bleeding, oral cavity bleeding, and GI bleeding. A higher score indicates higher risk of bleeding disorder [90, 91].

If a bleeding disorder is suspected after initial history taking and targeted physical exam, a series of laboratory tests is usually employed to determine whether the abnormality is caused by platelet insufficiency/dysfunction (primary hemostatic defect) or by coagulopathy (secondary hemostatic defect). Patients usually first receive tests including platelet count (normally 150–450 × 10^3/mL), morphology, activated partial thromboplastin time (30–40 seconds), and prothrombin time (9.5–13.5 seconds). Abnormality in platelet count and/or morphology can be reviewed from complete blood count. Skin bleeding time test was previously employed to assess platelet disorders; however, it is no longer commonly used because the results are poorly reproducible. Platelet function analyzer (PFA-100), as a replacement to bleeding time, simulates primary hemostasis of blood vessels in response to shear stress and is particularly sensitive to defects in von Willebrand factor [84, 92]. Von Willebrand disease (vWD) is the most common inherited bleeding disorder. It can be diagnosed with PFA-100 in conjunction with vWF activity and vWF antigen levels. It should be noted that in a rare type 2N vWD, factor VIII levels may be very low and the PFA-100 is normal; in type 2B vWD, patients may have varying degrees of thrombocytopenia.

Although PFA-100 is a useful tool to detect vWD, it has a poor sensitivity to many other platelet dysfunctions. Instead, platelet aggregation studies using light transmission aggregometry (LTA) have been widely implemented used in the diagnosis of platelet disorders [84]. Platelet aggregation is triggered by the addition of agonists (e.g., ADP, collagen, epinephrine, and thrombin), which causes the platelets to precipitate from solution. As a result, the turbidity of the solution decreases and allows increased light transmission. Light transmission is proportional to the extent of platelet aggregation induced by an agonist [93]. Application of specific agonists helps identify the underlying diseases. For example, in Glanzmann thrombasthenia due to defect in GPIIb-IIIa complex, platelets will only agglutinate in response to ristocetin; in Bernard-Soulier syndrome caused by a defect in GPIb-IX complex, platelets will aggregate in response to thrombin, collagen, epinephrine, and ADP, but not ristocetin.

Upon observation of abnormalities in the tests mentioned above, further investigation, if available, can be conducted with fresh blood samples. However, these tests can be expensive, time-consuming, and produce results that are dependent on the age of the samples. One example is flow cytometry with specific antibodies against important surface receptors (e.g., GPIIb/IIIa, GPIb/IX/V, GPIa/ IIa, and GPIIIb) and/or intra-platelet molecules that are crucial in aggregation signaling pathways. Flow cytometry provides both qualitative and quantitative analysis of platelet aggregation and thus helps to detect the specific defected molecules resulting in aggregation dysfunction [94]. Another example is transmission electron microscopy (TEM), which may be used to uncover the ultrastructure of platelet granules (alpha and delta granules) if a patient is suspected of having a platelet storage pool disease such as Chediak-Higashi syndrome or Hermansky-Pudlak syndrome [95]. Otherwise, these patients often present with normal platelet aggregometry and

PFA-100 results. TEM also helps with diagnosis of the non-muscle myosin heavy chain 9 (*MYH9*)-related disorders (i.e., May-Hegglin anomaly, Fechtner syndrome, Epstein syndrome, and Sebastian syndrome). Besides TEM, the content and secretion of platelet granules can also be evaluated by ELISA and luminometry based on release products such as platelet factor 4, PDGF, ATP/ADP, and serotonin [96]. Platelet adhesion and spreading disorders can be detected by adhesion and spreading tests, respectively. Surfaces made of different materials (e.g., collagen, fibrinogen, siliconized glass, and subendothelial matrix) serve to evaluate platelet adhesion function. Observation of platelet size and volume with light microscopy provides information about platelet spreading [84]. Finally, many platelet function disorders are inherited diseases. Therefore, genetic testing has been gaining popularity in the diagnosis of known platelet function disorders [97].

Management

There are several options to manage patients with platelet dysfunction disorders who have bleeding. This can vary from conservative management to drug therapy and platelet transfusions. Appropriate treatment depends on several factors including the causative agent, type of platelet disorder, severity of bleeding, and whether or not the patient is planned for an invasive procedure. A careful review of the patient's medical history is tantamount toward treatment. In general, the initial approach should involve identifying and removing any extrinsic causes of the thrombocytopathy. This could be the removal of certain medications or alteration in a patient's diet. In other cases, such as inherited or acquired platelet disorders, response to treatment can vary. In this section, we will discuss management and treatment of bleeding complications in patients with platelet disorders.

Desmopressin

Desmopressin is an analog to vasopressin. This medication is known to shorten bleeding time and decrease blood loss. Desmopressin induces the release of vWF from vascular endothelial cells which enhances platelet adhesion to the vessel walls [5]. It can be administered intravenously, subcutaneously, or as a nasal spray (Octostim) [53, 98]. The recommended parenteral dose is 0.3 micrograms/kilograms of body weight and the intranasal dose is 300 micrograms. It has been shown that desmopressin can shorten bleeding times in storage pool deficiencies among other thrombocytopathies. However, desmopressin response can be limited especially for patients with Glanzmann thrombasthenia or Bernard–Soulier syndrome [53, 98]. Furthermore, desmopressin does not shorten bleeding time in patients with thrombocytopenia. Because of this variation, it can be useful to give a trial dose. The side effect profile of this medication can vary and includes headache, flushing, blood pressure changes, hypersensitivity reaction (bronchospasm, fever, rash), fluid retention, and/or hyponatremia, which could increase the risk of seizures [53, 98].

Platelet Concentrates

Platelet concentrates concentrations are generally reserved for patients who have a defect in the production or consumption of platelets. Platelet concentrates are also used for patients who do not respond to desmopressin or those who experience severe bleeding complications after surgery/trauma.

Considering this, there are specific indications to the use of platelet concentrates. Platelet transfusions should be given to patients who suffer from bleeding complications secondary to Glanzmann thrombasthenia or Bernard–Soulier syndrome [5, 53, 98]. These platelet disorders are generally not responsive to desmopressin. A second indication is emergency therapy of bleeding for patients who have a defect in megakaryopoiesis or have an increase in platelet turnover secondary to DIC, liver disease, or immune thrombocytopenic purpura. A third indication is thrombocytopenia postmassive blood transfusion. The final indication for platelet transfusion is prophylaxis in patients determined to have high bleeding risk preoperatively [53, 98].

One unit of platelets contains approximately $2–4 \times 10^{11}$ platelets and in a normal response increases the platelet count by 20,000–30,000/μl in a 70 kg adult. For newborns and children, a 10 ml platelet concentrate/kg body weight is recommended. In general, patients can be given platelets prophylactically if their platelet count is below 5000/μl. However, if a patient has a superimposed qualitative defect, then platelet transfusion should be initiated at a platelet count above 20,000/μl [53].

Recombinant Activated Factor VII (rFVIIa)

Recombinant activated Factor VII is used for bleeding that cannot be treated by conventional means. It has been reported to be effective in patients with Glanzmann thrombasthenia and Bernard-Soulier syndrome for treatment of bleeding and in surgical intervention. Poon et al. determined that giving prophylactic rFVIIa was effective in 29 out of 31 patients with Glanzmann thrombasthenia [53]. rFVIIa is a viable alternative for patients who previously developed antibodies to platelet transfusions. In Europe, rFVIIa has been approved for patients with antibodies against GPIIb/IIIa and/or HLA and for those patients who do not respond to platelet transfusion [53].

Dosing includes a minimum of 3 bolus injections of 80–120 μg/kg body weight every 1.5–3 hours until hemostasis is achieved. This regiment has been shown to treat bleeding complications in patients with storage pool diseases, Bernard-Soulier syndrome, and several acquired platelet disorders. A single bolus of 270 g/kg has also been shown to be effective. Prior studies indicate that rFVIIa can be effective even when platelet counts are below <20,000/μl. However, it is more effective with higher platelet counts. Frequent administration of rFVIIa is recommended in patients who are less than 12 hours from the onset of acute bleeding episode [5, 53].

Antifibrinolytics

Antifibrinolytics such as aminocaproic acid and tranexamic acid are used to prevent further degradation of blood clots and therefore prevent rebleeding [98]. They are generally used to treat mucocutaneous bleeds, menorrhagia, or gastrointestinal bleeding. Antifibrinolytics combined with cryoprecipitate is the preferred treatment of von Willebrand disease. It can be given orally with a regiment of 2–3 times per day at a total of 1000–1500 mg daily. It can also be given intravenously or be made into a solution and placed on the mouth or nose. A known disadvantage to this medication is that it must be given frequently as bioavailability can be as low as 30% [98].

Hormonal Therapy

Birth control pills can be an option to control bleeding especially in women with significant menstrual bleeding. Another option is an intrauterine device that releases progesterone. This has been effective in women with bleeding disorders who have heavy menstrual bleeding.

Treatment of Nosebleeds

Nose bleeds can be treated by local measures. One method is to have the patient sit with their head tilted forward while pinching the soft part of their nose for 10 minutes until the bleeding stops. Individuals can apply petroleum jelly or propylene glycol to prevent drying of mucous membranes. Fibrin sealants containing fibrinogen, thrombin, factor XIII, and aprotinin can be used if bleeding is prolonged [98].

Bleeding Associated with Menstruation and Childbirth

Patients with heavy menstruation can use desmopressin, rFVIIa, and antifibrinolytics. These products are effective when used at the beginning and during each menstrual period. IUDs or birth control are used for long-term management [98].

For women who are pregnant are recommended to discuss a delivery plan with their physician. Approaches to bleeding can vary and depend on the specific platelet disorder, the person's experience with past bleeding, and whether delivery will be caesarian or vaginal. It is important to note that bleeding risk is elevated right after delivery and several weeks postpartum.

Dental Extraction

Individuals with platelet disorders undergoing dental extraction should be administrated desmopressin as part of their management. It should also be given to the patient prior to receiving a mandibular block which presents a bleeding risk. It is recommended that platelet function be corrected by desmopressin or another alternative before using performing a mandibular block. Antifibrinolytic therapy has been shown to reduce bleeding complications following tooth extraction and surgery. Timing is important when using these medications and should be initiated prior to surgery and continued for several days. Lastly, fibrin glue can be applied to the surgical site intraoperatively [98].

Medications to Avoid

Certain medications can cause platelet dysfunction and should be avoided if possible. Aspirin is commonly used as an antiplatelet medication. It irreversibly inhibits platelet cyclooxygenase impairing thromboxane A2. A dose of 200 mg is known to double bleeding time and can produce effects for as long as 4–10 days. Other NSAIDS such as phenylbutazone, indomethacin, fenoprofen, and ibuprofen have also been implicated [5].

Warfarin or heparin is commonly used and may worsen bleeding in these patients. Heparin in particular can cause heparin-induced thrombocytopenia. Antibiotics that have also been implicated in disruption of hemostasis include carbenicillin, ticarcillin, penicillin G, ampicillin, and cephalosporin.

Nutraceuticals and Foods to Avoid

Patients with thrombocytopathies should avoid certain foods, additives, and herbal products. These include alcohol, Chinese black tree fungus, ajoene (a component of garlic), feverfew, saw palmetto, and various plant barks.

There are several options for management of complicated bleeding in individuals who have platelet function disorders.

The approach depends on the offending agent (i.e., food, medications, etc.), the specific platelet disorder, severity of bleeding, and whether or not the patient is scheduled for an invasive procedure. Based on these factors, treatments can be conservative or may require medications and/or platelet transfusions. It is important to know the indications as well as the side effects of these treatment options, especially of agents such as desmopressin. Most patients with a platelet dysfunction disorder will not require regular treatment but may need medical management when determined to be at risk for bleeding complications.

Intraoperative Considerations

Type of Surgery and Prophylactic Treatments

Intraoperative bleeding disturbances can occur secondary to direct surgical manipulation of anatomy or due to hemostatic abnormalities [99]. Hemostatic abnormalities can be present at baseline or arise as a consequence of physiologic and pharmacologic changes associated with the perioperative period [99]. Baseline hematologic abnormalities, such as inherited platelet function disorders, present significantly higher intraoperative bleeding risk than inherited platelet number disorders [100]. There does not appear to be a linear relationship between platelet count and risk of spontaneous surgical bleeding, making this serious complication difficult to predict [101]. The Surgery in Platelet Disorders and Therapeutic Approach (SPATA) study showed that type of disorder impacts surgical bleeding risk, with biallelic Bernard-Soulier syndrome being associated with the highest occurrence of perioperative bleeding [100]. Bleeding history and sex are also determining factors of surgical bleeding risk, with female sex being associated with higher bleeding frequency [100]. Cardiovascular and urological surgery is associated with the highest incidence of intraoperative bleeding [100]. Use of laparoscopic versus open approaches and prophylactic establishment of access with two large-bore intravenous catheters have been shown to decrease frequency of hemostatic complications even in high-risk surgeries. Interestingly, the SPATA study demonstrated that the use of pro-hemostatic treatments as pre-operative prophylaxis decreases bleeding frequency in patients with inherited platelet function disorders but not inherited platelet number disorders [100]. Considering the substantial perioperative bleeding risk associated with inherited platelet disorders alone, prophylactic pre-operative pro-hemostatic treatments appear to be vital to decreasing bleeding incidence [100].

Traditionally, platelet transfusions have been used at the highest frequency in patients with established high bleeding risk [100]. While prophylactic platelet transfusions have been shown to decrease rates of clinically significant bleeding, they have not improved patient outcomes, decreased perioperative RBC requirements, or demonstrated overall mortality benefit [101]. Over time, platelet transfusions have been shown to be associated with significant negative outcomes such as higher rates of postoperative ICU admission and longer hospital stays [101]. In patients who experience acute spontaneous primary intracerebral hemorrhage while on antiplatelet therapy, platelet transfusions were associated with enlargement of hemorrhage and increased rates of infection [101]. Platelets have the highest risk of bacterial sepsis of any blood product [101]. Platelet transfusion has also been associated with transfusion-associated acute lung injury, immunomodulation, post-transfusion purpura, and alloimmunization [101]. These observations have paved the way for alternative prophylactic and reactive therapies such as desmopressin, antifibrinolytic agents (epsilon aminocaproic acid and tranexamic acid), procoagulant bypass agents (recombinant factor VIIIa and activated prothrombin complex concentrates), and thrombopoietin receptor agonists (romiplostim, eltrombopag, avatrombopag, and lusutrombopag), whose mechanisms have been described above [101]. Of note, thrombopoietin receptor agonists are currently used off-label except in patients with thrombocytopenia secondary to chronic liver disease [101].

Anesthesia and Anticoagulation

It has been demonstrated that anesthetic agents have the capacity to influence hemostasis [99]. In vitro, ketamine dose dependently inhibits platelet aggregation via action on platelet inositol 1,4,5-triphosphate formation, guanosine 5-triphosphatase activity, and calcium currents [99]. Inhibition by ketamine is most notable at doses that exceed concentrations used in clinical settings. This mechanism is important given that the specific effects of anesthetics on platelet function are poorly understood [99]. Anesthetic effects on platelets are difficult to evaluate because measurement of platelet function proves challenging [99]. At present, techniques such as bleeding time, platelet aggregometry, and thromboelastography can be used for measurement of platelet function, but there is no gold standard for accuracy and ease of use [99]. To this extent, platelet aggregometry has shown that not only ketamine but the majority of anesthetic agents including halothane and sevoflurane inhibit platelet function [99]. Propofol has been consistently associated with significant platelet inhibition [99]. Unfortunately, there are no data indicating that any one general anesthetic regimen is best for reducing perioperative bleeding [99]. So far, basic science reports have brought to the attention of clinicians the potential of hemostatic complications secondary to different anesthetics. Further investigation is needed to determine true clinical impact and the influences of genetic factors and perioperative conditions.

Temperature Regulation and the Coagulopathy of Hypothermia

Intraoperative hypothermia can be caused by a combination of multiple factors occurring simultaneously [102]. Upon entering the operating room, low ambient temperatures begin to externally cool the patient [102]. Following induction of anesthesia, the threshold at which the body perceives hypothermia drops from 37.5° to 34.5° [102]. Consequently, the body inappropriately initiates vasodilation, decreasing core temperature, and redistributing heat to the extremities [102]. As heat is continually lost due to the cold ambient temperature of the operating room, surface area of exposure during surgery is directly related to the amount of heat loss through convective and radiative pathways [103]. Heat loss further contributes to the depression of overall body temperature [103]. At approximately 34.5°C, the brain reinitiates thermoregulative control and induces vasoconstriction to protect against further core heat loss; however, this vasoconstriction occurs at the expense of the extremities, which continue to see decreasing temperatures [103]. Hypothermia can have a catastrophic effect on the coagulation cascade due to reflexive release of thromboxane A3 [104, 105]. This reversible impairment of platelet plug formation combined with the reduced coagulation cascade enzyme activity seen in hypothermic patients increases bleeding risk [104, 105]. A lethal triad of hypothermia, acidosis, and coagulopathy is seen in patients with traumatic injuries—in these cases the ineffectiveness of fibrinogen is explained through both hypothermia and acidosis mechanisms. Hypothermia prevents fibrinogen synthesis through a decrease in metabolic rate and acidosis causes an increase in degradation due to a pH that is incompatible with enzyme activity, together depleting the amount of fibrinogen available and causing coagulopathy [104, 105]. One meta-analysis showed that these mechanisms combine in hypothermic patients to cause a 20% increase in perioperative blood loss [106]. To combat hypothermia, upper and lower body forced-air warming devices for exposed skin and fluid warming devices for refrigerated blood product infusions should be liberally used to maintain normothermic temperatures that encourage adequate clotting capacity [105].

Postoperative Blood Loss and Transfusion Requirements

In the case of perioperative or postoperative blood loss, transfusion algorithms have been proposed to combat depressed clotting factors and hypovolemic shock without over-transfusing patients [105]. Intraoperatively, the most current transfusion protocol recommendations include sending the following labs every 30 minutes: PT/PTT, fibrinogen, CBC, ABG, and ROTEM [105]. Recommendations also include correction of a hemoglobin less than 7 g/dL, a platelet count less than 50,000, a fibrinogen level less than 200 mg/dL with a double dose given if the fibrinogen dips under 150 mg/dL, and a PT/INR greater than 150% of baseline [105]. If more than four units of packed RBCs are required to restore the hemoglobin concentration, it is recommended to follow a balanced resuscitation protocol that provides balanced units of blood cells and plasma with added platelets and cryoprecipitate. This transfusion protocol is used for non-traumatic patients and should not replace the accepted 1:1:1, pRBC:FFP:platelets protocol used in traumatic settings. These protocols offer more precise, guided treatments for non-traumatic settings of coagulopathic blood loss with the goal of replenishing the patient in a more balanced, physiologic manner that includes transfusion of platelets and fibrinogen more liberally than in other algorithms.

The type of procedure must also be considered in choosing a transfusion protocol; certain procedures inherently provide more coagulopathic risk [107]. When platelet count and function were examined in patients undergoing coronary cardiac surgery, platelet count and function were both found to decrease during cardiopulmonary bypass, which increased overall postoperative bleeding and transfusion requirements [107]. Due to the complexity of cardiac patients, an individualized algorithm has been established that varies slightly from the above recommendations; the main differences here include more aggressive fibrinogen correction that is recommended to occur before addressing other abnormalities [105].

Summary & Conclusion

Alteration in platelet number and function affects the body's clotting abilities. Platelet disorders can be inherited or acquired defects, which manifest as quantitative or qualitative abnormalities. Increased platelets (thrombocytosis and thrombocythemia) will increase the chances of a clot forming while decreased platelets (thrombocytopenia) will impair initial platelet plug formation. Altered platelet function with respect to adhesion, receptor function, secretion, enzyme activity, or signaling pathways can also contribution to dysfunctional formation of the platelet plug. Without adequate formation of the platelet plug individuals tend to experience increased bleeding, purpura, epistaxis, and mucocutaneous bleeding. It is important to differentiate these signs from those of the coagulopathies so that a platelet disorder can be identified and adequate hemostasis can be promoted.

Evaluation for a platelet disorder typically starts with the history and physical exam. A bleeding assessment tool (BAT) may also be included to screen for a bleeding disorder. If a bleeding disorder is suspected, then more formal testing can be done. Initial workup typically involves a complete blood count and light microscopy to assess platelet count and morphology. Coagulation studies are also ordered to evaluate for a coagulopathy. Bleeding time has been replaced by a platelet function analyzer to assess primary hemostasis. Other platelet disorders are typically tested for with light transmission aggregometry, which can detect platelet aggregation when different agonists are added, allowing the evaluator to narrow down the defect. Different surfaces can be used to evaluate platelet adhesion to various molecules in the body. Flow cytometry allows the detection of specific receptor defects once a differential of possible disorders has been established. Transmission electron microscopy, ELISA, and luminometry can all be used to assess platelet granules and secretion function. Finally, genetic testing can be pursued when an inherited disorder is suspected. Determining whether or not a platelet disorder is present and achieving the diagnosis frequently requires a combination of any of these tests. The approach to making the diagnosis is highly dependent on the given situation and the individual history of any given patient.

Once a platelet disorder has been discovered, management involves removing any identifiable causes, if applicable, and initiating treatment tailored to the given etiology. NSAIDs, heparin, antibiotics, alcohol, and several foods and herbs can all be culprits that contribute to the manifestation of platelet disorders. Administration of desmopressin can cause vasoconstriction to limit blood loss and release stores of vWF in a deficient patient. It is also used for bleeding associated with menses, childbirth, and dental extraction. Desmopressin is not helpful in situations where the receptors are defective or in patients with thrombocytopenia. In these cases, platelet transfusion may be considered. Transfusion is also used in cases of massive loss of platelets, such as that seen in consumptive disorders, or occasionally in those determined to be at a high risk of perioperative bleeding. In cases where this is ineffective, or in cases where the patient has been sensitized due to previous transfusions, recombinant activated Factor VII has been shown to be effective. Antifibrinolytics have shown to be efficacious in mucocutaneous bleeds and vWD, but the main limiting factor for their use is the required frequency of dosing. Choice of treatment is largely based on clinical judgment stemming from factors identified during workup.

Platelet disorders are important to consider in the operative setting. Platelet disorders increase the risk of intraoperative bleeding, with qualitative disorders presenting more risk than quantitative disorders. Preoperative prophylaxis with desmopressin, antifibrinolytics, procoagulant bypassing agents, and thrombopoietin receptor agonists can be used to reduce the risk of bleeding. Prophylactic platelet transfusions have fallen out of favor due to a high number of associated risks and limited benefit. The low transient temperature of the operating room combined with lowered thermoregulative control secondary to anesthesia can lead to perioperative hypothermia. Perioperative hypothermia affects the function of various coagulation enzymes and factors, which can lead to coagulopathy. These effects can be mitigated by using warming devices and warmed fluids as needed during the operation. Perioperative labs should be drawn every 30 minutes to monitor bleeding risk. Platelets can be given if concentrations fall below 50,000/μL or to maintain balanced physiology during larger blood transfusions. The type of surgery, the patient's history, and the situation surrounding the operation must all be considered by the clinical anesthesiologist and other members of the team when determining appropriate treatment for patients at risk of bleeding.

References

1. Krishnegowda M, Rajashekaraiah V. Platelet disorders: an overview. Blood Coagul Fibrinolysis. 2015;26(5):479–91.
2. D'Andrea G, Chetta M, Margaglione M. Inherited platelet disorders: thrombocytopenias and thrombocytopathies. Blood Transfus. 2009;7:278–92.
3. Freson K, Wijgaerts A, van Geet C. Update on the causes of platelet disorders and functional consequences. Int J Lab Hematol. 2014;36(3):313–25.
4. Ghoshal K, Bhattacharyya M. Overview of platelet physiology: its hemostatic and nonhemostatic role in disease pathogenesis. Scientific World Journal. Scientific World Ltd. 2014;2014:781857.
5. Huebsch LB, Harker LA. Disorders of platelet functions. Mechanisms, diagnosis and management. West J Med. 1981;134(2):109–27.
6. Krishnegowda M, Rajashekaraiah V. Platelet disorders: an overview. Blood Coagul Fibrinolysis. Lippincott Williams and Wilkins. 2015;26:479–91.
7. George JN. Platelets. Lancet. 2000;355(9214):1531–9.
8. Simon D, Kunicki T, Nugent D. Platelet function defects. Haemophilia. 2008;14(6):1240–9.
9. Gauer RL, Braun MM. Thrombocytopenia. Am Fam Physician. 2012;85:612–22.
10. Wolfromm A, Dallemagne J. Management of thrombocytopenia. Rev Med Brux. 2018;39(4):296–301.
11. Ali N, Auerbach HE. New-onset acute thrombocytopenia in hospitalized patients: pathophysiology and diagnostic approach. J Community Hosp Intern Med Perspect. 2017;7(3):157–67.

12. Wong EY, Rose MG. Why does my patient have thrombocytopenia? Hematol Oncol Clin North Am. 2012;26:231–52.
13. Moulis G, Christiansen CF, Darvalics B, Nørgaard M. Prevalence of thrombocytopenia and thrombocytosis upon acute hospital admission to internal medicine units. A cross-sectional study in Denmark. Eur J Intern Med. Elsevier B.V. 2018;57:e34–7.
14. Smock KJ, Perkins SL. Thrombocytopenia: an update. Int J Lab Hematol. 2014;36(3):269–78.
15. Warkentin TE, Warkentin AE. Acquired thrombocytopenia. In: Concise guide to hematology. Oxford, UK: Wiley-Blackwell; 2011. p. 154–73.
16. Dewitte A, Lepreux S, Villeneuve J, Rigothier C, Combe C, Ouattara A, et al. Blood platelets and sepsis pathophysiology: a new therapeutic prospect in critical ill patients? In: Annals of intensive care, vol. 7: Springer; 2017. https://www.ncbi.nlm.nih.gov/pmc/articles/PMC5709271/.
17. Venkata C, Kashyap R, Christopher Farmer J, Afessa B. Thrombocytopenia in adult patients with sepsis: incidence, risk factors, and its association with clinical outcome. J Intensive Care. 2013;1(1):9.
18. Sarode R, Nagalla S. Recent advances in understanding and management of acquired thrombocytopenia. F1000Research. Faculty of 1000 Ltd. 2018;7.
19. George JN, Aster RH. Drug-induced thrombocytopenia: pathogenesis, evaluation, and management. Hematology Am Soc Hematol Educ Program. 2009:153–8.
20. Patel N, VanDeWall H, Tristani L, Rivera A, Woo B, Dihmess A, et al. A comparative evaluation of adverse platelet outcomes among Veterans' Affairs patients receiving linezolid or vancomycin. J Antimicrob Chemother. 2012 Mar;67(3):727–35.
21. ten Berg MJ, Huisman A, Souverein PC, Schobben AFAM, Egberts ACG, van Solinge WW, et al. Drug-induced thrombocytopenia: a population study. Drug Saf. 2006;29(8):713–21.
22. Aster RH, Curtis BR, McFarland JG, Bougie DW. Drug-induced immune thrombocytopenia: pathogenesis, diagnosis, and management. J Thromb Haemost. 2009;7(6):911–8.
23. Reese JA, Li X, Hauben M, Aster RH, Bougie DW, Curtis BR, et al. Identifying drugs that cause acute thrombocytopenia: an analysis using 3 distinct methods. Blood. 2010;116(12):2127–33.
24. Pedersen-Bjergaard U, Andersen M, Hansen PB. Drug-specific characteristics of thrombocytopenia caused by non-cytotoxic drugs. Eur J Clin Pharmacol. 1998;54(9–10):701–6.
25. Pedersen-Bjergaard U, Andersen M, Hansen PB. Drug-induced thrombocytopenia: clinical data on 309 cases and the effect of corticosteroid therapy. Eur J Clin Pharmacol. 1997;52(3):183–9.
26. Pedersen-Bjergaard U, Andersen M, Hansen PB. Thrombocytopenia induced by noncytotoxic drugs in Denmark 1968-91. J Intern Med. 1996;239(6):509–15.
27. George JN, Raskob GE, Shah SR, Rizvi MA, Hamilton SA, Osborne S, et al. Drug-induced thrombocytopenia: a systematic review of published case reports. Ann Intern Med. 1998;129:886–90.
28. Von Drygalski A, Curtis BR, Bougie DW, McFarland JG, Ahl S, Limbu I, et al. Vancomycin-induced immune thrombocytopenia. N Engl J Med. 2007;356(9):904–10.
29. Arnold D, Cucker A. Drug-induced immune thrombocytopenia. Post TW, ed. UpToDate. Waltham: UpToDate Inc.
30. Vardiman JW, Arber DA, Brunning RD, Borowitz MJ, Porwit A, Harris NL, et al. The 2008 revision of the World Health Organization (WHO) classification of myeloid neoplasms and acute leukemia: rationale and important changes. Blood. 2009;114(5):937–51.
31. Alimeida JI, Coats R, Liem TK, Silver D, Sobel M. Reduced morbidity and mortality rates of the heparin-induced thrombocytopenia syndrome. J Vasc Surg. 1998;27(2):309–16.
32. Liebman HA. Thrombocytopenia in cancer patients. Thromb Res. 2014;133(Suppl 2):S63.
33. Ghanavat M, Ebrahimi M, Rafieemehr H, Maniati M, Behzad MM, Shahrabi S. Thrombocytopenia in solid tumors: prognostic significance. Oncol Rev. Page Press Publications. 2019;13:43–8.
34. Shahrabi S, Behzad MM, Jaseb K, Saki N. Thrombocytopenia in leukemia: pathogenesis and prognosis. Histol Histopathol. 2018;33:895–908.
35. Tefferi A, Hanson CA, Inwards DJ. How to interpret and pursue an abnormal complete blood cell count in adults. Mayo Clin Proc. Elsevier Ltd. 2005;80:923–36.
36. Assinger A. Platelets and infection - an emerging role of platelets in viral infection. Front Immunol. Frontiers Media S.A. 2014;5:649.
37. Chammard TB, Schepers K, Breurec S, Messiaen T, Destrem AL, Mahevas M, et al. Severe thrombocytopenia after zika virus infection, Guadeloupe, 2016. Emerg Infect Dis. 2017;23(4):696–8.
38. Olariu M, Olariu C, Olteanu D. Thrombocytopenia in chronic hepatitis C. J Gastrointestin Liver Dis. 2010;19(4):381–5.
39. Jelkmann W. The role of the liver in the production of thrombopoietin compared with erythropoietin. Eur J Gastroenterol Hepatol. 2001;13:791–801.
40. Dahal S, Upadhyay S, Banjade R, Dhakal P, Khanal N, Bhatt VR. Thrombocytopenia in patients with chronic hepatitis C virus infection. Mediterr J Hematol Infect Dis. 2017;9(1).
41. Chaudhary B, Imam Rabbani S. Thrombocytopenia and its causes. Available online www.jocpr.com. J Chem Pharm Res. 2016;8(2):184–9.
42. Navon L, Moritz E, Austin C, Wahl M, Aks S, Layden J. The public health response to a large poisoning outbreak involving an illicit substance: synthetic cannabinoids contaminated with a long-acting anticoagulant rodenticide, Illinois, March–July, 2018. J Public Heal Manag Pract. 9000;Publish Ah, Publish Ahead of Print.
43. Rahman K. Effects of garlic on platelet biochemistry and physiology. Mol Nutr Food Res. 2007;51:1335–44.
44. Harrison CN, Bareford D, Butt N, Campbell P, Conneally E, Drummond M, et al. Guideline for investigation and management of adults and children presenting with a thrombocytosis. Br J Haematol. 2010;149(3):352–75.
45. Skoda RC. Thrombocytosis. Hematol Am Soc Hematol Educ Progr. 2009;2009:159–67.
46. Bleeker JS, Hogan WJ. Thrombocytosis: diagnostic evaluation, thrombotic risk stratification, and risk-based management strategies. Thrombosis. 2011;2011:1–16.
47. Santhosh-Kumar CR, Yohannan MD, Higgy KE, al-Mashhadani SA. Thrombocytosis in adults: analysis of 777 patients. J Intern Med. 1991;229(6):493–5.
48. Griesshammer M, Bangerter M, Sauer T, Wennauer R, Bergmann L, Heimpel H. Aetiology and clinical significance of thrombocytosis: analysis of 732 patients with an elevated platelet count. J Intern Med. 1999;245(3):295–300.
49. Coon WW, Penner J, Clagett GP, Eos N. Deep venous thrombosis and postsplenectomy thrombocytosis. Arch Surg. 1978;113(4):429–31.
50. Buss DH, Stuart JJ, Lipscomb GE. The incidence of thrombotic and hemorrhagic disorders in association with extreme thrombocytosis: an analysis of 129 cases. Am J Hematol. 1985;20(4):365–72.
51. Kuku I, Kaya E, Yologlu S, Gokdeniz R, Baydin A. Platelet counts in adults with iron deficiency anemia. Platelets. 2009;20(6):401–5.
52. Koscielny J, Ziemer S, Radtke H, Schmutzler M, Kiesewetter H, Salama A, et al. [Preoperative identification of patients with impaired (primary) haemostasis. A practical concept]. Hamostaseologie. 2007;27(3):177–84.
53. Kirchmaier CM, Pillitteri D. Diagnosis and management of inherited platelet disorders. Transfus Med Hemother. 2010;37:237–46.

54. Rao AK. Congenital disorders of platelet function: disorders of signal transduction and secretion. Am J Med Sci. 1998;316(2):69–76.
55. Rao AK, Jalagadugula G, Sun L. Inherited defects in platelet signaling mechanisms. Semin Thromb Hemost. 2004;30:525–35.
56. Nurden AT, Nurden P. Inherited disorders of platelets: an update. Curr Opin Hematol. 2006;13(3):157–62.
57. Nurden P, Nurden AT. Congenital disorders associated with platelet dysfunctions. Thromb Haemost. 2008;99(2):253–63.
58. Malik MA, Masab M. Wiskott-Aldrich Syndrome. [Updated 2020 Jun 29]. In: StatPearls [Internet]. Treasure Island (FL): StatPearls Publishing; 2020 Jan-. Available from: https://www.ncbi.nlm.nih.gov/books/NBK539838/.
59. Villa A, Notarangelo L, Macchi P, Mantuano E, Cavagni G, Brugnoni D, et al. X–linked thrombocytopenia and Wiskott–Aldrich syndrome are allelic diseases with mutations in the WASP gene. Nat Genet. 1995;9(4):414–7.
60. Rodriguez V, Nichols WL, Charlesworth JE, White JG. Sebastian platelet syndrome: a hereditary macrothrombocytopenia. Mayo Clin Proc. 2003;78(11):1416–21.
61. Fechtner syndrome: physiologic analysis of macrothrombocytopenia. - PubMed - NCBI.
62. Untanu RV, Vajpayee N. May Hegglin anomaly. StatPearls. 2019.
63. Mhawech P, Saleem A. Inherited giant platelet disorders classification and literature review materials and methods. Am J Clin Pathol. 2000;113:176.
64. Bishop BN, Brady R. Velocardiofacial syndrome. StatPearls. 2019.
65. Berndt MC, Fournier DJ, Castaldi PA. Bernard-Soulier syndrome. Baillieres Clin Haematol. 1989;2(3):585–607.
66. Lanza F. Bernard-Soulier syndrome (hemorrhagiparous thrombocytic dystrophy). Orphanet J Rare Dis. 2006 Nov;1:46.
67. Savoia A, Balduini CL, Savino M, Noris P, Del Vecchio M, Perrotta S, et al. Autosomal dominant macrothrombocytopenia in Italy is most frequently a type of heterozygous Bernard-Soulier syndrome. Blood. 2001;97(5):1330–5.
68. Bragadottir G, Birgisdottir ER, Gudmundsdottir BR, Hilmarsdottir B, Vidarsson B, Magnusson MK, et al. Clinical phenotype in heterozygote and biallelic Bernard-Soulier syndrome – a case control studyfile:///Users/johannhauksson/Downloads/Bragadottir_et_al-2015-American_Journal_of_Hematology.pdf. Am J Hematol. 2015;90(2):149–55.
69. Matsubara Y, Murata M, Sugita K, Ikeda Y. Identification of a novel point mutation in platelet glycoprotein Ibalpha, Gly to Ser at residue 233, in a Japanese family with platelet-type von Willebrand disease. J Thromb Haemost. 2003;1(10):2198–205.
70. Franchini M, Montagnana M, Lippi G. Clinical, laboratory and therapeutic aspects of platelet-type von Willebrand disease. Int J Lab Hematol. 2008;30(2):91–4.
71. Othman M, Notley C, Lavender FL, White H, Byrne CD, Lillicrap D, et al. Identification and functional characterization of a novel 27-bp deletion in the macroglycopeptide-coding region of the GPIBA gene resulting in platelet-type von Willebrand disease. Blood. 2005;105(11):4330–6.
72. Giannini S, Cecchetti L, Mezzasoma AM, Gresele P. Diagnosis of platelet-type von willebrand disease by flow cytometry. Haematologica. 2010;95(6):1021–4.
73. Federici AB. Diagnosis of inherited von Willebrand disease: a clinical perspective. Semin Thromb Hemost. 2006;32(6):555–65.
74. Sadler JE, Budde U, Eikenboom JCJ, Favaloro EJ, Hill FGH, Holmberg L, et al. Update on the pathophysiology and classification of von Willebrand disease: a report of the Subcommittee on von Willebrand Factor. J Thromb Haemost. 2006;4(10):2103–14.
75. Nurden AT. Glanzmann thrombasthenia.
76. Ambrosio AL, Di Pietro SM. Storage pool diseases illuminate platelet dense granule biogenesis. Platelets. 2017;28(2):138–46.
77. Sandrock K, Zieger B. Current strategies in diagnosis of inherited storage pool defects. Transfus Med Hemother. 2010;37:248–58.
78. Nurden AT, Nurden P. The gray platelet syndrome: clinical spectrum of the disease. Blood Rev. 2007;21(1):21–36.
79. Huizing M, Anikster Y, Gahl WA. Hermansky-Pudlak syndrome and Chediak-Higashi syndrome: disorders of vesicle formation and trafficking. Thromb Haemost. 2001;86:233–45.
80. Gachet C. P2 receptors, platelet function and pharmacological implications. Thromb Haemost. 2008;99:466–72.
81. Arthur JF, Dunkley S, Andrews RK. Platelet glycoprotein VI-related clinical defects. Br J Haematol. 2007;139(3):363–72.
82. Wahlberg T, Blomback M, Hall P, Axelsson G. Application of indicators, predictors and diagnostic indices in coagulation disorders. II. Evaluation of laboratory variables with continuous test results. Methods Inf Med. 1980;19(4):201–5.
83. Wahlberg T, Blombäck M, Brodin U. Carriers and noncarriers of haemophilia A: I. Multivariate analysis of pedigree data, screening blood coagulation tests and factor VIII variables. Thromb Res. 1982;25:401.
84. Kirchmaier CM, Pillitteri D. Diagnosis and management of inherited platelet disorders. Transfus Med Hemother. 2010;37:3.
85. Lee CA. Women and inherited bleeding disorders: menstrual issues. Semin Hematol. 1999;36(3 Suppl 4):21–7.
86. Philipp CS, Faiz A, Bowling N, Dilley A, Michaels LA, Ayers G, et al. Age and the prevalence of bleeding disorders in women with menorrhagia. Obstet Gynecol. 2005;105:61.
87. Trasi SA, Pathare AV, Shetty SD, Ghosh K, Salvi V, Mohanty D. The spectrum of bleeding disorders in women with menorrhagia: a report from Western India. Ann Hematol. 2005;84:339.
88. Woo YL, White B, Corbally R, Byrne M, O'Connell N, O'Shea E, et al. von Willebrand's disease: an important cause of dysfunctional uterine bleeding. Blood Coagul Fibrinolysis. 2002;13:89.
89. Kadir RA, Economides DL, Sabin CA, Owens D, Lee CA. Frequency of inherited bleeding disorders in women with menorrhagia. Lancet. 1998;351:485.
90. Rodeghiero F, Tosetto A, Abshire T, Arnold DM, Coller B, James P, et al. ISTH/SSC bleeding assessment tool: a standardized questionnaire and a proposal for a new bleeding score for inherited bleeding disorders. J Thromb Haemost. 2010;8:2063.
91. Tosetto A, Castaman G, Plug I, Rodeghiero F, Eikenboom J. Prospective evaluation of the clinical utility of quantitative bleeding severity assessment in patients referred for hemostatic evaluation. J Thromb Haemost. 2011;9:1143.
92. Jilma B. Platelet function analyzer (PFA-100): a tool to quantify congenital or acquired platelet dysfunction. J Lab Clin Med. 2001;138:152.
93. Hvas AM, Favaloro EJ. Platelet function analyzed by light transmission aggregometry. Methods Mol Biol. 2017;1646:321–31.
94. Michelson AD, Barnard MR, Krueger LA, Frelinger AL, Furman MI. Evaluation of platelet function by flow cytometry. Methods. 2000;21:259.
95. Ahnadi CE, Chapman ES, Lépine M, Okrongly D, Pujol-Moix N, Hernández A, et al. Assessment of platelet activation in several different anticoagulants by the Advia 120 hematology system, fluorescence flow cytometry, and electron microscopy. Thromb Haemost. 2003;90(5):940–8.
96. Taaning E. Platelet immunology. ELISA for detection of platelet antibodies, platelet-specific antigens and platelet glycoproteins. Dan Med Bull. 1992;39(4):343–54.
97. Lentaigne C, Freson K, Laffan MA, Turro E, Ouwehand WH. Inherited platelet disorders: toward DNA-based diagnosis. Blood. 2016;127:2814.

98. Fuse I. Disorders of platelet function. Crit Rev Oncol Hematol. Elsevier Ireland Ltd. 1996;22:1–25.
99. Faraday N. Platelets, perioperative hemostasis, and anesthesia. Anesthesiology. 2002;96(5):1042–3.
100. Orsini S, Noris P, Bury L, Heller PG, Santoro C, Kadir RA, et al. Bleeding risk of surgery and its prevention in patients with inherited platelet disorders. Haematologica. 2017;102(7):1192–203.
101. Nagrebetsky A, Al-Samkari H, Davis NM, Kuter DJ, Wiener-Kronish JP. Perioperative thrombocytopenia: evidence, evaluation, and emerging therapies. Br J Anaesth. 2019;122(1):19–31.
102. Sun Z, Honar H, Sessler DI, Dalton JE, Yang D, Panjasawatwong K, et al. Intraoperative core temperature patterns, transfusion requirement, and hospital duration in patients warmed with forced air. Physiol Behav. 2015;122(2):276–85.
103. Kurz A, Sessler DI, Christensen R, Dechert M. Heat balance and distribution during the core-temperature plateau in anesthetized humans. Anesthesiology. 1995;83(3):491–9.
104. Martini WZ. Coagulopathy by hypothermia and acidosis: mechanisms of thrombin generation and fibrinogen availability. J Trauma - Inj Infect Crit Care. 2009;67(1):208–9.
105. Ghadimi K, Levy JH, Welsby IJ. Perioperative management of the bleeding patient. Br J Anaesth. 2016;117:iii18–30.
106. Reed RL, Johnston TD, Hudson JD, Fischer RP. The disparity between hypothermic coagulopathy and clotting studies. J Trauma - Inj Infect Crit Care. 1992;33:465–70.
107. Adeli EK, Alavi SM, Alizadeh-Ghavidel A, Bakhshandeh-Abkenar H, Pourfathollah AA. Perioperative changes in platelet count and function in patients undergoing cardiac surgery. Med J Islam Repub Iran. 2017;31(1):213–8.

Massive Transfusion Protocol

8

Mary Im, Usama Iqbal, Hong Yan, Jaime Sanders, and Henry Liu

Introduction

Massive transfusion in an adult has commonly been defined as 10 or more units of packed red blood cells (RBCs) in a 24-hour period, which almost replaces one blood volume based on the total blood volume of a 70-kg male [1]. Massive transfusion can also be defined if one of the following conditions is satisfied: blood loss exceeding circulating blood volume within a 24-hour period; blood loss of 50% of circulating blood volume within a 3-hour period; blood loss exceeding 150 ml/min; blood loss that necessitates plasma and platelets (PLTs) transfusion [2]. Hemorrhage is the main cause of death in major trauma patients surviving to the hospital admission [3]. In this review, we will discuss the indication of massive transfusion, components and strategies of a massive transfusion protocol (MTP), MTP for specific patient groups, and monitoring performance and outcomes.

Indication of Massive Transfusion

Perioperative massive hemorrhage can be caused by various etiologies, as illustrated in Table 8.1.

Table 8.1 Etiologies of massive perioperative bleeding [80]

Category	Etiologies
Surgical procedures	Major hepatic surgery
	Liver transplantation
	Cardiac/major vascular surgery
	Major cancer surgery
	Spine surgery
Coagulation abnormalities	Acute traumatic coagulopathy
	Clotting factor deficiencies
	An undiagnosed inherited bleeding disorder
	Dilutional coagulopathy
Obstetric diseases	Abnormal placentation
	Uterine atony
	Embryonic emboli-associated DIC

Trauma

Major Trauma is one of the leading causes of perioperative massive hemorrhage and hemorrhage is the main cause of death following major trauma in patients surviving to hospital admission with the highest incidence in 1–3 hours after admission [3]. Etiology of major trauma includes motor vehicle accidents, bullet injuries, blunt trauma injuries, fall from certain heights, glass injuries, blast injuries, etc. These traumatic injuries are potentially associated with major vascular laceration(s) or organ rupture, leading to extensive blood loss. Most of the patients die on their way to the hospital because of massive hemorrhage. Therefore, hemorrhage with hemorrhagic shock is still the leading cause of death in all major traumatic injuries worldwide [3].

Surgical Procedures

Liver Transplantation

In 1963, Starzl and colleagues performed the first liver transplantation procedure in human being. The first five patients all died of bleeding complications [4]. Liver transplantation

M. Im
Department of Anesthesiology, Lewis Katz School of Medicine Temple University, Temple University Hospital, Philadelphia, PA, USA

U. Iqbal
Department of Anesthesiology, NYU Langone School of Medicine, New York, NY, USA

H. Yan
Department of Anesthesiology, Wuhan Central Hospital, Wuhan, Hubei, China

J. Sanders
Drexel University College of Medicine, West Reading, PA, USA

H. Liu (✉)
Department of Anesthesiology and Perioperative Medicine, Milton S. Hershey Medical Center, Penn State College of Medicine, Hershey, PA, USA

© Springer Nature Switzerland AG 2021
C. S. Scher et al. (eds.), *Essentials of Blood Product Management in Anesthesia Practice*,
https://doi.org/10.1007/978-3-030-59295-0_8

Table 8.2 Consequences of liver disease on coagulation [80]

1. Thrombocytopenia
2. Accelerated or decreased fibrinolysis
3. Qualitative defects in platelets function
4. Predisposition to fibrinolysis

has usually been associated with massive bleeding and requires a considerable amount of blood transfusion. The etiologies of liver transplantation-associated bleeding can be multifactorial including preoperative liver failure, cirrhosis, cholestasis, and splenomegaly; intraoperative transaction of the fragile collateral vessels, release of heparin-like factors from the allograft, coagulopathy; and postoperative leaking at vascular anastomosis, graft-versus-host disease, thrombocytopenia, and coagulopathy [5]. Intraoperative management-related issues such as massive volume load and subsequent hypothermia & hypocalcemia secondary to citrate toxicity can also significantly worsen the pre-existing coagulopathy, thus further increase the perioperative hemorrhage [6]. Excessive blood loss and a large quantity of blood transfusion during orthotopic liver transplant are unfortunately associated with significantly decreased graft survival and markedly increased episodes of sepsis and prolonged ICU stay [6]. In principle, the degree of hemorrhage can be estimated based on the severity of preoperative liver disease and coagulation function, quality of the donor's liver, recipient's overall clinical status, and surgical skills and experience of the transplantation team [7]. There is a strong correlation between Model for End-Stage Liver Disease (MELD) score and transfusion requirements in patients undergoing orthotopic liver transplantation. Higher MELD scores (>30) were found to be significantly associated with increased bleeding and transfusion requirements when compared to patients with lower MELD scores (< 30) [8]. Massive bleeding may result from multiple clinical consequences, as illustrated in Table 8.2.

Cardiothoracic and Major Vascular Surgery

In cardiothoracic or major vascular surgeries, surgeons deal with main blood vessels like aorta, coronaries, femoral, tibial, brachial, or vertebral arteries. These procedures usually involve vascular anastomosis, therefore, there are higher chances of intraoperative and postoperative severe hemorrhage leading to significant adverse outcome.

Major Cancer and Spine Surgery

Reconstructive and multilevel procedures like spine surgery and spine fusion procedures are potentially complicated by significant intraoperative blood loss and the need for allogeneic blood transfusion. The unique prone position for spine surgery likely leads to increased intraabdominal pressure, which increases epidural venous pressure and consequently exacerbates intraoperative surgical bleeding. Raised intraabdominal pressure can be measured via a urinary bladder catheter [9]. The total blood loss is proportionate with the intraabdominal pressure, also proportionate with the patient's body mass index (BMI) [9]. In another study, the effects of prone versus jackknife position on intraabdominal pressure and intraoperative bleeding during lumbar disc herniation surgery were conducted, and intraabdominal pressure came out to be significantly higher in a prone position [10]. Anesthetic agents in spine and cancer surgeries can play an important role in exacerbating intraoperative blood loss like sevoflurane results in significantly greater intraoperative blood loss than Propofol [11]. Certain cancer surgeries also cause massive perioperative bleeding due to extensive intratumor blood vessel networks that lead to unpredictable internal bleeding during surgery. A case report of metastatic prostate adenocarcinoma described a patient who developed hyperfibrinolysis leading to widespread ecchymosis and disseminated intravascular coagulation (DIC). Any surgical attempt to resect this type of cancer can potentially lead to massive perioperative hemorrhage and other complications [12].

Coagulation Abnormalities

Acute Traumatic Coagulopathy

It could mainly be an iatrogenic or secondary coagulopathy, a condition in which various elements are thought to play a role, including consumption of clotting factors, hemodilution from a large quantity of crystalloid infusion, acidosis, and hypothermia. The exact mechanism of coagulopathy is still unknown. One theory believes that actual injury causes a release of certain tissue factors that result in thrombin and fibrin generation and utilization, leading to DIC [13]. Another theory describes that trauma-induced hypoperfusion and ischemia lead to a release of activated protein C, which leads to consumption of plasminogen activator inhibitor, inhibition of the clotting cascade, systemic anticoagulation, and hyperfibrinolysis [14].

Clotting Factors Deficiencies

Clotting factors deficiencies may be congenital or acquired. Congenital coagulation factor deficiency includes factor VIII deficiency called hemophilia A disease and deficiency of factor IX called hemophilia B. Another congenital bleeding disorder is Von Willebrand's disease caused by a deficiency of Von Willebrand's Factor (vWF). Acquired clotting factors deficiency also develops in selective individuals because of the autoantibodies affecting the activity or accelerating the clearance of clotting factors [15]. Such antibodies are usually directed against factor VIII and vWF. These acquired antibodies are IgG4 type targeting several epitopes of clotting factors [16].

Dilutional Coagulopathy

Dilutional coagulopathy is defined as a coagulation abnormality due to "loss, consumption, or dilution of coagulation factors that occurs when blood is replaced with fluids that do not contain adequate coagulation factors" [17]. This hemostatic disturbance is further deteriorated by continuous crystalloid administration, acidosis, fibrinolysis, and hypothermia. It is a multifaceted change that affects thrombin generation, clot firmness, and fibrinolysis. Acquired fibrinogen deficiency is considered the leading cause of dilutional coagulopathy [18]. High-molecular weight dextran is also linked to severe disturbances of clot formation [19]. This impact on clot formation was significantly reduced by introducing new low-molecular weight starches, but depending on the amount of fluid given, marked impairment of hemostasis can still be observed. Rotation Thromboelastometry (ROTEM) is the test of choice to evaluate perioperative coagulation status. Fresh frozen plasma (FFP) transfusion 30 ml/kg is the treatment of choice for dilutional coagulopathy and in massive transfusion scenarios [20].

Obstetric Diseases

Definition of massive obstetric hemorrhage includes a fall in hemoglobin concentration of >40 g/L or blood loss of >2500 mL or transfusion of >4 units of RBCs [21]. Postpartum hemorrhage (PPH) means more than 1000 mL blood loss from the genital tract within 24 hours of birth [22]. Common etiologies include uterine atony, placenta previa, placenta accreta, placental abruption, uterine rupture, or embryonic emboli-associated DIC. In parturient, fibrinogen levels are 4–6 g/L, almost twice the level when compared to nonpregnant females. And the concurrent drop in protein C and S promotes prothrombotic state resulting in shorter PT and aPTT values. Thus, the combined results may come out normal in massive hemorrhage [23].

Amniotic fluid embolism leading to DIC usually occurs at term pregnancy or immediate postpartum period [24]. Amniotic fluid contains surfactants and various pro and anticoagulants. Surfactant, a lipoprotein produced by fetal lungs and present in increasing amounts in amniotic fluid with increasing gestational age, is structurally like tissue thromboplastin and possesses significant thromboplastic activity. It also contains cysteine protease that directly activates factor X, and it directly inhibits the PLTs [25]. Newborn may develop tachypnea and cyanosis. A patient shows signs of hypotension, brief-generalized seizures, profuse vaginal bleeding followed by unconsciousness. PT, aPTT, and bleeding time all are prolonged while fibrinogen level falls drastically. Treatment strategy comprises of blood component replacement, including RBC, FFP, PLT, cryoprecipitate, and possibly fibrinogen concentrate. Recombinant-activated factor VIIa (rFVIIa) use is associated with increased mortality as compared to the patients who do not receive rFVIIa [26].

Massive Transfusion Protocol

The damage control resuscitation concept was first proposed in the mid-2000s as an alternative approach to manage the hemorrhagic shock. Damage control resuscitation components are shown in Table 8.3 [17, 27].

An MTP has been developed to provide a standard set of blood products to the unstable trauma patients immediately and in a sustained manner [28]. MTPs may have a predefined ratio of RBC, FFP, and PLT units in each pack for transfusion which is usually set to what would be found in whole blood [29, 30]. A set ratio of each component should be tailored to individual institution's needs that commonly deal with trauma, obstetrics, cardiac, and other major vascular surgeries.

While most institutions have developed own MTPs, the common theme of all such protocols is determining specific triggers for activation of an MTP, transfusion end targets, the logistics of blood product, and adjunct availability [31]. Once the protocol is adopted, it is necessary to approach as a multidisciplinary team, including surgeons, anesthesiologists, hematologists, and blood bank personnel [28]. A common component of MTP is shown in Table 8.4.

Table 8.3 Components of damage control resuscitation [80]

1. Rapid control of surgical bleeding
2. Early and increased use of red blood cells, plasma, and platelets in a 1:1:1 ratio
3. Hypotensive resuscitation strategies
4. Prevention and treatment of hypothermia, hypocalcemia, and acidosis
5. Limitation of excessive crystalloid use

Table 8.4 Common component of massive transfusion protocol [39, 68]

Common component of MTP
1. An MTP activation and deactivation process
2. Communication between the patient area and blood bank
3. Transfusion services processes for delivery of blood products
4. Consistent blood component packs
5. Disposition of unused blood components
6. Activation of adjunct therapies
7. Consistent and timely laboratory testing
8. Performance improvement monitoring

The Purpose of MTP

The main purpose of MTP is to provide blood products early in the resuscitation and to treat coagulopathy in an immediate and sustained manner [28, 32]. The hemostatic resuscitation can be achieved by providing a predefined ratio of RBC: FFP: PLT. Hemostatic resuscitation has been reported to be beneficial in the trauma setting. Although the evidence of benefits with a high transfusion ratio of plasma to RBC, this practice has spread to the nontrauma setting as well [33, 34].

Generally, MTP is activated after replacement of total blood volume in 24 h needing ≥10 units of packed RBCs, replacement of >4 units of packed RBCs in 1 h with the anticipation of continuous need for blood products or replacement of 50% of the total blood volume within 3 h. Blood loss up to 1.5 ml/kg/min for more than 20 min. In children, this is activated after transfusion of 4–10 units [35].

Emergency release of blood products can be universally compatible (i.e., group O, Rh(D) negative RBCs or AB plasma) or type-specific, if the patient's blood type is known [36]. Upon activation of MTP, sufficient types and volume of the blood can be delivered with short turnaround times [37]. Time delay in receiving blood products can significantly impact the resuscitation of massive hemorrhage and contribute to morbidity and mortality [38]. Protocols should include periodical laboratory tests to monitor coagulation status and hemostatic resuscitation. In some instances, point of care coagulation (POC) testing can provide the guidance to assess ongoing hemorrhage [39].

Optimal Ratios and Components of Blood Products

RBC, FFP, and PLT

The majority of the institutions have massive transfusion protocols provide 1:1:1 ratio of RBC:FFP: PLT since the early-mid 2000s. Retrospectively, the survival data from military and civilian trauma patients showed the benefit of transfusion with equal amounts of RBC, FFP, and PLT during the early phase of resuscitation [28, 40]. However, the optimal ratio of blood products remains debatable. Holcomb et al. conducted prospective cohort study which did not show that 1:1:1 or 2:1:1 has a clinical difference in mortality during the first 24 hours after admission [3]. This result was confirmed in a multisite, randomized clinical trial of 680 severely injured patients [41]. According to this study, there was no significant difference in mortality at 24 hours or at 30 days among patients with severe trauma and major bleeding with 1:1:1 or 2:1:1 RBC: FFP: PLT ratios. A recent systemic review of 16 randomized controlled trials concluded there is insufficient evidence of a difference in mortality and morbidity outcomes with a 2:1:1 (RBC: FFP: PLT) or 1:1:1 ratio of MTP [42]. In spite of the limited evidence of recommendation with 1:1:1 over 2:1:1 (RBC: FFP: PLT), most of the trauma centers of academic facilities in the United States use 1:1 ratio of RBC: FFP [43].

Fibrinogen Component

Low-plasma fibrinogen level has been observed in critical bleeding and associated with a risk of massive transfusion [33, 42, 44]. Fibrinogen supplementation during massive hemorrhage may be considered in addition to conventional MTP with RBCs, FFP, and PLTs. However, there is limited evidence of fibrinogen supplementation in terms of improving patient outcome. According to randomized controlled trials (RCTs) to determine the feasibility of cryoprecipitate or fibrinogen concentrates, RCTs did not show any difference in mortality or morbidity outcomes between the patients receiving fibrinogen components in addition to MTP [45, 46].

Whole Blood Compared to Component Therapy

Based on the experience in the military setting, whole blood use is associated with improved mortality outcome instead of component therapy with RBCs:FFP: PLT in a 1:1:1 ratio [47, 48]. One RCT to compare whole blood therapy with component therapy did not report any difference in 24-hour or 30-day mortality or morbidity outcomes between two groups. According to this study, the authors used leukodepleted cold stored whole blood which can reduce the safety concerns regarding whole blood transfusion [30].

Since the extensive military experience suggesting possible survival benefit, it may be warranted to conduct a multicenter RCT to evaluate the outcomes and adverse effect in massive hemorrhage [47].

Prediction of Massive Hemorrhage and Initiation of Protocol

Predicting massive bleeding and the decision to initiate an MTP can be challengeable. Foster et al. reviewed societal guidelines from the American Society of Anesthesiologists (ASA), American College of Surgeons (ACS), and European Society for Advanced Bleeding Care in Trauma (ABC-Trauma), and supporting literature with massive transfusion prediction scoring systems [49]. All three societies recommend using scoring systems to initiate a massive transfusion. The ASA and ACS recommend Assessment of Blood Consumption (ABC) Score Massive Hemorrhage and Initiation of Protocol, which is a 4-variable scoring system assessing massive transfusion risk in trauma patients shown in Table 8.5 [39, 50, 51].

Table 8.5 Assessment of bleeding consumption score [49]

Variable	Value	Points
Systolic blood pressure (mm Hg)	≤90	1
Heart rate (beats/min)	≥120	1
Focused Assessment with Sonography for Trauma examination (FAST)	Positive	1
Mechanism of injury	Penetrating	1
Score range	Positive score-threshold	0–49

Table 8.6 Shock index [52]

Shock index	HR (beats/min)/SBP (mmHg)
Positive-score threshold	SI ≥ 0.9 predicting massive hemorrhage (Olaussen) SI ≥ 0.8 predicting MTP (El-Menya)

While the American guidelines use ABC score activates the MTP, European guideline suggests that the shock index (SI) be used to assess the degree of hypovolemic shock [52]. SI is defined as the ratio of heart rate to systolic blood pressure, which has been used in massive transfusion risk assessments in the patients for critical bleeding [53–55]. SI with the prediction of massive transfusion is shown in Table 8.6.

Continuation of Massive Transfusion and Monitoring

In massive hemorrhage, clinicians should assess the extent of bleeding in consideration of the patient's physiology, injury pattern, mechanism of hemorrhage, and the initial response to the resuscitation [56]. Majority of the MTPs based on the fixed ratio of blood transfusion, however, it is necessary to reassess continuously ongoing changes and further resuscitation guided by hemodynamic monitoring and coagulation tests. Instead of focusing on applying one standardized protocol to all critical bleeding patients, MTP implementation should address specific factors of bleeding, source control, hemostatic monitoring, and physiologic responses following massive transfusion.

Laboratory Directed Transfusion Management in MTP

Prothrombin Time and Activated Partial Thromboplastin Time

Prothrombin Time (PT) is used to test Factor VII in the extrinsic factor pathway. Activated Partial Thromboplastin Time (aPTT) measures the integrity of the intrinsic system (Factor VIII, IX, XI, XII). Using the cut-off value of International Normalized Ratio (INR) of more than 1.5 times normal, PT demonstrates a sensitivity of 88% and a specificity of 88% in detecting at least one nonhemostatic coagulation factor level after trauma whereas prolongation of aPTT demonstrates a sensitivity of only 50% and a specificity of 100% because Factor VIII is often increased as an acute phase reactant in trauma and surgical patients [57]. The limitations of PT, aPTT are summarized in Table 8.7.

Table 8.7 Limitations of PT/aPTT [80, 81]

1. PT and aPTT do not provide any clue about in vivo interaction of platelets with coagulation factors
2. PT and aPTT remain prolonged even if thrombin generation is improved because of antithrombin or protein C deficiency
3. PT/aPTT does not tell about the overall stability of a hemostatic thrombus because both tests are terminated at very low thrombin levels and before fibrin is polymerized

Table 8.8 Advantages/disadvantages of POC testing [80, 82]

Advantages of POC testing	Disadvantages of POC testing
Small sample volume	Variation in performance between devices
Rapid test results	Lack of detailed guidelines for performance and quality controls
No transportation of samples	Overpriced tests
Portable devices and flexibilities to move to labs or exam rooms	Pre-existing coagulopathies or hypo/hyperthermia can affect the results

Point of Care Testing

POC testing is suggested in most of the trauma patients who have significant injuries to provide valuable information promptly. The advantages and disadvantages of POC are summarized in Table 8.8.

Thromboelastography and Rotational Thromboelastometry

Because PT and aPTT tests are usually performed in central laboratories of the hospital, there is a substantial time delay in getting the results. TEG or ROTEM can be performed as a POC hemostasis monitoring test. Both tests evaluate the speed and strength of clot formation as well as clot stability, but also help to diagnose hemophilia, fibrinogen deficiency, Factor XIII deficiency, and fibrinolytic state [33, 58].

Arterial Blood Gas Analysis

It includes basic electrolytes, glucose level, lactate measurement, arterial hemoglobin level as well as blood gas analysis. Timely measurement of these parameters facilitates in assessment of occurrence and severity of any disturbance and helps its management accordingly [39].

Termination of the Protocol

Based on PROPPR trial [41], the decision to terminate an MTP should include control of bleeding anatomically and physiologic recovery such as stable hemodynamic status. Laboratory values should be used additionally to guide further transfusion requirements. Once the ongoing bleeding is controlled, the fixed ratio MTP may be switched to the goal-directed protocol based on the laboratory finding. Frequent communication among the providers can facilitate the process of MTP to guide continuing blood transfusion, need for adjuncts, and determine the end of protocols [39].

Complications and Drawback of MTPs

Massive transfusion can lead to some complications such as acid-base disturbances, electrolyte abnormalities, and hypothermia, in addition to acute trauma coagulopathy, which is reviewed in Table 8.9.

The economic consequence of utilizing multiple blood products should be considered to minimize the wastage of unused products [32, 39]. It is crucial to ensure the MTP does not waste valuable resources by determining the initiation and termination process of the protocol [39].

MTP Strategies in Trauma and NonTrauma Settings

Hemostatic resuscitation with early transfusion with a higher ratio of plasma and PLTs to RBC has improved patient outcome, including mortality and morbidity in trauma setting [59]. Trauma-induced coagulopathy (TIC) is one of the complex phenomena in trauma patients causing critical bleeding. Early correction of TIC by an MTP activation plays a vital role in the initial resuscitation of trauma patients [60].

Although an MTP also applied to the patients with critical bleeding in the trauma and nontrauma settings, there is limited evidence that implementation of trauma MPT improves the outcome in nontrauma patients [61, 62]. Patel et al. conducted retrospective study to characterize blood utilization in a trauma MTP (6 units of RBCs, 5 units of FFP, and 1 unit apheresis PLTs) and a nontrauma MPT (6 units of RBCs and 3 units of FFP). In the nontrauma MTP group, majority of the patients did not require to switch to a trauma MTP and received lower numbers of transfusion with less wastage of unused blood products. A nontrauma MTP can optimize blood utilization instead of using universal MTP in trauma and nontrauma settings [62].

Table 8.9 Complications of massive transfusion [35]

Complications
Acute
Dilutional coagulopathy
Blood cells hemolysis
Metabolic acidosis
Electrolytes imbalances
Hyperkalemia
Hypocalcemia
Hypomagnesemia
Transfusion-related acute lung injury(TRALI)
Transfusion-associated circulatory overload (TACO)
Decreased oxygen distribution to tissues
Delayed
Postoperative bacterial infections
Microchimerism
Systemic inflammatory response syndrome
Immunosuppression
Longer hospital stays
Increased mortality

Massive Transfusion Protocol for Specific Patient Groups

Trauma

In trauma patients, MTPs have improved patient outcomes by providing blood product with the ratios closer to whole blood and early correction of coagulopathy. The implementation of MTPs improved efficiency in initial resuscitation of severely injured trauma patients such as quicker access to the first blood product, multidisciplinary team approach, and better communication among the providers. Based on PROPPR data, there is still benefit to use RBCs, FFP, and PLT in a 1:1:1 ratio in exsanguination which is prominent cause of death in 24 hours, however, there was no difference in mortality and morbidity compared to 2:1:1 group in mortality at 24 hours and 30 days [41]. Criteria to trigger the activation of the protocol and the subsequent process in trauma MTP are shown in Tables 8.10 and 8.11.

Major Hepatic Surgery and Liver Transplantation

Major hepatic surgery, including liver transplantation, is associated with massive hemorrhage during surgery. Hepatic surgery is performed in a mostly well-controlled setting and coagulation monitoring is available to guide transfusion.

Table 8.10 Criteria to trigger the activation of an MTP [39]

Criteria
ABC score ≥ 2
Persistent hemodynamic instability
Activates bleeding requiring operation or angioembolization
Blood transfusion in the trauma bay

Table 8.11 Sample massive transfusion protocol in trauma [39]

Transfuse Universal RBCs and FFP in a ratio between 1:1 or 2:1
Add one single donor apheresis PLT or random donor pool PLT every 6 units of RBCs
Automatically send a cooler with blood products in an established ratio by the blood bank
Subsequent coolers should be sent at 15-minutes intervals until termination of an MTP
Once major bleeding has been controlled, switch to a laboratory or POC-based transfusion
Once laboratory data available, resuscitation should be goal-directed based on clinical assessment and laboratory findings

POC coagulation monitors enable the accurate and rapid coagulation assessment intraoperatively to treat coagulopathy. In the uncontrolled hemorrhage, a fixed ratio MTP is still considered as a feasible option. Tune et al. reported the utilization of an MTP during liver resection with acute vascular bleeding [63]. An MTP is allowed to reduce the processing and transport time of blood products, and improve administration time in uncontrolled hemorrhage.

Although there is still limited evidence whether goal driven resuscitation guided by laboratory tests or fixed ratio MTPs, POC coagulation monitor-guided transfusion strategy would be recommended in the controlled setting such as major hepatic procedures. Ball et al. conducted a retrospective cohort study to evaluate the influence of a high plasma ratio MTP in major hepatic injury patients [64]. Overall, there was no difference in mortality; however, in MTP cohort, the rate of primary abdominal fascial closure was significantly higher than a preMTP cohort. The authors observed a decrease in crystalloid resuscitation following the use of an MTP. An MTP implementation and less crystalloid resuscitation led a decrease in both visceral and abdominal wall edema, which may improve the rate of definitive abdominal fascial closure [64].

Cardiac and Major Vascular Surgery

Cardiac surgery is one of the surgical settings requiring massive transfusion. Massive bleeding during cardiac surgery is associated with PLT dysfunction induced by cardiopulmonary bypass. However, the component of massive transfusion during cardiac surgery is not investigated. Delaney et al. analyzed data from a prospective RCT whether massive transfusion with a high ratio of FFP: RBC (1:1 or higher) or PLT: RBC (1:5 or higher) can impact the clinical outcomes in patients undergoing complex cardiac surgery [65, 66]. According to this study, less organ dysfunction was observed in the patients with a high ratio of FFP: RBC or PLT: RBC, and lower mortality in high ratio FFP: RBC group. TEG and ROTEM have been used successfully to predict excessive hemorrhage in cardiac surgery. However, their effect on mortality is still debatable [67].

Obstetric Hemorrhage

During pregnancy, the level of coagulation factors, including fibrinogen, vWF, and factor VIII, have increased that result in a prothrombotic state [68]. In obstetric hemorrhage, hemorrhage protocols or MTPs have been recommended to promote maternal safety [37, 69]. However, obstetric MTPs have been based on trauma experience without validating exclusively in obstetric hemorrhage. While ACOG recommended a fixed ratio of hemorrhage protocol, CMQCC recommendations include the emergency release of blood package with laboratory-guided transfusion strategy if time permits [32, 70].

Fibrinogen level during obstetric hemorrhage has been described as a biomarker for severe postpartum hemorrhage (PPH). A serum fibrinogen level below 200 mg/dL had a positive predictive value for severe PPH of 100% [71]. Although the appropriate fibrinogen level to maintain during PPH is not defined clearly, most of the societal guidelines recommend to replace fibrinogen when the level is between 125 and 200 mg/dL [22, 70, 72]. Cryoprecipitate (CRYO) is the most common form of fibrinogen replacement in the U.S. The usual dose of cryoprecipitates is 10 units expected to raise the serum fibrinogen 100 mg/dL in adult. Early fibrinolysis has been observed during childbirth [73]. Based on the trials from trauma and surgery, antifibrinolytic agent administration during PPH is recommended [32, 74]. The most recent international RCT to investigate the effect of early tranexamic acid (TXA) administration showed TXA-reduced death caused by PPH when it was used within 3 hours of giving birth especially [74]. Laboratory tests should be obtained as clinically indicated during an MTP activation. A suggested obstetric MTP is shown in Table 8.12.

Table 8.12 Sample obstetric hemorrhage MTP [32, 70]

Round	RBC (units)	FFP (units)	PLT (units)	CRYO (units)	TXA
1	6	6	6		
2	6	6	6		
3	6	6	6	8–10 repeat every third round	1 G IV over 10 min

Consider activating an MTP when 50% or more of blood volume needs to be replaced within 2 hours, bleeding continues after the transfusion of 4 units of RBCs within 1–2 hours, or systolic blood pressure is below 90 mm Hg and heart rate is above 120 beats per minute in the presence of uncontrolled bleeding. Cryoprecipitates may be considered to maintain the serum fibrinogen 150–200 mg/dL. After third round, if an MTP is not terminated, will repeat from round 1

Pediatric Population

In most of the pediatric population, the adult MTP can be applied as RBC: FFP: PLT ratio of 1:1:1. However, for smaller children, this protocol should be adjusted as a weight-based system [75, 76]. Dehmer et al. reviewed the transfusion management in pediatric trauma patients and suggested sample pediatric MTP in their recent publication [76]. The authors recommend including the following elements in pediatric MTPs in Table 8.13.

Outcomes, Performance, and Complication Monitoring

There is a good quality of evidence that the implementation of MTP improves patient outcomes, but also potential benefits enhancing the efficiencies of blood utilization, delivery of the care, and communication among the providers [33]. One study by Riskin et al. found a significant reduction in mortality despite unchanged blood component ratio and numbers of transfusion after the MTP implementation [77]. The authors conclude the improved survival was mainly achieved by the blood product availability promptly, and multidisciplinary team approaches concurrently.

Since the beginning of the implementation of MTPs, performance, and quality improvement review by a multidisciplinary committee for compliance were strongly recommended [28]. Performance indicators should include the time from activation of MTP to first RBC and plasma administration, adherence to a predetermined ratio or goal between 1–2 hours after initiation, informing the transfusion service within 1 hour of protocol termination, and wastage rate of blood products [39]. The example of performance indicators is shown in Table 8.14. According to the literature review, full compliance was significantly associated with survival rate [78, 79]. Bawazzer et al. measured compliance of MTP with their protocol criteria including timely activation and deactivation of the protocol, laboratory assessment in the trauma bay, communication with the blood bank, and prevention of wasting blood products. Based on the result of the study, noncompliance was observed more commonly in sending a complete hemorrhage panel from the trauma bay and monitoring blood work periodically. Also, discontinuation of the protocol following compliance was associated with a reduction in blood product wastage [79].

Massive transfusion could lead to a higher incidence of transfusion-related complications, including transfusion-related acute lung injury, immunomodulation, infectious disease, transfusion reactions, metabolic derangement, and circulatory overload. Therefore, it is recommended the trauma centers should review this massive transfusion-related complications in addition to the performance indicators [39].

Table 8.13 Suggested sample pediatric MTP [76]

Initiation	Persistent hemodynamic instability Ongoing bleeding after 40 ml/kg of crystalloid infusion More than 40 mL/kg packed red blood cells (PRBCs) transfused
Blood components	≥30 kg, 1:1:1 (RBC: FFP: PLT) with CRYO (4 ml/kg) in low-fibrinogen level (100–150 mg/dL) or ongoing bleeding after first round <30 kg, Wt-based 30:20:20 ratio EBL (ml/kg) 20–40: Crystalloid IV 20–40 ml/kg EBL 40 and above: RBC 30 ml/kg After 1 BV lost: RBC 30 ml/kg + FFP 20 ml/kg After 2 BV lost: RBC 30 ml/kg + FFP 20 ml/kg + PLT 20 ml/kg + CRYO 4 ml/kg
Monitoring	Body temperature Laboratory data including serum calcium and blood pH
rFVIIa	In extreme cases (i.e., after 3 BV lost), consider dose 90 mcg/kg

Table 8.14 An example of trauma massive transfusion protocol audit filters [28]

Initiation	Activated by the trauma surgeon
Blood product	Timely acquired of blood samples for type and screening process from ED
	PRBC: plasma administered in a ratio of 3:2
	PRBC: Platelets administered in a ratio of 5:1
	Timely response of required personnel and blood products from the blood bank
	Unused blood products are appropriately stored
Discontinuation	MTP discontinued when the active hemorrhage has been controlled

Summary

This chapter highlights the management of massive hemorrhage with MTPs. We discussed the implications of MTPs, including trauma, major hepatic, major vascular, cardiothoracic, spine surgery, and obstetric and pediatric patients. Activation and termination criteria of MTPs were discussed. Current evidence recommends using ratios either 2:1:1 or 1:1:1 of RBC:FFP:PLT, which is based on the trauma MTPs. Fibrinogen replacement is also indicated in obstetric hemorrhage and other uncontrolled, ongoing hemorrhage with fibrinogenemia. Initial massive transfusion with a fixed ratio of blood products can be switched as a laboratory-based protocol by POC tests or other coagulation studies when critical hemorrhage is controlled. Outcomes and compliance measurement are necessary to improve the performance and quality of MTPs. The implementation of an MTP has impacted the patient outcomes, but also improved the efficiencies in blood utilization and delivery of care. The multidisciplinary team approach plays a crucial role in the success of an MTPs.

References

1. Cleland S, Corredor C, Ye JJ, Srinivas C, McCluskey SA. Massive haemorrhage in liver transplantation: consequences, prediction and management. World J Transplant [Internet]. 2016;6(2):291; [cited 2019 May 19]. Available from: http://www.wjgnet.com/2220-3230/full/v6/i2/291.htm.
2. Hellstern P, Haubelt H. Indications for plasma in massive transfusion. Thromb Res [Internet]. 2002;107(Suppl 1):S19–22; [cited 2019 May 19]. Available from: http://www.ncbi.nlm.nih.gov/pubmed/12379288.
3. Holcomb JB, del Junco DJ, Fox EE, Wade CE, Cohen MJ, Schreiber MA, et al. The prospective, observational, multicenter, major trauma transfusion (PROMMTT) study: comparative effectiveness of a time-varying treatment with competing risks. JAMA Surg [Internet]. 2013;148(2):127–36; [cited 2019 May 14]. Available from: http://www.ncbi.nlm.nih.gov/pubmed/23560283.
4. Eiseman B. The puzzle people: memoirs of a transplant surgeon. Arch Surg [Internet]. 1992;127(9):1009–11; [cited 2019 May 28]. Available from: http://www.ncbi.nlm.nih.gov/pubmed/1514901.
5. Donohue CI, Mallett SV. Reducing transfusion requirements in liver transplantation. World J Transplant [Internet]. 2015;5(4):165; [cited 2019 May 19]. Available from: http://www.ncbi.nlm.nih.gov/pubmed/26722645.
6. Pandey CK, Singh A, Kajal K, Dhankhar M, Tandon M, Pandey VK, et al. Intraoperative blood loss in orthotopic liver transplantation: The predictive factors. World J Gastrointest Surg [Internet]. 2015;7(6):86; [cited 2019 May 19]. Available from: http://www.ncbi.nlm.nih.gov/pubmed/26131330.
7. Feltracco P, Brezzi M, Barbieri S, Galligioni H, Milevoj M, Carollo C, et al. Blood loss, predictors of bleeding, transfusion practice and strategies of blood cell salvaging during liver transplantation. World J Hepatol [Internet]. 2013;5(1):1–15; [cited 2019 May 19]. Available from: http://www.wjgnet.com/1948-5182/full/v5/i1/1.htm.
8. Perkins JD. Are we reporting the same thing? Liver Transpl [Internet]. 2007;13(3):465–6; [cited 2019 May 19]. Available from: http://www.ncbi.nlm.nih.gov/pubmed/17396292.
9. Han IH, Son DW, Nam KH, Choi BK, Song GS. The effect of body mass index on intra-abdominal pressure and blood loss in lumbar spine surgery. J Korean Neurosurg Soc [Internet]. 2012;51(2):81; [cited 2019 May 19]. Available from: http://www.ncbi.nlm.nih.gov/pubmed/22500198.
10. Akinci IO, Tunali U, Kyzy AA, Guresti E, Sencer A, Karasu A, et al. Effects of prone and jackknife positioning on lumbar disc herniation surgery. J Neurosurg Anesthesiol [Internet]. 2011;23(4):318–22; [cited 2019 May 19]. Available from: https://insights.ovid.com/crossref?an=00008506-201110000-00006.
11. Willner D, Spennati V, Stohl S, Tosti G, Aloisio S, Bilotta F. Spine surgery and blood loss. Anesth Analg [Internet]. 2016;123(5):1307–15; [cited 2019 May 19]. Available from: http://www.ncbi.nlm.nih.gov/pubmed/27749350.
12. Palma Anselmo M, Nobre de Jesus G, Lopes JM, Victorino RMM, Meneses Santos J. Massive bleeding as the first clinical manifestation of metastatic prostate cancer due to disseminated intravascular coagulation with enhanced fibrinolysis. Case Rep Hematol [Internet]. 2016;2016:7217915; [cited 2019 May 28]. Available from: https://www.hindawi.com/journals/crihem/2016/7217915/.
13. Gando S, Otomo Y. Local hemostasis, immunothrombosis, and systemic disseminated intravascular coagulation in trauma and traumatic shock. Crit Care [Internet]. 2015;19(1):72; [cited 2019 May 19]. Available from: http://www.ncbi.nlm.nih.gov/pubmed/25886801.
14. Brohi K, Cohen MJ, Ganter MT, Schultz MJ, Levi M, Mackersie RC, et al. Acute coagulopathy of trauma: hypoperfusion induces systemic anticoagulation and hyperfibrinolysis. J Trauma Inj Infect Crit Care [Internet]. 2008;64(5):1211–7; [cited 2019 May 19]. Available from: http://www.ncbi.nlm.nih.gov/pubmed/18469643.
15. Franchini M, Castaman G, Coppola A, Santoro C, Zanon E, Di Minno G, et al. Acquired inhibitors of clotting factors: AICE recommendations for diagnosis and management. Blood Transfus [Internet]. 2015;13(3):498–513; [cited 2019 May 19]. Available from: http://www.ncbi.nlm.nih.gov/pubmed/26192778.
16. Lindgren A, Wadenvik H, Tengborn L. Characterization of inhibitors to FVIII with an ELISA in congenital and acquired haemophilia A. Haemophilia [Internet]. 2002;8(5):644–8; [cited 2019 May 19]. Available from: http://www.ncbi.nlm.nih.gov/pubmed/12199673.
17. Ho AM-H, Dion PW, Yeung JHH, Holcomb JB, Critchley LAH, Ng CSH, et al. Prevalence of survivor bias in observational studies on fresh frozen plasma:erythrocyte ratios in trauma requiring massive transfusion. Anesthesiology [Internet]. 2012;116(3):716–28; [cited 2019 May 19]. Available from: http://anesthesiology.pubs.asahq.org/Article.aspx? https://doi.org/10.1097/ALN.0b013e318245c47b.
18. Innerhofer P, Kienast J. Principles of perioperative coagulopathy. Best Pract Res Clin Anaesthesiol [Internet]. 2010;24(1):1–14; [cited 2019 May 19]. Available from: http://www.ncbi.nlm.nih.gov/pubmed/20402166.
19. Fenger-Eriksen C, Tønnesen E, Ingerslev J, Sørensen B. Mechanisms of hydroxyethyl starch-induced dilutional coagulopathy. J Thromb Haemost [Internet]. 2009;7(7):1099–105; [cited 2019 May 19]. Available from: http://doi.wiley.com/10.1111/j.1538-7836.2009.03460.x.
20. Haas T, Mauch J, Weiss M, Schmugge M. Management of dilutional coagulopathy during pediatric major surgery. Transfus Med Hemother [Internet]. 2012;39(2):114–9; [cited 2019 May 19]. Available from: http://www.ncbi.nlm.nih.gov/pubmed/22670129.
21. Collis RE, Collins PW. Haemostatic management of obstetric haemorrhage. Anaesthesia [Internet]. 2015;70:78-e28; [cited 2019 May 19]. Available from: http://www.ncbi.nlm.nih.gov/pubmed/25440400.
22. Committee on Practice Bulletins-Obstetrics. Practice Bulletin No. 183. Obstet Gynecol [Internet]. 2017;130(4):e168–86; [cited 2017 Oct 24]. Available from: http://www.ncbi.nlm.nih.gov/pubmed/28937571.
23. Szecsi P, Jørgensen M, Klajnbard A, Andersen M, Colov N, Stender S. Haemostatic reference intervals in pregnancy. Thromb Haemost [Internet]. 2010;103(4):718–27; [cited 2019 May 19]. Available from: http://www.ncbi.nlm.nih.gov/pubmed/20174768.
24. Tamura N, Farhana M, Oda T, Itoh H, Kanayama N. Amniotic fluid embolism: Pathophysiology from the perspective of pathology. J Obstet Gynaecol Res [Internet]. 2017;43(4):627–32; [cited 2019 May 28]. Available from: http://www.ncbi.nlm.nih.gov/pubmed/28188959.
25. Harnett MJP, Hepner DL, Datta S, Kodali BS. Effect of amniotic fluid on coagulation and platelet function in pregnancy: an evaluation using thromboelastography. Anaesthesia [Internet]. 2005;60(11):1068–72; [cited 2019 May 19]. Available from: http://www.ncbi.nlm.nih.gov/pubmed/16229690.
26. Leighton BL, Wall MH, Lockhart EM, Phillips LE, Zatta AJ. Use of recombinant factor VIIa in patients with amniotic fluid embolism. Anesthesiology [Internet]. 2011;115(6):1; [cited 2019 May 28]. Available from: http://www.ncbi.nlm.nih.gov/pubmed/21720243.
27. del Junco DJ, Bulger EM, Fox EE, Holcomb JB, Brasel KJ, Hoyt DB, et al. Collider bias in trauma comparative effectiveness research: The stratification blues for systematic reviews. Injury [Internet]. 2015;46(5):775–80; [cited 2019 May 19]. Available from: http://www.ncbi.nlm.nih.gov/pubmed/25766096.
28. Nunez TC, Young PP, Holcomb JB, Cotton BA. Creation, implementation, and maturation of a massive transfusion protocol for the exsanguinating trauma patient. J Trauma [Internet].

2010;68(6):1498–505; [cited 2019 May 11]. Available from: http://www.ncbi.nlm.nih.gov/pubmed/20539192.

29. Patil V, Shetmahajan M. Massive transfusion and massive transfusion protocol. Indian J Anaesth [Internet]. 2014;58(5):590; [cited 2019 May 19]. Available from: http://www.ncbi.nlm.nih.gov/pubmed/25535421.
30. Cotton BA, Podbielski J, Camp E, Welch T, del Junco D, Bai Y, et al. A randomized controlled pilot trial of modified whole blood versus component therapy in severely injured patients requiring large volume transfusions. Ann Surg [Internet]. 2013;258(4):527–32; [cited 2019 May 22], discussion 532-3. Available from: https://www.facs.org/-/media/files/quality-programs/trauma/tqip/transfusion_guildelines.ashx.
31. Guerado E, Bertrand ML, Valdes L, Cruz E, Cano JR. Resuscitation of polytrauma patients: the management of massive skeletal bleeding. Open Orthop J [Internet]. 2015;9(1):283–95; [cited 2019 May 19]. Available from: http://www.ncbi.nlm.nih.gov/pubmed/26312112.
32. Pacheco LD, Saade GR, Costantine MM, Clark SL, GDV H. An update on the use of massive transfusion protocols in obstetrics. Am J Obstet Gynecol [Internet]. 2016;214(3):340–4; [cited 2019 Mar 25]. Available from: https://www-sciencedirect-com.ezproxy2.library.drexel.edu/science/article/pii/S0002937815010169.
33. Flint AWJ, McQuilten ZK, Wood EM. Massive transfusions for critical bleeding: is everything old new again? Transfus Med [Internet]. 2018;28(2):140–9; [cited 2019 Mar 25]. Available from: http://www.ncbi.nlm.nih.gov/pubmed/29607593.
34. Mesar T, Larentzakis A, Dzik W, Chang Y, Velmahos G, Yeh DD. Association between ratio of fresh frozen plasma to red blood cells during massive transfusion and survival among patients without traumatic injury. JAMA Surg [Internet]. 2017;152(6):574; [cited 2019 May 1]. Available from: http://archsurg.jamanetwork.com/article.aspx? https://doi.org/10.1001/jamasurg.2017.0098.
35. Guerado E, Medina A, Mata MI, Galvan JM, Bertrand ML. Protocols for massive blood transfusion: when and why, and potential complications. Eur J Trauma Emerg Surg [Internet]. 2016;42(3):283–95; [cited 2019 Apr 8]. Available from: http://www.ncbi.nlm.nih.gov/pubmed/26650716.
36. Main EK, Goffman D, Scavone BM, Low LK, Bingham D, Fontaine PL, et al. National partnership for maternal safety. Obstet Gynecol [Internet]. 2015;126(1):155–62; [cited 2019 May 1]. Available from: http://www.ncbi.nlm.nih.gov/pubmed/26091046.
37. Fung M, Harm S, Nester T. Transfusion management of the obstetrical patient: a clinical casebook. Cham: Springer; 2018. p. 39–45.
38. Shaylor R, Weiniger CF, Austin N, Tzabazis A, Shander A, Goodnough LT, et al. National and international guidelines for patient blood management in obstetrics. Anesth Analg [Internet]. 2017;124(1):216–32; [cited 2019 May 1]. Available from: http://www.ncbi.nlm.nih.gov/pubmed/27557476.
39. American College of Surgeons. ACS TQIP massive transfusion in trauma guidelines. 2013 [cited 2019 May 24]. Available from: https://www.facs.org/~/media/files/quality programs/trauma/tqip/massive transfusion in trauma guildelines.ashx.
40. Cannon JW, Khan MA, Raja AS, Cohen MJ, Como JJ, Cotton BA, et al. Damage control resuscitation in patients with severe traumatic hemorrhage. J Trauma Acute Care Surg [Internet]. 2017;82(3):605–17; [cited 2019 May 14]. Available from: http://www.ncbi.nlm.nih.gov/pubmed/28225743.
41. Holcomb JB, Tilley BC, Baraniuk S, Fox EE, Wade CE, Podbielski JM, et al. Transfusion of plasma, platelets, and red blood cells in a 1:1:1 vs a 1:1:2 ratio and mortality in patients with severe trauma: the PROPPR randomized clinical trial. JAMA [Internet]. 2015;313(5):471–82; [cited 2016 Nov 28]. Available from: http://www.pubmedcentral.nih.gov/articlerender.fcgi?artid=4374744&tool=pmcentrez&rendertype=abstract.
42. McQuilten ZK, Crighton G, Brunskill S, Morison JK, Richter TH, Waters N, et al. Optimal dose, timing and ratio of blood products in massive transfusion: results from a systematic review. Transfus Med Rev [Internet]. 2018;32(1):6–15; [cited 2019 Mar 25]. Available from: http://www.ncbi.nlm.nih.gov/pubmed/28803752.
43. Treml AB, Gorlin JB, Dutton RP, Scavone BM. Massive transfusion protocols. Anesth Analg [Internet]. 2017;124(1):277–81; [cited 2019 Apr 12]. Available from: http://www.ncbi.nlm.nih.gov/pubmed/27749352.
44. Lee DH, Lee BK, Noh SM, Cho YS. High fibrin/fibrinogen degradation product to fibrinogen ratio is associated with 28-day mortality and massive transfusion in severe trauma. Eur J Trauma Emerg Surg [Internet]. 2018;44(2):291–8; [cited 2019 May 22]. Available from: http://www.ncbi.nlm.nih.gov/pubmed/28921171.
45. Curry N, Rourke C, Davenport R, Beer S, Pankhurst L, Deary A, et al. Early cryoprecipitate for major haemorrhage in trauma: a randomised controlled feasibility trial. Br J Anaesth [Internet]. 2015;115(1):76–83; [cited 2019 May 22]. Available from: https://www.sciencedirect.com/science/article/pii/S0007091217312436.
46. Nascimento B, Callum J, Tien H, Peng H, Rizoli S, Karanicolas P, et al. Fibrinogen in the initial resuscitation of severe trauma (FiiRST): a randomized feasibility trial. Br J Anaesth [Internet]. 2016;117(6):775–82; [cited 2019 May 22]. Available from: https://www.sciencedirect.com/science/article/pii/S0007091217372008
47. Murdock AD, Berséus O, Hervig T, Strandenes G, Lunde TH. Whole blood: the future of traumatic hemorrhagic shock resuscitation. Shock [Internet]. 2014;41:62–9; [cited 2019 May 22]. Available from: http://www.ncbi.nlm.nih.gov/pubmed/24662782.
48. Nessen SC, Eastridge BJ, Cronk D, Craig RM, Berséus O, Ellison R, et al. Fresh whole blood use by forward surgical teams in Afghanistan is associated with improved survival compared to component therapy without platelets. Transfusion [Internet]. 2013;53(Suppl 1):107S–13S; [cited 2019 May 22]. Available from: http://doi.wiley.com/10.1111/trf.12044.
49. Foster JC, Sappenfield JW, Smith RS, Kiley SP. Initiation and termination of massive transfusion protocols. Anesth Analg [Internet]. 2017;125(6):2045–55; [cited 2019 Mar 25]. Available from: http://insights.ovid.com/crossref?an=00000539-201712000-00034.
50. Smith MC, Bauer AM, Pivalizza EG, Tanaka K, Boral L, Shander A, et al. Massive Transfusion ProtocoL (MTP) for hemorrhagic shock ASA Committee on Blood Management. 2012;1–11.
51. Cotton BA, Dossett LA, Haut ER, Shafi S, Nunez TC, Au BK, et al. Multicenter validation of a simplified score to predict massive transfusion in trauma. J Trauma [Internet]. 2010;69(Suppl 1):S33–9; [cited 2019 May 24]. Available from: https://insights.ovid.com/crossref?an=00005373-201007001-00006
52. Spahn DR, Bouillon B, Cerny V, Duranteau J, Filipescu D, Hunt BJ, et al. The European guideline on management of major bleeding and coagulopathy following trauma: fifth edition. Crit Care [Internet]. 2019;23(1):98; [cited 2019 May 21]. Available from: http://www.ncbi.nlm.nih.gov/pubmed/30917843.
53. Olaussen A, Blackburn T, Mitra B, Fitzgerald M. Review article: shock index for prediction of critical bleeding post-trauma: a systematic review. Emerg Med Australas [Internet]. 2014;26(3):223–8; [cited 2019 May 21]. Available from: http://doi.wiley.com/10.1111/1742-6723.12232.
54. El-Menyar A, Goyal P, Tilley E, Latifi R. The clinical utility of shock index to predict the need for blood transfusion and outcomes in trauma. J Surg Res [Internet]. 2018;227:52–9; [cited 2019 May 21]. Available from: https://linkinghub.elsevier.com/retrieve/pii/S0022480418300994.
55. Paladino L, Subramanian RA, Nabors S, Sinert R. The utility of shock index in differentiating major from minor injury. Eur J Emerg Med [Internet]. 2011;18(2):94–8; [cited 2019 May 28]. Available from: http://content.wkhealth.com/linkback/openurl?sid=WKPTLP:landingpage&an=00063110-201104000-00008.
56. Janelle GM, Shore-Lesserson L, Smith CE, Levy JH, Shander A. What is the PROPPR transfusion strategy in trauma resuscitation? Anesth Analg [Internet]. 2016;122(4):1216–9; [cited

2019 May 14]. Available from: http://www.ncbi.nlm.nih.gov/pubmed/26991624.
57. Yuan S, Ferrell C, Chandler WL. Comparing the prothrombin time INR versus the APTT to evaluate the coagulopathy of acute trauma. Thromb Res [Internet]. 2007;120(1):29–37; [cited 2019 May 28]. Available from: https://linkinghub.elsevier.com/retrieve/pii/S004938480600243X
58. Spiezia L, Radu C, Marchioro P, Bertini D, Rossetto V, Castelli M, et al. Peculiar whole blood rotation thromboelastometry (Rotem) profile in 40 sideropenic anaemia patients. Thromb Haemost [Internet]. 2008;100(6):1106–10; [cited 2019 May 22]. Available from: http://www.ncbi.nlm.nih.gov/pubmed/19132237.
59. McCullough J. Chapter 12: Transfusion therapy in specific clinical situations. In: Transfusion medicine. 4th ed. West Sussex: Wiley; 2017. p. 304–59.
60. Chang R, Cardenas JC, Wade CE, Holcomb JB. Advances in the understanding of trauma-induced coagulopathy. Blood [Internet]. 2016;128(8):1043–9; [cited 2019 May 22]. Available from: http://www.ncbi.nlm.nih.gov/pubmed/27381903.
61. Sommer N, Schnüriger B, Candinas D, Haltmeier T. Massive transfusion protocols in nontrauma patients. J Trauma Acute Care Surg [Internet]. 2019;86(3):493–504; [cited 2019 May 11]. Available from: http://www.ncbi.nlm.nih.gov/pubmed/30376535.
62. Patel EU, Ness PM, Marshall CE, Gniadek T, Efron DT, Miller PM, et al. Blood product utilization among trauma and non-trauma massive transfusion protocols at an Urban Academic Medical Center. Anesth Analg [Internet]. 2017;125(3):967–74; [cited 2019 Apr 8]. Available from: http://www.ncbi.nlm.nih.gov/pubmed/28719428.
63. Tune B. Utilization of a massive transfusion protocol during liver lobe resection: a case report [Internet]. AANA J. 2012;80:174; [cited 2019 May 16]. Available from: www.aana.com/aanajournalonline.
64. Ball CG, Dente CJ, Shaz B, Wyrzykowski AD, Nicholas JM, Kirkpatrick AW, et al. The impact of a massive transfusion protocol (1:1:1) on major hepatic injuries: does it increase abdominal wall closure rates? Can J Surg [Internet]. 2013;56(5):E128–34; [cited 2019 May 16]. Available from: http://www.ncbi.nlm.nih.gov/pubmed/24067528.
65. Steiner ME, Assmann SF, Levy JH, Marshall J, Pulkrabek S, Sloan SR, et al. Addressing the question of the effect of RBC storage on clinical outcomes: The Red Cell Storage Duration Study (RECESS) (Section 7). Transfus Apher Sci [Internet]. 2010;43(1):107–16; [cited 2019 May 23]. Available from: http://www.ncbi.nlm.nih.gov/pubmed/20655807.
66. Delaney M, Stark PC, Suh M, Triulzi DJ, Hess JR, Steiner ME, et al. Massive transfusion in cardiac surgery: the impact of blood component ratios on clinical outcomes and survival. Anesth Analg [Internet]. 2017;124(6):1777–82; [cited 2019 Mar 25]. Available from: http://www.ncbi.nlm.nih.gov/pubmed/28333704.
67. Petrou A, Tzimas P, Siminelakis S. Massive bleeding in cardiac surgery. Definitions, predictors and challenges. Hippokratia [Internet]. 2016;20(3):179–86; [cited 2019 May 16]. Available from: http://www.ncbi.nlm.nih.gov/pubmed/29097882.
68. Muirhead B, ADH W. Massive hemorrhage and transfusion in the operating room. Can J Anaesth [Internet]. 2017;64(9):962–78; [cited 2019 May 6]. Available from: http://link.springer.com/10.1007/s12630-017-0925-x.
69. O'Brien KL, Shainker SA, Lockhart EL. Transfusion management of obstetric hemorrhage. Transfus Med Rev [Internet]. 2018;32(4):249–55; [cited 2019 Mar 25]. Available from: https://www-sciencedirect-com.ezproxy2.library.drexel.edu/science/article/pii/S0887796318300130.
70. California Maternal Quality Care Collaborative. OB Hem Appendix D: sample massive transfusion protocol California Maternal Quality Care Collaborative [Internet]. [cited 2019 May 24]. Available from: https://www.cmqcc.org/resource/ob-hem-appendix-d-sample-massive-transfusion-protocol.
71. Charbit B, Mandelbrot L, Samain E, Baron G, Haddaoui B, Keita H, et al. The decrease of fibrinogen is an early predictor of the severity of postpartum hemorrhage. J Thromb Haemost [Internet]. 2007;5(2):266–73; [cited 2019 May 24]. Available from: http://doi.wiley.com/10.1111/j.1538-7836.2007.02297.x.
72. Royal College of Obstetricians and Gynaecologists. Postpartum haemorrhage, prevention and management (Green-top Guideline No. 52) [Internet]. 2016 [cited 2019 May 29]. p. Green-top Guidance No. 52. Available from: https://www.rcog.org.uk/en/guidelines-research-services/guidelines/gtg52/.
73. Kruithof EK, Tran-Thang C, Gudinchet A, Hauert J, Nicoloso G, Genton C, et al. Fibrinolysis in pregnancy: a study of plasminogen activator inhibitors. Blood [Internet]. 1987;69(2):460–6; [cited 2019 May 24]. Available from: http://www.ncbi.nlm.nih.gov/pubmed/2432970.
74. WOMAN Trial Collaborators H, Roberts I, Fawole B, Chaudhri R, El-Sheikh M, Akintan A, et al. Effect of early tranexamic acid administration on mortality, hysterectomy, and other morbidities in women with post-partum haemorrhage (WOMAN): an international, randomised, double-blind, placebo-controlled trial. Lancet (London, England) [Internet]. 2017;389(10084):2105–16; [cited 2019 May 24]. Available from: http://www.ncbi.nlm.nih.gov/pubmed/28456509.
75. Dressler AM, Finck CM, Carroll CL, Bonanni CC, Spinella PC. Use of a massive transfusion protocol with hemostatic resuscitation for severe intraoperative bleeding in a child. J Pediatr Surg [Internet]. 2010;45(7):1530–3; [cited 2019 May 16]. Available from: http://www.ncbi.nlm.nih.gov/pubmed/20638538.
76. Dehmer JJ, Adamson WT. Massive transfusion and blood product use in the pediatric trauma patient. Semin Pediatr Surg [Internet]. 2010;19(4):286–91; [cited 2019 May 29]. Available from: http://www.ncbi.nlm.nih.gov/pubmed/20889085.
77. Riskin DJ, Tsai TC, Riskin L, Hernandez-Boussard T, Purtill M, Maggio PM, et al. Massive transfusion protocols: the role of aggressive resuscitation versus product ratio in mortality reduction. J Am Coll Surg [Internet]. 2009;209(2):198–205; [cited 2019 May 11]. Available from: https://linkinghub.elsevier.com/retrieve/pii/S1072751509004670.
78. Cotton BA, Gunter OL, Isbell J, Au BK, Robertson AM, Morris JA, et al. Damage control hematology: the impact of a trauma exsanguination protocol on survival and blood product utilization. J Trauma Inj Infect Crit Care [Internet]. 2008;64(5):1177–83; [cited 2019 May 19]. Available from: http://www.ncbi.nlm.nih.gov/pubmed/18469638.
79. Bawazeer M, Ahmed N, Izadi H, McFarlan A, Nathens A, Pavenski K. Compliance with a massive transfusion protocol (MTP) impacts patient outcome. Injury [Internet]. 2015;46(1):21–8; [cited 2019 May 9]. Available from: https://linkinghub.elsevier.com/retrieve/pii/S0020138314004604.
80. Iqbal U, Sanders J, Yang L, Li M, Zebrower M, Liu H. Massive perioperative hemorrhage: considerations in clinical management. In: Catastrophic perioperative complications and management [Internet]. Cham: Springer International Publishing; 2019. p. 133–49; [cited 2019 May 29]. Available from: http://link.springer.com/10.1007/978-3-319-96125-5_10.
81. Bolliger D, Görlinger K, Tanaka KA. Pathophysiology and treatment of coagulopathy in massive hemorrhage and hemodilution. Anesthesiology [Internet]. 2010;113(5):1205–19; [cited 2019 May 22]. Available from: http://anesthesiology.pubs.asahq.org/Article.aspx?doi=10.1097/ALN.0b013e3181f22b5a
82. Weber CF, Zacharowski K. Perioperative point of care coagulation testing. Dtsch Aerzteblatt Online [Internet]. 2012; [cited 2019 May 22]. Available from: https://www.aerzteblatt.de/10.3238/arztebl.2012.0369.

New Biologicals to Assist Clotting

9

Liang Huang, Christopher Hoffman, Lin Chen, and Henry Liu

Introduction

Hemorrhage potentially results in significant morbidity and mortality. Hemorrhage occurs due to disruption of blood vessel integrity through trauma or as a result of some underlying medical conditions. The extent of cellular injury and organ dysfunction is a complex process dependent upon the duration and speed of bleeding and hypoperfusion [1]. These patients often require blood transfusion though there are many potential risks related to transfusion [2]. Transfusion-related risks may include transmission of infectious disease as hepatitis C and B, Human immunodeficiency virus (HIV), Creutzfeldt-Jakob disease, West Nile virus, cytomegalovirus; Bacterial contamination; Allergic reactions with symptoms including dyspnea, fever, chills, flushing, diaphoresis, tachycardia, and hypotension or hemodynamic instability; Transfusion-related acute lung injury (TRALI) can occur within 6 hours of blood transfusion, producing noncardiogenic pulmonary edema [3]; Acute immune hemolytic reaction occurs when the recipient develops antibodies against donor cells more than 24 hours after transfusion; Transfusion-associated graft-versus-host disease results when donor lymphocytes attack recipient antigen; Iron overload occurs when patient received large volume of blood transfusions, resulting in iron accumulation leading to liver, heart, pancreases, and testicular damage; Acute or delayed febrile reactions due to the response to white blood cells in donated blood [2, 3]. Transfusion-related risks and complications will be discussed in more detailed fashion in other chapters in this book.

The commonly used hemostatic techniques by the surgeons in the operating room include applying direct pressure, suture ligatures, and cautery. Newer intravenously administered pharmacological agents and topically applied hemostatic agents have also been developed in the last decades aiming to facilitate hemostasis by providing either extravascular substrate(s) or intravascular coagulation cascade component(s). External hemostatic dressings can be used to stop bleeding in emergency situations including combat injury or junctional (groin or axillary) hemorrhage. The aim of this chapter is to review and summarize newly developed hemostatic agent(s) in accordance with clinical setting, surgical scenario, and coagulation status.

Topical Hemostats

Topical hemostats are used as adjunctive measures to improve hemostasis during or after surgery, see Table 9.1 [4]. Biological topical hemostats include active or adhesive agents, mechanical hemostats, and sealant. Active agents contain fibrinogen and thrombin and actively trigger coagulation cascade and fibrin clot formation [5, 6]. These agents are especially useful in patients with coagulation disorders. They are supplied in liquid flowable form (fibrin glues) [7, 8] or in combination with collagen (fibrin patch) [9–11]. Sometimes these agents are called adhesive hemostats due to their hemostatic and sealing effect [12–15]. Mechanical hemostats contain porcine gelatin [16], oxidized cellulose [17], bovine collagen [18], and plant-derived polysaccharide spheres [19]. These products promote platelet activation and aggregation to form a clotting matrix at the site of bleeding. These agents are known as passive hemostats because their action enhances functional coagulation systems to achieve

L. Huang
Department of Anesthesiology, New York University Langone School of Medicine, New York, NY, USA

C. Hoffman
Department of Anesthesiology, Thomas Jefferson University Hospital, Philadelphia, PA, USA

L. Chen
Department of Anesthesiology, Hubei Women & Children's Hospital, Wuhan, Hubei, China

H. Liu (✉)
Department of Anesthesiology and Perioperative Medicine, Milton S. Hershey Medical Center, Penn State College of Medicine, Hershey, PA, USA

© Springer Nature Switzerland AG 2021
C. S. Scher et al. (eds.), *Essentials of Blood Product Management in Anesthesia Practice*,
https://doi.org/10.1007/978-3-030-59295-0_9

Table 9.1 Category of topical hemostats [4]

Category	Class	Brand
Topical Active Agent	Fibrin-Based Active Adhesives and Fibrin Patch	Tiesseel, Evicel, Tachosil
	Thrombin-Based Topical Hemostats	Thrombin JMI, Evithrom
	Combined Flowable Gelatin and Thrombin or Collagen-Based Topical Hemostats	Floseal, Surgiflo, Vitagel, Tachosil
Topical Mechanical Hemostats	Oxidized Cellulose	Surgicel, Nu-Knit, Surgicel Fibrillar
	Gelatin-Based Mechanical Hemostats	Gelfilm surgifoam and Gelfoam
	Bovine Collagen-Based Mechanical Hemostats	Avitene, Avitene, Ultrafoam, UltraWrap, Instat, Helitene, and Helistat.
	Polysaccharide-Based Mechanical Hemostats	Arista, Hemostase, Vitasure
Topical Synthetic Hemostatic Agents	Cyanoacrylates	Dermabond
	Polyethylene Glycol Hydrogel	CoSeal
	Glutaraldehyde Cross-Linked Albumin	BioGlue
	Synthetic Topical Hemostatic Nanomolecules	

Table 9.2 Intravenous hemostats

1 Intravenous Fibrin-Based agents	1.1 Artificial Platelet
	1.2 Fibrin-Binding Microgel Particles
2 Platelet-Derived Agents	
3 Liposome-Based Platelet Substitutes	
4 Polymeric Nanoparticles	
5 Tranexamic Acid (TXA)	
6 Recombinant Factor VIIa (rFVIIa)	
7 Aprotinin	

hemostasis. Sealants are usually supplied in the form of low-viscosity liquids that form a solid film through polymerization to connect tissue surfaces [20–23]. These can be categorized as synthetic (e.g., cyanoacrylate and polyethylene glycol-PEG sealants) [24–26], and semisynthetic (e.g., glutaraldehyde albumin-derived sealants) [27, 28]. The fast-developing nanotechnology is also being employed in products such as self-assembling peptide nanofibers and chitosan nanofibers.

Intravenous Hemostats

Blood products (e.g., fresh frozen plasma, cryoprecipitates, platelets) and recombinant clotting factors (NovoSeven) are intravenous hemostats utilized to restore clotting function in patients with coagulopathy due to large volume blood loss [29]. Biological agents present limitations including immunogenicity and viral transmission risk, particular storage conditions, short shelf-life, and manufacturing processes. Thus, synthetic intravenous hemostatic agents are very appealing. One major advantage of synthetic intravenous hemostats is the physical and chemical properties of synthetic polymers and polymeric nanoparticles can be modified to meet the clinical use. These agents require relatively straightforward manufacturing processes and have longer shelf-lives compared to biological products. Synthetic hemostats may be administered intravenously for resolution of bleeding occurring at inaccessible injury sites [30].

Products been introduced to facilitate blood clotting through fibrin formation and crosslinking are summarized in Table 9.2. Newly developing platelet substitutes can be prepared using drug delivery vehicles like modified liposomes and polylactic-co-glycolic acid (PLGA) nanoparticles to mimic platelet properties [30]. Platelet-like molecules have been made by using synthetic molecular cores such as a PLGA-poly-L-lysine (PLGA-PLL) block copolymer core with polyethylene glycol (PEG) arms including terminal with Arg-Gly-Asp (RGD) functionalities [31]. Other nanoparticles utilize poly-lactic acid (PLA) cores instead of PLGA [31].

Synthetic liposome nanoparticles coated with various moieties have also demonstrated improved hemostasis in bleeding models [32, 33]. Platelet-like nanoparticle (PLN) is another product manufactured to more closely mimic the function of human platelets [34]. The PLN circumference is comprised of poly-allylamine hydrochloride and bovine serum albumin (PAH/BSA) bilayers, providing a flexible shell to which collagen-binding peptides (CBP), vWF-binding peptides (VBP), and fibrinogen mimetic peptides (FMP) are attached. The deformability of these particles mimics platelet malleability, permitting them to move to and spread within fibrin matrices, and form to the contraction of a clot. A molecule, termed PolySTAT, was recently developed to cross-link fibrin and delay fibrinolysis [30].

Intravenous Fibrin-Based Hemostatic Agents

Fibrin-based hemostatic intravenous agent usually targets clotting stages downstream of initial platelet plug formations. Enhancing later-stage hemostasis relies on initial endogenous clotting and can potentially avoid undesired thrombotic activities. Clotting process starts with initial platelet plug formation during primary hemostasis which occurs when platelets adhere to the subendothelial matrix by binding of GPIbα and GPIa-IIa/GPVI to von Willebrand Factor and collagen. Multiple platelets binding to the same fibrinogen molecule lead to platelet aggregation. Then fibrin forms during secondary hemostasis with locally activated thrombin enzyme cleaving circulating fibrinogen to fibrin monomers to form protofibrils, which subsequently form fibrin fibers. These fibrin fibers form networks interspersed through the platelets plug composite to stop bleeding [35].

Artificial Platelet

The fibrinogen and RGD peptide-coated microparticles work as artificial platelets. During platelet activation, a conformational change of the platelet surface integrin GPIIb-IIIa enables its binding with any of the three peptide domains in fibrinogen (RGD motifs: RGDF, RGDS; H12 sequence) [36].

Commercial platelet substitutes were initially designed by coupling fibrinogen to the surface of platelets and erythrocytes and surface displaying RGD-containing peptide [37, 38]. Enhanced platelet aggregation occurred when delivered to thrombocytopenic rats. When human albumin microcapsules adsorbed with fibrinogen (marketed as Synthocytes) were used to treat severe thrombocytopenia in rabbit model and showed improved bleeding times were documented [39].

Purified fibrinogen has increased infectious contaminant risk. Erythrocytes with fibrinogen-mimetic peptides containing an RGD sequence are produced to avoid this risk. RGD peptides are binding sites to GPIIb-IIIa, which are smaller than fibrinogen molecules. Therefore, if combined with erythrocytes, a significantly greater number of RGD peptide binding sites can be produced (about 0.5–1.5 × 106 peptides per erythrocyte) compared to fibrinogen-modified erythrocytes (about 58 fibrinogens per erythrocyte) [38]. This product, termed as "thromboerythrocyte", represents one of the earliest uses of peptides in platelet engineering. There are also studies showing that thromboerythrocyte and Synthocyte ineffective at reducing bleeding and carrying the risk of adverse immunological response [40]. Other nano-engineered agents have shown promise in animal models achieving hemostasis with both topical and intravenous agents [41].

While these hemostatic agents were effective at inducing platelet aggregation, translation of these materials into clinical use is limited by possible immunogenic responses against the biologically derived components and difficulties in scale-up.

Fibrin-Binding Microgel Particles

Ultra-low cross-linked (ULC) poly-N-isopropylacrylamide-co-acrylic acid (pNIPAm-AAc) microgel particles show enhanced affinity for fibrin. These intravenous hemostats, named platelet-like particles (PLPs), are engineered with high deformability to mimic platelet malleability in secondary hemostasis. These PLPs have been tested in injured rat models and showed to halve the bleeding times in rat experimental models with femoral vein injury [42]. PLPs can also strengthen fibrin matrices and improve wound healing. However, clot retraction occurs more rapidly after clot formation when using PLPs [43].

Platelet-Derived Hemostatic Agents (PDHA)

Trauma-induced coagulopathy following severe hemorrhage leads to low-platelet counts and platelet dysfunction, necessitating balanced resuscitation with platelet transfusion [44]. The short shelf-life of fresh platelets, which is less than 1 week, highlights a need to develop new products [45]. One solution is to design platelet-like intravenous hemostatic agents as an alternative therapy to improve hemostasis. Platelet-derived hemostatic agents (PDHA) are substitutes prepared with liposomes or modified PLGA nanoparticles to obtain platelet features in size, shape, and flexibility [46] with platelet-like hemostatic capabilities [46]. Developing lyophilized platelets to prevent exsanguination and shock began in the 1950s, preserving platelets via freeze-drying to provide a stable infusible hemostatic agent used in combat casualties. Fixation by cross-linking agents can render platelets ability to withstand lyophilization, but can also cause loss of functionality. Fifty years of ongoing refinement of the fixation process has, to some extent, improved fundamental hemostatic properties with resultant product demonstrating efficacy in animal models [47]. Because the fixation process kills viruses and bacteria in suspension, lyophilized platelet is a sterile transfusion product. PDHA rehydrates with water, improving shelf life and ease of use.

Studies have shown mixed results with PDHAs though. A porcine hemorrhage model achieved hemostasis in 60% of animals [48]. However, Macko et al. used lyophilized platelets in a primate animal model and revealed no significant reduction in blood loss [49]. A new generation of PDHA (marketed as Stasix) using a proprietary process provides a foundation for future product. However, this new generation PDHA requires further evaluation of efficacy and dose-response reaction determination of therapeutic dosage range. Stasix was evaluated in rabbit models but has not yet been shown to improve hemostasis in a dose-dependent manner [46, 50]. Further refinement of new PDHAs is necessary before transitioning to human trials.

Intravenous Liposome-Based Platelet Substitutes

Liposomes are introduced as a key technology in the drug delivery field because liposome carries both hydrophobic and hydrophilic molecules. Modifications to polymer surface can potentially enhance functionalities and residence time in circulation [51]. Platelet-like liposomes contain more than 15 different platelet membrane proteins including GPIb,

GPIIb-IIIa, and GPVI/III. Platelet substitutes are functionalized with ligands such as vWF-binding and collagen-binding peptides to mimic platelet adhesion. Fibrinogen-mimetic peptides (e.g., H12 and RGD peptides) and P-selectin surface marker-binding peptides promote platelet aggregation and platelet plug formation. H12-targeted liposome-based platelets also deliver ADP for platelet activation [52].

Intravenous Polymeric Nanoparticles

One of the earliest synthetic polymer-based platelet substitutes is a hemostatic nanoparticle consisting of a PLGA-PLL copolymer core conjugated to a corona of PEG arms with RGD-peptide terminals [31]. RGD, RGDS, and GRGDS peptides are displayed by PEG linkers added with flanking residues. The combination of PEG 4600 linkers with GRGDS peptides leads to the greatest platelet aggregation and hemostatic effect by halving bleeding time in experimental models. Intravenous administration of these nanoparticles has been shown to reduce blood loss in a rat liver trauma model [40].

Tranexamic Acid

Tranexamic acid (TXA) is a synthetic analog of lysine that blocks lysine-binding sites of plasminogen, thus functioning as an antifibrinolytic agent. Intravenous administration of tranexamic acid has been found to reduce intraoperative bleeding and transfusion requirements in cardiac surgery and trauma [53]. Such studies showed considerable bleeding risk reduction, if TXA was given within the first 3 hours after trauma.

Recombinant Factor VIIa (rFVIIa)

Recombinant factor VIIa (rFVIIa) administration in severe blunt trauma has been shown to reduce the amount of massive transfusions required [54]. rFVIIa decreases blood product utilization in coagulopathic patients [55]. It remains unknown if rFVIIa administration will decrease hemorrhagic trauma mortality rates as of yet.

Aprotinin

Aprotinin is a trypsin inhibitor that demonstrates potent antifibrinolytic effect with reduction in blood loss during repeat cardiac surgery. Its use in open heart surgery was approved by the Food and Drug Administration in 1993. However, an increased risk of renal dysfunction was later reported [56, 57]. Additional trials found that in patients undergoing high-risk cardiac surgery, aprotinin was associated with a significantly higher 30-day mortality rate comparing to TXA or aminocaproic acid [58]. Aprotinin was subsequently withdrawn completely from the market. Later studies investigating the relationship between aprotinin use and blood loss in liver transplantation patients yielded mixed results [59, 60].

A recent Cochrane review compared aprotinin versus control, TXA versus control, and TXA versus aprotinin. No significant difference in 60-day mortality or thromboembolic episodes was revealed. Aprotinin did not confer any outcome benefit despite lower blood transfusion requirements [61]. Current practice still leans towards administration of TXA in the presence of fibrinolysis.

External Hemostatic Dressings

External hemostatic dressings are developed to stop severe hemorrhage in the battlefield or severe trauma inaccessible to surgical care in an emergent scenario. Severe hemorrhage still causes high-mortality rate in potentially survivable casualties in today's battlefield. Hemostatic dressings are aimed to be used for external hemorrhage at junctional sites (e.g., axilla, groin) when effective hemostasis failed by using tourniquet [62–65]. They are grouped as factor concentrators (zeolite), procoagulants (kaolin), and mucoadhesives (chitin) [65–67]. They come as granules, powders, or bandages [68]. These dressings are used to increase local concentration of platelets, clotting factors, and erythrocytes at the wound tissue [69]. Examples are shown in Table 9.3. Technological advancements have complicated wound type and severity. Military and civilian groups recommend external hemostatic agents for prehospital control of severe hemorrhage not amenable to control with a tourniquet. Significant improvements in hemostatic dressings for prehospital care have been introduced and many tactical and conventional care guidelines have been upgraded.

Table 9.3 External hemostatic dressings

Fibrinogen-based	Salmon Thrombin-Fibrinogen (STF)
Zeolites	QuikClot, Advanced Clotting Sponge, Advanced Clotting Sponge+
Clay-based gents	
Kaolin group	QuikClot Combat Gauze™(QCG), QuikClot Combat Gauze XL, QuikClot Combat Gauze TraumaPad, QuikClot interventional
Smectite	WoundStat group
Polysaccharide and polyelectrolyte	Celox Gauze (CEG), Celox Rapid (CR) Gauze, ChitoGauze, (HCG), HC ChitoFlex Pro

Fibrinogen-Based Hemostatic Dressings

These are attractive alternatives to current agents because of their ability to form clot in the absence of host coagulation proteins or in the presence of factors but in coagulopathic state such as hypothermia [70].

Zeolites

Zeolites are microporous crystalline aluminosilicate minerals which can be found in nature. Its structure is featured on tetrahedral units of $[SiO_4]^{4-}$and $[AlO_4]^{5-}$ that are coordinated via shared oxygen atoms. Zeolites possess cage-like cavities which can accommodate both water molecules and positively charged ions such as $Ca^{2+}$and Na^+. These cations can exchange with other cations in physiological solutions [71]. Zeolites contain a three-dimensional structure which helps the movement of water molecules in and out while remaining rigid [72]. Zeolite is commercially marketed as QuikClot granular powder and Advanced Clotting Sponge (Z-Medica Corporation, Wallingford, CT)). Case studies reported that QuikClot utilization to achieve hemostasis in a multiple gunshot victim and an uncontrollable pelvic bleed which were not amenable to conventional treatment [73].

QuikClot increases temperature at both wound surface and surrounding tissue and may cause thermal injury and necrosis [74]. Difficulty removing QuikClot once at the site of bleeding is an additional concern. QuikClot was removed from military inventory in 2008, but a newer generation of zeolite hemostats such as the Advanced Clotting Sponge and Advanced Clotting Sponge plus was approved by FDA for external use. Advanced Clotting Sponge is reported to be more effective than QuikClot for irregular cavities and profuse hemorrhage. It is also easier to remove than QuikClot [69]. Advanced Clotting Sponge plus causes minimal exothermic reaction and is easy to use and remove. The product is not as effective against arterial bleeding and generally replaced by second-generation dressings (e.g., clay materials).

Clay-Based Hemostatic Agents

Clay minerals consist of tetrahedral silicate and octahedral aluminate sheets [75]. Based on the ratio of tetrahedral to octahedral sheets, these clays can be classified into two groups, 1:1 and 2:1 [75, 76]. Clay 1:1 indicates one silica tetrahedral layer to one aluminum octahedral layer (e.g., kaolin). Clay 2:1 consists of one octahedral sheet between two tetrahedral sheets (e.g., smectite). Clays have thermal stability, small particle size, relatively large surface area, significant surface charge, and ion-exchange capability. Though Zeolites are similar to clay minerals (both are aluminosilicates), they are structurally different. Clay minerals have a layered crystalline structure that can shrink and swell when water is eliminated and absorbed between the layers [76].

Polysaccharide and Polyelectrolyte

Several third-generation chitosan-based dressings have been recently added as complimentary or replacement agents. As a popular biopolymer for development of drug delivery systems, chitosan is a unique positively charged polysaccharide. It possesses excellent biocompatibility, high biodegradability, little toxicity, and low-production cost [77, 78].

Both chitin and its deacetylated form chitosan have some hemostatic properties. Those properties of chitin dressing are believed to result from vasoconstriction and mobilization of erythrocytes, clotting factors, and platelets to the site of the injury. Thus, they induce hemostasis through direct interaction with erythrocytes and platelets. They are ideal dressings to stop bleeding in coagulopathic patients because their hemostasis mechanism is not dependent on host coagulation pathways [77]. Chitin dressings such as the Rapid Deployment Hemostat (RDH) is effective in treating minor wounds [78], and has been shown efficacy in swine models of splenic lacerations faster than the fibrin-based glue [79].

Chitosan dressing (marketed as HemCon) contains chitosan from shellfish, therefore it is not recommended for patients with shellfish allergies. However, testing showed no adverse reaction during bandage challenges in shellfish allergic patients [67]. The acidity of Chitosan (like in HemCon bandages, which include acetic acid) allows it to disrupt the membranes of Gram-negative bacteria, attributing to its natural highly microbicidal properties [80].

Delivery systems are usually fabricated from natural biopolymer-based polyelectrolyte complexes (PEC) which are formed by electrostatic interactions between two oppositely charged biopolymers. PECs using carboxymethyl starch and chitosan oligosaccharide were evaluated in a rabbit hepatic hemorrhage model. This study showed that the polyelectrolyte complexes could significantly activate and accelerate the coagulation cascade and showed antimicrobial activity against S. aureus (but failed against E. coli). Moreover, PECs have also displayed certain tissue compatibility in a rabbit liver model [81]. Different forms of chitosan-based PEC drug delivery systems have been developed for various specific applications (e.g., nanoparticles, microparticles, beads, gels, films, and membranes). Chitosan dressings appear to be functioning through mechanically sealing wounds and adhering to surrounding tissue. HemCon is currently in use by US Military Forces and has been successful in achieving hemostasis in the military and civilian emergency medical settings [82, 83]. HemCon will need hands-on training. The efficacy of HemCon depends on the bandage adhering well, and it is necessary to cut the bandage to adhere to awkwardly shaped wounds. This may prove challenging in emergencies and requires training and experience.

Summary

Applications of hemostatic agents can significantly reduce morbidity and mortality from hemorrhage. A variety of topical and intravenous agents are available for clinical applications. The majority is topically applied. The type of hemorrhage, the specific mechanism of agent, the patient's individual coagulation status, and the clinician's preference may determine which agent is the most appropriate to use. Current methods of resolving bleeding after trauma or during surgery include topical hemostats and transfusion of blood products or recombinant clotting factors to restore hemostatic function. Topical hemostats are limited to treating accessible sites. Biologically derived products can be effective but have many limitations such as short shelf-life, involved manufacturing processes, and risk of compression of surrounding tissues. Synthetic intravenous hemostatic agents can be used to stop bleeding in less accessible injuries. Numerous platelet substitutes have been developed using nanoparticles such as liposomes and PLGA and have shown some efficacy to mimic platelet margination, deformation, and adhesion to vessel walls. They can induce platelet aggregation and contraction. Fibrin has been utilized in intravenous hemostat development to stabilize clot structure. Optimized physical particle properties and binding component arrangement into one platelet construct might be the focus of future intravenous hemostat development. Hemostatic external dressing such as minerals and polysaccharides together with compression are somewhat effective to control severe bleeding. Kaolin-based agents may be recommended clinically.

In the future, hemostatic agents may be engineered to involve both primary and secondary hemostasis mechanisms for an enhanced and expedited hemostatic response.

References

1. Oklu R, Albadawi H, Jones JE, Yoo HJ, Watkins MT. Reduced hind limb ischemia-reperfusion injury in toll-like receptor-4 mutant mice is associated with decreased neutrophil extracellular traps. J Vasc Surg. 2013;58(6):1627–36.
2. Despotis GJ, Zhang L, Lublin DM. Transfusion risks and transfusion-related pro-inflammatory responses. Hematol Oncol Clin North Am. 2007;21(1):147–61.
3. Vamvakas EC, Blajchman MA. Transfusion-related mortality: the ongoing risks of allogeneic blood transfusion and the available strategies for their prevention. Blood. 2009;113(15):3406–17.
4. Chiara O, Cimbanassi S, Bellanova G, Chiarugi M, Mingoli A, Olivero G, et al. A systematic review on the use of topical hemostats in trauma and emergency surgery. BMC Surg. 2018;18(1):68. https://doi.org/10.1186/s12893-018-0398-z.
5. Dhillon S. Fibrin sealant (Evicel® [Quixil®/CrossealTM]): a review of its use as supportive treatment for haemostasis in surgery. Drugs. 2011;71(14):1893–915.
6. Echave M, Oyagüez I, Casado MA. Use of Floseal®, a human Gelatine-thrombin matrix sealant, in surgery: a systematic review. BMC Surg. 2014;14:111. https://doi.org/10.1186/1471-2482-14-111.
7. Saha SP, Muluk S, Schenk W 3rd, Dennis JW, Ploder B, Grigorian A, et al. A prospective randomized study comparing fibrin sealant to manual compression for the treatment of anastomotic suture-hole bleeding in expanded polytetrafluoroethylene grafts. J Vasc Surg. 2012;56(1):134–41.
8. Spotnitz WD. Fibrin sealant: the only approved hemostat, sealant, and adhesive-a laboratory and clinical perspective. ISRN Surg. 2014;2014:203943. https://doi.org/10.1155/2014/203943. eCollection 2014.
9. Colombo GL, Bettoni D, Di Matteo S, Grumi C, Molon C, Spinelli D, Mauro G, et al. Economic and outcomes consequences of TachoSil®: a systematic review. Vasc Health Risk Manag. 2014;10:569–75.
10. Genyk Y, Kato T, Pomposelli JJ, Wright JK Jr, Sher LS, Tetens V, et al. Fibrin sealant patch (TachoSil) vs oxidized regenerated cellulose patch (surgicel original) for the secondary treatment of local bleeding in patients undergoing hepatic resection: a randomized controlled trial. J Am Coll Surg. 2016;222(3):261–8.
11. Koea J, Baldwin P, Shen J, Patel B, Batiller J, Arnaud A, et al. Safety and hemostatic effectiveness of the fibrin pad for severe soft-tissue bleeding during abdominal, retroperitoneal, pelvic, and thoracic (non-Cardiac) surgery: A randomized, controlled, superiority trial. World J Surg. 2015;39(11):2663–9.
12. Cheng Y, Ye M, Xiong X, Peng S, Wu HM, Cheng N, et al. Fibrin sealants for the prevention of postoperative pancreatic fistula following pancreatic surgery. Cochrane Database Syst Rev. 2016;2:CD009621. https://doi.org/10.1002/14651858.CD009621.pub2. Review. Update in: Cochrane Database Syst Rev. 2018 6:CD009621.
13. Cormio L, Perrone A, Di Fino G, Ruocco N, De Siati M, de la Rosette J, et al. TachoSil ® sealed tubeless percutaneous nephrolithotomy to reduce urine leakage and bleeding: outcome of a randomized controlled study. J Urol. 2012;188(1):145–50.
14. Green AL, Arnaud A, Batiller J, Eljamel S, Gauld J, Jones P, et al. A multicentre, prospective, randomized, controlled study to evaluate the use of a fibrin sealant as an adjunct to sutured dural repair. Br J Neurosurg. 2015;29(1):11–7.
15. Kobayashi S, Takeda Y, Nakahira S, Tsujie M, Shimizu J, Miyamoto A, et al. Fibrin sealant with polyglycolic acid felt vs fibrinogen-based collagen fleece at the liver-cut surface for prevention of post-operative bile leakage and hemorrhage: a prospective, randomized, controlled study. J Am Coll Surg. 2016;222(1):59–64.
16. Ragusa R, Faggian G, Rungatscher A, Cugola D, Marcon A, Mazzucco A. Use of gelatin powder added to rifamycin versus bone wax in sternal wound hemostasis after cardiac surgery. Interact Cardiovasc Thorac Surg. 2007;6(1):52–5.
17. Wagenhäuser MU, Mulorz J, Ibing W, Simon F, Spin JM, Schelzig H, et al. Oxidized (non)-regenerated cellulose affects fundamental cellular processes of wound healing. Sci Rep. 2016;6:32238. https://doi.org/10.1038/srep32238.
18. Sabino L, Andreoni C, Faria EF, Ferreira PS, Paz AR, Kalil W, et al. Evaluation of renal defect healing, hemostasis, and urinary fistula after laparoscopic partial nephrectomy with oxidized cellulose. J Endourol. 2007;21(5):551–6.

19. Emmez H, Tonge M, Tokgoz N, Durdag E, Gonul I, Cevıker N. Radiological and histopathological comparison of microporous polysaccharide hemospheres and oxidized regenerated cellulose in the rabbit brain: a study of efficacy and safety. Turk Neurosurg. 2010;20(4):485–91.
20. Bruckner BA, Blau LN, Rodriguez L, Suarez EE, Ngo UQ, Reardon MJ, et al. Microporous polysaccharide hemosphere absorbable hemostat use in cardiothoracic surgical procedures. J Cardiothorac Surg. 2014;9:134. https://doi.org/10.1186/s13019-014-0134-4.
21. Imkamp F, Tolkach Y, Wolters M, Jutzi S, Kramer M, Herrmann T. Initial experiences with the Hemopatch® as a hemostatic agent in zero-ischemia partial nephrectomy. World J Urol. 2015;33(10):1527–34.
22. Lewis KM, Kuntze CE, Gulle H. Control of bleeding in surgical procedures: critical appraisal of HEMOPATCH (Sealing Hemostat). Med Devices (Auckl). 2015;9:1–10.
23. Xu D, Ren Z, Chen X, Zhuang Q, Sheng L, Li S. A randomized controlled trial on effects of different hemostatic sponges in posterior spinal fusion surgeries. BMC Surg. 2016;16(1):80.
24. Belletrutti PJ, Romagnuolo J, Hilsden RJ, Chen F, Kaplan B, Love J, et al. Endoscopic management of gastric varices: efficacy and outcomes of gluing with N-butyl-2-cyanoacrylate in a North American patient population. Can J Gastroenterol. 2008;22(11):931–6.
25. Dumville JC, Coulthard P, Worthington HV, Riley P, Patel N, Darcey J, et al. Tissue adhesives for closure of surgical incisions. Cochrane Database Syst Rev. 2014;(11):CD004287. https://doi.org/10.1002/14651858.CD004287.pub4.
26. Öllinger R, Mihaljevic AL, Schuhmacher C, Bektas H, Vondran F, Kleine M, et al. A multicentre, randomized clinical trial comparing the Veriset™ haemostatic patch with fibrin sealant for the management of bleeding during hepatic surgery. HPB (Oxford). 2013;15(7):548–58.
27. Miscusi M, Polli FM, Forcato S, Coman MA, Ricciardi L, Ramieri A, et al. The use of surgical sealants in the repair of dural tears during non-instrumented spinal surgery. Eur Spine J. 2014;23(8):1761–6.
28. Wright NM, Park J, Tew JM, Kim KD, Shaffrey ME, Cheng J, et al. Spinal sealant system provides better intraoperative watertight closure than standard of care during spinal surgery: a prospective, multicenter, randomized controlled study. Spine (Phila Pa 1976). 2015;40(8):505–13.
29. Spahn DR, Bouillon B, Cerny V, Coats TJ, Duranteau J, Fernández-Mondéjar E, et al. Management of bleeding and coagulopathy following major trauma: an updated European guideline. Crit Care. 2013;17(2):R76. https://doi.org/10.1186/cc12685.
30. Chan LW, White NJ, Pun SH. Synthetic strategies for engineering intravenous hemostats. Bioconjug Chem. 2015;26(7):1224–36.
31. Bertram JP, Williams CA, Robinson R, Segal SS, Flynn NT, Lavik EB. Intravenous hemostat: nanotechnology to halt bleeding. Sci Transl Med. 2009;1(11):11ra22.
32. Lashof-Sullivan MM, Shoffstall E, Atkins KT, Keane N, Bir C, VandeVord P, et al. Intravenously administered nanoparticles increase survival following blast trauma. Proc Natl Acad Sci U S A. 2014;111(28):10293–8.
33. Lashof-Sullivan M, Shoffstall A, Lavik E. Intravenous hemostats: challenges in translation to patients. Nanoscale. 2013;5(22):10719–28.
34. Anselmo AC, Modery-Pawlowski CL, Menegatti S, Kumar S, Vogus DR, Tian LL, et al. Platelet-like nanoparticles: mimicking shape, flexibility, and surface biology of platelets to target vascular injuries. ACS Nano. 2014;8(11):11243–53.
35. Lord ST. Molecular mechanisms affecting fibrin structure and stability. Arterioscler Thromb Vasc Biol. 2011;31(3):494–9.
36. Salsmann A, Schaffner-Reckinger E, Kabile F, Plançon S, Kieffer N. A new functional role of the fibrinogen RGD motif as the molecular switch that selectively triggers integrin alphaIIbbeta3-dependent RhoA activation during cell spreading. J Biol Chem. 2005;280(39):33610–9.
37. Agam G, Livne A. Passive participation of fixed platelets in aggregation facilitated by covalently bound fibrinogen. Blood. 1983;61(1):186–91.
38. Agam G, Livne AA. Erythrocytes with covalently bound fibrinogen as a cellular replacement for the treatment of thrombocytopenia. Eur J Clin Investig. 1992;22(2):105–12.
39. Davies AR, Judge HM, May JA, Glenn JR, Heptinstall S. Interactions of platelets with Synthocytes, a novel-platelet substitute. Platelets. 2002;13(4):197–205.
40. Shoffstall AJ, Atkins KT, Groynom RE, Varley ME, Everhart LM, Lashof-Sullivan MM, et al. Intravenous hemostatic nanoparticles increase survival following blunt trauma injury. Biomacromolecules. 2012;13(11):3850–7.
41. Annabi N, Tamayol A, Shin SR, Ghaemmaghami AM, Peppas NA, Khademhosseini A. Surgical materials: current challenges and nano-enabled solutions. Nano Today. 2014;9(5):574–89.
42. Brown AC, Stabenfeldt SE, Ahn B, Hannan RT, Dhada KS, Herman ES, et al. Ultrasoft microgels displaying emergent platelet-like behaviours. Nat Mater. 2014;13(12):1108–14.
43. Nandi S, Sproul EP, Nellenbach K, Erb M, Gaffney L, Freytes DO, et al. Platelet-like particles dynamically stiffen fibrin matrices and improve wound healing outcomes. Biomater Sci. 2019;7(2):669–82.
44. Saillant NN, Sims CA. Platelet dysfunction in injured patients. Mol Cell Ther. 2014;2:37. https://doi.org/10.1186/s40591-014-0037-8. eCollection 2014.
45. Dunbar NM, Dumont LJ, Szczepiorkowski ZM. How do we implement day 6 and day 7 platelets at a hospital-based transfusion service? Transfusion. 2016;56(6):1262–6.
46. Burdette AJ, Andrew Pratt G 3rd, Campagna MV, Sheppard FR. Evaluation of a new generation platelet-derived hemostatic agent in a rabbit thrombocytopenic model. Thromb Res. 2017;158:79–82.
47. Bode AP, Fischer TH. Lyophilized platelets: fifty years in the making. Artif Cells Blood Substit Immobil Biotechnol. 2007;35(1):125–33.
48. Hawksworth JS, Elster EA, Fryer D, Sheppard F, Morthole V, Krishnamurthy G, et al. Evaluation of lyophilized platelets as an infusible hemostatic agent in experimental non-compressible hemorrhage in swine. J Thromb Haemost. 2009;7(10):1663–71.
49. Macko AR, Crossland RF, Cap AP, Fryer DM, Mitchell TA, Pusateri AE, Sheppard FR. Control of severe intra-abdominal hemorrhage with an infusible platelet-derived hemostatic agent in a nonhuman primate (rhesus macaque) model. J Trauma Acute Care Surg. 2016;80(4):617–24.
50. Jy W, Johansen ME, Bidot C Jr, Horstman LL, Ahn YS. Red cell-derived microparticles (RMP) as haemostatic agent. Thromb Haemost. 2013;110(4):751–60.
51. Allen TM, Cullis PR. Liposomal drug delivery systems: from concept to clinical applications. Adv Drug Deliv Rev. 2013;65(1):36–48.
52. Okamura Y, Takeoka S, Eto K, Maekawa I, Fujie T, Maruyama H, Ikeda Y, Handa M. Development of fibrinogen gamma-chain peptide-coated, adenosine diphosphate-encapsulated liposomes as a synthetic platelet substitute. J Thromb Haemost. 2009;7(3):470–7.
53. Ramirez RJ, Spinella PC, Bochicchio GV. Tranexamic acid update in trauma. Crit Care Clin. 2017;33(1):85–99.
54. Khan AZ, Parry JM, Crowley WF, McAllen K, Davis AT, Bonnell BW, et al. Recombinant factor VIIa for the treatment of severe postoperative and traumatic hemorrhage. Am J Surg. 2005;189(3):331–4.
55. Martin JT, Alkhoury F, McIntosh BC, Fidler P, Schulz J. Recombinant factor VIIa: hemostatic adjunct in the coagulopathic burn patient. Eplasty. 2009;9:e27. PMID: 19649159.

56. Karkouti K, Beattie WS, Dattilo KM, McCluskey SA, Ghannam M, Hamdy A, et al. A propensity score case-control comparison of aprotinin and tranexamic acid in high-transfusion-risk cardiac surgery. Transfusion. 2006;46(3):327–38.
57. Mangano DT, Tudor IC, Dietzel C, Multicenter Study of Perioperative Ischemia Research Group, Ischemia Research and Education Foundation. The risk associated with aprotinin in cardiac surgery. N Engl J Med. 2006;354(4):353–65.
58. Fergusson DA, Hébert PC, Mazer CD, Fremes S, MacAdams C, Murkin JM, et al. A comparison of aprotinin and lysine analogues in high-risk cardiac surgery. N Engl J Med. 2008;358(22):2319–31.
59. Schofield N, Sugavanam A, Thompson K, Mallett SV. No increase in blood transfusions during liver transplantation since the withdrawal of aprotinin. Liver Transpl. 2014;20(5):584–90.
60. Trzebicki J, Kosieradzki M, Flakiewicz E, Kuzminska G, Wasiak D, Pacholczyk M, et al. Detrimental effect of aprotinin ban on amount of blood loss during liver transplantation: single-center experience. Transplant Proc. 2011;43(5):1725–7.
61. Gurusamy KS, Li J, Vaughan J, Sharma D, Davidson BR. Cardiopulmonary interventions to decrease blood loss and blood transfusion requirements for liver resection. Cochrane Database Syst Rev. 2012;5:CD007338. https://doi.org/10.1002/14651858.CD007338.pub3.
62. Bulger EM, Snyder D, Schoelles K, Gotschall C, Dawson D, Lang E, et al. An evidence-based prehospital guideline for external hemorrhage control: American College of Surgeons Committee on Trauma. Prehosp Emerg Care. 2014;18(2):163–73.
63. Te Grotenhuis R, van Grunsven PM, Heutz WM, Tan EC. Prehospital use of hemostatic dressings in emergency medical services in the Netherlands: a prospective study of 66 cases. Injury. 2016;47(5):1007–11.
64. Jacobs LM, Rotondo M, McSwain N, Wade DS, Fabbri WP, Eastman A, et al. Joint committee to create a national policy to enhance survivability from mass casualty shooting events: Hartford Consensus II. Conn Med. 2014;78(1):5–8.
65. Shina A, Lipsky AM, Nadler R, Levi M, Benov A, Ran Y, et al. Prehospital use of hemostatic dressings by the Israel Defense Forces Medical Corps: a case series of 122 patients. J Trauma Acute Care Surg. 2015;79(4 Suppl 2):S204–9.
66. Rhee P, Brown C, Martin M, Salim A, Plurad D, Green D, et al. QuikClot use in trauma for hemorrhage control: case series of 103 documented uses. J Trauma. 2008;64(4):1093–9.
67. Waibel KH, Haney B, Moore M, Whisman B, Gomez R. Safety of chitosan bandages in shellfish allergic patients. Mil Med. 2011;176(10):1153–6.
68. Kheirabadi BS, Mace JE, Terrazas IB, Fedyk CG, Estep JS, Dubick MA, et al. Safety evaluation of new hemostatic agents, smectite granules, and kaolin-coated gauze in a vascular injury wound model in swine. J Trauma. 2010;68(2):269–78.
69. Achneck HE, Sileshi B, Jamiolkowski RM, Albala DM, Shapiro ML, Lawson JH. A comprehensive review of topical hemostatic agents: efficacy and recommendations for use. Ann Surg. 2010;251(2):217–28. https://doi.org/10.1097/SLA.0b013e3181c3bcca.
70. Grissom TE, Fang R. Topical hemostatic agents and dressings in the prehospital setting. Curr Opin Anaesthesiol. 2015;28(2):210–6.
71. Mortazavi SM, Atefi A, Roshan-Shomal P, Raadpey N, Mortazavi G. Development of a novel mineral-based haemostatic agent consisting of a combination of bentonite and zeolite minerals. J Ayub Med Coll Abbottabad. 2009;21(1):3–7.
72. Pourshahrestani S, Zeimaran E, Djordjevic I, Kadri NA, Towler MR. Inorganic hemostats: the state-of-the-art and recent advances. Mater Sci Eng C Mater Biol Appl. 2016;58:1255–68.
73. Shanmugam V, Robinson MH. Case report of uncontrollable pelvic bleeding--managed by a previously unreported method (QuikClot). Color Dis. 2009;11(2):221–2.
74. Wright JK, Kalns J, Wolf EA, Traweek F, Schwarz S, Loeffler CK, et al. Thermal injury resulting from application of a granular mineral hemostatic agent. J Trauma. 2004;57(2):224–30.
75. Rosales-Landeros C, Barrera-Díaz CE, Bilyeu B, Guerrero VV, Núñez FU. A review on Cr(VI) adsorption using inorganic materials. Am J Anal Chem. 2013;4:8–16.
76. Williams LB, Haydel SE. Evaluation of the medicinal use of clay minerals as antibacterial agents. Int Geol Rev. 2010;52(7/8):745–70.
77. Khan MA, Mujahid M. A review on recent advances in chitosan-based composite for hemostatic dressings. Int J Biol Macromol. 2019;124:138–47.
78. Kulling D, Vournakis JN, Woo S, Demcheva MV, Tagge DU, Rios G, et al. Endoscopic injection of bleeding esophageal varices with a poly-N-acetyl glucosamine gel formulation in the canine portal hypertension model. Gastrointest Endosc. 1999;49(6):764–71.
79. Chan MW, Schwaitzberg SD, Demcheva M, Vournakis J, Finkielsztein S, Connolly RJ. Comparison of poly-N-acetyl glucosamine (P-GlcNAc) with absorbable collagen (Actifoam), and fibrin sealant (Bolheal) for achieving hemostasis in a swine model of splenic hemorrhage. J Trauma. 2000;48(3):454–7; discussion 457-8.
80. Tsai GJ, Su WH. Antibacterial activity of shrimp chitosan against Escherichia coli. J Food Prot. 1999;62(3):239–43.
81. Chen X, Yan Y, Li H, Wang X, Tang S, Li Q, et al. Evaluation of absorbable hemostatic agents of polyelectrolyte complexes using carboxymethyl starch and chitosan oligosaccharide both in vitro and in vivo. Biomater Sci. 2018;6(12):3332–44.
82. Wedmore I, McManus JG, Pusateri AE, Holcomb JB. A special report on the chitosan-based hemostatic dressing: experience in current combat operations. J Trauma. 2006;60(3):655–8.
83. Brown MA, Daya MR, Worley JA. Experience with chitosan dressings in a civilian EMS system. J Emerg Med. 2009;37(1):1–7.

Herbal Substances that Affect Hemostasis

10

Craig Lilie, Phillip Morris, and J. Clint Tippett

Abbreviations

AA	Arachidonic Acid
ADP	Adenosine Diphosphate
aPTT	Activated Partial Thromboplastin Time
CAM	Complementary and Alternative Medicine
CBD	Cannabidiol
CBN	Cannabinol
COX	Cyclooxygenase
FDA	Food and Drug Administration
INR	International Normalized Ratio
NO	Nitric Oxide
NSAIDS	Nonsteroidal Anti-inflammatory Drugs
PAF	Platelet-Activating Factor
PAI-1	Plasminogen Activator Inhibitor-1
PT	Prothrombin Time
PTT	Partial Thromboplastin Time
THC	Tetrahydrocannabinol

Background

The use of naturally occurring plants to heal ailments in man dates to approximately 5000 years ago. The practice spanned multiple geographically distinct civilizations and remains engrained in many cultures today. According to the World Health Organization, approximately 80% of the world's population uses traditional medicine, consisting primarily of plants and their components [1]. The traditional purported healing effects of these natural substances are wide-ranging and include treatment for fever, cardiovascular disease, gastrointestinal disease, pain, and wound healing [2]. Today, the use of nutritional and herbal supplementation has become a popular option for self-treatment of ailments and the use has steadily increased in the United States over the past several decades [3]. Nutritional supplements represent a component of complementary and alternative medicine (CAM) that exists outside of what is generally accepted to be conventional practice. CAM is generally not taught in US or UK medical schools and is generally not practiced in hospitals [4]. CAM therapies additionally include homeopathic preparations, chiropractic manipulations, massage, acupuncture, meditation, and prayer, [5] which are outside of the scope of this chapter. Nutritional and herbal supplementation represents an opportunity to take charge in improving one's own health and is often marketed as natural or homeopathic. Therefore, the consumption of these pharmacologically active products is often perceived by consumers as low risk and may explain the observed underreporting of their use to care providers, use without expert consultation, and concurrent use with other medications where interactions may exist.

Herbal dietary supplements have continued to have an upward trend in sales in recent years and surpassed $8 billion in sales in the United States in 2017. Combination preparations of herbal supplements, in contrast with defined single product herbal supplements, represented 41.1% of these sales [6]. Herbal medicines represent a $60 billion industry worldwide [7]. Approximately 38 million adults in the United States (18.9% of the population) use herbal or other natural supplements, but only one-third tell their physician about this use [8]. This trend of increasing sales of herbal and nutritional supplements, the differing rules of regulation by the United States Food and Drug Administration (FDA), and the potential complexity of each preparation requires the perioperative physician be educated about these substances and their potential perioperative implications.

Despite the prevalent use of herbal supplements, there remains a relative paucity of high-quality evidence to support the use of these pharmacologically active substances in improving morbidity and mortality. The risks of these therapies are often poorly defined as high-quality clinical research

C. Lilie (✉) · P. Morris · J. C. Tippett
Baylor Scott and White Medical Center – Temple, Department of Anesthesiology, Temple, TX, USA
e-mail: Craig.lilie@bswhealth.org; Jason.tippett@bswhealth.org

© Springer Nature Switzerland AG 2021
C. S. Scher et al. (eds.), *Essentials of Blood Product Management in Anesthesia Practice*,
https://doi.org/10.1007/978-3-030-59295-0_10

to further advance this body of knowledge is expensive and difficult to perform, especially given the lack of financial motivation for industry to pursue randomized, placebo-controlled trials [5]. Much of the available literature regarding safety of herbal supplements is dependent upon in vitro studies, in vivo animal studies, and clinical case reports. The case reports themselves may be somewhat limited in their conclusions as people commonly ingest more than one herbal supplement [9, 10].

Regulation of the nutritional and herbal supplement industry is necessary to protect consumers from potential adverse effects of these substances and ensure proper marketing and labeling. Current regulation of dietary supplements by the FDA is largely defined by the Dietary Supplement Health and Education Act, passed into law in 1994. It considers dietary supplements as foods which decreases the regulatory review and scientific evaluation required prior to being marketed and sold. It requires that any dietary supplement or ingredient be unadulterated and properly identified and states that the FDA is responsible for taking action if this is violated by a manufacturer. Subsequent legislation passed in 2006 requires supplement manufacturers to notify the FDA within 15 days of being notified of a serious adverse event by a consumer. Additionally, a standard for Good Manufacturing Practices passed in 2007 is designed to ensure the quality of supplements being sold, including accuracy of ingredients, lack of contaminants, and proper labeling. This differs from the regulations by which other food products and drugs, such as pharmaceuticals, are regulated [11, 12]. Despite these efforts, the herbal and supplement industry lacks mandated standardization of production of nutritional supplements such that variability in final product exists between manufacturers [13]. Ideally, herbal supplements should contain the supplement on its label with purity, be accurate to the dosage reported, and be devoid of contaminants. Challenges with meeting these expectations have been reported in the literature. In one study, Ginkgo biloba DNA was verifiable in only 83.8% of Ginkgo biloba supplements tested [14]. Also, contaminants have been demonstrated in herbal supplements which have led to patient harm [15, 16]. Thus, ensuring the safety of these preparations is of ongoing importance and newer technologies are being validated and utilized to evaluate the quality and effect of herbal preparations [17, 18]. The National Institutes of Health National Center for Complementary and Integrative Health (formerly known as National Center for Complementary and Alternative Medicine) has funded many research projects to scientifically explore complementary and alternative medicine to improve consumer information and safety [11].

In order to properly counsel patients regarding their use of supplements in the perioperative period, accurate disclosure of their use must first be achieved. A study of patients in the clinic setting revealed that only 21.3% of patients disclosed their herbal supplement use to their physicians [19]. In one study in the ambulatory surgery setting, 32% of patients admitted to using a dietary supplement, though 70% of patients failed to disclose their supplement use when a routine preoperative assessment was performed [20]. Thus, it is critical for perioperative physicians to inquire about both conventional medication use as well as nutritional supplement use. It may be prudent to request patients bring either a list or the medications themselves for their preoperative evaluation, since combination herbal supplements are commonly used. A recent review suggests that 52% of adults in the United States used supplements at some point between 1999–2012 [3]. Further, some patient populations in particular have a high incidence of ongoing herbal medication use. Selected patient populations include the elderly [21], solid organ transplant recipients [11], chronic pain patients [22], breast and gynecologic cancer patients [23], cosmetic surgery patients [10], and pediatric Down syndrome patients [24] (Table 10.1).

Over 90 dietary supplements may possess pharmacodynamic antiplatelet and anticoagulant effects [13]. Many of these are some of the top-selling herbal supplements and may increase the risk for perioperative hemorrhage. Supplements also have indirect interactions with other medications that may either increase or decrease the efficacy of a patient's pharmaceutical anticoagulant or antiplatelet medication by inhibition or induction of CYP450 isoenzymes. Finally, these herbal medications may cause organ dysfunction which could increase the risk for hemorrhage [25, 26]. Supplement-induced hepatic injury has been described to have multiple causes [26, 27]. This could manifest as an isolated coagulation disturbance due to impaired hepatic synthesis of coagulation factors, though they may also have other signs of organ dysfunction which would prompt an investigation of the cause of hepatic failure. Regardless of mechanism, perioperative hemorrhage is a risk associated with the use of many nutritional supplements and providers must have an awareness of this potential in the perioperative period.

Table 10.1 Incidence of supplement use in select patient populations

Patient population	Reported incidence of supplement use
Elderly (62–85 years of age)	63.7%
Renal, Liver, Combined Renal/Heart transplant recipients	58%
Chronic pain patients	52%
Breast and ovarian cancer patients	52% and 45%
Cosmetic surgery patients	49%
Pediatric down syndrome	49%

Herbs and Herbal Extracts

Due to the global diversity of plants and the propensity of humans in different cultures to explore the possible uses of these plants, there are a very large number of herbs utilized for a variety of medicinal purposes. At present, many of the most commonly utilized herbs do not appear to result in a bleeding diathesis and are excluded from this discussion. The following selected herbal preparations were chosen for discussion based on both their propensity to cause bleeding and their popular use (Table 10.2).

Table 10.2 Herbal supplements, multivitamin and non-herbal vitamin supplements

Herbal supplements			
Supplement	Marketed uses/Effects	Anticoagulant/Antiplatelet effect	Drug interactions (if known)/ Miscellaneous
Andrographis *Andrographis paniculata*	Immunostimulatory, antiviral, antibacterial, anti-inflammatory, antitumor, antidiabetic, antimalarial, hepatoprotective, cardiovascular disease, infertility	Inhibits PAF-induced platelet aggregation	–
Ashwagandha *Withania somnifera*	Anti-arthritic, antirheumatic, anti-inflammatory	Inhibition of platelet aggregation	–
Boswellia *Boswellia serrata*	Osteoarthritis, rheumatoid arthritis, inflammatory bowel disease, asthma	Prolongs PT and aPTT, inhibition of Factor Xa and XIa	–
Bromelain *Bromeliaceae* spp.	Anti-edema, anti-inflammatory, antithrombotic, fibrinolytic	Inhibition of ADP-induced platelet aggregation, reduced platelet endothelial adhesion, prolongs PT and PTT	Chemical burn debridement agent
Cannabinoids *Cannabis* spp.	Multiple sclerosis, chronic pain, nausea/vomiting, others	CBN and THC inhibit thrombin-induced clot formation, prolong clotting times	CBD may increase warfarin concentrations
Cranberry *Vaccinium macrocarpon*	Improve urinary tract infection, metabolic profile, antioxidant	Component compounds inhibit platelets, no data supporting cranberry juice itself inhibiting platelets	Increased INR in those taking warfarin
Danshen *Salvia miltiorrhiza*	Atherosclerosis, hypercholesterolemia, arthritis, insomnia, menstrual disorders	Inhibits ADP-induced platelet aggregation, thrombosis formation	Significantly increases concentrations of warfarin
Devil's Claw *Harpagophytum procumbens*	Analgesic, antipyretic	COX-1 and COX-2 inhibition	–
Dong Quai *Angelicae sinensis*	Menstrual cramping, menstrual regulation, migraine, antispasmodic	Inhibits platelet aggregation	May potentiate warfarin effect
Evening Primrose Oil *Oenothera biennis*	Anti-inflammatory, women's health conditions	Antiplatelet effects, coumarin constituents	May potentiate warfarin effect
Fenugreek *Trigonella foenum-graecum*	Increase milk production, antidiabetes, anticancer, anticholesterol, antioxidant, anti-inflammatory, antimicrobial, hepato- and neuro-protective	Contains Vitamin K antagonist coumarins	Should be avoided in those taking warfarin
Feverfew *Tanacetum parthenium*	Fever, migraine, rheumatoid arthritis, menstrual problems	Reduced ADP-induced platelet aggregation, decreased COX production	–
Garlic *Allium sativum*	Atherosclerosis, hypertension, thrombus formation, and lower serum lipid and cholesterol levels	Inhibit platelet aggregation in vivo in dose-dependent fashion	Warfarin use increases bleeding risk, rich in sulfur-containing compounds allicin and alliin
Ginger *Zingiber officinale*	Arthritis, rheumatism, muscular aches, pains, sore throats, cramps, constipation, indigestion, nausea, vomiting, motion sickness, hypertension, dementia, fever, infectious diseases, helminthiasis	Inhibit AA-induced human platelet serotonin release and aggregation	–
Ginkgo *Ginkgo biloba*	Cognitive disorders, peripheral vascular disease, erectile dysfunction	Inhibition of PAF-induced platelet aggregation	–
Ginseng *Panax* spp.	Improve energy and alertness, aphrodisiac, diabetic blood sugar control	Inhibits in vitro thromboxane synthesis, increased blood clotting time, PAF inhibition	Increased warfarin clearance

(continued)

Table 10.2 (continued)

Herbal supplements			
Supplement	Marketed uses/Effects	Anticoagulant/Antiplatelet effect	Drug interactions (if known)/ Miscellaneous
Green Tea *Camelia sinensis*	Cardiovascular benefits, antioxidant, anti-inflammatory, antidiabetic, antiviral	Inhibits AA, collagen, and ADP-induced platelet aggregation	Contains Vitamin K, may decrease warfarin effect
Hawthorn *Crataegus* spp.	Digestive disorders, gall bladder disease, asthma	Inhibition of ADP-induced platelet aggregation, reduction in thromboxane A2 biosynthesis	–
Horse Chestnut *Aesculus hippocastanum*	Chronic venous insufficiency, hemorrhoids, anti-inflammatory, antioxidant, anti-edema	Inhibits ADP-induced platelet aggregation, arterial and venous contraction mediated by 5HT(2A) receptor	Plant contains esculin, a poison that can cause death if eaten raw
Kava *Piper methysticum*	Anxiolytic, sedative	Inhibits COX, Dose-dependent decrease in platelet aggregation	May result in liver toxicity
Motherwort *Leonurus japonicus*	Menstrual disorders, blood stasis, analgesia	Inhibition of ADP-induced platelet aggregation	–
Oregano *Origanum vulgare*	Respiratory and gastrointestinal disorders, others	Prolongs aPTT	–
Policosanol	Cardiovascular benefits, claudication pain relief	Reduces AA, collagen and ADP-induced platelet aggregation	Increases effect of omega-3 fatty acids and aspirin, extracted from sugar cane and beeswax plants
Resveratrol	Anti-inflammatory, anticancer, anti-Alzheimer's, antidiabetes	Increases platelet NO, inhibits PAI-1	May partially explain cardiovascular effects of wine consumption
Saw Palmetto *Serenoa repens*	Benign prostatic hypertrophy, anti-inflammatory	Inhibits COX	–
Skullcap *Scutellaria baicalensis*	Antioxidant, antibacterial, antiviral, antitumor, others	Prolongs aPTT, PT, inhibits fibrin polymerization and platelet aggregation	Healing effects are described in the oldest Chinese medicinal book in existence
St. John's Wort *Hypericum perforatum*	Depression, anxiety, sleep disturbances	CYP3A4 isoenzyme induction	Decreased warfarin efficacy, enhances clopidogrel efficacy
Turmeric *Curcuma longa*	Skin conditions, respiratory illness, analgesic, liver dysfunction	Inhibition of ADP and GPVI-induced platelet aggregation	–
Willow Bark *Salix alba*	Anti-inflammatory, analgesic, antirheumatic, antipyretic	Inhibits AA-induced platelet aggregation	Contains precursor to salicylic acid
Wintergreen Oil (methyl salicylate)	Arthralgia, skin irritation	Structurally similar to aspirin	Elevated INR when combined with warfarin
Multivitamins and non-herbal vitamin supplements			
Coenzyme Q10	Cardiovascular benefit, possibly improve liver, muscle, and brain health	–	Possible elevated bleeding risk if taking warfarin
Fish Oil (omega-3 long chain fatty acids)	Cardiovascular benefits	May decrease ADP-induced platelet aggregation and prolong bleeding time	Bleeding risk elevated in those also taking warfarin or aspirin/NSAIDS
Glucosamine/ Chondroitin Sulfate	Cartilage health in osteoarthritis	Glucosamine inhibits ADP-induced platelet activation	May increase INR in those taking warfarin
Vitamin E	Antioxidant, anti-atherosclerosis, cancer prevention	Antagonizes Vitamin K effect and inhibit thrombin-induced platelet aggregation	Bleeding risk may be elevated if dose is high or taking anticoagulants
Others: Magnesium, Lycopene, Selenium, Taurine	Various	May inhibit platelet function	Selenium may increase warfarin activity

Andrographis

The herbaceous plant *Andrographis paniculata* has many pharmacological effects which could be used for a number of disease states including protection from cardiovascular disease, infertility, and potentially many others. It contains the herbal compound andrographolide which is shown to inhibit platelet-activating factor (PAF)-induced human platelet aggregation in a dose-dependent manner and exhibits its antiplatelet activity through other molecular mechanisms [28].

Ashwagandha

Ashwagandha is an important Indian medicinal plant which may have anti-arthritic, antirheumatic, anti-inflammatory, and other properties. Extracts are shown to have some inhibitory effects on platelet aggregation [29].

Boswellia

Boswellia serrata, or Indian frankincense, is classically used as an anti-inflammatory agent for the treatment of arthritis. There is evidence of substantial antithrombotic properties from the extract causing prolonged prothrombin time (PT) and activated partial thromboplastin time (aPTT) that appears linked directly to Factor Xa and XIa inhibition [30].

Bromelain

Bromelain extract is produced from pineapples and confers anti-edema, anti-inflammatory, antithrombotic, and fibrinolytic activities. It contains a number of proteases which may prevent adenosine diphosphate (ADP)-induced platelet aggregation and adhesion of platelets to blood vessel endothelial cells. In high doses, it may also prolong the PT and partial thromboplastin time (PTT). It may be utilized clinically as a chemical burn debridement or anti-edema agent and has not yet had a reported occurrence of the adverse effect of bleeding in humans [31].

Cannabinoids

Cannabis extract is used as a therapy for multiple sclerosis, chronic pain, nausea/vomiting, and others. Cannabinol (CBN) and tetrahydrocannabinol (THC) appear to inhibit thrombin-induced clot formation in vitro and prolong clotting times in vivo in a rat model [32]. Another component, cannabidiol (CBD), inhibits P450 (CYP) 3A enzymes (and other isoenzymes), and it may decrease the metabolism of warfarin as a result [33].

Cranberry

Cranberry juice or supplements are taken to improve urinary tract infections, improve metabolic profile, and as an antioxidant. Clinical data do not currently report cranberry having an effect on platelet aggregation, despite several of its components having been shown to do so [34]. Case reports demonstrate an interaction between cranberry and warfarin resulting in an elevated international normalized ratio (INR) [35, 36].

Danshen

Danshen is an herb used for centuries to improve cardiovascular health. An extract contacting several constituents has been shown to inhibit thrombosis formation and platelet aggregation [37]. At least one active component of Danshen inhibits platelet aggregation induced by ADP [38]. Danshen enhances anticoagulation in patients taking warfarin by directly increasing plasma concentrations of warfarin [39].

Devil's Claw

Devil's Claw is a plant of the sesame family used as an analgesic and anti-pyretic. The active ingredient harpagoside has been implicated in previous in vitro studies that show altered platelet function [40]. Further studies have confirmed that cyclooxygenase (COX)-1 and COX-2 inhibition by this active ingredient are likely responsible [41]. The clinical implication of this remains questionable.

Dong Quai

Dong quai is an ancient Chinese herbal medication which is taken largely for its benefits with menstrual cramping, menstrual regulation, and migraine headache. It has also been used as an antispasmodic [42]. It possesses several constituents which are known to decrease platelet aggregation by inhibiting thromboxane A_2 synthesis and a clinical study supports this action in select patients [43, 44]. A case report suggests dong quai may potentiate the effect of warfarin [42].

Evening Primrose Oil

Evening primrose oil originates from the evening primrose plant and is used as an anti-inflammatory and in women's health conditions. It is postulated to have antiplatelet effects and contains coumarin constituents which could lead to an interaction with warfarin [45, 46].

Fenugreek

Fenugreek is an ancient herbal which possesses many vitamins and active compounds which have been used for the treatment of increasing milk production, diabetes, cancer, and hypercholesterolemia. It possesses antioxidant, anti-inflammatory, antimicrobial, and hepato- and neuroprotective properties [47]. Fenugreek contains a high content of coumarin-like compounds which can lead to increased risk of bleeding. Excessive intake of fenugreek has been shown to cause a Vitamin K reversible prolongation of INR with coagulation failure in a susceptible patient. It may be advisable to avoid this medication in patients taking warfarin [48].

Feverfew

Feverfew has classically been used as an antipyretic and in the treatment of migraines. Feverfew's active constituent of sesquiterpene lactones is suspected to be responsible for its effect on platelets. The primary effect is a reduction in ADP-mediated platelet aggregation [49]. It has also been shown to decrease COX production leading to reduction in thromboxane synthesis [50].

Garlic

Garlic is a plant bulb and species of the onion family that is well known for its culinary applications, but it has also been used medicinally for several millenia. Today, it is used principally for the treatment of atherosclerosis, hypertension, thrombus formation, and to lower serum lipid and cholesterol levels [51]. Primary chemical components of garlic, ajoene and volatile oil, have been implicated in irreversibly potentiating platelet inhibitors, including prostacyclin, indomethacin, and dipyridamole [52]. Garlic reportedly inhibits platelet aggregation in vivo in a dose-dependent fashion [53, 54], mainly through the effects of sulfur-containing compounds alliin and allicin which inhibit the production and release of thromboxane and adenosine [55]. However, these antiplatelet results have not been reproducible in all clinical trials [56–58]. Some studies report that aged garlic extract has been found to significantly reduce adrenaline-induced platelet aggregation and to a lesser extent collagen-induced platelet aggregation, with no effect on ADP-induced platelet aggregation [59, 60]. There are several cases in the literature of excessive dietary garlic intake or use of garlic as a medicine associated with coagulation alterations [61]. One case report describes an elevated INR, reportedly due to an interaction between garlic and warfarin [62]. At recommended doses, it appears that garlic supplements do not have anticoagulant properties in individuals not taking concomitant anticoagulant medications. However, when consumed in higher than recommended doses or when used in combination with anticoagulants, garlic may be a factor for increased risk of bleeding.

Ginger

Ginger is the rhizome of the *Zingiber officinale* plant with widespread uses ranging from the treatment of arthritis and inflammatory conditions to hypertension and dementia. It is commonly utilized in the treatment of nausea and gastrointestinal discomfort [63, 64]. Gingerols are the key active component of ginger and have been shown to inhibit arachidonic acid (AA)-induced human platelet serotonin release and aggregation [65]. In vitro studies have also shown COX-1 inhibition leading to antiplatelet activity more potent than aspirin alone [66]. Despite these findings, further experiments have failed to demonstrate significant changes in clotting status or coagulation in individuals taking warfarin [67].

Ginkgo

Ginkgo biloba is marketed for improvement in peripheral vascular disease, erectile dysfunction, and has gained traction for Alzheimer's disease and multi-infarct dementia treatment. Ginkgolides are one of the more widely studied active ingredients and have been shown to have dose-dependent, rapid onset, potent inhibition of PAF-induced platelet aggregation [68]. Several case reports exist implicating gingko as the cause of unexpected hemorrhage in the perioperative period including unprovoked intracranial hemorrhage [69, 70].

Ginseng

Ginseng (*Panax ginseng*) has a long history of use in eastern Asian culture to boost the immune system. Today, it is a prominent additive to energy drinks for increased alertness and focus [71]. One of ginseng's bioactive component, gensinosides, seems to be responsible for anticoagulation effects and may reduce platelet volume through PAF inhibition. Ginseng has also been shown to inhibit in vitro thromboxane synthesis and lead to increased blood clotting time [72]. Despite the effective inhibition of the coagulation cascade, a clinical trial showed that warfarin clearance was increased with concomitant use of ginseng, leading to less effective anticoagulation as shown by a corresponding difficulty in achieving the desired therapeutic INR [73].

Green Tea

Green Tea, the second most consumed beverage in the world, has many purported benefits including improved cardiovascular health, antioxidant, anti-inflammatory, antidiabetic, and antiviral effects [27, 42]. Components of green tea, including polyphenols and catechins, have been shown to inhibit AA, collagen, and ADP-induced platelet aggregation [74]. In vivo studies have supported this with significantly prolonged bleeding time in conscious mice after green tea and catechin administration [75]. Additionally, Vitamin K is present in green tea in a significant quantity and may decrease the anticoagulant effect of warfarin [34].

Hawthorn

Hawthorn is classically used for gastrointestinal disorder treatment. There are many active ingredients in hawthorn and some interact with platelet function. In vitro studies have shown that hawthorn extract and inhibits ADP-induced platelet aggregation and causes a significant reduction in biosynthesis of thromboxane A2 [76].

Horse Chestnut

Horse chestnut is an herbal medication historically taken for chronic venous insufficiency and is purported to have anti-inflammatory, antioxidant, and anti-edema properties. Extracts have been shown to inhibit ADP-induced human platelet aggregation and cause contraction of both veins and arteries [77]. One clinical study has shown it is as effective as compression stockings in chronic venous insufficiency. The potential for drug interactions with other antiplatelet drugs needs further study [74].

Kava

Kava is a substance with predominantly psychomotor activities and is used as an anxiolytic and sedative. It inhibits COX with a similar potency to nonsteroidal anti-inflammatory drugs (NSAIDS), causes a dose-dependent decrease in platelet aggregation and may also cause hepatotoxicity [78].

Motherwort

Motherwort is classically used to treat menstrual disorders such as amenorrhea and dysmenorrhea but applications extend to other conditions of blood stasis and analgesia. Studies have shown decreased platelet aggregation after intravenous administration [79]. Further in vitro studies have isolated an active ingredient bis-spirolabdane diterpenoid that has the ability to significantly reduce ADP-induced platelet aggregation [80].

Oregano

Oregano is an herbal supplement purportedly utilized for respiratory disorders, gastrointestinal disorders, and many others and has been shown to prolong aPTT in an in vitro study [81].

Policosanol

Policosanol is taken for its purported ability to improve lipid profile and for its cardiovascular health benefits, policosanol is shown to inhibit platelet aggregation response to AA, collagen, and ADP [82]. It seems to have an additive antiplatelet effect when taken along with aspirin and omega-3 fatty acids, though no reports have identified policosanol as a contributor to clinical bleeding [83, 84].

Resveratrol

Resveratrol is a phenolic antioxidant present in grape skin, which may explain part of the beneficial cardiovascular effects of wine consumption. The compound increases the production of nitric oxide (NO) by stimulated platelets and, thus, blunts platelet function through inhibition of the pro-inflammatory pathway [85]. It also decreases plasminogen activator inhibitor-1 (PAI-1) which may increase a patient's fibrinolytic state [86]. Case reports of clinically significant bleeding due to resveratrol are lacking.

Saw Palmetto

Saw palmetto is a commonly used herbal supplement which improves symptoms of benign prostatic hypertrophy [87]. Presumably through its ability to inhibit COX, it has been implicated in a case report of reported severe bleeding during craniotomy, as well as a cause of hematuria and coagulopathy [27]. The true clinical impact on coagulation remains unclear.

Skullcap

Skullcap is a traditional Chinese herbal medicine with many purported medicinal benefits, perhaps most notably as an antioxidant, antibacterial, antiviral, and antitumor agent. It is a component of dozens of Chinese medicinal preparations and its constituents are being widely researched to define medicinal benefits [88]. One of its major components, oroxylin A, is shown to prolong the aPTT and PT, inhibit fibrin polymerization, and platelet aggregation [89].

St. John's Wort

St. John's wort is a widely used supplement, particularly in the treatment of depression, anxiety, and sleep disturbances. Most of the effects on coagulation come through potent cytochrome isoenzyme modulation. St. John's wort reduces plasma warfarin concentrations through induction of CYP3A4 and possibly other CYP isoforms because warfarin, which exists as a racemic mixture of R- and S-enantiomers, is metabolized by CYP1A1 and CYP3A4 (R-warfarin) and CYP2C9 (S-warfarin). Such interactions have been confirmed in clinical trials showing decreased plasma concentrations of warfarin and phenprocoumon [90]. In contrast, the efficacy of clopidogrel is enhanced with coadministration of St. John's wort. The induction of CYP3A4 enhances conversion of the prodrug clopidogrel to its active form resulting in demonstrable decreases in ADP-induced platelet aggregation [91].

Turmeric

Turmeric is a commonly used spice in cooking on the Indian subcontinent and particularly in curry dishes, but it is also marketed as a treatment for aches, respiratory conditions, skin conditions, and liver dysfunction [92]. Curcumin has been identified as the active ingredient with anti-inflammatory properties and data are limited on its effect on platelet function. In vitro studies have found evidence of ADP and glycoprotein VI inhibition leading to reduced platelet aggregation [93, 94]. Despite the demonstrated in vitro platelet inhibitory effects, clinical data to investigate and substantiate this effect in vivo are lacking [34].

Willow Bark

Willow tree bark extract is an ancient supplement historically utilized for the treatment of inflammation and additionally is an analgesic, antirheumatic, and antipyretic substance. The primary pharmacologically active compound is salicin, which once oxidized becomes salicylic acid [34]. In a double-blinded, randomized controlled trial of 35 patients receiving willow bark extract or placebo and 16 patients receiving acetylsalicylate, willow bark extract was shown to have a statistically significant inhibition of AA-induced platelet aggregation compared to placebo. However, this inhibition was not as great as those who had received acetylsalicylate [95].

Wintergreen Oil

Wintergreen oil, or methyl salicyclate, is most commonly used as a topical ointment for the treatment of arthritis and other skin irritation. The active compound methyl salicyclate is structurally very similar to aspirin and even topical absorption can lead to substantial blood concentrations. Several cases of increased INR have been reported when wintergreen is used by patients on a stable warfarin regimen [96, 97].

Numerous other herbal compounds may have some effect on blood coagulation. Berberine has been shown in an in vitro study to inhibit thrombin-induced platelet aggregation as a direct thrombin inhibitor [98]. Boldo may have interactions with warfarin causing increased INR [99]. Chinese Peony has been reported to have anticoagulant properties. Analysis of extracts reveal chemical structural similarities to animal heparin [100]. *Corydalis yanhusuo* has been shown to inhibit platelet aggregation [101]. Cyanidin-3-Glucoside is a plant-based anthocyanin that is shown to inhibit platelet function at multiple points including platelet activation, aggregation, secretion, and thrombus formation [102]. Persimmon leaf ethanol extract is shown to prolong aPTT and inhibit platelet activation, while ethanol extract of persimmon leaf and *Citrus junos* (Yuzu) prolongs aPTT and PT in mice [103, 104]. Poncitrin is often taken for gastrointestinal problems, contains coumarin compounds, and has been shown to inhibit the aggregation of rabbit platelets induced by ADP, PAF, AA, and collagen [105]. Piper wallichii possesses compounds which inhibit platelet aggregation induced by PAF [106]. Rhus verniciflua stokes is a traditional herbal supplement which decreases platelet aggregation to collagen in vivo [107]. Safflower extract and some of its components have significant antiplatelet and anticoagulation activity [108]. Of note, a number of herbals contain a large amount of vitamin K and may decrease the effectiveness of warfarin, including stinging nettle *(Urtica dioica)*, noni fruit *(Morinda citrifolia)*, dandelion *(Taraxacum officinale)*, and horsetail *(Equisetum arvense)* [109].

When multiple supplements that have been identified as inhibiting coagulation or platelet function are taken together, this will likely further increase the risk of perioperative bleeding [110]. Traditional herbal preparations are often prepared as combination herbal supplements which are shown to possess antithrombotic and antiplatelet effects [111]. For instance, treatment of rats with reduction of Sheng-Nao-Kang decoction, comprised of six herbal components, prolongs aPTT, PT, thrombin time, and decreases fibrinogen [112].

Multivitamins and Vitamin Supplements

Multivitamins/minerals, calcium, and individual vitamins (B, D, C, E) are among the most common nutritional supplements people take [21]. Clinicians should be aware of their potential bleeding concerns in the perioperative setting (Table 10.2).

Coenzyme Q10

Coenzyme Q10 supplementation may have cardiovascular benefits and may provide some benefit to liver, muscle, and brain health. It does not appear to increase bleeding when taken in isolation [71]. Coenzyme Q10 has a complex interaction with warfarin. It appears to increase the clearance of both R- and S-enantiomers of warfarin without decreasing the therapeutic effects of warfarin. Coadministration of warfarin and coenzyme Q10 may lead to a mild increased risk of bleeding in patients taking warfarin, though this interaction is poorly understood and lacks definitive support [27].

Fish Oil

Omega-3 fatty acids are found naturally in certain fish and these supplements are typically taken for their purported cardiovascular benefits. Ingestion of supplemental omega 3 long-chain polyunsaturated fatty acid reduces risk for myocardial infarction and coronary artery disease at 1 g/day, perhaps even more importantly for those with low fish intake [3]. Standard dosage of fish oil has recently been shown to decrease platelet aggregation and clot formation when assessed by multiplate aggregometry and viscoelastic rotational thromboelastometry [113]. Other studies reporting a decrease in platelet aggregation and a prolonged bleeding time are reported, though, fish oil alone did not appreciably cause abnormal surgical bleeding or abnormal bleeding time or platelet aggregation [71]. Bleeding time appears to be increased when this supplement is taken concurrently with warfarin or aspirin/NSAIDS [27].

Glucosamine/Chondroitin Sulfate

Often taken concurrently, glucosamine and chondroitin sulfate supplements are utilized for the improvement of cartilage health for those with osteoarthritis. Interestingly, chondroitin shares a similar glycosaminoglycan structural makeup with heparin [114]. Glucosamine is shown to reduce platelet function via inhibition of ADP-induced platelet activation in humans [115]. In isolation, these supplements have not been convincingly shown to increase clinical bleeding. The use of glucosamine or glucosamine-chondroitin sulfate with warfarin may result in increased INR and bruising [116].

Vitamin E

Vitamin E supplements are purported to provide antioxidant and anti-atherosclerosis benefit as well as cancer prevention [114]. Vitamin E may antagonize the effect of Vitamin K and inhibit the production of Vitamin K-dependent factors, although this typically occurs only at high doses [117]. Vitamin E has been shown to inhibit the intrinsic coagulation pathway and may inhibit platelet aggregation and adhesion in patients with thrombocytopenia or diabetes [118]. In vitro reports and several clinical studies suggest a significant increase in bleeding risk due to Vitamin E-induced inhibition of platelet aggregation or interaction with aspirin or warfarin, though subsequent clinical studies have been unable to consistently replicate these results. Thus, any anticoagulant effects of Vitamin E may be dose-dependent and there may be elevated bleeding risk if they are co-administered with anticoagulants [27, 114].

Others

Magnesium, lycopene, selenium, and taurine may inhibit platelet function [71, 118]. Selenium may increase warfarin activity as shown in an animal model, possibly by displacing warfarin from albumin [119].

Supplement Interaction with Prescription Medication

One mechanism of nutritional supplement-associated hemorrhage is related to interaction with prescription medications. Perhaps the best studied prescription medication with such a risk is warfarin [34]. In general, the use of any previously mentioned nutritional supplement which independently exhibits an antiplatelet or anticoagulant effect, along with a pharmaceutical with antiplatelet or anticoagulant effects, should be expected to increase the risk of perioperative hemorrhage.

Perioperative Considerations

Routine questioning of patients about nutritional supplement usage is both reasonable and practical. Recommendations by several societies and care groups have been reported regarding the suggested time to avoid taking nutritional supplements in anticipation of surgery. These recommendations are limited by the clinical data available and should not replace clinical judgment in different patient care scenarios. The American Society of Anesthesiologists has previously recommended discontinuation of all herbal medications 2–3 weeks before an elective surgical procedure [120]. The Swedish Medical Products Agency recommends the discontinuation of some of the most commonly taken naturopathic medicines 2 weeks prior to surgery [113]. Dental professionals suggest discontinuation of herbal supplements 14 days prior to receiving invasive surgical procedures, though supplements may not need to be held prior to routine dental and dental hygiene procedures [121]. Others suggest discontinuation of any supplement around 15 days before an elective urologic extracorporeal shockwave lithotripsy procedure [122]. This seems prudent given ongoing effects of some herbals even at 14 days after administration [123]. The American Society of Regional Anesthesia and Pain Medicine has published updated guidelines addressing the risks of bleeding-related complications associated with regional anesthesia in patients receiving any antithrombotic or thrombolytic therapy. The authors recommend against required discontinuation of herbal supplements prior to neuraxial procedures and that regional anesthesia should not be withheld in those patients using these therapies. There is not a need to cancel a surgery or procedure if patients have not already discontinued these supplements [124].

Until more rigorous scientific studies related to bleeding risks associated with herbal medications and supplements exists, 2 weeks seems to be both a reasonable and consensus time period for discontinuing herbal medications prior to elective surgery. In isolated circumstances, such as prior to urgent or emergent surgery where bleeding poses a risk, it may be prudent to investigate the effects of a patient's nutritional supplements with standard coagulation tests in order to guide treatment for hemorrhage.

References

1. Craig WJ. Health-promoting properties of common herbs. Am J Clin Nutr. 1999;70(3,Suppl):491S–9S.
2. Petrovska BB. Historical review of medicinal plants' usage. Pharmacogn Rev. 2012;6:1–5.
3. Khan SU, Khan MU, Riaz H, Valavoor S, Zhao D, Vaughan L, et al. Effects of nutritional supplements and dietary interventions on cardiovascular outcomes: an umbrella review and evidence map. Ann Intern Med. 2019;9. Epub ahead of print
4. Mohan A, Lahiri A. Herbal medications and plastic surgery: a hidden danger. Aesthet Plast Surg. 2014;38(2):479–81.
5. Miller FG, Emanuel EJ, Rosenstein DL, Straus SE. Ethical issues concerning research in complementary and alternative medicine. JAMA. 2004;291(5):599–604.
6. Smith T, Kawa K, Eckle V, Morton C, Stredney R. Herbal supplement sales in US increased 8.5% in 2017, Topping $8 Billion. Herbal Gram. 2018;119:62–71.
7. Kirk J, Dunker KS. Dietary counseling: the ingredient for successfully addressing the use of herbal supplements and probiotics in chronic kidney disease. Adv Chronic Kidney Dis. 2014;21(4):377–84.
8. Kennedy J, Wang CC, Wu CH. Patient disclosure about herb and supplement use among adults in the US. Evid Based Complement Alternat Med. 2008;5(4):451–6.
9. Wang L, Lanka L, Chen D, Pruthi RK. Severe postoperative hemorrhage in a patient on dietary and herbal supplements. J Perioper Pract. 2018;28(10):263–6.
10. Zwiebel SJ, Lee M, Alleyne B, Guyuron B. The incidence of vitamin, mineral, herbal, and other supplement use in facial cosmetic patients. Plast Reconstr Surg. 2013;132(1):78–82.
11. Corey RL, Rakela J. Complementary and alternative medicine: risks and special considerations in pretransplant and posttransplant patients. Nutr Clin Pract. 2014;29(3):322–31.
12. Cohen MH. Complementary and integrative medical therapies, the FDA, and the NIH: definitions and regulation. Dermatol Ther. 2003;16(2):77–84.

13. Abe A, Kaye AD, Gritsenko K, Urman RD, Kaye AM. Perioperative analgesia and the effects of dietary supplements. Best Pract Res Clin Anaesthesiol. 2014;28(2):183–9.
14. Little DP. Authentication of Ginkgo biloba herbal dietary supplements using DNA barcoding. Genome. 2014;57(9):513–6.
15. Amster E, Tiwary A, Schenker MB. Case report: potential arsenic toxicosis secondary to herbal kelp supplement. Environ Health Perspect. 2007;115(4):606–8.
16. Buettner C, Mukamal KJ, Gardiner P, Davis RB, Phillips RS, Mittleman MA. Herbal supplement use and blood lead levels of Unites States adults. J Gen Intern Med. 2009;24(11):1175–82.
17. Yan G, Zhu Z, Jin L, Chen J, Xie H, Miozzi J, et al. Study on the quality evaluation of compound Danshen preparations based on the xCELLigence real-time cell-based assay and Pharmacodynamic authentication. Molecules. 2018;23(9):2090.
18. Vaclavik L, Krynitsky AJ, Rader JI. Mass spectrometric analysis of pharmaceutical adulterants in products labeled as botanical dietary supplements or herbal remedies: a review. Anal Bioanal Chem. 2014;406(27):6767–90.
19. Aykan DA, Aykan AC. Factors associated with the concomitant use of cardiovascular drugs and dietary herbal products: a cross-sectional study. J Cardiovasc Pharmacol Ther. 2018;27:1074248418794938. Epub ahead of print
20. Kaye AD, Clarke R, Sabar R, Vig S, Dhawan KP, Hofbauer R, Kaye AM. Herbal medicines: current trends in anesthesiology practice – a hospital survey. J Clin Anesth. 2000;12(6):468–71.
21. Qato DM, Wilder J, Schumm LP, Gillet V, Alexander GC. Changes in prescription and over-the-counter medication and dietary supplement use among older adults in the United States, 2005 vs 2011. JAMA Intern Med. 2016;176:473–82.
22. Rosenberg EI, Genao I, Chen I, Mechaber AJ, Wood JA, Faselis CJ, et al. Complementary and alternative medicine use by primary care patients with chronic pain. Pain Med. 2008;9(8):1065–72.
23. Navo MA, Phan J, Vaughan C, Palmer JL, Michaud L, Jones KL, et al. An assessment of the utilization of complementary and alternative medication in women with gynecologic or breast malignancies. J Clin Oncol. 2004;22(4):671–7.
24. Lewanda AF, Gallegos MF, Summar M. Patterns of dietary supplement use in children with down syndrome. J Pediatr. 2018;201:100–5.
25. Shaikh SA, Tischer S, Choi EK, Fontana RJ. Good for the lung but bad for the liver? Garlic-induced hepatotoxicity following liver transplantation. J Clin Pharm Ther. 2017;42(5):646–8.
26. Medina-Caliz I, Garcia-Cortes M, Gonzalez-Jimenez A, Cabello MR, Robles-Diaz M, Sanabria-Cabrera J. et al; Spanish DILI registry. Herbal and dietary supplement-induced liver injuries in the Spanish DILI registry. Clin Gastroenterol Hepatol. 2018;16(9):1495–502.
27. Wang CZ, Moss J, Yuan CS. Commonly used dietary supplements on coagulation function during surgery. Medicines. 2015;2(3):157–85.
28. Jayakumar T, Hsieh CY, Lee JJ, Sheu JR. Experimental and clinical pharmacology of Andrographis paniculata and its major bioactive Phytoconstituent Andrographolide. Evid Based Complement Alternat Med. 2013;2013:846740.
29. Madhusudan M, Zameer F, Naidu A. M N Nagendra Prasad, Dhananjaya BL, Hegdekatte R. Evaluating the inhibitory potential of Withania somnifera on platelet aggregation and inflammation enzymes: an in vitro and in silico study. Pharm Biol. 2016;54(9):1936–41.
30. Kokkiripati PK, Bhakshu LM, Marri S, Padmasree K, Row AT, Raghavendra AS, et al. Gum resin of Boswellia serrata inhibited human monocytic (THP-1) cell activation and platelet aggregation. J Ethnopharmacol. 2011;137(1):893–901.
31. Maurer HR. Bromelain: biochemistry, pharmacology and medical use. Cell Mol Life Sci. 2001;58(9):1234–45.
32. Coetzee C, Levendal RA, van de Venter M, Frost CL. Anticoagulant effects of a Cannabis extract in an obese rat model. Phytomedicine. 2007;14(5):333–7.
33. Yamaori S, Ebisawa J, Okushima Y, Yamamoto I, Watanabe K. Potent inhibition of human cytochrome P450 3A isoforms by cannabidiol: role of phenolic hydroxyl groups in the resorcinol moiety. Life Sci. 2011;88(15–16):730–6.
34. McEwen BJ. The influence of herbal medicine on platelet function and coagulation: a narrative review. Semin Thromb Hemost. 2015;41(3):300–14.
35. Paeng CH, Sprague M, Jackevicius CA. Interaction between warfarin and cranberry juice. Clin Ther. 2007;29(8):1730–5.
36. Hamann GL, Campbell JD, George CM. Warfarin-cranberry juice interaction. Ann Pharmacother. 2011;45(3):e17.
37. Fei YX, Wang SQ, Yang LJ, Qiu YY, Li YZ, Liu WY, et al. Salvia miltiorrhiza Bunge (Danshen) extract attenuates permanent cerebral ischemia through inhibiting platelet activation in rats. J Ethnopharmacol. 2017;207:57–66.
38. Maione F, De Feo V, Caiazzo E, De Martino L, Cicala C, Mascolo N. Tanshinone IIA, a major component of Salvia mlthorriza Bunge, inhibits platelet activation via Erk-2 signaling pathway. J Ethnopharmacol. 2014;155(2):1236–42.
39. Chan TY. Interaction between warfarin and danshen (Salvia miltiorrhiza). Ann Pharmacother. 2001;35(4):501–4.
40. Bermejo Benito P, Diaz Lanza AM, Silvan Sen AM, De Santos GJ, Fernandez Matellano L, Sanz Gomez A, et al. Effects of some iridoids from plant origin on arachidonic acid metabolism in cellular systems. Planta Med. 2000;66(4):324–8.
41. Anauate MC, Torres LM, de Mello SB. Effect of isolated fractions of Harpagophytum procumbens D.C. (devil's claw) on COX-1, COX-2 activity and nitric oxide production on whole-blood assay. Phytother Res. 2010;24(9):1365–9.
42. Page RL 2nd, Lawrence JD. Potentiation of warfarin by dong quai. Pharmacotherapy. 1999;19(7):870–6.
43. Dong WG, Liu SP, Zhu HH, Luo HS, Yu JP. Abnormal function of platelets and role of angelica sinensis in patients with ulcerative colitis. World J Gastroenterol. 2004;10(4):606–9.
44. Norred CL, Brinker F. Potential coagulation effects of preoperative complementary and alternative medicines. Altern Ther Health Med. 2001;7:58–67.
45. Bayles B, Usatine R. Evening primrose oil. Am Fam Physician. 2009;80(12):1405–8.
46. Werneke U, Earl J, Seydel C, Horn O, Crichton P, Fannon D. Potential health risks of complementary alternative medicines in cancer patients. Br J Cancer. 2004;90(2):408–13.
47. Ahmad A, Alghamdi SS, Mahmood K, Afzal M. Fenugreek a multipurpose crop: potentialities and improvements. Saudi J Biol Sci. 2016;23(2):300–10.
48. Philips CA, Augustine P. Rare cause of isolated severe coagulation failure in cirrhosis: traditional healing with fenugreek. BMJ Case Rep. 2018;12:2018.
49. Groenewegen WA, Heptinstall S. A comparison of the effects of an extract of feverfew and parthenolide, a component of feverfew, on human platelet activity in-vitro. J Pharm Pharmacol. 1990;42(8):553–7.
50. Heptinstall S, White A, Williamson L, Mitchell JR. Extracts of feverfew inhibit granule secretion in blood platelets and polymorphonuclear leucocytes. Lancet. 1985;1(8437):1071–4.
51. Stevinson C, Pittler MH, Ernst E. Garlic for treating hypercholesterolemia. A meta-analysis of randomized clinical trials. Ann Intern Med. 2000;133(6):420–9.
52. Apitz-Castro R, Escalante J, Vargas R, Jain MK. Ajoene, the antiplatelet principle of garlic, synergistically potentiates the antiaggregatory action of prostacyclin, forskolin, indo-

methacin and dypiridamole on human platelets. Thromb Res. 1986;42(3):303–11.
53. Chan KC, Yin MC, Chao WJ. Effect of diallyl trisulfide-rich garlic oil on blood coagulation and plasma activity of anticoagulation factors in rats. Food Chem Toxicol. 2007;45(3):502–7.
54. Fukao H, Yoshida H, Tazawa Y, Hada T. Antithrombotic effects of odorless garlic powder both in vitro and in vivo. Biosci Biotechnol Biochem. 2007;71(1):84–90.
55. Makheia AN, Vanderhoek JY, Bailey JM. Inhibition of platelet aggregation and thromboxane synthesis by onion and garlic. Lancet. 1979;1(8119):781.
56. Scharbert G, Kalb ML, Duris M, Marschalek C, Kozek-Langenecker SA. Garlic at dietary doses does not impair platelet function. Anesth Analg. 2007;105(5):1214–8.
57. Macan H, Uykimpang R, Alconcel M, Takasu J, Razon R, Amagase H, et al. Aged garlic extract may be safe for patients on warfarin therapy. J Nutr. 2006;136(3 Suppl):793S–5S.
58. Mohammed Abdul MI, Jiang X, Williams KM, Day RO, Roufogalis BD, Liauw WS, et al. Pharmacodynamic interaction of warfarin with cranberry but not with garlic in healthy subjects. Br J Pharmacol. 2008;154(8):1691–700.
59. Steiner M, Lin RS. Changes in platelet function and susceptibility of lipoproteins to oxidation associated with administration of aged garlic extract. J Cardiovasc Pharmacol. 1998;31(6):904–8.
60. Beckert BW, Concannon MJ, Henry SL, Smith DS, Puckett CL. The effect of herbal medicines on platelet function: an in vivo experiment and review of the literature. Plast Reconstr Surg. 2007;120(7):2044–50.
61. Borrelli F, Capasso R, Izzo AA. Garlic (Allium sativum L.): adverse effects and drug interactions in humans. Mol Nutr Food Res. 2007;51(11):1386–97.
62. Sunter W. Warfarin and garlic. Pharm J. 1991;246:722.
63. Al-Suhaimi EA, Al-Riziza NA, Al-Essa RA. Physiological and therapeutical roles of ginger and turmeric on endocrine functions. Am J Chin Med. 2011;39:215–31.
64. Saenghong N, Wattanathorn J, Muchimapura S, Tongun T, Piyavhatkul N, Banchonglikitkul C, et al. Zingiber officinale improves cognitive function of the middle-aged healthy women. Evid Based Complement Alternat Med. 2012;2012:383062.
65. Koo KL, Ammit AJ, Tran VH, Duke CC, Roufogalis BD. Gingerols and related analogues inhibit arachidonic acid-induced human platelet serotonin release and aggregation. Thromb Res. 2001;103(5):387–97.
66. Nurtjahja-tjendraputra E, Ammit AJ, Roufogalis BD, Tran VH, Duke CC. Effective anti-platelet and COX-1 enzyme inhibitors from pungent constituents of ginger. Thromb Res. 2003;111(4–5):259–65.
67. Jiang X, Williams KM, Liauw WS, Ammit AJ, Roufogalis BD, Duke CC, et al. Effect of ginkgo and ginger on the pharmacokinetics and pharmacodynamics of warfarin in healthy subjects. Br J Clin Pharmacol. 2005;59(4):425–32.
68. Koch E. Inhibition of platelet activating factor (PAF) - induced aggregation of human thrombocytes by ginkgolides: considerations on possible bleeding complications after oral intake of Ginkgo biloba extracts. Phytomedicine. 2005;12(1–2):10–6.
69. Rowin J, Lewis SL. Spontaneous bilateral subdural hematomas associated with chronic Ginkgo biloba ingestion. Neurology. 1996;46(6):1775–6.
70. Vale S. Subarachnoid haemorrhage associated with Ginkgo biloba. Lancet. 1998;352(9121):36.
71. Stanger MJ, Thompson LA, Young AJ, Lieberman HR. Anticoagulant activity of select dietary supplements. Nutr Rev. 2012;70(2):107–17.
72. Teng CM, Kuo SC, Ko FN, Lee JC, Lee LG, Chen SC, et al. Antiplatelet actions of panaxynol and ginsenosides isolated from ginseng. Biochim Biophys Acta. 1989;990(3):315–20.
73. Janetzky K, Morreale AP. Probable interaction between warfarin and ginseng. Am J Health Syst Pharm. 1997;54(6):692–3.
74. Jagroop IA. Plant extracts inhibit ADP-induced platelet activation in humans: their potential therapeutic role as ADP antagonists. Purinergic Signal. 2014;10(2):233–9.
75. Kang WS, Lim IH, Yuk DY, Chung KH, Park JB, Yoo HS, et al. Antithrombotic activities of green tea catechins and (−)-epigallocatechin gallate. Thromb Res. 1999;96(3):229–37.
76. Vibes J, Lasserre B, Gleye J, Declume C. Inhibition of thromboxane A2 biosynthesis in vitro by the main components of Crataegus oxyacantha (hawthorn) flower heads. Prostaglandins Leukot Essent Fatty Acids. 1994;50(4):173–5.
77. Felixsson E, Persson IA, Eriksson AC, Persson K. Horse chestnut extract contracts bovine vessels and affects human platelet aggregation through 5-HT(2A) receptors: an in vitro study. Phytother Res. 2010;24(9):1297–301.
78. Raduege KM, Kleshinski JF, Ryckman JV, Tetzlaff JE. Anesthetic considerations of the herbal, kava. J Clin Anesth. 2004;16(4):305–11.
79. Zou QZ, Bi RG, Li JM, Feng JB, Yu AM, Chan HP, et al. Effect of motherwort on blood hyperviscosity. Am J Chin Med. 1989;17(1–2):65–70.
80. Xiong L, Zhou QM, Peng C, Xie XF, Guo L, Li XH, et al. Sesquiterpenoids from the herb of Leonurus japonicus. Molecules. 2013;18(5):5051–8.
81. Alikhani Pour M, Sardari S, Eslamifar A, Azhar A, Rezvani M, Nazari M. Cheminformatics-based anticoagulant study of traditionally used medicinal plants. Iran Biomed J. 2017;21(6):400–5.
82. Arruzazabala ML, Molina V, Mas R, Fernandez L, Carbajal D, Valdes S, et al. Antiplatelet effects of policosanol (20 and 40 mg/day) in healthy volunteers and dyslipidaemic patients. Clin Exp Pharmacol Physiol. 2002;29(10):891–7.
83. Arruzazabala ML, Valdes S, Mas R, Carbajal D, Fernandez L. Comparative study of policosanol, aspirin and the combination therapy policosanol-aspirin on platelet aggregation in healthy volunteers. Pharmacol Res. 1997;36(4):293–7.
84. Castaño G, Arruzazabala ML, Fernández L, Mas R, Carbajal D, Molina V, et al. Effects of combination treatment with policosanol and omega-3 fatty acids on platelet aggregation: a randomized, double-blind clinical study. Curr Ther Res Clin Exp. 2006;67(3):174–92.
85. Gresele P, Pignatelli P, Guglielmini G, Carnevale R, Mezzasomoa AM, Ghiselli A, et al. Resveratrol, at concentrations attainable with moderate wine consumption, stimulates human platelet nitric oxide production. J Nutr. 2008;138(9):1602–8.
86. Tomé-Carneiro J, Gonzálvez M, Larrosa M, Yáñez-Gascón MJ, García-Almagro FJ, Ruiz-Ros JA, et al. One-year consumption of a grape nutraceutical containing resveratrol improves the inflammatory and fibrinolytic status of patients in primary prevention of cardiovascular disease. Am J Cardiol. 2012;110(3):356–63.
87. Oki T, Suzuki M, Nishioka Y, Yasuda A, Umegaki K, Yamada S. Effects of saw palmetto extract on micturition reflex of rats and its autonomic receptor binding activity. J Urol. 2005 Apr;173(4):1395–9.
88. Zhao T, Tang H, Xie L, Zheng Y, Ma Z, Sun Q, et al. Scutellaria baicalensis Georgi. (Lamiaceae): a review of its traditional uses, botany, phytochemistry, pharmacology and toxicology. J Pharm Pharmacol. 2019;71(9):1353–69.
89. Ku SK, Lee IC, Bae JS. Antithrombotic activities of oroxylin a in vitro and in vivo. Arch Pharm Res. 2014;37(5):679–86.
90. Borrelli F, Izzo AA. Herb-drug interactions with St John's wort (Hypericum perforatum): an update on clinical observations. AAPS J. 2009;11(4):710.
91. Lau WC, Welch TD, Shields T, Rubenfire M, Tantry US, Gurbel PA. The effect of St John's wort on the pharmacody-

namic response of clopidogrel in hyporesponsive volunteers and patients: increased platelet inhibition by enhancement of CYP3A4 metabolic activity. J Cardiovasc Pharmacol. 2011;57(1):86–93.
92. Aggarwal BB, Sundaram C, Malani N, Ichikawa H. Curcumin: the Indian solid gold. Adv Exp Med Biol. 2007;595:1–75.
93. Shah BH, Nawaz Z, Pertani SA, Roomi A, Maymood H, Saeed SA, et al. Inhibitory effect of curcumin, a food spice from turmeric, on platelet-activating factor- and arachidonic acid-mediated platelet aggregation through inhibition of thromboxane formation and Ca2+ signaling. Biochem Pharmacol. 1999;58(7):1167–72.
94. Mayanglambam A, Dangelmaier CA, Thomas D, Damodar Reddy C, Daniel JL, Kunapuli SP. Curcumin inhibits GPVI-mediated platelet activation by interfering with the kinase activity of Syk and the subsequent activation of PLCgamma2. Platelets. 2010;21(3):211–20.
95. Krivoy N, Pavlotzky E, Chrubasik S, Eisenber E, Brook G. Effect of salicis cortex extract on human platelet aggregation. Planta Med. 2001;67(3):209–12.
96. Yip AS, Chow WH, Tai YT, Cheung KL. Adverse effect of topical methylsalicylate ointment on warfarin anticoagulation: an unrecognized potential hazard. Postgrad Med J. 1990;66(775):367–9.
97. Joss JD, Leblond RF. Potentiation of warfarin anticoagulation associated with topical methyl salicylate. Ann Pharmacother. 2000;34(6):729–33.
98. Wang X, Zhang Y, Yang Y, Wu X, Fan H, Qiao Y. Identification of berberine as a direct thrombin inhibitor from traditional Chinese medicine through structural, functional and binding studies. Sci Rep. 2017;7:44040.
99. Lambert JP, Cormier J. Potential interaction between warfarin and boldo-fenugreek. Pharmacotherapy. 2001;21(4):509–12.
100. Liapina LA, Novikov VS, Pastorova VE, Uspenskaia MS, Smolina TI, Liapin GI. An anticoagulant from extracts of peony roots: its isolation and properties. Izv Akad Nauk Ser Biol. 1995;2:249–51.
101. Li CH, Chen C, Zhang Q, Tan CN, Hu YJ, Li P, et al. Differential proteomic analysis of platelets suggested target-related proteins in rabbit platelets treated with Rhizoma Corydalis. Pharm Biol. 2017;55(1):76–87.
102. Yao Y, Chen Y, Adili R, McKeown T, Chen P, Zhu G, et al. Plant-based food Cyanidin-3-glucoside modulates human platelet glycoprotein VI signaling and inhibits platelet activation and thrombus formation. J Nutr. 2017;147(10):1917–25.
103. Kim AH, Kim HJ, Ryu R, Han HJ, Han YJ, Lee MK, et al. A mixture of ethanol extracts of persimmon leaf and citrus junos sieb improves blood coagulation parameters and ameliorates lipid metabolism disturbances caused by diet-induced obesity in C57BL/6J mice. J Microbiol Biotechnol. 2016;26(2):295–308.
104. Ryu R, Kim HJ, Moon B, Jung UJ, Lee MK, Lee DG, et al. Ethanol extract of persimmon tree leaves improves blood circulation and lipid metabolism in rats fed a high-fat diet. J Med Food. 2015;18(7):715–23.
105. Teng CM, Li HL, Wu TS, Huang SC, Huang TF. Antiplatelet actions of some coumarin compounds isolated from plant sources. Thromb Res. 1992;66(5):549–57.
106. Shi YN, Shi YM, Yang L, Li XC, Zhao JH, Qu Y, et al. Lignans and aromatic glycosides from Piper wallichi and their antithrombotic activities. J Ethnopharmacol. 2015;162:87–96.
107. Lee JH, Kim M, Chang KH, Hong CY, Na CS, Dong MS, et al. Antiplatelet effects of Rhus verniciflua stokes heartwood and its active constituents-fisetin, butein, and sulfuretin-in rats. J Med Food. 2015;18(1):21–30.
108. Yao D, Wang Z, Miao L, Wang L. Effects of extracts and isolated compounds from safflower on some index of promoting blood circulation and regulating menstruation. J Ethnopharmacol. 2016;191:264–72.
109. Fasinu PS, Bouic PJ, Rosenkranz B. An overview of the evidence and mechanisms of herb-drug interactions. Front Pharmacol. 2012;3:69.
110. Bedi HS, Tewarson V, Negi K. Bleeding risk of dietary supplements: a hidden nightmare for cardiac surgeons. Indian Heart J. 2016;68(Suppl 2):S249–50.
111. Kim TH, Lee KM, Hong ND, Jung YS. Anti-platelet and anti-thrombotic effect of a traditional herbal medicine Kyung-ok-Ko. J Ethnopharmacol. 2016;178:172–9.
112. Dang X, Miao JJ, Chen AQ, Li P, Chen L, Liang JR, et al. The antithrombotic effect of RSNK in blood-stasis model rats. J Ethnopharmacol. 2015;173:266–72.
113. Bagge A, Schott U, Kander T. Effects of naturopathic medicines on Multiplate and ROTEM: a prospective experimental pilot study in healthy volunteers. BMC Complement Altern Med. 2016;16:64.
114. Wong WW, Gabriel A, Maxwell GP, Gupta SC. Bleeding risks of herbal, homeopathic, and dietary supplements: a hidden nightmare for plastic surgeons? Aesthet Surg J. 2012;32(3):332–46.
115. Hua J, Suguro S, Iwabuchi K, Tsutsumi-Ishii Y, Sakamoto K, Nagaoka I. Glucosamine, a naturally occurring amino monosaccharide, suppresses the ADP-mediated platelet activation in humans. Inflamm Res. 2004;53(12):680–8.
116. Knudsen JF, Sokol GH. Potential glucosamine-warfarin interaction resulting in increased international normalized ratio: case report and review of the literature and MedWatch database. Pharmacotherapy. 2008;28(4):540–8.
117. Booth SL, Golly I, Sacheck JM, Roubenoff R, Dallal GE, Hamada K, et al. Effect of vitamin E supplementation on vitamin K status in adults with normal coagulation status. Am J Clin Nutr. 2004;80(1):143–8.
118. Grisa A, Florio S, Bellia E, Cho SC, Froum SJ. The role of dietary supplements in postsurgical bleeding: an update for the practitioner. Compend Contin Educ Dent. 2016;37(10):690–5.
119. Davila JC, Edds GT, Osuna O, Simpson CF. Modification of the effects of aflatoxin B1 and warfarin in young pigs given selenium. Am J Vet Res. 1983;44(10):1877–83.
120. Frost EA. Herbal medicines and interactions with anesthetic agents. Middle East J Anaesthesiol. 2006;18(5):851–78.
121. Spolarich AE, Andrews L. An examination of the bleeding complications associated with herbal supplements, antiplatelet and anticoagulant medications. J Dent Hyg. 2007;81(3):67.
122. Gravas S, Tzortzis V, Rountas C, Melekos MD. Extracorporeal shock-wave lithotripsy and garlic consumption: a lesson to learn. Urol Res. 2010;38(1):61–3.
123. Morihara N, Hino A. Aged garlic extract suppresses platelet aggregation by changing the functional property of platelets. J Nat Med. 2017;71(1):249–56.
124. Horlocker TT, Vandermeulen E, Kopp SL, Gogarten W, Leffert LR, Benzon HT. Regional anesthesia in the patient receiving antithrombotic or thrombolytic therapy. Reg Anesth Pain Med. 2018;43:263–309.

Ultrasound for Bleeding Disorders

11

Chrissy J. Cherenfant

Principles of Ultrasound

Ultrasound imaging, also known as sonography, is the use of high-frequency sound waves to visualize the body internally [1, 2]. The frequency of ultrasound (US) is above 20,000 Hertz, which is beyond what can be heard by humans [1]. A concept important to understanding ultrasound imaging is resolution. Resolution is sonography's ability to differentiate between two points amidst a certain tissue depth. Lateral resolution is the minimal distance differentiated between two points located perpendicular to the ultrasound beam and is determined by beam width. Axial or longitudinal resolution is the minimal distance distinguished between two points parallel to the direction of the ultrasound beam [3–5]. Axial resolution is dependent on frequency. High-frequency probes, also known as transducers, have shorter wavelengths with less penetration and higher resolution. In contrast, low-frequency probes have longer wavelengths, less resolution, and better penetration, which is more suitable in viewing deeper structures [1, 3, 4].

Tissue echogenicity is another concept that is essential to the value of ultrasound. Echogenicity is a bodily tissue's ability to transmit and reflect waves compared to surrounding tissues. Favorably, differences in echogenicity of structures allows for a visible contrast on image display. Descriptions of echogenicity include hyperechoic, isoechoic, hypoechoic, and anechoic. Hyperechoic describes brighter echoes that appear white compared to surrounding structures, isoechoic are echoes equal in comparative appearance, hypoechoic depicts darker echoes that appear gray, and anechoic characterization is completely black on imaging. For instance, ascitic fluid and blood are anechoic, which attribute to sonography's usefulness in detecting fluid among solid hyperechoic or hypoechoic structures [1]. Echogenicity may also encompass imaging texture description, as heterogeneous being nonuniform and homogenous indicating uniform texture [3, 6].

Acquiring ultrasound imaging involves placing a probe (transducer) onto skin or into a body opening such as vagina or rectum. The purpose of the transducer is to convert electrical energy into the mechanical energy of sound waves that are directed into the patient. The transducer also receives the reflected echoes of waves bouncing off of body tissues and sends them to the computer for processing and image display [5, 7]. To aid in image acquisition, a layer of gel is placed onto the skin as a means of ultrasound wave transmission from the probe into the body. The three most commonly used probes are curved array, phased array, and linear. Curved array, also known as curvilinear, is a low-frequency transducer with a wedge-shaped US beam. It has a large field of view due to its large footprint, which is the surface that ultrasound waves are emitted from. Its low-frequency leads to greater tissue penetration, which contributes to the curved array being known as the abdominal probe, as it is more suitable for abdominal imaging. Compared to a curvilinear probe, the phased array probe also has a low-frequency, but with a smaller footprint. Its small footprint is fitting for visualizing cardiac and intrathoracic structures between ribs and echocardiography. Lastly, the linear probe has high-resolution and frequency, and preserved lateral resolution, making it better for procedural guidance and viewing superficial structures like vessels, nerves, and lung apices [3–6, 8–10] (Fig. 11.1). Of note, although probe choice is reliant on the particular objective, it is encouraged to choose the probe that will achieve the best resolution for the required depth. Nevertheless, probe selection and preference is ultimately user dependent [6].

Mode selection significantly impacts the quality and usefulness of ultrasound imaging. Amplitude or a-mode is the simplest ultrasound type showing a one-dimensional image. As a product of early ultrasonography, a-mode is used to assess the depth of a structure by exhibiting echo amplitude

C. J. Cherenfant (✉)
NYU Langone Health, NYU Langone Orthopedic Hospital, Department of Anesthesiology, Perioperative Medicine, and Pain Medicine, New York, NY, USA

© Springer Nature Switzerland AG 2021
C. S. Scher et al. (eds.), *Essentials of Blood Product Management in Anesthesia Practice*,
https://doi.org/10.1007/978-3-030-59295-0_11

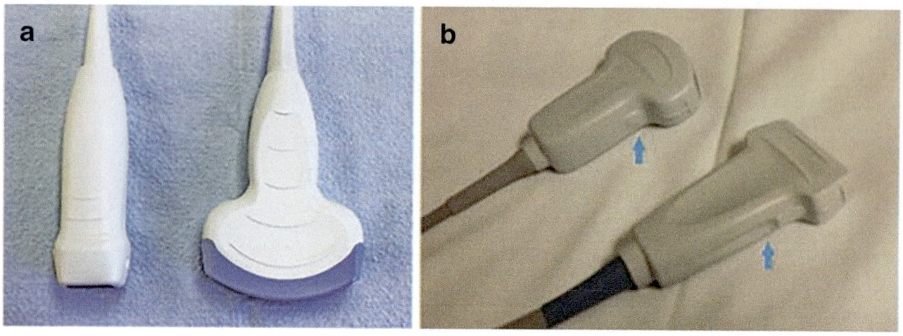

Fig. 11.1 (a) Phased array (left), curvilinear probe (right) (Reprinted with permission from Bornemann et al. [58]:9); (b): curvilinear (left), high-frequency linear (right) (Reprinted with permission from dela Cruz et al. [59], p. 175)

over distance. A-mode is commonly used in ophthalmology and therapeutic ultrasound as treatment for soft lesions, calculus, or tumor ablation [1, 11, 12]. Brightness mode which is also known as b-mode or gray scale or 2D is two-dimensional black and white imaging that is usually the default on ultrasound machines. B-mode/2D also displays echogenicity in shades of gray images, and allows the chosen plane, sagittal, transverse, cornal or oblique, to be visualized. Motion mode or m-mode is used to measure or display movement over time with a line on the screen that is adjustable. M-mode is mostly used in echocardiography and lung evaluation for pathologies such as pleural effusion and pneumothorax [1, 3, 13]. Spectral doppler ultrasound modality displays flow velocity over time in continuous and pulsed waves, which is beneficial for cardiac evaluation. Color doppler demonstrates velocity and direction of flow by color, with the usual convention of red symbolizing flow toward the probe and blue being away from the probe. There are additional modes such as three dimensional and four dimensional that are often used in obstetrics; however, the modes most commonly used in medical imaging have been mentioned [3].

Additional features that may impact ultrasound imaging include probe orientation, manipulation, angle of incidence, sliding/alignment, and pressure application. These skills and techniques are fundamentally dependent on the provider's education, clinical exposure, and clinical experience. Yet, it is important to note that they may impact the usefulness of ultrasound and consequently patient clinical management [3, 6].

Point-of-Care Ultrasound (PoCUS): What Is It?

Point-of-care ultrasound (PoCUS) is the real-time, goal-oriented use of ultrasound performed and interpreted by a healthcare provider at a patient's bedside, with the intention of improving patient outcomes. By its quality of rapid imaging that could be correlated with a patient's symptoms, PoCUS is the application of ultrasound for answering a specific diagnostic question, narrowing differentials, screening, and ultimately aiding in clinical decision making as an adjunct to physical examination [1, 8, 14–17]. PoCUS has the feature of being easily repeatable, which is advantageous in monitoring patients as their condition change [1]. Additionally, it serves as a means of acute intervention and therapeutic guidance, while also having the capacity to guide invasive procedures [14, 18]. The fundamental difference between PoCUS and regular ultrasonography is that regularly ultrasound can assess anatomy, bodily functions, and procedural guidance, while PoCUS encompasses these features with the addition of being goal-oriented and providing immediate clinical information at the bedside [19].

Indications

Within anesthesiology and its subspecialties, ultrasound is used in many ways, including central venous catheter (CVC) guidance, intravenous access, US-guided peripheral nerve blockade, facet joint and transforaminal nerve root injections, and echocardiography. PoCUS has the ability to execute these existing features and further assist in diagnostic and procedural elements at the patient's bedside in perioperative, intraoperative, and postoperative settings [1, 14, 20–23]. Furthermore, point-of-care ultrasound possesses value in evaluating the whole body, from head to toe (Table 11.1).

Ophthalmology/Neurology

Optic nerve sheath diameter (ONSD) measured by PoCUS has been found to be associated with intracranial pressure [20] (Fig. 11.2). In continuity with the brain subarachnoid space, the optic nerve sheath can be reflective of intracranial pressure (ICP). Although diameter measuring 5–7 mm can be normal, ONSD greater than 5 mm has been associated with evidence of increased ICP evident on CT [23–25]. In obstetric populations, there have been findings of thicker optic nerve sheath among patients with preeclampsia [26]. In pediatric population with neurological pathology, enlarged

Table 11.1 Ultrasound application in anesthesiology: Critical care and perioperative medicine

Objective	PoCUS Application
Airway	Procedural: Endotracheal tube placement, double lumen placement, cricoid membrane puncture, cricothyroidotomy, upper airway regional block, tracheostomy Diagnostic: Cervical spine, anterior neck fat tissue, vocal cord mobility, diaphragmatic movement, predicting extubation failure,
Abdominal	Procedural: TAP /truncal blockade guidance, paracentesis Diagnostic: Free fluid (FAST), gastric volume and content
Cardiology	Procedural: Pacing capture detection, pericardiocentesis Diagnostic: Echocardiography, ventricular and valvular function, hemodynamics, fluid status, pericardial effusion
Ophthalmology/neurology	Diagnostic: ICP estimation by optic nerve sheath diameter, foreign bodies, retinal detachment, lens dislocation, vitreous hemorrhage,ocular hematoma
Pulmonary	Procedural: endobronchial/double lumen tube placement, thoracentesis Diagnostic: Dyspnea, pleural effusion, pneumothorax, pulmonary edema, pneumonia, severe interstitial disease
Regional anesthesia/pain medicine	Procedural: Peripheral nerve blockade, neuraxial blockade, trunk blockade,transforaminal/interlaminar nerve root injections
Shock	Diagnostic: Fluid status monitoring, hemodynamic evaluation
Urinary	Procedural: Foley catheterization confirmation Diagnostic: Renal obstruction
Vascular	Procedural: Guidance for venous and arterial access (central and peripheral), central venous catheterization Diagnostic: arterial and venous patency, aortic dissection, aortic aneurysm, IVC collapsibility, Doppler flow across peripheral arteries and LVOT, vascular compression for DVT
Other	Procedural: Abscess drainage Diagnostic: Cellulitis and abscess assessment

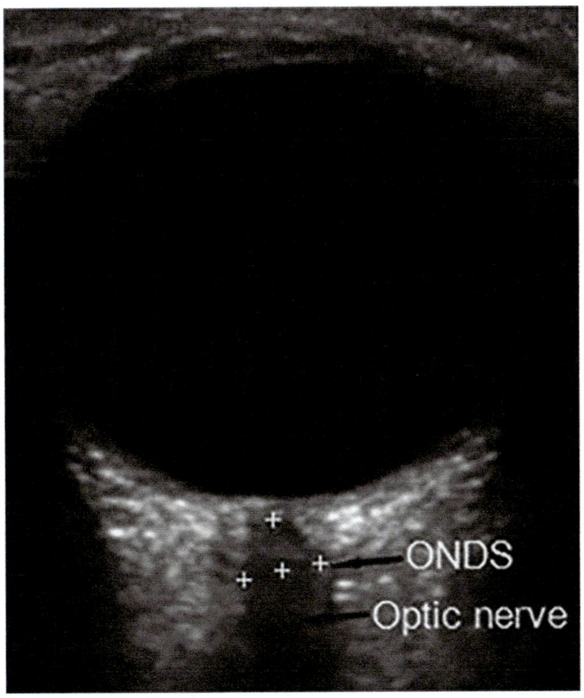

Fig. 11.2 Optic nerve sheath diameter (Reprinted with permission from Jeong [60], p. 151)

ONSD has also been correlated with increased ICP [27]. Thus, in patients with symptoms of or pathologies susceptible to increased intracranial pressure, PoCUS can be used diagnostically, especially in the acute setting.

Airway Evaluation

Ultrasound has the existing role of procedural guidance for upper airway regional blocks [23]. Airway assessment and management is an emerging application of PoCUS that poses usefulness to intensivists and anesthesiologists, preoperatively and intraoperatively. PoCUS can confirm placement of endotracheal and double lumen tubes and can differentiate between endobronchial, tracheal, and esophageal intubations [23, 28]. Linear probe use at the suprasternal notch has been found to have high specificity and sensitivity in determining endotracheal tube placement [21]. US can also be used at the patient's bedside preoperatively for airway examination. Compared to regular airway screening tests such as, mouth opening and neck mobility, US measured reduced mandibular condylar mobility is correlated with difficult laryngoscopy, with limited mobility defined as less than 10 mm in one study [29, 30]. PoCUS can also aid in identifying potential difficult laryngoscopies by measuring anterior neck soft tissue thickness at the level of the hyoid bone and thyrohyoid membrane [15]. Another study found US measured anterior neck soft tissue thickness at the level of the vocal cords greater than 0.23 cm to be a possible predictor of challenging intubation [31]. Other US airway measurements and imaging that may predict difficult intubations prior to induction of anesthesia include hyomental distance, tracheal diameter, vocal cord pathologies or dysfunctions, and anatomic variations [23, 28]. PoCUS may also reduce risk of failure or complications from emergency surgical airway, where US has been found to be more reliable than manually locating the cricothyroid membrane in obese patients [32]. In the setting of possible airway complications, point-of-care ultrasound can serve as a valuable tool that benefits patient care [14, 18, 26, 28, 32].

Pulmonary

In the fields of emergency medicine and critical care, ultrasound has the established role of diagnosing pneumothorax by the absence of lung sliding [16, 33, 34]. Lung sliding is visualized from US as an artifact of parietal pleura moving against visceral pleura during respiration. The sliding is prohibited with a pneumothorax because air is between the visceral and parietal pleura [8, 35]. As a consequence of trauma or an iatrogenic complication from central venous catheterization or peripheral nerve blockade, determining the occurrence of pneumothorax is very important. PoCUS is beneficial among patients concerning for pneumothorax due to it providing rapid critical imaging that can be immediately interpreted and managed by the clinician at the bedside. Using B-mode or M-mode and a linear transducer with higher frequency and better resolution (Fig. 11.3), pneumothorax can be diagnosed via PoCUS. The imaging will demonstrate the absence of lung sliding on B-mode, while on M-mode, pneumothorax displays as a uniform linear pattern above and below the pleural line that is known as "barcode or stratosphere sign." In contrast, a normal lung ultrasound on M-mode would show "seashore sign" pattern linear to granular pattern change at the visceral pleural line [8, 26, 35] (Fig. 11.4). In evaluating trauma patients, US has been shown to be twice as more sensitive at detecting occult pneumothorax than supine chest radiography [1, 36]. However, it is important to note that the absence of lung sliding indicating pneumothorax must be in the presence of no other concurrent lung disease and in the appropriate clinical context. The lack of lung sliding is not specific for pneumothorax, as any lung disease process, such as pneumonia, atelectasis, or contralateral endobronchial intubation, can manifest as absent lung sliding. Also, small pneumothorax may be missed by US and blebs or scarring may cause false positives [1, 20, 21, 35].

Lung ultrasound having high accuracy in diagnosing hypoxia strengthens PoCUS's diagnostic role in pulmonary presentations [38]. Pathological conditions that can be discovered by PoCUS include pulmonary edema, pulmonary effusion, consolidations reflective of pneumonia, dynamic air bronchograms concerning for pneumonia, chronic obstructive pulmonary disease, pulmonary embolism, pulmonary fibrosis, and alveolar interstitial disease [9, 14, 35, 37, 38]. One of the common ultrasound findings are B lines, which may represent fluid overload, pleural effusion, lung consolidation due to pneumonia, or interstitial disease [1, 21, 35]. After detecting pleural effusion, PoCUS can further serve as a diagnostic and therapeutic aid in procedural guidance for thoracentesis [23]. There have also been some suggestions for use of PoCUS to detect atelectasis preoperatively and to address desaturation on pulse oximetry intraoperatively [18]. Due to its sensitive, specific, and expeditious

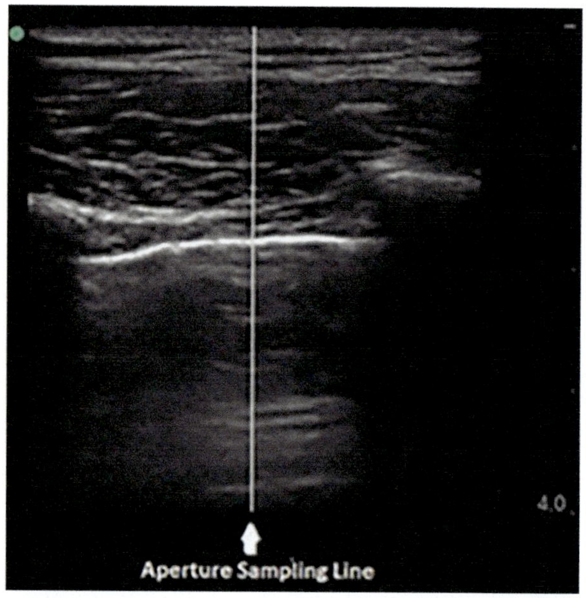

Fig. 11.3 M-mode with sampling line in the intercostal space (Reprinted with permission from dela Cruz et al. [59], p. 180)

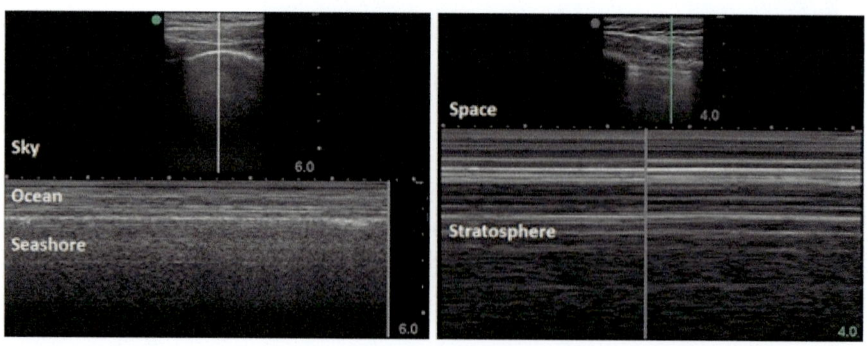

Fig. 11.4 Normal M-mode seashore sign (left) and barcode/stratosphere sign indicating pneumothorax (right) (Reprinted with permission from dela Cruz et al. [59], p. 181)

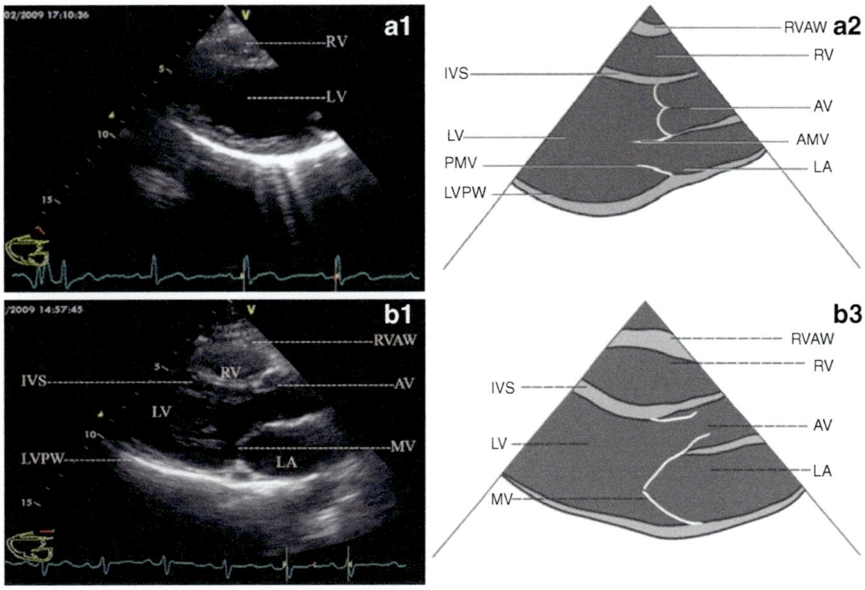

Fig. 11.5 Parasternal left ventricular long axis view (**a**) Diastole (**b**) Systole IVS Interventricular septum, LV Left ventricle, PMV Pulmonary valve, LVPW Left ventricular posterior wall, LA left atrium, AMV Anterior mitral valve, AV Aortic valve, RV Right ventricle, RVAW Right ventricle anterior wall (Reprinted with permission from He [61], p. 75)

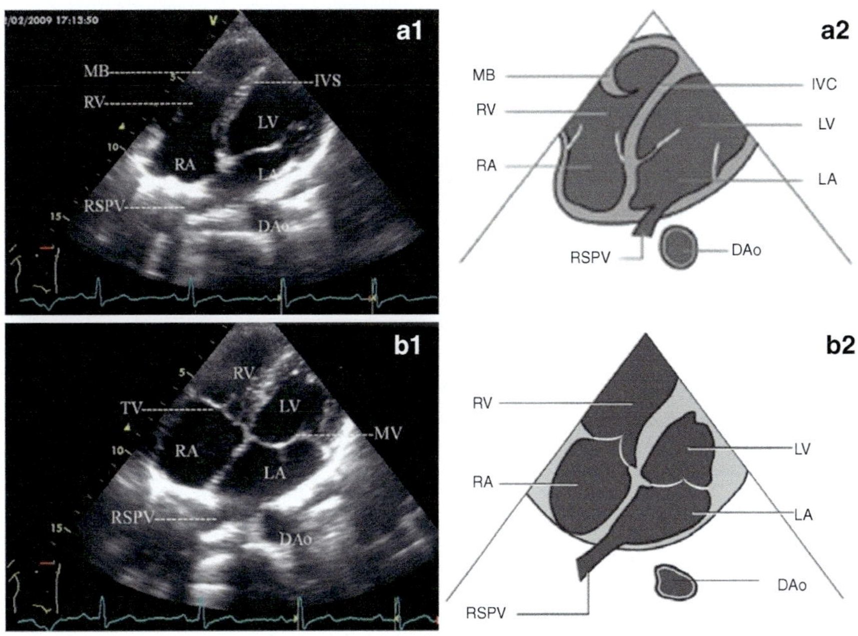

Fig. 11.6 Parasternal four chamber view (**a**) Diastole (**b**) Systole MB Moderator band, RV Right ventricle, RA Right atrium, RSPV Right superior pulmonary vein, DAo Descendign aorta, LA left atrium, LV left ventricle, IVC Inferior vena cava (Reprinted with permission from He [61], p. 84)

detection of a wide array of lung pathologies, especially during times of acute patient deterioration, lung ultrasound is considered to be an essential PoCUS skill [9, 39].

Cardiology

Cardiac ultrasound is utilized by anesthesiologists diagnostically. Transesophageal echocardiography (TEE) is an established practice in cardiac surgeries and is a PoCUS skill that has standard guidelines [14, 21, 40]. At the bedside in the intensive care unit (ICU), focused cardiac ultrasound (FoCUS) with transthoracic echocardiography (TTE) is used to determine ventricular failure and pericardial effusions [15, 27]. PoCUS can augment cardiac physical examination performed by an anesthesiologist. For instance, a murmur heard on examination can be rapidly correlated with valvular pathology [40]. Cardiac pathologies detected by PoCUS include pericardial effusion, tamponade, pulmonary emboli, severe hypovolemia, postpartum cardiomyopathy, myocardial thickness, and dilated heart chambers [15, 26, 29]. PoCUS can also serve as procedural guidance for pericardiocentesis and detect pacing capture [23]. Of note, PoCUS differs from TTE performed by cardiologists by being less comprehensive and more goal-oriented with the aim of assisting physicians to quickly rule out or in diagnoses [21]. The phased array probe, also known as the cardiac probe, in 2D or M-mode is more suitable for cardiac evaluation [3, 9, 41, 42] (Figs. 11.5, 11.6, 11.7, and 11.8).

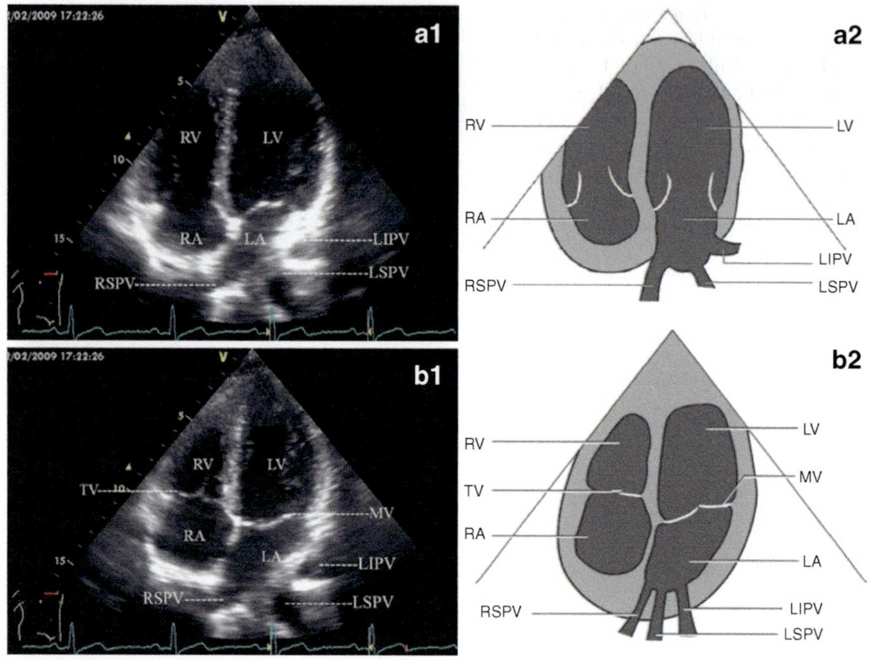

Fig. 11.7 Apical four chamber view (**a**) Diastole (**b**) Systole RV Right ventricle, RA Right atrium, LV Left ventricle, LA Left atrium, RSPV Right superior pulmonary vein, LSPV Left superior pulmonary vein, LIPV Left inferior pulmonary vein, TV Tricuspid valve, MV Mitral valve (Reprinted with permission from He [61], p. 85)

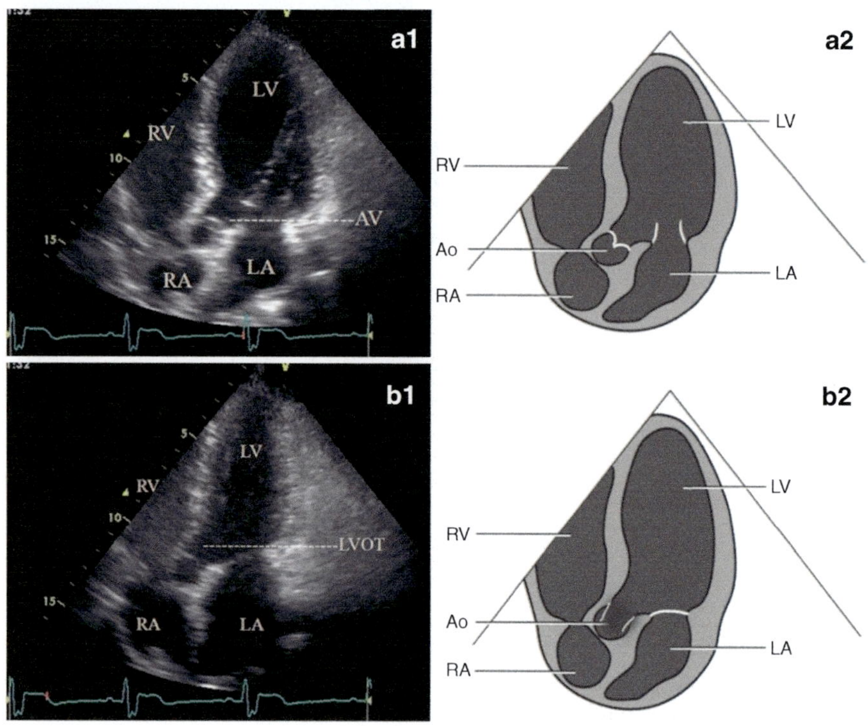

Fig. 11.8 Apical five chamber view (**a**) Diastole (**b**) Systole RV Right ventricle, Ao Aorta, RA Right atrium, LA Left atrium, LV Left ventricle (Reprinted with permission from He [61], p. 93)

Cardiac PoCUS, which essentially is a focused TTE, also has the ability to identify and monitor ventricular dysfunction and severe valvular pathology, not only during cardiac procedures but also during non cardiac surgeries, periods of hemodynamic instability, and preoperatively [1, 14, 23]. Focused TTE has been found to change patient management and impact perioperative care. Studies have shown that preoperative TTE in patients at risk for cardiac disease or with periods of hemodynamic instability can diagnose low ejection fraction, aortic and mitral valve disease, hypovolemia, tamponade, and ventricular failure. These findings often resulted in changed anesthetic management such as medication changes, cancellations, fluid boluses or restrictions, and implementation of invasive monitoring [15, 29, 40, 43]. This effect supports the need for cardiac PoCUS use preoperatively.

PoCUS during pulse checks of cardiac arrests can also be valuable in aiding decision making. This is due to PoCUS providing further information such as detecting a potential etiology like pericardial effusion or hypovolemia and displaying an absence of systolic contractions, which suggests minimal likelihood for return of spontaneous circulation after three rounds of cardiopulmonary resuscitation medication administration [16, 44]. In addition, focused assessment with sonography for trauma (FAST) examination includes obtaining a pericardial view to diagnose cardiac free fluid such as blood, in trauma patients [16]. This also exhibits PoCUS's practicality in determining cardiac injury.

Abdominal

Abdominal point-of-care ultrasound aids in the immediate visualization of abdominal tissues and organs [2]. This is advantageous in the setting of abdominal trauma, symptoms, or procedures. Curvilinear or curved array probe is better suited for abdominal imaging due to its low-frequency and greater penetrance [3, 8]. The FAST exam is well known in emergency medicine as a focused abdominal assessment for free fluid. FAST encompasses evaluation of the hepatorenal space, perisplenic space, subcostal/subxiphoid space, and suprapubic area [8, 16, 21] (Fig. 11.9).

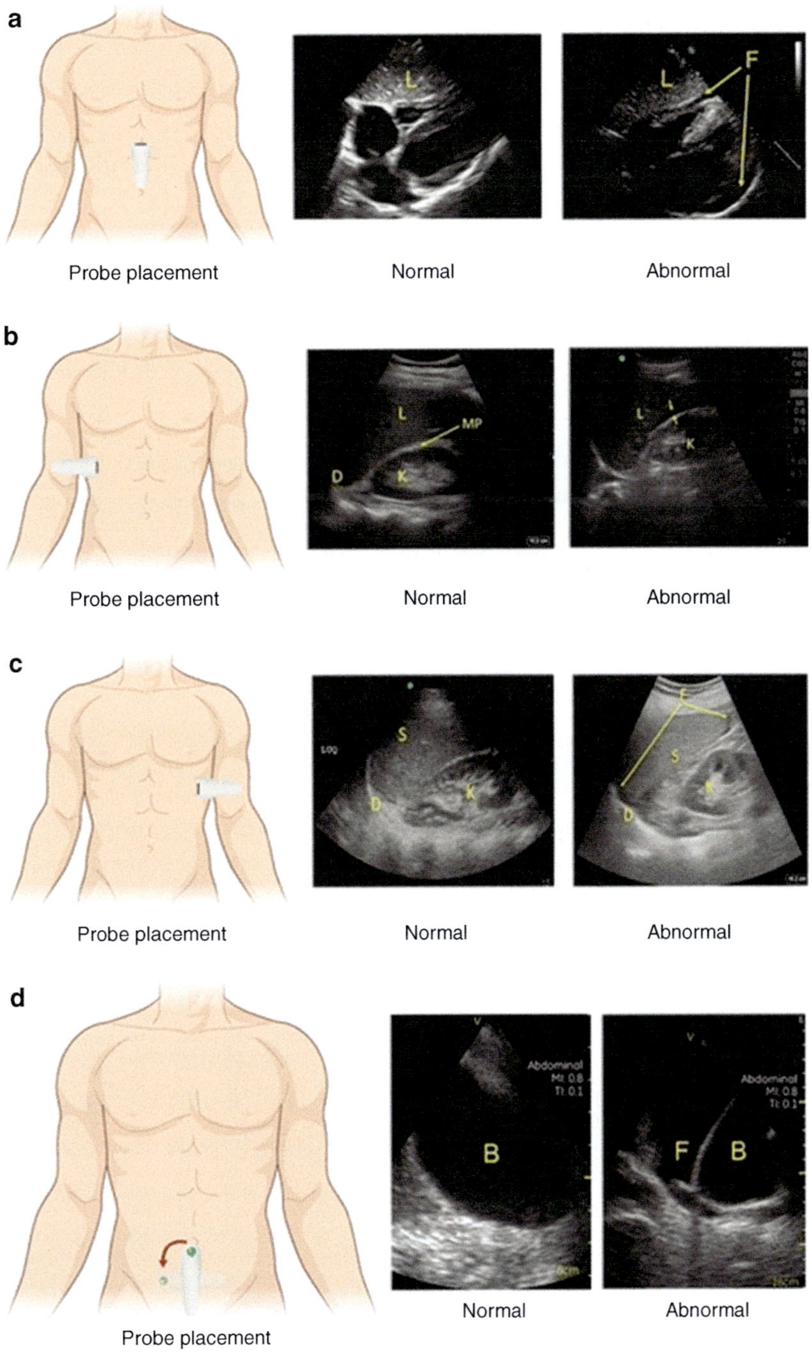

Fig. 11.9 FAST examination. (**a**) Probe to subxiphoid with liver (L) showing presence of absence of pericardial fluid (F). (**b**) Probe to RUQ, showing absence or presence of free fluid in Morrison's Pouch (MP) between liver and kidney (K). (**c**) Probe to LUQ, showing absence or presence of free fluid (F) near spleen (S) and kidney. (**d**) Long axis pelvic view with normal bladder (B) on left and free fluid posterior to bladder on left. B bladder, D diaphragm, F fluid, K kidney, L liver, MP Morrison's pouch, S Spleen (Reprinted with permission from Bornemann et al. [58], p. 15)

Abdominal PoCUS can acutely evaluate disease processes and diagnose etiologies of sepsis. Cholethiasis is identified by rounded, hyperechoic structures and common bile duct dilation, and cholecystitis displays as gallbladder wall thickening and pericholecystic fluid. US can detect intestinal obstruction by loops of bowel >3 cm, extra-luminal fluid, luminal air, and bowel wall thickening. PoCUS can also evaluate etiologies of renal colic by displaying stones and hydronephrosis and identify abdominal aortic aneurysms [16]. Abdominal US is also used at the bedside in medicine for diagnosis of ascites, and therapeutically by facilitating procedural guidance for paracentesis [23].

In pain management of abdominal surgeries, ultrasound is used for procedural guidance of nerve blockades like rectus main sheath and transversus abdominis plane (TAP) blocks. Ultrasound use has decreased complications and improved anesthesia placement [26, 39, 45, 46]. Abdominal PoCUS has further applications that can be beneficial to care provided by anesthesiologists. Preoperatively, PoCUS can aid in decreasing the risk of aspiration, by examining gastric content and volume [17, 21, 23, 27, 41]. Ultrasound measurement of gastric antrum cross-sectional area and stomach content volume are indicators of aspiration risk at induction, where a patient in right lateral decubitus position having a cross-sectional area < 4 cm is 95% specific for an empty stomach [20–22]. Gastric PoCUS can therefore lead to anesthetic management changes in patients who do not follow fasting instructions [22]. Postoperatively, abdominal PoCUS examination can detect intra-abdominal fluid extravasation (IAFE) that has correlated to increased pain scores in the postanesthesia care unit [29, 47]. Another indication of abdominal PoCUS is confirming gastric tube placement in the ICU, which reduces x-ray exposure [20]. Overall, with its many applications, abdominal PoCUS can enhance perioperative care.

Regional Anesthesia

Ultrasound guidance in regional anesthesia is conventionally used for peripheral nerve and truncal blockade and in interventional pain medicine with a comparable effectiveness to fluoroscopy [20, 23, 48].Ultrasound has made regional anesthesia safer, more efficient and effective, and easier to teach [20, 21, 26, 29, 41, 45, 46, 49–52]. Although not replacing the gold standard of radiographs, musculoskeletal PoCUS can diagnose dislocated shoulder and reduction [8]. US-guided neuraxial anesthesia can be beneficial in the setting of obesity, edema, previous spinal surgery, scoliosis, lordosis, and difficult landmark identification by locating vertebral spaces, interspinous spaces, angulation, and epidural depth, better than palpitation [18, 26, 48, 53]. The American Society of Regional Anesthesia and Pain Medicine (ASRA) has supported the recommendation that neuraxial ultrasound increases lumbar neuraxial anesthesia efficiency and is more accurate in predicting depth to target than palpation [52]. Despite these advantages, US-guided neuraxial anesthesia is not widely utilized due to the success of palpitating lumbar spinous processes [41].

Vascular/Shock

Ultrasound is often used by healthcare providers as guidance for venous and arterial access, with examples of intravenous line placement and central venous catheterization [1, 18, 21, 23, 26, 39, 41]. PoCUS can be used by intensivists in the ICU and anesthesiologists in the perioperative period to rapidly characterize shock. Ultrasound can differentiate between hypovolemic, cardiogenic, and distributive etiologies of shock by evaluating the heart, lungs, inferior vena cava (IVC), and abdomen [9, 44]. PoCUS has been found to aid clinicians in narrowing their differential diagnosis in patients with undifferentiated hypotension in the emergency department [16]. Thus, PoCUS can lead to faster diagnosis and consequently sooner treatment, while also providing a platform for monitoring treatment results [44]. PoCUS has also been shown to assess for fluid administration response preoperatively and in the PACU. This is done by IVC measurement during spontaneous ventilation, which is correlated to intravascular volume [27] (Figs. 11.10 and 11.11). Additionally, ultrasound is the screening modality for abdominal aortic aneurysm in men with smoking history of ages 65–75 and can be used to evaluate for aneurysm in patients with symptoms of aortic rupture [20] (Fig. 11.12).

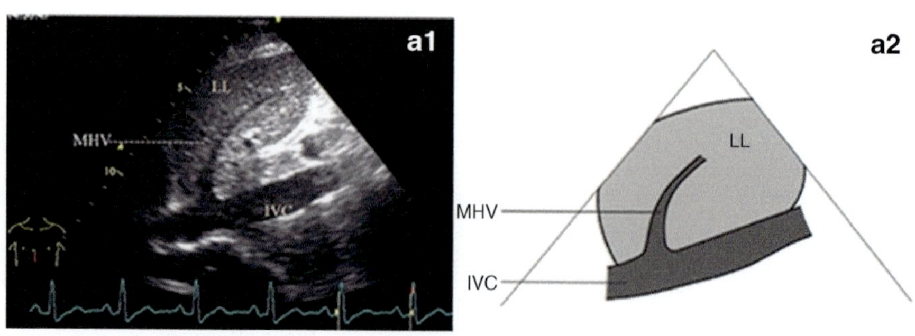

Fig. 11.10 Short axis view of IVC MHV middle hepatic vein, LL liver, IVC inferior vena cava (Reprinted with permission from He [61], p. 94)

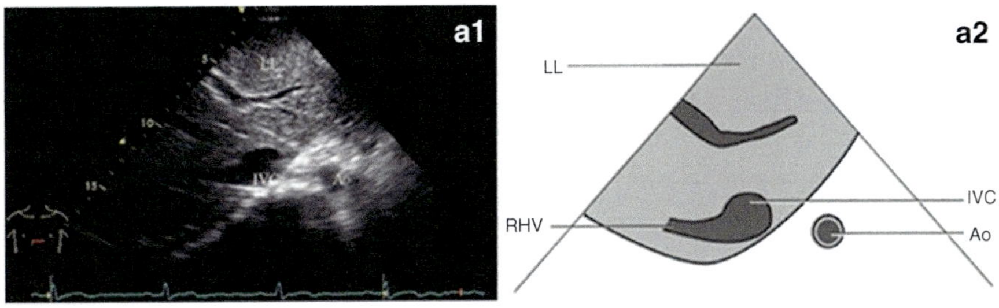

Fig. 11.11 Long axis view of IVC IVC inferior vena cava, LL Liver, RHV right hepatic vein, Ao Aorta (Reprinted with permission from He [61], p. 95)

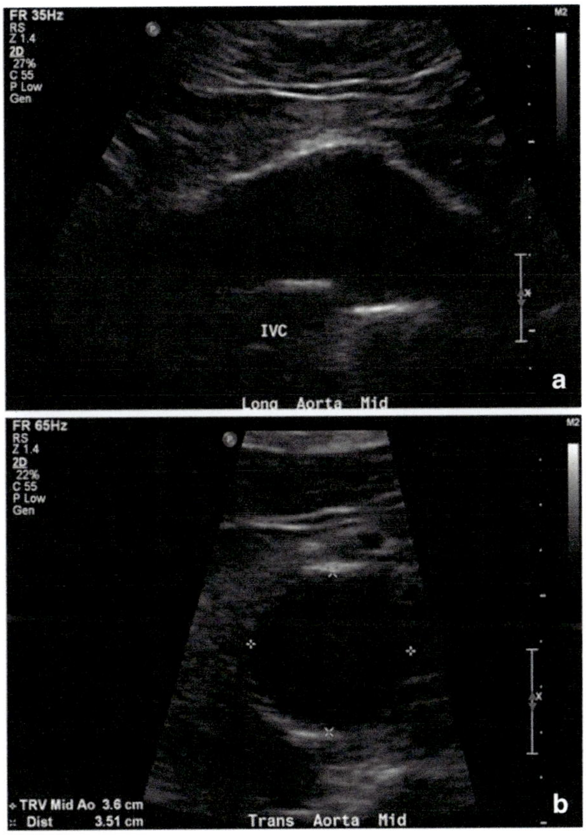

Fig. 11.12 Abdominal aortic aneurysm (**a**) short axis (**b**) long axis (Reprinted with permission from Bornemann et al. [58], p. 29)

Ultrasound Views

Depending on its objective, PoCUS is optimally utilized in certain views. Generally, structures can be viewed in short axis, long axis, and oblique views. Vessels, nerves, and other anatomical structures are commonly viewed in short axis, while a long-axis approach is preferred for needle vascular access, so the needle can be visualized during the procedure. Yet, it may be easier for the vessel and needle to both be in view in short axis [1, 6]. For cardiac PoCUS, parasternal long- and short-axis views are recommended. To further evaluate valvular pathology, apical or subcostal chamber views and color Doppler are useful [40]. FAST examination is composed of pericardial view, also described as subcostal or subxiphoid, right upper quadrant or perihepatic view, left upper quadrant or perisplenic view, and suprapubic or pelvic view. The extended FAST also includes bilateral anterior chest wall views to assess for lung sliding usually at the mid-clavicular line in M-mode [1, 8, 16, 21]. Fundamentally, multiple views and modes can be easily selected and are ultimately user dependent.

Benefits and Drawbacks

The major advantage of point-of-care testing is improved speed of diagnostic testing with accuracy. The time between onset of symptoms and therapy initiation is decreased, resulting in better patient outcomes [16]. The benefits of point-of-care ultrasound are that it is reliable and time saving since immediate clinician interpretation eliminates the waiting on radiologists and cardiologists readings, which is favorable for acute issues [1, 18]. PoCUS is also easily repeatable which is ideal for monitoring [1]. With no ionizing radiation, diagnostic ultrasound is safe, especially in obstetric and pediatric populations [1, 20]. PoCUS used for procedural guidance decreases number of attempts and complication rates and improves safety and quality of care [20, 21]. PoCUS equipment is also becoming less expensive and portable, making it more accessible and suitable for low resource settings [1, 20, 21].

The major drawback of PoCUS is that the provided information is user dependent, relying on the user's skills with the transducer and ability to accurately identify findings while avoiding artifacts. In the hands of an unskilled user, PoCUS may not be beneficial to patient care since an inaccurate diagnosis can lead to complications or inappropriate therapies [1, 5, 54]. Ultrasound imaging may also be negatively impacted by patient immobility [37]. In certain scenarios, although PoCUS provides rapid imaging, it does not replace diagnostic imaging interpreted by radiologists [20]. There is also a concern that PoCUS use on multiple patients may increase disease transmission if not disinfected. PoCUS may also be overused, leading to unnecessary interventions due to false-positive findings or inadequate further assessment due to false negatives that can be harmful and expensive [1, 21]. Furthermore, many anesthesiology PoCUS applications have no guidelines for education, training, or appropriate use. This contributes to the concern of PoCUS utility without substantial knowledge or proficiency demonstration [54].

The Future

The main barrier to widespread point-of-care ultrasound use in anesthesiology is the deficit of PoCUS education and training in the field, especially when compared to emergency medicine. In the USA, most anesthesiologists have not had any training in PoCUS, and there is no standard PoCUS curriculum in most anesthesiology residencies [14, 55]. However, there has been many calls for action to create a curriculum and develop guidelines for perioperative PoCUS use [14, 23, 54, 55].

In 2015, a perioperative PoCUS special interest group was created within ASRA. In 2016, they held their first meeting and continue to have a growing membership today [14, 56]. One paper discusses the perioperative anesthesiology ultrasonographic evaluation (PAUSE) approach during perioperative management. It is a tool for anesthesiologists to "pause" various times and use PoCUS to assess patients and extend upon information from physical examination and vitals monitoring [40]. With increasing interest in PoCUS, there have been many discussions and investigations on the possible methods of institutionalizing perioperative PoCUS and evaluating its existing and additional applications. There is a need for a multipurpose curriculum to be reflective of the many settings anesthesiology is practiced [15]. There have been suggestions of implementing PoCUS via many modalities such as e-learning, didactic teaching, practical sessions, and human model or stimulation practicing. Among anesthesiology residents, online didactics, hands-on training, and simulation-based curriculum have resulted in increased knowledge, improved image acquisition and manual dexterity, high participant satisfaction, and clinical transferability of skills. It has been suggested that teaching and training should be longitudinal, across years and rotations, to decrease the likelihood of diminished skills that occurs without reinforcement and continued use [34, 39, 54, 57]. PoCUS curriculum must also continue to have the goal of improving patient care [34, 56]. Fundamentally, there continues to be a need for research on point-of-care ultrasound effect on patient care and outcomes, applications, and how to implement effective PoCUS training.

Summary

Point-of-care ultrasound is a tool and skill that can optimize clinical evaluation, beyond physical examinations. PoCUS is advantageous due to its abundance, diverse applications in cardiac, pulmonary, abdominal, neurological, airway, hemodynamic, and vascular systems. Its role of safely and immediately answering specific diagnostic questions, directing therapy, and guiding procedures further validates its significance. As point-of-care ultrasound positively impacts patient care, there continues to be a need for development of curriculum and guidelines for PoCUS education and training, as well as research to provide further evidence of its benefits and uses. Just as ultrasound is commonly known to be employed in regional anesthesia and for central venous catheterization, it is conceivable that in the future point-of-care ultrasound may also be used ubiquitously.

References

1. Moore CL, Copel JA. Point-of-care ultrasonography. N Engl J Med. 2011;364(8):749–57.
2. Center for Devices and Radiological Health. Ultrasound imaging. U.S. Food and Drug Administration. https://www.fda.gov/radiation-emitting-products/medical-imaging/ultrasound-imaging. Published 8 Aug 2019. Accessed 5 Sept 2019.
3. Baston CM, Moore C, Krebs EA, Dean AJ, Panebianco N, editors. Physics and knobology. In: Pocket guide to POCUS: point-of-care tips for point-of-care ultrasound. New York: McGraw-Hill. http://accessmedicine.mhmedical.com.ezproxy.med.nyu.edu/content.aspx?bookid=2544&sectionid=210344236. Accessed 5 Sept 2019.
4. Ng A, Swanevelder J. Resolution in ultrasound imaging. Contin Educ Anaesth Crit Care Pain. 2011;11(5):186–92. https://doi.org/10.1093/bjaceaccp/mkr030.
5. Rumack CM, Levin D, editors. Diagnostic ultrasound. 5th ed. Philadelphia: Elsevier; 2018.
6. Ihnatsenka B, Boezaart AP. Ultrasound: basic understanding and learning the language. Int J Shoulder Surg. 2010;4(3):55–62. https://doi.org/10.4103/0973-6042.76960.
7. NCI Dictionary of Cancer Terms. National Cancer Institute. https://www.cancer.gov/publications/dictionaries/cancer-terms/def/ultrasound-transducer. Accessed 5 Sept 2019.
8. Gleeson T, Blehar D. Point-of-care ultrasound in trauma. Semin Ultrasound CT MR. 2018;39(4):374–83.
9. Díaz-gómez JL, Via G, Ramakrishna H. Focused cardiac and lung ultrasonography: implications and applicability in the perioperative period. Rom J Anaesth Intensive Care. 2016;23(1):41–54.
10. Coté CJ, Lerman J, Anderson BJ, Karmakar MK, Kwok WH. Ultrasound-guided regional anesthesia. In: A practice of anesthesia for infants and children. 6th ed. Philadelphia: Elsevier; 2019. p. 988–1022. https://www.sciencedirect.com/science/article/pii/B9780323429740000434. Accessed 5 Sept 2019.
11. Silverman RH. Focused ultrasound in ophthalmology. Clin Ophthalmol. 2016;10:1865–75. Published 2016 Sep 27. https://doi.org/10.2147/OPTH.S99535.
12. Miller DL, Smith NB, Bailey MR, et al. Overview of therapeutic ultrasound applications and safety considerations. J Ultrasound Med. 2012;31(4):623–34.
13. Carovac A, Smajlovic F, Junuzovic D. Application of ultrasound in medicine. Acta Inform Med. 2011;19(3):168–71. https://doi.org/10.5455/aim.2011.19.168-171.
14. De marchi L, Meineri M. POCUS in perioperative medicine: a North American perspective. Crit Ultrasound J. 2017;9(1):19.
15. Jasudavisius A, Arellano R, Martin J, Mcconnell B, Bainbridge D. A systematic review of transthoracic and transesophageal echocardiography in non-cardiac surgery: implications for point-of-

care ultrasound education in the operating room. Can J Anaesth. 2016;63(4):480–7.
16. Adhikari S, Zeger W, Schmier C, et al. Pilot study to determine the utility of point-of-care ultrasound in the assessment of difficult laryngoscopy. Acad Emerg Med. 2011;18(7):754–8.
17. Haskins SC, Feldman D, Fields KG, et al. Teaching a point-of-care ultrasound curriculum to anesthesiology trainees with traditional didactic lectures or an online E-learning platform: a pilot study. J Educ Perioper Med. 2018;20(3):E624.
18. Mok D, Schwarz SKW, Rondi K. Point-of-care ultrasonography in Canadian anesthesiology residency programs: a national survey of program directors. Can J Anaesth. 2017;64(10):1023–36.
19. Smallwood N, Dachsel M. Point-of-care ultrasound (POCUS): unnecessary gadgetry or evidence-based medicine? Clin Med (Lond). 2018;18(3):219–24.
20. Roche D, Iohom G. Point-of-care ultrasound in anaesthesia and intensive care medicine. Rom J Anaesth Intensive Care. 2018;25(2):95–6.
21. Ursprung E, Oren-grinberg A. Point-of-care ultrasound in the perioperative period. Int Anesthesiol Clin. 2016;54(1):1–21.
22. Alakkad H, Kruisselbrink R, Chin KJ, et al. Point-of-care ultrasound defines gastric content and changes the anesthetic management of elective surgical patients who have not followed fasting instructions: a prospective case series. Can J Anaesth. 2015;62(11):1188–95.
23. Meineri M, Bryson GL, Arellano R, Skubas N. Core point-of-care ultrasound curriculum: what does every anesthesiologist need to know? Can J Anaesth. 2018;65(4):417–26.
24. Blaivas M, Theodoro D, Sierzenski PR. Elevated intracranial pressure detected by bedside emergency ultrasonography of the optic nerve sheath. Acad Emerg Med. 2003;10(4):376–81.
25. Baston CM, Moore C, Krebs EA, Dean AJ, Panebianco N, editors. Ocular ultrasound. In: Pocket guide to POCUS: point-of-care tips for point-of-care ultrasound. New York: McGraw-Hill. http://accessmedicine.mhmedical.com.ezproxy.med.nyu.edu/content.aspx?bookid=2544&sectionid=210344762. Accessed 16 Sept 2019.
26. Su E, Dalesio N, Pustavoitau A. Point-of-care ultrasound in pediatric anesthesiology and critical care medicine. Can J Anaesth. 2018;65(4):485–98.
27. Ramsingh D, Rinehart J, Kain Z, et al. Impact assessment of perioperative point-of-care ultrasound training on anesthesiology residents. Anesthesiology. 2015;123(3):670–82.
28. You-ten KE, Siddiqui N, Teoh WH, Kristensen MS. Point-of-care ultrasound (POCUS) of the upper airway. Can J Anaesth. 2018;65(4):473–84.
29. Ramsingh D, Gudzenko V, Martin RD. Point-of-care ultrasound: novel technology to routine perioperative assessment tool. Anesth Analg. 2017;124(3):709–11.
30. Yao W, Zhou Y, Wang B, et al. Can mandibular condylar mobility sonography measurements predict difficult laryngoscopy? Anesth Analg. 2017;124(3):800–6.
31. Reddy PB, Punetha P, Chalam KS. Ultrasonography – a viable tool for airway assessment. Indian J Anaesth. 2016;60(11):807–13.
32. You-ten KE, Desai D, Postonogova T, Siddiqui N. Accuracy of conventional digital palpation and ultrasound of the cricothyroid membrane in obese women in labour. Anaesthesia. 2015;70(11):1230–4.
33. Melgarejo S, Schaub A, Noble VE. Point of care ultrasound: an overview. American College of Cardiology. https://www.acc.org/latest-in-cardiology/articles/2017/10/31/09/57/point-of-care-ultrasound. Published 31 Oct 2017. Accessed 5 Sept 2019.
34. Deshpande R, Montealegre-gallegos M, Matyal R, Belani K, Chawla N. Training the anesthesiologist in point-of-care ultrasound. Int Anesthesiol Clin. 2016;54(1):71–93.
35. Baston CM, Moore C, Krebs EA, Dean AJ, Panebianco N, editors. Lung ultrasound: parenchyma and lung sliding. In: Pocket guide to POCUS: point-of-care tips for point-of-care ultrasound. New York: McGraw-Hill. http://accessmedicine.mhmedical.com.ezproxy.med.nyu.edu/content.aspx?bookid=2544&sectionid=210367900. Accessed 5 Sept 2019.
36. Kirkpatrick AW, Sirois M, Laupland KB, et al. Hand-held thoracic sonography for detecting post-traumatic pneumothoraces: the Extended Focused Assessment with Sonography for Trauma (EFAST). J Trauma. 2004;57(2):288–95.
37. Adler AC, Greeley WJ, Conlin F, Feldman JM. Perioperative Anesthesiology UltraSonographic Evaluation (PAUSE): a guided approach to perioperative bedside ultrasound. J Cardiothorac Vasc Anesth. 2016;30(2):521–9.
38. Volpicelli G, Elbarbary M, Blaivas M, et al. International evidence-based recommendations for point-of-care lung ultrasound. Intensive Care Med. 2012;38(4):577–91.
39. Lee A, Loughrey JPR. The role of ultrasonography in obstetric anesthesia. Best Pract Res Clin Anaesthesiol. 2017;31(1):81–90.
40. Bøtker MT, Vang ML, Grøfte T, Kirkegaard H, Frederiksen CA, Sloth E. Implementing point-of-care ultrasonography of the heart and lungs in an anesthesia department. Acta Anaesthesiol Scand. 2017;61(2):156–65.
41. Pulton D, Feinman J. Hocus POCUS: making barriers to perioperative point-of-care ultrasound disappear. J Cardiothorac Vasc Anesth. 2019;33(9):2419–20.
42. Baston CM, Moore C, Krebs EA, Dean AJ, Panebianco N, editors. Cardiac ultrasound. In: Pocket guide to POCUS: point-of-care tips for point-of-care ultrasound. New York: McGraw-Hill. http://accessmedicine.mhmedical.com.ezproxy.med.nyu.edu/content.aspx?bookid=2544&sectionid=210344444. Accessed 5 Sept 2019.
43. Canty DJ, Royse CF, Kilpatrick D, Bowman L, Royse AG. The impact of focused transthoracic echocardiography in the preoperative clinic. Anaesthesia. 2012;67(6):618–25.
44. Kimura BJ. Point-of-care cardiac ultrasound techniques in the physical examination: better at the bedside. Heart. 2017;103(13):987–94.
45. Blanco R, Ansari T, Girgis E. Quadratus lumborum block for postoperative pain after caesarean section: a randomised controlled trial. Eur J Anaesthesiol. 2015;32(11):812–8.
46. Abrahams M, Derby R, Horn JL. Update on ultrasound for truncal blocks: a review of the evidence. Reg Anesth Pain Med. 2016;41(2):275–88.
47. Haskins SC, Desai NA, Fields KG, et al. Diagnosis of intraabdominal fluid extravasation after hip arthroscopy with point-of-care ultrasonography can identify patients at an increased risk for postoperative pain. Anesth Analg. 2017;124(3):791–9.
48. Lawson W, Uy M, Strike K, et al. Point of care ultrasound in haemophilia: building a strong foundation for clinical implementation. Haemophilia. 2017;23(5):648–51.
49. Champaneria R, Shah L, Wilson MJ, Daniels JP. Clinical effectiveness of transversus abdominis plane (TAP) blocks for pain relief after caesarean section: a meta-analysis. Int J Obstet Anesth. 2016;28:45–60.
50. Børglum J, Gögenür I, Bendtsen TF. Abdominal wall blocks in adults. Curr Opin Anaesthesiol. 2016;29(5):638–43.
51. Ranganath A, Srinivasan KK, Iohom G. Ultrasound guided axillary brachial plexus block. Med Ultrason. 2014;16(3):246–51.
52. Neal JM, Brull R, Horn JL, et al. The second American society of regional anesthesia and pain medicine evidence-based medicine assessment of ultrasound-guided regional anesthesia: executive summary. Reg Anesth Pain Med. 2016;41(2):181–94.
53. Srinivasan KK, Lee PJ, Iohom G. Ultrasound for neuraxial blockade. Med Ultrason. 2014;16(4):356–63.
54. Haskins SC, Boublik J, Wu CL. Point-of-care ultrasound for the regional anesthesiologist and pain specialist: a series introduction. Reg Anesth Pain Med. 2017;42(3):281–2.
55. Mahmood F, Matyal R, Skubas N, et al. Perioperative ultrasound training in anesthesiology: a call to action. Anesth Analg. 2016;122(6):1794–804.

56. Boublik J, Haskins S. Introducing the Perioperative Point-of-Care Ultrasound (PoCUS) Special Interest Group (SIG). American Society of Regional Anesthesia eand Pain Medicine. https://www.asra.com/news/129/introducing-the-perioperative-point-of-c. Published November 25, 2016. Accessed 10 Sept 2019.
57. Weiniger CF, Sharoni L. The use of ultrasound in obstetric anesthesia. Curr Opin Anaesthesiol. 2017;30(3):306–12.
58. Bornemann P, Wagner MS, Barron KR. Abdomen. In: Daniels JM, Hoppmann RA, editors. practical point-of-care medical ultrasound. Cham: Springer; 2016.
59. dela Cruz J, Cowley B, Patel C, Yeghiazarian S. The Thorax. In: Daniels JM, Hoppmann RA, editors. Practical point-of-care medical ultrasound. Cham: Springer; 2016.
60. Jeong DH, Chitturi S. Eye (Ocular). In: Daniels JM, Hoppmann RA, editors. Practical point-of-care medical ultrasound. Cham: Springer; 2016.
61. He S. Echocardiography. In: Zhang M, editor. Atlas of human body ultrasound scanning. Singapore. Singapore: Springer; 2018.

12 Complications of Blood Transfusion

Joseph Cassis and Robert Gaiser

As any procedure in medicine, the transfusion of blood products to the patient involves benefits and risks. The benefits of increased oxygen carrying capacity with the ability to deliver oxygen to the tissue are clear in the setting of severe hemorrhage. The risks are not as clear. While patients are mainly concerned with infectious risks, there are other risks that must be considered by the provider.

Transfusion-Related Acute Lung Injury

Transfusion-related acute lung injury (TRALI) is an acute lung injury that occurs within 6 hours of blood transfusion; the entity was first described in 1951 [1]. The actual syndrome and its link to the administration of blood products did not occur until 1983. In a case series of 3130 consecutive blood transfusions, five patients developed respiratory distress in close association to the transfusion [2]. The lung injury was linked to the transfusion with term TRALI being used. TRALI occurs in both women and men and occurs in patients of any age, except neonates. The reason for the concern with TRALI is the significant morbidity and mortality. Survival from TRALI is estimated at 50%. All plasma-containing blood and blood components have been implicated in the development of TRALI. A common theme to the cases of TRALI is the receipt of blood products 6 hours prior to the development of pulmonary symptoms. Other symptoms that also may occur include fever and hypotension.

A consensus panel was convened in 2004 to establish the criteria for the diagnosis of TRALI [3]. TRALI was defined as a new acute lung injury that occurred during or within 6 hours of a completed transfusion that was not related to another cause for the lung injury. While the diagnosis requires the administration of the blood products within 6 hours, the overwhelming majority of patients will have the onset of symptoms within 1–2 hours following the transfusion. The diagnosis was to be based upon clinical symptoms combined with a radiographic diagnosis. The diagnostic criteria for TRALI are outlined in Table 12.1. The chest x-ray should show bilateral infiltrates that may be patchy or diffuse suggestive of alveolar or interstitial disease [4].

Possible TRALI is a diagnosis used when it is difficult to determine whether the actual etiology of the lung injury is TRALI or another cause of the acute lung injury [5]. Sometimes it is difficult to determine whether the lung injury is from the blood transfusion. In patients meeting the diagnosis of TRALI but with another reason to explain the acute lung injury, the alternative diagnosis of "possible TRALI" is used. Possible TRALI refers to transfusion-related lung injury in a patient with a preexisting lung injury prior to the transfusion. This term is not universally accepted, with many feeling that possible TRALI is simply ARDS or TRALI type II (TRALI in a patient with risk factor for ARDS) [6].

Postmortem tissue examination of patients with TRALI demonstrates pulmonary edema, diffuse alveolar damage, and granulocytes in the alveoli. The pulmonary vasculature contains neutrophil aggregates when examined postmortem. The major finding in patients with TRALI is increased pulmonary microvascular permeability with protein in the fluid. Patients with TRALI have chest x-rays that demonstrate bilateral infiltrates that suggest cardiac failure with no evidence for cardiac causes of the findings.

The pathogenesis is poorly understood. The most common theory for TRALI is the two hit model in the transfused donor [1]. In this theory, a patient who had an increase in

Table 12.1 Diagnostic criteria for TRALI

1. Abrupt onset
2. No evidence of left atrial hypertension
3. Bilateral infiltrates on chest x-ray
4. Hypoxemia as defined PaO2/FiO2 ≤ 300 mmHg or oxygen saturation ≤ 90% on room air

J. Cassis (✉) · R. Gaiser
University of Kentucky, Department of Anesthesiology, Lexington, KY, USA
e-mail: Jsca246@uky.edu; Robert.gaiser@uky.edu

© Springer Nature Switzerland AG 2021
C. S. Scher et al. (eds.), *Essentials of Blood Product Management in Anesthesia Practice*,
https://doi.org/10.1007/978-3-030-59295-0_12

Table 12.2 Risk Factors for Development of TRALI

Cardiac Surgery
Mechanical ventilation with increased peak airway pressure
Chronic alcohol use
Current smoker
End-stage liver disease
Liver transplantation
Hematologic malignancy

neutrophil responsiveness receives a stimulus from the transfusion itself. The possible risk factors (Table 12.2) that may cause the first hit include chronic alcohol abuse, sepsis, mechanical ventilation, shock, surgery, smoking, inflammation, and fluid overload. The inflammatory proteins that are elevated in patients with TRALI include interleukin-6 and interleukin-8 as well as protein C-reactive protein. The second hit comes from the antibodies in the transfused blood products. In the two-hit model, a certain threshold from the initial insult must be present in a patient who receives a sufficient amount of volume and titer of antibody. If the amount of antibody is insufficient to initiate antibody-antigen activation, TRALI will not occur. In the critically ill patient, the neutrophils are primed and ready to be activated from the antibodies in the transfused blood, which leads to pulmonary edema.

Approximately 80% of cases of TRALI are due to the presence of donor antibodies such as antihuman leukocyte or antihuman neutrophil antibodies. The implicated antibodies include cognate anti-HLA-Class II and anti-human neutrophil antigen (HNA)-positive antibodies. Antibodies are the second hit for TRALI. Antibodies to leukocyte antigen Class I or II or neutrophil antigen can be detected in the transfused blood of patients who develop TRALI. These antibodies in the donor product activate neutrophils in the recipient lung causing pulmonary damage and capillary leak. Donors have developed these antibodies when the immune system comes into contact with foreign HNA or HLA during pregnancy, transfusion, or transplantation [7].

The remaining 20% of cases of TRALI are related to biolipids of the blood products or components from aging blood. These microparticles occur in blood products and activate inflammatory mediators resulting in plasma leak within the lung. The microparticles may be generated from any cell, including platelets, red blood cells, and white blood cells. The exact mechanism for TRALI from this etiology is poorly understood [7].

Given the role of human leukocyte antigen antibodies in the development of TRALI, blood banks have moved toward the use of male-predominant plasma. Multiparous women have a high exposure to fetal HLA antigens and other granulocyte-borne antigens from the fetus. This knowledge has led to the practice of eliminating donor plasma from multiparous women or the screening of female donors for HLA antibodies. This practice was instituted in 2004. Prior to this change, the estimated incidence of TRALI was 1 in 5000 blood and blood components, 1 in 2000 plasma-containing components, 1 in 7900 units of fresh frozen plasma, and 1 in 432 units of whole blood-derived platelets [8]. Since the introduction of male-predominant plasma, the incidence of TRALI has decreased. The University of Texas Health Science Center in Houston evaluated the incidence of TRALI as this center uses plasma in the setting of trauma, and the use is early and aggressive [9]. Over a 10-year period, a total of 714,757 units of blood products were transfused with seven cases of TRALI, giving an incidence of 1 in 102,000. As compared to the screening and discarding of blood based on the presence of antibodies, another approach is the use of pooled solvent-detergent-treated plasma instead of fresh frozen plasma. This treatment with solvent and detergent was done to inactivate lipid-enveloped viruses. This approach has been shown to be effective in eliminating the antibodies [10].

No specific treatment exists for TRALI. The provision of increased concentrations of oxygen is required in all, and mechanical ventilation is required in most [7]. Given the lung injury component of TRALI, it is recommended that lung protective strategies be used for ventilation. Also, these patients should not be treated with diuretics as fluid overload is not the precipitating factor. TRALI may be differentiated from transfusion-associated circulatory overload by obtaining a B-type natriuretic peptide level, which is elevated in overload. Other factors that differentiate TRALI from transfusion-associated circulatory overload include the elevated pulmonary capillary wedge pressure and the positive response to diuretics in overload. Given the two-hit theory, managing the patient's underlying risk factors as well as decreasing transfusion would decrease the incidence of TRALI.

Transfusion-Associated Circulatory Overload

Transfusion-associated circulatory overload (TACO) is the most common type of transfusion-related pulmonary complication with an estimated incidence estimate of 1–8% (although some estimating it to be as high as 11%) [11]. TACO was first observed in the 1930s, but became recognized as a distinct clinical entity in the 1990s [12]. The incidence of TACO varies by study, with data from passive surveillance showing a very low incidence while studies with active surveillance reporting a higher incidence. This point highlights the general consensus that TACO is vastly underreported and lacks a clear, established defining set of criteria, as evidenced by the variation in the reported incidence among studies with active surveillance. Data from the Serious Hazards of Transfusion UK reporting system suggest that the understanding of TACO has improved as reports of TACO increased each year between 2007 and 2013 [13]. TACO was more likely to occur with the transfusion of packed red blood cells (1/8000), as compared to plasma (1/15,000) or platelets (1/48,000) [14]. Various other studies have supported this relationship between volume transfused and TACO although the impact of the rate of transfusion on the incidence remains unknown.

TACO is defined as acute cardiogenic pulmonary edema associated with volume overload occurring within 6 hours of receiving a blood transfusion [15]. This temporal relationship between transfusion of blood products and pulmonary edema is a key feature of TACO (as well as TRALI) distinguishing it from other forms of pulmonary edema. The pulmonary edema caused by TACO is thought to be due to increased hydrostatic pressure (i.e., cardiogenic pulmonary edema) as opposed to capillary leak (i.e., noncardiogenic pulmonary edema), the latter being associated with transfusion-related acute lung injury [16]. Although there is no consensus on standardized criteria for TACO, the Centers for Disease Control's Hemovigilance Module Surveillance Protocol proposed possible criteria for recognizing and diagnosing TACO (Table 12.3) [17]. The CDC criteria state that a patient must have 3 or more of the following findings within 6 hours of cessation of transfusion:

- Acute respiratory distress
- Elevated brain natriuretic peptide(BNP)
- Elevated CVP
- Evidence of left heart failure
- Evidence of positive fluid balance
- Radiographic evidence of pulmonary edema

Table 12.3 Comparison of diagnostic criteria transfusion-associated circulatory overload based upon organization

	CDC Biovigilance Surveillance Protocol	International Society of Blood Transfusion
Timing/onset	Within 6 hours of cessation of transfusion	During/up to 12 hours
Criteria based on observed signs/ symptoms or measured values	Three or more of the following:	Acute or worsening respiratory distress and/or evidence of pulmonary edema and three or more of the following criteria:
	Acute respiratory distress Radiographic evidence of pulmonary edema Evidence of left heart failure Evidence of positive fluid balance Elevated brain natriuretic peptide Elevated CVP	Acute or worsening respiratory distress Evidence of acute or worsening pulmonary edema (based on physical exam, CXR, or echocardiogram Evidence of cardiovascular system changes that are unrelated to their underlying condition (HTN, tachycardia, JVD, Enlarged cardiac silhouette, peripheral edema, widened pulse pressure Evidence of fluid overload: Positive fluid balance, change in weight in the peri-transfusion period, response to diuretic therapy(medication or dialysis) Biomarker: increase in BNP or NT-pro BNP above age-adjusted reference range and greater than 1.5 times pretransfusion value. Normal BNP level most transfusion is not consistent with TACO diagnosis

Since TACO is a form of cardiogenic pulmonary edema related to the transfusion of blood products, understanding the pathophysiology of pulmonary edema will aide in the management of TACO. In the normal lung, fluid that is filtered out of circulation into the alveolar interstitial space does not enter the alveoli due to tight junctions that prevent passage; this fluid is removed via the lymphatics. The hydrostatic force for fluid filtration between the capillaries and alveoli microcirculation is roughly equal, with the osmotic pressure of the capillaries tipping the balance slightly in favor of capillary circulation [14]. In TACO, the hydrostatic pressure increases due to the rapid increase in circulatory volume resulting in an imbalance. There is an increase in fluid filtration (edema into the interstitial space), and the tight junctions of the epithelium are overcome allowing protein poor fluid to enter the alveolar space thus causing pulmonary edema.

There are multiple risk factors for TACO, with age, cardiovascular dysfunction, and renal disease being the major risk factors. Although TACO can occur at any age, advanced age appears to be the greatest risk with most studies reporting the highest incidence in patients aged greater than 70 years. Patients with cardiovascular dysfunction also have a higher incidence of TACO. In particular, patients with CHF (especially NYHA Class 4), atrial fibrillation, a history of coronary artery disease, use of diuretics (and lack of use when there is evidence of TACO), and amiodarone all have a higher risk of developing TACO [16]. Chronic renal failure has also been shown to be a risk factor. Other risk factors include positive fluid status (fluids other than blood products can contribute to TACO), number of units transfused, type of product transfused (likely related to volume), rate of transfusion, preexisting pulmonary disease, female sex (although the evidence is not conclusive), patients of small stature, shock, anemia, and hospitalized patients (especially OR and ICU) [12, 14, 15]. Many of the risk factors lend credence to the hypothesis that TACO occurs when the body's ability to manage intravascular volume status is overwhelmed, especially when intravascular volume is increased by a large amount or at higher infusion rates. For example, the incidence of TACO correlates with the number of units of blood products transfused, and there is evidence that higher rates of infusion lead to higher incidence of TACO [12, 18].

Respiratory distress/worsening pulmonary status within 6 hours of receiving a blood transfusion is the principle manifestation of TACO. A patient's respirations, oxygen saturation, heart rate, temperature, blood pressure, and fluid balance should all be monitored closely during transfusion. Increasing oxygen requirement and decreasing oxygen saturation on pulse oximetry should warrant further investigation including a chest x-ray and physical exam. Consideration should be given to close monitoring for 24 hours after transfusion as multiple studies show clear evidence that active surveillance yields higher rates of recognition of TACO. Supplemental oxygen which is common in the OR and ICU can mask evidence for worsening pulmonary status, especially if the patient is intubated. Arterial blood gas monitoring measures the ratio of the partial pressure of oxygen to fractional inspired oxygen (PaO2/FiO2) which is used in ARDS and TRAILI and could prove useful in TACO. [14] Potential respiratory manifestations include the following:

- Dyspnea
- Tachypnea
- Hypoxia
- Pulmonary edema – CXR (possible enlarged cardiac silhouette, pleural effusions, enlarged vascular pedicle, distribution of edema is even/central
- Orthopnea
- Crackles

In addition to respiratory status, patients should be monitored for cardiac dysfunction before, during, and after transfusion. Hypertension is sometimes, though not always, a distinguishing feature from the noncardiogenic pulmonary edema associated with TRALI. Physical examination of the patient may reveal jugular venous distention and peripheral edema. A patient's fluid balance should be determined before a transfusion is started as studies demonstrating overall positive volume status contribute to the development of TACO. Chart review, urine output, patient's weight, response to diuretics, and volume removed through dialysis can all be used to determine fluid balance. Bedside echocardiography may be utilized to determine cardiac function as well as volume status.

B-type natriuretic peptide (BNP) and NT-pro-BNP have been studied as a way to diagnose TACO and differentiate it from TRALI to aide in clinical decision making. Unfortunately, the evidence is mixed as to whether or not BNP is an effective biomarker for distinguishing TACO from TRALI. The evidence is weaker for differentiating TACO from other forms of pulmonary edema [19]. The most significant problem with these biomarkers is the vast differential and large number of factors that can explain elevations. Heart failure, renal dysfunction, age, gender, sepsis, and ACE inhibitors affect BNP and NT-pro-BNP levels.

Management of TACO is essentially the same as managing patients with other causes of cardiogenic pulmonary edema. If TACO is suspected, the initial step in treatment is to stop the transfusion. Treatment should begin with supplemental oxygen and elevating the head of the bed to 30 degrees. Supplemental oxygen may be delivered via nasal canula; however, positive pressure may be required if the pulmonary edema is severe; BiPap or high flow nasal canula can be useful. Diuretic use has shown a significant decrease in not only the incidence of TACO but also the mortality when it occurs. In cases of severe renal failure, CRRT or hemodialysis is used to reduce volume overload. Reduction of afterload as tolerated by the patient may also prove useful in decreasing workload and increasing cardiac output. In the most severe cases, intubation, vasopressors, and inotropes are necessary.

Transfusion Reactions

The understanding of the antigen/antibody cause for the blood group system was developed by Dr. Karl Landsteiner when he noted that mixing red blood cells with different plasma and different patterns of agglutination was obtained [20]. He termed the first pattern A and the second pattern B. There were other individuals who did not achieve any pattern of agglutination, which was termed C. The first two patterns led to the nomenclature of Type A and Type B; it was the lack of a pattern of agglutination that led to Type O. Furthermore, it was these observations that led Dr. Landsteiner to postulate that whichever ABO antigens are lacking on a red blood cell will result in the corresponding antibody. This theory has been termed Landsteiner's Law. The antigens for the ABO system are produced by various enzymes that add sugars to the oligosaccharide chain. The source of the antibodies is less clear; it may due to inherited antibodies or due to classical immune-mediated reactions. When ABO incompatible blood is administered, hemolysis may occur.

For the transfusion of red blood cells, patients may receive group O red blood cells as these cells lack A and B antigens and are compatible with plasma. For plasma, all patients may receive AB plasma as these lack anti-A and anti-B antibodies. Of note, while ABO compatibility is vital for red blood cells to prevent a fatal acute hemolytic transfusion reaction, it is not vital and frequently not followed for plasma and platelets. Although plasma may contain anti-A or anti-B antibodies, the presence of A and B antigens on endothelial cells, dilution in the patient blood volume, and the presence of soluble A and B antigen in the plasma of secretors provide protection [21].

The presence of D antigen on the donor and recipient also must be considered. Antibody to the D antigen is not naturally occurring, requiring exposure to develop the antibody. Exposure to D+ red blood cells in a D- patient will result in the development of antibodies in 1 out of every 5 exposures. The formation of D antibodies is most important in women of childbearing age where the antibody may complicate the pregnancy. As such, men and women who are beyond childbearing typically receive D+ packed red blood cells, due to the shortage of D- blood. In fact, D- blood has become so low that many transfusion services provide D+ blood, even for women of childbearing age [21].

A febrile nonhemolytic transfusion reaction is defined as an increase in temperature of 1 degree Celsius above 37 degrees that occurs during or after the transfusion of blood products. This reaction is the most common during transfusion. The reaction may occur without the symptoms of chills, rigors, and rash or may occur with it. The most common blood product to produce a non-hemolytic transfusion reaction is platelets. Initially, it was felt that the reaction was due to the presence of white blood cells in the patient's plasma that reacted with the white cells in the blood product. This explanation mainly applies to red blood cells; platelets have a different explanation. The reaction is more likely to occur the older the platelets are. Within the stored platelets, there is the generation of cytokines during storage. These cytokines are responsible for the reaction [22]. The most important point when a patient develops a febrile response to a transfusion is to insure that it is not due to an acute hemolytic reaction or transfusion of a contaminated product.

There is always the risk of administering the wrong blood product to the patient. While infectious disease transmission has decreased, mistransfusion remains a constant risk to the patient [23]. In an effort to prevent this error of incompatible blood products, an institution conducted a quality improvement project with the introduction of a cognitive aid. This cognitive aid was a simple card that was worn with the participants' badge, as demonstrated in Table 12.4. Based upon a quiz, there was a marked improvement in ABO compatibility.

Table 12.4 ABO compatibility based upon blood product type

Group	O	B	A	AB
ABO group of compatible RBCs				
AB	•	•	•	•
A	•		•	
B	•	•		
O	•			
ABO group of compatible FFP				
AB				•
A			•	•
B		•		•
O	•	•	•	•

Hemolytic transfusion reactions occur when the antibodies within the recipient react to the antigens on the red blood cell surface. These reacts are classified as acute or delayed. An acute reaction occurs during the transfusion, while a delayed reaction occurs within days or weeks of transfusion. The most common reason for a hemolytic transfusion reaction is misidentification of the patient or mislabeling the blood sample. When the IgM antibody binds to the antigen, the red cell membrane is destroyed resulting in the release of contents within the red blood cell into the circulation. The free hemoglobin damages the kidney, while the complement activation leads to disseminated intravascular coagulation [24]. Management includes stopping the transfusion and administering fluids, vasopressors, and blood products for the coagulopathy. A delayed reaction occurs from antibodies developed from a previous transfusion. These antibodies are not present in a detectable level at the time of the testing and appear days after the transfusion. Typical manifestations of a delayed reaction include anemia and jaundice.

Infectious Complications

Transfusion-transmitted infection due to viral and bacterial contamination decreased dramatically with the transition to closed, sterile systems for collection and storage. John Elliott developed the first vacuum bottle for blood collection in 1940 [25, 26]. In addition, the testing of blood donations has further contributed to a dramatic reduction in transfusion-transmitted infections. By 1947, every unit of blood collected was tested for syphilis followed by hepatitis B in 1971, hepatitis C in 1990, and HIV-1 and 2 by 1992 [26]. Over time viral infections related to transfusion have seen a significant drop; transfusion-transmitted bacterial infection has not seen the same reduction over the last 30 years. According to studies from the US FDA, French Hemovigilance study, and the British SHOT study, the incidence for bacterial contamination/sepsis has not decreased (in fact, has not changed) to the same degree as viral infection [25].

Bacterial contamination is the most common cause of transfusion-transmitted infection, with an estimated overall prevalence of 0.2% [27, 28]. Bacterial infection is more common than viral or fungal infection. It is estimated that bacterial contamination is approximately 1 in 3000 units [29]. Transfusion-transmitted bacterial infections accounted for the most reports transfusion-related fatality, accounting for 20% of fatalities (second to ABO errors) [25, 30]. The actual incidence of transfusion-transmitted bacterial infection varies based on the study (Table 12.5). This variation is likely due to differences in the processing and storage of blood products [30]. The FDA reports mortality from transfusion-related infections to range from 1 in 6,000,000 to

Table 12.5 Risk of Bacterial Transmission Through Transfusion

French Bacthem Case-Control Study [4]		Transfusion-transmitted bacterial infection in the US [5]	
Summary of Transfusion-transmitted Bacterial Infection Incidence Rates		Rate of transfusion-transmitted bacteremia (in events/million units)	
Blood Products	Rate	Blood Products	Rate
Packed red blood cells (PRBCs)	5.8	PRBCs	0.21
Pooled Platelets	71.8	Single Unit Platelets	9.98
Single Unit Platelets	9.4	Pooled Platelets	10.64
Apheresis Platelets	31.8		
FFP	7.4		
Total Units Transfused: 5,423,597		Patients who received gram negative bacteria were at greatest risk of death Transfusion-transmitted bacterial infections accounted for the most reports transfusion related fatality after hemolytic reactions (>10% from 1985–1999)	

1 in 9,000,000 when examining all blood products together and 1 in 1,000,000 for platelets [30].

Though the incidence of bacterial contamination and transfusion-transmitted bacterial infections varies, the highest risk of contamination and infection occurs with platelets. This incidence is due to storage as platelets are stored at room temperature, allowing bacteria to grow that would otherwise remain dormant at lower levels with refrigeration. In countries where platelets are screened using BacT/ALERT culture system, the incidence of transfusion-transmitted bacterial infections is lower [31]. The detection of bacterial contamination in platelet samples is largely dependent on bacterial concentration as tests where resampling of a previously positive BacT/ALERT screenings has yielded negative results [32]. Unlike viruses, bacteria have the ability to multiply during storage making the duration of their storage another factor in the incidence of transfusion-related bacterial infection. One study found that the incidence of contamination and the bacterial levels measured were both significantly less for units transfused in under 4 days compared with units that were 5 days and older [33].

The infectious concern with the transfusion of red blood cells is primarily viral. The risk depends upon which testing is performed. Current testing of red blood cells includes Hepatitis B (antibody in 1987; nucleic acid in 2009), Hepatitis C (antibody in 1990; nucleic acid in 1999), Human Immunodeficiency Virus (antibody in 1985; nucleic acid in 2000), West Nile Virus, and Zika Virus [34]. The risk of viral infection occurs when a virus emerges in which testing does not occur, as happened with Zika Virus, which was added in 2016 [35]. Currently, blood is not tested for Hepatitis A, malaria, or new variants of Creutzfeld-Jacob disease prions.

Conclusion

The transfusion of blood products has risk to the patient. There is always the risk of misidentification resulting in the administration of the wrong blood product. Even when the patient is properly cross-matched, there are infectious risks from both known and unknown agents. There is also the risk of transfusion-related acute lung injury and transfusion-associated circulatory overload. While the risks may be mitigated, they cannot be removed completely. These concerns help one understand the continually evolving transfusion thresholds and administer products only when truly indicated.

References

1. Semple JW, McVey MJ, Kim M, Rebetz J, Kuebler WM, Kapur R. Targeting transfusion-related acute lung injury: the journey from basic science to novel therapies. Crit Care Med. 2018;46:e452–8.
2. Popovsky MA, Moore SB. Diagnostic and pathogenetic considerations in transfusion-related acute lung injury. Transfusion. 1985;25:573–7.
3. Kleinman S, Caulfield T, Chan P, Davenport R, McFarland J, et al. Toward an understanding of transfusion-related acute lung injury: statement of a consensus panel. Transfusion. 2004;44:1774–89.
4. Goldman M, Webert KE, Arnold DM, Freedman J, Hannon J, Blaichman MA, Consensus Panel TRALI. Proceedings of a consensus conference towards an understanding of TRALI. Transfus Med Rev. 2005;19:2–31.
5. Friedman T, Javidroozi M, Lobel G, Shander A. Complications of allogeneic blood product administration, with emphasis on transfusion-related acutelung injury and transfusion-associated circulatory overload. Adv Anesth. 2017;35:159–73.
6. Vlaar APJ, Toy P, Fung M, Looney MR, Juffermans NP, et al. A consensus redefinition of transfusion-related acute lung injury. Transfusion. 2019;1111:1–12.
7. Peters AL, Van Stein D, APJ V. Antibody-mediated transfusion-related acute lung injury; from discovery to prevention. Br J Haematol. 2015;170:597–614.
8. Toy P, Popovsky MA, Abraham E, et al. Transfusion-related acute lung injury: definition and review. Crit Care Med. 2005;33:721–6.
9. Meyer DE, Reynolds JW, Hobbs R, Bai Y, Hartwell B, Pommerening MJ, Fox EE, Wade CE, Holcomb JB, Cotton BA. The incidence of transfusion-related acute lung injury at a large,urban tertiary medical center: a decade's experience. Anesth Analg. 2018;127:444–9.
10. Lorello GR, Alam A. Perioperative transfusion-related acute lung injury. Int Anesth Clin. 2018;56:47–67.
11. Bachowski G, et al. A compendium of transfusion practice guidelines. 3rd ed. Washington, DC: American Association Blood Banks; 2017.
12. Piccin A, Cronin M, Murphy C, Eakins E, Lawlor E. Transfusion associated circulatory overload (TACO) incidence and risk factors. Blood. 2009;114:3157.
13. Ware LB, Matthay MA. Clinical practice. Acute pulmonary edema. N Engl J Med. 2005;353:2788–96.
14. Centers for Disease Control. National healthcare safety network biovigilance component hemovigilance module surveillance protocol. Accessed 30 July 2019. www.cdc.gov/nhsnm
15. Murphy EL, Kwaan N, Looney MR, et al. Risk factors and outcomes in transfusion-associated circulatory overload. Am J Med. 2013;126:e29–38.

16. Bolton-Maggs PH, Cohen H. Serious Hazards of Transfusion (SHOT) haemovigilance and progress is improving transfusion safety. Br J Haematol. 2013;163:303–14.
17. Semple JW, Rebetz J, Kapur R. Transfusion-associated circulatory overload and transfusion-related acute lung injury. Blood. 2019:epub.
18. International Society of Blood Transfusion Working Party on Haemovigilance Transfusion-associated circulatory overload (TACO) Definition (2018). Accessed 30 July 2018. http://www.aabb.org/research/hemovigilance/Documents/TACO-2018-Definition.pdf.
19. Li G, Daniels CE, Kojicic M, et al. The accuracy of natriuretic peptides (BNP and NT-pro-BNP) in the differentiation between Transfusion Related Acute Lung Injury (TRALI) and Transfusion Related Circulatory Overload (TACO) in the critically ill. Transfusion. 2009;49:13–20.
20. Branch DR. Anti-A and anti-B: what are they and where do they come from? Transfusion. 2015;55:S74–9.
21. Harm SK, Dunbar NM. Immunologic risks of whole blood: ABO compatibility, D alloimmunization, and transfusion-related acute lung injury. Transfusion. 2019;59:1507.
22. Heddle NM. Pathophysiology of febrile nonhemolytic transfusion reactions. Curr Opin Hematol. 1999;6:420–6.
23. MacDougall N, Dong F, Broussard L, Comunale ME. Preventing mistransfusions: an evaluation of institutional knowledge and a response. Anesth Analg. 2018;126:247–51.
24. Panch SR, Montemayor-Garcia C, Klein HG. Hemolytic transfusion reactions. NEJM. 2019;381:150–62.
25. Wagner SJ. Transfusion-transmitted bacterial infection: risks, sources, and interventions. Vox Sang. 2004;86:157–63.
26. AABB. Highlights of transfusion medicine history. Accessed 31 July 2019. http://www.aabb.org/tm/Pages/highlights.aspx.
27. Fuller AK, Uglik KM, Savage WJ, Ness PM, King KE. Bacterial culture reduces but does not eliminate the risk of septic transfusion reactions to single donor platelets. Transfusion. 2009;49:2588–93.
28. Perez P, Rachid-Salmi L, Follea G, et al. Determinants of transfusion-associated bacterial contamination: results of the French Bacthem Case-Control Study. Transfusion. 2001;41:862–72.
29. Blajichman MA, Goldman M. Bacterial contamination of platelet concentrates: incidence, significance, and prevention. Sem Hematol. 2001;38:S20–6.
30. Kuehnert MJ, Roth VR, Haley NR, et al. Transfusion-transmitted bacterial infection in the United States, 1998 through 2000. Transfusion. 2001;41:1493–9.
31. Kreuger AL, Middelburg RA, Kerkhoffs JLH, et al. Storage medium of platelet transfusions and the risk of transfusion-transmitted bacterial infections. Transfusion. 2017;57:657–60.
32. Mueller TH, Montag T, Seltsam AW. Laboratory evaluation of the effectiveness of pathogen reduction procedures for bacteria. Transfus Med Hemother. 2011;38:242–50.
33. Yomtovian R, Lazarus HM, Goodnough LT, et al. A prospective microbiologic surveillance program to detect and prevent the transfusion of bacterially contaminated platelets. Transfusion. 1993;33:902–9.
34. Goodnough LT, Ranigrahi AK. Blood transfusion therapy. Med Clin North Am. 2017;101:431–47.
35. Fauci AS, Morens DM. Zika virus in the Americas – yet another arbovirus threat. N Engl J Med. 2016;374:601–4.

Diseases of the Coagulation System: Hemophilia, Von Willebrands Disease, Cryoglobulinemia, and Inborn Errors of Factor Synthesis

13

Pierre Alex Casthely and Shruthima Thangada

Hemophilia A

There are three major types of hemophilias, A, B, and C. They are classified based on their deficient coagulation factor. Hemophilias A and B are X-linked recessive disorders caused by a mutation in the long arm of chromosome X at the F8 and F9 genes. Males are affected, and females are carriers [1]. Hemophilia A is the most common X-linked genetic disease and the second most common factor deficiency after von Willebrand disease (vWD). The worldwide incidence of hemophilia A is approximately 1 out of 5000 males [2]. The exact number of people living with hemophilia A is not known [3]. The prevalence of hemophilia A varies by country and ranges 5.4–14.5 cases per 100,000 males. In the United States, the prevalence of hemophilia A is 20.6 cases per 100,000 males, and the number of people in the United States with hemophilia was estimated to be about 20,000 in 2016 [4].

Etiology of Hemophilia A

Hemophilia A can be caused by a factor VIII deficiency, dysfunctional factor VIII, or even factor VIII inhibitors leading to the disruption of the normal intrinsic coagulation cascade. Any defect or absence in factor VIII will cause a decrease in thrombin production by FIXa and FVIIIa in the intrinsic pathway of the coagulation cascade. The factor VIII gene is large and comprises 0.1% of the DNA in the X chromosome. A defect in the normal factor VIII coding sequence caused by a mutation can result in an inability to properly transcribe the complete, normal factor VIII protein, resulting in the loss of its normal function [4].

Signs and Symptoms

Bleeding is the number one sign of hemophilia A. The severity of symptoms depends on the amount of factor VIII in the plasma. Normal plasma levels of factor VIII range from 50% to 150% (0.5–1.5 IU/ml). Levels below 50%, or half of what is needed to form a clot, determine a person's symptoms. Those with mild hemophilia have 6–49% of factor VIII. These account for 25% of all cases. They generally experience bleeding only after serious injury, trauma, or surgery. In many cases, mild hemophilia is not diagnosed until after an injury has occurred and results in prolonged bleeding. Women with mild hemophilia often experience heavy menstrual periods and are at risk for hemorrhage during childbirth [5].

Patients with moderate hemophilia A have 1–5% of factor VIII in the blood. This accounts for 15% of all cases. They may have bleeding episodes after injuries, but rarely bleed spontaneously.

Severe hemophilia A occurs in patients with less than 1% of factor VIII and accounts for 60% of cases. In addition to bleeding following an injury, they may experience frequent spontaneous bleeding into their joints (hemarthrosis) and muscles [5]. Chronic bleeding into the joints, particularly the knees, elbows, and ankles, can lead to decreased range of motion, contractures, and muscle hypertrophy. Over time, degenerative joint disease, osteoarthritis, and osteophyte formation can occur, necessitating surgery [6].

In addition to bleeding into the joint space, bleeding can also occur in the gastrointestinal tract. Infections such as Helicobacter pylori can increase the frequency of GIB in patients with hemophilia [7]. Intracranial hemorrhage is a rare occurrence, but a serious cause of morbidity and mortality in patients with hemophilia, thirty percent, result in death.

P. A. Casthely · S. Thangada (✉)
NYU Langone Medical Center, NYU Department of Anesthesiology, Perioperative Care, & Pain Medicine, New York, NY, USA
e-mail: casthp02@nyulmc.org; Shruthima.Thangada@nyulangone.org

© Springer Nature Switzerland AG 2021

C. S. Scher et al. (eds.), *Essentials of Blood Product Management in Anesthesia Practice*,
https://doi.org/10.1007/978-3-030-59295-0_13

Hypotension, lethargy, and anemia may all present as non-specific manifestations of intracranial bleeding. More severe signs and symptoms include painful headaches, repeated vomiting, double vision, or seizures [7].

Diagnosis

About 70% of children who have a positive history of hemophilia A in the family are diagnosed at birth. Performing a complete history and physical exam in suspected cases and collecting demographic data are all important in diagnosis. It should be followed by appropriate hemostasis assays to confirm the diagnosis. Screening tests include the following: complete blood cell count, activated partial thromboplastin time (aPTT), prothrombin time (PT), and vWF:Ag tests. In hemophilia A, the PT and platelet count are normal. The aPTT is prolonged in moderate and severe disease. In mild cases, however, aPTT can be normal if factor levels are above 15 percent [8]. Therefore, a normal aPTT does not rule out mild hemophilia, and specific factor VIII assay is necessary for the diagnosis of hemophilia A.

Acquired Hemophilia A (AHA)

Acquired hemophilia A (AHA) occurs when a patient develops autoantibodies to factor VIII. These autoantibodies can inhibit the function of factor VIII. This condition is rare and affects approximately 1.5 per million population per year. Patients tend to be older in age (median age 70), and males have a higher incidence than females [9]. The disease presentation is similar to congenital hemophilia A and is characterized by spontaneous bleeding. The difference is, however, that the patient does not have a family history of bleeding. Like in congenital hemophilia A, the patient may have extensive skin hematomas, severe muscle bleeding, retroperitoneal bleeding, epistaxis, hematuria, gastrointestinal bleeding, and even intracerebral bleeds. Bleeding into the joints however is not as common. Malignancy, pregnancy (postpartum inhibitors), infections, medications, and autoimmune diseases have all been associated with AHA. Laboratory testing shows a prolonged activated partial thromboplastin time (aPTT) with normal prothrombin time, fibrinogen level, and platelet counts. Quantifying the inhibitor titer is complicated in AHA but can be achieved using the classical Bethesda assay. The inhibitor titer levels are important because they can determine the type of treatment needed to best suit the patient. In patients with high factor VIII inhibitor titers (> 5 BU/mL), simple replacement with human factor VIII concentrates may be ineffective. Bypassing agents and recombinant porcine factor VIII are approved for the treatment of acute bleeding in AHA [9]. These bypassing agents include recombinant factor VIIa, factor VIII inhibitor bypassing activity (FEIBA). Inhibitor titer reduction by immune tolerance reduction is also a possible mode of treatment [6].

Hemophilia B

Hemophilia B, or Christmas disease, is an inherited, X-linked, recessive disorder that results in deficiency of plasma coagulation factor IX. All ethnic groups are affected equally [10]. It occurs in approximately 1 in 30,000 live males and accounts for 20% of hemophilia cases [8]. The prevalence of hemophilia B is 5.3 cases per 100,000 male individuals and 44% have severe disease.

Etiology

Hemophilia B is caused by mutations in the *F9* gene on the X chromosome. Several hundred mutations with different amino acid substitutions have been described, including partial and total deletions and missense mutations. This results in the decreased or abnormal production of factor IX and, therefore, insufficient production of thrombin via the intrinsic pathway of the coagulation cascade [11].

Signs and Symptoms

The signs and symptoms of hemophilia B are similar to that of hemophilia A, and they can vary from one person to another depending on factor IX levels. In mild cases of hemophilia B, individuals may have easy bruising and prolonged bleeding after surgery or trauma. Patients with moderate hemophilia B may have spontaneous hemarthrosis and bleeding into the muscles as well. In cases of severe hemophilia B, spontaneous joint bleeding is the most common reported symptom [11].

Diagnosis

Like hemophilia A, diagnosing hemophilia B is made through the patient's history and laboratory testing. An activated partial thromboplastin time (aPTT) should be obtained. If aPTT is elevated, more specific blood tests should be drawn to determine if the cause of the elevated aPTT is from a deficiency of factor IX/hemophilia B or another clotting factor. If hemophilia B is suspected, a specific factor IX activity level should then be performed [11]. A factor IX activity level below 40 percent of normal will confirm the diagnosis [8].

Hemophilia C (Rosenthal's Disease)

While hemophilias A and B are X-linked recessive disorders, hemophilia C is an autosomal recessive genetic disorder. Autosomal disorders are disorders caused by variations in genes located on non-sex chromosomes. Because of this, hemophilia C affects both males and females equally [11]. It is characterized by a deficiency of factor XI and has a higher prevalence in Ashkenazi Jews. Estimated prevalence is 1: 1,000,000 [12]. Bleeding is the most common presentation, and similarly, the condition is classified as either mild or severe depending on the degree of factor XI protein deficiency. Regardless of the severity of the protein deficiency, most affected individuals have mild bleeding problems if any. A recent survey concluded that, of the known congenital coagulation factor deficiencies, the correlation between factor level and symptoms is poorest for factor XI [13]. The common features of factor XI deficiency are prolonged bleeding after trauma or surgery, especially involving the inside of the mouth and nose or genitourinary tract. Other symptoms include frequent nosebleeds, easy bruising, bleeding gums, prolonged menstrual bleeding (menorrhagia), or prolonged bleeding after childbirth. Spontaneous bleeding into the urine (hematuria), gastrointestinal tract, or skull is not common in factor XI deficiency, but they can still occur in severe cases [13].

Treatment of Hemophilias

The primary goal of hemophilia treatment and management is the prevention of bleeding that can lead to painful and disabling joint arthropathy. Prophylactic treatment with clotting-factor concentrates is, therefore, the standard of care for hemophilias A and B [14]. The theory behind prophylaxis is that patients with mild or moderate hemophilia rarely have spontaneous bleeding or develop chronic joint arthropathy. Therefore, increasing factor levels preemptively will convert patients with severe hemophilia to levels of patients with mild to moderate hemophilia, which can help decrease spontaneous bleeding [6].

In a US multicenter trial of young boys with severe hemophilia A, prophylaxis with regular infusions of recombinant factor VIII was compared to enhanced on-demand infusion at the time of a joint hemorrhage. When the boys were evaluated a few years later, 93% of those in the prophylaxis group had normal index-joint (elbows, knees, and ankles) structure on magnetic resonance imaging (MRI) compared to only 55% of those in the on-demand therapy group [15]. Though these findings significantly favor prophylactic therapy, there are disadvantages. One major drawback is the frequency in which the treatment must be given. Factor replacement must be administered 2–3 times per week due to their short half-life (10–14 hours for factor VIII and 15–24 hours for factor IX) [6].

Factor replacement products were initially derived from human plasma, which is the liquid part of blood containing antibodies, albumin, and clotting factors. In 1992, the US Food and Drug Administration (FDA) approved recombinant factor VIII concentrate, which does not come from human plasma. This concentrate was genetically engineered using DNA technology and does not contain plasma or albumin and, therefore, cannot spread bloodborne viruses, rendering it much safer than factors derived from human plasma [16].

Recombinant factor VIII (Fc fusion protein) and Recombinant factor IX (Fc fusion protein) are two examples of these recombinant factors. Recombinant factor IX Fc fusion protein received FDA approval in March 2014 for patients with hemophilia B. The B-LONG study which evaluated the safety and efficacy of recombinant, long-acting coagulation factor IX Fc fusion protein (rFIXFc) in patients with severe hemophilia B showed a reduction in bleeding episodes in those receiving weekly rFIXfc. Furthermore, the drug demonstrated an increased half-life in subjects thereby extending circulation time of rFIXfc in the body and lengthening the intervals between prophylactic infusions [6].

The FDA also approved recombinant factor VIIIFc for the control and prevention of bleeding, perioperative management, and routine prophylaxis in adults and children with hemophilia A. It also has an extended half-life and extends the interval between prophylactic infusions [6].

Several different treatments are available for factor XI deficiency. These include fresh frozen plasma (preferably pathogen-inactivated), factor XI concentrates, and antifibrinolytics. Affected individuals usually only require preventive therapy before surgical procedures. In the United States, fresh frozen plasma is the most widely used treatment and is effective in treating individuals with factor XI deficiency. FFP does have the risk of infection and allergic reaction, but the risk of infection is small. Factor XI concentrate is NOT available in the United States [17].

Purified factor products (virally inactivated plasma-derived concentrates or recombinant products) should be used whenever possible, to avoid potential transfusion-transmitted infection and transfusion reactions. However, if they are NOT available, fresh frozen plasma (FFP) or cryoprecipitate (for hemophilia A) can be used. [8].

Treatment of Patients with Factor Inhibitors

All patients should be screened for inhibitors to factor VIII and IX. Depending on the amount of inhibitors present, patients are classified as either low risk (< 5 Bethesda units/ml) or high risk (>5 Bethesda units/ml) [1]. The low-risk group can be treated with higher doses of factor concentrates, while in the high-risk group bypassing agents such as recombinant factor VIIa (rfVIIa) and activated prothrombin complex concentrates (aPCC) [18]. Recombinant factor VIIa directly activates factor X leading to improved thrombin formation. It is effective in about 80% of cases [1, 18]. It may even play a role in bleeding prophylaxis with rfVIIa but so far has shown limited success [18].

Activated prothrombin complex (aPCC) is a mixture of factors II, VII, IX, and X and protein C and S. The dose is 50 units/kg. Its half-life is 8–12 hours and has a 62% overall reduction in bleeding frequency [18].

Other Modes of Treatment

In addition to factors and blood products, other pharmacologic options are available for the control of bleeding in patients with hemophilia. The synthetic vasopressin analog desmopressin acetate (DDAVP) has been used to manage mild bleeding episodes in patients with mild hemophilia A. A single dose (0.3 μg kg − 1) given over 20–30 minutes can increase the FVIII level threefold to sixfold 1 h after administration [2, 19].

Tranexamic acid (TXA) has also been found as a helpful adjunct in hemophilia. It is a synthetic analog of the amino acid lysine. TXA competitively inhibits the conversion of plasminogen to plasmin which degrades fibrin (antifibrinolytic). The half-life is 2 hours. It can be used orally (15–25 mg/kg every 8 hours) or i.v. (10 mg/kg every 8 hours) [1, 19].

Anesthetic Considerations

Patients with hemophilia require a detailed history and physical. Information about transfusion history, prior response to DDAVP, and the use of recombinant factors must all be assessed. Preoperative labs should include a complete blood count, coagulation profile, fibrinogen level, and factor specific assays [1]. Preoperative screening for factor alloantibodies is also imperative [2, 18]. Patients with hemophilia A require 80–100% correction of their factor VIII prior to major surgery [1]. Postoperatively, those levels should be maintained for up to 6 weeks after orthopedic surgery and 1–2 weeks for other procedures [1]. In severe acute bleeding, the factor activity level should be maintained above 50 percent at all times. An immediate dose of factor should be given to raise the peak factor level to 80 to 100 percent. An initial dose of 50 U/kg of factor VIII or 100 U/kg of factor IX should be given to raise the factor levels to 100%. Each factor VIII unit per kilogram of body weight infused i.v. will raise the plasma level by approximately 2%. The number of units of factor VIII required = wt of patient × % factor level desired x 0.5. Each factor IX unit per kilogram of body weight infused i.v will raise plasma factor IX levels approximately 1%. The number of units of factor IX required = weight of patient × % factor level desired [1]. Plasmapheresis may be useful in patients with a high titer inhibitor to lower the inhibitor titer and allow replacement factors to given. This is usually done in patients with life-threatening bleeding and an inhibitor titer >5 BU [20].

There are no guidelines for the use of regional anesthesia in patients with hemophilia. Factor levels should be corrected, and the risk-benefit ratio must be evaluated before proceeding with a regional anesthetic. Unfortunately, there is no safe factor level recommended for neuraxial blockade in either the obstetric or general population. For the obstetric patient, factor VIII and IX levels must be measured immediately before delivery and postpartum and maintained above 50% of pooled plasma to minimize the risk of life-threatening hemorrhage [1].

Von Willebrand's Disease

Von Willebrand's disease (VWD) is the most common congenital disorder of hemostasis. The pattern of transmission is autosomal inheritance, carried on the short arm of chromosome 12, in which females and males can be equally affected. Prevalence ranges from 3 to 4 per 100,000 to as high as 1.3% of the population [21]. The characteristic feature of this disease is a dysfunction or deficient von Willebrand factor (vWF), which is needed to mediate platelet adhesion at injured sites as well as act as a carrier protein for coagulation factor VIII. Von Willebrand factor is a clotting protein synthesized in megakaryocytes and endothelial cells and circulates in plasma as multimers of different sizes. Platelet adhesion is only activated by large multimeric forms of vWF [22]. Binding of vWF to factor VIII and platelets in blood vessels contribute in the formation of a platelet plug during the clotting process. Any impairment of vWF can result in an ineffective platelet plug and the inability to maintain hemostasis.

Etiology

There are three main types of VWD which are differentiated on the basis of having qualitative or quantitative defects in vWF. A fourth type, acquired VWD, is not hereditary. Type 1 VWD, found in 60%–80% of patients, has a quantitative decrease in vWF and inherited in an autosomal dominant pattern. Levels of vWF in the blood range from 20% to 50% of normal levels. Symptoms are usually mild. Type 2 VWD, found in 15–30% of patients, has a qualitative deficiency in their VWF and is also inherited in an autosomal dominant pattern. Symptoms of type 2 VWD can range from mild to moderate. Type 2 VWD is further broken down into four subtypes based on the presence and behavior of multimers of vWF. The four subtypes include type 2A, type 2B, type 2 M, and type 2 N. Type 2A is characterized by a qualitative abnormality in protein where only small multimers exist rather than the large forms that are needed to mediate platelet adhesion. Type 2B VWD is characterized by platelets clumping together prematurely in the bloodstream rather than at the site of injury. Type 2 M is seen when there is low activity of vWF causing less interaction with platelets. Type 2 N VWD is characterized by inability of vWF to transport factor VIII to the site of injury resulting in reduced factor VIII levels in the blood [23]. Type 3 VWD is a rare autosomal recessive form, found in 5–10% of patients, and has a qualitative deficiency of vWF where the factor is nearly absent. This is the most severe form of hereditary VWD, in which symptoms can include spontaneous bleeding episodes into joints and muscles. Acquired VWD is diagnosed alongside a diagnosis of an autoimmune disease, heart disease, some types of cancer, or after consumption of certain medications.

Signs and Symptoms

Symptoms of Von Willebrand's disease are generally mild in which most bleeding is mucosal (epistaxis, gingival bleeding, menorrhagia) or even asymptomatic. Gastrointestinal bleeding can occur, but is less common. Incisional bleeding after surgery or dental extractions is common and is exacerbated bleeding after aspirin consumption. Bleeding decreases during pregnancy or estrogen use. This is thought to be from an increase in vWF and factor VIII levels gradually throughout the course of pregnancy [24].

Diagnosis

Laboratory findings include normal platelets with the likelihood of an increased bleeding time. Type 1 VWD, the most common, is characterized by reduced vWF levels in plasma. This can indirectly be measured by factor VIII antigen, which measures the immunologic presence of vWF, or by ristocetin cofactor activity, which measures functional properties of vWF in mediating platelet adhesion and aggregation.

Treatment

Although many cases of VWD have mild symptoms in which treatment is not necessitated, ultimately severity of the disease determines treatment. VWD patients that are to receive surgical or dental procedures should be prepared and optimized appropriately by a hematologist prior to the procedure. The best indicator of treatment prior to a procedure is bleeding time. If bleeding time is normal and the patient is undergoing a minor procedure, treatment is usually not given. Recommendations of the National Heart, Lung, and Blood Institute are to maintain levels of vWF and factor VIII activity at a minimum of 30% and preferably over 50% for 1–5 days for minor surgery [25]. Desmopressin acetate (DDAVP), a synthetic version of the natural hormone vasopressin, is used to treat mild forms of type I VWD and can be given as an injectable or nasal form. The mechanism of action of desmopressin acetate is release of stored vWF from endothelial cells, which also indirectly increases factor VIII. DDAVP is an antidiuretic, so caution should be taken to fluid restrict appropriately when DDAVP is given to prevent hyponatremia [26]. Anesthesiologists must be aware not to fluid overload a patient resulting in hyponatremia and electrolyte imbalance in patients that have been treated with DDAVP prior to a procedure especially in the elderly and patients with heart disease, hypertension, or stroke. The Medical and Scientific Advisory Council (MASAC) has issued guidelines in treatment of the various forms of VWD. Patients with symptomatic type 1 VWD should be treated with DDAVP (1.5 mg/ml injectable form or nasal spray). For any situation that can potentially cause increased bleeding, if bleeding is not controlled with DDAVP, consider a factor VIII concentrate rich in vWF. Patients with type 2A, 2 M, and 2 N should be treated with DDAVP if previously shown to be responsive to a DDAVP trial. Patients with type 2B, type 3, and those with type 1, 2A, 2 M, and 2 N who are not responsive to DDAVP should be treated with factor VIII concentrates [22]. DDAVP treatment should be given once every 24 hours as vWF stores become depleted and should not be used for more than 3 consecutive days unless recommended by the hemophilia treatment staff [22]. In more severe forms of VWD, factor VIII concentrates or cryoprecipitate can be given to replace factor. Some of these products contain functional vWF and screened for transmittable diseases as HIV and hepatitis A, B, and C. Humate-P (Armour), a human plasma-derived product, is one such product. Baxaltas Vonvendi is the first recombinant vWF product approved in 2015 by the FDA. This product only contains vWF and is approved to treat on demand and for bleeding control in adults 18 and older [22]. Cryoprecipitate should only be used in a life-threatening emergency situation where DDAVP, factor 8 concentrates, or a recombinant vWF is unavailable, due to potential transmission of diseases. One must be aware if factor concentrates or cryoprecipitate is given of the potential risk of allergic reactions, thrombotic complications, and the transmission of blood borne pathogens. Tranexamic acid and aminocaproic acid are antifibrinolytic agents that can be used during dental procedures and treatment of mucosal bleeds. The recommended treatment in such cases includes initial administration of a clotting factor to form clot followed by an antifibrinolytic to sustain clot and prevent clot breakdown. In the pediatric and adolescent population where bleeding may not be obvious a diagnosis of vWD may be challenging. Investigative laboratory tests and studies are typically done on a patient of this subset with a family history of vWD, coagulopathies, or abnormal lab tests that were done prior to a procedure.

Cryoglobulinemia

Etiology

Cryoglobulinemia is a rare form of vasculitis where abnormal immunoglobulins known as cryoglobulins form causing blood flow restriction resulting in harm to key organs and tissues.

The etiology of the disease is unknown, but some inciting triggers are infections/viruses, genetics, medications, and environmental factors. The estimated prevalence is thought to be 1 in 1,000,000 worldwide where female adults over 50 years of age are affected more than males of similar age [27]. Cryoglobulins are abnormal blood proteins that clump together in cold temperatures and can cause multisystemic damage especially to the kidneys. Cryoglobulins can be classified into three types based on serology. Type I can be described as monoclonal immunoglobulins without rheumatoid factor activity seen in severe malignant conditions of the immune system, and workup for hematological malignancies should also be performed. Manifestations of type I often present as intravascular obstruction. Type II has polyclonal IgG and monoclonal IgM rheumatoid factors. Lastly, type III has polyclonal IgG and rheumatoid factors. Types II and III due to their composition are frequently described as mixed cryoglobulins [28]. These are often seen as true immune complex-mediated vasculitis [29]. This disease state is most commonly seen alongside a diagnosis of hepatitis C, but can also be seen with inflammatory and connective tissue disease states. Prompt treatment of hepatitis C is necessary as 90% of mixed cryoglobulinemia cases are associated with hepatitis C.

Signs and Symptoms

The presentation of cryoglobulinemia can be variable. Symptoms may include kidney damage presenting as a membranoproliferative glomerulonephritis, cutaneous rash with red spots, purplish discoloration from bleeding under the skin (purpura), myalgia and joint pain, peripheral neuropathy, weakness, and respiratory difficulties. In severe forms, the brain and heart can be involved [27].

Diagnosis

Diagnosis of cryoglobulinemia is multifold, but a blood test detecting cryoglobulins is the mainstay for diagnosis. Thorough history and physical, clinical presentation, specialized imaging, urinalysis, nerve conduction tests of extremities, and a biopsy of an affected tissue or organ may be ordered to help with diagnosis and treatment plan.

Treatment

Symptoms of this disease state may be mild in which conservative treatments as avoiding cold temperatures and NSAID's can improve symptoms to more symptomatic severe symptoms that can be treated with immunosuppressive drugs. Being an immunologic disorder, cryoglobulinemia is most often treated with corticosteroids and other medications that suppress the immune system when necessary. In most cases, once the underlying disease process is treated, cryoglobulinemia improves. When seen with hepatitis C, antivirals are given as well. Follow-up after remission of disease state is important as recurrence can occur. Anesthetic considerations in a patient with cryoglobulinemia are continuous temperature monitoring. Cryoglobulins precipitate at temperatures below 37.0 °C and can cause an increase in blood viscosity and organ dysfunction due to microangiopathy. In particular, patients undergoing cardiopulmonary bypass performed under hypothermic considerations should be treated appropriately prior to surgery. Perioperative treatment measures as plasmapheresis and steroid pulse therapy have shown to reduce blood viscosity in such cases [30].

References

1. Shah U, Narayanan M, Graham SJ. Anaesthetic considerations in patients with inherited disorders of coagulation. Contin Educ Anaesth Critic Care Pain. 2015;15(1):26–31.
2. Mensah PK, Gooding R. Surgery in patients with inherited bleeding disorders. Anaesthesia. 2015;70:112–20. https://doi.org/10.1111/anae.12899.
3. Hemophilia: Data & Statistics. Centers for Disease Control and Prevention. Available at http://www.cdc.gov/ncbddd/hemophilia/data.html. 12 Apr 2017. Accessed 5 Aug 2019.
4. Drelich, Douglass A. Hemophilia A. Practice essentials, background, pathophysiology. 26 Feb 2019. emedicine.medscape.com/article/779322-overview#a4.
5. Hemophilia A. National Hemophilia Foundation, 15 July 2015. www.hemophilia.org/Bleeding-Disorders/Types-of-Bleeding-Disorders/Hemophilia-A. Date Accessed: 5 Aug 2019.
6. Bauer K. Current challenges in the management of Hemophilia. Am J Manag Care. 2015;21(6 Suppl):S112–22.
7. Mansouritorghabeh H. Clinical and laboratory approaches to Hemophilia A. Iran J Med Sci. 2015;40(3):194–205.
8. Hoots, W Keith, and Amy Shapiro. Clinical manifestations and diagnosis of hemophilia. UpToDate, 16 July 2019, https://www.

uptodate.com/contents/clinical-manifestations-and-diagnosis-of-hemophilia/print.
9. Knoble P. Prevention and management of bleeding episodes in patients with acquired Hemophilia A. Drugs. 2018;78(18):1861–72. https://doi.org/10.1007/s40265-018-1027-y.
10. Zaiden, R. Hemophilia B. Medscape https://emedicine.medscape.com/article/779434-overview. Date Accessed: 5 Aug 2019.
11. Shapiro, A. National organization for rare diseases. Hemophilia B. https://rarediseases.org/rare-diseases/hemophilia-b/. Date Accessed 6 Aug 2019.
12. Peyvandi F, Duga S, Akhaven S, Mannucci PM. Rare coagulation deficiencies. Haemophilia. 2002;8:208.
13. Wheeler AP, Gailani D. Why factor XI deficiency is a clinical concern. Expert Rev Hematol. 2016;9(7):629–37. https://doi.org/10.1080/17474086.2016.1191944. Epub 2016 Jun 24. Citation on PubMed or Free article on PubMed Central.
14. Acharya S. Advances in hemophilia and the role of current and emerging prophylaxis. Am J Manag Care. 2016;22(5 Suppl):s116–25. PMID: 27266808
15. Manco-Johnson MJ, Abshire TC, Shapiro AD, et al. Prophylaxis versus episodic treatment to prevent joint disease in boys with severe hemophilia. N Engl J Med. 2007;357(6):535–44.
16. Hemophilia: treatment of Hemophilia. Centers for Disease Control and Prevention. Available at http://www.cdc.gov/ncbddd/hemophilia/data.html. 11 Mar 2019. Accessed 6 Aug 2019.
17. Factor XI Deficiency. NORD (National Organization for Rare Disorders). https://rarediseases.org/rare-diseases/factor-xi-deficiency/.
18. Kempton, Christine L., and Shannon L. Meeks. Toward optimal therapy for inhibitors in Hemophilia. Blood J Am Soc Hematol. 27 Nov 2014. http://www.bloodjournal.org/content/bloodjournal/124/23/3365.
19. Peyvandi F, Garagiola I, Biguzzi E. Advances in the treatment of bleeding disorders. J Thromb Haemost. 2016;14(11):2095–106.
20. Hoots, W Keith, and Amy D Shapiro. Treatment of bleeding and perioperative management in Hemophilia A and B. UpToDate, 26 Nov 2018. https://www.uptodate.com/contents/treatment-of-bleeding-and-perioperative-management-in-hemophilia-a-and-b.
21. Oshika H, Koyama Y. Perioperative management of a pediatric patient with suspected type 1 von Willebrand disease undergoing tonsillectomy: a case report. JA Clin Rep. 2019;5:54.
22. Von Willebrand Disease. National Hemophilia Foundation. www.hemophilia.org/Bleeding-Disorders/Types-of-Bleeding-Disorders/Von-Willebrand-Disease. Date Accessed 1 Aug 2019.
23. Von Willebrand Disease. National Organization for Rare Disorders, https://rarediseases.org/rare-diseases/von-willebrand-disease/. Date Accessed 1 Aug 2019.
24. Kadir R. Chapter 6: Von Willebrand Disease. In: Inherited bleeding disorders in women. 2nd ed. Newark: John Wiley & Sons; 2018. p. 83–91.
25. Nichols WL, Hultin MB. Von Willebrand disease (WD): evidence based diagnosis and management guidelines, the National Heart, Lung, and Blood Institute (NHLBI) Expert Panel Report (USA). Hemophilia. 2008;14:171–232.
26. Mannucci PM. Desmopressin (DDAVP) for treatment of disorders of hemostasis. Prog Hemost Thromb. 1986;8:19–45.
27. Cryoglobulinemia. Vasculitis Foundation. https://www.vasculitisfoundation.org/education/forms/cryoglobulinemia/#1545061618025-a76f8b6a-11d8. Date Accessed 8 Aug 2019.
28. Agnello V, Chung R, Kaplan L. A role for hepatitis C virus infection in type II Cryoglobulinemia. N Engl J Med. 1992;327:1490–5.
29. Desbois A, Cacoub P, Saadoun D. Cryoglobulinemia: An update in 2019. Elsevier. 2019;86(3):241–8.
30. Satomi S, Kasai A, Hamaguchi E. Normothermic cardiopulmonary bypass in patient with Waldenstrom's macroglobulinemia and cryoglobulinemia: a case report. A A Case Rep. 2017;9(6):162–3.

Blood Conservation Strategies and Bloodless Medicine

14

Eric Gomez, Mario DeAngelis, and Henry Liu

Introduction

Multiple studies have shown anemia and allogeneic blood transfusion (ABT) as independent risk factors for adverse perioperative outcomes [1]. The World Health Organization (WHO) defines anemia as a hemoglobin (Hb) concentration <13 g/dl for men and <12 g/dl for women [2]. Anemia has been shown to correlate strongly with morbidity and mortality in the preoperative non-cardiac surgical patients. Anesthesiologists and surgeons make the decision to transfuse patients with blood products every day. Intraoperative blood product transfusions occur in approximately 9% of major non-cardiac surgeries [3]. However, they will have to face the challenge in some clinical scenarios during their career whether to cancel the surgical procedure due to patients' religious beliefs or lack of resources in blood products. There are many well-documented deleterious effects of blood transfusions, and several international campaigns from major hematological societies to promote proper blood utilization and/or conservation [4]. Patients may refuse ABT for various reasons, and appropriate blood product may be unavailable for a specific patient after the cross-matching process is completed. Blood conservation strategies are developed to address these situations [3]. Recent studies have demonstrated that by adopting appropriate blood conservation management, patients who refuse ABT may achieve similar clinical outcomes comparing to those who accept ABT [5]. Given the many risks associated with ABT, and a growing population of patients who refuse blood transfusions, an increasing number of medical centers have implemented the so-called "bloodless medicine" programs [5].

"Bloodless medicine" programs are multidisciplinary patient-centered care models that implement strategies for blood conservation for patients who would prefer no blood products. These programs require teams of surgeons, anesthesiologists, hematologists, nurses, laboratory technicians, perfusionists, as well as the patient. Which products or factors an individual may be willing to receive vary greatly from person to person. An individual discussion with a patient regarding their preference in a very detailed fashion should be made prior to the scheduled surgical procedure. "Bloodless medicine" programs begin preparing patients for surgery preoperatively by enhancing blood production, intraoperatively by implementing various blood conservation techniques and minimizing surgical blood loss, and postoperatively by adopting policies to decrease blood loss and improve hemostasis. Anesthetic techniques and appropriate hemodynamic management, new point of care testing modalities, autologous blood salvage, and normovolemic hemodilution are commonly applied strategies that decrease intraoperative loss of red blood cells [1]. In cardiac surgery, blood conservation strategies have been increasingly implemented and benefit patients with decreased morbidity and mortality [6]. As the evidence of benefits from blood conservation techniques is accumulating, more and more other strategies to avoid or minimize ABT are emerging and maturing, such as use of antifibrinolytics, noninvasive surgical techniques/instruments, and blood substitutes [6, 7].

Transfusion-Related Risks

As discussed in other chapter(s) in this book, blood transfusion is not a completely benign procedure. There can be significant morbidity and mortality from blood transfusions (Table 14.1). According to an FDA database (FDA/CBER),

E. Gomez
Department of Anesthesiology, Thomas Jefferson University Hospital, Philadelphia, PA, USA

M. DeAngelis
Department of Anesthesiology, Methodist Division, Thomas Jefferson University Hospital, Philadelphia, PA, USA

H. Liu (✉)
Department of Anesthesiology and Perioperative Medicine, Milton S. Hershey Medical Center, Penn State College of Medicine, Hershey, PA, USA

© Springer Nature Switzerland AG 2021
C. S. Scher et al. (eds.), *Essentials of Blood Product Management in Anesthesia Practice*,
https://doi.org/10.1007/978-3-030-59295-0_14

Table 14.1 Transfusion-related risks

Infectious	–
Viral	HIV, HCV, HBV, West Nile virus
Bacterial	Microbial contamination, sepsis
Immunological	–
TRALI, TRIM, TACO	Pulmonary edema, oncological promotion
Hemolytic transfusion reaction	ABO vs non-ABO incompatibility
Graft versus host disease	Transplant rejection
Viral transmission	CMV, Ebstein Barr, HTLV
Anaphylaxis	Hypotension
Febrile	Benign
Physiological	–
Electrolyte derangement	Potassium, calcium chelation
Hypothermia	–

from 2012 to 2016, transfusion-related acute lung injury (TRALI), transfusion-associated circulatory overload (TACO), hemolytic transfusion (HTR) reaction due to non-ABO incompatibility, and microbial contamination account for 84% of transfusion-related mortality. Complications of blood transfusions are explained in greater detail in Chap. 12. Despite the advancements and systems-based safety protocols already in place to decrease transfusion-related risks, the only way to completely mitigate risks is to avoid transfusion of blood products completely [8].

Blood Conservation Strategies and Benefits

Preoperative Management

To minimize the need for perioperative transfusions, surgical patients should have a history and physical examination performed a week or more prior to surgery to allow some time for correction of preoperative anemia. Patients who have preoperative anemia carry a higher risk of requiring a blood transfusion. The preoperative prevalence of anemia in surgical patients, when defined as a hemoglobin level of less than 13 g/dL in men or 11.5 g/dL in women, has been estimated to be as high as 60% in some studies [9]. In the face of preoperative anemia for elective procedures, postponement until correction of anemia may be considered [9].

The most common cause of preoperative anemia is iron deficiency [10]. Iron, vitamin B12, and folate can be administered to these patients aiming to correct anemia secondary to respective deficiencies. Erythropoietin may also be used to correct anemia perioperatively, usually under the guidance and monitoring of a hematology team. Low-dose recombinant erythropoietin administered just 4 days before surgery may induce rapid erythropoiesis significant enough to halve the blood transfusion requirements in cardiac surgery [11]. Patients scheduled for myomectomy/hysterectomy for fibroids may have anemia secondary to uterine bleeding. Administration of Lupron Depot concomitantly with iron in these patients has been demonstrated in increase in hemoglobin by >2 g/dL in 3 months [12].

Careful attention and thorough history review should focus on any bleeding history and the use of anticoagulant/antiplatelet medications. Patients with hematological disorders, such as those with von Willebrand's disease or uremic platelet dysfunction, should be identified preoperatively. Patients on long-acting anticoagulants (like warfarin) may need to be switched to short-acting bridging medications in the perioperative setting, and in some cases, reversal of anticoagulation may even be necessary, especially in the case of emergency surgery [8].

Preoperative autologous blood donation can be used to transfuse autologous blood instead of allogeneic blood. According to an American Society of Anesthesiologists (ASA) task force, when autologous blood is preferred, patients may be offered the opportunity to donate prior to admission and adequate time for erythropoietic reconstitution if surgical schedule allows. Preoperative autologous blood donation can potentially increase rates of preoperative anemia, costs, so it is not routinely practiced. Autologous blood transfusions may still have adverse effects, including transfusion reaction secondary to clerical error and even bacterial contamination [8].

Intraoperative Management

Intraoperatively, surgical technique, delicate anesthetic/hemodynamic management, and blood conservation strategies work together to minimize loss of red blood cells and subsequent need of ABT. Minimally invasive surgical techniques, endovascular techniques, and interventional radiology can have profound impacts on blood conservation when compared to open surgery [13, 14]. Interventional radiologists can help decrease the amount of intraoperative blood loss significantly with preoperative embolization of specific feeding arteries [15]. Topical hemostatic agents can also be used as an adjunct in achieving adequate surgical hemostasis. There are several currently available commercial products which use gelatin, collagen, thrombin, and other materials as the core ingredients respectively. Continued interest in improving surgical hemostasis has led to the development of improved electrocautery in the form of the radiofrequency bipolar hemostatic sealer (RHBS). RHBS uses saline-cooled energy which seals blood vessels without burning them. Studies have shown reduction in blood transfusion requirements using this technology in liver resections, total hip arthroplasty, total knee arthroplasty, and multilevel spinal fusion surgery [16].

Anesthetic and hemodynamic management may potentially have significant impact on blood transfusion requirement. As physiologist, anesthesiologists should have a thorough understanding of the importance of ensuring optimal conditions for blood coagulation and hemostasis in surgical patients. Platelet aggregation and activation are impaired with hypothermia, acidosis, and severe hypocalcemia [17]. Reviews of case reports of trauma patients with refractory coagulopathy revealed the importance of correction/avoidance of hypothermia and acidosis [18]. The manipulation of physiological parameters has historically been used for specific types of surgical operations as well. Controlled hypotension has been used to decrease the total blood loss and improve the surgical field in a variety of surgical procedures. Several studies have demonstrated the benefit in reducing the blood transfusion requirement in major spine surgery [19]. A recent Cochrane review of the use of propofol for controlled hypotension in functional endoscopic sinus surgery revealed that there is insufficient evidence to show a clear benefit of hypotension for decreasing blood loss, but there may be some benefit in improving the surgical field. This review was limited in that there were only four published trials with a small number of participants at the time of publishing [20]. The maintenance of a low central venous pressure using anesthetic techniques and infusions has been used in hepatic resections for decreasing blood loss and transfusion requirements, as well [21].

There is a significant role for point-of-care testing in perioperative blood conservation. Viscoelastic hemostatic assays, specifically thromboelastography (TEG) and rotational thromboelastometry (ROTEM), when used in conjugation with transfusion protocols, have been shown to decrease the incidence and total volume of ABT in cardiac surgery [22]. TEG analysis can provide information on the speed of clot formation, platelet function, and fibrinolysis. With this information, medical practitioners can correct specific coagulation abnormalities and improve hemostasis. TEG-directed therapy can help determine which patients may benefit from administration of fresh frozen plasma, platelets, or antifibrinolytics. In patients who may have rapid changes in hemoglobin intraoperatively, assessment with point-of-care testing of hemoglobin can help reduce unnecessary transfusions as well. To minimize frequent blood sampling and allow for accurate assessment of hemoglobin, noninvasive continuous hemoglobin monitors can be used as well. Furthermore, there are point-of-care devices that can measure PT/PTT and platelet function [23].

Intraoperative Blood Salvage

Intraoperative blood salvage or cell salvage is the process in which blood shed during surgery is collected and returned to the same patient. Blood is aspirated using low-pressure suction as it is mixed with an anticoagulant. Once a sufficient amount is retrieved, it is washed, concentrated, and filtered prior to transfusion back to the patient. Recovered shed blood can have a hematocrit of 45% or higher after processing [24].

Cell salvage should be used for patients who may experience significant surgical blood loss, patients who may not have cross-matched blood available, and patients who refuse allogeneic blood transfusion but will accept autologous blood (as in the Jehovah's Witness). Cell salvage may be indicated in cardiothoracic, major orthopedic, vascular, obstetric, gynecological, urological, neurosurgical, and other procedures [25]. In situations where there is uncertainty over the possible blood loss, cell salvage can be used in a "stand-by" or "collection" mode; if blood is collected in sufficient amount, it can be processed for transfusion. Of note, cell salvage does not eliminate allogeneic blood transfusion-related complications but just decrease it. There are still significant benefits from decreased overall exposure to allogeneic blood. However, salvaged blood does not have to be transfused back if the patient is not anemic since it may still cause some complications.

Patient refusal may be the only absolute contraindication to intraoperative cell salvage. In the case of the Jehovah's Witness, patient care should be tailored to the individual wishes of the patient. Some patients are willing to accept autologous blood that remains in circuit with them in a "closed loop." This has allowed for some patients to accept cardiopulmonary bypass [26]. A thorough discussion should be held with patients prior to admission to determine the best course of action.

With the use of a leukocyte depletion filter (LDF) and washing, cell salvage has reduced or minimized the risks associated with many of its relative contraindications [25]. These include bacterial contamination, obstetrics, and malignancy. Bacterial contamination of cell salvage product is common, but after filtration and washing, a 99% decrease in bacterial load can be observed [27]. Historically, because of the theoretical risk of amniotic fluid embolism or Rh sensitization from fetal hemoglobin exposure, cell salvage in obstetrics practice was almost completely avoided. With the development of cell salvage washing and better filtration, a multitude of case reports in obstetric hemorrhage have been reported and changed the standards of obstetric practice. Currently, the American College of Obstetricians and Gynecologists advocates for the use of cell salvage. In patients with malignancy, filtration removes tumor cells from cell salvage product decreasing the risk of diffuse tumor cell dissemination [28].

Normovolemic Hemodilution

Acute normovolemic hemodilution (ANH) is the process in which a few units of blood are removed from a patient after induction of anesthesia and replaced with crystalloid and/or colloid. The objective is to decrease the patient's hemoglobin concentration during the surgery, so as to decrease the amount of hemoglobin lost in surgical blood loss. The blood that was withdrawn is returned to the patient during or after the surgical operation.

ANH is most effective in decreasing or eliminating allogeneic blood transfusions in patients who have a high initial/preoperative hematocrit, a low transfusion trigger hematocrit value, and a high blood loss. It is best used in healthy patients who can tolerate the initial decrease in hematocrit [29]. ANH can be used in a closed loop system, allowing for some Jehovah's witnesses to accept this procedure as well [30]. Studies of ANH in cardiothoracic surgery have shown that the decreased viscosity that comes from hemodilution may have certain cardioprotective effects [31]. Another advantage of using ANH is its relatively low cost, compared to intraoperative cell salvage.

Postoperative Management

Blood conservation techniques should continue in the postoperative period and are usually tailored to the specific needs of individual patients. In patients who have uncontrolled bleeding, interventional radiology may be employed to embolize source arteries. Iatrogenic blood loss from postoperative hypertension and frequent laboratory testing should be minimized, and sometimes blood samples may be collected in smaller "pediatric" tubes. Arterial and venous blood gasses can be used to obtain some electrolyte and hemoglobin values from less than 1 ml of blood. Blood conservation can also include the use of postoperative blood salvage. Surgical drains can collect significant amounts of blood, and this can be processed through blood salvage machines.

Blood Conservation in Orthopedic Surgery

There are several orthopedic procedures that can have large volumes of blood loss, and multiple strategies have been employed in total joint surgery. Induced hypotension has demonstrated significant reductions in blood loss and blood transfusion requirements, specifically with epidural anesthesia [32, 33]. Hypotensive epidural anesthesia also decreases the risk of deep vein thrombosis and provides a relatively "dryer" surgical field for cementing of joints [34].

Antifibrinolytics, such as tranexamic acid (TXA), are employed in total joint surgery as well for blood conservation [7]. TXA has been used intravenously and topically. There is ongoing debate on the true contraindications of TXA. While TXA is historically avoided in patients with venous thromboembolism, recent studies may categorize this risk as negligible [35]. More detailed information on antifibrinolytics and their mechanism of action can be found in other chapters of this book.

Outcomes of Blood Conservation in Cardiac Surgery

The majority of perioperative blood transfusions occur in patients undergoing cardiothoracic surgery. The Society of Thoracic Surgeons and the Society of Cardiovascular Anesthesiologists have identified that there are certain characteristics that define a patient as high risk for blood transfusion. These include advanced age, preoperative anemia, small body size, non-CABG or urgent surgery, preoperative antithrombotic drugs, coagulation abnormalities, and multiple patient comorbidities (insulin-dependent diabetes, sepsis, liver failure, peripheral vascular disease). Surgical patients categorized as high risk for blood transfusion should undergo appropriate blood conservation strategies (pharmacological intervention, intraoperative blood salvage, normovolemic hemodilution, institution-specific blood transfusion algorithms supplemented by POC testing, and a multimodality approach to blood conservation). Studies regarding the safety and efficacy of permissive anemia (hemoglobin of 6–7 g/dL) as a component of blood conservation have already demonstrated safety and effectiveness in reducing transfusions and complications including death [6].

The Future of Bloodless Medicine

Artificial blood substitutes are currently under very active research and development, but none are currently FDA-approved. Artificial blood substitutes are either perfluorochemical-based (PFC) or hemoglobin-based. PFCs are inert, non-toxic substances with oxygen-carrying capacity. Hemoglobin-based blood substitutes can be human derived (from old bags), animal, or recombinant. The hemoglobin from the earthworm Lumbricus terrestris (LtEc) is another very attractive blood substitute candidate. One of the features is its resistance to oxidation and aggregation during storage. Some investigations have been aiming to optimize the thermal and oxidative stability of LtEc during storage by manipulating pH, antioxidant supplements, and deoxygenation. A technique for the reduction of fully oxidized LtEc with antioxidants has also been developed. LtEc was shown to have the highest thermal stability in Ringer's modified lactate solution with 10 mM HEPES at pH 7.0. Deoxygenation of the LtEc was shown to significantly reduce oxidation of the ferrous heme iron. The oxygen transport properties of LtEc were believed to be unaffected by storage at high temperatures or oxidation [36]. The stability of Lumbricus terrestris erythrocruorin can also be increased via poly(acrylic acid) conjugation [37]. The development of red blood cells from stem cells is currently also underway. The use of pluripotent stem cells could allow for the mass production of red blood cells in the future. High production cost is the strongest limiting factor, and this could diminish over time [38].

Summary

Blood transfusions, while potentially life-saving, are fraught with risks and refusal by patients and sometimes unavailable. Blood transfusions can cause significant morbidity and mortality. Bloodless medicine involves preoperative assessment of anemia and minimization of iatrogenic/surgical blood loss. Strategies are readily employed in a variety of patients including the Jehovah's witness, the orthopedic patient, and the cardiac patient. Many blood substitutes are being developed to provide red blood cells' oxygen-carrying capability. As bloodless medicine continues to advance, the need for blood transfusions will decrease.

References

1. Blaudszun G, Butchart A, Klein AA. Blood conservation in cardiac surgery. Transfus Med. 2018;28(2):168–80. https://doi.org/10.1111/tme.12475.
2. Rivilla Marugán L, Lorente Aznar T, Molinero Rodriguez M, García-Erce JA. Anaemia and the elderly: critical review of its definition and prevalence. Rev Esp Geriatr Gerontol. 2019 Jul - Aug;54(4):189–94. https://doi.org/10.1016/j.regg.2019.02.008.
3. Chen A, Trivedi AN, Jiang L, Vezeridis M, Henderson WG, Wu WC. Hospital blood transfusion patterns during major noncardiac surgery and surgical mortality. Medicine (Baltimore). 2015;94(32):e1342. https://doi.org/10.1097/MD.0000000000001342.
4. Callum JL, Waters JH, Shaz BH, et al. The AABB recommendations for the choosing wisely campaign of the American Board of Internal Medicine. Transfusion. 2014;54:2344–52.
5. Frank SM, Wick EC, Dezern AE, Ness PM, Wasey JO, Pippa AC, et al. Clinical outcomes for bloodless patients. Transfusion. 2004;54:2668–77. https://doi.org/10.1111/trf.12752.
6. Moskowitz DM, McCullough JN, Shander A, Klein JJ, Bodian CA, Goldweit RS, et al. The impact of blood conservation on outcomes in cardiac surgery: is it safe and effective? Ann Thorac Surg. 2010;90(2):451–8. https://doi.org/10.1016/j.athoracsur.2010.04.089.
7. Álvarez JC, Santiveri FX, Ramos I, Vela E, Puig L, Escolano F. Tranexamic acid reduces blood transfusion in total knee arthroplasty even when a blood conservation program is applied. Transfusion. 2008;48:519–25. https://doi.org/10.1111/j.1537-2995.2007.01564.x.
8. American Society of Anesthesiologists Task Force on Perioperative Blood Management. Practice guidelines for perioperative blood management: an updated report by the American Society of Anesthesiologists Task Force on perioperative blood management. Anesthesiology. 2015;122(2):241–75. https://doi.org/10.1097/ALN.0000000000000463.
9. Shander A, Knight K, Thurer R, Adamson J, Spence R. Prevalence and outcomes of anemia in surgery: a systematic review of the literature. Am J Med. 2004;116(Suppl 7A):58S–69S. https://doi.org/10.1016/j.amjmed.2003.12.013.
10. Kansagra AJ, Stefan MS. Preoperative anemia: evaluation and treatment. Anesthesiol Clin. 2016;34(1):127–41. https://doi.org/10.1016/j.anclin.2015.10.011.
11. Yazicioğlu L, Eryilmaz S, Sirlak M, Inan MB, Aral A, Taşöz R, et al. Recombinant human erythropoietin administration in cardiac surgery. J Thorac Cardiovasc Surg. 2001;122(4):741–5. https://doi.org/10.1067/mtc.2001.115426.
12. Abbvie Inc. Lupron Depot 3.75 mg and –3 Month 11.25 mg: Highlights of prescribing information. https://www.rxabbvie.com/pdf/lupron3month11_25mg.pdf. Accessed 18 Apr 2019.
13. Patel AA, Zfass-Mendez M, Lebwohl NH, Wang MY, Green BA, Levi AD, et al. Minimally invasive versus open lumbar fusion: a comparison of blood loss, surgical complications, and hospital course. Iowa Orthop J. 2015;35:130–4.
14. Kiran RP, Delaney CP, Senagore AJ, Millward BL, Fazio VW. Operative blood loss and use of blood products after laparoscopic and conventional open colorectal operations. Arch Surg. 2004;139(1):39–42. https://doi.org/10.1001/archsurg.139.1.39.
15. Dumousset E, Chabrot P, Rabischong B, Mazet N, Nasser S, Darcha C, et al. Preoperative uterine artery embolization (PUAE) before uterine fibroid myomectomy. Cardiovasc Intervent Radiol. 2008;31(3):514–20. https://doi.org/10.1007/s00270-005-0342-3.
16. Frank SM, Wasey JO, Dwyer IM, Gokaslan ZL, Ness PM, Kebaish KM. Radiofrequency bipolar hemostatic sealer reduces blood loss, transfusion requirements, and cost for patients undergoing multilevel spinal fusion surgery: a case control study. J Orthop Surg Res. 2014;9:50. https://doi.org/10.1186/s13018-014-0050-2.
17. De Robertis E, Kozek-Langenecker SA, Tufano R, Romano GM, Piazza O, Zito MG. Coagulopathy induced by acidosis, hypothermia and hypocalcaemia in severe bleeding. Minerva Anestesiol. 2015;81(1):65–75.
18. Ferrara A, MacArthur JD, Wright HK, Modlin IM, McMillen MA. Hypothermia and acidosis worsen coagulopathy in the patient requiring massive transfusion. Am J Surg. 1990;160(5):515–8. https://doi.org/10.1016/S0002-9610(05)81018-9.
19. Dutton RP. Controlled hypotension for spinal surgery. Eur Spine J. 2004;13(Suppl 1):S66–71. https://doi.org/10.1007/s00586-004-0756-7.
20. Boonmak P, Boonmak S, Laopaiboon M. Deliberate hypotension with propofol under anaesthesia for functional endoscopic sinus surgery (FESS). Cochrane Database Syst Rev. 2016;(10) Art. No.: CD006623 https://doi.org/10.1002/14651858.CD006623.pub3.
21. Hughes MJ, Ventham NT, Harrison EM, Wigmore SJ. Central venous pressure and liver resection: a systematic review and meta-analysis. HPB (Oxford). 2015;17(10):863–71. https://doi.org/10.1111/hpb.12462.
22. Shore-Lesserson L, Manspeizer HE, DePerio M, Francis S, Vela-Cantos F, Ergin MA. Thromboelastography-guided transfusion algorithm reduces transfusions in complex cardiac surgery. Anesth Analg. 1999;88(2):312–9.
23. Van Cott EM. Coagulation point-of-care testing. Clin Lab Med. 2001;21(2):337–50.
24. AuBuchon JP, Puca K, Saxena S, Shulman IA, Waters JH. Getting started in patient blood management. [Internet]. AABB; 2011. Available from: https://www.aabb.org/pbm/Documents/112024DB.pdf. Accessed 10 May 2019.

25. Esper SA, Waters JH. Intra-operative cell salvage: a fresh look at the indications and contraindications. Blood Transfus. 2011;9(2):139–47. https://doi.org/10.2450/2011.0081-10.
26. Lawson T, Ralph C. Perioperative Jehovah's witnesses: a review. Br J Anaesth. 2015;115(5):676–87. https://doi.org/10.1093/bja/aev161.
27. Waters JH, Tuohy MJ, Hobson DF, Procop G. Bacterial reduction by cell salvage washing and leukocyte depletion filtration. Anesthesiology. 2003;99(3):652–5.
28. Kongsgaard UE, Wang MY, Kvalheim G. Leucocyte depletion filter removes cancer cells in human blood. Acta Anaesthesiol Scand. 1996 Jan;40(1):118–20.
29. Jamnicki M, Kocian R, van der Linden P, Zaugg M, Spahn DR. Acute normovolemic hemodilution: physiology, limitations, and clinical use. J Cardiothorac Vasc Anesth. 2003;17(6):747–54.
30. Lindstrom E, Johnstone R. Acute normovolemic hemodilution in a Jehovah's witness patient: a case report. AANA J. 2010;78(4):326–30.
31. Licker M, Ellenberger C, Sierra J, Kalangos A, Diaper J, Morel D. Cardioprotective effects of acute normovolemic hemodilution in patients undergoing coronary artery bypass surgery. Chest. 2005;128(2):838–47.
32. Sharrock NE, Salvati EA. Hypotensive epidural anesthesia for total hip arthroplasty. Acta Orthop Scand. 1996;67:91–107.
33. Juelsgaard P, Larsen UT, Sorensen JV, Madsen F, Soballe K. Hypotensive epidural anesthesia in total knee replacement without tourniquet: reduced blood loss and transfusion. Reg Anesth Pain Med. 2001;26:105–10.
34. Sambandam B, Batra S, Gupta R, Agrawal N. Blood conservation strategies in orthopedic surgeries: a review. J Clin Orthop Trauma. 2013;4(4):164–70. https://doi.org/10.1016/j.jcot.2013.11.002.
35. Goobie SM, Frank SM. Tranexamic acid: what is known and unknown, and where do we go from here? Anesthesiology. 2017;127:405–7. https://doi.org/10.1097/ALN.0000000000001788.
36. Muzzelo C, Neely C, Shah P, Abdulmalik O, Elmer J. Prolonging the shelf life of Lumbricus terrestris erythrocruorin for use as a novel blood substitute. Artif Cells Nanomed Biotechnol. 2018;46(1):39–46. https://doi.org/10.1080/21691401.2017.1290645.
37. Spivack K, Tucker M, Zimmerman D, Nicholas M, Abdulmalik O, Comolli N, Elmer J. Increasing the stability of Lumbricus terrestris erythrocruorin via poly(acrylic acid) conjugation. Artif Cells Nanomed Biotechnol. 2018;46(sup2):1137–44. https://doi.org/10.1080/21691401.2018.1480491.
38. Moradi S, Jahanian-Najafabadi A, Roudkenar MH. Artificial blood substitutes: first steps on the long route to clinical utility. Clin Med Insights Blood Disord. 2016;9:33–41.

When Blood Is Not an Option: Care of the Jehovah's Witness Patient

15

Justin B. Feit and Seth Perelman

Clinical Case Description

A fifty eight-year-old female Jehovah's Witness with medical history significant for ESRD not yet on dialysis, COPD, presenting with worsening shortness of breath, found to have severe mitral regurgitation and severe tricuspid regurgitation. After consultation with surgeons, decision was made to proceed with an open mitral valve and tricuspid valve replacements. She is referred to presurgical testing for medical and surgical optimization prior to surgery.

Introduction

Perioperative blood management is a crucial aspect of the anesthesiologist's clinical duties. While it is important to avoid/prevent perioperative anemia due to its morbidity and mortality [1], blood product administration has its own consequences [2], including transfusion reactions [3], pathogen transmission [4], immunomodulation [5], transfusion-related acute lung injury (TRALI) [6], and transfusion-associated circulatory overload (TACO) [7]. There are indications for specific blood product transfusions, including need for increased oxygen-carrying capacity and tissue oxygenation and treatment of coagulopathy secondary to factor deficiencies or platelet dysfunction, for example [8, 9].

Despite situations in which blood product transfusion is indicated (and withholding of these products can be fatal), there are certain patients that will refuse blood product transfusion based on religious beliefs; among these patients, the most notable population includes patients of the Jehovah's Witness faith. These patients pose a particular challenge among anesthesiologists with respect to perioperative blood management due to their refusal of certain blood products and limited intraoperative treatment options.

Blood Transfusions

The modern history of blood transfusions began in the mid-1660s when English physician Richard Lower experimented with transfusing blood between dogs shortly before physician Jean Denis experimented with transfusing humans using blood taken from dogs [10]. In the late eighteenth century, Joseph Priestley described red blood cells as capable of carrying oxygen [11], shortly before French chemist Antoine Lavoisier described the importance of oxygen in respiration [12]. Further advances in blood transfusion occurred in the early nineteenth century with English obstetrician James Blundell, the "Father of Autotransfusion"; it was discovered that giving back blood lost during surgery was not only safer than transfusing animal blood to humans, but also that autotransfusion improved mortality in massive surgical hemorrhages [13].

Despite improved outcomes demonstrated by Blundell with human transfusion in the nineteenth century, there were many issues that needed additional research including transfusion reactions and blood product storage. In the early twentieth century, Karl Landsteiner, a German physician, began elucidating the ABO red blood cell antigen system which helped decrease the amount of deadly transfusion reactions significantly [14]. Storage of blood products was increased to almost 3 weeks through the discovery of adding citrate (by Richard Weil) [15] and dextrose (by Peyton Rous and JR Turner) [16]. Blood transfusions became more practical for humans after World War II with the creation of the modern blood bank by Drs. Bernard Fantus and Lindon Seed out of Chicago, IL [17].

J. B. Feit
NYU Langone Health, NYU School of Medicine, Department of Anesthesiology, Perioperative Care, and Pain Medicine, New York, NY, USA
e-mail: Justin.Feit@nyulangone.org

S. Perelman (✉)
NYU Grossman School of Medicine, Department of Anesthesiology, Perioperative Care and Pain Medicine, New York, NY, USA
e-mail: Seth.perelman@nyulangone.org

© Springer Nature Switzerland AG 2021
C. S. Scher et al. (eds.), *Essentials of Blood Product Management in Anesthesia Practice*, https://doi.org/10.1007/978-3-030-59295-0_15

Over the 300 years since Dr. Lower began his experimentation, there have been numerous further advances in transfusion medicine with respect to efficacy and safety. To this day, blood transfusions are the most common invasive procedure performed in the United States across all of medicine [18]. Blood transfusions can be lifesaving in many surgical environments, especially with increased morbidity and mortality associated with anemia, coagulopathy, and catastrophic surgical bleeding. However, despite well-recognized indications for blood transfusion, patients who receive a blood transfusion during their hospital stay for whatever reason are also more likely to have increased length of stays and mortality within 28 days [19], and the efficacy of allogeneic transfusion has come into question.

It is important for anesthesiologists to know what types of products are available to administer and their specific indications. The four most common blood products given in the perioperative period are red blood cells, platelets, fresh frozen plasma, and cryoprecipitate [20]. Red blood cells are used to increase the oxygen-carrying capacity in patients with anemia or with significant blood loss that impacts tissue oxygenation [21]. Platelets are commonly administered to treat or prevent bleeding in patients with low platelet counts or with platelet dysfunction [22]. Fresh frozen plasma (FFP) is the frozen version of the fluid portion of whole blood; FFP includes all of the coagulation factors with the exception of platelets [23]. FFP administration is commonly indicated in the setting of coagulation factor deficiency in the presence of active bleeding [24]; other situations include planned surgery in the setting of abnormal coagulation and thrombotic thrombocytopenic purpura. If FFP is thawed at 4 °C as opposed to its normal 37 °C, cryoprecipitate is created [25]. While FFP contains all coagulation factors, cryoprecipitate is made up of fibrinogen, factor VIII, factor XIII, and Von Willebrand's factor [25]. Cryoprecipitate is commonly administered in the setting of massive hemorrhages associated with hypofibrinogenemia, most commonly seen in cardiac surgery, obstetrics, and liver transplantation [25].

There are other blood product derivatives that are also used in the perioperative period including albumin, individual clotting factors, prothrombin complex concentrate (PCC), and immunoglobulins.

Jehovah's Witnesses

The Jehovah's Witness faith was founded in 1881 by Charles Taze Russell, a Pittsburgh-based Christian minister [26]. Russell began disseminating his beliefs in *Zion's Watch Tower and Herald of Christ's Presence*, a monthly religious magazine publication that was used to spread the teachings that would eventually become the main principles of the Jehovah's Witness faith [26]. With respect to their beliefs regarding blood management, their teachings are based on specific passages in the bible, namely, Genesis 9:4, which states, "Only, you shall not eat flesh with its life, that is, its blood" [27], and Leviticus 17:10, saying, "If anyone of the house of Israel or of the aliens who reside among them eats any blood, I will set my face against that person who eats blood, and will cut that person off from the people" [27]. These passages are interpreted to form one of the main tenets of the JW religion: their refusal of numerous types of blood products. As a result, these beliefs have led to multiple challenges in the medical and surgical care of Jehovah's Witnesses.

The JW religion includes 2,000,000 followers in the United States and over 8,000,000 worldwide [18]; it is likely that an anesthesiologist will encounter a Jehovah's Witness as a patient and possibly in a clinical situation where blood transfusion may be clinically indicated, but patient beliefs may make this scenario medically and legally challenging.

Legality

With respect to any patient population, it is important to understand each specific patient's requests/beliefs with regards to their medical care. Regarding blood management and Jehovah's Witness patients, their refusal/acceptance of various blood products is deeply rooted in ancient Biblical scriptures and subsequently passed down from generation to generation [26]. With these reasons for refusing certain blood products even in life-threatening situations, it is imperative as anesthesiologists that we understand and respect the wishes of this patient population. Even with the widely believed notion that Jehovah's Witnesses refuse all types of blood products, it is important to have an individualized conversation with each patient and clearly delineate which products are acceptable and which products are not acceptable as they may differ from patient to patient. Generally speaking, most JW patients will refuse "major blood fractions," namely, red blood cells, white blood cells, plasma, and platelets, while some will accept "minor blood fractions," including hemoglobin-based oxygen carriers, interferons, albumin, cryoprecipitate, and specific clotting factors [28]. Most JW patients will accept fluids (crystalloids/colloids), synthetic stimulating agents (erythropoietin, thrombopoietin), recombinant factor VIIa, and artificial blood substitutes [28].

The reason why certain patients within this population may accept or refuse certain blood products differs from patient to patient based on their interpretation of the scriptures, and it is important to document their specific wishes in order to come up with an acceptable plan for both the provider and patient before undergoing surgery. Documenting these wishes in the medical record is of tantamount importance before taking care of this patient population. Consulting your institution's risk management or the JW HLS (Hospital Liaison Services) may also be of assistance prior to planned surgical interventions. Not only institutions have legal/risk management services available for the perioperative period, but also there are specific blood consent forms that include each type of blood product/substitute and allow the patient to delineate which products are acceptable or objectionable.

During most patient encounters, there is enough time to have this discussion with the patient, and it is clear what products the patient will and will not accept; what about when there is an emergency or if the patient does not have capacity to have this conversation? Many Jehovah's Witnesses carry a Durable Power of Attorney (DPA) card that may delineate which products are and are not acceptable in the event of an emergency, but also may designate a person who will be able to make clear their wishes in the event that they cannot make their wishes known at that specific time [29]. In the event of a DPA card and health-care proxy with conflicting opinions on treatment options, the DPA card will ultimately override the health-care proxy. If no card or health-care proxy is immediately available in an emergency life-threatening situation, a medical provider should treat as according to the standard of care, including transfusion of any clinically indicated blood products or derivatives [29].

Acceptable and Unacceptable Treatments

As previously mentioned, there are "major blood fractions" that are generally not accepted by JW patients, and there are "minor blood fractions" that may be accepted by most JW patients. There are also products that are often accepted by most Jehovah's Witness patients which include fluids (crystalloids and colloids), synthetic stimulating agents (erythropoietin and thrombopoietin), recombinant factor VII, and artificial blood substitutes [28]. All of these agents refer to intravenous "blood substitutes" that are part of overall blood. Topical hemostatic agents (Avitene™, Tisseel™, etc.) are generally accepted and may be used as part of surgical hemostasis; these agents typically work by directly activating platelets and promoting thrombin formation, thus stabilizing blood clot formation during surgical bleeding. As with other products, these topical agents should be part of the blood refusal consent process as some JW may refuse thrombin-containing products.

Additional available treatments for JW patients include extracorporeal closed loop techniques—acute normovolemic hemodilution (ANH), cardiopulmonary bypass (CPB), and dialysis [28]; many of these procedures are acceptable, given that the circuit is maintained in a closed loop configuration. ANH involves preemptive removal of blood from a patient followed by replacement with acellular fluid, typically crystalloid or colloid [30]; this process leads to decreased red blood cell loss during surgery. At the end of surgery, the removed blood is then transfused back to the patient [31].

Preoperative Assessment

Perioperative assessment is crucial in optimizing this specific patient population. Traditionally, anesthesiologist's roles with respect to patient blood management exclusively occurred in the operating room setting, but it has become more prevalent over the last 15–20 years for the anesthesiologist to be involved in the patient's optimization in the presurgical period as part of a multidisciplinary team including surgeons, internists, and hematologists [32].

Part of the preoperative assessment requires an open conversation regarding what specific products and procedures will be acceptable and which would be objectionable. This discussion is critical in planning for the perioperative management of the JW especially in situations where blood products may be administered based on clinical indications. Ideally, this respectful discussion should happen early in the care of the patient, without the need to repeat it with each health-care provider encounter, which could be viewed as disrespectful or at worst coercion.

While there are indications for preoperative transfusion for all types of major blood products, red blood cell transfusion is the most common product transfused preoperatively [18]. Perioperative anemia is not only a risk factor for increased morbidity/mortality in the perioperative period [33] but also a predictor of intraoperative and postoperative red blood cell transfusions[1]; this makes correction of anemia in the Jehovah's Witness population particularly crucial to improving their postoperative outcomes. However, there are opportunities to optimize their hemoglobin levels without using blood products [34]. There are numerous etiologies of anemia that should be identified and treated, such as iron-deficiency anemia (iron), megaloblastic anemia (Vitamin B12, folate), or inadequate erythropoietin synthesis (erythropoietin-stimulating agents) [35]. There are various formulations for these acceptable alternatives, including oral, intravenous, intramuscular, and subcutaneous, that give this population options to allow for preoperative optimization without the need for allogeneic transfusion. The importance of the early evaluation and treatment of preoperative anemia should not be limited to the JW population and should be part of the preoperative evaluation of all patients, but in the JW patient, it is critical.

Perioperative Blood Management Strategies

There are many opportunities in the perioperative period to provide optimal medical/surgical care for these patients while simultaneously respecting their specific beliefs. Our obligation as physicians is not limited to a patient's physical ailments but also extends to respecting their spiritual beliefs. In collaboration with the surgeons, it is important to minimize blood loss when possible. For example, use of minimally invasive procedures, intraoperative cell salvage, arterial tourniquets, acute normovolemic hemodilution, and permissive hypotension are all strategies that can be employed in collaboration with our surgical colleagues to minimize blood loss intraoperatively [1]. Use of interventional radiology when applicable, compared to open techniques, can also minimize blood loss [1].

Maintaining euvolemia is crucial to allow the physiological response to anemia tolerance which includes increased tissue oxygen extraction, increased cardiac output, and increased sympathetic response to maintain oxygen delivery [36]. Supplemental oxygen, along with aggressively optimizing preoperative lung function can help maximize oxygen delivery, especially in low hemoglobin states [28]. Aggressively treating high metabolic demand states both intraoperatively and postoperatively (i.e., antibiotics for septic shock, mechanical support for cardiogenic shock, fluids/vasopressors for hypovolemic shock, paralysis) minimizes oxygen demand and thus compensates for potentially lower oxygen-carrying capacities [28].

Coagulation defects are often easily treated with plasma and/or platelets, but those products are usually restricted in the Jehovah's Witness population. One of the least invasive, yet most important opportunities to minimize coagulopathies as anesthesiologists is by maintaining normothermia—hypothermia impairs thrombin generation as part of coagulation initiation and thus by maintaining normothermia, or more importantly avoiding hypothermia, can avoid unnecessary coagulopathies [37]. There are also many pharmacologic treatments of coagulopathy that can potentially obviate the need for plasma/platelets; these treatments include prothrombin complex concentrate (PCC), calcium, vitamin K, tranexamic acid (TXA)/aminocaproic acid, desmopressin, and recombinant factors among others [36]. Perioperative consultation with a hematologist can provide further guidance on how to use these treatments should certain reversible coagulopathies arise intra- or postoperatively.

Minimizing phlebotomy perioperatively minimizes HAA (hospital acquired anemia), which although may seem inconsequential compared to possibly large intraoperative blood losses has been shown to lead to worse outcomes compared with patients with less iatrogenic blood loss [38]. While it is important to assess a patient's overall clinical status using laboratory tests, similar information can be acquired using more efficient techniques. POC (point-of-care) tests and the availability of pediatric test tubes can also limit hospital acquired anemia. Additionally, routine arterial blood gases for ventilated patients can be replaced by using continuous end-tidal carbon dioxide monitoring and noninvasive oximetry to assess respiratory status, thus potentially limiting the need for frequent blood draws [39].

Anemia Tolerance and Patient Outcomes

While it is important to understand how anesthesiologists can use alternate therapies rather than using "major blood products," it is also imperative to understand transfusion thresholds and how that corresponds to patient outcomes, especially in the JW population. There are situations during major hemorrhage and coagulopathy when most providers will empirically give blood products before getting any lab tests, as per widely accepted standards of care. However, there are other instances when time allows for goal-directed therapy based on POC testing, and it is up to the anesthesiologist to decide how to proceed with this information and whether a transfusion is indicated. With well-documented side effects, potential complications, and questionable efficacy of blood transfusions [40], transfusions should not be threshold based but should be based on clinical symptoms of anemia or coagulopathy.

What do we tell our patient when she comes to pre-surgical testing and asks how her religious beliefs will affect her overall outcome? Compared to patients without personal transfusion restrictions, Jehovah's Witness patients undergoing cardiac surgery who refuse all major blood products have similar short-term and long-term mortality [41]. Similarly, for Jehovah's Witness patients undergoing cardiac surgery who refuse blood transfusions, there has been a lower incidence of postoperative myocardial infarction, shorter time to extubation, shorter length of stay, and reduced costs in both the intensive care unit and the hospital [42]. With careful attention paid to these patients from the moment they are scheduled for surgery to when they leave the hospital, it is possible to have outcomes similar to those patients who are less restricted in their blood product acceptance. While these studies may indicate similar/better outcomes for JW patients compared to the general population, it is important to recognize their limitations, namely, that most of these studies are observational and that there are no randomized-control trials that have looked at similar information. Additionally, it is possible and that these JW patients were not randomized that there were both conscious and subconscious modifications of surgical technique knowing that there are limitations for blood transfusion in the event of uncontrolled surgical bleeding.

Summary

With respect to our patient scheduled for cardiac surgery, there are many options for optimization despite the possibility of a high blood-loss surgery. While the surgery is not elective, it is also not emergent such that there is adequate time for optimization. Presurgical consultation with an anesthesiologist is imperative and crucial for minimizing perioperative morbidity. Patients who are dialysis-dependent are often chronically anemic due to impaired erythropoietin production in interstitial cells found in the renal cortex. Other etiologies of anemia in patients with end-stage renal disease include uremic-induced inhibitors of red blood cell production and nutritional deficiencies (iron, folate, vitamin B12). Improvement in anemia for this patient can be accomplished by targeting each of the previously mentioned causes of anemia—use of erythropoiesis-stimulating agents (ESA- examples including Aranesp™, Epogen™), strict dialysis and use of desmopressin to address uremic platelet dysfunction, and importantly intravenous iron, folate, and vitamin B12 to address possible nutritional deficiencies. Intraoperatively, strategies to minimize blood loss include ANH, cell saver, and the use of permissible "minor blood products," if indicated. Postoperative strategies involve minimization of blood draws, use of vasopressors if indicated, and continued treatment of postoperative anemia.

Blood management in the Jehovah's Witness patient poses particular challenges for the anesthesiologist most notably their refusal of certain blood products due to religious beliefs. Patients having surgeries in which there is a high likelihood of moderate blood loss should be evaluated as soon as possible to assess for the presence and treatment of preoperative anemia but also to set out expectations for both the patient and the physician. There are many tools in our arsenal to deal with this challenging clinical scenario in high-risk, high blood-loss surgeries within the confines of honoring a patient's religious beliefs; with the knowledge of available institutional resources along with a clear understanding of the patient's specific wishes, it is possible to have good surgical outcomes while avoiding transfusions.

References

1. Resar LMS, Frank SM. Bloodless medicine: what to do when you can't transfuse. ASH Educ Program Book. 2014;2014(1): 553–8.
2. Vincent J-L, et al. Efficacy of allogeneic red blood cell transfusions. Best Pract Res Clin Anaesthesiol. 2007;21(2):209–19.
3. Siddon AJ, et al. Delayed haemolytic and serologic transfusion reactions: pathophysiology, treatment and prevention. Curr Opin Hematol. 2018;25(6):459–67.
4. Busch MP, Kleinman SH, Nemo GJ. Current and emerging infectious risks of blood transfusions. JAMA. 2003;289(8):959–62.
5. Blajchman MA. Immunomodulation and blood transfusion. Am J Ther. 2002;9(5):389–95.
6. Bux J, Sachs UJH. The pathogenesis of transfusion-related acute lung injury (TRALI). Br J Haematol. 2007;136(6):788–99.
7. Gilliss BM, Looney MR, Gropper MA. Reducing noninfectious risks of blood transfusion. Anesth J Am Soc Anesth. 2011;115(3):635–49.
8. Crosby ET. Perioperative haemotherapy: I. indications for blood component transfusion. Can J Anaesth. 1992;39(7):695–707.
9. Yaddanapudi S, Yaddanapudi LN. Indications for blood and blood product transfusion. Indian J Anaesth. 2014;58(5):538.
10. Giangrande PLF. The history of blood transfusion. Br J Haematol. 2000;110(4):758–67.
11. Schofield RE. The enlightened Joseph Priestley: a study of his life and work from 1773 to 1804. University Park, PA: Penn State Press; 2004.
12. Karamanou M, Tsoucalas G, Androutsos G. Hallmarks in the study of respiratory physiology and the crucial role of Antoine-Laurent de Lavoisier (1743–1794). Am J Phys Lung Cell Mol Phys. 2013;305(9):L591–4.
13. Blundell J. Experiments on the transfusion of blood by the syringe. Med Chir Trans. 1818;9(Pt 1):56.
14. Landsteiner K. Uber agglutinationserscheinungen normalen menschlichen blutes. Wien Klin Wshr. 1901;14:1132–4.
15. Weil R. Sodium citrate in the transfusion of blood. J Am Med Assoc. 1915;64(5):425–6.
16. Rous P, Turner JR. The preservation of living red blood cells in vitro: I. Methods of preservation. J Exp Med. 1916;23(2):219–37.
17. Strauss RG. Elmer L. DeGowin, MD: blood transfusions in war and peace. Transfus Med Rev. 2006;20(2):165–8.
18. Jorgenson TD, et al. When blood is not an option: the case for a standardized blood transfusion consent form. ASA Newsl. 2017;81(6):48–50.
19. Vincent JL, et al. Anemia and blood transfusion in critically ill patients. JAMA. 2002;288(12):1499–507.
20. Beliën J, Forcé H. Supply chain management of blood products: a literature review. Eur J Oper Res. 2012;217(1):1–16.
21. Suresh S. Mechanical response of human red blood cells in health and disease: some structure-property-function relationships. J Mater Res. 2006;21(8):1871–7.
22. Weiss HJ. Platelet physiology and abnormalities of platelet function. N Engl J Med. 1975;293(11):531–41.
23. Dara SI, et al. Fresh frozen plasma transfusion in critically ill medical patients with coagulopathy. Crit Care Med. 2005;33(11):2667–71.
24. Khawar H, Kelley W, Guzman N. Fresh Frozen Plasma (FFP). Stat Pearls [Internet]. Treasure Island, FL: Stat Pearls Publishing; 2019.
25. Callum JL, Karkouti K, Lin Y. Cryoprecipitate: the current state of knowledge. Transfus Med Rev. 2009;23(3):177–88.
26. Knox Z. Writing witness history: the historiography of the Jehovah's witnesses and the watch tower bible and tract Society of Pennsylvania. J Relig Hist. 2011;35(2):157–80.
27. The Holy Bible: New International Version. Zondervan; 1984.
28. Lawson T, Ralph C. Perioperative Jehovah's witnesses: a review. Br J Anaes. 2015;115(5):676–87.
29. Remmers PA, Speer AJ. Clinical strategies in the medical care of Jehovah's witnesses. Am J Med. 2006;119(12):1013–8.
30. Bryson GL, Laupacis A, Wells GA. Does acute normovolemic hemodilution reduce perioperative allogeneic transfusion? A meta-analysis. Anesth Analg. 1998;86(1):9–15.
31. Segal JB, et al. Preoperative acute normovolemic hemodilution: a meta-analysis. Transfusion. 2004;44(5):632–44.
32. Gupta A. Preoperative screening and risk assessment in the ambulatory surgery patient. Curr Opin Anesthesiol. 2009;22(6):705–11.

33. Wu W-C, et al. Preoperative hematocrit levels and postoperative outcomes in older patients undergoing noncardiac surgery. JAMA. 2007;297(22):2481–8.
34. SABM. Anemia prevention and management program implementation guide. 2015.
35. Scharman CD, et al. Treatment of individuals who cannot receive blood products for religious or other reasons. Am J Hematol. 2017;92(12):1370–81.
36. Crookston KP. The approach to the patient who declines blood transfusion. In: Post TW, editors. UpToDate. Waltham: UpToDate Inc. https://uptodate.com. Accessed on 28 Mar 2019.
37. Eddy VA, Morris JA Jr, Cullinane DC. Hypothermia, coagulopathy, and acidosis. Surg Clin N Am. 2000;80(3):845–54.
38. Fischer DP, Zacharowski KD, Meybohm P. Savoring every drop–vampire or mosquito? Crit Care. 2014;18(3):306.
39. Koch CG, et al. Hospital-acquired anemia: prevalence, outcomes, and healthcare implications. J Hosp Med. 2013;8(9):506–12.
40. Fung YL, et al. To transfuse, or not to transfuse: that is the question. Crit Care Resusc. 2009;11(1):71.
41. Reyes G, et al. Bloodless cardiac surgery in Jehovah's witnesses: outcomes compared with a control group. Revista Española de Cardiología (English Edition). 2007;60(7):727–31.
42. Pattakos G, et al. Outcome of patients who refuse transfusion after cardiac surgery: a natural experiment with severe blood conservation. Arch Intern Med. 2012;172(15):1154–60.

Blood Substitutes and Artificial Oxygen Carriers

16

Jacob Tiegs

History

Experiments using substances to deliver oxygen to tissues have been conducted since the seventeenth century [1]. Initially, hemoglobin solutions were injected into humans with very poor results. Morbidity likely arose from free hemoglobin particles and their negative effects on the GU system and kidneys in particular. A number of factors contributed to a rebirth in interest for artificial oxygen carriers including increased warfare during the twentieth century and the identification of blood-born infectious diseases. As blood transfusion became safer and methods for decreasing the risk of transfusion-related infections developed, the impetus for breakthroughs in blood substitutes may have waned. However, soon a number of companies had promising products that were in the later phases of clinical trials. Unfortunately, these trials soon ended due to concerns over ability to get regulatory approval while funding became scarce [2]. Despite this, the need for blood substitutes and artificial oxygen carriers still exists, and some products continue to be in development.

Ideal Characteristics of Oxygen Carriers

There are a number of characteristics that would be part of an ideal artificial oxygen carrier. First, it would be readily available and able to be mass produced. It would also need to be safe. This would mean minimal side effects, ability to interact in a non-detrimental way with nitric oxide, and it would be sterile. The substance would ideally be portable and easily stored while having a long or manageable shelf life. The compound would be able to be given universally to all patients and be cost effective. This list may seem unattainable and lengthy; however, there are at least two compounds currently that satisfy most of these requirements.

Current Types of Oxygen Carriers

To date, there are two main categories of oxygen carriers. Hemoglobin-based oxygen carriers, or HBOCs, are derived from bovine or human blood. First, hemoglobin is separated from the red cell structure by ultrafiltration and purification [3]. A number of processes exist to then stabilize the hemoglobin compound and prepare it for use. These include cross-linking, pyridoxylation, polymerization, or pegylation. These processes prevent the dissociation of hemoglobin's four chain configuration into its basic alpha and beta dimers [4]. Unfortunately, preparations have been limited by side effects. Early formulations caused nephrotoxicity thought to be secondary to red cell stromal fragments in the hemoglobin. Encapsulated HBOCs were attempted but ran into problems with the host-defense systems (reticuloendothelial system) [5]. Most recently, hypoxic vasodilation that normally occurs in hypoxic states has been theorized to be limited by HBOCs due to the deactivation of this reflex by the scavenging of nitric oxide by the HBOC compounds causing problematic vasoconstriction. Because of these drawbacks, there is not currently a HBOC that can replace our current standard of care using transfusion of red blood cells. However, each trial has given us new information to use and incorporate into the next possible product. There is still hope and products in the pipeline (Table 16.1).

Perfluorocarbons, or PFCs, are chemically inert compounds where fluorine replaces hydrogen atoms. They are water insoluble which requires a lipid emulsification system to be utilized. PFCs act as solvents for oxygen, and unlike the coupling reaction and relationship of hemoglobin, the amount of oxygen that can be dissolved follows a linear

J. Tiegs (✉)
NYU Langone Medical Center, Department of Anesthesiology, New York, NY, USA
e-mail: Jacob.tiegs@nyulangone.org

© Springer Nature Switzerland AG 2021
C. S. Scher et al. (eds.), *Essentials of Blood Product Management in Anesthesia Practice*,
https://doi.org/10.1007/978-3-030-59295-0_16

Table 16.1 Examples of HBOCs

Name	Description
Diaspirin crosslinked Hb, HemAssist	Chemically cross-linked Hb alpha chains
Hemopure (HBOC-201)	Polymerized bovine Hb
PolyHeme	Pyridoxylated polymerized Hb from outdated human blood
MP4OX	PEG-conjugated human Hb
rHb1.1, rHb2.0	Recombinant human Hb (from E.coli)
Sanguinate	PEG carboxylated bovine Hb

progression and obeys Henry's law and is related directly with PO_2 [6]. However, PFCs have fairly short half-lives (2–4 h), and the necessary emulsion limits how quickly the compound can be administered. A number of side effects were seen in early clinical trials with PFCs, but the etiology of the problems is unclear. A flu-like illness was often seen after administration as well as thrombocytopenia, which likely occurred due to the emulsion's effects on the platelets' surface [6]. Initially, one PFC was approved for use in ischemic tissue situations (Fluosol); however, it was later pulled due to lack of profitability [7]. Currently, there does not appear to be many trials in the pipeline for PFCs.

Most Beneficial Uses for Oxygen Carriers Currently

There are currently no oxygen carriers approved by the FDA for use in the USA Right now, the only way to obtain one is through the US Food and Drug Administration (FDA) Expanded Access Protocol. Specifically, the use of the unlicensed OC HBOC-201 (Hemopure) may be approved for life-threatening anemia in patient populations where allogenic red blood cell transfusion is not an option [8]. Of note, Hemopure is currently used in Russia and South Africa [9].

Side Effects and Challenges of Oxygen Carriers

The issues surrounding HBOCs have led to most trials being discontinued and preventing further studies from taking off. Some of the side effects were mentioned earlier, but a number of different complications have been noted. One of the main and most seen effects of HBOCs given at therapeutic doses is systemic hypertension. Blood pressure seems to increase without a corresponding increase in cardiac output. This hypertension also occurs in the pulmonary vasculature. So, in sum, increases are seen in SVR, PVR, MAP, and pulmonary vasculature resistance index, and a concomitant decrease is seen in cardiac output. The most commonly accepted explanation is that HBOCs interact with and inactivate endothelial nitric oxide, which is a potent vasodilator [10].

Other effects on the cardiovascular system have also been seen. One of these effects is an increase in myocardial infarctions in patients receiving HBOCs. Obviously, this is a worrisome complication, but the etiology is not fully known. It does not appear that the scavenging of nitric oxide compounds is fully responsible for this phenomenon. In fact, in studies where HBOCs were infused directly into coronary arteries, no increase in vasoconstriction was seen [11].

Changes in coagulation and concern for coagulopathy also have surrounded the use of HBOCs. Possible etiologies for coagulopathy include dilutional coagulopathy and hypocalcemia, oxidation of the compound to methemoglobin and subsequently inhibiting platelet aggregation, large molecular weight molecules (HBOCs) complexing with von Willebrand factor and speeding its elimination, and lastly nitric oxide scavenging as mentioned previously [12].

One side effect that has been seen in early trials that may be improved or eliminated in more recent trials is nephrotoxicity. Stroma-free hemoglobin caused excess glomerular filtration of hemoglobin dimers, resulting in acute tubular necrosis and oliguria.

In addition to the above concerns, HBOCs and free hemoglobin have been implicated in a multitude of other possible complications: interference of macrophage function, GI distress, iron deposition, neurotoxicity, antigenicity, and alterations on a number of clinical laboratory tests (bilirubin, creatinine kinase, magnesium, uric acid, and gamma-glutamyltransferase) [13].

The main side effects of PFCs were flu-like reactions and symptoms likely secondary to the cytokine-mediated effects of the compounds and platelet sequestration in the spleen and liver [3].

Outlook and Future Development

Unfortunately, no current oxygen carriers are FDA approved for use in the United States. Although there are some companies pursuing this avenue for oxygen delivery, the side effects and inability for previous products to be proven safe and effective have limited further development. Further HBOC compounds will have to address the nitric oxide scavenging and molecular size and properties of the hemoglobin molecule. It is not currently known whether PFCs will have a role in the future blood substitute world.

One exciting and new possibility is the culturing of red blood cells in vitro. Advances using hematopoietic progenitor cells from sources such as umbilical cord blood and stem cells make this theoretically possible. As does the prospect of creating immortalized adult erythroid progenitor cells. However, many roadblocks exist from the science and regulatory aspects before this can become a real possibility [14].

HBOCs continue to offer a glimpse of what can be possible. A future without the need for blood donation and blood transfusion may be a lofty but still worthwhile goal. With continued research and study, it is possible to come up with a compound that can at the very least reduce our reliance on blood product administration, which will benefit the healthcare system and most importantly the patient tremendously.

References

1. Winslow RM. Blood substitutes, a moving target. Nature Med. 1995;1:1212–5.
2. Fridey JL, Silvergleid AJ, Tirnauer JS editors. Oxygen carriers as alternatives to red blood cell transfusion. Up to Date. Accessed 30 Aug 2019. https://www-uptodate-com.proxy1.lib.tju.edu/contents/oxygen-carriers-as-alternatives-to-red-blood-cell-transfusion?search=oxygen%20carriers%20as%20alternatives%20to%20red%20blood%20cell%20transfusion&source=search_result&selectedTitle=1~150&usage_type=default&display_rank=1
3. Scott MG, Kucik DF, Goodnough LT, Monk TG. Blood substitutes: evolution and future applications. Clin Chem. 1997;43(9):1724.
4. Natanson C, Kern SJ, Lurie P, Banks SM, Wolfe SM. Cell-free hemoglobin-based blood substitutes and risk of myocardial infarction and death: a meta-analysis. JAMA. 2008;299(19):2304. Epub 28 Apr 2008.
5. Szebeni J, Wassef NM, Hartman KR, Rudolph AS, Alving CR. Complement activation in vitro by the red cell substitute, liposome-encapsulated hemoglobin: mechanism of activation and inhibition by soluble complement receptor type 1. Transfusion. 1997;37(2):150.
6. Scott MG, Kicik DF, Goodnough LT, Monk TG. Blood substitutes: evolution and future applications. Clin Chem. 1997;43(9):1724–31.
7. Kerins DM. Role of the perfluorocarbon Fluosol-DA in coronary angioplasty. Am J Med Sci. 1994;307(3):218.
8. Donahue LL, Shapira I, Shander A, Kolitz J, Allen S, Greenburg G. Management of acute anemia in a Jehovah's witness patient with acute lymphoblastic leukemia with polymerized bovine hemoglobin-based oxygen carrier: a case report and review of literature. Transfusion. 2010;50(7):1561.
9. Mer M, Hodgson E, Wallis L, Jacobson B, Levien L, Snyman J, Sussman MJ, James M, van Gelder A, Allgaier R, Jahr JS. Hemoglobin glutamer-250 (bovine) in South Africa: consensus usage guidelines from clinician experts who have treated patients. Transfusion. 2016;56(10):2631. Epub 2016 Sep 23
10. Kim HW. Acellular hemoglobin-based oxygen carrier mediated blood pressure elevation and vasoconstriction: a review of proposed mechanisms and contributing factors. In: Kim H, Greenburg A, editors. Hemoglobin-based oxygen carriers as red cell substitutes and oxygen therapeutics. Berlin/Heidelberg: Springer; 2013.
11. Estep TN. HBOCs and cardiac integrity. In: Kim H, Greenburg A, editors. Hemoglobin-based oxygen carriers as red cell substitutes and oxygen therapeutics. Berlin/ Heidelberg: Springer; 2013.
12. Jahr JS, Chung M, Anvarhosseini A, Kim HW. Effects of hemoglobin-based oxygen carriers on blood coagulation. In: Kim H, Greenburg A, editors. Hemoglobin-based oxygen carriers as red cell substitutes and oxygen therapeutics. Berlin/Heidelberg: Springer; 2013.
13. Smani Y. HBOC interferences with routine clinical laboratory tests. In: Kim H, Greenburg A, editors. Hemoglobin-based oxygen carriers as red cell substitutes and oxygen therapeutics. Berlin/Heidelberg: Springer; 2013.
14. Trakarnsanga K, Griffiths R, Wilson M, Blair A, Satchwell T, Meinders M, Cogan N, Kupzig S, Kurita R, Nakamura Y, Toye A, Anstee D, Frayne J. An immortalized adult human erythroid line facilitates sustainable and scalable generation of functional red cells. Nature Communications. 2017;8:14750.

Preoperative Therapy for Anemia

17

Larry R. Hutson Jr, John C. Cargile, and Garrett D. Starling

Definition and Prevalence of Anemia

Any discussion of anemia and its correction must include a definition of anemia. For the past several decades, the World Health Organization (WHO) has been the authority on global anemia prevalence, tracking rates of anemia, and the most common causes [7]. The WHO defines anemia as a hemoglobin concentration of less than 13.0 g per 100 milliliters (g/dL) in adult men (15 years of age and up), less than 12 g/dL in children ages 12–14 and in nonpregnant women, less than 11.5 g/dL in children ages 5–11, and less than 11 g/dL in children under the age of 5 years and in pregnant women. The WHO further breaks down anemia into mild, moderate, and severe categories (Table 17.1) [8]. Adult women with a hemoglobin of 12 g/dL are twice as likely as men with 13 g/dL of hemoglobin to require a transfusion – usually due to lower circulating blood volumes – therefore their threshold for anemia is set 1 g/dL less than for men [9].

In the latest examination of anemia from the WHO, the overall rate globally was 32.9% [8]. In some high-risk populations, the incidence of anemia may range from 50% to 80%, with 10–20% suffering from moderate to severe anemia [10]. Those at highest risk are individuals low in socioeconomic status, low in body weight, and experiencing post-partum [11]. Of course, the rate and cause of anemia vary across countries. Iron deficiency is most common, followed by parasitic infections (malaria, schistosomiasis, and hookworms), then hemoglobinopathies, and obstetric/gynecologic disorders [7].

In the United States, studies demonstrate that anemia is present in 5.1–6.1% of the overall population, with a rate of moderate to severe anemia of 1.4–1.7% (excluding pregnant women). Women have double the risk of men and five times the risk for moderate to severe anemia until the age of 80 years old, at which point the rate is equal for both genders [12]. It is present at triple the frequency in African Americans [13]. While the data demonstrates that the general US population would be classified as having a mild public health issue, anemia is a more serious health concern for certain subgroups due to their higher rates of both anemia and moderate to severe anemia: African Americans, Hispanics, adults over 60 years of age, nonpregnant women of reproductive age, and pregnant women [8, 12]. Iron deficiency anemia is present at a lower rate in the United States compared with other countries around the globe, which means that a higher proportion of anemia causes can be attributed to hemoglobinopathies, chronic kidney disease, and gastrointestinal bleeding than in lower income countries, though iron deficiency anemia is still the most common kind in the United States [7, 12].

Table 17.1 Definitions of anemia

Population	Severe	Moderate	Mild
Children 6–59 months	<7	7–9.9	10–10.9
Children 5–11 years	<8	8–10.9	11–11.4
Children 12–14 years	<8	8–10.9	11–11.9
Non-pregnant women	<8	8–10.9	11–11.9
Pregnant women	<7	7–9.9	10–10.9
Men (over 15 years)	<8	8–10.9	11–12.9

Anemia definitions (in g/dL) by population group [10]

As people increase in age, so too does the prevalence of anemia. Those aged 75–84 years old had a rate of 13%; this almost doubles to 23% above the age of 85 [14]. Overall, this gave a prevalence of 17%, with roughly a third categorized as moderate to severe [15].

For patients who are hospitalized, anemia rates are increased over the general population, with 19% of admitted patients presenting with anemia. More interesting, 60% of those who were not anemic on admission developed hospital-acquired anemia [16]. A European study of cancer patients demonstrated that those undergoing radiation therapy had an

L. R. Hutson Jr · J. C. Cargile · G. D. Starling (✉)
Texas A&M University – College of Medicine, Bryan, TX, USA

Baylor Scott and White Medical Center – Temple, Department of Anesthesiology, Temple, TX, USA
e-mail: Larry.hutson@bswhealth.org; John.cargile@bswhealth.org; Garrett.starling@bswhealth.org

© Springer Nature Switzerland AG 2021
C. S. Scher et al. (eds.), *Essentials of Blood Product Management in Anesthesia Practice*,
https://doi.org/10.1007/978-3-030-59295-0_17

anemia frequency of 29%, while cis-platinum-based chemotherapy patients had almost triple that at 75% [17]. Congestive heart failure patients are commonly anemic (17%), resulting in worsening survival [18, 19].

In noncardiac surgical patients overall, the rate of anemia was around 34%, with three quarters of that due to iron deficiency [20]. Certain surgical cohorts face their own anemia challenges. Orthopedic patients present with anemia at a frequency of 10.5%, with the major causes split between nutritional deficiencies and anemia of chronic inflammation [21]. In patients scheduled for colorectal cancer resection, more than half present with iron deficiency, though not necessarily with anemia [22].

In terms of trends, the global prevalence decreased from 40.2% when studied by the WHO in 1990, to the most recent rate of 32.9% in the report published in 2011 [8]. Most of these gains occurred in women and children, who have been the focus of an action plan related to improving nutrition in these populations from the World Health Assembly, as well as other programs – such as the UN Secretary-General's Every Woman Every Child initiative and the Global Strategy for Women's and Children's Health – that have emphasized a reduction in risk factors that adversely affect these two groups [23]. In the United States, the prevalence of both anemia and moderate to severe anemia almost doubled between 2003 and 2012 for reasons that are unclear [12].

Risks of Anemia for Surgery

Preoperative anemia imposes increased risks of morbidity and mortality for surgical patients [24]. While the severity and cause of anemia are important determinants of risk level, any degree of anemia may negatively impact a patient's risk for perioperative transfusion, intraoperative and postoperative complications, as well as length of hospital stay and readmission rate [25–27]. In fact, a preoperative hemoglobin lower than 10 g/dL is associated with an almost threefold increase in postoperative pulmonary complications [28, 29]. While morbidity increases with hemoglobin levels less than 10 g/dL, mortality rate increases with hemoglobin levels below 7, and as levels approach 2.5 g/dL without transfusion, mortality is 50% [30, 31]. The current recommendation for transfusion threshold is 7 g/dL in stable, hospitalized adult patients; however considerations such as preexisting cardiac disease, ongoing or expected blood loss, and type of surgery may necessitate a higher threshold [32, 33].

Preoperative anemia increases the chance of red blood cell transfusion, and while red blood cell transfusion is the most effective and immediate way of increasing oxygen-carrying capacity in an anemic patient at risk for ischemia, it is itself associated with increased risks. Transmission of infection, transfusion-related acute lung injury (TRALI), transfusion-associated circulatory overload (TACO), and numerous types of hypersensitivity and hemolytic reactions remain real concerns [34].

The world blood supply is safer than ever before, but certain bacteria, viruses, prions, and parasites still may be transmitted through transfusion of blood products. All donors are risk screened with a questionnaire and all blood units tested for various infectious agents. There is a comprehensive list of pathogens and the tests used to screen them on the US Food and Drug Agency website. Despite this, there remains a risk that an emerging pathogen – not yet identified as a threat to be tested – may still be transmitted during transfusion.

As discussed in a separate chapter on complications of blood transfusions, transfusion-related acute lung injury (TRALI) is a potential life-threatening reaction to donor unit(s) that manifest as dyspnea, hypotension, and fever. The vast majority of cases are due to multiparous, female donors that have anti-HLA and/or anti-granulocyte antibodies. While red blood cell units have little plasma in them, there may still be enough donor antigens present to react with recipient antibodies. Transfusion-related circulatory overload (TACO) results from overwhelming of the body's ability to compensate for the increased volume introduced into the circulatory system with transfusion. Susceptibility to this varies with patient preexistent comorbidities, acute/chronic illness, and the volume transfused. Treatment consists of diuretics and judicious use of transfusion products.

Hypersensitivity reactions are due to allergens, primarily IgA and haptoglobin. The rate is approximately 0.15% for red blood cell transfusion [35]. TRALI and TACO are included in this category, but many others occur. Treatment is generally symptomatic. Mild reactions may be treated with an antihistamine and steroids. More serious reactions may require stabilization with epinephrine. When a suspected allergic reaction to transfusion occurs, serum tryptase levels may be drawn as a confirmatory test. Tryptase is released in large amounts from granulocytes during an allergic reaction and remains high for as long as 2 h after release.

Hemolytic reactions – the destruction of red blood cells during or after a transfusion – may be immune or nonimmune mediated. Immune-mediated hemolytic reactions are caused by transfusing red blood cells that are incompatible with the patient's anti-A, anti-B, or other red blood cell antibodies. Sometimes, this reaction may be delayed. If a patient develops antibodies after a transfusion, the level of those antibodies may diminish over time. These antibodies may, in fact, be undetectable by standard crossmatching techniques. Then, after a subsequent transfusion, through an anamnestic response, the antibody levels may increase leading to a delayed hemolytic transfusion reaction.

There have been studies that demonstrate increased rates of hepatic cancer and non-Hodgkins lymphoma among patients who received blood transfusions, though the concept is controversial, as there has never been a study showing direct causation. Theories exist that suggest a link to transmission of viruses that cause cancer, or due to a direct transfer of cancer cells through blood transfusion. Immunomodulation has also been suggested as a mechanism. There are previously described models where this happens, such as how the hepatitis C virus can be a precipitating factor for hepatocellular carcinoma and how the E virus is associated with lymphoma. However, for every theory there are multiple confounding variables that limit the logic of the argument [36]. The risk of cancer may just be related to the corresponding risk of transmission of any offending virus. This is discussed in greater detail in another chapter.

Preoperative Anemia Clinic

There was a time when patients would donate their own blood weeks in advance of surgery for their own use. This autologous blood prevented issues with type compatibility, but is nevertheless on the decline as institutions find that costs are high, about half of the units go to waste instead of being used, and patients often arrived for surgery anemic as a result of the donation, thus increasing their risk [37]. Correcting anemia through (non-autologous) blood transfusion introduces the previously described risks, resulting in detrimental effects to the surgical outcome as well as longer lengths of hospital stay postoperatively, higher rates of ICU admission, and increased rates of in-hospital mortality [38–42].

Instead, hospitals are increasingly turning to the use of a preoperative anemia clinic (PAC) in the hope of resolving anemia in patients who can afford to delay surgery. One of the earliest and best described PACs was created at Duke University's School of Medicine. Flowing out of the early success of enhanced recovery after surgery protocols (ERAS), in July 2013, they created a multidisciplinary team – the Perioperative Enhancement Team (POET) – in order to optimize patients bound for surgery, which included a PAC [43]. The PAC portion started as a pilot program for orthopedic patients intended to receive lower extremity total joint replacement due to the high relative rate of blood transfusion for this service line despite aggressive use of antifibrinolytics, cell salvage when appropriate, and restrictive transfusion practices [44].

There is currently no level-one evidence for improved outcomes in the treatment of preoperative anemia [45]. On the other hand, it stands to reason that the use of PACs for those at higher risk for perioperative transfusion might lead to a reduction in those same transfusions, thus allowing for better overall management of the blood supply, especially since blood collection historically has fallen behind the demand [46].

One institution reported a significant reduction of 36% in length of stay (from 5.5 days down to 3.5 days) for those patients with anemia who were referred to their PAC, as well as a 48% reduction in the number of units of blood transfused in that same cohort [47]. Another institution reported a similar decrease in length of stay for patients who were treated in their PAC, as well as a 37% reduction in the number of patients who were transfused perioperatively. Their initial calculated cost savings were estimated to be $200,000 per year for their hospital, a figure which did not include length of stay savings [48]. The financial modeling of the Duke POET program projected net savings of $2.5 million over 5 years, a result of decreased transfusion rates, improved outcomes, and revenue generation from preoperative infusions, all despite the costs associated with the PAC and increased preoperative testing [44].

Being the most prevalent type, most of the published data around preoperative correction of anemia relates specifically to iron deficiency anemia. A study of colorectal surgery patients demonstrated an average reduction in length of stay by a little over 2 days, as well as cost savings (both direct and indirect) of between $300 and $500, depending on the formulation of intravenous iron used [49]. Another institution reduced their transfusion rate in lower extremity total joint patients from 26.4% to 11.5%, also using intravenous iron in patients with IDA [50]. A longer ranging, far larger study – the PREVENTT trial, designed to provide sufficient study power to demonstrate the effects of intravenous iron on preoperative anemia before major open abdominal operations – is currently underway in the United Kingdom, with enrollment in the study to be completed in late 2019 [51].

Each institution must decide on their own path to creating a PAC, as patient populations, hospital resources, and surgical cases done at that institution can vary greatly. To start a program with the entire surgical population would be daunting. Furthermore, not all anemic patients need a delay and aggressive therapy for their condition, given that minor procedures are unlikely to result in transfusion [46]. Guinn et al. in a publication regarding the creation of POET described beginning with a pilot population, one that had significant rates of anemia amenable to treatment, high perioperative transfusion rates, consistent follow-up, and a surgical team willing to delay an operation in favor of preoperative hemoglobin optimization. Some institutions utilize point-of-care testing equipment to allow for initial screening for anemia in the surgical clinics before the patient leaves from the consultation at which surgery was arranged [44].

Laboratory testing should occur as early as possible to allow for progression down an algorithm, to determine whether anemia is present, and if so the nature of the anemia. Additionally, it takes time for anemia to correct without the use of transfusion. For example, in IDA, maximal effect of intravenous iron takes 2–3 weeks [52, 53]. Ultimately, success of a PAC relies upon institutional support and multidisciplinary cooperation between surgery, internal medicine, and anesthesiology.

Iron Deficiency Anemia

Iron deficiency anemia (IDA) is the most common type of anemia worldwide, comprising roughly one half of the anemia burden [7]. IDA affects 1–2% of the US population and up to 12% of women aged 20–49 [54]. The primary causes of IDA are inadequate intake of iron, malabsorption, and blood loss [55]. According to a systematic analysis for the Global Burden of Disease Study 2016, IDA was the fourth highest cause of years lived with disability, demonstrating the significant health consequences of this type of anemia [56]. In the perioperative setting, specific undesired outcomes include increased risk of perioperative transfusion, morbidity (acute myocardial infarction, ischemic stroke, or kidney injury), and hospital and 30-day mortality [57]. For these reasons, preoperative IDA should be diagnosed and properly treated before major surgery [58, 59].

Though diagnosis and treatment of anemia is often performed by primary care physicians, perioperative physicians must be familiar with the basics of evaluating IDA. An appropriate history should be obtained from patients in whom anemia is suspected, detailing symptoms that occur in IDA. These include fatigue, dyspnea on exertion, dysphagia, glossitis, cheilosis, pallor, koilonychias, palpitations, headaches, tinnitus, taste disturbances, and pica; physical findings include a fatigued appearance, conjunctival or lingual pallor, angular stomatitis, glossitis, tachycardia, systolic flow murmur, pulmonary edema, hepatomegaly, splenomegaly, koilonychias, skin pallor, and poor capillary refill [55, 60, 61]. Chronic blood loss is commonly associated with menstruation and gastrointestinal diseases; therefore a gastrointestinal and gynecologic history should also be obtained. Additionally, patients should be questioned regarding symptoms or a history of inflammatory bowel disease, celiac disease, and gastrointestinal surgery [62]. A thorough medication review is important, as certain medications – such as antacids, H2 blockers, proton pump inhibitors, nonsteroidal anti-inflammatory drugs, and zinc and manganese supplements – can contribute to iron malabsorption and thus IDA [55].

For patients with suspected anemia based on the history and physical exam, diagnosis confirmation should be performed with laboratory analysis. A complete blood count (CBC) both confirms and details the degree of the anemia. It also includes several red blood cell indices that can be helpful in attempting to diagnose IDA. The mean corpuscular volume (MCV) is 97.6% sensitive for IDA with values typically below 80 μm when it is present [63, 64]. A CBC also provides the red cell distribution width, which is normally increased in IDA [55]. A reticulocyte count may also be helpful and is typically low in IDA [65]. Other relevant laboratory tests and their relative values in IDA are as follows: serum iron levels (low), total iron binding capacity (high), transferrin saturation (low), and ferritin levels (low) [63, 66]. A transferrin receptor assay can be particularly helpful in distinguishing between IDA (high) and anemia of chronic disease (normal) [55].

The gold standard for diagnosis of IDA is iron staining of a bone marrow aspirate. In IDA, staining would be absent or decreased. This study is more expensive than the earlier described studies and is generally unnecessary [55]. Many patients will require minimal studies to establish the diagnosis. For instance, an otherwise healthy woman of reproductive age will likely only need a history, physical examination, CBC, and ferritin to diagnose IDA [66]. In the perioperative patient, a CBC and transferrin saturation are often the most reliable way to determine the need for iron [48].

Despite the multiple complications of IDA, routine screening by primary care physicians is not recommended in the asymptomatic and nonpregnant patient population [59]. Additionally, not all surgical patients require a preoperative hemoglobin, hematocrit, or complete blood count. Clinical judgement must therefore be used in determining which patients require preoperative testing for IDA. It is recommended that all hospitals performing major surgical procedures have a clear perioperative anemia management pathway, including guidelines for preoperative testing. Patients undergoing procedures in which the transfusion risk is ≥10% and/or estimated blood loss ≥500 mL should undergo an appropriate laboratory workup for anemia [48].

Once IDA has been diagnosed, it is important to determine and treat the underlying cause. The severity of anemia, urgency of surgical intervention, and likelihood of perioperative bleeding will determine whether this determination and treatment should take place preoperatively or postoperatively. The anemia itself should be treated with oral iron or intravenous iron, with or without recombinant human erythropoietin (rHuEPO), depending on the patient's hemoglobin levels, anemia tolerance, and comorbidities [58]. Red blood cell transfusion (RBCT) should only be used for severe or hemodynamically significant anemia.

The National Institute for Health and Care Excellence in the UK (NICE) recommends offering oral iron either before or after surgery to patients with IDA [67]. Gastrointestinal adverse effects may reduce tolerance and compliance with oral iron supplementation [68]. Low once daily or alternate day dosing may reduce these adverse effects and maximize fractional absorption [69]. A retrospective study of primary hip replacement showed that, compared to no iron supplementation, liposome-encapsulated ferric pyrophosphate iron (30 mg/day for 3–4 weeks preoperatively) was well tolerated, reduced transfusion requirements, reduced length of hospital stay, and resulted in higher hemoglobin levels 30 days after discharge [70]. Preoperative oral iron supplementation requires several weeks to result in modest increases in hemoglobin; therefore, it may be appropriate for treatment of mild-to-moderate IDA when a sufficient time interval prior to surgery exists [48]. The current evidence is unsupportive for postoperative oral iron supplementation. A review of seven RCTs involving orthopedic and cardiac surgical patients demonstrated that high-dose oral iron therapy was not superior to placebo in correcting postoperative anemia or reducing transfusions and was associated with significant gastrointestinal side effects [71].

Intravenous iron is the preferred route in cases of severe intolerance to oral iron, moderate-to-severe anemia, ongoing blood loss, inflammatory status, use of erythropoiesis-stimulating agents, short time to surgery, or nonelective procedures [48]. It is also superior to oral iron for the management of postoperative anemia [71]. Intravenous iron has been shown to reduce transfusion requirements in the gynecological setting, as well as in colorectal cancer patients [72, 73]. It is also effective in those with both solid organ and hematological malignancies [74]. In one prospective study of anemic colorectal cancer patients, a 2-week preoperative course of intravenous iron resulted in a mean hemoglobin increase of 1.1 g/dL [75]. Most professional association guidelines recommend intravenous iron for the management of perioperative IDA.

Anemia of Chronic Disease

Anemia of chronic disease (ACD) is a hypoproliferative anemia resulting from systemic illness and/or inflammation and is the second most common type of anemia, behind IDA [76]. It is associated with a variety of conditions including infections, malignancies, autoimmune disease, chronic renal failure, and chronic heart failure. It is the result of impaired production of erythropoietin (EPO), blunted marrow erythroid response to EPO, iron-restricted erythropoiesis, and a decreased number of EPO-responsive cells [77]. Low serum iron levels are common in ACD and are a result of increased hepcidin, a hormone produced primarily by hepatocytes that causes decreased gastrointestinal absorption of iron and decreased release of the iron stores within the body [78].

Diagnosis of ACD can be challenging. In addition to a detailed history and physical exam, the anemia itself is usually confirmed with a complete blood count. ACD typically produces a normochromic and normocytic anemia, though it may become microcytic further in the disease progression. Common laboratory findings used to assess for inflammation include neutrophilia, monocytosis, thrombocytosis, elevated C-reactive protein, and elevated erythrocyte sedimentation rate. Distinguishing between ACD and IDA is difficult because the two conditions often co-exist, and a functional iron deficiency is a common occurrence in ACD. Transferrin levels can be helpful in distinguishing the two as they are increased in IDA but normal or decreased in ACD [77]. Other tests, such as new red blood cell indices and hepcidin assays, are being investigated as possible ways to aid in the diagnosis of ACD, but further study is needed [79].

The treatment of ACD should involve targeting the underlying cause of inflammation or malignancy as well as improving the anemia. The most common pharmacologic regimen for the treatment of the anemia involves combining erythropoiesis-stimulating agents (ESA) and iron supplementation. Recombinant human EPO (rHuEPO) is a commonly used ESA and has been shown in numerous studies on patients with ACD of various causes to significantly improve hemoglobin levels beyond the levels in patients treated with iron alone. There is concern that EPO administration may increase the risk of cardiovascular events and thrombosis, as well as possibly modulate tumor growth via cytoprotective effects [77].

The FDA has published warnings regarding the usage of EPO related to both adverse effects and has specifically recommended that it not be used in certain tumor types [80]. Functional iron deficiency is part of the pathogenesis of ACD, and IDA frequently occurs with ACD. For these reasons, iron supplementation is often effective at improving the anemia in patients with ACD [79]. Intravenous iron has been shown to be more effective than oral iron in certain types of ACD, such as the anemia caused by chronic renal disease [81]. Additionally, there is evidence that intravenous iron enhances the effects of ESAs in patients with other types of ACD [82]. The American Society of Hematology guidelines recommend monitoring of iron status in patients receiving ESAs but currently do not make a recommendation for supplementing ESAs with intravenous iron to improve the response [83].

Sickle Cell Disease

Sickle cell disease (SCD) is the most common inherited red blood cell disorder and is the result of a chromosomal mutation leading to an abnormal β-globin subunit of the hemoglobin molecule [84]. In response to various triggers, including hypoxemia, hypothermia, and dehydration, the abnormal hemoglobin molecule forms insoluble globin polymers, a process known as sickling, which causes red blood cells (RBC) to stick to each other and to vascular endothelium. This results in vascular endothelial damage and inflammation, causing further sickling. Ultimately, this process ends in sludging of blood and vascular occlusion [85]. It is this vascular occlusion that forms the basis for the myriad sequelae of SCD.

Sickled RBCs have a lifespan of 10–20 days, as opposed to the 120-day lifespan of normal RBCs. They are fragile and easily hemolyzed, which can lead to megaloblastic or aplastic anemia. Chronic hemolysis results in patients adapting to new "normal" hemoglobin levels, often as low as 6–9 g/dL [86]. Other sequelae of SCD, such as splenic sequestration of RBCs, can lead to profound anemia, requiring transfusion in any presenting setting, perioperative or otherwise [87]. The chronic, long-term anemia often associated with SCD can cause chronic high cardiac output and result in cardiovascular complications, including left ventricular hypertrophy, cardiomegaly, and hypertrophic cardiomyopathy [86].

The perioperative treatment of the chronic anemia in SCD relies primarily on RBCT. There are three basic perioperative transfusion strategies: exchange transfusions, "top-up" transfusions, and non-routine transfusions. Exchange transfusions attempt to decrease the abnormal hemoglobin to <30% of the total hemoglobin. Alternatively, the goal of "top-up" transfusions is to simply increase the hemoglobin to a pre-set goal. A non-routine transfusion strategy declines to have automatic transfusion requirements for patients with SCD [88]. Numerous studies have been done comparing the various transfusion strategies with widely mixed results [89]. A recent Cochrane Database review of the existing randomized controlled trials found insufficient evidence to make determinations regarding the relative effectiveness of each strategy. That review did find very low-quality evidence that preoperative blood transfusion may prevent the development of acute chest syndrome [90]. Despite the lack of evidence, the current consensus in the United States is "to bring the hemoglobin level to 10 g/dL prior to undergoing a surgical procedure involving general anesthesia" [91]. A recent international review recommends that "transfusion decisions need to be selective and individualized based on the type of SCD, the baseline hemoglobin, the baseline cardiopulmonary reserve, and the risk of the surgical procedure" [89].

Pernicious Anemia

Pernicious anemia is caused by deficiencies of vitamin B_{12} and/or folate. These are necessary for the transfer of a methyl group from N5-methyltetrahydrofolate to cobalamin. The resulting megaloblastic red blood cells can be identified on a CBC by an increased mean corpuscular volume and on peripheral smear by the hypersegmented neutrophils. When vitamin B^{12} levels are low, there are increased levels of methylmalonic coenzyme A (MMA) and homocysteine. In fact, levels of MMA and homocysteine begin to increase even before vitamin B^{12} levels fall below the lower limit of normal on a lab assay. Therefore, they are considered early indicators of vitamin B^{12} deficiency [92]. Antibodies to intrinsic factor have a very high specificity (near 100%), but sensitivity is only 70% [93]. Folate deficiency may cause increased homocysteine levels. Treatment of pernicious anemia is vitamin B^{12} and folate supplementation. These should be taken together because it can be difficult to differentiate between the two deficiencies, and a deficiency in one can lead to a deficiency in the other.

Other Causes of Anemia

Some causes of anemia require further evaluation before elective surgery. A thorough preoperative history and physical exam many times will reveal concern for gastrointestinal bleeding, renal dysfunction or a variety of symptoms that could reveal a hematological or oncological diagnosis. Not only would many of these diseases require treatments that could be complicated by an elective surgery, but these comorbidities could increase the morbidity and/or mortality of operative and recovery phases of an elective procedure.

References

1. Mantilla CB, Wass CT, Goodrich KA, et al. Risk for perioperative myocardial infarction and mortality in patients undergoing hip and knee arthroplasty: the role of anemia. Transfusion. 2011;51:82–91.
2. Wu WC, Schifftner TL, Henderson WG, et al. Preoperative hematocrit levels and postoperative outcomes in older patients undergoing noncardiac surgery. JAMA. 2007;297:2481–8.
3. Carabini LM, Zeeni C, Moreland NC, et al. Development and validation of a generalizable model for predicting major transfusion during spine fusion surgery. J Neurosurg Anesthesiol. 2014;26:205–15.
4. Rosencher N, Kerkkamp HE, Macheras G, et al. Orthopedic surgery transfusion Hemoglobin European overview (OSTHEO) study: blood management in elective knee and hip arthroplasty in Europe. Transfusion. 2003;43:459–69.
5. Beattie WS, Karkouti K, Wijeysundear DN, et al. Risk associated with preoperative anemia in noncardiac surgery: a single-center cohort study. Anesthesiology. 2009;110:574–81.
6. Hebert PC, Wells G, Blajchman MA, et al. A multicenter, randomized, controlled clinical trial of transfusion requirements in critical care. Transfusion requirements in critical care investigators, Canadian critical care trials group. N Engl J Med. 1999;340:409–17.
7. Kassebaum NJ, Jasrasaria R, Naghavi M, et al. A systematic analysis of global anemia burden from 1990 to 2010. Blood. 2014;123:615–24.
8. WHO. The global prevalence of anemia in 2011. Geneva: World Health Organization; 2015.
9. WHO. Haemoglobin concentrations for the diagnosis of anaemia and assessment of severity. WHO/NMH/NHD/MNM/11.1. http://www.who.int/vmnis/indicators/haemoglobin.pdf.
10. WHO. The prevalence of anemia in women: a tabulation of available information. 2nd ed. Geneva: WHO; 1992.
11. Bentley ME, Griffiths PL. The burden of anemia among women in India. Eur J Clin Nutr. 2003;57(1):52–60.

12. Le CCH. The prevalence and anemia and moderate-severe anemia in the US population (NHANES 2003-2012). PLoS One. 2016;11(11):e0166635. https://doi.org/10.1371/journal.pone.0166635.
13. Zakai NA, McClure LA, Prineas R, et al. Correlates of anemia in American blacks and whites: the REGARDS renal ancillary study. Am J Epidemiol. 2009;160(3):355–64.
14. Gurlanik JM, Einsenstaedt RS, Ferrucci L, et al. Prevalence of anemia in person 65 years and older in the United States: evidence for a high rate of unexplained anemia. Blood. 2004;104:2263–8.
15. Gaskell H, Derry S, Andrews Moor R, Mcquay HJ. Prevalence of anemia in older persons: systematic review. BMC Geriatr. 2008;8:1.
16. Koch CG, Li L, Sun Z, et al. From bad to worse: anemia on admission and hospital acquired anemia. J Patient Saf. 2014; https://doi.org/10.1097/PTS.0000000000000142.
17. Ludwig H, Van Belle S, Barrett-Lee P, et al. The European Cancer Anaemia Survey (ECAS): a large, multinational, prospective survey defining the prevalence, incidence, and treatment of anemia in cancer patients. Eur J Cancer. 2004;40:2293–306.
18. Horwich TB, Fonarow GC, Hamilton MA, MacLellan WR, Borenstein J. Anemia is associated with worse symptoms, greater impairment in functional capacity and a significant increase in mortality in patients with advanced heart failure. J Am Coll Cardiol. 2002;39(11):1780–6.
19. Ezekowitz JA, McAlister FA, Armstrong PW. Anemia is common in heart failure and is associated with poor outcomes: insights from a cohort of 12065 patients with new onset heart failure. Circulation. 2003;107(2):223–5.
20. Garca-Erce JA, Laso-Morales MJ, Gomez-Ramrez S, et al. Analysis of the prevalence and causes of low preoperative haemoglobin levels in a large multicenter cohort of patients undergoing major noncardiac surgery. Transfus Med. 2016;26(Suppl 1):48.
21. Jans O, Jorgensen C, Kehlet H, Johansson PI. Role of preoperative anemia for risk of transfusion and postoperative morbidity in fast track hip and knee arthroplasty. Transfusion. 2014;54:717–26.
22. Diaz Espallardo C, Laso Morales MJ, Colilles Calvert C, et al. The multidisciplinary approach is useful for optimizing preoperative hemoglobin in colorectal cancer surgery. Cir Esp. 2011;89:392–9.
23. Stevens GA, Finucane MM, De-Regil LM, et al. Global, regional, and national trends in hemoglobin concentration and prevalence of total and severe anemia in children and pregnant and nonpregnant women for 1995-2011: a systematic analysis of population-representative data. Lancet Glob Health. 2013;1(1):e16–25.
24. Glance LG, Dick AW, Mukamel DB, Fleming FJ, Zollo RA, Wissler R, Salloum R, Meredith UW, Osler TM. Association between intraoperative blood transfusion and mortality and morbidity in patients undergoing noncardiac surgery. Anesthesiology. 2011;114(2):283–92.
25. Abdullah HR, Sim YE, Hao Y, Lin GY, Liew GHC, Lamoureux EL, Tan MH. Association between preoperative anaemia with length of hospital stay among patients undergoing primary total knee arthroplasty in Singapore: a single-Centre retrospective study. BMJ Open. 2017;7(6):e016403.
26. Viola J, Gomez MM, Restrepo C, Maltenfort MG, Parvizi J. Preoperative anemia increases postoperative complications and mortality following total joint arthroplasty. J Arthroplast. 2015;30(5):846–8.
27. Hare GM, Freedman J, David MC. Review article: risks of anemia and related management strategies: can perioperative blood management improve patient safety? Can J Anaesth. 2013;60(2):168–75.
28. Canet J, Gallart L, Gomar C, et al. Prediction of postoperative pulmonary complications in a population-based surgical cohort. Anesthesiology. 2010;113(6):1338–50.
29. Lee JY, Lee SH, Jung MJ, Lee JG. Perioperative risk factors for in-hospital mortality after emergency gastrointestinal surgery. Medicine (Baltimore). 2016;95(35):e4530.
30. Shander A, Javidroozi M, Aregbeyen O, et al. An update on mortality and morbidity in patients with very low postoperative hemoglobin levels who decline blood transfusion. Transfusion. 2014;54(10 Pt 2):2688–95.
31. Weiskopf RB, Silverman TA. Balancing potential risks and benefits of hemoglobin-based oxygen carriers. Transfusion. 2013;53:2327–33.
32. Shander A, Lobel GP, Javidroozi M. Anesthesia for Patients with Anemia. Anesthesiol Clin. 2016;34(4):711–30.
33. Carson JL, Guyatt G, Heddle NM, et al. Clinical practice guidelines from the AABB: red blood cell transfusion thresholds and storage. JAMA. 2016;316(19):2025–35.
34. Connell NT. Transfusion medicine. Prim Care. 2016;43(4):651–9.
35. Delaney M, Wendel S, Bercovitz RS, et al. Biomedical excellence for safer transfusion (BEST) collaborative. Transfusion reactions: prevention, diagnosis, and treatment. Lancet. 2016;388(10061):2825–36.
36. Yang TO, Cairns BJ, Reeves GK, Green J, Beral V. Million women study collaborators. Cancer risk among 21st century blood transfusion recipients. Ann Oncol. 2017;28(2):393–9.
37. Kumar A. Perioperative management of anemia: limits of blood transfusion and alternatives to it. Cleve Clin J Med. 2009;76(4):S112–8.
38. Hogan M, Klein AA, Richards T. The impact of anaemia and intravenous iron replacement therapy on outcomes in cardiac surgery. Eur J Cardiothorac Surg. 2015;4:218–26.
39. Carson JL, Duff A, Poses RM, et al. Effect of anaemia and cardiovascular disease on surgical mortality and morbidity. Lancet. 1996;348:1055–60.
40. Ferraris VA, Davenport DL, Saha SP, et al. Surgical outcomes and transfusion of minimal amounts of blood in the operating room. Arch Surg. 2012;147:49–55.
41. Musallam KM, Tamil HM, Richards T, et al. Preoperative anemia and postoperative outcomes in noncardiac surgery: a retrospective cohort study. Lancet. 2011;378:1396–407.
42. Baron DM, Hochrieser H, Posch M, et al. European Surgical Outcomes Trials (EuSOS) group for trials groups of European Society of Intensive Care; European Society of Anesthesiology. Preoperative anemia is associated with poor clinical outcome in noncardiac surgery patients. Br J Anaesth. 2014;113(3):416–23.
43. Aronson S, Westover J, Guinn N, et al. A perioperative medicine model for population health: an integrated approach for an evolving clinical science. Anesth Analg. 2018;126(2):682–90.
44. Guinn NR, Guercio JR, Hopkins TJ, et al. How do we develop and implement a preoperative anemia clinic designed to improve perioperative outcomes and reduce cost? Transfusion. 2016;56:297–303.
45. Munoz M, Acheson AG, Auerbach M, et al. International consensus statement on the perioperative management of anaemia and iron deficiency. Anaesthesia. 2017;72:233–47.
46. US Department of Health and Human Services. The 2007 National Blood Collection and Utilization Survey. Available at: http://www.aabb.org/Documents/Programs_and _Services/Data_Center/07nbcusrpt.pdf.
47. Lentendre P, Coberly E, Dettenwanger K, et al. Patient Blood Management: Implementation of a Preoperative anemia clinic for elective orthopedic surgical patients. Poster presentation ASH Annual meeting 2018.
48. Perepu US, Leitch AM, Reddy S. Implementation of a preoperative anemia management clinic in a tertiary academic medical center. Blood. 2016;128:1004.
49. Calvet X, Gene E, Ruiz MA, et al. Cost-minimization analysis favors intravenous ferric carboxymaltose over ferric sucrose or oral iron as preoperative treatment in patients with colon cancer and iron deficiency anemia. Technol Health Care. 2016;24:111–20.
50. Munoz M, Gomez-Ramirez S, Martin-Montanez E, et al. Cost of post-operative intravenous iron therapy in total lower limb arthro-

plasty: a retrospective matched cohort study. Blood Transfus. 2014;12:40–9.
51. Richards T, Clevenger B, Kiedan J, et al. PREVENTT: preoperative intravenous iron to treat anemia in major surgery: study protocol for a randomized control trial. Trials. 2015;16:254.
52. Theussinger OM, Leyvraz PF, Schanz U, et al. Treatment of iron deficiency anemia in orthopedic surgery with intravenous iron: efficacy and limits: a prospective study. Anesthesiology. 2007;107:923–7.
53. Jin L, Kapadia TY, Gehr AV, et al. Feasibility of a preoperative anemia protocol in a large integrated health care system. Perm J. 2019;23:17–200.
54. Centers for Disease Control and Prevention (CDC). Iron deficiency - United States, 1999–2000. MMWR Morb Mortal Wkly Rep. 2002;51:897–9.
55. Hempel EV, Bollard ER. The evidence-based evaluation of iron deficiency anemia. Med Clin N Am. 2016;100(5):1065–75.
56. Vos T, Abajobir AA, Abate KH, et al. GBD 2016 disease and injury incidence and prevalence collaborators. Global, regional, and national incidence, prevalence, and years lived with disability for 328 diseases and injuries for 195 countries, 1990-2016: a systematic analysis for the global burden of disease study 2016. Lancet. 2017;390(10100):1211–59.
57. Fowler AJ, Ahmad T, Phull MK, et al. Meta-analysis of the association between preoperative anaemia and mortality after surgery. Br J Surg. 2015;102(11):1314–24.
58. Gomez-Ramirez S, Bisbe E, Shander A, et al. Management of perioperative iron deficiency anemia. Acta Haematol. 2019;142:21–9.
59. McCarthy M. Evidence for iron deficiency screening "inadequate" US panel concludes. BMJ. 2015;350:1841.
60. Clark SF. Iron deficiency anemia. Nutr Clin Pract. 2008;23:128–41.
61. Frewin R, Henson A, Provan D. ABC of clinical haematology. Iron deficiency anemia. BMJ. 1997;314:360–3.
62. Bermeja J, Garcia-Lopez S. A guide to diagnosis of iron deficiency and iron deficiency anemia in digestive diseases. World J Gastroenterol. 2009;15:4638–43.
63. Ioannou GN, Spector J, Scott K, et al. Prospective evaluation of a clinical guideline for the diagnosis and management of IDA. Am J Med. 2002;113:281–7.
64. Killip S, Bennett J, Chambers M. Iron deficiency anemia. Am Fam Physician. 2007;75:671–8.
65. Means. Iron deficiency anemia. Hematology. 2013;18:305–6.
66. Punnonen K, Irjala K, Rajamaki A. Serum transferrin receptor and its ratio to serum ferritin in the diagnosis of iron deficiency. Blood. 1997;89:1052–7.
67. NICE. guideline (NG24). Blood transfusion. National Institute for Health and Care Excellence. Available from: https://www.nice.org.uk/guidance/ng24/chapter/Recommendations#alternatives-to-blood-transfusion-for-patients-having-surgery-2.
68. Tolkien Z, Stecher L, Mander AP, et al. Ferrous sulfate supplementation causes significant gastrointestinal side-effects in adults: a systematic review and meta-analysis. PLoS One. 2015;10(2):e0117383.
69. Stoffel NU, Cercamondi CI, Brittenham G, et al. Iron absorption from oral iron supplements given on consecutive versus alternate days and as single morning doses versus twice-daily split dosing in iron-depleted women: two open-label, randomised controlled trials. Lancet Haematol. 2017;4(11):e524–33.
70. Scardino M, Di Matteo B, Martorelli F, et al. Improved patient blood management and cost saving in hip replacement surgery through the implementation of pre-operative Sucrosomial® iron supplementation: a quality improvement assessment study. Int Orthop. 2019;43(1):39–46.
71. Munoz M, Acheson AG, Bisbe E, et al. An international consensus statement on the management of postoperative anaemia after major surgical procedures. Anaesthesia. 2018;73(11):1418–31.
72. Van Wyck DB, Mangione A, Morrison J, et al. Large-dose intravenous ferric carboxymaltose injection for iron deficiency anaemia in heavy uterine bleeding: a randomised, controlled trial. Transfusion. 2009;49:2719–28.
73. Munoz M, Garcia-Erce JA, Diez-Lobo AI, et al. Usefulness of the administration of intravenous iron sucrose for the correction of preoperative anemia in major surgery patients. Med Clin (Barc). 2009;132:303–6.
74. Henry DH, Dahl NV, Auerbach M, et al. Intravenous ferric gluconate significantly improves response to epoetin alfa versus oral iron or no iron in anemic patients with cancer receiving chemotherapy. Oncologist. 2007;12:231–42.
75. Simpson JAD, Ng SL, Brookes MJ, Acheson AG. Single dose preoperative administration of intravenous iron corrects iron deficiency anaemia in colorectal cancer. J Blood Disord Transfus. 2010;1(1):101.
76. Dallman PR, Yip R, Johnson C. Prevalence and causes of anemia in the United States, 1976 to 1980. Am J Clin Nutr. 1984;39:437–45.
77. Cullis JO. Diagnosis and management of anaemia of chronic disease: current status. Br J Haematol. 2011;154:289–300.
78. Brasse-Lagnel C, Karim Z, Letteron P, et al. Intestinal DMTI cotransporter is downregulated by hepcidin via proteasome-internalization and degradation. Gastroenterology. 2011;140:1261–71.
79. Goodnough LT, Nemeth E, Ganz T. Detection, evaluation, and management of iron-restricted erythropoesis. Blood. 2010;116:4754–61.
80. Jenkins JK. Erythropoiesis-stimulating agents (ESA). 2007. Available at: http://www.fda.gov/NewsEvents/Testimony/ucm110908.htm.
81. Locatelli F, Covic A, Eckardt KU, et al. Anaemia management in patients with chronic kidney disease: a position statement by the anaemia working Group of European Renal Best Practice (ERBP). Nephrol Dial Transplant. 2009;24:348–54.
82. Littlewood TJ, Alikhan R. The use of intravenous iron in patients with cancer-related anaemia. Br J Haematol. 2008;141:751–6.
83. Rizzo JD, Brouwers M, Hurley P, et al. American Society of Clinical Oncology/American Society of Hematology clinical practice guideline update on the use of epoetin and darbepoetin in adult patients with cancer. Blood. 2010;116:4045–59.
84. Yawn BP, Buchanan GR, Afenyi-Annan AN, et al. Management of sickle cell disease: summary of the 2014 evidence-based report by expert panel members. JAMA. 2014;312:1033–48.
85. Farrell K, Dent L, Nguyen ML, et al. The relationship of oxygen transport and cardiac index for the prevention of sickle cell crises. J Natl Med Assoc. 2010;102:1000–7.
86. Khurmi N, Gorlin A, Misra L. Perioperative considerations for patients with sickle cell disease: a narrative review. Can J Anesth. 2017;64:860–9.
87. Manci EA, Culberson DE, Yang YM, et al. Causes of death in sickle cell disease: an autopsy study. Br J Haematol. 2003;123:359–65.
88. Howard J, Malfroy M, Llewelyn C, et al. The transfusion alternatives preoperatively in sickle cell disease (TAPS) study: a randomised, controlled, multicentre clinical trial. Lancet. 2013;381:930–8.
89. Adjepong KO, Otegbeye F, Adjepong YA. Perioperative management of sickle cell disease. Mediterr J Hematol Infect Dis. 2018;10(1):e2018032.
90. Estocourt LJ, Fortin PM, Trivella M, Hopewell S. Preoperative blood transfusions for sickle cell disease. Cochrane Database Syst Rev. 2016;4(4):CD003149.
91. Yawn BP, Buchanan GR. Elective surgery in children with sickle cell disease without preoperative blood transfusion. J Pediatr Surg. 1993;28(5):681–5.
92. Klee GG. Cobalamin and folate evaluation: measurement of methylmalonic acid and homocysteine vs vitamin B(12) and folate. Clin Chem. 2000;46(8 Pt 2):1277–83.
93. Hvas AM, Nexo E. Diagnosis and treatment of vitamin B12 deficiency--an update. Haematologica. 2006 Nov;91(11):1506–12.

Blood Deployment in Natural Disasters and a Military in Conflict

18

Christa L. Riley and Joseph Dean

Abbreviations

AABB	American Association of Blood Banks
ARC	American Red Cross
ASBP	Armed Services Blood Program
BSCM	Blood supply chain management
CDC	Centers for Disease Control
DCR	Damage control resuscitation
DCS	Damage control surgery
DHSS	Department of Health and Human Services
EDP	Emergency donor pool
FDA	Food and Drug Administration
FFP	Fresh frozen plasma
FLYP	French lyophilized plasma (freeze dried plasma)
FWB	Fresh whole blood
ICU	Intensive care unit
JTS CPG	Joint Trauma System Clinical Practice Guideline
MCE	Mass casualty event
MERT	Medical Emergency Response Team
MTF	Military treatment facility
RBC	Red blood cells
SAMU	Service d'Aide Medicale Urgente
SWB	Stored whole blood
TTD	Transfusion-transmitted disease
WBB	Walking blood bank

C. L. Riley (✉)
VCU Health, Department of Anesthesiology, Richmond, VA, USA

J. Dean
Virginia Commonwealth University School of Medicine, Richmond, VA, USA
e-mail: deanjc@vcu.edu

Disaster Preparedness, Resuscitation, and the Anesthesiologist

Since the terrorist attacks on the World Trade Center on 9/11, the public health sector has increased focus on disaster preparedness and response and recovery efforts. National and state organizations have focused primarily on prehospital and emergency room preparedness to handle a surge of patients that would occur during a mass casualty event (MCE). Hospitals must also be prepared to manage an influx of patients and provide advanced care to those requiring urgent intervention such as damage control surgery or intensive care. By definition, a mass casualty event is an incident(s) that results in large numbers of severely injured patients which overwhelm available resources, limiting the ability to deliver optimal care [1]. The term mass casualty event often refers to terrorist attacks or mass shootings. Natural disasters such as hurricanes or earthquakes and military conflict also can result in a mass casualty event that additionally includes interruption of infrastructure increasing the difficulty of response.

Anesthesiologists are perioperative and resuscitative physicians and are uniquely skilled to provide advanced care in a variety of settings. Anesthesiologists also are skilled in directing teams of personnel in the management of surgical patients and therefore can be utilized to lead teams both in preparing for emergencies and in responding to those events [2]. For these reasons, anesthesiologists are an obvious but often untapped resource for prehospital and hospital emergency or disaster preparedness. Although anesthesiologists in the United States have not been traditionally included as a resource in emergency preparedness planning and exercises, their skill set is valued and routinely utilized in other countries. The Royal Air Force has a long history of providing forward aeromedical evacuation and developed the Medical Emergency Response Team (MERT) in 2006 to manage the high levels of trauma casualties in Afghanistan [3]. MERT is a multidisciplinary medical team led by an anesthetist (British

© Springer Nature Switzerland AG 2021
C. S. Scher et al. (eds.), *Essentials of Blood Product Management in Anesthesia Practice*,
https://doi.org/10.1007/978-3-030-59295-0_18

anesthesiologist) or emergency medicine physician. The team provides hospital level care to patients in flight after recovering them from the battlefield in potentially non-permissive areas (hostile) while transporting them to more definitive care [3]. Anesthesiologists in France have been part of the disaster response system for several decades and are a key element of the French emergency medical service, Service d'Aide Medicale Urgente (SAMU) [2]. Anesthesiologists are often the lead clinician sent with SAMU to mass casualty events to provide an advanced level of care near the site of the disaster and coordinate with fire and police. In this arrangement, prehospital disaster management and hospital disaster management are integrated [2].

Hemorrhage is the leading cause of potentially preventable mortality in MCEs [1, 4–7]. Mortality from terrorist attacks increased 500% between 2000 and 2014. Although mortality from terrorist attacks has dropped to 27% since 2014, terrorism is more widespread affecting more countries than in 2014 [8]. While only modest numbers of patients following MCEs require transfusion, a small number of patients with critical injuries and polytrauma will require immediate transfusion as part of damage control resuscitation (DCR). Damage control resuscitation is a resuscitation strategy to prevent death from catastrophic hemorrhage and refers to US military guidelines developed for combat casualties with massive bleeding in Iraq and Afghanistan. DCR is well described throughout trauma and resuscitation literature and involves multiple interventions including earlier and balanced transfusion of plasma and platelets with initial red blood cell (RBC) transfusion. DCR evolved from the earlier concept of damage control surgery (DCS), the practice of rapid and abbreviated surgery after initial resuscitation to control bleeding and reduce infection risk by removing debris, fecal matter, and body fluids followed by continued resuscitation and physiological stabilization in the intensive care unit (ICU) [9]. Definitive surgical repair could be deferred for several days as DCS emphasized avoiding the lethal triad of acidosis, hypothermia, and coagulopathy. However, direct treatment of coagulopathy was not a primary focus of DCS because coagulopathy had been presumed to be due primarily to initial resuscitation, hemodilution, and hypothermia rather than the physiological response to trauma and hemorrhage [10]. Damage control resuscitation is a comprehensive approach (incorporating DCS) from the point of trauma to definitive treatment to minimize blood loss, maintain tissue oxygenation, and correct the lethal triad at the earliest moment after the occurrence of trauma [9, 10]. Intravascular treatment of bleeding and coagulopathy are integral to damage control resuscitation, and more recent DCR research has shown that prehospital initiation of resuscitation, including transfusion of packed RBCs, thawed plasma, and platelets, decreases morbidity and mortality in trauma patients at risk of shock [11–15] (Fig. 18.1).

The surge in demand for blood products during a mass casualty event and the earlier and higher number of blood products required for DCR demand that transfusion emergency preparedness be integrated into the medical emergency preparedness planning process [16, 17]. Effective and timely deployment of blood products during natural and man-made disasters and in military conflict requires the integration of research from multiple specialties including industrial engineering and operations research, emergency

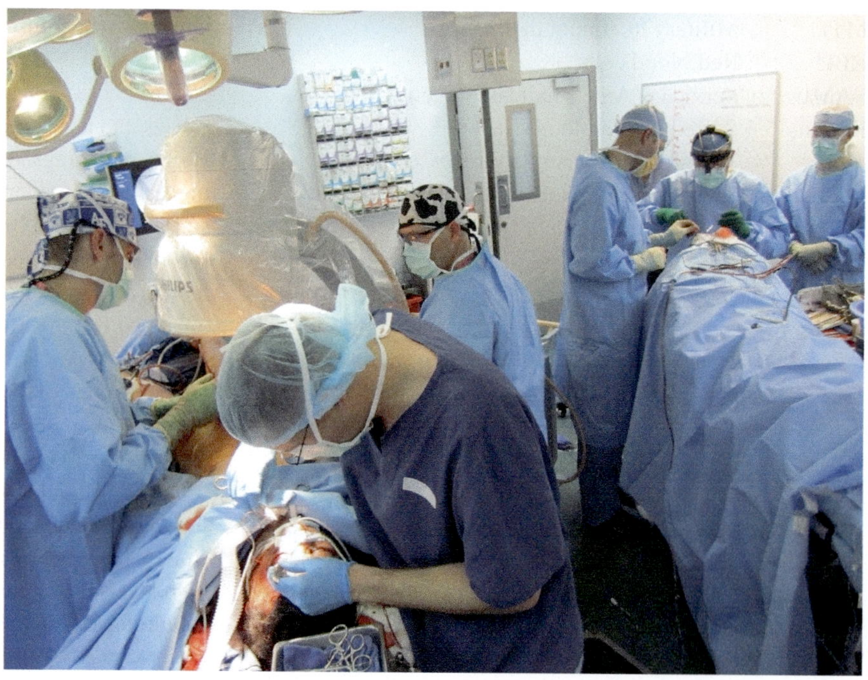

Fig. 18.1 Mass casualty event at Bagram air base 2011 – single operating room used for two simultaneous surgeries after a mass casualty event (Photograph from author's private collection)

preparedness, blood banking, transfusion medicine, as well as emergency and trauma medicine. As anesthesiologists assume larger roles in hospital and community emergency preparedness, a basic understanding of blood transfusion emergency preparedness across the continuum of care is valuable.

The US Blood Supply System and Current Challenges to Sustainability and Resiliency

Organization

The US blood supply system is comprised of many organizations with different structures and philosophies and all function to meet the nation's blood needs for component therapy and plasma. This chapter focuses on the collection of whole blood for processing into component therapy (RBCs, plasma, platelets, cryoprecipitate) used in transfusion because these components are the primary therapies required in MCEs. Although plasma collected by plasmapheresis can be used for transfusion, this collection process is separate, and the plasma collected is generally used as raw material to manufacture plasma derivatives such as fibrinogen, Factor IX, anti-thrombin III, etc. The blood collection system in the USA is heterogeneous because it developed on the free market without consideration of patient referral patterns [18]. Blood collection is performed by a network of federally regulated nonprofit organizations and supplied by donors that are all financially uncompensated volunteers. Nearly half of all blood is collected by the American Red Cross (ARC) collection centers. The remainder of blood collection in areas not represented by the ARC is performed by independent nonprofit community blood centers and hospital blood banks. Most geographical areas are served by only one blood collection organization. Although blood is collected from volunteers by nonprofit collections centers, blood and its fractionated products are commodities with processing and distribution costs as well as a fluctuating "market price" depending on supply and demand. Areas with high supply and low demand can export their oversupply to areas with high demand and lower supply through blood resource sharing. "Spot" markets exist for urgent purchases where prices are based on current market supply and immediate delivery. Blood collection centers compete on blood component price for contracts to supply hospitals and other health-care organizations [18].

Regulation

Blood centers are licensed and regulated by the US Food and Drug Agency (FDA). Other Federal organizations involved in maintaining the health and safety of the blood supply include the Department of Health and Human Services (DHHS), the Public Health Service (PHS), and the Centers for Disease Control (CDC) providing direction, oversight, and surveillance. The American Association of Blood Banks (AABB) is a nonprofit association that performs inspections and accreditation of blood banks and blood centers; establishes standards for blood collection, processing, and storage; and participates in the National Blood Exchange Program, facilitating movement of blood products from surplus areas to shortage areas.

Challenges in the US Blood Supply System

Over the last decade, the demand for blood products has decreased significantly. Between 2009 and 2016, the number of units of blood collected and distributed by the American Red Cross decreased by >25% [19]. This decline is largely due to several advances in clinical medical practice and hospital cost-containment efforts. Less invasive surgeries, pharmacological alternatives to transfusion, non-myeloablative treatment of malignancies, and comprehensive patient blood management strategies have reduced the demand for blood [20]. Patient blood management has been motivated by the need to improve blood safety and patient outcomes, preserve the blood inventory, and constrain escalating hospital costs [21]. Blood management strategies promote appropriate use of blood components with the goal of minimizing their use and promote transfusion alternatives.

Despite the decreased demand for blood products, the number of blood centers collecting, processing, and distributing blood has remained nearly the same. Costs for these blood centers have remained constant or increased. New testing for specific diseases and broader pathogen-reduction technologies add production and testing costs to the blood centers that are difficult to pass on to hospitals [22]. For example, the emergence of the Zika virus in Puerto Rico required development and implementation of additional testing at additional cost to blood centers. Additionally, blood products from non-affected areas had to be transported to Puerto Rico to maintain a safe blood supply prior to development of Zika testing. Other blood center cost increases include more selective donor criteria, expensive information systems for data analysis, and leukocyte reduction of RBCs. All of this has made blood transfusion safer but also more expensive. Hospital consolidation has shifted negotiating power away from blood centers and kept blood component prices low. Private and government insurers do not treat blood as a distinct reimbursable product or service in hospitalized patients resulting in no direct linkage between hospital reimbursement and the true cost of providing blood components. Approximately 80% of all transfusions occur in hospitals.

The blood center response to these challenges has been predictable but concerning for the ability of the US blood supply system to remain resilient especially in the face of a prolonged disaster. Many blood centers have removed excess capacity by reducing collections to a minimum, reducing staff, limiting availability of specialty blood products, and reducing or eliminating uncompensated services like surveillance and education [23]. In response to the changing economic landscape of blood centers, the Department of Health and Human Services (DHHS) contracted the RAND Corporation to study the sustainability of the blood supply in the United States. The RAND (Research ANd Development) Corporation is an American nonprofit global policy think tank created in 1948 by Douglas Aircraft Company to offer research and analysis to the US Armed Forces. Their report *Toward a Sustainable Blood Supply in the United States: An Analysis of the Current System and Alternatives for the Future* [22] concluded that the current blood supply system is robust, operating efficiently most of the time, but that continued market contraction will likely result in more widespread shortages in the future. Recommendations for improving the resiliency of the US blood supply include both market solutions and government intervention. Their conclusions include the following:

1. Separate payments for blood products may mitigate pressures on the blood system.
2. Assess emerging technologies for maximum benefit and incentivize the adoption of these technologies.
3. Develop a vision of appropriate levels of surge capacity.
4. Distinguish between the costs of maintaining a surge capacity and the normal costs of doing business and finance the surge capacity.
5. Build relationships across blood brokerages (ARC, Armed Services Blood Program) to address short-term and local shortages.
6. Implement emergency use authorizations by DHHS for replacement supplies in the event of a shortage.

Review of the literature also suggests that international blood product sharing agreements could support longer-term blood supply challenges such as infectious disease emergencies like Zika virus outbreak [24].

Other ongoing challenges to the blood supply include donor dependence, perishability of blood products, and costly transit. The size of the donor pool is dwindling due to increased donor exclusions and the aging population. Minorities are also underrepresented in the donor pool due to higher donor deferral rates, mistrust of the medical community, and lack of awareness of the blood donation process and the need for rare blood [25]. The shelf life of blood products is short, and therefore there is great potential for waste which further burdens the cost of producing the product. Blood products require careful temperature control, and therefore shipping blood products is costly with added weight of insulation and ice.

Armed Services Blood Program

Organization and Regulation

The US military maintains its own blood supply under the Armed Services Blood Program (ASBP). The ASBP represents all three branches of military, and its components collect, process, store, transport, and transfuse blood to service members and their families worldwide. Like civilian blood centers, the ASBP is governed by the FDA guidelines for maintaining safety and quality of blood products. The ASBP also follows the standards, procedures, recommendations, and guidelines of the AABB. Any service member receiving blood or blood products in a combat area will receive blood through the ASBP. Although the ASBP does work with the ARC and other blood centers during civilian emergencies, the two blood supplies are usually distinct. The ASBP sends all blood collected at military blood donation centers (on military bases and civilian locations) to two Armed Services Whole Blood Processing Laboratories (ASWBPLs). Blood reaches combat theater either by pre-positioning frozen blood at Blood Product Depots or by sending blood and blood components to Expeditionary Blood Transshipment Systems which move the blood products to Blood Supply Units in theater. From there, blood is moved in theater to forward deployed surgical units, theater hospitals, US Navy ships, and Allied/Coalition hospitals. Forward surgical units and theater hospitals provide blood and blood products to first responders at the individual unit level [26].

Challenges in the Joint Service Blood Supply Chain

The military blood supply chain faces different challenges especially in some operating environments. Large-scale combat operations can potentially result in a significant demand surge for blood products while simultaneously reducing freedom of movement for US forces and limiting the capacity to transport blood products to forward operating locations. A sustained conflict successful at targeting critical military infrastructure such as command centers, runways, and fuel depots could limit the movement of blood into theater from donation centers. Blood stored in medical treatment facilities (MTFs) would become depleted interrupting care to combat casualties [27]. The Defense Advanced Research Projects Agency (DARPA) has focused on developing approaches to augment operational resiliency. Three principles of operational resiliency have been integrated in the joint service blood supply chain. Fractionation enables the scaling of elements within the supply chain to deploy downrange as needs require. For example, a small expeditionary blood collection center could be deployed until a larger capability was established or restored. Composition enables tailoring capabilities to best suit the needs downrange. Although a deploying Army brigade may not have the capability to thaw and process frozen blood, the Air Force has a small deployable capability that offers these services. The Air Force capability can be tasked to deploy with the Army. Functional substitution enables amending current capabilities with substitutes better suited for operational needs such as stocking frozen packed red blood cells that have a longer shelf life than packed red blood cells [27].

Transfusion Disaster Preparedness

Transfusion Disaster Plan

Transfusion support is critical in the health-care response to MCEs, and every hospital should include transfusion disaster preparedness in its overall emergency planning. The overall goals of transfusion disaster preparedness should be holistic and include the following aims [28]:

1. To protect the delivery of key products and services
2. To manage the incident within regulatory requirements
3. To strive for recovery of normal business as soon as possible
4. To safeguard the health, safety, and welfare of staff and donors

After September 11, 2001, the American Society of Anesthesiologists (ASA) formed the Committee on Trauma and Emergency Preparedness (COTEP). Recognizing the unique skill set anesthesiologists have, COTEP collaborated with different organizations to create a resource center for anesthesiologists to learn about emergency preparedness. COTEP developed the Emergency Preparedness Manual for Anesthesia Department Organization and Management that emphasizes the importance of care coordination within the hospital in order to successfully manage the surge of patients requiring intervention. Core concepts of any hospital emergency preparedness plan should include the following:

1. Integration – It is of private and public medical capabilities with public health systems.
2. Medical preparedness – Increase the response capabilities and surge capacities.
3. At-risk populations – Identify populations most at-risk after an event and determine their needs.
4. Continuity of operations – Maintain adequate public health and medical services.

More specific details should include process and outcome objectives with identification of surveillance methods. Chain of command and expected flow of information should be determined including methods for communicating with the public. Personnel response timing and phasing should be established including clinical and administrative leaders. Equipment needs should be identified. Anesthesiologists can provide airway and resuscitation expertise in a first responder role in the emergency department as well as liaison with staff in the operating room to facilitate appropriate operating room utilization. Figure 18.2 details a general checklist for operating room readiness in a mass casualty event.

The AABB has developed a disaster operations handbook to help blood centers, hospital blood banks, and transfusion services respond to disasters affecting the blood supply or the distribution of blood products [29]. The handbook is intended to facilitate coordination among blood centers, hospital transfusion services, national blood organizations, and government officials to determine the medical need for blood, to establish transportation of blood from one facility to another, and to communicate a common message to the national blood community and the public about the status of the blood supply in the disaster-affected area. The AABB defines a disaster as any event that:

1. Suddenly requires a much larger amount of blood than usual
2. Temporarily restricts/eliminates a blood collector's ability to collect, test, process, and distribute blood
3. Temporarily restricts/prevents local population from donating blood
4. Temporarily restricts/prevents use of available inventory of blood products requiring immediate replacement
5. Creates a sudden influx of donors requiring accelerated drawing of blood to meet an emergent need elsewhere

This definition of disaster is broad and focuses attention on any disruption however brief to the blood supply chain. The broad definition encourages early communication between all points in the blood supply chain to ensure early response to interruptions in blood product supply. Communication up and down the blood supply chain is probably the single most important component of any transfusion disaster preparedness plan and should include hospital physicians involved in emergency response. See Fig. 18.3.

Another important element in any transfusion disaster preparedness plan is a business continuity plan to prevent loss of function if routine infrastructure is disrupted (computer networks, blood processing centers), maintain services through event, and initiate disaster recovery [30]. Disaster plans should

Fig. 18.2 Operating room procedures for mass casualty – management step by step (Reprinted with permission of the American Society of Anesthesiologists, 1061 American Lane, Schaumburg, Illinois 60,173–4973)

OPERATING ROOM PROCEDURES FOR MASS CASUALTY

MANAGEMENT STEP BY STEP

Objective

To be able to manage the flow of patient care in the OR's during a mass casualty situation.

Steps (Indicate date and time for each item)

☐**Refer to facility's Operation's Manual**

Open up appropriate annex

☐**Activate call-in tree**

Assign an individual to activate. Use clerical personnel or automatic paging system, if available

☐**Assess status of operating rooms**

Determine staffing of OR's 0-2, 2-12 and 12-24 hours. Hold elective cases.

☐**Alert current OR's**

Finish current surgical procedures as soon as possible and prepare to receive trauma

☐**Assign staff**

Set up for trauma/emergency cases

☐**Anesthesia Coordinator should become OR Medical Director**

Work with OR Nursing Manager to facilitate communication and coordination of staff and facilities

☐**Report OR status to Hospital Command Center (HCC)**

Enter telephone, email address of HCC

☐**Ensure adequate supplies**

Coordinate with anesthesia techs/supply personnel to ensure adequate supplies of fluids, medications, disposables, other

☐**Contact PACU**

Accelerate transfer of patients to floors/ICU's in preparation for high volume of cases

☐**Anesthesiologist should act as liaison in Emergency Department (ED)**

Send an experienced practitioner to the ED to act as a liaison (your eyes & ears) and keep communications open to Anesthesia Coordinator

☐**Consider assembly of Stat Teams**

Combination of anesthesia, surgical, nursing, respiratory personnel to triage, as needed

☐**HAZMET/WMD event**

Review special personal protective procedures, such as DECON & isolation techniques. Consider if part of the OR or hallways should be considered "hot" or should have ventilation altered. Good resources include CHEMM/REMM websites

☐**Coordinate with blood bank**

Verify blood availability

☐**Coordinate with other patient care areas**

ICU's, OB, Peds, etc to ensure continuity of care for new and existing patients

Developed by the Committee on Trauma and Emergency Preparedness

be rehearsed [28, 29] regularly. Exercises can be simple tabletop exercises and do not require extensive simulation equipment. Low fidelity exercises can challenge current assumptions and reveal inadequate or inefficient processes [28]. Previous assumptions are based on past data and do not reflect future challenges so transfusion emergency planning should be viewed as dynamic and iterative. For example, the last decade has seen both a change in resuscitation and transfusion practice and increased lethality in many events including terrorist attacks and mass shootings [1, 31].

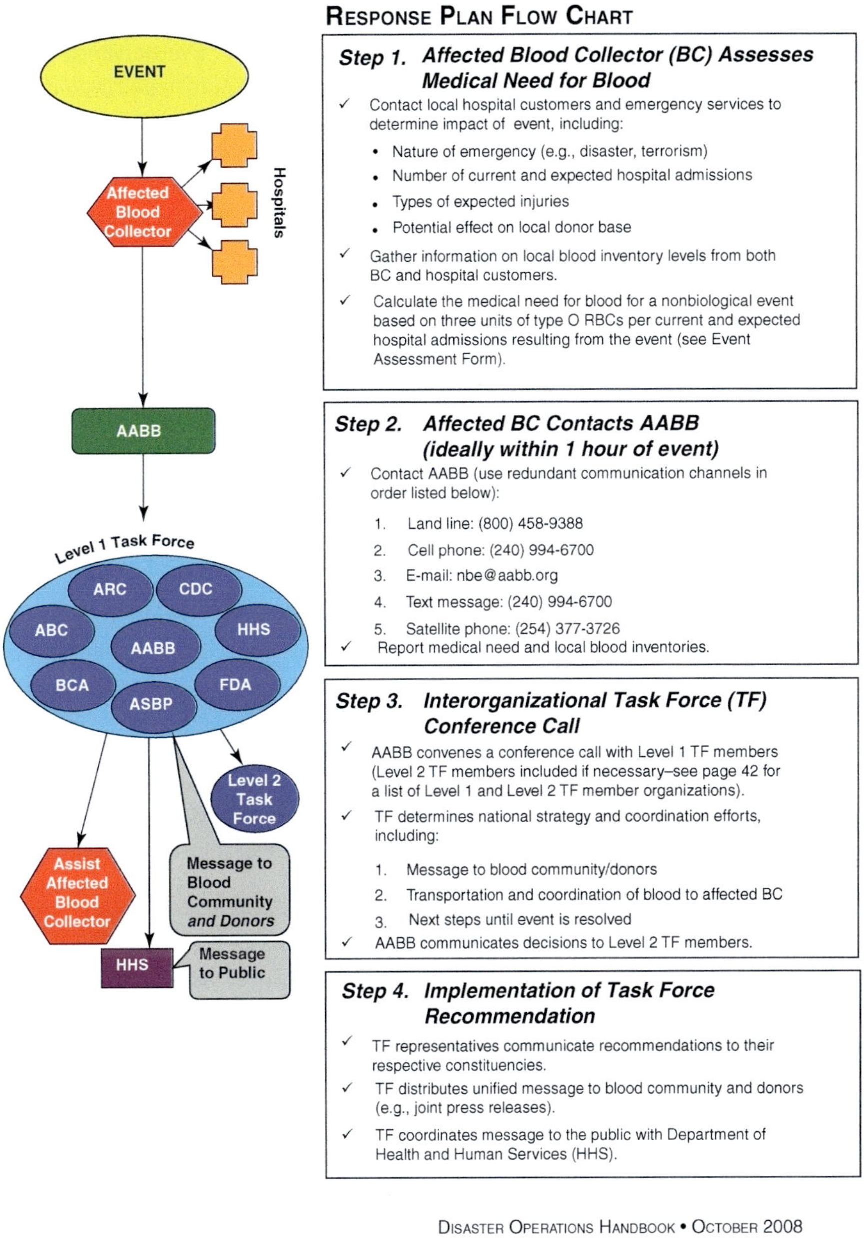

RESPONSE PLAN FLOW CHART

Step 1. Affected Blood Collector (BC) Assesses Medical Need for Blood

✓ Contact local hospital customers and emergency services to determine impact of event, including:

- Nature of emergency (e.g., disaster, terrorism)
- Number of current and expected hospital admissions
- Types of expected injuries
- Potential effect on local donor base

✓ Gather information on local blood inventory levels from both BC and hospital customers.

✓ Calculate the medical need for blood for a nonbiological event based on three units of type O RBCs per current and expected hospital admissions resulting from the event (see Event Assessment Form).

Step 2. Affected BC Contacts AABB (ideally within 1 hour of event)

✓ Contact AABB (use redundant communication channels in order listed below):

1. Land line: (800) 458-9388
2. Cell phone: (240) 994-6700
3. E-mail: nbe@aabb.org
4. Text message: (240) 994-6700
5. Satellite phone: (254) 377-3726

✓ Report medical need and local blood inventories.

Step 3. Interorganizational Task Force (TF) Conference Call

✓ AABB convenes a conference call with Level 1 TF members (Level 2 TF members included if necessary–see page 42 for a list of Level 1 and Level 2 TF member organizations).

✓ TF determines national strategy and coordination efforts, including:

1. Message to blood community/donors
2. Transportation and coordination of blood to affected BC
3. Next steps until event is resolved

✓ AABB communicates decisions to Level 2 TF members.

Step 4. Implementation of Task Force Recommendation

✓ TF representatives communicate recommendations to their respective constituencies.

✓ TF distributes unified message to blood community and donors (e.g., joint press releases).

✓ TF coordinates message to the public with Department of Health and Human Services (HHS).

DISASTER OPERATIONS HANDBOOK • OCTOBER 2008

Fig. 18.3 Response plan flow chart – this flowchart shows the bidirectional communication flow for transfusion response during a disaster. ARC American Red Cross, CDC Centers for Disease Control, HHS Health and Human Services, AABB American Association of Blood Banks, BCA Blood Centers of America, ABC America's Blood Centers, ASBP Armed Services Blood Program, FDA Food and Drug Administration

Blood Supply Chain Management (BSCM)

Glasgow et al. [1] showed that there are relationships between casualty statistics and RBC use but that reporting of blood use is often inconsistent and incomplete. Understanding how the blood supply chain operates during the surge conditions of an MCE is challenging because data collection and experimentation are low priority during an event. Furthermore, the blood supply chain is dynamic with irregular supply, stochastic demand, perishable commodities, expensive and technical processing, and costly transportation. Operational research techniques offer an approach to investigate this complex system as these techniques provide models that can interact and experiment with the numerous variables involved in the delivery of transfusion services during an MCE [32]. Operational research models can evaluate BSCM along each of the four main processes: procurement, production, inventory, and distribution [33]. Other models can evaluate for efficiency (minimize cost) and effectiveness (minimize delivery time) and effects of pandemics on blood supply regionally [34, 35]. Dynamic supply chain modeling can consider adjustments in location and capacity of facilities at different time periods representing different periods of an MCE. In-hospital MCE response modeling has shown perceived hospital ability to manage MCEs to be overly optimistic and specifically identified blood resources as a limiting factor in event response time [36] and recommend early automatic restocking during an MCE to preserve red cell supply. BSCM modeling offers additional techniques to prepare for MCEs that do not interrupt patient care and can consider the large number of variables that impact the complex blood supply chain. This area of research is promising as resuscitation and transfusion practices evolve, and MCE planning must include supply of coagulation components both in the hospital and prehospital response.

Transfusion Demand Forecasting and Planning

The greatest challenge in transfusion disaster preparedness is balancing demand and supply especially the demand for universal components such as group O RBCs in an MCE. Transfusion services must assess the event and predict the likelihood for extensive use of blood components and rapidly obtain more components if necessary. Transfusion demand planning is increasingly important for MCE planning, and the literature is evolving. Transfusion demand planning has been informed by civilian MCEs globally as well as by changing trends in trauma care. Evidence from these global MCEs suggests only a modest number of MCE victims admitted to the hospital require transfusion. The mean blood use per patient is consistently calculated at 2–3 units PRBC per patient or 6–7 units PRBC per moderately and severely injured patient. Most of that product is transfused within the first 6–12 h [1, 28, 37, 38]. Blood use reporting however is inconsistent following MCEs, and reporting standardization would improve data validation. Additionally, much of the data used to derive the above estimates was gathered before the introduction of damage control resuscitation. Blood use has changed over the last decade with the increased use of hemostatic components [1] including in the prehospital period. While this may reduce the demand on RBCs, there will likely be strain on supplies of plasma, platelets, and cryoprecipitate in the future. A recent attempt to correlate transfusion needs with injury mechanisms and severity found that while the demand for components correlated with the number of casualties, injury mechanism was less useful in prediction of blood requirements [28, 31] possibly because response and evacuation times for events were very different.

Early Blood Grouping and Transfusion Triage

Massive transfusion protocol use in treatment of hemorrhage has led to increased demand for group O Rh negative RBCs and AB plasma. Activation of massive transfusion protocols for multiple patients in an MCE can quickly lead to a demand that exceeds supply of universal components and hemostatic components if these practices are not incorporated into local demand planning. Transfusion triage of patients by age and gender can identify patients that are able to receive alternative universal blood products (O Rh positive RBCs for all men and women over 50 years old). Use of anti-D immunoglobulin can also reduce the risk from alternative universal blood products. The use of group A plasma in patients with unknown blood type instead of group AB plasma has not been shown to increase morbidity and mortality in patients with group B blood [39]. Similarly, group A and B platelets have been used in lieu of group O platelets in patients with unknown blood types. Although red cell contamination can increase the risk of alloimmunization, platelet additive solutions may reduce the risk of hemolysis [40, 41]. Transfusion triage also can identify patients in whom transfusion is not immediately required. Early blood grouping of these less acute patients can help preserve the supply of universal components [28]. It is important to mention that blood grouping during an MCE increases the risk of ABO blood group incompatible transfusion and any blood grouping plan should include a clear emergency plan for identifying, sampling, and labeling patients and their blood group. Glasgow et al. [32] described simulation modeling of deliberate RBC, and emergency group O blood transfusion restriction during an MCE increased overall patient treatment rates. Red blood cell transfusion restriction especially in combination with hemorrhage control, early use of tranexamic acid, and prehospital plasma transfusion offers another potential tool to extend blood supply in an MCE.

Management of Blood Donation and Stock

Management of blood stock and blood donation during an MCE is critical to disaster preparedness. Maintaining large stock holdings leads to wastage due to perishability, but insufficient stock may interrupt the ability to provide clinical care to patients. Immediate demand for blood should be met by existing stocks although this may require movement of stock. Shortages should be expected during any unplanned event, and blood shortage plans should be prepared. More rural areas may not be able to depend on immediate stock. In a prolonged MCE or an event with large numbers of casualties or an event in remote areas, replacement will be required. Blood collection agencies should work closely with donors to ensure continued supply of blood but also not overwhelm the collection system during a disaster. After the World Trade Center and Pentagon attacks on September 11, 2001, over 475,000 units of blood were collected of which only 258 were used [42]. Blood collection centers need to appeal to that altruism during non-disaster periods to meet collection targets that will ensure capacity when emergency events occur. Most blood services prefer to hold sufficient replacement stock rather than accept emergency donations, but a prolonged MCE may require a variety of approaches to restocking supplies including stock movement, use of an emergency/high-readiness donor pool, increase collection targets, adjustments in testing and processing, and support from other blood services [16]. Transportation should also be a consideration in blood stock planning. Interruption of usual transportation modes and routes must be considered in contingency plans for continued re-supply. Emerging technologies such as aerial drone technology offer transportation alternatives for delivery of blood products to austere or remote locations. Any transportation alternative must consider the cold chain management required for blood products to ensure safe use. Widespread use of aerial drones for a variety of tasks is accelerating the development of improved drone capability with an associated reduction in cost. This includes increased speed and increased payload capacity. This technology holds promise for blood stock resupply in a disaster [43].

Emergency Donors and Whole Blood

Development of blood component therapy focused primarily on medical indications for transfusion therapy for specific patient groups. Component therapy enables targeted treatment for patients with a single blood cell or factor deficiency as in sickle cell disease or hemophilia. Component therapy also optimizes storage of a limited resource that is dependent on volunteers for sourcing. In contrast to medical patients, hemorrhaging patients become deficient in all components of blood, and our current balanced mass transfusion practice attempts to replace all of these components.

The US military has been using whole blood transfusion in resuscitation of severe traumatic hemorrhage since World War I [44, 45]. Whole blood (WB) transfusion can provide oxygen-carrying capacity to military personnel injured in austere environments and has been used extensively during the wars in Iraq and Afghanistan by the US military and NATO Coalition Forces [44, 46–48]. The current US military Joint Trauma System Clinical Practice Guideline (JTS CPG) for whole blood transfusion provides guidelines for both cold-stored whole blood (SWB) and fresh whole blood (FWB) transfusion [49]. Whole blood in one of the anticoagulant citrate solutions is an FDA-approved product when it is collected, stored, and tested for transfusion-transmitted disease (TTD). It can be stored for 21–35 days depending on the citrate solution at 1–6°C and is referred to as SWB. The hemostatic function of SWB is adequate and stable for the first 2 weeks after collection but may require supplementation with other blood components (platelets, FFP) for adequate hemostasis after 2 weeks. FWB refers to whole blood collected on an emergency basis from a "walking blood bank" (WBB), a group of pre-screened donors that respond to an emergency call from the military treatment facility (MTF). FWB can be stored at room temperature for up to 24 h before it must be discarded. If refrigerated within 8 h of collection and submitted for complete transfusion-transmitted disease testing, FWB becomes SWB. FWB has full hemostatic function and usually does not undergo full FDA-approved TTD testing prior to transfusion. For this reason, FWB transfusion is not FDA-approved and is reserved for when tested blood products are unavailable and the need for transfusion is urgent [49]. See Fig. 18.4 for a sample emergency donor panel questionnaire for FWB donor.

The most important safety factor when transfusing WB is donor RBC compatibility with the recipient's pre-formed anti-A or anti-B antibodies. WB from group O donors contain RBCs compatible with all recipients, but the plasma in group O WB may cause hemolysis if the anti-A or anti-B antibody titers are high. This challenge can be addressed by transfusing only same-group WB (A to A, B to B, AB to AB, and O to O) or using low titer anti-A and anti-B group O WB (LTOWB) [50, 51]. LTOWB is considered the universal donor WB, and low titer SWB is the preferred resuscitation product for the prehospital treatment of patients in hemorrhagic shock [52]. If the situation permits, rapid infectious disease testing (HIV, HBV, HCV) is performed on donor specimens prior to transfusion, and retrospective samples on all donors are sent for FDA-approved TTD testing.

Clinical data suggests that the use of WB to treat hemorrhage results in outcomes at least as favorable as those with component therapy including RBCs, plasma, and platelets [14]. WB mitigates some of the challenges of adequate stored components and supplies hemostatic components with a smaller anticoagulant load [53]. Infection risk in a properly prescreened donor group appears to be low. The ASBP sponsored an epidemiological study to characterize transfusion-transmitted infection associated with emergently collected blood product transfusion [54]. The study looked at 761 recipients of emergently collected blood product transfusion and found no HIV or HBV transmission. One HCV transmission was identified. The study estimated the transfusion-transmitted infection prevalence in potential walking blood bank donors to be 8 in 1000 for HCV and 4 in 1000 for HBV. This non-zero risk requires a risk-benefit analysis prior to use of FWB by experienced clinicians capable of assessing risk of withholding transfusion. A robust "walking blood bank" (WBB) with practiced collection and testing can provide a more agile and resilient emergency transfusion response to a major incident especially in isolated regions. The Immunology and Transfusion Medicine Department of Haukeland University Hospital in Bergen, Norway, in collaboration with the Norwegian Naval Special Operation Commando establishes a WBB for military settings. The collaboration led to a mass casualty event contingency plan for the hospital that includes the use of low titer anti-A and anti-B FWB from established or pre-tested blood group O donors

[55]. The contingency plan was exercised in July 2018 when a critically ill patient received over 200 units of blood products, exhausting the supply of stored LTOWB. Collection of FWB was considered the fastest way to obtain platelet-containing blood product for immediate transfusion [53]. Norway has geography and population density that pose numerous transportation challenges especially in the long winter periods. Blood transfusion programs are therefore regional rather than national. Blood banks are run by local and regional hospitals and blood stock is maintained to meet usual hospital needs. This decentralized management of the Norwegian blood supply is similar to the independent blood center management of much of the US blood supply system. Locally developed transfusion disaster preparedness plans that include the development of a walking blood bank will increase the resiliency and responsiveness of their blood supply especially in a major incident.

Future of Transfusion Disaster Preparedness: The Golden Hour of Trauma

Military trauma care has transformed civilian trauma care in the last decade. Military practice has also impacted mass casualty event planning in the civilian sector because current trauma care is dependent on networks of first responders trained in damage control resuscitation, blood centers responsive to the need for massive transfusion for major hemorrhage, and experienced clinicians leading emergency and surgical teams in triage and resource allocation for maximum treatment capability in a major incident. The development of trauma registries has facilitated collaborative translational research that has improved overall survival in trauma patients.

Emergency donor panels (EDPs) and whole blood, tourniquets and hemostatic dressings, and early tranexamic

Fig. 18.4 Proposed field emergency donor panel questionnaire (Reproduced with permission from Wiley)

Field Emergency Donor Panel Questionnaire and Triage Tool

- **Give blood donor briefing to potential donor group**
- **Confirm blood group(s) required**
- **Exclude air crew, HGV drivers and key machinery operators**

Primary Triage (Question as a group)

Serial	Question	Yes	No	Action
1	**Do you want to give blood?**			Disqualify if NO
2	**Have you given blood before**			If yes - Consider early selection

Secondary Triage (Question individually)

Serial	Question	Yes	No	Action
3	**Are you unwell now?** New Fever/ Diarrhea / Vomiting Chronic medical condition and not well			Disqualify if YES
4	**Are you taking medication for blood pressure; stroke or heart, lung, kidney, cancer or blood conditions?**			Disqualify if YES
5	**Have you had a blood transfusion or blood products in the last year**			Disqualify if YES Accept after 1 year
6	**Are you living with HEP B,C / HIV / AIDS – OR living with anyone with these conditions**			Disqualify if YES
7	**Have you ever been refused as a donor or told not to donate blood** (a past history of treated anemia may be acceptable)			Disqualify if YES
8	**Male donors only.** Have you ever had sex with another male?			Disqualify if YES
9	**Have you ever taken illegal drugs with a needle (even steroids)**			Disqualify if YES
11	**Are you currently pregnant or breast-feeding?**			Disqualify if YES
12	**Conduct a physical examination** **Check: Temperature / Rash / Malnutrition, / Pallor / Jaundice / Cyanosis / Shortness of breath / Intoxication from alcohol or drugs / Veins**			Disqualify any potentially unwell donor or donors with very difficult veins

- **The remaining group form the Emergency Donor Panel (EDP)**
- **Use the Risk Triage Screen to risk score the potential donors**

Fig. 18.4 (continued)

Risk Triage (Question Individually)

Score	Questions	Subtotal	Notes
	Blood donation history		
1	Regular Donor		Optimum
2	Previous Donor		
3	Non Donor		
	Veins and body weight		
1	Good lateral (outer) vein		Optimum
3	Poor or difficult vein		
3	Under 60 kg		Risk of fainting
	Infection		
1	> 21 Days Well		Optimum
3	< 21 Days Well		
	Travel		
1	No travel in the countries below in the last 6 months		Optimum
2	South America		
4	Asia and Africa		
	Life style:		
1	Sex with one partner		Optimum
3	Sex with multiple partners but protected		
-	Sex with a sex worker or in exchange for money/drugs		Avoid for 12 months
	Serious medical conditions		
1	None		Optimum
3	Past or present serious medical conditions but managed and well		
3	Untreated current medical conditions but well		
	TOTAL		

- **Add up score and record: Lowest score = Lowest Risk**
- **Use Point of Care Test for TTI's – Eliminate and counsel any positives**
- **Blood type donors and document results**

acid and hemostatic components are trauma practices that have been incorporated into civilian trauma care in the last decade. Despite the changes in trauma care and improvement in overall trauma patient survival, the mortality for trauma patients undergoing laparotomy that arrive at the emergency department (ED) with hypotension has remained unchanged and is approximately 48% [56].

Efforts to reduce that mortality risk are now focused on early hemorrhage control in the prehospital period, sometimes referred to as the golden hour of trauma. Controlling hemorrhage before a patient is in shock reduces the risk of the lethal triad of acidosis, hypothermia, and coagulopathy. Transfusion of pre-thawed plasma has been incorporated into many ED transfusion stocks because it reduces plasma thaw time and patients receive balanced transfusion ratio of 1:1 plasma to RBCs earlier. In 2018, the FDA granted emergency use authorization to the Department of Defense to use pathogen-reduced leukocyte-depleted freeze-dried plasma. Freeze-dried plasma, known as French FDP or French lyophilized plasma (FLYP) because it is manufactured by the French Military Blood Institute, has been used in the European Union (EU) for almost two decades. FLYP can be stored at room temperature for 2 years without deterioration of coagulation factors, and the hemostatic properties of FLYP are comparable to those of fresh frozen plasma [57, 58]. The immediate availability of FLYP translates to earlier balanced transfusion of plasma and RBCs and may reduce the need for massive transfusion in trauma patients [59]. The storage capabilities of this product could potentially simplify the supply chain challenges for plasma. Alternative storage methods for blood components and development of synthetic blood components (platelets and oxygen carrying molecules) continue to be researched [60–62] with the goal of reducing mortality from traumatic hemorrhage.

Summary

Transfusion capability is critical to the health-care response to MCEs with the key challenge being to match supply and demand. Hospitals and the community health-care services should include transfusion planning in their emergency preparedness plans. Review of historical events can provide guidance for future planning, but each new event offers new insight for transfusion management. Transfusion emergency preparedness is necessary to provide a timely, safe, and sustainable blood supply. Transfusion emergency preparedness plans need to include modeling frameworks to understand supply chain operations. Operations research is a research area that offers opportunity to model various scenarios including blood product demand changes, transportation interruption, and supply effects of restriction transfusion. Stressors that may challenge the supply chain should be understood, and therefore after-event analysis and periodic MCE exercises should be included in any plan. Low fidelity tabletop exercises can expose areas of weakness in preparedness and should involve representative health-care workers across the continuum of care. Gaps in current capabilities of the system should be identified, and mitigation approaches should be considered. Delay of blood arrival to the operating room (OR) may be related to supply, communication between the OR and transfusion services, or deficiencies in transportation between sites, but the gap will persist without evaluation. Evolving technologies and alternative transfusion practices should be evaluated for applicability to improve resiliency. Finally, one technology or mitigation approach may not be adequate to cover gaps in supply, but combined mitigation approaches may cover those gaps. Use of tranexamic acid, pre-thawed plasma, and SWB earlier may reduce the overall number of blood component products needed and reduce the strain on supply.

Anesthesiologists are well qualified to participate and lead emergency planning in their hospitals. Their expertise in resuscitation practices and their participation in care across many departments in the hospital give them a unique understanding of the challenges in managing multiple critically ill patients at once.

References

1. Glasgow S, Davenport R, Perkins Z, Tai N, Brohi K. A comprehensive review of blood product use in civilian mass casualty events. J Trauma Acute Care Surg. 2013;75(3):468–74.
2. Mangunta VR, Patel D. The era of mass casualty events: perspectives on care paradigms from Mangunta a critical care anesthesiologist. Mo Med. 2019;116(1):49–52.
3. Thomas A. An overview of the medical emergency response team (MERT) in Afghanistan: a paramedic's perspective. J Paramed Pract. 2014;6(6):296–302.
4. Eastman AB. Wherever the dart lands: toward the ideal trauma system. J Am Coll Surg. 2010;211(2):153–68.
5. Zink KA, Sambasivan CN, Holcomb JB, Chisholm G, Schreiber MA. A high ratio of plasma and platelets to packed red blood cells in the first 6 hours of massive transfusion improves outcomes in a large multicenter study. Am J Surg. 2009;197(5):565–70.
6. John HB, Neil MR, Lisa PE, Jim CR, Charles WK, Lynne O-GK, et al. Causes of death in US special operations forces in the global war on terrorism: 2001–2004. Ann Surg. 2007;245(6):986–91.
7. Brian EJ, Robert ML, Peter SE, Joyce CK, Terrill TS, Paul UB, et al. Death on the battlefield (2001–2011): implications for the future of combat casualty care. J Trauma Acute Care Surg. 2012;73(6 Suppl 5):S431–7.
8. Institute for Economics and Peace. Global Terrorism Index 2018: measuring the impact of terrorism. Institute for Economics and Peace: Sydney; 2018.
9. Oakley P, Dawes R, Rhys Thomas GO III. The consultant in trauma resuscitation and anaesthesia. Br J Anaesth. 2014;113(2):207–10.
10. John HB, Don JD, Peter RJ, Jay JJ, Peter MF, Sumeru MW, et al. Damage control resuscitation: directly addressing the early coagulopathy of trauma. J Trauma Inj Infect Crit Care. 2007;62(2):307–10.
11. Brown JB, Guyette FX, Neal MD, Claridge JA, Daley BJ, Harbrecht BG, et al. Taking the blood bank to the field: the design and rationale of the Prehospital Air Medical Plasma (PAMPer) trial. Prehosp Emerg Care. 2015;19(3):343–50.
12. Sperry JL, Guyette FX, Brown JB, Yazer MH, Triulzi DJ, Early-Young BJ, et al. Prehospital plasma during air medical transport in trauma patients at risk for hemorrhagic shock. N Engl J Med. 2018;379(4):315–26.
13. Joshua BB, Mitchell CJ, Joseph MP, Ronald MV, Michaela WA, Timothy BR, et al. Pretrauma center red blood cell transfusion is associated with reduced mortality and coagulopathy in severely injured patients with blunt trauma. Ann Surg. 2015;261(5):997–1005.
14. Shackelford SA, Del Junco DJ, Powell-Dunford N, Mazuchowski EL, Howard JT, Kotwal RS, et al. Association of prehospital blood product transfusion during medical evacuation of combat casualties in Afghanistan with acute and 30-day survival. JAMA. 2017;318(16):1581.
15. Holcomb JB, Del Junco DJ, Fox EE, Wade CE, Cohen MJ, Schreiber MA, et al. The prospective, observational, multicenter, major trauma transfusion (PROMMTT) study: comparative effectiveness of a time-varying treatment with competing risks. JAMA Surg. 2013;148(2):127.
16. Doughty H, Glasgow S, Kristoffersen E. Mass casualty events: blood transfusion emergency preparedness across the continuum of care. Transfusion. 2016;56(S2):S208–16.
17. Rackham R, Kelly A. Emergency planning and business continuity: why blood services must plan for both. How the EBA working group (WG) is assisting blood services. ISBT Sci Ser. 2018;13(1):51–8.
18. Klein HG, Hrouda JC, Epstein JS. Crisis in the sustainability of the US blood system. N Engl J Med. 2017;377(15):1485–8.
19. Ellingson KD, Sapiano MRP, Haass KA, Savinkina AA, Baker ML, Chung K, et al. Continued decline in blood collection and transfusion in the United States–2015. Transfusion. 2017;57(S2):1588–98.
20. Hébert PC, Carson JL. Transfusion threshold of 7 g per deciliter — the new normal. N Engl J Med. 2014;371(15):1459–61.
21. Murphy WG. Of mad cows and bolted horses: the economics of blood safety. Transfusion. 2012;52(11):2278–81.
22. Mulcahy AW, Kapinos KA, Briscombe B, Uscher-Pines L, Chaturvedi R, Case SR, Hlavka JP, Miller BM. Building a more sustainable US blood system. Santa Monica: RAND Corporation, RB-9939-DHHS; 2016. As of December 12, 2019: https://www.rand.org/pubs/research_briefs/RB9939.html
23. Snyder EL, Stramer SL, Benjamin RJ. The safety of the blood supply — time to raise the bar. N Engl J Med. 2015;372(20):1882–5.
24. Ravi SJ. Strengthening health systems through international blood product sharing agreements. Health Secur. 2017;15(1):11–117.
25. Frye V, Caltabiano M, Kessler DA, Schaffler H, Reboza M, Hillyer CD, et al. Evaluating a program to increase blood donation among racial and ethnic minority communities in New York City. Transfusion. 2014;54(12):3061–7.
26. Armed Services Blood Distribution Chart Text Version. https://www.militaryblood.dod/about/distrib_chart_text.aspx. Accessed 6 Sept 2019 and again 12 Mar 2019.
27. Thomas B, Anania K, DeCicco A, Hamm JA. Toward resiliency in the joint blood supply chain. Santa Monica: RAND Corporation, RR-2482-DARPA; 2018. As of December 10, 2019: https://www.rand.org/pubs/research_reports/RR2482.html
28. Doughty H, Rackham R. Transfusion emergency preparedness for mass casualty events. ISBT Sci Ser. 2019;14(1):77–83.
29. Disaster Operations Handbook – Coordinating the nation's blood supply during disasters and Biological events, AABB, Maryland. 2008. Available from: http://www.aabb.org/programs/disasterresponse/Documents/disastophndbkv2.pdf.

30. Morgan SJ, Rackham RA, Penny S, Lawson JR, Walsh RJ, Ismay SL. Business continuity in blood services: two case studies from events with potentially catastrophic effect on the national provision of blood components. Vox Sang. 2015;108(2):151–9.
31. Ramsey G. Blood component transfusions in mass casualty events. Vox Sang. 2017;112(7):648–59.
32. Glasgow SM, Perkins ZB, Tai NRM, Brohi K, Vasilakis C. Development of a discrete event simulation model for evaluating strategies of red blood cell provision following mass casualty events. Eur J Oper Res. 2018;270(1):362–74.
33. Mansur A, Vanany I, Arvitrida NI. Modified allocation capacitated planning model in blood supply chain management. IOP Conf Ser Mater Sci Eng. 2018;337(1):012028.
34. Fahimnia B, Jabbarzadeh A, Ghavamifar A, Bell M. Supply chain design for efficient and effective blood supply in disasters. Int J Prod Econ. 2017;183(PC):700–9.
35. Simonetti A, Ezzeldin H, Walderhaug M, Anderson SA, Forshee RA. An inter-regional US blood supply simulation model to evaluate blood availability to support planning for emergency preparedness and medical countermeasures. Disaster Med Public Health Prep. 2018;12(2):201–10.
36. Abir M, Davis MM, Sankar P, Wong AC, Wang SC. Design of a model to predict surge capacity bottlenecks for burn mass casualties at a large academic medical center. Prehosp Disaster Med. 2013;28(1):23.
37. Eilat SG, Vered YG, Barbara SG. Meeting blood requirements following terrorist attacks: the Israeli experience. Curr Opin Hematol. 2006;13(6):452–6.
38. Glasgow SM, Allard S, Doughty H, Spreadborough P, Watkins E. Blood and bombs: the demand and use of blood following the London bombings of 7 July 2005--a retrospective review. Transf Med (Oxford, England). 2012;22(4):244–50.
39. Stevens TW, Bryan MC, Andrew BL, Daniel DG, Valerie SD, Michael GM, et al. Incompatible type a plasma transfusion in patients requiring massive transfusion protocol: outcomes of an Eastern Association for the surgery of trauma multicenter study. J Trauma Acute Care Surg. 2017;83(1):25–9.
40. Lozano M, Heddle N, Williamson LM, Wang G, Aubuchon JP, Dumont LJ. Practices associated with ABO-incompatible platelet transfusions: a BEST collaborative international survey. Transfusion. 2010;50(8):1743–8.
41. Eastcourt LJ, Birchall J, Allard S, Bassey SJ, Hersey P, Kerr JP, et al. Guidelines for the use of platelet transfusions. Br J Haematol. 2017;176(3):365.
42. Schmidt PJ. Blood and disaster—supply and demand. N Engl J Med. 2002;346(8):617.
43. Ling G, Draghic N. Aerial drones for blood delivery. Transfusion. 2019;59(S2):1608–11.
44. Spinella PC, Dunne J, Beilman GJ, O'Connell RJ, Borgman MA, Cap AP, et al. Constant challenges and evolution of US military transfusion medicine and blood operations in combat. Transfusion. 2012;52(5):1146–53.
45. David KS, John HB, Gary NC, John HR. Fresh whole blood transfusion: a controversial military practice. J Trauma Inj Infect Crit Care. 2006;61(1):181–4.
46. Miller BT, Lin AH, Clark SC, Cap AP, Dubose JJ. Red tides: mass casualty and whole blood at sea. J Trauma Acute Care Surg. 2018;85(1S Suppl 2):S134–9.
47. Beckett A, Callum J, da Luz LT, Schmid J, Funk C, Glassberg E, et al. Fresh whole blood transfusion capability for special operations forces. Can J Surg. 2015;58(3 Suppl 3):S153–6.
48. Garcia Hejl C, Martinaud C, Macarez R, Sill J, Le Golvan A, Dulou R, et al. The implementation of a multinational "walking blood bank" in a combat zone: the experience of a health service team deployed to a medical treatment facility in Afghanistan. J Trauma Acute Care Surg. 2015;78(5):949–54.
49. Joint Trauma System Clinical Practice Guideline (JTS CPG ID:21) – Whole Blood Transfusion. 15 May 2018. Available on the Internet at the following address: https://jts.amedd.army.mil/assets/docs/cpgs/JTS_Clinical_Practice_Guidelines_(CPGs)/Whole_Blood_Transfusion_15_May_2018_ID21.pdf.
50. Tamara BR, Mark YH, Michael MA, Roland FL, Wilbur MW, James SR, et al. An evaluation of methods for producing low-titer group O whole blood to support military trauma resuscitation. J Trauma Acute Care Surg. 2017;82(6S Suppl 1):S79–86.
51. Yazer MH, Seheult J, Kleinman S, Sloan SR, Spinella PC. Who's afraid of incompatible plasma? A balanced approach to the safe transfusion of blood products containing ABO-incompatible plasma. Transfusion. 2018;58(2):532–8.
52. Cap AP, Beckett A, Benov A, Borgman M, Chen J, Corley JB, et al. Whole blood transfusion. Mil Med. 2018;183(suppl 2):44–51.
53. Doughty H, Strandenes G. Whole blood in disaster and major incident planning. ISBT Sci Ser. 2019;14(3):323–31.
54. Hakre S, Peel S, O'Connell R, Sanders-Buell E, Jagodzinski L, Eggleston C, et al. Transfusion—transmissible viral infections among US military emergency transfusion recipients. Prehosp Disaster Med. 2010;25(S2):s99.
55. Kaada SH, Apelseth TO, Hagen KG, Kristoffersen EK, Gjerde S, Sønstabø K, et al. How do I get an emergency civilian walking blood bank running? Transfusion. 2019;59(S2):1446–52.
56. Max MM, Rich CG, Lalin NM, Iain SRM, Jowan P-BM, Luke KM, et al. Outcomes following trauma laparotomy for hypotensive trauma patients: a UK military and civilian perspective. J Trauma Acute Care Surg. 2018;85(3):620–5.
57. Beaume S, Prunet B, Cotte J, Guyen CN, Aguillon P, Vinciguerra D, et al. Utilisation du plasma lyophilisé (PLYO) en salle d'accueil des urgences vitales (SAUV) pour l'accueil des traumatisés graves. Annales francaises d'anesthesie et de reanimation. 2014;33:A125.
58. Sailliol A, Martinaud C, Cap A, Civadier C, Clavier B, Deshayes A, et al. The evolving role of lyophilized plasma in remote damage control resuscitation in the French armed forces health service. Transfusion. 2013;53(s1):65S–71S.
59. Nguyen C, Bordes J, Cungi P-J, Esnault P, Cardinale M, Mathais Q, et al. Use of French lyophilized plasma transfusion in severe trauma patients is associated with an early plasma transfusion and early transfusion ratio improvement. J Trauma Acute Care Surg. 2018;84(5):780–5.
60. Gould SA, Moore EE, Moore FA, Haenel JB, Burch JM, Sehgal H, et al. Clinical utility of human polymerized hemoglobin as a blood substitute after acute trauma and urgent surgery. J Trauma. 1997;43(2):325.
61. Moore EE, Moore FA, Fabian TC, Bernard AC, Fulda GJ, Hoyt DB, et al. Human polymerized hemoglobin for the treatment of hemorrhagic shock when blood is unavailable: the USA multicenter trial. J Am Coll Surg. 2009;208(1):1–13.
62. Hickman DA, Pawlowski CL, Shevitz A, Luc NF, Kim A, Girish A, et al. Intravenous synthetic platelet (SynthoPlate) nanoconstructs reduce bleeding and improve 'golden hour' survival in a porcine model of traumatic arterial hemorrhage. Sci Rep. 2018;8(1):1–14.

Commonly Prescribed Medications that Affect Clotting: A Comprehensive Overview

19

Anitha Shelvan, Allyson L. Spence, Anne Lee Parsiola, Prathima Anandi, Harish Siddaiah, Dustin Latimer, J. Arthur Saus, Amit Prabhakar, Daniel E. Core, Elyse M. Cornett, and Alan David Kaye

Introduction

Within our vasculature, blood must maintain fluidity while still clotting quickly during times of vascular injury. When a blood vessel is damaged, the finely regulated hemostasis process repairs the vascular injury to limit blood loss. Under normal circumstances, hemostasis maintains the intricate balance between coagulation and fibrinolysis. Dysregulation of this pathway can lead to two extremes: thrombosis or hemorrhage [1].

A thrombosis, or blood clot, can occur in veins or arteries, and both types of blood clots can be deadly. Thromboembolic diseases are also the leading cause of death in developed countries [2]. A coronary arterial thrombosis can lead to a heart attack and a cerebral thrombosis can lead to a stroke – two of the leading causes of death in the United States [3]. Venous thrombosis frequently develops in the deep veins of the leg (deep vein thrombosis, or DVT). These clots can break free and enter the arteries of the lungs, resulting in a pulmonary embolism (PE) [4]. DVTs are the source of more than 90% of patients who suffer from a PE [5]. Furthermore, venous thromboembolisms (VTEs) are common, affecting nearly 900,000 people in the United States every year and killing up to one-third of these individuals [6]. Estimates have shown that VTEs cost the United States healthcare system approximately $7–10 billion each year [7]. Despite these alarming statistics, incidences involving VTEs have persisted for the past few decades. Thrombosis is primarily associated with events that can result in a dysregulation of the hemostatic pathway, such as prolonged immobility, obesity, cancer, and surgery. As the prevalence of these events continues to increase, there are surmounting fears that the incidence of VTEs will also increase [8].

Antithrombotic therapies have been used to prevent blood clots for nearly 80 years [2]. The two classes of antithrombotic drugs include anticoagulants, which block various steps in the coagulation cascade, and antiplatelet drugs, which attenuate platelet activation and clot formations [9]. The type and dose of medication administered vary according to each patient's risk of thrombosis, bleeding complications and cost [10].

The most extensively prescribed and studied anticoagulants for the prevention of VTEs include heparin and its derivatives and vitamin K antagonists, such as warfarin [2]. Heparin, which is found in the secretory granules of mast cells, can be extracted from animal sources, such as bovine and porcine. Unfractionated heparin (UFH) and the low-molecular-weight heparins (LMWHs) indirectly alter anticoagulant activity through their activation of antithrombin, which is a naturally occurring blood thinner and inactivates

A. Shelvan · A. L. Parsiola · P. Anandi · H. Siddaiah · D. Latimer
J. A. Saus · E. M. Cornett
Department of Anesthesiology, LSU Health Shreveport, Shreveport, LA, USA
e-mail: ashelv@lsuhsc.edu; aparsi@lsuhsc.edu; panan4@lsuhsc.edu; hbanga@lsuhsc.edu; dlatim@lsuhsc.edu; jsaus@lsuhsc.edu; ecorne@lsuhsc.edu

A. L. Spence
Department of Pharmaceutical Science, Regis University, Denver, CO, USA
e-mail: aspence002@regis.edu

A. Prabhakar
Emory University School of Medicine, Department of Anesthesiology, Atlanta, GA, USA

D. E. Core
LSU Health Shreveport School of Medicine, Shreveport, LA, USA
e-mail: dcore@lsuhsc.edu

A. D. Kaye (✉)
Department of Anesthesiology and Pharmacology, Toxicology, and Neurosciences, Louisiana State University School of Medicine-Shreveport, Shreveport, LA, USA

LSU Health Shreveport School of Medicine, New Orleans, LA, USA

Tulane School of Medicine, New Orleans, LA, USA
e-mail: akaye@lsuhsc.edu

© Springer Nature Switzerland AG 2021
C. S. Scher et al. (eds.), *Essentials of Blood Product Management in Anesthesia Practice*,
https://doi.org/10.1007/978-3-030-59295-0_19

enzymes associated with the coagulation pathway [11]. These drugs are commonly prescribed following orthopedic surgeries of the lower extremities to prevent VTEs [2]. Warfarin is another anticoagulant that protects against VTEs. Heparin is parenterally administered and warfarin can be orally administered. Since the coagulation pathway involves a vitamin K-dependent step, warfarin produces its anticoagulant activity through its ability to block the activation of vitamin K in the body [12].

While anticoagulants interfere with the enzymes involved in the coagulation cascade, antiplatelet drugs interfere with the binding of platelets, thus preventing the actual formation of blood clots [9]. For decades, aspirin (acetylsalicylic acid) has been considered the "gold standard" for preventing arterial thromboses [13, 14]. Although aspirin is efficacious in reducing the risk of recurrent VTE, warfarin and other anticoagulants are more effective [15, 16].

In contrast to the action of preventing or retarding blood clot formation by use of antithrombotic therapies, antifibrinolytic agents reduce excessive bleeding by reducing the rate of clot breakdown. They are used to prevent excessive bleeding and induce the formation of blood clots [17]. Fibrin is an important protein in the coagulation cascade system and is crucial during the formation of blood clots [18]. By inhibiting fibrinolysis, or the enzymatic breakdown of fibrin within blood clots, antifibrinolytic agents can significantly reduce bleeding. They are commonly administered during surgeries associated with a high risk of bleeding, such as cardiac surgeries [19]. Tranexamic acid has exhibited significant efficacy in reducing the number of patients that require blood transfusions following cardiac and orthopedic surgeries [17, 20]. Tranexamic acid is also effective in treating hemophilia and cyclic heavy menstrual bleeding [21].

Coagulation modifiers must be carefully monitored, and doses properly adjusted to ensure efficacious therapy, while reducing potentially dangerous and life-threatening adverse effects. Although antithrombotic therapies are relatively effective they produce a highly variable anticoagulant effect in patients and require thorough monitoring and ongoing patient education. Many commonly prescribed anticoagulants (e.g., warfarin and heparin) have a narrow therapeutic window, and careful monitoring must occur to lower the risk of blood clots and, avoid bleeding complications [22]. Just as antithrombotic therapies must be closely monitored to reduce the risk of adverse bleeding events, coagulants must be closely monitored as they increase the risk of VTE [17, 23].

Furthermore, patients who are prescribed coagulation modifiers must be educated on the potential drug and herb interactions that can exacerbate the side effects of these medications [24]. NSAIDs, such as ibuprofen, are some of the most commonly administered over-the-counter medications, but these drugs are contraindicated in individuals who are taking antithrombotic agents as the co-administration of these drugs can increase the risk of gastrointestinal (GI) bleeding [25]. Herbal products, such as garlic and ginkgo biloba, can increase the risk of hemorrhage when combined with antithrombotic drugs. Other herbal products, including St. John's wort and ginseng, are contraindicated. They can decrease the efficacy of anticoagulants and antiplatelet drugs [26]. Other combinations of drugs must also be closely monitored. For example, if antidepressants, such as selective serotonin reuptake inhibitors (SSRIs), are added to warfarin therapy, the patient must be carefully monitored for bleeding [27, 28].

Although coagulation modifiers have important implications for therapeutic use, these drugs require careful monitoring, thorough patient education, and a good relationship between healthcare providers and patients. This will ensure effective therapeutic results and reduce complications. In this paper, we will discuss anticoagulants, antifibrinolytics, and antiplatelets and interactions that can occur with these medications.

Anticoagulants

Several common anticoagulants have important intraoperative implications. New oral anticoagulants, such as the direct thrombin inhibitors (dabigatran) and Factor Xa inhibitors (rivaroxaban, apixaban, edoxaban, and betrixaban), have been approved by FDA for various clinical indications. They are efficacious in treating thromboprophylaxis and preventing deep vein thrombosis (DVT). Additionally, these medications have favorable pharmacodynamic and pharmacokinetic properties.

Although warfarin has been the "standby" medication for oral anticoagulation for many years, warfarin exerts anticoagulant activity through a different mechanism of action than "direct oral anticoagulants" (DOAC, formerly known as novel oral anticoagulants) [29, 30]. Compared with traditional oral anticoagulants like warfarin, DOACs have better safety profile, can be administered in fixed daily doses, do not require periodic monitoring of the international normalized ratio (INR), and have less drug-drug interactions. This makes the administration of these drugs easier and safer [31–34].

To properly manage the effects of anticoagulants during the intraoperative or perioperative period, medical personnel should be familiar with the mechanism of action, indications, contraindications, dosing, side effects, and drug interactions associated with these medications. Currently, there are four different mechanisms of action associated with anticoagulants:

- vitamin K antagonist (coumarin, warfarin)
- Heparin and the low-molecular-weight heparins (LMWH)
- Direct thrombin inhibitors

- Factor Xa inhibitors

A diagram of the coagulation cascade demonstrating the conversion of prothrombin to thrombin, and the central role of thrombin in not only converting fibrinogen to fibrin but also of its enzymatic role in stabilizing the fibrin clot is shown in Fig. 19.1 [35].

The formation of Factors II, VII, IX, and X, all of which are necessary in the intrinsic and extrinsic coagulation cascade, depends on the presence of vitamin K. Factor II (prothrombin), which has such a critical role in coagulation, has 10 glutamic acids in the amino-terminal region of the protein, which are carboxylated. Without vitamin K, the carboxylation does not occur, and the proteins that are synthesized to become prothrombin are biologically inactive [36].

While vitamin K is found in several foods, including leafy green vegetables, cauliflower, and calves' liver, in most cases the absence of dietary vitamin K is not deleterious. Bacteria found in the large intestine synthesize vitamin K; this is the primary source of vitamin K in the human body. vitamin K is a fat-soluble vitamin. Both vitamin K consumed in the diet and vitamin K formed by microbial action are absorbed into intestinal lymph along with other lipids. Since vitamin K is a fat-soluble material, intestinal absorption depends upon bile secretion into the intestine. Liver disease that results in decreased bile synthesis leads to impaired vitamin K absorption; in turn, this results in a vitamin K deficiency. Additionally, a majority of clotting factors are synthesized almost exclusively in the liver. Liver disease can cause defects in blood clotting by several mechanisms. Both reduced absorption of vitamin K and reduced synthesis of other factors necessary for coagulation by the diseased liver predisposes to the bleeding tendency often seen in patients with severe hepatic cirrhosis [36].

In pregnancy, the fetus obtains vitamin K from its mother through the placenta. The liver in the neonate has essentially no reserve of vitamin K, and deficiency of vitamin K in human infants can lead to the hemorrhagic disease of vitamin K deficiency bleeding (VKDB) of the newborn [37–39].

Newborn infants have low vitamin K reserves. Some explanations for this low vitamin K are below.

1. Vitamin K transport across the placental barrier is limited.
2. The liver storage of vitamin K is very low.
3. The vitamin K cycle may not be fully functional in newborns, especially premature infants.
4. The vitamin K content of breast milk is low.
5. Infants whose mothers are on antiseizure medications are at risk for vitamin K deficiency.

Lack of vitamin K intake, or situations, which interfere with absorption of vitamin K synthesized by bacteria, may result in a vitamin K deficiency in the newborn, leading to death or permanent brain damage [40]. Newborn babies who are exclusively breast-fed are at increased risk for vitamin K deficiency, because human milk is relatively low in vitamin K, compared to formula. Because VKDB is life threatening and easily prevented, the American Academy of Pediatrics and a number of similar international organizations recom-

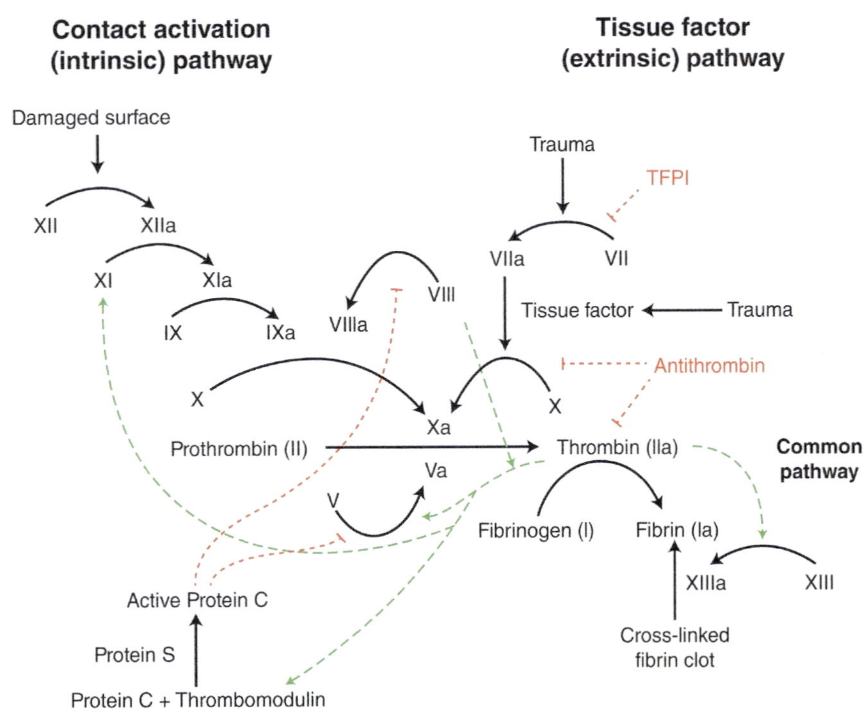

Fig. 19.1 Coagulation cascade (Modified from [35])

mend that an intramuscular dose of phylloquinone (vitamin K_1) be administered to all newborns [38].

In the formation of the active coagulation factors II, VII, IX, and X, the chemically reduced form of vitamin K reacts with the target protein containing a glutamic acid to create a gamma carboxy glutamic acid. The chemically reduced form of vitamin K becomes an oxidized version (vitamin K oxide). The vitamin K oxide is then reduced back to the original vitamin K to once again react with the target protein to form more active coagulation factors. Coumarin derivatives such as dicumarol and warfarin provide anticoagulation effects by interfering with the recycling of vitamin K and thereby with the production of Factors II, VII, IX, and X, all of which are necessary for the clotting cascade to occur. This interference results in a lower concentration of these proteins and interferes with the coagulation process, See Fig. 19.2 [36].

Heparin administration has been the primary injectable anticoagulant for many years. Heparin and the newer low-molecular-weight heparin medications, enoxaparin (Lovenox), and dalteparin (Fragmin), function as anticoagulants by blocking the action of Factors X and II (prothrombin); this action provides anticoagulation by inhibiting the conversion of fibrinogen to fibrin.

Direct Factor Xa Inhibitors (The Four Drugs with Names Ending in -Aban)

Activated Factor X (Factor Xa) enzymatically cleaves two sites on prothrombin to produce thrombin. In turn, thrombin acts as a serine protease to convert soluble fibrinogen into insoluble strands of fibrin and to also convert Factor XIII to the activated Factor XIIIa. This thrombin-induced activation of Factor XIIIa cross-links strands of fibrin to form the more stable fibrin clot (as can be easily seen in the drawing of the coagulation cascade illustrated in Fig. 19.1), thrombin, acting as a serine protease, functions in a "positive feedback manner" (follow the green arrows in the drawing) to enhance further thrombin formation and to enhance cross-linked fibrin clot formation.

As a result, any agent that interferes with the conversion of prothrombin to thrombin, such as Factor Xa inhibitors, is a very potent anticoagulant [41]. Medications which directly inhibit the action of Factor Xa do not require other cofactors, such as antithrombin, to exert their anticoagulation effects.

Currently, there are four oral medications available, which function as selective, direct inhibitors of Factor Xa: rivaroxaban (Xarelto), apixaban (Eliquis) and edoxaban (Savaysa), and betrixaban (Bevyxxa). These direct inhibitors of Factor Xa reduce thrombin generation and thrombus formation by inhibiting free and clot bound Factor Xa, prothrombinase activity, and thrombin-induced platelet aggregation. Whenever these medications are used changes are observed in prothrombin time (PT), international normalized ratio (INR), and activated partial thromboplastin time (aPTT). However, evaluations of these parameters are not useful to moniter the anticoagulant effect induced by Factor Xa inhibitors.

Rivaroxaban

Rivaroxaban (Xarelto) is an orally administered, direct Factor Xa inhibitor and was the first oral direct Factor Xa inhibitor to gain approval for human use. It targets both free and clot-bound Factor Xa and Factor Xa in the prothrombinase complex, thereby prolonging clotting times [41]. This effect is significantly different than the effects exerted by indirect Factor Xa inhibitors. Rivaroxaban binds directly and reversibly to Factor Xa and exerts action by competitively inhibiting the activity of Factor Xa. It is more than 10,000-fold more selective for Factor Xa than for other related serine proteases, and it does not inhibit other serine proteases at concentrations up to 20 μM [42]. Thrombin generation was almost completely inhibited at therapeutically relevant concentrations (80–100 nM) of rivaroxaban [43, 44]. The onset of action of rivaroxaban is rapid; maximum PT prolongation was seen 1–4 h after tablet intake, and PT prolongation correlated with plasma rivaroxaban concentrations (up to 500 μg/L) in an almost linear fashion [45].

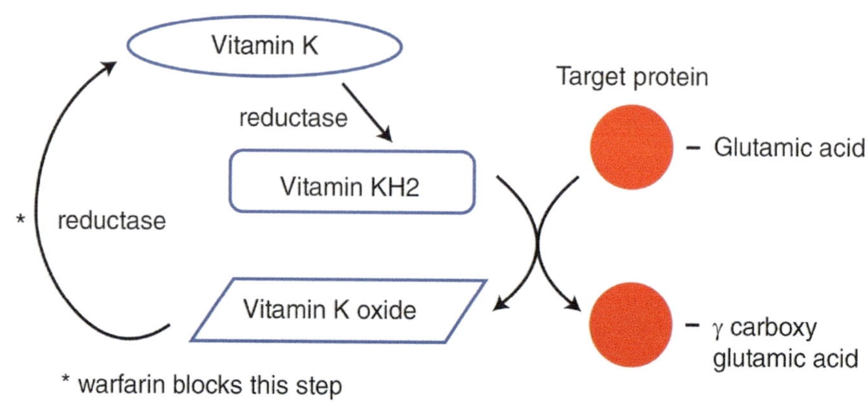

Fig. 19.2 Vitamin K and warfarin (Modified from [36])

Rivaroxaban is used for thromboembolic prophylaxis, such as venous thromboembolism (VTE) prophylaxis after total knee replacement (TKR) or total hip replacement (THR). Rivaroxaban has also been used as secondary prevention after recent acute coronary syndrome (ACS) and for stroke prevention in patients who have atrial fibrillation [42]. When used for the prevention of venous thromboembolism following hip or knee replacements, extended therapy for at least 3 months or longer is usually recommended [46]. In the presence of significant renal or hepatic impairment, the use of rivaroxaban may be contraindicated, or at least significant reduction in the dosage may be needed [41, 46]. Clearance of rivaroxaban depends on the cytochrome P3A4 system. Use is not recommended in patients receiving concomitant systemic treatment with strong inhibitors of CYP3A4 and P-glycoprotein–azole-antimycotics (e.g., ketoconazole) or HIV protease inhibitors (e.g., ritonavir) because they may increase rivaroxaban plasma concentrations to a clinically relevant degree. Since rifampin strongly induces CYP3A4, co-administration with rifampin led to a decrease in effect and more rapid clearance of the administered dose. Co-administration with naproxen (500 mg), aspirin (500 mg followed by 100 mg), clopidogrel (300 mg followed by 75 mg), enoxaparin (40 mg), and warfarin (titrated to and INR of 2.0–3.0) did not affect the pharmacokinetics of rivaroxaban [42].

Adverse side effects of rivaroxaban include intracranial hemorrhage, gastrointestinal bleeding, and an increased risk of PE or DVT. The most common adverse reaction (>5%) is bleeding, increased risk of stroke after discontinuation in nonvalvular atrial fibrillation, and spinal/epidural hematoma [47]. When compared to other direct oral anticoagulants (DOAC), rivaroxaban has the highest proportion of reported adverse events. The risk of breakthrough venous thromboembolism appears higher than for other DOACs, but this appears to be more likely when other underlying disease processes are also present [42, 48].

Apixaban

Apixaban (Eliquis), another orally administered direct Factor Xa inhibitor, has similar indications to rivaroxaban. Similar to other anticoagulants, the most significant side effect is a dose-dependent increased risk of bleeding [31, 47]. Of all Factor Xa inhibitors, apixaban demonstrates the least dependence on renal metabolism, but current guidelines still advise dose modifications depending on creatinine clearance, age, and body weight [41]. Dosing of apixaban is dependent on the clinical scenario; for VTE prophylaxis in surgical patients, 2.5 mg twice daily for 12–25 days is recommended. For secondary prevention or treatment of VTE, the recommendation generally is administration of 10 mg twice daily for 7 days followed by 5 mg twice daily. For prevention of cerebrovascular accidents due to thromboembolism in patients who have atrial fibrillation and any two of the following: age ≥80 years, body weight ≤60 kg, or serum creatinine ≥1.5 mg/dL, dosing of 2.5 mg or 5 mg twice daily is recommended [41]. When compared to other DOACs, apixaban appeared to show the lowest rate of adverse event occurrence [47].

Edoxaban

Like rivaroxaban and apixaban, edoxaban (Savaysa) is an oral direct Factor Xa inhibitor. Additionally, edoxaban has a >10,000-fold selectivity for Factor Xa as compared to thrombin, which makes it efficient as an anticoagulation medication [49]. The indications for use of edoxaban include venous thromboembolism treatment and prevention of stroke and systemic embolism in patients who have atrial fibrillation [50]. Use of Edoxaban is not recommended in individuals who are pregnant, those who have mechanical heart valves, or those who have creatinine clearances >95 mL/min or <15 mL/min. When used for patients who have atrial fibrillation the most common adverse reaction is bleeding and anemia (≥5%). When used in patients with DVT and pulmonary embolism the risk of bleeding, rash, or abnormal liver function tests is reported to be ≥1% [51]. Again, like rivaroxaban and apixaban, major side effects include increased risk of bleeding and increased risk of spinal or epidural hematoma following spinal puncture or administration of neuraxial anesthesia. In those undergoing treatment for Venous Thromboembolism, the recommended edoxaban dosing is 30–60 mg once daily following 5 days of parenteral anticoagulation [41].

Betrixaban

Betrixaban (Bevyxxa) is also an orally administered Factor Xa inhibitor. It is dosed only once a day and is excreted primarily in the bile, with very low (approximately 17%) renal excretion [52]. Betrixaban selectively blocks the active site of Factor Xa and does not require a cofactor (such as Antithrombin III) for activity. Betrixaban inhibits free and prothrombinase bound Factor Xa in a concentration-dependent manner, thereby decreasing thrombin generation [53]. Studies demonstrate that betrixaban provides more potent inhibition of the thrombin–antithrombin complex, and F1 + 2 generation when compared with fondaparinux. Betrixaban has no direct effect on platelet aggregation.

Similar to other Factor Xa inhibitors, its indications are primarily prophylactic to prevent venous thromboembolism (VTE) in adult patients hospitalized for an acute medical illness, and who are at risk for thromboembolic complications due to moderate or severe restricted mobility, and have other risk factors for VTE. Currently, it is the only FDA-approved direct oral anticoagulant for extended-duration prophylaxis of VTE in acute medically ill patients. While studies did not demonstrate superiority to enoxaparin in the prevention of major and non-major bleeding in total knee replacement patients in the phase 2 EXPERT trial, effective antithrombotic activity was demonstrated at 15-mg and 40-mg doses, and these doses were well tolerated. In the phase 2 EXPLORE-Xa trial in patients with nonvalvular atrial fibrillation, betrixaban doses of 40, 60, and 80 mg demonstrated the lowest occurrence of any bleeding events. The risk of bleeding was comparable to well-controlled warfarin in patients with atrial fibrillation at risk for stroke. The use of Betrixaban was associated with higher rates of diarrhea than with use of warfarin [52].

Although there is no data recommending the use of betrixaban in pregnant women, it is expected that use of this medication (and all direct Factor Xa inhibitors) would increase the risk of hemorrhage during labor and delivery. Additionally, patients with severe renal impairment (creatinine clearance greater than 15 ml/min but less than 30 ml/min) may have an increased risk of bleeding events. No dosage adjustment is needed for patients with creatinine clearance greater than 30 ml/min. Patients with hepatic impairment frequently have intrinsic coagulation abnormalities. Betrixaban has not been tested in patients with hepatic impairment and therefore, use in these patients is not recommended. The safety and effectiveness in pediatric patients have not been established. Betrixaban is supplied as 40 and 80 mg capsules.

Fondaparinux

Fondaparinux is a synthetic anticoagulant based on the pentasaccharide sequence, which makes up the minimal antithrombotic binding region of heparin. Fondaparinux functions by mimicking the site where heparin binds to Antithrombin III, thereby enhancing the anticoagulant action of ATIII [54]. It is a highly selective, indirect inhibitor of activated Factor X. Fondaparinux has no interaction with platelets, and it has a longer half-life than heparin. It does not actually inhibit thrombin, but instead functions as an indirect inhibitor of Factor Xa. Initial studies in patients following total hip replacements demonstrated that at minimum doses of 1.5 mg/day, less venous thromboembolism occurred than in patients who were treated with Fondaparinux than in those treated with 30 mg enoxaparin injections each 12 h. However, excessive bleeding was also noted in these patients when they received daily injections of 6 or 8 mg per day. Use of Fondaparinux has been recommended in the situation when anticoagulation effects are desirable, yet the patient exhibits a hypersensitivity to low molecular weight and unfractionated heparins [55]. Further studies suggested that when Fondaparinux was administered to a patient during her pregnancy, there was no detectable effect in the fetus, implying that there was no placental transfer of the medication [56].

Direct Thrombin Inhibitors

Dabigatran

Another DOAC, dabigatran (Pradaxa), has some similarities and some differences when compared to direct Factor Xa inhibitors. Like these medications, dabigatran is used for venous thromboembolic prophylaxis and treatment, and for secondary prevention after the occurrence of an acute coronary syndrome. Unlike the direct Factor Xa Inhibitors, dabigatran is a reversible, oral, direct thrombin (Factor IIa) inhibitor with a half-life of approximately 12–14 h [30]. Dabigatran usually exerts a maximum anticoagulation effect within 2–3 h of ingestion, but while not affecting the bioavailability of the drug, fatty foods delay its absorption. Dabigatran inhibits both free and clot-bound thrombin; it also inhibits thrombin-induced platelet aggregation. Dabigatran inhibits the conversion of fibrinogen into fibrin during the coagulation cascade and prevents development of a thrombus. As a result, dabigatran prolongs coagulation markers such as aPTT, ecarin clotting time (ECT), and thrombin time (TT). The degree of anticoagulant activity can be assessed by ECT and aPTT [33, 57].

The use of dabigatran is not recommended in patients with renal insufficiency [41]. Use of dabigatran carries a major risk of gastrointestinal bleeding and intracranial hemorrhage. Dabigatran had the highest reported rates of ischemic stroke [47]. Other contraindications to use of dabigatran include obesity and concurrent use of p-glycoprotein inhibitors or inducers such as ketoconazole, verapamil, or rifampin. The most common adverse reactions with dabigatran (>15%) are gastritis-like symptoms and bleeding, increased risk of thrombotic events after premature discontinuation, and thromboembolic and bleeding events in patients with prosthetic heart valves [58].

When used as VTE prophylaxis in surgical patients, dosing for dabigatran is 110 mg one to four hours after surgery, followed by 220 mg once daily for 28–35 days (total hip replacement) or 10 days (total knee replacement). If being used for VTE treatment, 5–10 days of parenteral anticoagulation should be administered initially; then dabigatran is administered at a dose of 150 mg twice daily [41].

Indications for Use

Currently, DOACs are approved for the following indications:

1. Prevention of stroke and systemic embolism in patients with non-valvular atrial fibrillation (NVAF)
2. Treatment of deep vein thrombosis (DVT) and pulmonary embolism (PE) and prevention of recurrence of these conditions
3. Prevention of venous thromboembolism (VTE) in patients undergoing hip and knee replacement surgery

Administration and Dosing Recommendations for DOACs

When considering DOAC use, periodically assess renal function as clinically indicated and adjust therapy accordingly [52]. FDA recommended dosing is for the following indications: [39, 59, 60].

1. Prevention of stroke and systemic embolism in patients with non-valvular atrial fibrillation (NVAF):
   Dabigatran 150 mg orally, twice daily (BID) in patients with creatinine clearance (CrCl) >30 mL/min and 75 mg orally, BID in patients with CrCl 15–30 mL/min.
   Rivaroxaban 20 mg orally, once daily (OD) with the evening meal in patients with CrCl >50 mL/min and 15 mg orally, OD with the evening meal in patients with CrCl 15–50 mL/min.
   Apixaban 5 mg orally BID and 2.5 mg orally BID in patients with at least two of the following characteristics: age ≥80 years, body weight ≤60 kg, or serum creatinine ≥1.5 mg/dL.
   Edoxaban 60 mg OD in patients with CrCl >50 to ≤95 mL/min and avoid in patients with CrCl >95 mL/min, 30 mg OD in patients with CrCl 15–50 mL/min.
2. Treatment of DVT and PE and prevention of recurrence of these conditions:
   Dabigatran 150 mg orally, BID after previous treatment in patients with CrCl >30 mL/min.
   Rivaroxaban 15 mg orally BID with food for the first 21 days followed by 20 mg orally OD with food, for prevention of recurrence 10 mg OD after at least 6 months of standard anticoagulant treatment [61]. Apixaban 10 mg BID for 7 days and 5 mg BID afterward [62].
   Edoxaban 60 mg OD and 30 mg OD for patients with CrCl 15–50 mL/min or body weight ≤60 kg or who use certain P-gp inhibitors
3. Prevention of VTE in patients undergoing hip and knee replacement surgery.
   Dabigatran 110 mg orally first day, then 220 mg OD in patients with CrCl >30 mL/min.
   Rivaroxaban 10 mg orally OD with or without food.
   Apixaban 2.5 mg BID. Treatment is recommended for 35 days in hip and 12 days in knee replacement surgery.

Side Effects and Contraindications

The most common adverse reactions with dabigatran (>15%) are gastritis-like symptoms and bleeding, increased risk of thrombotic events after premature discontinuation, and thromboembolic and bleeding events in patients with prosthetic heart valves [63, 64]. With rivaroxaban, the most common adverse reaction (>5%) was bleeding, increased risk of stroke after discontinuation in nonvalvular atrial fibrillation, and spinal/epidural hematoma [65, 66]. With edoxaban, the most common adverse reactions when used for NVAF are bleeding and anemia (≥5%), and when used for DVT and PE are bleeding, rash, abnormal liver function tests, and anemia (≥1%) [67, 68]. With apixaban, the most common adverse reactions (>1%) are related to bleeding and increased risk of thrombotic events after premature discontinuation [69]. Dabigatran and Factor Xa inhibitor drugs are contraindicated in patients with active pathological bleeding, a history of a serious hypersensitivity reaction to dabigatran, and mechanical prosthetic heart valve [39, 59, 60].

IV Administered Direct Thrombin Inhibitors

Bivalirudin (Angiomax) and argatroban also function as inhibitors of coagulation but are not considered as "DOACs" since they must be administered by the IV route, not the oral route. Bivalirudin is a synthetic derivative of Hirudin, a compound found in the salivary glands of the medicinal leech (Hirudo medicinalis). As such, sometimes it is humorously referred to as "snail spit." Bivalirudin is a potent and highly specific inhibitor of thrombin (Factor IIa). Following IV administration, it inhibits both circulating and clot-bound thrombin and also inhibits thrombin-mediated platelet activation and aggregation. Due to its quick onset of action and short half-life, its antithrombotic response is very predictable. While bivalirudin directly inhibits thrombin, it is not related to heparin and therefore presents no risk of heparin-induced thrombocytopenia (HIT). It may be used in those patients susceptible to HIT. Although there is currently no medication that can be administered to terminate or inhibit bivalirudin's action, it is cleared by a combination of renal mechanisms (approximately 20%) and proteolytic cleavage (approximately 80%) by proteins present in blood serum and liver.

The expected half-life of bivalirudin anticoagulation action is about 25 min in patients with normal renal function, and return to baseline coagulation times can be expected to occur within about an hour after discontinuation of a bivalirudin infusion; this may be prolonged to just under an hour in patients with severe renal dysfunction. When administered to a patient with severe renal impairment, dose adjustments are needed [70]. The half-life of anticoagulation activity may be prolonged to about 3.5 h in patients who are dialysis dependent.

In the United Sates, typical dosing for bivalirudin is an initial IV bolus of 0.75 mg/kg of patient body weight, followed by an infusion of 1.75 mg/kg/hr. Although not approved for cardiac surgery or other perioperative use, bivalirudin is the only "alternative anticoagulant", which has been prospectively studied in cardiac surgery for use in HIT and non-HIT patients [71]. When used as the anticoagulant for cardiac surgery in which cardiopulmonary bypass will be used, often the recommended initial dose is 1.5 mg/Kg administered by IV bolus, and an additional 50 mg of bivalirudin is added to the cardiopulmonary bypass pump priming fluid. Following administration of the initial dose, an activated clotting time (ACT) can be used to monitor anticoagulation provided by bivalirudin. Adequate anticoagulation for cardiopulmonary bypass is documented by achieving an ACT of at least 500 s and over 200 s for a vascular surgery procedure such as an "off-pump" cardiopulmonary bypass. There is currently no "reversal agent" to terminate the action of bivalirudin, so termination of the anticoagulation effect depends on the patient's intrinsic clearance mechanisms.

Argatroban

Argatroban is a direct thrombin inhibitor. The FDA initially licensed it for prophylaxis or thrombosis treatment in patients with heparin-induced thrombocytopenia (HIT). It is currently used both in the management of HIT and for anticoagulation. Argatroban is metabolized in the liver, and clearance is primarily by hepatic metabolism. In patients who have hepatic dysfunction, adjustments in the dose of argatroban may be necessary [72]. Argatroban has a half-life of about 45–50 min in patients with normal hepatic function. In patients with hepatic impairment, clearance was approximately one-fourth that of healthy patients, and the half-life of an administered dose increased by two-to threefold [73].

To achieve adequate anticoagulation for vascular surgery, when argatroban is used, an infusion is often started with a bolus injection of 350 mcg/kg over 3–5 min and continued with an infusion of 25 mcg/kg/min. Argatroban is a direct thrombin inhibitor with a half-life of approximately 40–50 min. This makes it less suitable as an anticoagulant for cardiac surgery requiring cardiopulmonary bypass since frequent monitoring and re-dosing would be required. If used for an "off-pump CABG," an ACT of greater than 200 s should be confirmed. An activated clotting time (ACT) should be checked approximately 5–10 min following the bolus injection to assure anticoagulation is adequate for the planned procedure. Like bivalirudin, there is currently no "reversal agent" to terminate the anticoagulation effects following the administration of argatroban. Either bivalirudin or argatroban may be used to achieve anticoagulation for cardiac surgery in patients who have persistent heparin-induced thrombocytopenia IgG antibodies.

Monitoring Anticoagulation Effects

Monitoring the anticoagulation effects, to titrate the doses to the desired effect may be challenging whenever using either bivalirudin or argatroban for anticoagulation. Although viscoelastic testing (such as TEG or ROTEM) is used extensively to guide therapy at the "point of care" with procoagulants and hemostatic agents, there is little data describing its use for parenteral direct thrombin inhibitors. Direct thrombin inhibitors, including argatroban and bivalirudin, can increase the clot formation time but may have only a minor effect on the maximum clot strength [74]. Use of the ecarin clotting time can measure the concentrations of direct thrombin inhibitors more accurately [75].

Traditionally Used Anticoagulants: Warfarin and Heparin

Warfarin

Warfarin has been used in human medicine since 1954 and is the most widely used anticoagulant in the world. The history of warfarin's discovery dates back more than 30 years earlier. In the 1920s, cattle in the Northern United States and Canada suddenly demonstrated an unusual disease characterized by fatal bleeding, either spontaneously or from minor injuries. It was recognized that these cattle had been eating moldy silage made from sweet clover [39]. Scientific examinations demonstrated this moldy clover contained a factor causing hemorrhage by decreasing the activity of prothrombin. It took until 1940 when Karl Link, an American biochemist at the University of Wisconsin–Madison, and his student Harold Campbell were able to isolate the hemorrhagic compound and later discovered that the identity of the anticoagulant in the sweet clover disease was dicoumarol (3,3'-methylenebis-(4-hydroxy coumarin)) [59]. With further research, by 1945, Link synthesized and patented warfarin. It was initially approved in the United States in 1952 as a rodenticide and then was later approved as a human anticoagulant in 1954. The name warfarin derives from the initials of the "Wisconsin Alumni Research Foundation" (the business entity which held the patent on the compound), WARF, and *-arin* from the ending of the scientific name of the primary compound "coumarin" [39].

In comparison to the DOAC medications discussed previously, warfarin is an oral anticoagulant that exerts its action by competitively inhibiting subunit 1 of a multi-unit vitamin K epoxide reductase complex. This decreases the carboxylation of vitamin K-dependent proteins (as presented earlier in this chapter) and inhibits activation of clotting Factors II (with a half-life of 59 h), VII (with a half-life of 6 h), IX, and X. Warfarin also reduces the activities of regulatory anticoagulant protein C and protein S resulting in an initial procoagulant state. Since it has no effect on fully carboxylated molecules in circulation, it takes days for the establishment of an antithrombotic effect. Warfarin has been used as thromboembolic prophylaxis in individuals who have a history of atrial fibrillation, acute coronary syndrome, heart failure, prosthetic heart valve, stroke, deep venous thrombosis (DVT), pulmonary embolism (PE), or antiphospholipid syndrome.

Warfarin exists as two optically active isomers, R and S, which are highly protein-bound (99%). Oral bioavailability is around 90%. Warfarin is metabolized by oxidative metabolism in the liver, which involves several cytochrome P450 isoenzymes; the elimination of warfarin is almost entirely by hepatic microsomal enzyme metabolism. S-Warfarin is five times more potent than R warfarin and is metabolized primarily by CYP2C9, while R- warfarin is metabolized primarily by CYP2C19, CYP1A2, and CYP3A4. Certain individuals carry allele variations of CYP2C9, which reduces the rate of warfarin metabolism. These variations are estimated to occur in up to 11% of the Caucasian population. Warfarin half-life ranges from 25 to 60 h (mean – 40 h), and duration of effect can be 2–5 days [76].

Warfarin has a narrow therapeutic index and variable dose requirements. This combination of variable dose requirements, and variable rates of metabolism and clearance makes it difficult to maintain patients within a defined range of anticoagulation. Maintaining the patient in the ideal INR target range of greater than 2 but less than 3 is challenging; an INR of less than 2 increases the risk of thrombotic events, while INR greater than 3 increases the risk of bleeding [39]. These bleeding events can range from ecchymosis, occult bleeding, or hemorrhage and from upper or lower gastrointestinal tract, microscopic or macroscopic hematuria, epistaxis, or intracranial hemorrhage. The use of warfarin has the highest fatal intracranial bleeding risk when the risk is compared to the newer DOAC medications [42]. Additionally, warfarin administration carries associated risks of teratogenicity, cholesterol embolization, vascular calcification, nephropathy, and skin necrosis in patients with protein C deficiency. On the other side of the spectrum, subtherapeutic INR can result in life-threatening thromboembolic events.

Similar to concerns with the use of other anticoagulant agents, contraindications to use of warfarin include active bleeding, severe thrombocytopenia (defined as platelet count <50,000/L), significant trauma, invasive procedures, obstetric delivery, history of intracranial hemorrhage, intracranial or spinal tumor, administration of neuraxial anesthesia, and severe, uncontrolled hypertension. Other contraindications that are more specific to warfarin include thyroid disease and renal insufficiency [39]. Patients who are beginning warfarin therapy; usually start with 5 mg daily on days 1 and 2 of therapy; then on day 3, the dose is usually adjusted based on results of PT/INR. Patients who are elderly, frail, malnourished, or with preexisting liver, heart, or kidney disease usually use 2.5 mg daily or 2.5 mg alternating with 5 mg daily [59]. Several factors affect the warfarin dose, including age, body mass index, gender, race, concomitant drug use, comorbidities, and genetic variables that affect warfarin pharmacokinetics and pharmacodynamics. Saleh et al. have proposed application of artificial neural network (ANN) to develop a warfarin dosing algorithm, and they were able to predict ideal warfarin dosage in 48% of patients [77].

Heparin

Unlike the other oral and IV anticoagulants discussed previously, which do not depend on antithrombin activity to provide anticoagulation effects, heparin is an antithrombin-dependent, indirect Factor Xa inhibitor [60]. Heparin may be administered via the subcutaneous or intravenous route, but it is not administered via an oral route. Indications for the use of heparin include prophylaxis and treatment of thromboembolic disorders (VTE, PE) and thrombotic complications associated with atrial fibrillation, prevention of clotting during vascular and cardiac surgery, and as an anticoagulant for extracorporeal circulation and dialysis procedures. Contraindications of heparin include hypersensitivity to heparin, severe thrombocytopenia, history of heparin-induced thrombocytopenia (HIT), and uncontrolled active bleeding except when that bleeding is due to diffuse intravascular coagulation (DIC) [66]. Initiation of heparin anticoagulation often starts with an initial bolus of 80 units/kg followed by 18 units/kg/hr as a therapeutic dose or 5000 units subcutaneously 2 h preoperatively and then every 8–12 h postoperatively as a prophylactic dose [78]. Side effects associated with heparin use include thrombocytopenia, HIT, chest pain, shock, thrombosis, vasospasm, hemorrhage, and increased liver enzymes [66]. Unlike warfarin, heparin does not cross the placenta, so when anticoagulation is needed during pregnancy, it is considered to be a more useful anticoagulation medication and associated with a significantly reduced risk. Heparin can be used for treatment of thromboembolic disease during pregnancy [65].

Warfarin, heparin, and the newer DOACs may be used to provide prophylaxis against and treatment of major thromboembolic complications that may arise in the peri-operative period. While these medications each have specific side effects, common to all anticoagulants is the risk of major bleeding. Since patients who are using any of these anticoagulation medications are often concurrently taking medications that can affect the metabolism of anticoagulants, they often have an increased risk of experiencing adverse events. Clinicians who prescribe these medications or administer them should be well-informed about the various drug-drug interactions that exist. Interactions that occur between anticoagulants and antidepressants, antiplatelets, antibiotics, NSAIDs, and herbal supplements are clearly documented [60–63, 78].

Drug-Drug Interactions: Drug Classes

Antidepressants and SSRIs

Warfarin is metabolized by the cytochrome P450 enzymes. One of these enzymes, cytochrome P450 2C9 (abbreviated as CYP2C9), demonstrates a major role in the oxidation of xenobiotic and endogenous compounds. This enzyme is inhibited by the antidepressants fluoxetine and fluvoxamine. Whenever a patient using one of these antidepressants also has warfarin administered, the warfarin is not metabolized as efficiently. This leads to increased warfarin levels and enhanced warfarin effects. Other antidepressants, such as citalopram, nefazodone, and sertraline, have not demonstrated such associations with warfarin [69]. Similarly, a severely elevated INR was found with the concomitant use of duloxetine and warfarin. This was hypothesized to be the result of metabolism by various cytochrome P450 enzymes or competitive binding of both substances at protein-binding sites [63].

Antiplatelet Drugs

Several studies have demonstrated that combining antiplatelet drugs and anticoagulants can lead to detrimental synergistic reactions that ultimately lead to increased bleeding. One such example is detailed in a paper by So and Eckman; they state, "multiple studies examining outcomes of combined antiplatelet and anticoagulant therapy in patients with indications for both have demonstrated an increased risk of major hemorrhage compared with either treatment alone" [79]. Similarly, a meta-analysis of 25,307 patients demonstrated that the combination of antiplatelets and anticoagulants in individuals with ACS does not reduce major adverse cardiac events (MACE), such as all-cause death, nonfatal MI, and nonfatal thromboembolic stroke, but it does increase the risk of major bleeding. Due to the negative clinical outcomes associated with concomitant use of full-dose warfarin and aspirin, this combination is not preferred for long-term treatment of coronary artery disease or peripheral artery disease [63]. "Medications affecting platelet function have a synergistic pharmacodynamic interaction with warfarin; concomitant use, therefore, can result in significant increases in PT-INR and, in turn, in an increased risk of bleeding" [68]. A study done in 278,074 Australian veterans who had been using warfarin demonstrated that approximately 7.2% received co-administration of nonsteroidal anti-inflammatory agents and 5.9% received antiplatelet medications such as NSAIDs. This study, however, did not assess harm associated with these potentially hazardous interactions and noted that their study could not assess concomitant purchase of over-the-counter medications such as aspirin and some NSAIDs [80].

Antibiotics

Antibiotics, like antidepressants, are heavily metabolized by CYP450 enzymes, most notably CYP3A4, and have also been found to interact with permeability glycoproteins. Because many anticoagulants interact with both CYP3A4 and permeability glycoproteins, drug-drug interactions may arise and affect the metabolism of these drugs. Notably, the bioavailability of dabigatran is decreased with concurrent use of clarithromycin and rifampicin. Clarithromycin, erythromycin, fluconazole, and ketoconazole affect the bioavailability of rivaroxaban. Because apixaban and edoxaban are newer drugs, less drug-drug interaction data is available [62]. As detailed in a table from Minno et al., plasma DOAC concentrations can be increased with concurrent use of common antifungals and antibiotics due to inhibition of permeability glycoproteins (P-gp) and CYP450 enzymes [68]. Those that inhibit P-gp and CYP3A4 are the "-conazole" antibiotics: ketoconazole, itraconazole, voriconazole, and posaconazole. those that inhibit P-gp and CYP450 are the "-mycin" antibiotics: erythromycin, clarithromycin, and azithromycin.

NSAIDs

A synergistic effect, which led to increased bleeding, has been noted with the concomitant use of NSAIDs and warfarin. Other commonly used anti-inflammatory drugs, such as acetaminophen, allopurinol, celecoxib, dextropropoxyphene, indomethacin, methyl-prednisolone, piroxicam, sulindac, and tramadol, were all found to increase PT/INR, while mesalazine and sulfasalazine lowered PT/INR [68]. Adverse drug-drug interactions have been noted to occur between NSAIDs and a variety of concomitantly administered medications such as aspirin, alcohol, some antihypertensives, antidepressants, and other commonly used medications [81].

Herbal Supplements/Ginkgo

Like medications discussed previously, many herbal supplements have drug-drug interactions with anticoagulants and may, therefore, contribute to increased bleeding risks. Compared to vitamin K antagonists, such as warfarin, DOAC effects have proven to be more stable and less influenced by herbal supplements or differences in diet [68]. Additionally, the quantity of herbal supplements taken by patients already taking warfarin also influences the risk of bleeding; Chan et al. found that "warfarin patients taking no herbal medications or only 1 herbal <4 times per week were more likely to have PT-INR values within the optimal therapeutic range of 2.0–3.0 compared to those taking >1 type of herbal ≥ 4 times per week (58.1% vs 51.1%, $P = 0.046$)" [60]. Consumption of Ginkgo can also increase the risk of bleeding; in vitro studies have shown that flavanol aglycones like amentoflavone, which are components of Ginkgo, can inhibit CYP2C9 and thereby increase plasma concentrations of anticoagulants metabolized by this enzyme [68].

Drug-Drug Interactions: Specific Drugs

Amiodarone

Since warfarin is used to prevent or reduce the risk of stroke in patients with atrial fibrillation, prosthetic valves, and patients with a history of thromboembolic disorders, both amiodarone and warfarin have been used concurrently. When concerns of ventricular or supraventricular arrhythmias exist, amiodarone (as a Vaughan-Williams class III antiarrhythmic agent with a long half-life) may be administered concurrently with warfarin. It is essential to be aware of the resulting interactions when a patient uses both of these medications. Amiodarone is metabolized by CYP3A4 and CYP2C8 to desethylamiodarone, and these hepatic enzymes are also involved to some extent in warfarin metabolism. Amiodarone decreases CYP2C9 1A2 and 3A4 enzymes and thereby inhibits warfarin hydroxylation [82–84]. This reduces clearance of the more potent S- warfarin. In patients receiving the drug combination of amiodarone and warfarin, the anticoagulation effect is increased from this reduction in hepatic clearance whenever both drugs are administered. Anticoagulation is potentiated since the dose of warfarin required to achieve a therapeutic INR is reduced. Some studies have also suggested altered protein binding as a contributor to this effect.

Multiple factors affect these interactions, such as the patient's specific genetics, and the presence of comorbidities from cardiac, hepatic, or renal systems, thyroid dysfunction, GI bleed, or cancer. The specific interactions affecting the rate of metabolism and clearance may also relate to specific other medications used. These interactions are patient specific and not clearly predictable. Advanced patient age may also reduce the clearance of both medications and increase the potential for adverse interactions.

Drug interaction between warfarin and amiodarone results in a potentiation of warfarin's effect and prolonged INR due to prolonged half-life. In a Swedish retrospective study conducted by Holm et al., more than one in three patients receiving both warfarin and amiodarone revealed supratherapeutic anticoagulative effect within 3 weeks to an INR of around 3.07 [82].

There is an increased bleeding risk when a patient uses both amiodarone and warfarin. After initiation of amiodarone, close monitoring of INR once every 3–4 days to maintain therapeutic level of anticoagulation, and timely dose adjustment, is vital to prevent life-threatening bleeding episodes and thus hospitalizations. A study by Sanoski et al. to determine the dosage relationship in patients on long-term amiodarone indicates that the magnitude of interaction peaks at 7 weeks and is associated with a 44% mean maximum reduction in warfarin dose; the warfarin requirement gradually increased thereafter. Additionally, they report that the interaction is dependent on the maintenance dose of amiodarone [83]. Lam et al., in a retrospective study on older patients found a greater risk of hemorrhage among patients who received amiodarone compared with patients receiving warfarin alone and encountered mortality of 12.5% following initiation of amiodarone [85].

When initiating amiodarone therapy, there are many recommendations. Holm et al. recommend an initial reduction of the mean dose of warfarin by 25% [82]. A study by Sanoski recommends reducing dose of warfarin by 40% when using 400 mg/d of amiodarone and additional 55% reduction in warfarin dose when amiodarone dose is tapered to achieve INR of 2–3 [83]. Family practice physicians were cautioned about the interaction between amiodarone and warfarin in 2002; a percentage reduction in the administered warfarin dose based on the administered amiodarone dose was recommended [86]. Carpenter et al. suggested an empiric warfarin dose reduction of 30–50% upon initiation of amiodarone and weekly INR monitoring [84].

Ciprofloxacin (Cipro)

In a population-based study, Fischer et al. stated that concomitant use of warfarin and ciprofloxacin in older patients increased the risk of hospital admission with upper gastrointestinal hemorrhage [87]. Lane and colleagues found that 42.6% of antimicrobial prescriptions among warfarin users were for medications (TMP/SMX, ciprofloxacin, levofloxacin, metronidazole and fluconazole) that presented risk for excessive bleeding [88].

A study of all 66 cases reported to the FDA spontaneous reporting system (SRS) database from 1987 through 1997, including the two that occurred at his institution, Ellis et al. report that patients previously anticoagulated with warfarin, who have ciprofloxacin administered, may develop an exaggerated hypoprothrombinemic response and bleeding diathesis. In 50 of these patients, this coagulopathy was recognized within 5.5 days following initial administration of ciprofloxacin. The ciprofloxacin–warfarin coagulopathy occurred most commonly in patients in their seventh decade of life and in those who required polypharmacy. Additionally, they reported a more rapid resolution of the coagulopathy when the patients received active treatment for the coagulopathy, rather than simply withholding the medications involved and keeping the patients under medical observation while the coagulopathy spontaneously resolved. This study by Ellis suggests that INR should be checked within 4–5 days following initiation of ciprofloxacin, especially in older patients [89].

Clarithromycin (Biaxin)

Clarithromycin is a macrolide antibiotic. As described by Lane et al., this drug is a high-risk antibiotic that interacts with warfarin and increases the risk of serious bleeding that requires hospitalization [90]. Clarithromycin inhibits warfarin metabolism particularly via CYP3A and P-glycoprotein. It may also eliminate vitamin K-producing bacteria in the intestines to further alter the therapeutic effect of warfarin and prolong the international normalized ratio (INR). INR monitoring is essential within 3–14 days of the prescription to reduce the risk of serious bleeding event. A case report published in Emergency Medicine Journal, 2006, reports a case of retroperitoneal hematoma in a 69-year-old woman who had been on chronic warfarin and was prescribed clarithromycin for lower respiratory infection [91].

Erythromycin, and Quinidine

Both erythromycin and quinidine are known to affect cytochromes P1A2 and P3A4. Al-Jundi and Rubin have described a rare presentation of spontaneous hemopericardiac tamponade in a patient on warfarin who was treated with erythromycin for a chest infection [92].

Rifampin (Rifadin, Rimactane)

Administration of rifampin is known to induce CYP2C9 and CYP3A4, and it therefore increases clearance of warfarin. This may result in a decrease of the INR, unless the dose of warfarin is concomitantly increased by 25–40% when therapy with rifampin is initiated. Poon et al. reported a warfarin-rifampin drug interaction in a 20-month-old-female where the warfarin management posed a challenge due to dramatic increase in warfarin dosing requirement [93].

Metronidazole (Flagyl)

Metronidazole decreases CYP2C9 activity and therefore interferes with metabolism of S-warfarin. This results in an increase in the INR when metronidazole is added to the medications a patient takes, when the patient is using warfarin. This increased INR is likely to be clinically important as the risk for intracranial hemorrhage doubles for each 1.0 increase in the INR. Even if intracranial hemorrhage does not occur, it appears that the risk for other minor bleeding complications increases. It is recommended that the warfarin dose should be reduced by 25–40% when metronidazole (Flagyl) therapy is initiated [94]. A retrospective study by Holt et al., recommends 30–35% reduction in mean daily dose (a preemptive dose reduction) to maintain therapeutic anticoagulation while on metronidazole. However, while considering a preemptive dose reduction of warfarin, the risk of subtherapeutic INR and risk of thromboembolic events should be weighed against risk of bleeding. INR should be monitored no later than 72 h after initiation of both medications in such instances where risk of thromboembolism is high [94].

Trimethoprim/Sulfamethoxazole (Bactrim)

Bactrim is a potent antimicrobial that interacts with warfarin. Antimicrobials can inhibit CYP450 isozymes, alter protein binding, and alter the gut flora, thereby reducing vitamin K absorption. Several studies illustrate that this drug significantly and rapidly elevates INR in patients taking warfarin and significantly increases risks of undesired bleeding, especially in elderly patients. Concomitant use of warfarin and cotrimoxazole was discussed in the Annals of Internal Medicine in 2010. This article clearly states that few drug interactions are as well established as the interactions between these two medications. These interactions were felt to markedly increase risk of upper GI hemorrhage, which qualifies as a "never event" by the National Quality Forum [95]. Bactrim decreases CYP2C9 activity; this is primarily due to the sulfamethoxazole component, rather than from trimethoprim. Concurrent use of warfarin and trimethoprim/sulfamethoxazole is associated with two to fivefold increase in bleeding risk [96]. When initiating bactrim therapy in a patient who is also using warfarin, the INR should be monitored within 3–4 days of starting the antimicrobial. When bactrim is initiated, the recommended dose reduction of warfarin is by 10–20% to avoid potentially dangerous increase in INR prior to the INR follow-up [97]. Dose titration should be slower due to longer half-life of warfarin. It is equally important to adjust the warfarin dose once the antimicrobial is discontinued to avoid subtherapeutic INR. Fischer et al. recommend that in older patients receiving warfarin, it is better to prescribe alternative antibiotics as patients are at high risk for upper GI hemorrhage when cotrimoxazole is administered along with warfarin [87].

Fluvastatin (Lescol)

HMG-CoA (3-hydroxy-3-methylglutaryl coenzyme A) reductase inhibitors are effective in both primary and secondary prevention of ischemic heart disease. Since they are usually prescribed in older patients for a prolonged duration, the drug interactions must always be borne in mind. Fluvastatin is a synthetic HMG Co-A reductase inhibitor and a lipid-regulating drug. Patients with cardiovascular disease are often prescribed warfarin and statins concurrently. In an investigation of the interaction between the two, it was found that fluvastatin significantly displaced the plasma protein binding of warfarin [98]. Fluvastatin inhibits *CYP2C9* and the formation of 7-hydroxy warfarin. This increased warfarin concentrations and increased bleeding risk. Other "statin" medications, lovastatin, rosuvastatin, and simvastatin, exert a similar effect. Although the combination therapy of a "statin" and warfarin is frequently considered useful, the INR should be closely monitored after initiation therapy or a change in the dose of the medication.

Atorvastatin (Lipitor)

Another HMG-CoA reductase inhibitor is often prescribed for both primary and secondary prevention of ischemic heart disease. Since this class of medications is usually prescribed in older patients for a prolonged duration, the drug interactions must always be borne in mind. In addition to the interactions already noted that occur with this class of medications, atorvastatin inhibits *CYP3A4 isozymes,* which metabolizes the less active R isomer and creates the same concerns noted previously with use of itraconazole (Sporanox). An observational study by Schelleman et al. reported that initiation of statins in chronic warfarin users increases the potential risk of gastrointestinal bleeding, especially during the first antihyperlipidemic prescription [99]. A case report in the British Journal of Hospital Medicine describes the rare event of acute rhabdomyolysis following initiation of warfarin in a patient on stable atorvastatin therapy [100]. The mechanism of this appears to be that warfarin administration increased the bioavailability of the statin, resulting in acute rhabdomyolysis. Close monitoring of INR, serum creatine kinase levels, and constant vigilance is required when these drugs are co-prescribed as there is potential for increased bioavailability of either drug.

Carbamazepine (Tegretol)

Carbamazepine is an antiseizure medication of the iminostilbene class, indicated for use in the management of temporal lobe epilepsy/complex partial seizures. Additionally, carbamazepine has been used as a first-line medication for trigeminal neuralgia. It enhances warfarin metabolism by induction of the cytochrome P450 group, primarily CYP2C9 and CYP3A4. A Swedish retrospective study reports that patients on warfarin who were co-administered carbamazepine experienced a subtherapeutic anticoagulation effect within 3–5 weeks. The average warfarin dose was subsequently increased by 49.2% (95% CI 42.8–55.9) to maintain the desired level of anticoagulation [101]. Clarke et al. also found that warfarin dose requirement increased by 32% after carbamazepine initiation. The onset of interaction with warfarin was chronic and with a variable onset ranging from 16 to 30 days in this study. Therefore, the authors did not make a recommendation for a predicted preemptive dose adjustment [102].

Close INR monitoring is essential when carbamazepine is initiated or withdrawn during warfarin therapy, to meet the anticipated change in dose demand and to prevent ischemic stroke and thrombosis.

Fluvoxamine (Luvox)

Concomitant use of fluvoxamine or other selective serotonin reuptake inhibitors (SSRIs) and warfarin is very common, as cardiovascular disease and depression often coexist. In theory, SSRIs could inhibit platelet aggregation by preventing platelet reuptake of serotonin. Fluvoxamine maleate has the potential to inhibit multiple cytochromes (CYP1A2, CYP2C9, CYP2C19, and CYP3A4) to a significant degree. It is a potent CYP2C9 inhibitor with a half-life of 17–22 h after a single dose. This is an important consideration because CYP2C9 is the main metabolizing enzyme of the more active (S)- enantiomer of coumadin. This would appear to increase the risk of excessive anticoagulant effect of warfarin when these medications are co-administered.

A multi-database cohort study by Dong et al. followed 52,129 patients for up to 180 days and analyzed the bleeding and thromboembolic events and mortality in patients exposed to SSRIs and warfarin. They concluded that patients concomitantly treated with warfarin and SSRIs that are potent CYP2C9 inhibitors had comparable rates of bleeding events, ischemic or thrombotic events, and mortality. This study suggests that SSRI inhibition of CYP2C9 does not appear to affect major safety or effectiveness outcomes of warfarin treatment in clinical practice, where patients may be closely monitored [103]. A possible explanation for less impact on pharmacokinetic interaction than expected, and hence minimal effects on clinical outcome, could be upregulation of other enzymes that metabolize warfarin.

In contrast to the Dong study however, a few years prior to its publication, Quinn et al. reported that SSRI exposure was associated with major hemorrhage risk in patients taking warfarin [104]. Almost 2 years earlier Hackam et al. also described an increased risk of intracerebral and intracranial hemorrhage with concomitant use of SSRI and oral anticoagulants when compared to patients with oral anticoagulants alone [105]. It would certainly appear that caution is advised when managing patients using both SSRI medications and warfarin, even though there may be no clear "cause and effect" relationship.

Fluoxetine (Prozac)

Fluoxetine is a selective serotonin reuptake inhibitor, which ranks 14th on the list of medications used concomitantly with warfarin [76]. Fluoxetine hydrochloride is a potent CYP2C9 inhibitor and inhibits oxidative metabolism of S-warfarin. This drug has high affinity for plasma albumin. SSRIs might hinder platelet aggregation by depletion of platelet serotonin levels and could result in an increased therapeutic response and an increase in INR. Recognizing the narrow therapeutic index of warfarin, and the potential for multiple medications used in psychiatry to interfere with it, an analysis of data published in 2009 recommended that while fluvoxamine and fluoxetine pose the highest potential risks, sertraline and citalopram appear to be the safest antidepressant medications to use in patients who concomitantly use warfarin [106].

Itraconazole (Sporanox)

Itraconazole is a broad-spectrum triazole antifungal agent for prophylaxis and treatment of aspergillosis, endemic mycoses, onychomycosis, and vaginal candidiasis. It inhibits CYP3A4, which metabolizes R (+) warfarin (the less biologically active enantiomer of warfarin) and P-glycoprotein, and therefore, interactions are less severe than other azole antifungals [107]. It is recommended to monitor for increased anticoagulant effects (e.g., INR, bleeding) if itraconazole is initiated/dose increased, and decreased effects if itraconazole is discontinued/dose decreased [107].

Fluconazole (Diflucan)

Fluconazole inhibits the metabolism of S-warfarin via CYP2C9 and 8-hydroxylation of R-warfarin through CYP2C19 [108]. UpToDate recommends empiric reduction in warfarin dose of 10–20% along with INR monitoring for dosing titrations [109].

Miconazole (Monistat)

Miconazole is a broad-spectrum antifungal agent and is the strongest inhibitor of CYP2C9 and CYP2C19, followed by voriconazole and fluconazole. Due to the strong inhibition of CYP2C9 and therefore, inhibition of the conversion of (S) warfarin to (S) 7-hydroxywarfarin, PT-INR increases [108]. Elderly patients on warfarin usually have comorbidities and increased risk of oral candidiasis. Systemic absorption after topical administration decreases total body clearance of both (R) and (S) warfarin. A study reports the pro-hemorrhagic effects of ecchymosis, subcutaneous hematomas, and hematuria after two weeks of concomitant use with warfarin [68]. Another case report describes intestinal intramural hematoma presenting as acute abdomen after initiation of topical miconazole for vaginal candidiasis [110]. In patients using warfarin, nystatin appears to be a safer choice for oral candidiasis treatment [111].

Voriconazole (Vfend)

Voriconazole is a triazole with broad-spectrum antifungal activity. It is metabolized by CYP450 enzymes, primarily by CYP2C19, CYP2C9, and CYP3A4 [108]. It is also a strong inhibitor of CYP3A4. The (S) form is the more pharmacologically active isomer. Since the CYP2C9 pathway is involved in its metabolism, the interactions with anticoagulation medications are clinically significant. This involvement results in a prolongation of the prothrombin time. Purkins et al. performed a double-blind randomized controlled study and noted that voriconazole potentiates warfarin-induced prothrombin time prolongation. Without a reduction in warfarin dose, the peak anticoagulation effect at 40–50 h following a voriconazole dose appears to be approximately 50% greater. This enhanced anticoagulation effect can still be seen even at 144 h following co-administration with voriconazole. They recommended regular monitoring of the prothrombin time if voriconazole and warfarin are co-administered [112].

Zafirlukast (Accolate)

Zafirlukast is a selective peptide leukotriene receptor antagonist of three leukotriene C4, D4, and E4 (LTC4, LTD4 and LTE4), which are components of the slow-reacting substance of anaphylaxis (SRSA). Cysteinyl leukotriene production and receptor occupation have been correlated with the pathophysiology of asthma, including airway edema, smooth muscle constriction, and altered cellular activity associated with the inflammatory process, which contribute to the signs and symptoms of asthma. In vitro studies demonstrated that Zafirlukast antagonized the contractile activity of three leukotrienes (LTC_4, LTD_4, and LTE_4) in conducting airway smooth muscle from laboratory animals and humans. It also prevented intradermal LTD_4-induced increases in cutaneous vascular permeability and inhibited inhaled LTD_4-induced influx of eosinophils into animal lungs. In humans, zafirlukast inhibited bronchoconstriction caused by several kinds of inhalational challenges. The bronchodilation, anti-inflammatory properties, and steroid-sparing effects provide significant benefits to patients with allergic and exercise-induced asthma. Pretreatment with single oral doses of zafirlukast inhibited the bronchoconstriction caused by sulfur dioxide and cold air in patients with asthma. It usually takes weeks before maximal benefit is seen when this class of medication is administered. As such, these medications are primarily used for prophylaxis and treatment of allergic and exercise-induced asthma. Zafirlukast exhibits a peak plasma concentration within 3 h after oral administration and exhibits a plasma protein binding of >99% to albumin. Its mean terminal elimination half-life is ~10 h. It is cleared by hepatic metabolism involving hydroxylation by the CYP450 system, primarily utilizing CYP2C9. In vivo studies have demonstrated that zafirlukast inhibits CYP3A4 and CYP2C9 isoenzymes [113]. In patients with significant hepatic impairment (e.g., biopsy proven cirrhosis), there is a reduced clearance resulting in 50–60% greater maximum concentration and a prolonged area under the curve in clearance studies, when compared to normal subjects [114]. If co-administered to a patient on warfarin therapy, Zafirlukast impairs the normal clearance of warfarin, and enhanced antithrombotic effects result. This is demonstrated by an increase in PT and INR values demonstrated on coagulation studies.

Cimetidine (Tagamet)

Use of cimetidine does not appear to be of significant concern to patients taking warfarin. The cytochrome isoenzymes involved in cimetidine metabolism, CYP1A2 and CYP3A4, are primarily involved in the metabolism of the less potent R-warfarin isomer. Interactions and inhibition of metabolism are usually of less magnitude than when co-administered medications affect the CYP2C9 isoenzyme.

Patients with HIV Infections

Patients who suffer from HIV are prone to venous thrombosis. Antiretroviral drug interactions are mediated through the cytochrome P450 pathway and through P-glycoproteins to a lesser extent. Anti-HIV medications are protease inhibitors and therefore demonstrate inhibition of the cytochrome P450 system; they also tend to induce CYP2C9. This tends to enhance the metabolism of warfarin. The extent of this effect and the specific CYP450 isoenzymes involved vary from one anti-HIV medication to another. The INR response from the administration of any of these medications should be monitored when a patient is also using any anti-HIV medications concurrent with the use of anticoagulation medications.

Indinavir (Crixivan)

Indinavir is a protease inhibitor and an inhibitor of CYP3A4. Even though indinavir demonstrates mild to moderate hepatic impairment, there is less concern about excessive inhibition of warfarin metabolism when indinavir is co-administered, because the CYP2C9 isoenzyme is not involved.

Ritonavir (Norvir)

Liedtke and Rathbun found that intermittent ritonavir use may result in inhibition of CYP2C9 and CYP3A4, rather than induction [115].

Prednisone (Deltasone, Sterapred, Preds, Etc.)

Prednisone is a frequently used anti-inflammatory agent. Prednisone and warfarin have been used together in idiopathic hypereosinophilic syndrome (IHES), a rare disease associated with cardiac thrombosis and endocardial wall thickness. They are also prescribed together in the management of peripheral vascular disease associated with autoimmune disease, systemic lupus erythematosus (SLE), multiple myeloma, Behcet's disease, etc. Case reports indicate an increased INR response after the addition of prednisone to warfarin [116].

A randomized controlled trial by Dowd et al. compared a 10–20% preemptive dose reduction vs. a reactive adjustment and found that the preemptive warfarin dose reduction resulted in a nonsignificant reduction in supratherapeutic INR but, contrary to expectations, increased the chances of subtherapeutic INR [117]. These studies demonstrate that an increase in INR within 3–10 days after corticosteroid initiation may be expected. Timely INR monitoring is essential when these two medications are co-prescribed. A therapeutic dose adjustment may be expected but should be based on INR response.

Nonsteroidal Anti-inflammatory Drugs (NSAIDs)

NSAIDs are commonly used to control musculoskeletal pain. NSAIDs are known to interact with warfarin due to their high protein binding and their cytochrome P450 dependent clearance mechanism. Additionally, they also have antiplatelet effects. NSAIDs may cause gastric ulcers by erosion of the stomach lining and increase the risk of significant gastrointestinal bleeding when the anticoagulant effect of warfarin is superimposed. Yildirim et al. have described a rare complication in an 80-year-old female on stable chronic warfarin therapy for the previous ten years and who was tested regularly for anticoagulation status. Her last INR values prior to this emergency presentation had been 2.1. Following use of a non-steroidal anti-inflammatory medication for arthritis pain three days earlier, she presented to the emergency department with complaints of the sudden onset of severe abdominal pain but had not noted melena or hematochezia. CT evaluation demonstrated findings of distal jejunum and proximal ileal transmural thickening along with extensive free peritoneal fluid. During her observation in the emergency department, her hemoglobin level dropped to 3 g/dL and she developed hemorrhagic shock, despite no clear evidence of external bleeding or intraluminal intestinal bleeding. On admission, she had a prothrombin time of 68.9 s and INR of 12. She was given fresh frozen plasma, vitamin K supplements, and red blood cells to normalize INR and hemoglobin level [118].

Chronic Ethanol Use or Abuse

Chronic ethanol ingestion increased warfarin clearance via induction of CYP2E1, while acute ethanol use inhibits warfarin metabolism.

Vitamin K

Many foods contain significant amounts of vitamin K. The average person in the United States takes in 60–80 micrograms (mcg) of vitamin K per day. Dietary vitamin K can alter the effectiveness of warfarin. Consistency in dietary intake of food containing high amounts of potassium is also important for patients on warfarin. Dietary supplements that contain vitamin K or metabolites related to vitamin K-coenzyme Q10 have the potential to reduce the effects of warfarin. Other dietary constituents which may affect a patient's coagulation status, especially when using anticoagulation medications, include weight-loss diets (rich in green vegetables), multivitamins/dietary supplements, broccoli, brussels sprouts, cabbage, collard greens, endive, kale, lettuce, mustard greens, parsley, spinach, swiss chard, turnip greens, watercress, lentils, garbanzo beans, soybeans, soybean, canola oil, olive oil, liver (from beef, pork, or chicken), avocados, dried basil, thyme, oregano, dill pickle, green peas, foods packed in oil, snack foods fortified with vitamin

K, grapefruit, grapefruit juice (the component furanocoumarin in grapefruit and grapefruit juice decreases warfarin metabolism by inhibiting CYP3A4), store-bought margarine, store-bought mayonnaise, and store-bought salad dressings (due to vegetable oil content).

St. John's Wort (Hypericum perforatum)

Herbal supplements, which are not FDA-approved medications can often be overlooked. It is not always easy to elicit the history of ingestion of herbal supplements from the patients, as they might mistakenly think that they are herbs and hence innocuous. Herbs have the potential to cause adverse effects when used concomitantly with medications as they contain bioactive compounds. Patients should be educated regarding the possible interactions, risks, and consequences with drugs and supplements. St. John's Wort is notably used for depression, sleep disorders, anxiety, and pain. It is documented to interact with 147 medications [119]. Its decreases the plasma concentration of warfarin by inducing CYP2C9 and CYP3A4 [120, 121]. This increases the clearance of both R and S enantiomers of warfarin. Thus, concurrent use of St John's Wort reduces the efficacy of warfarin, putting the patient at a greater risk for a decrease in the INR and the development of a thrombotic event.

In summary, many drug-drug interactions between anticoagulants and other medications exist, and careful consideration of these interactions is recommended during the peri-operative period. If physicians are not diligent about attention to detail, serious, avoidable complications related to excessive or inadequate anticoagulation may arise.

When considering them as a group, anticoagulants are an exceptional class of medications that help to provide life-saving prophylaxis and treatment for thromboembolic events. Many individuals are prescribed anticoagulation for the remaining duration of life. Without these medications, complications such as blood clots, DVTs, PEs, and strokes would be much more common and would have much higher mortality rates. Anticoagulants are effective, cost-efficient, and used all over the world. However, risks of side effects and other adverse effects are associated with the use of medications, which provide anticoagulation effects. Many drug-drug interactions exist, which may adversely impact the safe and effective use of these medications. Due to the often fast-paced and trauma-associated nature of their specialties, anesthesiologists and physicians working in Emergency Rooms should be well-informed about potential risks associated with the various medications, which have anticoagulation properties. When using anticoagulation medications, patients should keep readily found information with them (e.g., Medic-Alert bracelets or other identification cards), which will quickly alert medical personnel to use of these agents. Proper management by medical personnel can be achieved only when they readily know, which anticoagulant medication, or combination of anticoagulation medications, is being used.

Antifibrinolytics

Under normal physiologic conditions, both the coagulation and fibrinolytic systems are intimately related allowing for balanced hemostasis. Fibrinolysis is a tightly controlled enzymatic process that is responsible for blood clot regulation and breakdown. These processes are regulated by a vast array of receptors, inhibitors, and cofactors [122]. Fibrin is a central component and serves as the main conduit for both thrombus breakdown and formation. Plasminogen is converted to plasmin via two primary serine proteases, tissue plasminogen activator (tPA), and urokinase plasminogen activator (uPA). Plasmin acts as the primary fibrinolysin for thrombus breakdown. tPA is synthesized and released by endothelial cells and is found intravascularly [122, 123]. When compared to tPA, uPA has a lower affinity to plasminogen, is primarily extravascular, and is located in the urinary epithelium, macrophages, and monocytes [122]. In vivo, both have very short half-lives of 4–8 min and are hepatically cleared. This brief half-life is attributable to the high concentrations of circulating serine protease inhibiting factors like plasminogen activator-inhibitor-1(PAI-1). Serine protease inhibitors play a pivotal role to inhibit excess and unregulated plasmin activity. Our understanding and appreciation of fibrinolysis has been greatly improved with the advent of rotational thromboelastography (ROTEM). ROTEM allows for a visual representation of fibrinolysis and can indicate normal, hyper, or hypoactive fibrin breakdown. A detailed description of the many components of the fibrinolytic pathway is beyond the scope of this paper. A review of the most common antifibrinolytics is below.

Antifibrinolytics act by inhibiting the fibrinolytic cascade and preventing the breakdown of blood clots. Their use has been broadly studied for control of hemorrhage in trauma, cardiac surgery, traumatic brain injury, and numerous other clinical situations. Examples of antifibrinolytics include aprotinin, tranexamic acid (TXA), and epsilon-aminocaproic acid. Aprotinin is a serine protease inhibitor that is no longer used in clinical practice. Results from the blood conservation using antifibrinolytics in a randomized trial (BART) found an increased risk of 30-day mortality after use in cardiac surgery [123, 124]. Subsequent studies have also shown that patients given aprotinin have an increased risk of kidney failure, stroke, heart failure, and 5-year mortality [123–125]. As a result of these findings, clinical focus has shifted to the lysine analogs, TXA, and epsilon-aminocaproic acid.

Both tranexamic acid (TXA) and epsilon-aminocaproic acid are synthetic lysine analogs that work by competitively inhibiting the activation of plasminogen to plasmin [125]. The inhibition of plasminogen maintains fibrin integrity and prevents clot degradation. TXA is 6–10 times more potent than its counterpart epsilon-aminocaproic acid [126]. Unlike aprotinin, both lysine analogs have been shown to increase thrombus formation by increasing ADP content in platelets without resulting in increased thromboembolic events like a pulmonary embolus [126]. TXA has also been found to have anti-inflammatory properties by mitigating cytokine release. A randomized controlled trial consisting of 50 patients undergoing cardiopulmonary bypass (CPB) found that patients who received TXA had a significantly lower levels of inflammatory markers compared to those that received placebo [127]. Decreased levels of inflammatory cytokines translate to less severe vasoplegic shock, less time requiring vasopressor support, and decreased time for mechanical respiratory support in the postoperative period [127]. In patients undergoing cardiac surgery with CPB, either TXA or epsilon-aminocaproic acid is routinely given to reduce perioperative bleeding and also subsequently decrease transfusion of blood products.

Lysine analogs have also shown significant benefits in noncardiac surgery. A recent meta-analysis included over 10,000 patients and found that those who received TXA had a 38% reduction in probability to require a blood transfusion compared to those patients who did not receive TXA [128]. The landmark CRASH-2 study looked at TXA administration in over 20,000 hemorrhagic trauma patients [129]. Patients who received TXA upon initial presentation were found to have a significant reduction in all-cause mortality and death due to bleeding compared to those that did not get TXA [128]. Even more recently, the CRASH-3 trial looked at TXA administration within 3 h in patients with traumatic brain injury [130]. Findings were significant for a reduction in injury-related death in those that received TXA compared to those that did not [130]. Both TXA and epsilon-aminocaproic acid have also been found to be beneficial for reducing blood loss in orthopedic surgery, facilitating control of gastrointestinal hemorrhage and pulmonary hemorrhage [126].

TXA and epsilon-aminocaproic acid have a half-life of 2–3 h and are primarily cleared renally. Clinicians need to be cognizant of potential adverse effects associated with lysine analogs. High-dose TXA is associated with a dose-dependent increase in seizures [131]. Epsilon-aminocaproic acid may also have an increased risk of renal dysfunction; however, more research needs to be done for confirmation.

Antiplatelets

Antiplatelet drugs work by inhibiting the capacity of platelets to participate in the clotting process. There are several discrete mechanisms by which platelets activate and aggregate. Thus, there are several pharmacologic targets. A growing area of concern and research are the various interactions antiplatelet drugs can participate in with other drugs and commonly consumed substances.

When vessel endothelium is damaged, platelets are exposed to subendothelial matrix, which triggers multiple intracellular signaling pathways that lead to glycoprotein IIb/IIIa complexes on platelets activating and binding to fibrinogen, which results in platelet aggregation. One of these intracellular pathways is activated by thromboxane A2, which is produced by activated of cyclooxygenase-1 [132]. The antiplatelet action of aspirin is primarily mediated through its inhibition of COX-1 and consequently its inhibition of the thromboxane A2 pathway to platelet activation. Aspirin is unique among the NSAIDs in that it irreversibly inhibits COX by acetylating serine residues. It is readily absorbed in the acidic gastric environment where it can inhibit the protective effects of prostaglandins on the stomach lining [133]. Thromboxane A2 inhibition within platelets is cumulative with repeated low doses of aspirin due to the irreversible enzyme inactivation via acetylation throughout the 7–10-day lifetime of platelets. This allows for aspirin to be given once daily and be effective despite its very short half-life (15–20 min) [132]. For patients with ACS, a recommended 150–325 mg of oral aspirin is chewed to achieve rapid inhibition of thromboxane A2 [134]. Frequently aspirin is used for treatment and prophylaxis of pathologic thrombus formation. 100 mg/day is sufficient for prevention of thrombus formation in the coronary circulation; higher doses may be required for the prevention of vascular events in the cerebral and peripheral circulation [13].

Aspirin has numerous interactions with various drugs. While non-aspirin NSAIDs also inhibit COX, they are not useful for platelet inhibition due to their reversible mode of action, which does not ensure permanent platelet inhibition. Most NSAIDs including, celecoxib, dipyrone (active metabolite), ibuprofen, flufenamic acid, naproxen, nimesulide, oxaprozin, and piroxicam significantly interfere with the antiplatelet activity of aspirin. Diclofenac, ketorolac, and acetaminophen do not interfere with aspirin. This is thought to be due to interfering with NSAIDs forming hydrogen bonds with the aspirin binding site [135]. There is also evidence that co-administration can lead to an increased risk of myocardial infarction [81]. Alcohol consumption with aspirin is associated with an increased risk of GI bleeding [136], and smoking cigarettes increases platelet aggregation and suppressing the effect of aspirin [137]. When administered with tamoxifen, aspirin decreases the angiogenic potential of some breast cancers [138]. There is evidence which shows that aspirin can blunt the effect with ACE-inhibitors, but paradoxically, there is evidence of reduced mortality with co-administration [139]. Triple therapy with ACE-inhibitors, diuretics, and NSAIDs, including aspirin, has been associated with an increased risk of acute kidney injury [140]. Serotonergic agents, such as selective serotonin reuptake inhibitors, can increase risk of bleeding when combined with any oral anticoagulant, including antiplatelets and aspirin [141].

P2Y12 is an adenosine diphosphate (ADP) receptor that, once activated, propagates intracellular signals that increase intracellular calcium, alter platelet shape, and increase platelet aggregation [142]. P2Y12 antagonists block these receptors. The use of aspirin and a P2Y12 receptor antagonist, known as dual antiplatelet therapy, is the basis of treatment in patients with ACS and those undergoing coronary stenting [132]. Clopidogrel and prasugrel are both prodrugs that need biotransformation in the liver to become active [143]. These two drugs irreversibly inhibit the P2Y12 receptor. Steady-state inhibition of platelet function is noted after 5–7 days of clopidogrel maintenance dosing, accounting for the role of a loading dose to achieve more rapid inhibition. For clopidogrel, the recommended loading dose is 600 mg, and maintenance dose is 75 mg [132].

Clopidogrel is the most popular P2Y12 inhibitor and has numerous interactions with other substances. Proton-pump inhibitors (PPIs), such as omeprazole and esomeprazole (both substrates and inhibitors of CYP2C19), are associated with decreased inhibition of platelet aggregation by clopidogrel [144, 145]. However, more research remains on whether this affects clinical outcomes. Unlike aspirin, nicotine was found to increase the antiplatelet activity of clopidogrel [146], while grapefruit juice and ketoconazole decrease antiplatelet activity [147] due to the induction and inhibition of liver cytochrome enzymes respectively. Clopidogrel, aspirin, and warfarin have increased risk of GI bleeding when taken in combination than when any is taken alone [148].

Ticagrelor, another P2Y12 inhibitor, acts by reversibly binding P2Y12 away from the active site [132]. Ticagrelor is not a prodrug, and the recommended loading and maintenance doses are 180 mg once and 90 mg twice per day [132]. Ticagrelor is more effective than clopidogrel in preventing major cardiovascular events in patients with acute coronary syndromes, but is associated with increased bleeding events, ventricular pauses, and dyspnea [142]. Some research has shown evidence that administration of high doses of aspirin can blunt ticagrelor's effects [142, 149]. Ticagrelor is an inhibitor of CYP3A4 and consequently can increase plasma concentrations of simvastatin and lovastatin. This could potentially catalyze rhabdomyolysis and myopathy in vulnerable patients [150]. Statins and ticagrelor are commonly co-administered for long-term maintenance of ACS patients, and more research needs to be conducted to stratify risk and monitor long-term patient outcomes.

The intracellular signals generated by the stimulation of platelet receptors results in conformational change of the major platelet adhesion receptor, GPIIb/IIIa (integrin-$\alpha_{IIb}\beta_3$) [151]. GPIIb/IIIa exists in a low-affinity conformation on the resting platelet, which can bind immobilized, but not soluble, fibrinogen. When platelets are activated, signals are propagated from within the platelet, which leads to a change in the conformation of GPIIb/IIIa from a low-affinity to a high-affinity state that enables binding to soluble plasma proteins. These protein ligands include vWF, fibronectin, and the primary GPIIb/IIIa ligand fibrinogen [151, 152]. Thus, this integrin receptor is the crux of stable platelet aggregation and thrombus formation, making it an excellent target for pharmacotherapy.

GPIIb/IIIa inhibitors prevent fibrinogen from binding to activated platelets, thus directly inhibiting their aggregation. Three agents are currently in use: abciximab, a humanized antigen-binding fragment of a mouse monoclonal antibody; eptifibatide, a cyclic heptapeptide with a motif mimicking the fibrinogen binding sequence within GPIIb/IIIa; and tirofiban, a nonpeptidic small molecule also mimicking the fibrinogen binding site [153]. However, except in high-risk patients, the clinical use of integrin αIIbβ3 antagonists has recently decreased due to the increased use of ADP receptor antagonists. This replacement stems from the demonstrated benefit of ADP receptor antagonists [154]. Therefore, the clinical benefit derived from GPIIb/IIIa inhibitors seems to be restricted to particular high-risk subgroups, such as patients with MI undergoing PCI without pretreatment with a P2Y12 antagonist [152]. GPIIb/IIIa inhibitors are potent antithrombotic drugs and can cause bleeding complications in up to 50% of patients [155].

There are other less well-known and less studied drugs that affect platelet function. Cilostazol inhibits phosphodiesterase III and increases levels of cyclic AMP, which leads to vasodilation, reduction of vascular smooth muscle proliferation, and inhibition of platelet aggregation. Cilostazol is suggested for symptomatic management of peripheral vascular disease and has been used after percutaneous coronary intervention and for secondary prevention of non-cardioembolic stroke or TIA. Its effects are strongly potentiated by ketoconazole and likely by other CYP3A4 inhibitors such as itraconazole, fluconazole, miconazole, fluvoxamine, fluoxetine, nefazodone, sertraline, and macrolides [156]. There is evidence that it is moderately inhibited by lovastatin [156].

Dipyridamole blocks the uptake of adenosine, which acts on the platelet A_2-receptor to activate platelet adenylate cyclase, reducing platelet aggregation. Dipyridamole also inhibits phosphodiesterase. This drug is used for prevention of postoperative thromboembolic complications associated

Table 19.1 Common antiplatelets and their actions

Drug	Mechanism of action	Interactions
Aspirin	Inhibits COX and the formation of thromboxane A2	NSAIDs (except diclofenac, ketorolac), alcohol, cigarettes, tamoxifen, ACE-inhibitors, diuretics, serotonergic agents (SSRIs)
Clopidogrel	Irreversibly inhibits the ADP P2Y12 receptor	Omeprazole, esomeprazole, nicotine, grapefruit juice, ketoconazole, warfarin, serotonergic agents (SSRIs)
Ticagrelor	Reversibly inhibits P2Y12 receptor	Statins, serotonergic agents (SSRIs)
Cilostazol	Blocks phosphodiesterase	Ketoconazole, itraconazole, fluconazole, miconazole, fluvoxamine, fluoxetine, nefazodone, sertraline, macrolides, serotonergic agents (SSRIs), lovastatin
Dipyridamole	Blocks adenosine receptor	Adenosine, LMWH, warfarin, clopidogrel, serotonergic agents (SSRIs)

with cardiac valve replacement and for prevention of secondary stroke [132]. Dipyridamole has multiple drug interactions. Dipyridamole potentiates the effects of adenosine likely because the inhibition leads to increased intravascular adenosine concentration and could cause symptomatic bradycardia [157]. It may also increase bleeding risk with low molecular weight heparin, ticagrelor, and warfarin.

Metformin has been shown to decrease thrombosis by inhibiting platelet activation through a novel pathway involving mitochondrial DNA release [158]. Fish oil has some evidence of antiplatelet effect and may potentiate the effect of antiplatelet drugs [159].

Platelet aggregation and coagulation is a complex phenomenon with multiple pharmacologic targets for antithrombus therapy. Despite the complexity, two main drug classes make up the bulk of antiplatelet therapy, aspirin, and P2Y12 inhibitors. These drugs also interact with a variety of other drugs and commonly ingested compounds. Common antiplatelet drugs, their mechanisms of action, and main drug interactions are summarized in Table 19.1.

Summary and Future Directions

Anticoagulant, antiplatelet, and antifibrinolytic drugs are some of the most commonly prescribed drugs in the world, and their concurrent use with other popular drugs may cause effects that are undesirable. The list of indications for anticoagulant therapy is extensive and warranted for those with concerns for clotting, but the interactions of these drugs with other prescription pharmaceuticals or over-the-counter supplements may be associated with an increased risk of bleeding or clotting. Recent studies have begun to uncover drug-drug interactions with some of the most commonly prescribed medications, such as antidepressants that have serotonin reuptake inhibition as their main mechanism of action, being associated with an increased risk of bleeding when taken with aspirin or other NSAIDs [160]. The current CDC recommends that all adults 50–69 years old with a ≥10% risk of cardiovascular disease take a low-dose aspirin daily to prevent cardiovascular disease and colorectal cancer [161]. In recent years, it has been reported that one in eight Americans have taken antidepressants within the last month, and that number has continued to increase consistently since the 1990s [162]. Ideally, every patient would understand each medication they are taking, the reason why they are prescribed the medication, and would have informed their primary care physician of every medication and supplement they are currently taking to decrease drug-drug interactions. Asking the general population to fully understand the complexity of their medications and disease processes is not feasible, but continually exploring the interactions of popular medications is of the utmost importance to progress the field of medicine and decrease the number of complications that patients experience.

New commonly used anticoagulants such as rivaroxaban, dabigatran, apixaban, warfarin, and heparin are a mainstay treatment for a plethora of afflictions, and it is a relatively common occurrence for these medications to be taken alongside other popular medications. Antidepressants, antiplatelet, antibiotics, and herbal supplements are very common among the general population, and these drugs can interact with anticoagulants to make them function outside of their therapeutic range. Warfarin's mechanism of action is unique in that it works by competitively inhibiting the vitamin K epoxide reductase complex 1, an essential enzyme for activating the vitamin K available in the body [12]. The action of warfarin is based on having a consistent amount of vitamin K in the individual's diet, and any change in diet or drugs that alter the amount of available vitamin K changes the efficacy of warfarin [12]. Bactrim, prednisone, and various SSRIs are some of the most commonly prescribed medications that alter the function of warfarin and make obtaining the therapeutic index more difficult.

Antifibrinolytics are used to obtain optimal coagulation, especially in the setting of surgical intervention. Antifibrinolytics inhibit the conversion of plasminogen to plasmin, which removes excess fibrin to promote fibrin clot forming and wound healing [163]. Aprotinin, tranexamic acid, and epsilon-aminocaproic acid are a few examples of antifibrinolytics that are used to prevent blood loss in patients having surgery [164]. These drugs are commonly used in surgery and also in the setting of acute trauma with blood loss [165]. Some drugs that affect antifibrinolytic therapy are anti-inhibitor coagulant complex, chlorpromazine, tretinoin, nicotine, and alcohol. Nicotine and alcohol are some of the most commonly used substances in the world, and their interactions with coagulation pharmaceuticals do not stop at antifibrinolytic therapy. Antiplatelet drugs are also affected by an array of commonly prescribed medication.

Antiplatelet therapy works by inhibiting the ability of platelets to participate in the clotting process and some of the most common antiplatelet drugs being aspirin, clopidogrel, and ticagrelor. Aspirin has long been recommended by the CDC as prophylaxis to prevent pathologic thrombus formation and is commonly used on an "as-needed" basis for common aches and pains. Alcohol can cause an increased risk of GI bleeding in patients taking aspirin, while cigarette smoking can increase platelet aggregation and suppress the effects of aspirin [136, 137]. Commonly prescribed hypertension medications can have drug-drug interactions with antiplatelet drugs, which can hinder both drugs in acting therapeutically [139]. Proton pump inhibitors, metformin, and antidepressants, (specifically selective serotonin reuptake inhibitors) may affect the efficacy of antiplatelet therapy when these drugs are given together [158, 166]. With the high rate of drug-drug interactions with antiplatelet, anticoagulant, and antifibrinolytic therapies, progress is being made to develop newer therapies that decrease the rate of drug-drug interaction.

A 2017 study looked at the possibility of targeting mast cell granular content as it plays a role in the formation of deep venous thrombosis [167]. Current therapies available for deep venous thrombosis target the coagulation cascade, and complications can arise from altering this homeostasis maintenance process. Inflammation has been proven to play a role in triggering deep venous thrombosis, and mast cells are known to play a major role in allergic inflammation, a risk factor for deep venous thrombosis [167]. Granules within mast cells are filled with anticoagulants such as heparin and tissue-type plasminogen activator, endothelial activators, and many other enzymes that aid in the anticoagulation process [167]. In this recent study, the authors looked at the possibility of targeting mast cells to prevent deep vein thrombosis from occurring as an alternative means to conventional therapy for patients with anticoagulation concerns. The study looked at mast cell-deficient mice versus wild-type mice, and their results proved mast cells play a definite role in the development of deep venous thrombosis [167]. The results of their study showed that the two strains of mice that were deficient in mast cells were protected from deep vein thrombosis while maintaining their bleeding homeostasis under the control of the coagulation cascade [167]. The mast cells' effect was proven to be a combination of release of histamine and mast cell granule constituents [167]. While more research is needed to determine the efficacy that this study would have in the human population, this study shows the potential of a new target in human deep venous thrombosis prevention [167]. See Fig. 19.3.

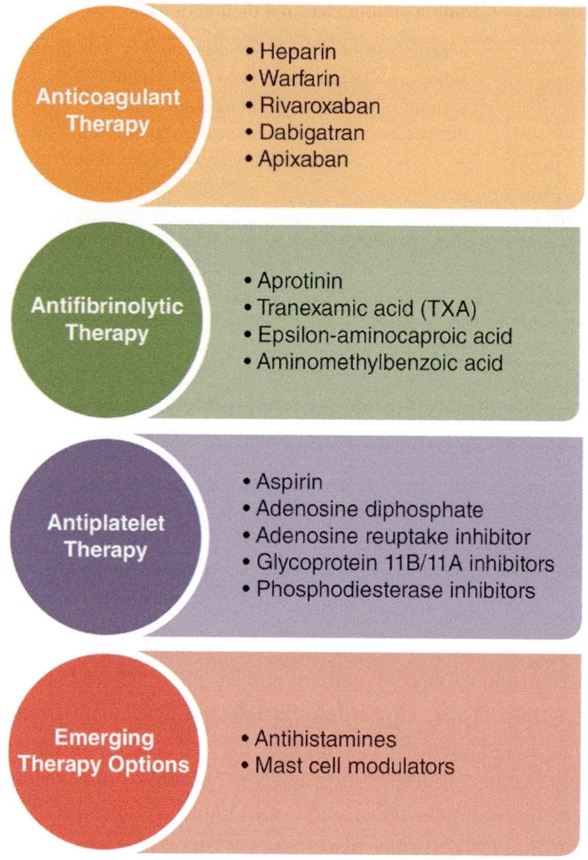

Fig. 19.3 Summary of anticoagulant, antifibrinolytic, antiplatelet, and emerging therapies

References

1. Dahlbäck B. Advances in understanding pathogenic mechanisms of thrombophilic disorders. Blood. 2008;112(1):19–27.
2. Franchini M, Liumbruno GM, Bonfanti C, Lippi G. The evolution of anticoagulant therapy. Blood Transfus. 2016;14(2):175–84.
3. Benjamin EJ, Muntner P, Alonso A, Bittencourt MS, Callaway CW, Carson AP, Chamberlain AM, Chang AR, Cheng S, Das SR, Delling FN, Djousse L, Elkind MSV, Ferguson JF, Fornage M, Jordan LC, Khan SS, Kissela BM, Knutson KL, Kwan TW, Lackland DT, Lewis TT, Lic VS. Heart disease and stroke statistics-2019 at-a-glance heart disease, stroke and other cardiovascular diseases. Am Hear Assoc. 2019;139:1–5.
4. Raskob GE, Silverstein R, Bratzler DW, Heit JA, White RH. Surveillance for deep vein thrombosis and pulmonary embolism. Recommendations from a national workshop. Am J Prev Med. 2010;38(4 SUPPL):S502–9.
5. Moser KM, LeMoine JR. Is embolic risk conditioned by location of deep venous thrombosis? Ann Intern Med. 1981;94(4 pt 1):439–44.
6. Heit JA, Spencer FA, White RH. The epidemiology of venous thromboembolism. J Thromb Thrombolysis. 2016;41(1):3–14.
7. Grosse SD, Nelson RE, Nyarko KA, Richardson LC, Raskob GE. The economic burden of incident venous thromboembolism in the United States: a review of estimated attributable healthcare costs. Thromb Res. 2016;137:3–10. [Internet]. Available from: https://linkinghub.elsevier.com/retrieve/pii/S0049384815302097

8. Heit JA, Ashrani AA, Crusan DJ, McBane RD, Petterson TM, Bailey KR. Reasons for the persistent incidence of venous thromboembolism. Thromb Haemost. 2017;117(2):390–400.
9. Kearon C, Akl EA, Ornelas J, Blaivas A, Jimenez D, Bounameaux H, et al. Antithrombotic therapy for VTE disease. Chest. 2016;149(2):315–52.
10. Lauw MN, Büller HR. Treatment of deep vein thrombosis. In: Current approaches to deep vein thrombosis. Future medicine, 2014. https://www.futuremedicine.comhttps://doi.org/10.2217/fmeb2013.13.98.
11. Gray E, Mulloy B, Barrowcliffe TW. Heparin and low-molecular-weight heparin. Thromb Haemost. 2008;99(5):807–18.
12. DeLoughery TG. Warfarin. In: Hemostasis and thrombosis. 3rd ed. Springer, Cham; 2015. https://doi.org/10.1007/978-3-319-09312-3.
13. Schrör K. Aspirin and platelets: the antiplatelet action of aspirin and its role in thrombosis treatment and prophylaxis. Semin Thromb Hemost. 1997;23(4):349–56.
14. Wakefield TW, Obi AT, Henke PK. An aspirin a day to keep the clots away. Circulation. 2014;130(13):1031–3.
15. Marik PE, Cavallazzi R. Extended anticoagulant and aspirin treatment for the secondary prevention of thromboembolic disease: a systematic review and meta-analysis. PLoS One. 2015;10(11):1–12.
16. Mant J, Hobbs FR, Fletcher K, Roalfe A, Fitzmaurice D, Lip GY, et al. Warfarin versus aspirin for stroke prevention in an elderly community population with atrial fibrillation (the Birmingham atrial fibrillation treatment of the aged study, BAFTA): a randomised controlled trial. Lancet. 2007;370(9586):493–503.
17. Levy JH, Koster A, Quinones QJ, Milling TJ, Key NS. Antifibrinolytic therapy and perioperative considerations. Anesthesiology. 2018;128(3):657–70.
18. Kattula S, Byrnes JR, Wolberg AS. Fibrinogen and fibrin in hemostasis and thrombosis. Arterioscler Thromb Vasc Biol. 2017;37(3):e13–21.
19. Dhir A Antifibrinolytics in cardiac surgery. Ann Card Anaesth. 2013;16(2):117–25.
20. Dunn CJ, Goa KL. Tranexamic acid: a review of its use in surgery and other indications. Drugs. 1999;57(6):1005–32. https://doi.org/10.2165/00003495-199957060-00017.
21. Lumsden MA, Wedisinghe L. Tranexamic acid therapy for heavy menstrual bleeding. Expert Opin Pharmacother. 2011;12(13):2089–95.
22. Vojacek J. Clinical monitoring of the antithrombotic treatment. Cor Vasa. 2012;54(2):e97–103.
23. Weinberger J. Adverse effects and drug interactions of antithrombotic agents used in prevention of ischaemic stroke. Drugs. 2005;65(4):461–71.
24. Hicks RW, Wanzer LJ, Goeckner B. Perioperative pharmacology: blood coagulation modifiers. AORN J. 2011;93(6):726–36.
25. Moore N. Ibuprofen: a journey from prescription to over-the-counter use. J R Soc Med. 2007;100(Suppl 48):2–6.
26. Tsai HH, Lin HW, Lu YH, Chen YL, Mahady GB. A review of potential harmful interactions between anticoagulant/antiplatelet agents and Chinese herbal medicines. PLoS One. 2013;8(5):e64255.
27. Serebruany VL. Selective serotonin reuptake inhibitors and increased bleeding risk: are we missing something? Am J Med. 2006;119(2):113–6.
28. Schalekamp T, Klungel OH, Souverein PC, De Boer A. Increased bleeding risk with concurrent use of selective serotonin reuptake inhibitors and coumarins. Arch Intern Med. 2008;168(2):180–5.
29. Barnes GD, Ageno W, Ansell J, Kaatz S. Recommendation on the nomenclature for oral anticoagulants: communication from the SSC of the ISTH. J Thromb Haemost. 2015;13(6):1154–6.
30. Kane S. NOAC, DOAC, or TSOAC: what should we call novel oral anticoagulants? Pharm Times. 2016.
31. Easton JD, Lopes RD, Bahit MC, Wojdyla DM, Granger CB, Wallentin L, et al. Apixaban compared with warfarin in patients with atrial fibrillation and previous stroke or transient ischaemic attack: a subgroup analysis of the ARISTOTLE trial. Lancet Neurol. 2012;11(6):503–11.
32. Giugliano RP, Ruff CT, Braunwald E, Murphy SA, Wiviott SD, Halperin JL, et al. Edoxaban versus warfarin in patients with atrial fibrillation. N Engl J Med. 2013;369(22):2093–104.
33. Patel MR, Mahaffey KW, Garg J, Pan G, Singer DE, Hacke W, et al. Rivaroxaban versus warfarin in nonvalvular atrial fibrillation. N Engl J Med. 2011;365(10):883–91.
34. Connolly SJ, Ezekowitz MD, Yusuf S, Eikelboom J, Oldgren J, Parekh A, et al. Dabigatran versus warfarin in patients with atrial fibrillation. N Engl J Med. 2009;361(12):1139–51.
35. Joe D. More in-depth version of the coagulation cascade. Wikimedia Commons. 2007; p. N/A
36. Bowen R. vitamin K. Vivo Pathophysiology. 2019. p. N/A.
37. Shearer MJ. vitamin K deficiency bleeding (VKDB) in early infancy. Blood Rev. 2009;23(2):49–59.
38. Controversies concerning vitamin K and the newborn. American academy of pediatrics committee on fetus and newborn. Pediatrics. 2003;112(1 Pt 1):191–2.
39. Pirmohamed M. Warfarin: almost 60 years old and still causing problems. Br J Clin Pharmacol. 2006;62(5):509–11.
40. Higdon J. vitamin K. Linus Pauling Institute. Miconutrient Information Center. 2000. p. N/A.
41. Leung, LLK, Mannucci, PM, Tirnauer JS. Direct oral anticoagulants and parenteral direct thrombin inhibitors: dosing and adverse effects - UpToDate. UpToDate. 2019. p. N/A.
42. Mueck W, Stampfuss J, Kubitza D, Becka M. Clinical pharmacokinetic and pharmacodynamic profile of rivaroxaban. Clin Pharmacokinet. 2014;53(1):1–16.
43. Gerotziafas GT, Elalamy I, Depasse F, Perzborn E, Samama MM. In vitro inhibition of thrombin generation, after tissue factor pathway activation, by the oral, direct factor Xa inhibitor rivaroxaban. J Thromb Haemost. 2007;5(4):886–8.
44. Samama MM. The mechanism of action of rivaroxaban – an oral, direct factor Xa inhibitor – compared with other anticoagulants. Thromb Res. 2011;127(6):497–504.
45. Mueck W, Lensing AWA, Agnelli G, Decousus H, Prandoni P, Misselwitz F. Rivaroxaban: population pharmacokinetic analyses in patients treated for acute deep-vein thrombosis and exposure simulations in patients with atrial fibrillation treated for stroke prevention. Clin Pharmacokinet. 2011;50(10):675–86.
46. Kearon C, Akl EA. Duration of anticoagulant therapy for deep vein thrombosis and pulmonary embolism. Blood. 2014;123(12):1794–801.
47. DeLoughery EP, Shatzel JJ. A comparative analysis of the safety profile of direct oral anticoagulants using the FDA adverse event reporting system. Eur J Haematol. 2019 May;103(1):ejh.13240.
48. Shah R, Patel MR. Primary and key secondary results from the ROCKET AF trial, and their implications on clinical practice. Ther Adv Cardiovasc Dis. 2017;11(3):105–20.
49. Camm AJ, Bounameaux H. Edoxaban: a new oral direct factor xa inhibitor. Drugs. 2011;71(12):1503–26.
50. Stacy ZA, Call WB, Hartmann AP, Peters GL, Richter SK. Edoxaban: a comprehensive review of the pharmacology and clinical data for the Management of Atrial Fibrillation and Venous Thromboembolism. Cardiol Ther. 2016;5(1):1–18.
51. Zelniker TA, Ruff CT, Wiviott SD, Blanc J-J, Cappato R, Nordio F, et al. Edoxaban in atrial fibrillation patients with established coronary artery disease: insights from ENGAGE AF-TIMI 48. Eur Hear J Acute Cardiovasc care. 2019;8(2):176–85.
52. Connolly SJ, Eikelboom J, Dorian P, Hohnloser SH, Gretler DD, Sinha U, et al. Betrixaban compared with warfarin in patients with atrial fibrillation: results of a phase 2, ran-

domized, dose-ranging study (Explore-Xa). Eur Heart J. 2013;34(20):1498–505.
53. Skelley JW, Thomason AR, Nolen JC, Candidate P. Betrixaban (Bevyxxa): a direct-acting Oral anticoagulant factor Xa inhibitor. P T. 2018;43(2):85–120.
54. Turpie AG, Gallus AS, Hoek JA. A synthetic pentasaccharide for the prevention of deep-vein thrombosis after total hip replacement. N Engl J Med. 2001;344(9):619–25.
55. Parody R, Oliver A, Souto JC, Fontcuberta J. Fondaparinux (ARIXTRA) as an alternative anti-thrombotic prophylaxis when there is hypersensitivity to low molecular weight and unfractionated heparins. Haematologica. 2003;88(11):ECR32.
56. Lagrange F, Vergnes C, Brun JL, Paolucci F, Nadal T, Leng JJ, et al. Absence of placental transfer of pentasaccharide (Fondaparinux, Arixtra) in the dually perfused human cotyledon in vitro. Thromb Haemost. 2002;87(5):831–5.
57. Halton JML, Lehr T, Cronin L, Lobmeyer MT, Haertter S, Belletrutti M, et al. Safety, tolerability and clinical pharmacology of dabigatran etexilate in adolescents. Thromb Haemost. 2016;116(09):461–71.
58. Eriksson B, Dahl O, Huo M, Kurth A, Hantel S, Hermansson K, et al. Oral dabigatran versus enoxaparin for thromboprophylaxis after primary total hip arthroplasty (RE-NOVATE II). Thromb Haemost. 2011;105(04):721–9.
59. Campbell HA, Link KP. Studies on the hemorrhagic sweet clover disease. IV. The isolation and crystallization of the hemorrhagic agent. J Biol Chem. 1941;138(1):21–33.
60. Chan H-T, So L-T, Li S-W, Siu C-W, Lau C-P, Tse H-F. Effect of herbal consumption on time in therapeutic range of warfarin therapy in patients with atrial fibrillation. J Cardiovasc Pharmacol. 2011;58(1):87–90.
61. Wells PS, Prins MH, Levitan B, Beyer-Westendorf J, Brighton TA, Bounameaux H, et al. Long-term anticoagulation with rivaroxaban for preventing recurrent VTE: a benefit-risk analysis of EINSTEIN-extension. Chest. 2016;150(5):1059–68.
62. Lippi G, Favaloro E, Mattiuzzi C. Combined Administration of Antibiotics and Direct Oral Anticoagulants: a renewed indication for laboratory monitoring? Semin Thromb Hemost. 2014;40(07):756–65.
63. Glueck CJ, Khalil Q, Winiarska M, Wang P. Interaction of duloxetine and warfarin causing severe elevation of international normalized ratio. JAMA. 2006;295(13):1517–8.
64. Gurbel PA, Fox KAA, Tantry US, Ten Cate H, Weitz JI. Combination antiplatelet and Oral anticoagulant therapy in patients with coronary and peripheral artery disease. Circulation. 2019;139(18):2170–85.
65. Turrentine MA, Braems G, Ramirez MM. Use of thrombolytics for the treatment of thromboembolic disease during pregnancy. Obstet Gynecol Surv. 1995;50(7):534–41.
66. Lexicomp. Heparin (unfractionated): Drug information. UpToDate. 2019. p. N/A.
67. Hull, RD, Garcia, DA, Burnett AE. Heparin and LMW heparin: dosing and adverse effects. UpToDate. 2019. p. N/A.
68. Di Minno A, Frigerio B, Spadarella G, Ravani A, Sansaro D, Amato M, et al. Old and new oral anticoagulants: food, herbal medicines and drug interactions. Blood Rev. 2017;31:193–203.
69. Sayal KS, Duncan-McConnell DA, McConnell HW, Taylor DM. Psychotropic interactions with warfarin. Acta Psychiatr Scand. 2000;102(4):250–5.
70. Chew DP, Bhatt DL, Kimball W, Henry TD, Berger P, McCullough PA, et al. Bivalirudin provides increasing benefit with decreasing renal function: a meta-analysis of randomized trials. Am J Cardiol. 2003;92(8):919–23.
71. Koster A, Faraoni D, Levy JH. Argatroban and Bivalirudin for perioperative anticoagulation in cardiac surgery. Anesthesiology. 2018;128(2):390–400.
72. Di Nisio M, Middeldorp S, Büller HR. Direct thrombin inhibitors. N Engl J Med. 2005;353(10):1028–40. [Internet] [cited 2016 Dec 14]. Available from: http://www.nejm.org/doi/abs/10.1056/NEJMra044440
73. Swan SK, Hursting MJ. The pharmacokinetics and pharmacodynamics of argatroban: effects of age, gender, and hepatic or renal dysfunction. Pharmacotherapy. 2000;20(3):318–29.
74. Young G, Yonekawa KE, Nakagawa PA, Blain RC, Lovejoy AE, Nugent DJ. Recombinant activated factor VII effectively reverses the anticoagulant effects of heparin, enoxaparin, fondaparinux, argatroban, and bivalirudin ex vivo as measured using thromboelastography. Blood Coagul Fibrinolysis. 2007;18(6):547–53.
75. Carroll RC, Chavez JJ, Simmons JW, Snider CC, Wortham DC, Bresee SJ, et al. Measurement of patients' bivalirudin plasma levels by a thrombelastograph ecarin clotting time assay: a comparison to a standard activated clotting time. Anesth Analg. 2006;102(5):1316–9.
76. Teles JS, Fukuda EY, Feder D. Warfarin: pharmacological profile and drug interactions with antidepressants. Einstein (Sao Paulo). 2012;10(1):110–5.
77. Saleh MI, Alzubiedi S. Dosage individualization of warfarin using artificial neural networks. Mol Diagn Ther. 2014;18(3):371–9.
78. Hull R, D. Garcia, David A, Vazquez SR. Warfarin and other VKAs: dosing and adverse effects. UpToDate. 2019. p. N/A.
79. So CH, Eckman MH. Combined aspirin and anticoagulant therapy in patients with atrial fibrillation. J Thromb Thrombolysis. 2017;43(1):7–17.
80. Roughead EE, Kalisch LM, Barratt JD, Gilbert AL. Prevalence of potentially hazardous drug interactions amongst Australian veterans. Br J Clin Pharmacol. 2010;70(2):252–7.
81. Moore N, Pollack C, Butkerait P. Adverse drug reactions and drug–drug interactions with over-the-counter NSAIDs. Ther Clin Risk Manag. 2015;11:1061.
82. Holm J, Lindh JD, Andersson ML, Mannheimer B. The effect of amiodarone on warfarin anticoagulation: a register-based nationwide cohort study involving the Swedish population. J Thromb Haemost. 2017;15(3):446–53.
83. Sanoski CA, Bauman JL. Clinical observations with the amiodarone/warfarin interaction: dosing relationships with long-term therapy. Chest. 2002;121(1):19–23.
84. Carpenter M, Berry H, Pelletier AL. Clinically relevant drug-drug interactions in primary care. Am Fam Physician. 2019;99(9):558–64.
85. Lam J, Gomes T, Juurlink DN, Mamdani MM, Pullenayegum EM, Kearon C, et al. Hospitalization for hemorrhage among warfarin recipients prescribed amiodarone. Am J Cardiol. 2013;112(3):420–3.
86. Miller KE. Amiodarone and warfarin interaction. Am Fam Physician. 2002;65(8):1669–70.
87. Fischer HD, Juurlink DN, Mamdani MM, Kopp A, Laupacis A. Hemorrhage during warfarin therapy associated with cotrimoxazole and other urinary tract anti-infective agents: a population-based study. Arch Intern Med. 2010;170(7):617–21.
88. Lane MA, Devine ST, McDonald JR. High-risk antimicrobial prescriptions among ambulatory patients on warfarin. J Clin Pharm Ther. 2012;37(2):157–60.
89. Ellis RJ, Mayo MS, Bodensteiner DM. Ciprofloxacin-warfarin coagulopathy: a case series. Am J Hematol. 2000;63(1):28–31.
90. Lane MA, Zeringue A, McDonald JR. Serious bleeding events due to warfarin and antibiotic co-prescription in a cohort of veterans. Am J Med. 2014;127(7):657–63. e2
91. Phillips S, Barr A, Wilson E, Rockall TASJF. Two cases of retroperitoneal haematoma caused by interaction between antibiotics and warfarin. Emerg Med J. 2006;23(1):e08.
92. Al-Jundi W, Rubin N. Cardiac tamponade secondary to haemopericardium in a patient on warfarin. BMJ Case Rep. 2010;2010.
93. Poon M, Moffett BS, Yee DL. Warfarin-Rifampin drug interaction in a Pediatric patient. J Pediatr Pharmacol Ther: JPPT Off J PPAG United States. 2017;22:375–7.

94. Holt RK, Anderson EA, Cantrell MA, Shaw RF, Egge JA. Preemptive dose reduction of warfarin in patients initiating metronidazole. Drug Metabol Drug Interact. 2010;25(1–4):35–9.
95. Fischer HD. ACP journal Club: concomitant use of warfarin and cotrimoxazole or ciprofloxacin increased risk for admission for upper GI hemorrhage. Ann Intern Med. 2010;153(6):JC3–13.
96. Hale SF, Lesar TS. Interaction of vitamin K antagonists and trimethoprim-sulfamethoxazole: ignore at your patient's risk. Drug Metabol Drug Interact. 2014;29(1):53–60.
97. Ahmed A, Stephens JC, Kaus CA, Fay WP. Impact of preemptive warfarin dose reduction on anticoagulation after initiation of trimethoprim-sulfamethoxazole or levofloxacin. J Thromb Thrombolysis. 2008;26(1):44–8.
98. Shaik AN, Bohnert T, Williams DA, Gan LL, LeDuc BW. Mechanism of drug-drug interactions between warfarin and statins. J Pharm Sci. 2016;105(6):1976–86.
99. Schelleman H, Bilker WB, Brensinger CM, Wan F, Yang Y-X, Hennessy S. Fibrate/statin initiation in warfarin users and gastrointestinal bleeding risk. Am J Med. 2010;123(2):151–7.
100. Mackay JW, Fenech ME, Myint KS. Acute rhabdomyolysis caused by combination therapy with atorvastatin and warfarin. Br J Hosp Med (Lond). 2012;73(2):106–7.
101. Mannheimer B, Andersson ML, Jarnbert-Pettersson H, Lindh JD. The effect of carbamazepine on warfarin anticoagulation: a register-based nationwide cohort study involving the Swedish population. J Thromb Haemost. 2016;14(4):765–71.
102. Clark NP, Hoang K, Delate T, Horn JR, Witt DM. Warfarin interaction with hepatic cytochrome P-450 enzyme-inducing anticonvulsants. Clin Appl Thromb Hemost. 2018;24(1):172–8.
103. Dong Y-H, Bykov K, Choudhry NK, Donneyong MM, Huybrechts KF, Levin R, et al. Clinical outcomes of concomitant use of warfarin and selective serotonin reuptake inhibitors. J Clin Psychopharmacol. 2017;37(2):200–9.
104. Quinn GR, Singer DE, Chang Y, Go AS, Borowsky LH, Udaltsova N, et al. Effect of selective serotonin reuptake inhibitors on bleeding risk in patients with atrial fibrillation taking warfarin. Am J Cardiol. 2014;114(4):583–6.
105. Hackam DG, Mrkobrada M. Selective serotonin reuptake inhibitors and brain hemorrhage: a meta-analysis. Neurology. 2012;79(18):1862–5.
106. Sansone RA, Sansone LA. Warfarin and antidepressants: happiness without Hemorrhaging. Psychiatry (Edgmont). 2009;6(7):24–9.
107. Lexicomp® Drug Interactions - UpToDate. vitamin K Antagonists / Itraconazole. UpToDate. 2019.
108. Niwa T, Shiraga T, Takagi A. Effect of antifungal drugs on cytochrome P450 (CYP) 2C9, CYP2C19, and CYP3A4 activities in human liver microsomes. Biol Pharm Bull. 2005;28(9):1805–8.
109. Lexicomp® Drug Interactions - UpToDate. vitamin K Antagonists / Fluconazole. UpToDate. 2019.
110. Pendlimari R, Anaparthy R, Sugumar A. Drug interaction presenting as acute abdomen. World J Gastrointest Pharmacol Ther. 2010;1(1):40–2.
111. Hellfritzsch M, Pottegard A, Pedersen AJT, Burghle A, Mouaanaki F, Hallas J, et al. Topical Antimycotics for Oral candidiasis in warfarin users. Basic Clin Pharmacol Toxicol. 2017;120(4):368–72.
112. Purkins L, Wood N, Kleinermans D, Nichols D. Voriconazole potentiates warfarin-induced prothrombin time prolongation. Br J Clin Pharmacol. 2003;56(Suppl 1):24–9.
113. Dekhuijzen PNR, Koopmans PP. Pharmacokinetic profile of zafirlukast. Clin Pharmacokinet. 2002;41(2):105–14.
114. U.S. Food and Drug Administration. Accolate - zafirlukast. 2009. p. 1–9.
115. Liedtke MD, Rathbun RC. Warfarin-antiretroviral interactions. Ann Pharmacother. 2009;43(2):322–8.
116. Stading JA, Chock A, Faulkner MA, Skrabal MZ. Effects of prednisone on the international normalized ratio. Am J Health Syst Pharm. 2006;63(23):2354–6.
117. Dowd MB, Vavra KA, Witt DM, Delate T, Martinez K. Empiric warfarin dose adjustment with prednisone therapy. A randomized, controlled trial. J Thromb Thrombolysis. 2011;31(4):472–7.
118. Yıldırım F, Kara İ, Bilaloğlu B, Erbaş G, Türkoglu M, Aygencel G. A rare complication with the concomitant use of warfarin and nonsteroidal anti-inflammatory drugs: Hemoperitoneum and intramural small bowel hematoma. Iran J Med Sci. 2016;41(4):359–60.
119. Tsai H-H, Lin H-W, Simon Pickard A, Tsai H-Y, Mahady GB. Evaluation of documented drug interactions and contraindications associated with herbs and dietary supplements: a systematic literature review. Int J Clin Pract. 2012;66(11):1056–78.
120. Markowitz JS, Donovan JL, DeVane CL, Taylor RM, Ruan Y, Wang J-S, et al. Effect of St John's Wort on drug metabolism by induction of cytochrome P450 3A4 enzyme. JAMA. 2003;290(11):1500.
121. Greenblatt DJ, von Moltke LL. Interaction of warfarin with drugs, natural substances, and foods. J Clin Pharmacol. 2005;45(2):127–32.
122. Chapin JC, Hajjar KA. Fibrinolysis and the control of blood coagulation. Blood Rev. 2015;29(1):17–24. [Internet]. [cited 2019 Oct 24]. Available from: http://www.ncbi.nlm.nih.gov/pubmed/25294122
123. Székely A, Lex DJ. Antifibrinolytics. Hear lung Vessel. 2014;6(1):5–7. [Internet]. [cited 2019 Oct 24] Available from: http://www.ncbi.nlm.nih.gov/pubmed/24800192
124. Fergusson DA, Hébert PC, Mazer CD, Fremes S, MacAdams C, Murkin JM, et al. A comparison of aprotinin and lysine analogues in high-risk cardiac surgery. N Engl J Med. 2008;358(22):2319–31.
125. Koster A, Faraoni D, Levy JH. Antifibrinolytic therapy for cardiac surgery: an update. Anesthesiology. 2015;123:214–21. Lippincott Williams and Wilkins
126. Ng W, Jerath A, Wąsowicz M. Tranexamic acid: a clinical review. Anaesthesiol Intensive Ther. 2015;47(4):339–50. [Internet]. [cited 2019 Oct 24] Available from: http://www.ncbi.nlm.nih.gov/pubmed/25797505
127. Jimenez JJ, Iribarren JL, Lorente L, Rodriguez JM, Hernandez D, Nassar I, et al. Tranexamic acid attenuates inflammatory response in cardiopulmonary bypass surgery through blockade of fibrinolysis: a case control study followed by a randomized double-blind controlled trial. Crit Care. 2007;11(6):R117. [Internet]. [cited 2019 Oct 24]; Available from: http://www.ncbi.nlm.nih.gov/pubmed/17988379
128. Ker K, Edwards P, Perel P, Shakur H, Roberts I. Effect of tranexamic acid on surgical bleeding: systematic review and cumulative meta-analysis. BMJ (Online). 2012;344.
129. Shakur H, Roberts I, Fawole B, Chaudhri R, El-Sheikh M, Akintan A, et al. Effect of early tranexamic acid administration on mortality, hysterectomy, and other morbidities in women with post-partum haemorrhage (WOMAN): an international, randomised, double-blind, placebo-controlled trial. Lancet. 2017;389(10084):2105–16.
130. Cap AP. CRASH-3: a win for patients with traumatic brain injury. Lancet [Internet]. 2019 Oct [cited 2019 Oct 24]; Available from: https://linkinghub.elsevier.com/retrieve/pii/S0140673619323128.
131. Manji RA, Grocott HP, Leake J, Ariano RE, Manji JS, Menkis AH, et al. Seizures following cardiac surgery: the impact of tranexamic acid and other risk factors. Can J Anaesth. 2012;59(1):6–13. Available from: http://www.ncbi.nlm.nih.gov/pubmed/22065333. [Internet]. [cited 2019 Oct 24].
132. Mega JL, Simon T. Pharmacology of antithrombotic drugs: an assessment of oral antiplatelet and anticoagulant treatments. Lancet. 2015;386(9990):281–91.
133. Dubois RN, Abramson SB, Crofford L, Gupta RA, Simon LS, Van De Putte LB, et al. Cyclooxygenase in biology and disease. FASEB J. 1998;12(12):1063–73.

134. O'Gara PT, Kushner FG, Ascheim DD, Casey DE, Chung MK, de Lemos JA, et al. 2013 ACCF/AHA guideline for the management of ST-elevation myocardial infarction: executive summary: a report of the American College of Cardiology Foundation/ American Heart Association task force on practice guidelines. J Am Coll Cardiol. 2013;61(4):485–510.
135. Saxena A, Balaramnavar VM, Hohlfeld T, Saxena AK. Drug/drug interaction of common NSAIDs with antiplatelet effect of aspirin in human platelets. Eur J Pharmacol. 2013;721(1–3):215–24.
136. Strate LL, Singh P, Boylan MR, Piawah S, Cao Y, Chan AT. A prospective study of alcohol consumption and smoking and the risk of major gastrointestinal bleeding in men. PLoS One. 2016;11(11):e0165278.
137. Li W-J, Zhang H-Y, Miao C-L, Tang R-B, DU X, Shi J-H, et al. Cigarette smoking inhibits the anti-platelet activity of aspirin in patients with coronary heart disease. Chin Med J. 2011;124(10):1569–72.
138. Holmes CE, Jasielec J, Levis JE, Skelly J, Muss HB. Initiation of aspirin therapy modulates Angiogenic protein levels in women with breast cancer receiving tamoxifen therapy. Clin Transl Sci. 2013;6(5):386–90.
139. Colwell JA, Nesto RW. The platelet in diabetes: focus on prevention of ischemic events. Diabetes Care. 2003;26:2181–8.
140. Lapi F, Azoulay L, Yin H, Nessim SJ, Suissa S. Concurrent use of diuretics, angiotensin converting enzyme inhibitors, and angiotensin receptor blockers with non-steroidal anti-inflammatory drugs and risk of acute kidney injury: nested case-control study. BMJ. 2013;346:e8525.
141. Vazquez SR. Drug-drug interactions in an era of multiple anticoagulants: a focus on clinically relevant drug interactions. Hematology. 2018;2018(1):339–47.
142. Cattaneo M. P2Y $_{12}$ receptors: structure and function. J Thromb Haemost. 2015;13:S10–6.
143. Savi P, Pereillo JM, Uzabiaga MF, Combalbert J, Picard C, Maffrand JP, et al. Identification and biological activity of the active metabolite of clopidogrel. Thromb Haemost. 2000;84(5):891–6.
144. Angiolillo DJ, Gibson CM, Cheng S, Ollier C, Nicolas O, Bergougnan L, et al. Differential effects of omeprazole and pantoprazole on the pharmacodynamics and pharmacokinetics of Clopidogrel in healthy subjects: randomized, placebo-controlled. Crossover Comparison Studies Clin Pharmacol Ther. 2011;89(1):65–74.
145. Sukhovershin RA, Cooke JP. How may proton pump inhibitors impair cardiovascular health? Am J Cardiovasc Drugs. 2016;16(3):153.
146. Gurbel PA, Bliden KP, Logan DK, Kereiakes DJ, Lasseter KC, White A, et al. The influence of smoking status on the pharmacokinetics and pharmacodynamics of Clopidogrel and Prasugrel: the PARADOX study. J Am Coll Cardiol. 2013;62(6):505–12.
147. Holmberg MT, Tornio A, Neuvonen M, Neuvonen PJ, Backman JT, Niemi M. Grapefruit juice inhibits the metabolic activation of Clopidogrel. Clin Pharmacol Ther. 2014;95(3):307–13.
148. Delaney JA, Opatrny L, Brophy JM, Suissa S. Drug drug interactions between antithrombotic medications and the risk of gastrointestinal bleeding. CMAJ. 2007;177(4):347–51.
149. Cattaneo M, Lecchi A. Inhibition of the platelet P2Y $_{12}$ receptor for adenosine diphosphate potentiates the antiplatelet effect of prostacyclin. J Thromb Haemost. 2007;5(3):577–82.
150. Danielak D, Karaźniewicz-Łada M, Główka F. Assessment of the risk of Rhabdomyolysis and myopathy during concomitant treatment with Ticagrelor and statins. Drugs. 2018;78(11):1105–12.
151. Bennett JS. Structure and function of the platelet integrin alphaIIbbeta3. J Clin Invest. 2005;115(12):3363–9.
152. McFadyen JD, Schaff M, Peter K. Current and future antiplatelet therapies: emphasis on preserving haemostasis. Nat Rev Cardiol. 2018;15(3):181–91.
153. Michelson AD. Antiplatelet therapies for the treatment of cardiovascular disease. Nat Rev Drug Discov. 2010;9(2):154–69.
154. Mukherjee D, Roffi M. Glycoprotein IIb/IIIa receptor inhibitors in 2008: do they still have a role? J Interv Cardiol. 2008;21(2):118–21.
155. Serebruany VL, Malinin AI, Eisert RM, Sane DC. Risk of bleeding complications with antiplatelet agents: meta-analysis of 338,191 patients enrolled in 50 randomized controlled trials. Am J Hematol. 2004;75(1):40–7.
156. PLETAL. (PLAY-tal) (cilostazol) (sil-OS-tah-zol) Tablets.
157. Mader TJ. Adenosine: adverse interactions. Ann Emerg Med. 1992;21(4):453.
158. Huang W, Xin G, Wei Z, Ji C, Zheng H, Gu J, et al. Metformin uniquely prevents thrombosis by inhibiting platelet activation and mtDNA release. Sci Rep. 2016;6:36222.
159. Li XL, Steiner M. Fish oil: a potent inhibitor of platelet adhesiveness. Blood. 1990;76(5):938–45.
160. Morriss R. Antidepressants are associated with hospital admitted intracranial bleeds in people taking other medication associated with bleeding. Evid Based Ment Health. 2016;19(1):24.
161. Dehmer SP, Maciosek MV, Flottemesch TJ. Aspirin use to prevent cardiovascular disease and colorectal cancer. Aspirin use to prevent cardiovascular disease and colorectal cancer: a decision analysis: technical report. 2015.
162. Pratt LA, Brody DJ, Gu Q. Antidepressant use among persons aged 12 and over:United States,2011–2014. NCHS Data Brief. 2017;283:1–8.
163. Antifibrinolytic Drugs. In: Encyclopedia of molecular Pharmacology. Springer; 2008. p. 130. https://doi.org/10.1007/978-3-540-38918-7.
164. Ker K, Roberts I, Shakur H, Coats T. Antifibrinolytic drugs for acute traumatic injury. Sao Paulo Med J. 2015;129(5):CD004896.
165. Hobbs JC, Welsby IJ, Green CL, Dhakal IB, Wellman SS. Epsilon aminocaproic acid to reduce blood loss and transfusion after total hip and total knee arthroplasty. J Arthroplast. 2018;33(1):55–60.
166. Furuta T, Sugimoto M, Kodaira C, Nishino M, Yamade M, Uotani T, Sahara S, et al. Influence of low-dose proton pump inhibitors on anti-platelet function of clopidogrel. Gastroenterology. 2012;142:S215.
167. Ponomaryov T, Payne H, Fabritz L, Wagner DD, Brill A. Mast cells granular contents are crucial for deep vein thrombosis in mice. Circ Res. 2017;121(8):941–50.

Blood Transfusion in the Severe Trauma Patient

20

Jose C. Humanez, Oladapo Oshikoya, Albert Hsu, and Amie L. Hoefnagel

Initial Trauma Bay Management

A systematic and organized approach is required for the immediate management of any trauma patient irrespective of the injury's severity. The Advanced Trauma Life Support® (ATLS®) program developed by the American College of Surgeons (ACS) teaches a standardized approach for the treatment of the trauma patient. It has been adopted at trauma centers in the United States and worldwide and is recognized as the standard of care in the treatment of multiply injured patients. The underlying foundation of the ATLS program is that life-threatening conditions should be treated expeditiously. Furthermore, a detailed and accurate history is not essential to begin the initial evaluation of a patient with acute injuries [2].

The initial assessment and management of injured patients begins with the primary survey. The purpose of the primary survey is to rapidly assess and initiate treatment of life-threatening conditions in a prioritized sequence so that the greatest threat to life is treated first. The following ABCDE algorithm constitutes the sequential steps of the primary survey.

- **A**irway maintenance with cervical spine protection
- **B**reathing and ventilation
- **C**irculation with bleeding control
- **D**isability/neurologic assessment
- **E**xposure and environmental control

Performing the primary survey is a coordinated effort among all members of the medical team. The steps are frequently performed simultaneously when medical providers are well experienced with treating trauma patients. The airway is assessed first for patency. The airway may need to be suctioned, and any foreign bodies should be removed. The chin lift and jaw thrust maneuvers can help maintain airway patency. A prompt decision is made to secure a definitive airway if it is required. The presence of a tension pneumothorax, massive hemothorax, rib fractures with flail chest and pulmonary contusion, or open pneumothorax is rapidly identified and treated as those conditions can severely impair ventilation and oxygenation.

Hemorrhage is the leading cause of preventable death in trauma patients. Hemorrhagic shock has to be recognized promptly and the source of bleeding identified and addressed as soon as possible. External bleeding should be controlled with direct pressure or a tourniquet. Resuscitation begins with obtaining adequate intravenous access in the form of two large bore peripheral lines or a large bore central line, preferably above the diaphragm. The massive transfusion protocol may need to be activated and the use of hemostatic adjuncts such as tranexamic acid should be considered. A sample of blood is obtained from the patient and sent to the blood bank so that cross-matched blood may be administered when feasible. The decision to transfer the patient to the operating room to address the source of hemorrhage also needs to be made expediently.

At the end of the survey, a rapid and basic neurologic evaluation is performed to determine the level of consciousness and the presence of any focal neurologic deficits. The primary survey concludes with completely undressing the patient to facilitate a thorough assessment and then covering the patient in warm blankets to prevent hypothermia.

J. C. Humanez · O. Oshikoya · A. L. Hoefnagel (✉)
University of Florida – Jacksonville, Department of Anesthesiology, Jacksonville, FL, USA
e-mail: Jose.humanez@jax.ufl.edu; oladapo.oshikoya@jax.ufl.edu; amie.hoefnagel@jax.ufl.edu

A. Hsu
University of Florida – Jacksonville, Department of Surgery, Jacksonville, FL, USA
e-mail: albert.hsu@jax.ufl.edu

© Springer Nature Switzerland AG 2021
C. S. Scher et al. (eds.), *Essentials of Blood Product Management in Anesthesia Practice*,
https://doi.org/10.1007/978-3-030-59295-0_20

Transfusion Strategies

The strategy of damage control resuscitation of a trauma patient in hemorrhagic shock involves preserving end-organ perfusion and preventing any further progression of the lethal triad of death. The triad of death in the setting of trauma describes the combination of hypothermia, acidosis, and coagulopathy that is commonly associated with hemorrhagic shock [1]. Patients with severe hypothermia despite warming maneuvers, persistent metabolic acidosis despite massive resuscitation, and coagulopathy with bleeding not amenable to surgical control have a high mortality rate of 20–50% [3]. Packed red blood cells should be transfused to maintain oxygen-carrying capacity and other blood components transfused to optimize hemostasis. Administration of crystalloids should be minimized as its use is associated with increased morbidity as demonstrated by a multi-institutional analysis from Duchesne et al. [4] Infusion of large volumes of crystalloid can also worsen coagulopathy by diluting coagulation factors. In this setting, the trauma surgeon may elect to perform a damage control operation to limit the surgical intervention, to control only hemorrhage and contamination, and to minimize the amount of time spent in the operating room. The patient is then further resuscitated in the ICU setting prior to returning to the OR.

For a patient in hemorrhagic shock requiring large volume resuscitation, a massive transfusion protocol (MTP) that was developed and implemented by the institution should be followed. The benefits of a massive transfusion protocol in improving mortality and reducing the usage of blood products are discussed separately in this text (Chap. 8). The protocol defines the target ratio of blood products that should be transfused during the initial phase of resuscitation. Many centers have adopted the practice of administering plasma, platelets, and red blood cells in a balanced 1:1:1 transfusion ratio. This was largely the result of the publication of the landmark Pragmatic, Randomized Optimal Platelet and Plasma Ratios (PROPPR) trial. The multicenter randomized controlled PROPPR trial, published in 2015, was designed to determine the safety and efficacy of a balanced 1:1:1 transfusion ratio in patients predicted to require massive transfusion. The study compared a 1:1:1 transfusion ratio with a 1:1:2 ratio [5]. Though the study found no difference in all cause 24 h or 30 day mortality comparing the 1:1:1 with the 1:1:2 ratio, there was a significant decrease in 24 h mortality due to exsanguination in the 1:1:1 group. The physiology supporting a balanced transfusion strategy is that the 1:1:1 transfusion ratio mimics the composition of whole blood. Furthermore, an unbalanced transfusion ratio where more of one blood component is administered will serve to dilute the other two components and may lead to inadequate hemostasis [6]. The practice of a 1:1:1 transfusion ratio in the initial phase of resuscitation was also incorporated into a recently published clinical practice guideline on damage control resuscitation [7].

More recently, whole blood transfusion in trauma patients has been gaining in popularity. Our institution has recently made whole blood available for use in the Trauma Resuscitation Unit. The benefits of whole blood transfusion are that the blood components are more concentrated, and it is simpler to administer compared to blood component therapy. The indications, interactions, and adverse effects of whole blood transfusion are discussed separately. Further research, however, is needed before it can be determined that whole blood should be included as part of the standard practice for damage control resuscitation.

Tranexamic Acid

Tranexamic acid (TXA) is an antifibrinolytic lysine analog used to prevent the enzymatic breakdown of fibrin blood clots. TXA has a structural similarity to lysine, which allows TXA to competitively inhibit plasminogen conversion to plasmin and reduces the rate of fibrin degradation [8]. TXA also partially prevents fibrinogenolysis induced by tissue factor [9]. The administration of TXA has been shown to decrease the amount of intraoperative blood loss and associated blood transfusion for patients undergoing either elective or emergency surgery [8]. TXA has been shown to decrease blood loss by one-third, regardless of surgery type or amount of expected blood loss, when given intraoperatively to surgical patients just prior to incision [10, 11].

When given within 3 h of trauma to a bleeding trauma patient, TXA reduces the risk of death from bleeding. TXA actually increases mortality risk when given longer than 3 h post-traumatic incident so its administration should be as close to the traumatic event as possible, potentially suggesting prehospital administration [12]. For all of its antifibrinolytic properties and ability to reduce blood loss, TXA has not been shown to increase the risk of thrombosis and has actually shown reduced odds of fatal and non-fatal vascular occlusive events [13, 14].

Administration of TXA in trauma patients is typically a 1 g loading dose over 10 min, followed by an infusion of 1 g over 8 h [12]. Alternative dosing regimens exist, including bolus injection of 10 mg/kg over 30 min followed by an infusion of 1 mg/kg/h. TXA is a pregnancy category B medication, with no harm found in animal models, so its use in parturients involved in bleeding trauma should be considered. A dose reduction is required in mild to moderate renal impairment and contraindicated in severe renal impairment due to 95% renal excretion. No such dose reduction exists for liver impairment [15].

Cell Saver and Autologous Blood Transfusion

Trauma patients utilize large amounts of hospital resources, including the use of approximately 70% of all blood transfused at a trauma center, [16] which can have a financial and resource burden for the institution. Transfusion protocols from donated cross-matched blood and the use of MTP remain the standard treatment for the patient in hemorrhagic shock due to trauma. Transfusion of donated blood does not come without risks; the potential for citrate toxicity, hyperkalemia, disease transmission, hypothermia, acidosis, hypomagnesemia, sepsis, acute respiratory failure (TRALI, TACO, ARDS), and thrombotic side effects pose a significant risk [17–20]. Auto-transfusion has been widely used as an alternative or adjunct to transfusion of donated blood to reduce or avoid the number of transfusions and the associated risks and costs, with fewer side effects.

Autotransfusion was first documented in 1818 by Dr. James Blundell. He experimented with auto-transfusion in canine models and later tried on humans, but with significant mortality [21]. In 1874, Dr. William Highmore at the Yeatman Hospital in the United Kingdom proposed the idea of reinfusing shed blood. He described a case of a woman that suffered a postpartum hemorrhage. The patient died with "several pounds of blood in a vessel and in the bed, which, could have been used to save her life had he been able to transfuse it back into her veins" [22]. In 1883, at the Roosevelt Hospital in New York, William Halsted described a technique for "reinfusion blood" to treat carbon monoxide poisoning. His method included defibrination and straining of blood removed from the patient prior to reinfusion [23]. Other successful cases of autotransfusion were reported by Duncan and Miller in 1885 at the Royal Infirmary in Edinburgh, Scotland, where a patient with crush injury was retransfused his own blood after it had been treated with phosphate of soda [24]. In 1914, the German gynecologist H. J. Thies treated removed blood with citrate and strained it through gauze before returning it to his patients [25]. In 1943, Griswold and Ortner published 100 patients in the first case series [26]. However, autotransfusion fell out of favor in the 1940s and 1950s with progress in blood donation, blood storage, and advances in blood banking that simplified and increased the safety of allogeneic transfusion. In the 1960s and 1970s, there was renewed interest in autotransfusion when Dyer, Klebanof, and Pathak developed techniques and new devices for the reinfusion of salvaged unwashed blood. Their research provided data on hemolysis reduction, contaminant filtration, and most important clinical outcomes. Klebanoff's device consisted of a cardiotomy reservoir and a roller pump, which was known as the Bentley autotransfuser [27]; its use decreased after the report of several cases of air embolism. In 1968, Wilson and Taswell from the Mayo Clinic developed a prototype machine that collected and washed the salvaged blood. Technological advances in the 1970s resulted in the availability of several commercial devices [28]. In 1974, Haemonetics (Braintree, MA) developed a device that could collect, wash, and concentrate autologous red blood cells and make them available for reinfusion. They called it the "cell saver" device. Subsequently, the term "cell saver" refers generically any blood salvage device used perioperatively.

Indications and Contraindications

Cell saver or autologous blood transfusion should be considered in every trauma patient with active bleeding. In order to make it worthwhile, there should be a blood loss of at least 1000 mL [14]. Other reported indications include the need for immediate blood, inability to obtain or provide cross-matched blood, and if the patient is unwilling to receive cross-matched blood [30]. The American Association of Blood Banks recommends the use of cell saver if the expected surgical blood loss is either 20% of the patient's estimated blood volume, or greater than 1000 mL, or if the average transfusion for the procedure is greater than 1 unit of blood. Further indications are patient refusal of allogenic transfusion or lack of availability of cross-matched blood [32].

More than the indication, one important question is the consideration of contraindications for the use of cell saver. One contraindication is if the blood has suffered contamination either by an infectious or non-infectious source. An example of an infectious source is the mix of blood with gastrointestinal contents or purulent material. Non-infectious sources involve the mixing of blood with solutions such as iodine, sterile water, alcohol, chlorhexidine, irrigation solutions, or hemostatic agents such as thrombin [31, 32].

Other contraindications for autologous blood transfusion include sickle cell disease, presence of malignancy (risk of reinfusion of cancer cells and development of metastasis), and cesarean delivery (theoretical risk of amniotic fluid embolism) Table 20.1 summarizes the indication and contraindication for the use of a cell saver device.

Table 20.1 Indications and relative contraindications to autologous blood salvage

Indications for cell salvage
Surgery with ≥1000 ml (or 20% of total blood volume) anticipated blood loss
To reduce or avoid exposure to allogeneic blood
When crossmatch compatible blood is difficult to find
Patients with red cell alloantibodies
Patients who do not accept allogeneic blood
Low preoperative red cell mass and high bleeding risk
Contraindications to cell salvage
Sickle cell disease
Drug and other contaminants (betadine, alcohol, prep solutions)
Thrombin, fibrin and other hemostatic agents
Bone cement (methyl methacrylate)
Relative contraindications to cell salvage
Caesarean section (amniotic fluid contamination)
Cancer surgery
Bacterial contamination

The Cell Saver Equipment and Process

The cell saver process has three phases: cell salvage or collection, washing, and reinfusion. The final product has a hematocrit that varies between 50% and 80%, has a storage time of less than 6 h, and requires the use of a filter to provide leukocyte reduction.

Blood is collected via suction from the surgical field and transferred into a canister where it is mixed with an anticoagulant. The process involves centrifugation of the blood and then removal of the supernatant. To remove residual harmful contaminants, copious amounts of normal saline and further centrifugation are used to wash the blood. The red cells are then resuspended in normal saline for infusion. Figure 20.1 depicts the different components that are part of the autotransfusion device.

The composition of the salvaged blood has physiologic differences from circulating blood due to chemical and physical contaminants from the surgical field and cellular breakdown products from the operative field and blood contact with the artificial surfaces in the cell saver device. Finally, washing of the salvaged blood removes the contaminants and plasma proteins that would not be removed by simple filtration.

Once blood is collected, it must be anticoagulated. There are two primary anticoagulants used for this purpose: heparin and citrate. Heparin anticoagulated salvaged blood leads to lower levels of free hemoglobin, improved osmotic fragility, and oxidative reserve capacity [33]; however, for patients with heparin-induced thrombocytopenia, citrate is the anticoagulant of choice.

Once the final product is obtained, it is passed through a leukoreduction filter resulting in 99.6–100% removal of bacteria. Though not routinely practiced, the addition of antibiotics may reduce bacterial load even further [33].

The use of cell saver and autotransfusion does not come without risk or development of complications. The most common complication of autotransfusion is loss of ability to return blood if the setup is not properly connected. The more serious complication includes blood contamination, resulting in infection and development of sepsis [29] which can be prevented by following sterile guidelines. Other less common complications include hemodilution, hemolysis due to suction or degradation, air embolism, contamination of activated leukocytes, and thrombocytopenia [29]. Overall complications are avoidable with the use of sterile technique and if less than 3000 mL of blood is reinfused.

In conclusion, cell saver and autotransfusion should be considered in trauma patients without contraindications in whom significant blood loss is anticipated. It can be used in addition to cross-matched blood or can be used as a temporizing measure while waiting for the arrival of cross-matched blood. The use of cell saver can reduce the risk of transfusion reactions for the patient as may provide cost-saving benefits compared with allogeneic blood transfusion.

Thromboelastography (TEG) in Trauma Resuscitation

Thromboelastography (TEG) is a test of whole blood coagulation. There is an entire chapter in this text dedicated to this subject, so we will touch on it only briefly here. The test results are available within an hour; however, there is computer software that will allow clinicians to watch the tracing form in real time. This tracing is frequently displayed within the trauma

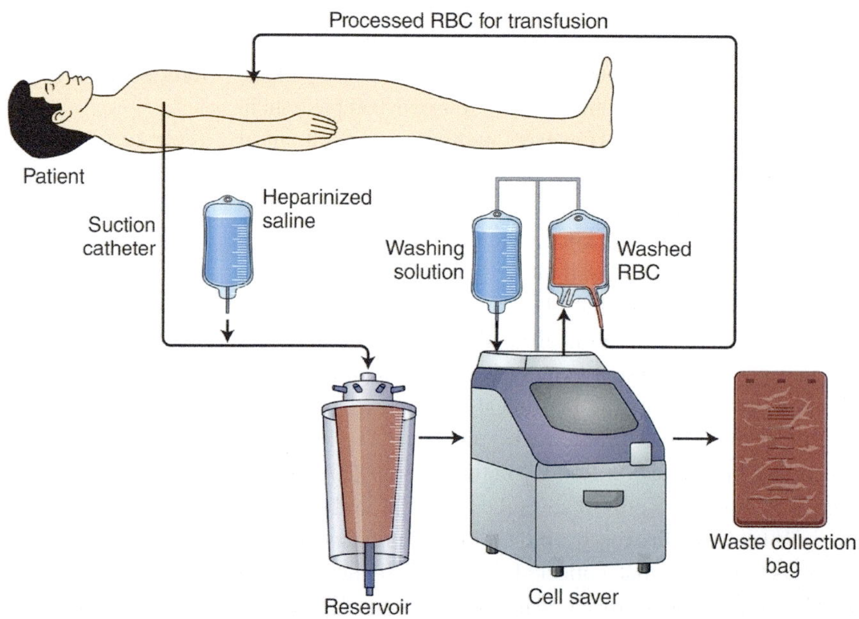

Fig. 20.1 Components of the autotransfusion device

resuscitation center or the operating room. Hemorrhagic shock due to severe blood loss is a major factor in trauma-related deaths. A contributing factor to ongoing hemorrhage is the development of trauma-induced coagulopathy (TIC), which is an intrinsic dysregulation of the coagulation pathway [34, 35]. The intrinsic coagulopathy in TIC seems to be driven by endothelial hypoxemia, pathological activation of protein C, platelet dysfunction, and fibrinolytic dysregulation. The development of TIC is associated with increased mortality (4X) [36] and with the development of serious events such as uncontrolled bleeding, ongoing massive transfusion requirements, and multiorgan failure, which can lead to longer intensive care unit (ICU) and hospital length of stay [37, 38]. Prior to 2000, resuscitation was based mainly on the transfusion of packed red blood cells (PRBCs) and synthetic fluids to maintain intravascular volume and tissue oxygen delivery. With the use of conventional coagulation tests (CCTs), specific coagulation defects were identified leading to the addition of other blood component products such as fresh frozen plasma (FFP) and platelets during trauma resuscitation [39].

Traditional laboratory testing offers valuable information on varying aspects of coagulation, but they were originally designed for the monitoring of therapeutic anticoagulation in a laboratory setting, rather than identification of TIC. There are several limitations of CCTs: They are imprecise in the delineation of the complex nature of TIC and require significant time for final result reporting and therefore may have limited clinical relevance in the quickly changing trauma patient [35, 40]. With these limitations of CCTs in mind, viscoelastic assays such as thromboelastography (TEG) or rotational thromboelastometry (ROTEM) are alternative diagnostic methods for the timely identification of specific coagulation defects which could enable individualized resuscitation.

TEG can be used in trauma patients to predict the need for blood component therapy or the use of hemostatic agents (PCC, rFVIIa, fibrinogen, and TXA) in hypocoagulable and coagulopathic patients. Also, it can help to identify that subset of trauma patients are hypercoagulable and may benefit from early deep vein thrombosis (DVT) prophylaxis [41].

Individualization in administration of blood component therapy with the use of TEG helps to address the immediate needs of the bleeding trauma patient. Therefore, minimizing the overuse and waste of blood products and decreasing the appearance of complications such as DVT, TRALI, TACO, acute respiratory distress syndrome (ARDS), infections, and allergic reactions [42–44].

Adverse Transfusion Outcomes in Severe Trauma

The major life-threatening complication for massive transfusion in severe trauma is transfusion-related acute lung injury (TRALI). While TRALI is the primary cause of transfusion-related morbidity and mortality [45], the overall rate of TRALI in the setting of massive resuscitation for hemorrhagic shock is low [46]. Still, an extensive literature review published by Patel et al. revealed that the odds of ARDS/ALI and death increased with each additional unit of red blood cells transfused (odds ratio [OR] 1.06 and 1.07, respectively) [47]. The use of older blood for massive transfusion may also contribute to increased mortality and adverse events [48]. The epidemiology, pathogenesis, risk factors, and management of TRALI are discussed separately within this text.

Other physiologic derangements that may occur with massive transfusion include acid-base disturbance in the form of metabolic alkalosis and electrolyte abnormalities such as hypocalcemia and hyperkalemia [49]. A substantial amount of citrate is delivered to the patient during massive transfusion since citrate is used as an anticoagulant in stored blood. The citrate is metabolized to bicarbonate, and the excess bicarbonate is excreted in the urine. Metabolic alkalosis may develop when bicarbonate excretion is reduced in the setting of renal failure. There may also be associated hypokalemia when hydrogen ions move out of cells in exchange for potassium ions moving into cells to compensate for the metabolic alkalosis. A clinically significant metabolic alkalosis is not a common event as the patient in hemorrhagic shock likely already has a metabolic acidosis due to end-organ hypoperfusion. Another adverse effect of the citrate is that it chelates calcium and decreases ionized calcium levels. Profound hypocalcemia may lead to seizures or arrhythmias and cardiac arrest. Calcium is a critical component for the proper functioning of the coagulation cascade, and hypocalcemia can worsen the coagulopathy that is frequently associated with hemorrhagic shock. Patients undergoing massive transfusion are also at risk for hyperkalemia. The risk is increased with the use of older red blood cells and irradiated blood [50]. The potassium concentration in the supernatant of red blood cells increases linearly by 1 mEq/day and approximates the number of days in storage. The most critical complication of this electrolyte abnormality is the potential for transfusion-associated hyperkalemic cardiac arrest. Arterial blood gases, potassium, and ionized calcium levels should be obtained to guide the management of the patient.

As part of the lethal triad of hemorrhagic shock, hypothermia can be worsened by massive transfusion, and this can exacerbate any ongoing coagulopathy. Coagulation begins to become impaired when the core body temperature decreases to less than 37°C [51, 52]. Furthermore, a rapid decline in body temperature can lead to bradycardia, ventricular fibrillation, and subsequent cardiac arrest. The risk can be reduced by using a rapid infuser that has the capability of warming blood during rapid transfusion.

Rapid Infusion Devices

There are several medical devices currently on the market to provide warming for intravenous fluids and blood products. The simplest of devices utilize heating plates, water baths, or countercurrent heat exchange to warm fluid. While these devices provide excellent warming of fluids and blood products during routine care, they are limited in their ability warm blood products at rapid flow due to insufficient contact time with cold blood products. Newer devices designed specifically for the rapid infusion of blood products utilize electromagnetic induction, microwave technology, and dry thermal transfer to rapidly warm blood products. Table 20.2 compares three commercially available rapid infusion devices [53–55].

When evaluating rapid infusion devices, several factors should be taken into consideration. For the purposes of this chapter, we will focus on the Level 1, the Belmont, and the ThemaCor1200. The Level 1 system provides warming via countercurrent heat exchange through warmed water. Delivery of blood products is based on dual pneumatic pressure infusers with the ability to infuse one unit while loading another unit on the opposite side (Fig. 20.2). The Belmont and ThermaCor1200 both utilize a mechanical pump to deliver blood products rapidly from a large reservoir. The Belmont heats via electromagnetic microwave warming, while the ThermaCor1200 relies on dry thermal heat transfer.

During the rapid administration of large volumes of cold blood, there is a risk for venous air embolism and hypothermia; therefore, rapid infusion systems should be able to reliably detect and purge air and warm cold blood products at

Table 20.2 Comparison of infusion devices

	Level-1 H-1000	ThermaCor 1200	Belmont rapid infuser
Manufacturer	Smith's medical	Smission-Cartledge biomedical, LLC	Belmont instrument corporation
Footprint	Medium	Small	Medium
Heat mechanism	Countercurrent	Dry thermal	Microwave warming
Transfusion rate	~500 mL/min	10 mL/h–1.2 L/min	2.5 mL/min–1 L/min
Weight (kg)	32	9.5	12
Air removal	Manual	Automatic	Automatic
Ease of fluid loading	No reservoir for blood products. Air must be expelled from each unit to prevent air embolization	3 spike inflow set, fluid reservoir available	3 or 4 spike inflow set, 3 L fluid reservoir
Ease of set-up	Easy	Primes in <60 s	Primes in <60 s
Battery capability	No	Yes	Yes
Other	Ability to heat blood products dependent on infusion rate		Does not heat until flow is 10 mL/min

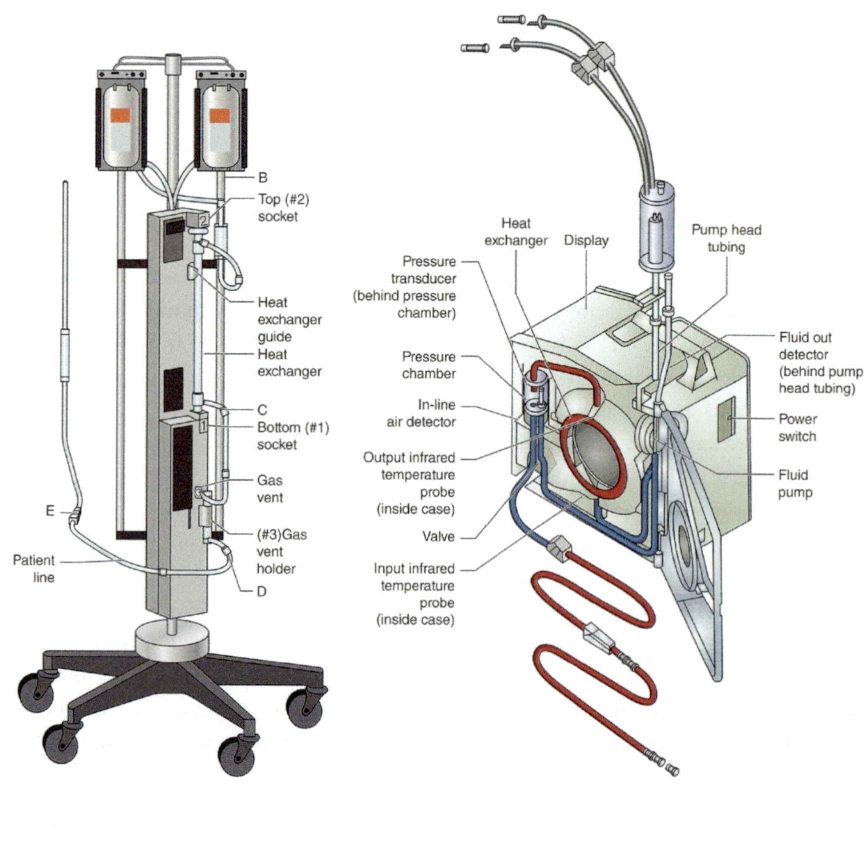

Fig. 20.2 The level 1 H1025 (**a**) and the Belmont FMS 2000 (**b**) (Modified from: Comunale [56])

rapid rates. The Level 1 system has a gas vent which automatically eliminates microbubbles within the system. On newer models, there is an optional integrated air detector and clamp that will alert the clinician to the presence of air and stop flow to the patient [54]. The ThermaCor1200 has four air sensors built into the disposable cassette although the exact mechanism is proprietary [53]. On the Belmont, there are two ultrasonic air detectors which detect as little as 0.1 mL of air [56]. Cumunale, in a comparative study between the Level 1 and Belmont device, injected 10 mL of air into each system proximal to the heat exchanger and found that the air bolus was able to pass through the delivery tubing in the level 1 system. The air was detected and purged by the Belmont [56]. This same study compared the warming abilities of each device at a rapid flow rate of 500 mL/min. While both devices warmed to physiologic temperatures at low flow, at high flow rates the blood delivered by the Level 1 averaged 32°C [56, 57]. Current peer reviewed literature comparing the ThermaCor1200 to either the Level 1 or Belmont is not available at this time.

All of the rapid infusion devices have the availability to deliver fluid at a very high rate; however, what is delivered to the patient will be based on the intravenous (IV) access present. For the three devices above, an 18 gauge IV is the minimum size for infusion. Theoretically, the maximum flow rate of fluids in an IV catheter is predicted by Poiseuille's law (Fig. 20.3) where flow is related to fluid viscosity, the pressure gradient across the catheter, and the length and diameter of the IV catheter. Doubling the diameter of a catheter increases the flow rate by 16-fold. However, this only applies to laminar flow. When rapidly infusing blood, the actual flow rate cannot fully be predicted by Poiseulle's law due to the development of turbulence [57]. However, we do know that larger and shorter IV catheters provide superior flow rates over smaller and/or longer IV catheters.

It is very difficult to find studies showing the difference in flow rates through standard IV catheters and large bore central infusion lines. A study published by Wrenn et al. [58] compared flow rates between several catheters comparing both hetastarch and normal saline (NS) as delivered by the ThermaCor1200 rapid infusion device. This study compared flow rates between 18-gauge, 16-gauge, 14-gauge, 7.0 Fr and 8.5 Fr rapid infusion catheter (RIC), 14-gauge double lumen central line, 8.5 Fr sheath introducer, and a multilumen access catheter (MAC) introducer. With similar driving pressures from the ThermaCor1200, they found that the 8.5 Fr RIC and the MAC catheter were superior at rapid transfusion with both NS and hetastarch, each providing flow rates exceeding 1 L/min with driving pressures of 300 mmHg. The double lumen central line performed the worst, followed by the 18-gauge peripheral IV delivering 180 mL/min and 210 mL/min of hetastarch, respectively. While hetastarch is no longer used clinically in the United States, it is more viscous than NS and therefore is more predictive of flow rates with blood products than NS.

Q	Flow Rate
P	Pressure
r	Radius
η	Fluid Viscosity
l	Length of tubing

$$Q = \frac{\pi P r^4}{8 \eta l}$$

Fig. 20.3 Poiseuilles' equation

Table 20.3 Common IV catheter sizes and infusion time for 1000 mL of normal saline [59]

Size	Type	1000 mL infusion time (min)
8.5 Fr	RIC	0.46
7.0 Fr	RIC	1.0
8.5 Fr	Sheath introducer	1.05
14 Ga	Standard IV cannula	1.30
16 Ga	Standard IV cannula	2.20
18 Ga	Standard IV cannula	4.23
14 Ga	4 lumen central line	5.20
20 Ga	Standard IV cannula	6.47

RIC rapid infusion catheter

Andrew Buck ran a similar experiment where he determined the time it took to infuse 1 liter of NS on a pneumatic rapid infusion device through several commonly used intravenous catheters [59]. In this study, the 8.5 Fr RIC was also shown to be the quickest transfusion method with a 1 L infusion time of 46 s. The 8.5 Fr sheath introducer took 1:05 min, a 14-gauge 4 lumen central venous catheter took 5:20, and a standard 20 gauge peripheral IV took 6:47 min to infuse a liter of NS (Table 20.3).

Both of these studies support the use of large diameter short cannulas for IV access to facilitate rapid infusion of volume. Central venous access may not be the best method for volume administration, especially given the complexity of placement and the frequency of other tasks that need simultaneous attention in a severe trauma patient.

Conclusion

Hemorrhage is the leading preventable cause of death in trauma patients. The initial management of trauma patient involves ATLS protocols with a focus of treating life-threatening injuries first. The strategy of damage control resuscitation of a trauma patient in hemorrhagic shock involves preserving end-organ perfusion and preventing any further progression of the lethal triad of death. Volume resuscitation in the bleeding trauma patient should focus on replacement of blood volume with blood products in a 1:1:1 ration and minimal crystalloid. Use of cell salvaged blood should be considered to minimize the amount of allogenic product when possible. Targeted blood product replacement utilizing TEG or ROTEM is recommended if possible. Trauma patients that require blood transfusion should also be given TXA within the first 3 h after injury. Complications associated with large volume transfusion include TRALI, TACO, hyperkalemia, hypocalcemia, and hypothermia. Hypothermia can be minimized warming blood products prior to administration. Utilization of a rapid infusion device improves the ability to rapidly deliver warmed blood products to the patient. Intravenous access to accommodate high rates of transfusion is best accomplished with large diameter short length catheters.

References

1. Schreiber MA. Coagulopathy in the trauma patient. Curr Opin Crit Care. 2005;11:590.
2. American College of Surgeons Committee on Trauma. ATLS advanced trauma life support student course manual. 10th ed. Chicago: American College of Surgeons; 2018.
3. Moore EE, Feliciano DV, Mattox KL. Trauma. 8th ed. New York: McGraw-Hill; 2017.
4. Duchesne JC, Heaney J, Guidry C, et al. Diluting the benefits of hemostatic resuscitation: a multi-institutional analysis. J Trauma Acute Care Surg. 2013;751:76.
5. Holcomb JB, Tilley BC, Baraniuk S, et al. Transfusion of plasma, platelets, and red blood cells in a 1:1:1 vs a 1:1:2 ratio and mortality in patients with severe trauma: the PROPPR randomized clinical trial. JAMA. 2015;313:471.
6. Kornblith LZ, Howard BM, Cheung CK, et al. The whole is greater than the sum of its parts: hemostatic profiles of whole blood variants. J Trauma Acute Care Surg. 2014;77:818.
7. Cannon JW, Khan MA, Raja AS, et al. Damage control resuscitation in patients with severe traumatic hemorrhage: a practice management guideline from the Eastern Association for the surgery of trauma. J Trauma Acute Care Surg. 2017;82:605.
8. Roberts I. Tranexamic acid in trauma: how should we use it? J Thromb Haemost. 2015;13(Suppl. 1):S195–S9.
9. Takada A, Makino Y, Takada Y. Effects of tranexamic acid on fibrinolysis, fibrinogenolysis and amidolysis. Thromb Res. 1986;42:39–47.
10. Ker K, Edwards P, Perel P, Shakur H, Roberts I. Effect of tranexamic acid on surgical bleeding: systematic review and cumulative meta-analysis. BMJ. 2012;344:e3054.
11. Ker K, Prieto-Merino D, Roberts I. Systematic review, meta-analysis and meta-regression of the effect of tranexamic acid on surgical blood loss. B J Surg. 2013;100:1271–9.
12. Roberts I, Shakur H, Coats T, et al. The CRASH-2 trial: a randomized controlled trial and economic evaluation of the effects of tranexamic acid on death, vascular occlusive events and transfusion requirement in bleeding trauma patients. Health Technol Assess. 2013;17(10):1–79. https://doi.org/10.3310/hta17100.
13. CRASH-2 Collaborators I, Roberts HS, Afolabi A, et al. The importance of early treatment with tranexamic acid in bleeding trauma patients: an exploratory analysis of the CRASH-2 randomized controlled trial. Lancet. 2011;377(9771):1096–101. 21439633.
14. Roberts I, Pablo P, David P-M, Haleema S, Tim C, Hunt Beverley J, et al. Effect of tranexamic acid on mortality in patients with traumatic bleeding: prespecified analysis of data from randomized controlled trial. BMJ. 2012;345:e5839.
15. "Lysteda (tranexamic acid) Package Insert" (PDF). accessdata.FDA.gov. Retrieved 20 June 2019.
16. Kauvar DS, Lefering R, Wade CE. Impact of hemorrhage on trauma outcome: an overview of epidemiology, clinical presentations, and therapeutic considerations. J Trauma. 2006;60(6 Suppl):S3–11.
17. Perez P, Salmi LR, Folléa G, Schmit JL, de Barbeyrac B, Sudre P, Salamon R, BACTHEM Group. French haemovigilance network. Determinants of transfusion-associated bacterial contamination: results of the French BACTHEM case-control study. Transfusion. 2001 Jul;41(7):862–72.
18. Williamson LM, Lowe S, Love EM, Cohen H, Soldan K, McClelland DB, Skacel P, Barbara JA. Serious hazards of transfusion (SHOT) initiative: analysis of the first two annual reports. BMJ. 1999;319(7201):16–9.
19. Kuehnert MJ, Roth VR, Haley NR, Gregory KR, Elder KV, Schreiber GB, Arduino MJ, Holt SC, Carson LA, Banerjee SN, Jarvis WR. Transfusion-transmitted bacterial infection in the United States, 1998 through 2000. Transfusion. 2001;41(12):1493–9.
20. Menis M, Forshee RA, Anderson SA, McKean S, Gondalia R, Warnock R, Johnson C, Mintz PD, Worrall CM, Kelman JA, Izurieta HS. Febrile non-haemolytic transfusion reaction occurrence and potential risk factors among the U.S. elderly transfused in the inpatient setting, as recorded in Medicare databases during 2011-2012. Vox Sang. 2015 Apr;108(3):251–61.
21. Blundell J. Experiments on the transfusion of blood by the syringe. Med Chir Trans. 1818;9(Pt 1):56–92.
22. Highmore W. Practical remarks on an overlooked source of blood supply for transfusion in post-partum haemorrhage suggested by a recent fatal case. Lancet. 1874;103:89–90.
23. Halsted WS. Refusion in carbonic-oxide poisoning. New York J Med. 1883;38:625–9.
24. Duncan J. On re-infusion of blood in primary and other amputations. Br Med J. 1886;1:192–3.
25. Thies HJ. Zur Behandlung der Extrauteringravidität. Zentralbl Gynäkol. 1914;38:1191–3.
26. Griswald RA, Ortner AB. Use of autotransfusion in surgery of serous cavities. Surg Gynecol Obstet. 1943;77:167–77.
27. Klebanoff G. Early clinical experience with a disposable unit for the intraoperative salvage and reinfusion of blood loss (intraoperative autotransfusion). Am J Surg. 1970;120:718–22.
28. Wilson JD, Taswell HF. Autotransfusion: historical review and preliminary report on a new method. Mayo Clin Proc. 1968;43(1):26–35.
29. Carless PA, Henry DA, Moxey AJ, O'Connell D, Brown T, Fergusson DA. Cell salvage for minimizing perioperative allogeneic blood transfusion. Cochrane Database Syst Rev. 2010;4:CD001888.
30. Garcia JH, Coelho GR, Feitosa Neto BA, Nogueira EA, Teixeira CC, Mesquita DF. Liver transplantation in Jehovah's witnesses patients in a center of northeastern Brazil. Arq Gastroenterol. 2013;50(2):138–40.
31. Waters JH. Indications and contraindications of cell salvage. Transfusion. 2004;44(12 Suppl):40S–4S.
32. Esper SA, Waters JH. Intra-operative cell salvage: a fresh look at the indications and contraindications. Blood Transfus. 2011;9(2):139–47.
33. Sikorski RA, Rizkalla NA, Yang WW, Frank SM. Autologous blood salvage in the era of patient blood management. Vox Sang. 2017;112:499–510.
34. White NJ. Mechanism of trauma-induced coagulopathy. Hematology Am Soc Hematol Educ Program. 2013;2013:660–3.

35. Mohamed, et al. Scand J Trauma Resusc Emerg Med 2017: 25:99.
36. Adelfattah K, Cripps MW. Thromboelastography and rotational thromboelastometry use in trauma. Int J Surg. 2016;33:196–201.
37. Brohi K, Singh J, Heron M, Coats T. Acute traumatic coagulopathy. J Trauma Acute Care Surg. 2003; Jun 1;54(6):1127–30.
38. Khan S, Brohi K, Chana M, Raza I, Stanworth S, Gaarder C, Davenport R. Hemostatic resuscitation is neither hemostatic nor resuscitative in trauma hemorrhage. J Trauma Acute Care Surg. 2014;76(3):561–8.
39. Howley IW, Haut ER, Jacobs L, et al. Is thromboelastography (TEG)-based resucitation better than empirical 1:1 transfusion? Trauma Surg Acute Care Open. 2018;3:1–3.
40. Schochl H, Maegele M, Solomnon C, Gorlinger K, Voelckel W. Early and individualized goal-directed therapy for trauma induced coagulopathy. Scand J Trauma Resusc Emerg Med. 2012;20:15.
41. Kashuk J, Moore E, Sawyer M, et al. Post injury coagulopathy management: goal directed resuscitation via POC thromboelastography. Ann Surg. 2010;251(4):604–14.
42. Massaro A, Doerfler S, Nawalinski K, et al. Thromboelastography defines late hypercoagulability after TBI: a pilot study. Neurocrit Care. 2015;22:45–51.
43. Mitra B, Cameron P, Gruen R. Aggressive fresh frozen plasma (FFP) with massive blood transfusion in the absence of acute traumatic coagulopathy. Injury. 2012;43(1):33–7.
44. Gruen R, Jacobs I, Reade M. Trauma and tranexamic acid. Med J Aus. 2013;199(5):310–1.
45. Walsh M, Fritz S, Hake D, Son M, et al. Targeted Thromboelastographic (TEG) blood component and pharmacologic hemostatic therapy in traumatic and acquired coagulopathy. Curr Drug Targets. 2016;17:954–70.
46. Benson AB, Moss M, Silliman CC. Transfusion-related acute lung injury (TRALI): a clinical review with emphasis on the critically ill. Br J Haematol. 2009;147:431.
47. Meyer DE, Reynolds JW, Hobbs R, et al. The incidence of transfusion-related acute lung injury at a large, Urban Tertiary Medical Center: a decade's experience. Anesth Analg. 2018;127:444.
48. Patel SV, Kidane B, Klingel M, et al. Risks associated with red blood cell transfusion in the trauma population, a meta-analysis. Injury. 2014;45:1522.
49. Jones AR, Patel RP, Marques MB, et al. Older blood is associated with increased mortality and adverse events in massively transfused trauma patients: secondary analysis of the PROPPR trial. Ann Emerg Med. 2019;73:650.
50. Vraets A, Lin Y, Callum JL. Transfusion-associated hyperkalemia. Transfus Med Rev. 2011;25:184.
51. Sihler KC, Napolitano LM. Complications of massive transfusion. Chest. 2010;137:209.
52. Perlman R, Callum J, Laflamme CA, et al. A recommended early goal-directed management guideline for the prevention of hypothermia-related transfusion, morbidity, and mortality in severely injured trauma patients. Crit Care. 2016;20:107.
53. ThermaCor 1200 rapid infusion device website. https://www.thermacor1200.com/company-info.cms. Accessed 10 Jul 2019.
54. Level 1 rapid infusion device website. https://www.smiths-medical.com/products/temperature-management/blood-and-fluid-warming-systems/fast-flow-fluid-warming-trauma/level-1-h1200-fast-flow-fluid-warmer-with-integrated-air-detectorclamp. Accessed 10 Jul 2019.
55. Belmont rapid infusion device website. http://www.eostip.com/imgs/pdf/pdf_1_10.pdf. Accessed 10 Jul 2019.
56. Cumunale ME. A laboratory evaluation of the level 1 rapid infuser (H1025) and the Belmont instrument fluid management system (FMS 2000) for rapid transfusion. Anesth Analg. 2003;97:1064–9.
57. Barcelona SL, Vilich F, Cote CJ. A comparison of flow rates and warming capabilities of the level 1 and rapid infusion system with various-size intravenous catheters. Anes Analg. 2003;97:358–63.
58. Wrenn EA, Wohlers R, Montgomery M, et al. Comparison of flow dynamics of peripherally and centrally inserted intravenous catheters using a rapid infusion system (ThermaCor1200). AANA. 2017;85(4):256–60.
59. Buck A. Large bore IV access showdown: do you know which IV cannula can deliver fluid to your patient the fastest? ETM Course. https://etmcourse.com/large-bore-iv-access-showdown/. Accessed 15 Jul 2019.

Point-of-Care Tests in for Blood Coagulation in the Perioperative Period

21

Sarah Leavitt, Shairko Missouri, Divya Patel, and Corey S. Scher

Thromboelastography utilizing the TEG® analyzer systems (*Haemonetics Corporation, Boston, MA*) and thromboelastometry utilizing the Rotem® analyzer systems (*Instrumentation Laboratory, Bedford, MA*) are presently benchmark tests for goal-directed blood component transfusions, in scenarios of bleeding and hemorrhage in cardiac, obstetrical, blunt, and penetrating trauma, brain trauma, and solid organ transplantation. It isis essential to know that there are no studies to compare Rotem and TEG. The choice between the two lies in which product was deployed by a department or hospital administration. Both tests rely on the concept of viscoelasticity. A substance is thought of as just a solid or just a liquid. One that is viscoelastic may have both properties. Elastic substances may undergo strain when stretched but will return to its normal state once that stressing factor is removed. Viscosity gives the material more stability and resists stretching [1]. Blood is a viscoelastic substance. Plasma demonstrates pure viscous behavior, while other components of blood are elastic. The viscoelasticity of blood is under the influence of four factors: (1) the environment (temperature), (2) interplay (RBC orientation and aggregation), (3) plasma factors (osmotic pressure, pH, concentration of fibrinogen and other plasma proteins), and (4) RBC factors (viscoelasticity and deformability of erythrocytes and their membranes).

There is little difference in blood viscoelasticity among normal cases but becomes significant with certain pathological states or surgical interventions. The formation of a clot results from the polymerization of factors that generate fibrin. The ongoing reactions generate a three-dimensional polymer network. This network changes the viscoelasticity prior and through the phase of fibrin generation. The changes in viscoelasticity during the clotting phase can be measured and presented to the anesthesiologist as a computerized tracing) [2].

The thromboelastogram (TEG®) tracing is nonlinear, and while valuable, it lacks a mathematical way to determine accuracy of the curves. Viscoelastic testing (TEG® and Rotem) has more than stood the test of time and remains an essential part of goal-directed blood product administration. Their utility is now in question as new tests based on different sciences are making their way to the market and appear to be more accurate due to the measurements that are linear.

Figure 21.1 is a TEG 5000 (Haemonetics Corporation®). To generate test results utilizing a TEG® 5000 analyzer, a small sample of whole blood (native, citrated or heparinized depending on tests run) is placed in a 37-degree cuvette (Fig. 21.2). A disposable pin is suspended from a torsion wire into the cup. The cup rotates through an angle of 4° for 45 min with each cycle lasting approximately10 s (Fig. 21.2). As the blood begins to clot and it adheres to both the pin and the cuvette, the clot will begin to transmit the rotation of the cup to the pin. The pin is suspended by a torsional spring which adds an elastic element to the system. The extent of resulting pin rotation is directly proportional to the strength of the clot. The corresponding numeric results and tracing represent all of the phases of clot formation and lysis [2].

Figures 21.3 and 21.4 illustrate all of the components of a TEG tracing to understand rate, strength, and stability or sustainability of a clot. The R reflects the "Reaction Time" and represents the coagulation pathways resulting in the initial thrombin burst and generation of fibrin or factor IIa.

A long "R" time may denote that factors are deficient and goal-directed fresh frozen plasma, or newly developed synthetic factors (10,9,7,2-KCENTRA®) [3]. Utilization of a

S. Leavitt · S. Missouri · D. Patel · C. S. Scher (✉)
NYU-Grossman School of Medicine, Department of Anesthesiology, New York, NY, USA
e-mail: sarah.leavitt@nyumc.org; Corey.Scher@nyulangone.org

© Springer Nature Switzerland AG 2021
C. S. Scher et al. (eds.), *Essentials of Blood Product Management in Anesthesia Practice*,
https://doi.org/10.1007/978-3-030-59295-0_21

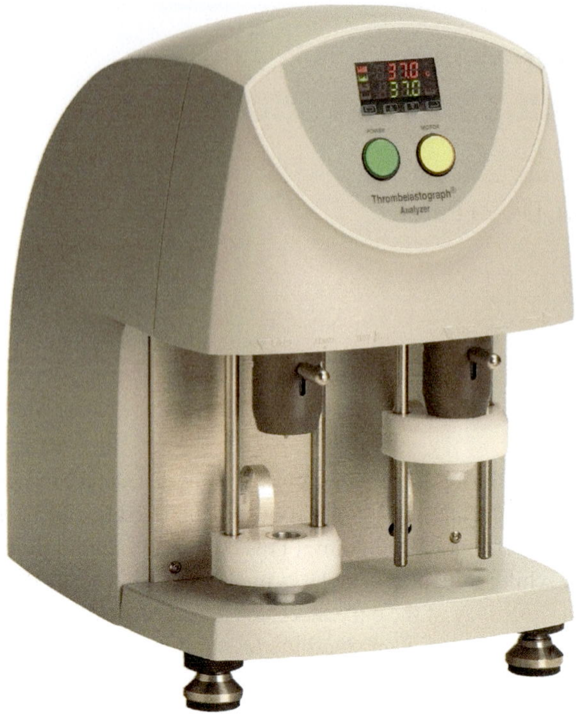

Fig. 21.1 TEG 5000. (With permission from Haemonetics Corporation)

cuvette impregnated with heparinase (identified with a blue colorant in the disposable plastic cup) can help determine if systemic heparin is responsible for the observed delay in clot formation.

Depending on the coagulation status of the patient and on the type of test run, it takes minutes or longer for the entire body of the TEG results to be displayed (Figs. 21.3 and 21.4).

The alpha (α), angle parameter is the slope of the line beginning at the point that the tracing diverges from the baseline line and is tangential to the TEG tracing. This represents the acceleration of fibrin buildup and cross-linking.

Critical information of the TEG analysis lies in the MA or maximum amplitude. It is the widest component of the TEG and represents the platelet fibrinogen interaction and overall clot strength. A general rule of thumb is that 80% of clot strength is contributed by platelets and 20% to fibrinogen [4, 6–8]. The clinician might surmise that if the MA is narrow, platelets are most likely deficient or not functioning. However, a TEG Functional Fibrinogen Assay measures the fibrinogen contribution to clot strength and provide greater specificity to guide therapy. The TEG Platelet Mapping® [5, 6] is an adjunctive test run on the same TEG analyzer that can assess platelet function of the MA if it is suboptimal.

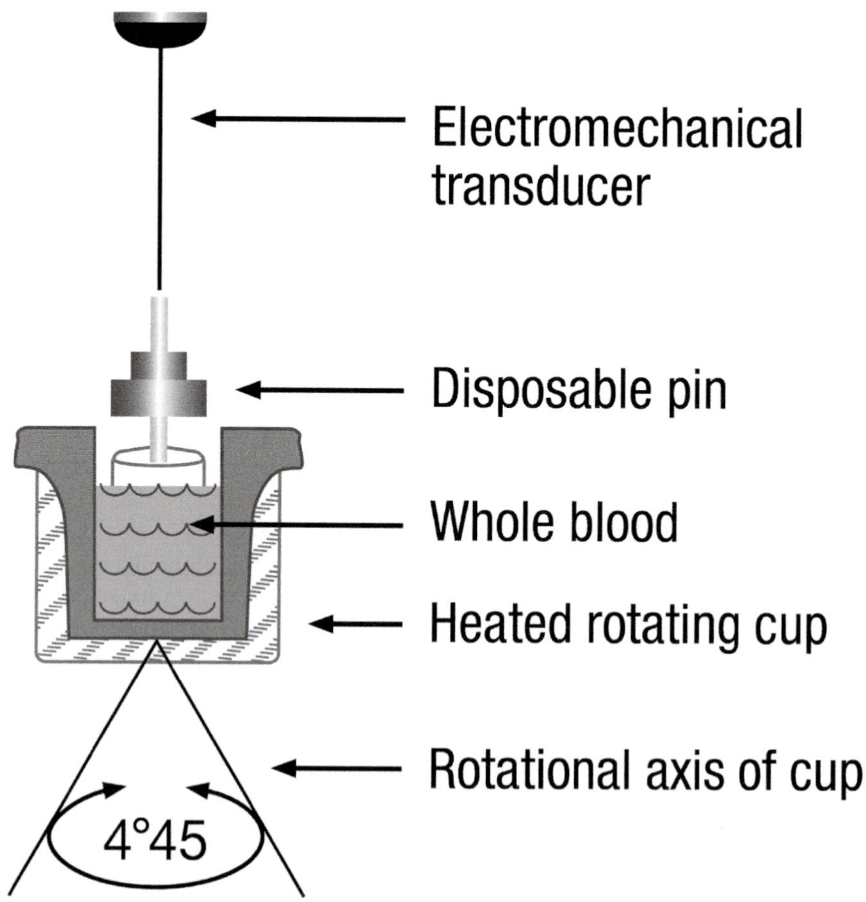

Fig. 21.2 The technology of TEG where the cup rotates. (With permission from Haemonetics Corporation)

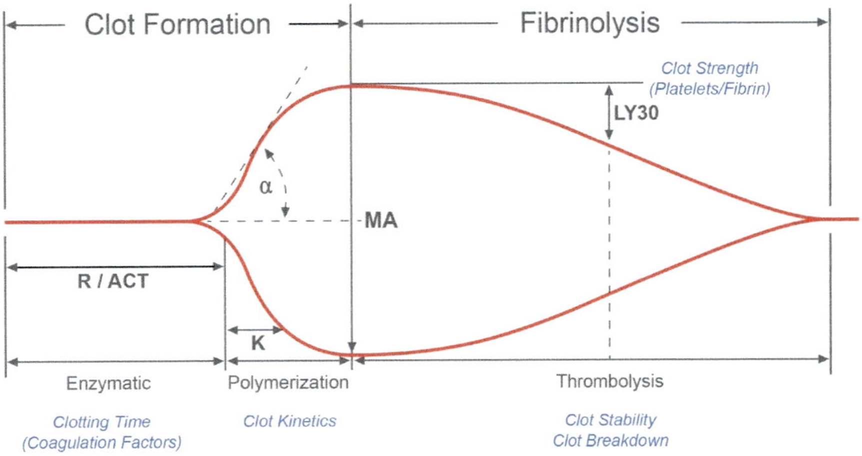

Fig. 21.3 TEG components. (With permission from Haemonetics Corporation)

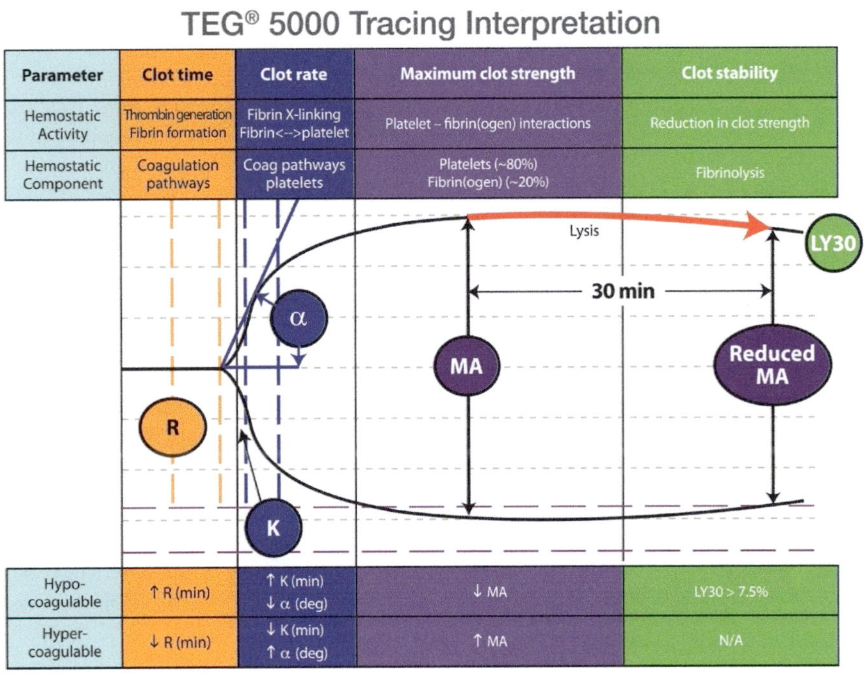

Fig. 21.4 Detailed figure demonstrating each component of a TEG using the TEG 5000. (With permission from Haemonetics Corporation)

The platelet function analyzer measures the speed of platelet adhesion.

Clot instability (Figs. 21.3 and 21.4) appears in this illustration as the MA declines near the end of the TEG tracing. The clot loses its stability as the amplitude of the tracing declines. This reflects fibrinolysis in the blood sample. Fibrinolytic inhibitors may be used prophylactically in some settings, such as CV surgery and some trauma setting. In settings where the hazard of thrombosis is much greater, and prophylactic anti-fibrinolytics are not desired, those drugs can quickly correct hyperfibrinolysis when it is detected. Fibrinolytic inhibitors, to have maximal effect, should be administered before hemorrhage begins for maximal prophylaxes. Once fibrinolysis begins, fibrinolytic inhibitors like aminocaproic acid and tranxamic acid are not helpful.

D-dimers are more useful as a tool of exclusion for VTE but can be elevated by a number of inflammatory states related to fibrinolysis. Even if a clot is confirmed, the D-dimer shows what has already happened in terms of clot breakdown. The TEG tracing shows the presence of active fibrinolysis by elevated clot lysis (LY30) or the lack of fibrinolysis by a stable MA.

Assays Available on the TEG 5000 Analyzer System Include

Kaolin (+/− heparinase) - An intrinsic pathway activated assay. This thrombin-generated tracing identifies underlying hemostatic characteristics and risk of bleeding or thrombosis.

RapidTEG (+/− heparinase) - An intrinsic and extrinsic pathway activated assay increases the coagulation process rapidly assess coagulation properties.

Functional Fibrinogen - An extrinsic pathway activated assay uses a potent GPIIb/IIIa platelet inhibitor to isolate fibrin contribution to clot strength. Used in conjunction with Kaolin, TEG can assess relative contribution of platelets and fibrin to overall clot strength.

Platelet Mapping (Haemonetics Corporation©) includes a thrombin-generated tracing (kaolin) and platelet receptor-specific tracing(s) (ADP/AA). Identifies the level of platelet function and inhibition using the patient's underlying hemostatic potential from the Kaolin TEG as the reference point.

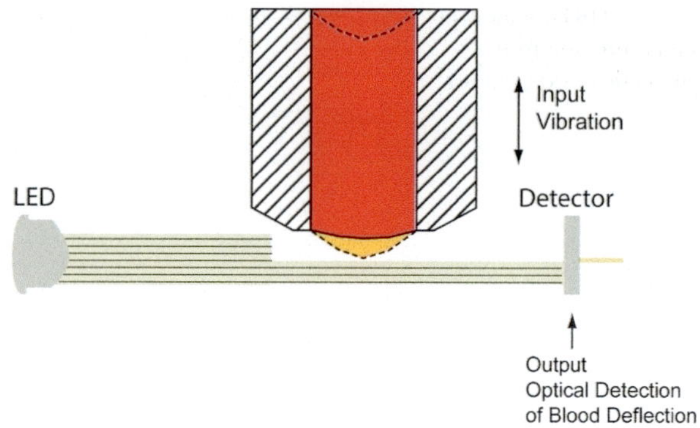

Fig. 21.6 The new technology of TEG 6000. (With permission from Haemonetics Corporation)

The TEG® 6s Analyzer System

TEG 6s (Haemonetics Corp, Boston MA) (Fig. 21.5) is the newest platform in the thrombelastography portfolio. It is a cartridge-based system which dramatically increases the ease of operation and the reproducibility of results [5, 6, 8]. All reagents are already in the cartridge and are mixed with the blood when a sample is added to the cartridge by means of a simple transfer pipette. Another benefit is a reduction in the amount of blood required to obtain the results. A cartridge with four assays can be run with 340 mcl of blood. These changes make the device well suited to use in a variety of care settings [1]. Each cartridge provides results from multiple tracings to provide data using a variety of assays to provide the quickest, most specific results to guide treatment decisions.

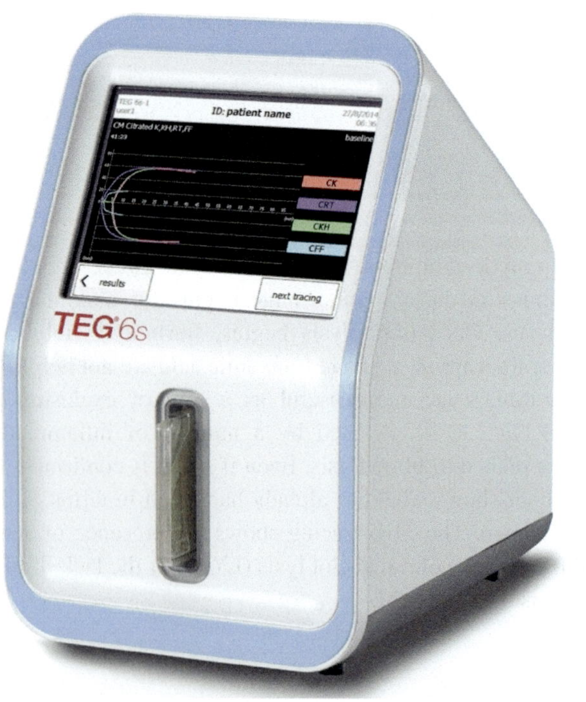

Fig. 21.5 The cartridge-based TEG® 6s analyzer. (With permission from Haemonetics Corporation)

Because it is a cartridge design, it no longer uses a cup and pin methodology, instead uses resonant frequency to assess the clot (Figs. 21.6 and 21.7). Each assay occupies a separate channel of the cartridge, to a total of four channels. Blood is added to the cartridge, where it is mixed with the reagents, then channeled into a capillary tube with a meniscus of blood at the testing chamber end of the capillary tube. A range of radiofrequencies are applied to the tube. The frequency which causes the blood to distend the furthest into the test chamber, blocking light from a photodetector, is the resonant frequency. Each resonant frequency is associated with a specific clot strength. As the clot moves through the process of clot initiation, reaches maximum clot strength, and potentially begins to break down, those changing resonant frequencies are plotted to produce the familiar TEG tracing (Figs. 21.6 and 21.7).

There are currently three cartridges available for the TEG 6s system. A Global Hemostasis cartridge provides four assays: citrated kaolin, citrated kaolin with heparinase, citrated rapid TEG, and citrated functional fibrinogen. This cartridge is FDA cleared for use in CV surgery and cardiology procedures. The Platelet Mapping® cartridge uses the same reagents as the Platelet Mapping (Haemonetic Corporation) assays in TEG 5000 to provide information on percent inhibition/aggregation and residual platelet reactivity, using ADP and arachidonic acid as the agonists (Figs. 21.6 and 21.7). This is used to assess the patient's response to antiplatelet therapies. The most recent cartridge is approved for use in trauma. It includes assays for citrated kaolin, citrated

RapidTEG™, and citrated functional fibrinogen. Using these assays in combination, it is possible to more specifically address hemostatic defects between platelets, fibrinogen, factors, heparin effect, and fibrinolysis (Figs. 21.8 and 21.9).

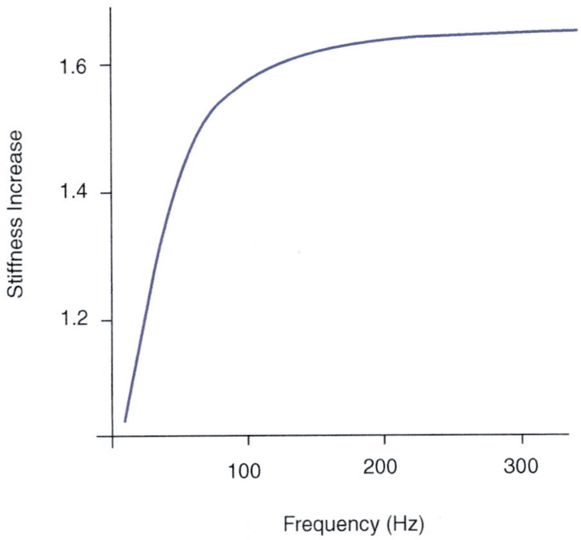

Fig. 21.7 New to the TEG system technology is the measurement of clot viscoelasticity using a resonance method. To measure the clot strength with the resonance method, the sample is exposed to a fixed vibration frequency. With LED illumination, a detector measures up/down motion of the blood meniscus. The frequency leading to resonance is identified and then converted to the TEG system readout. Stronger clots have higher resonant frequencies and higher TEG readouts. (With permission from Haemonetics Corporation)

Educational Tools

Rotational Thromboelastometry

ROTEM® or rotational thromboelastometry (**TEM** ®) is an alternative method of viscoelastic testing (Fig. 21.10). The cups in TEM determine the interaction of normal coagulation factors of blood with inhibitors, anticoagulant drugs, platelets, red blood cells, and fibrinolytics. ROTEM as in TEG utilizes a whole blood to assess clotting. Only the heparinase cups which are available for TEG have reactive agent.

Blood (300 μl) anticoagulated with citrate is placed into a cuvette using an electronic pipette. A disposable pin is attached to a shaft which is connected with a thin spring (the equivalent to Hartert's torsion wire in thrombelastography) and slowly oscillates back and forth. The signal of the pin suspended in the blood sample is transmitted via an optical detector system. The developing clot slows down the pin as the clot forms.

The test starts by adding appropriate reagents. The instrument measures and graphically displays the changes in elasticity at all stages of the developing clot. It is essential to know that the clot formed may become unstable by activating those factors that generate fibrinolysis. The typical test temperature is 37°C, but different temperatures can be selected, as in patients with hypothermia (Fig. 21.11).

By adding specific reagents, TEM like TEG can find specific points in the coagulation cascade where a problem exists.

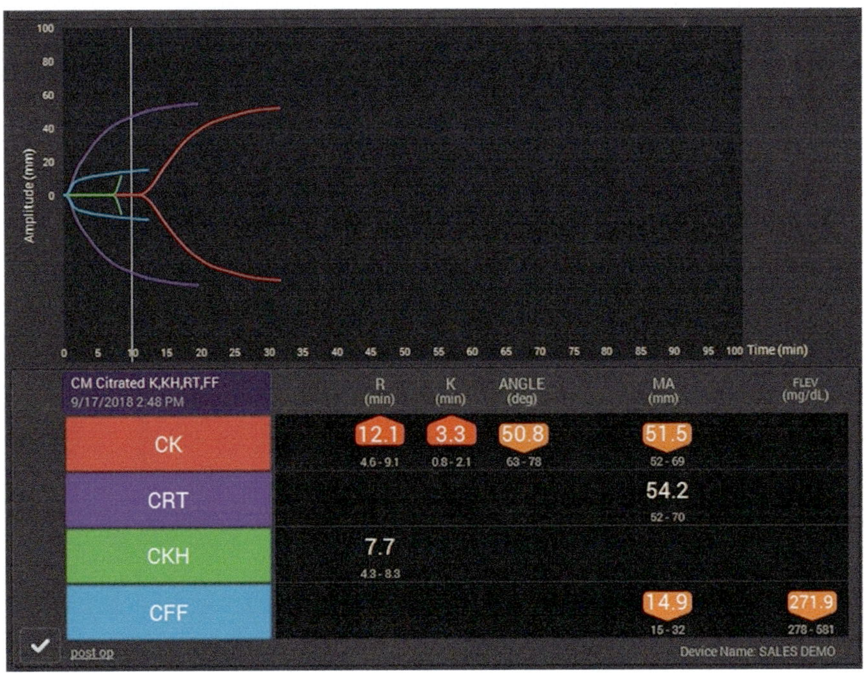

Fig. 21.8 Tracings on the left from the Global Hemostasis cartridge. CK citrated kaolin, CKH citrated kaolin with heparinase, CRT citrated RapidTEG, CFF citrated functional fibrinogen. The *white line* is a 10 min marker, by which time several parameters are already available to guide decision-making

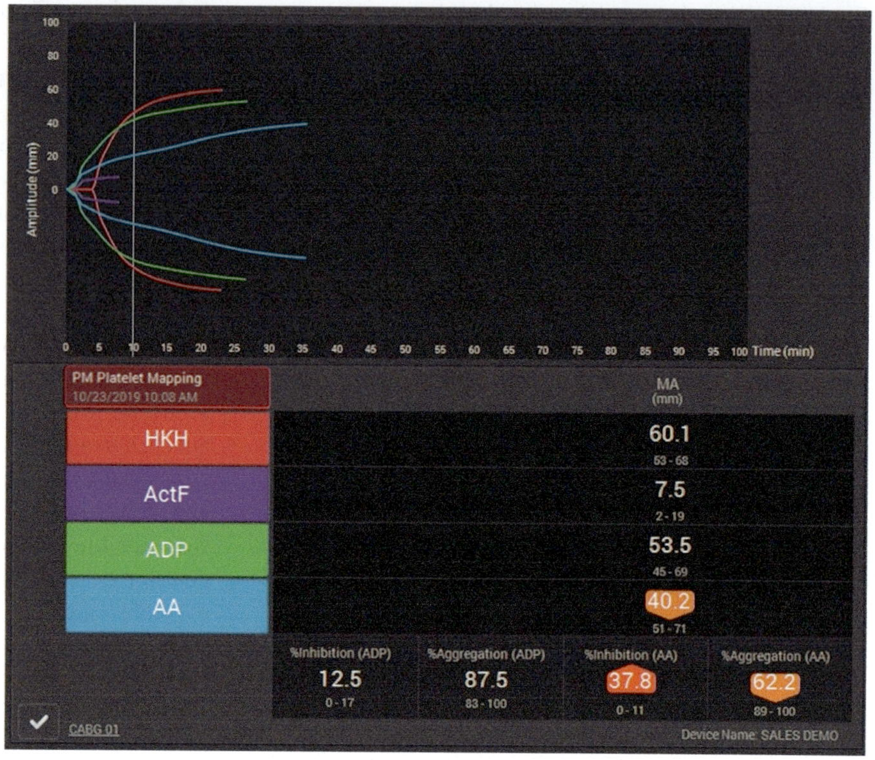

Fig. 21.9 Tracings above are from the Platelet Mapping cartridge. *HKH* heparinized kaolin with heparinase, represents maximum platelet activation, or no inhibition. *ActF* represents clot without platelet contribution, or 100% inhibition. ADP and AA tracings reflect strength of clot when those agonists are added to the activator. These last two are the patient's residual platelet reactivity after inhibition is assessed

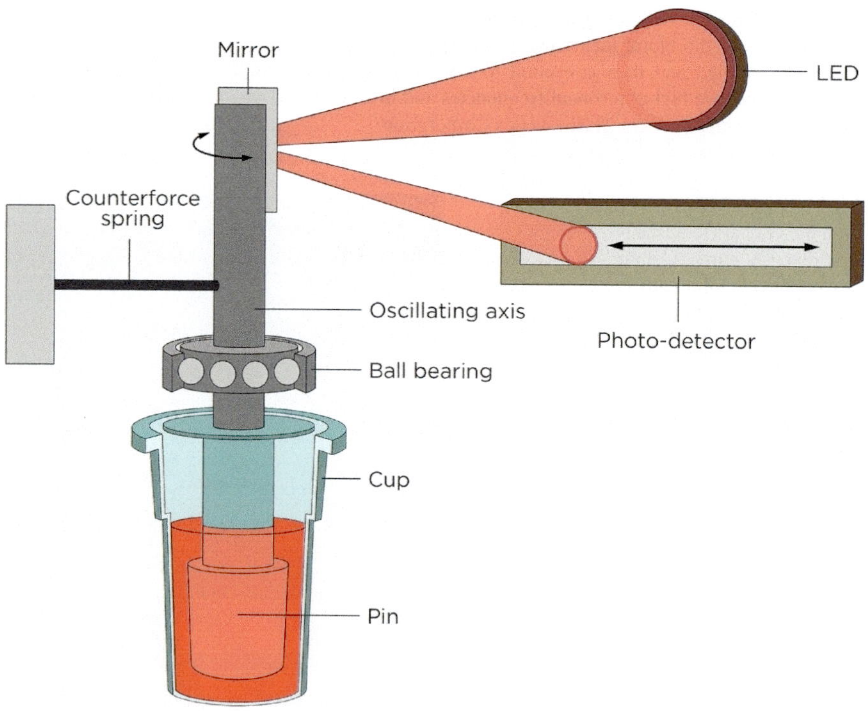

Fig. 21.10 The technology of ROTEM. Opposite from TEG, the torsion wire moves due to viscoelastic forces of clotting. In TEG the cup moves

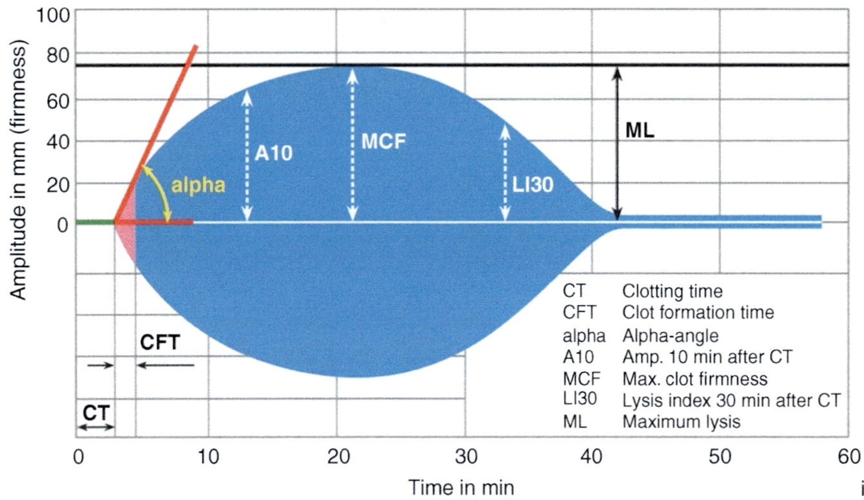

Fig. 21.11 This figure is the final result of ROTEM. While similar to TEG, the parameters measured for clot formation are different. Compare Fig. 21.3 to this Figure

As explained by Instrumentation Laboratories Worldwide (Fig. 21.12):

1. INTEM – Contains phospholipid and elagic acid which are activators and provides information similar to that of the aPTT
2. EXTEM – Contains tissue factor as an activator and provides information similar to that of the PT
3. HEPEM – Contains lyophilized heparinase for neutralizing heparin
4. APTEM – Contains aprotinin for inhibiting fibrinolysis
5. IBTEM – Utilizes cytochalasin D, **a** platelet inhibitor which blocks the platelet contribution to clot formation, allowing qualitative analysis of the functional fibrinogen component

TEG and TEM measurements, for the most part, are not interchangeable. The time of initial fibrin formation is the R time in TEG or clotting time in TEM. Clotting time or CT is the time from the test beginning until the amplitude of 2 mm is reached (Fig. 21.5). The CT time is increased or prolonged by hereditary or acquired inhibitors, (hemophilia or warfarin), factor deficiencies, or when factor function becomes impaired as with the direct thrombin inhibitors. Simply stated, when the CT line increases, coagulation factors are needed. In hemophilia, TEG/TEM monitoring is helpful when factor 10a activity is blocked as seen with apixaban with resumed activity when this drug was discontinued [7, 8].

Application of the TEG® System in Trauma

Trauma is the second leading cause of death worldwide with 40% mortality associated with massive hemorrhage. The balance between hemostasis and fibrinolysis is disrupted by acidosis, hypothermia and hemodilution, tissue damage, exposure, and fluid/blood product administration tip scales away from hemostasis. Acute traumatic coagulopathy, mediated by activation of the thrombomodulin-protein C system, further promotes fibrinolysis.

The Prospective, Observational, Multicenter, Major Trauma Transfusion Trial (PROMMTT) investigated the "Comparative Effectiveness of a Time-varying Treatment with Competing Risks [9], which recognized coagulopathy in 42% of trauma patients. Management of DIC typically involved conventional coagulation analysis to guide transfusion protocol. Since the utilization of TEG in Germany, it has become increasingly popular in the acute monitoring of coagulation for cardiac and liver transplantation cases and has expanded into other medical specialties, other than trauma.

One of the earliest prospective studies [10] investigating the utility of TEG in the assessment of trauma patients demonstrated that of the parameters measured, (demographics, medical history of coagulopathy, medications, TEG indices, platelet count, PT/PTT, revised trauma score, and injury severity score), only TEG and injury severity score were accurate predictors of early transfusion [10]. The Injury Severity Score assesses trauma severity. It correlates with mortality, morbidity, and hospitalization time after trauma.

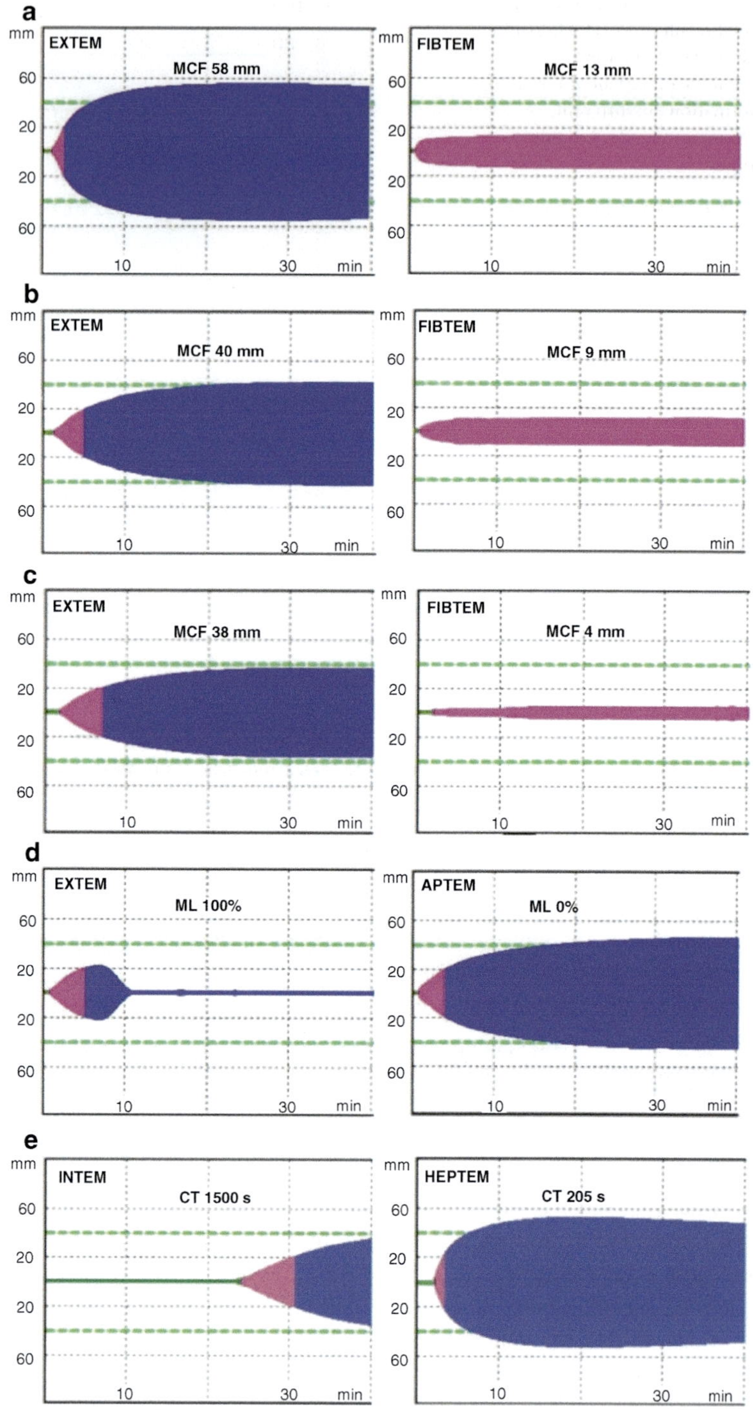

Fig. 21.12 INTEM This test activates the contact phase of hemostasis. The result is influenced by coagulation factors, platelets, fibrinogen, and heparin. In the absence of heparin, INTEM is a screening test for the hemostasis system. It is used for therapeutic decisions regarding the administration of fresh frozen plasma, coagulation factors, fibrinogen, or platelets HEPTEM. This assay represents an INTEM assay performed in the presence of heparinase, a heparin (or LMWH)-degrading enzyme. The difference between HEPTEM and INTEM CT-value comparison confirms the presence of heparin.
EXTEM test activates hemostasis via the physiological activator tissue factor. The result is influenced by extrinsic coagulation factors, platelets, and fibrinogen. EXTEM represents the extrinsic pathway. This assay is not influenced by heparin (heparin inhibitor included in the EXTEM reagent). It guides goal-directed therapy with the deployment of coagulation factors, fibrinogen, or platelets.
FIBTEM test is an EXTEM-based assay for the fibrin part of the clot. FIBTEM eliminates the platelet contribution of clot formation by inhibiting the platelets irreversibly with cytochalasin D, a potent inhibitor of actin polymerization which disrupts actin microfilaments, an essential part of a cytoskeleton-mediated contractibility apparatus of the platelet. The use of cytochalasin is more favorable than using glycoprotein IIb/ IIIa inhibitors which block platelet incompletely.
FIBTEM allows for the detection of fibrinogen deficiency or fibrin polymerization disorders, e.g., induced by certain plasma expanders, and may identify rapidly the need to substitute fibrinogen.
APTEM test is an EXTEM-based assay for fibrinolysis. APTEM compared to EXTEM allows to detect fulminant hyperfibrinolysis.

It is used to define the term major trauma. A major trauma is defined as the Injury Severity Score being greater than 15.

Consistent with the PROMMTT trial, 75% of the trauma patients were diagnosed with coagulopathy. Of those, 87% were hypercoagulable and the remaining hypocoagulable. By design, this study did not allow for TEG coagulation analysis to alter clinical decision-making. The authors noted that TEG data can predict the magnitude of hemostasis derangement and may be implemented into the approach for transfusion.

A subsequent porcine study [11] compared PT, PTT, and activated clotting time against TEG indices in hypothermia versus hemorrhagic shock. Hypothermia directly results in inhibition of platelet function and reduction of clotting factor activity. This caused a hindrance to initial clot formation. In contrast, hemorrhage elicits massive bleeding, disseminated intravascular coagulation, and thrombotic/embolic complications; all impairing clot strength and stability. In this investigation, pigs were subjected to sham, hypothermic, hemorrhagic, or hypothermia and hemorrhagic conditions.

PT and PTT lacked sensitivity and activated clotting time lacked specificity in identifying the condition associated with the coagulopathy. TEG accurately differentiated between the conditions due its comprehensive assessment of the coagulation process. The authors recommended implementing TEG data into treatment of hypothermia- and hemorrhagic shock-related coagulopathy [11].

Adding to the pre-existing literature, a study published in 2012 [12] evaluated nearly 2000 trauma patients with a median injury severity score of 17. Twenty-five percent of these patients presented with overt shock, and of these, 28% were transfused. After controlling for age, mechanism of injury, weighted-revised trauma score, base excess, and hemoglobin, the investigators deduced that the TEG r-time predicted RBC transfusion with greater superiority than PT/PTT/INR. The TEG α angle predicted plasma transfusion with greater superiority than fibrinogen; and, the TEG maximum amplitude predicted platelet transfusion with greater superiority than platelet count. These correlations improved in transfusion, shock, and head injury cases. Additionally, the cost of r-TEG was only marginally greater than that of the five conventional tests (PT, PTT, INR, platelet count, fibrinogen) [12].

In a prospective study of 272 trauma patients [13], TEG r and k time were available within 5 min and maximum amplitude and α angle within 15 min as compared to conventional coagulation tests that were not available until 48 min. r-TEG values, ACT k-time, and r values predicted red blood cell, plasma, and platelet transfusion within 2 h of arrival; specifically, ACT > 128 predicted massive transfusion, whereas ACT < 105 predicted no transfusion.

Investigators at Ben Taub General in Houston [14] published a study following the hospital's transition from massive transfusion protocol guided by TEG to a 1:1:1 ratio of blood, plasma, and platelets [14]. Their data demonstrated no difference in resuscitation strategy in patients receiving greater than 6 units of red blood cells or in patients with blunt trauma receiving greater than 10 units of red blood cells. The 1:1:1 protocol had greater mortality rates than the TEG protocol in cases of penetrating trauma with transfusion of 10 or more units of red blood cells. This suggests that the 1:1:1 protocol may not be extrapolated and hemostatic to all patients.

Following this investigation, the Denver Health Medical Center [15] with a level 1 trauma center published a randomized clinical trial to test the hypothesis that massive transfusion protocol guided by TEG improves clinical outcomes compared with massive transfusion protocol goal directed by conventional coagulation assays (CCA, PT, PTT, fibrinogen, platelet count, and d-dimers). A total of 111 patients with a median injury severity score of 30 were enrolled and of whom 27% presented with penetrating trauma. As compared to 36% mortality in CCA-guided transfusion group, the TEG-guided transfusion group had a 19% mortality rate. This difference was believed to be secondary to decreased early hemorrhagic death in the TEG group. There were significantly more plasma and platelet transfusions within 2 h of arrival and overall more cryoprecipitate transfusions in the CCA guided transfusion arm. There were no differences in the volume of crystalloid or red blood cell units transfused. The TEG-guided transfusion group was also associated with decreased ventilator dependence and ICU hospitalization.

In summary, acute traumatic coagulopathy is associated with greater transfusion requirements, prolonged ICU hospitalization, and increased incidence of multi-organ complications. As compared to patients without coagulopathy, those diagnosed with coagulopathy have 3–4 times greater mortality rate overall and 8 times greater mortality rate within the first 24 h of injury.

Given these statistics, rapid identification and treatment, with modalities such as TEG, improved and ongoing coagulopathy.

Application of Thromboelastography/Thromboelastometry in Obstetric Hemorrhage

The 2017 American College of Obstetricians and Gynecologist guidelines define postpartum hemorrhage (PPH) as bleeding with signs and symptoms of hypovolemia or cumulative blood loss of >1000 mL within the first 24 h of delivery. The national incidence of PPH varies between 1% and 10% of all deliveries, and PPH remains one of the top 5 causes of obstetric morbidity and mortality globally.

While pregnancy induces a hypercoagulable state, the postpartum period elicits fibrinolysis. Hyperfibrinolysis is associated with the consumption and depletion of coagulation factors (particularly fibrinogen) and inhibition of clot formation. This phenomenon is critical to the development of acquired coagulopathy of PPH and is targeted in the management of PPH [16]. Conventional laboratory tests for hyperfibrinolysis (D-dimer, fibrinogen) reflect indirect measures of coagulopathy through report of historical events and may take 60–90 min to result [17]. This either delays goal-directed transfusion therapy or, in emergent cases, unnecessarily promotes empiric treatment of suspected hyperfibrinogenemia. Point-of-care TEG analyses allow for early identification of the hemostatic derangements during pregnancy. A recent prospective longitudinal study comparing TEG parameters demonstrated a hypercoagulable profile with increased clot strength and decreased fibrinolysis during pregnancy as compared to 8 weeks postpartum [18]. A subsequent study, investigating TEG parameters in massive obstetric hemorrhage, (MOH; defined as >2 L estimated blood loss) reported rapid initiation of clotting, decreased clot strength, and decreased fibrinolysis in MOH as compared to normal delivery. The same study also compared TEG to conventional coagulopathy analyses (PT, PTT, fibrinogen, antithrombin, D-dimer) and suggested integration of viscoelastic assays into transfusion protocol can rapidly diagnose etiology of bleeding and thereby improve response time [19].

Rotational thromboelastometry (ROTEM) provides the FIBTEM assay as a measure of clot strength; this analysis is available within 10 min and accurately differentiates among hypofibrinogenemia, hypofibrinogenesis, and hyperfibrinolysis, thereby theoretically informing fibrinogen replacement therapy [20]. A prospective, observational study compared the utility of FIBTEM (TEM surrogate for plasma fibrinogen level) and conventional fibrinogen in 356 women with 1–1.5 L PPH. The investigators recognized FIBTEM, but not fibrinogen/PTT/PT, as an independent predictor of progression of bleeds >2.5 L, ≥4 U packed red blood cells (PRBCs), and 8 U allogeneic products [20]. It was noted that FIBTEM was an early biomarker for PPH severity/progression. Fibrinogen <2 g/L and FIBTEM <10 mm were associated with prolonged bleeding, increased frequency of invasive procedures, and earlier transfusion. Based on these findings, the authors deduced ROTEM has the potential to markedly improve clinical outcomes via early administration of fibrinogen concentrate and decreased transfusion of high-volume blood products, including RBCs, FFP, and platelets. These results were replicated with similar findings in subsequent investigations with one observational study showing a 1.8-fold reduction in total MOH transfusions with integration of a ROTEM-guided transfusion protocol [21].

A recent multicenter, double-blinded, randomized controlled trial studied the efficacy of early fibrinogen replacement guided by visco-elastometric measures. The trial enrolled 55 females with PPH of 1–1.5 L. Participants with FIBTEM <15 mm were randomized to fibrinogen concentrate or placebo transfusion with the primary outcome comparing total number of blood products transfused. The results indicated no statistically significant reduction in transfusion requirements between the two groups. These findings also suggested FIBTEM of 15 mm as too high as an interventional trigger. The authors further concluded that at FIBTEM A5 > 12 mm or fibrinogen >2 g/L, normal physiologic hemostasis still occurs and does not warrant fibrinogen replacement [21].

The utility of TEG [22] expands beyond PPH to include recognition and management of catastrophic amniotic fluid embolism, gray platelet syndrome, Glanzmann's thrombasthenia, hemophilia, platelet storage pool disorder, placental abruption, disseminated intravascular coagulation, and HELLP syndrome. Despite these findings, the primary limitation to widespread integration of TEG/TEM-guided transfusion protocols remains the lack of large randomized controlled trials. Further investigations with high-power and multicenter involvement are needed.

New Technologies for Clot Assessment and Clot Stability

- Sonorheometry
- Microfluidic devices
- Quartz crystal microbalance
- Laser speckle rheology

Sonorheometry

Sonic Estimation of Elasticity via Resonance (SEER) or sonorheometry is a technology that employs ultrasound waves to measure changes in viscoelastic properties during the process of coagulation. This identifies and qualifies clot formation [23].

Repetitive high-frequency ultrasound signals propagate through the blood sample in an air-sealed cartridge generating gentle nudging on the blood clot early in the process of its formation. Clot displacement (i.e., shear modulus) will occur which will generate series of returning frequency echoes (Fig. 21.13 *left panel*). Tracking and analyzing the returning echoes can estimate the sample motion over time and creating a displacement curve. The shape of the displacement curve is directly related to the shear modulus of the sample at any point time [24].

Changes over time in shear modulus is a direct physical measure of clot stiffness. Repeating signals over time creates a signature time-displacement curve. Figure 21.13 reflects the dynamic changes in shear modulus of the sample during coagulation at any given point in time.

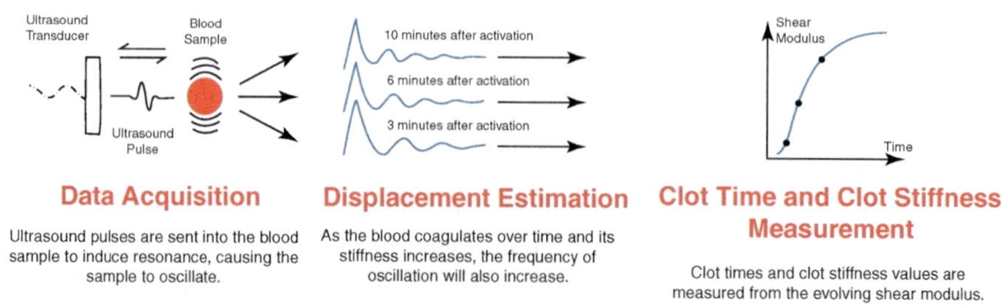

Fig. 21.13 Sonorheometry technology. (Copy permitted by Quantra HemoSonics)

The shear modulus is the elastic properties of materials [25]. It is a parameter of materials to resist displacement when exhibiting external forces, and it is measured by Pascal (Pa). For example, bone tissue has a shear force of 3.3 GPa shear, while natural rubber has 600 Pa and liquids has 0 Pa. The "Quantra Hemostasis Analyzer," designed by HemoSonics, is a point-of-care (POC) test that provides quick results in a critical care environment. It generates complete test results within 15 min of test initiation [24].

The analysis cartridge allows a small sample to be collected, provides no physical contacts with the blood sample, and will permit detection of early soft clots identification. It has been demonstrated that a large shear stress applied by instruments during measurements like ROTAM [26] did disrupt clot formation. The lack of disruption to the sample during the processing provides high sensitivity to detect soft/weak clots which are often associated with clinical bleeding [27]. The "Quantra" analyzer cartridge is a multi-channeled and a single-use disposable plastic component (Fig. 21.14). It has four independent channels, each containing pre-filled lyophilized reagents that enable simultaneous differential testing without the need for any reagent preparation or pipetting. Lyophilization of the reagents provides stability at room temperature [28].

The cartridge is the only component of the device that is in direct contact with blood which prevents potential biohazard spills. The cartridge protects the sample from environmental factors interference, such as temperature, vibration, or evaporation.

Cartridges

The QPlus Cartridge was designed to evaluate a patient's functional coagulation status in major surgeries. The cartridge can be stored at room temperature and immediately available for acute bleeding situations without warming or special preparation. This cartridge provides all the parameters of Quantra analyzer (Fig. 21.15) except for clot stability to lysis (CSL) which can be measured by the QStat® Cartridge [28]. CSL measures changes to clot stiffness change in the presence of tranexamic acid which is the function of fibrinogen. It is useful in level 1 traumas, liver transplantation, complicated obstetrics, cardiac surgery, and critical care units.

Fig. 21.14 Measured parameters on hemosonics analyzer (QPlus Cartridge)

QPlus Cartidge Measurements

Parameter	units	Description	Measurement
Clot Time (CT)	Seconds	Clot time citrated whole blood.	Clot time measured in Channel #1 with activator of the intrinsic pathway (kaolin).
Heparinase Clot Time (CTH)	Seconds	Clot time in citrated whole blood with heparin neutralization.	Clot time measured in Channel #2 with activator of the intrinsic pathway (kaolin) and heparinase.
Clot Time Ratio (CTR)	No units	The CTR parameter may indicate the prolongation of the intrinsic pathway clotting time that is likely due to the influence of unfractionated heparin. CTR values are not directly correlated with heparin levels in the sample; if CTR is > 1.4, it is only indicative of heparin in the sample.	Calculated as the ratio of clot time values of Channel #1 over Channel #2 (CT/CTH).
Clot Stiffness (CS)	hecto Pascals (hPa)	Stiffness of the whole blood clot.	Clot stiffness measured in Channel #3 with an activator of the extrinsic pathway (thromboplastin) and heparin inhibitor (polybrene).
Fibrinotgen Contribution to Clot Stiffness (FCS)	hecto Pascals (hPa)	Contribution of functional fibrinogen to overall clot stiffness.	Clot stiffness measured in Channel #4 with an activator of the extrinsic pathway (thromboplastin) and heparin inhibitor (polybrene) and platelet inhibitor (abciximab).
Platelet Contribution to Clot Stiffness (PCS)	hecto Pascals (hPa)	Contribution of platelet activity to overall clot stiffness.	Calculated by subtracting clot stiffness value of Channel #4 from Channel #3.

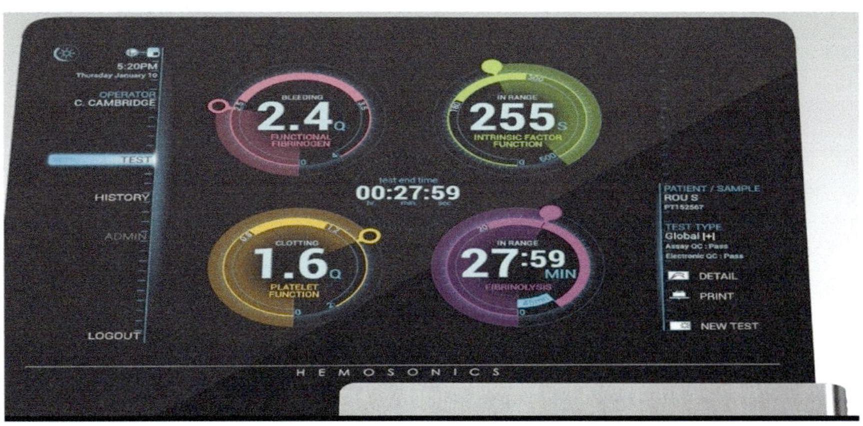

Fig. 21.15 Test results as displayed on hemosonics analyzer

Microfluidic Devices

The Wyss Institute team led by Wyss Institute Founding Director Donald Ingber, M.D., Ph.D., has developed a novel microfluidic device in which blood flows through a life like network of small "vessels," where it is subjected to true-to-life shear stresses and force gradients of the human vascular network. Using automated pressure sensors and a proprietary algorithm developed by the Wyss team, data acquired from the device is analyzed in real time, precisely predicting the time at which a certain blood sample will obstruct. The hemostasis monitoring microdevice mimics rapid changes in blood flow dynamics associated with stenosis or narrowing of small blood vessels by pumping pressurized blood flow through the device's microfluidic channels [29].

In this schematic and series of magnified insets (Fig. 21.16) from left to right, the microfluidic channels progress from pre-stenosis, to stenosis, to post-stenosis, simulating the narrowing of blood vessels that can often occur in patients as a result of medical conditions or treatments. The effects of stenosis on blood clotting tendency are visible: blood clotting protein fibrin (green) and blood platelets (red) are seen coagulating as they progress through the device, and most notably in the post-stenotic region.

By combining Wyss's fabricated microfluidic device that mimics blood flow dynamics of small arterioles with their novel data analysis software, a quantitate hemostasis in real-time and predict if blood clots will develop in an individual or in a blood sample. The integrated low-cost miniaturized equipment requires less than 1.0 ml of blood sample and have made it ideal as a bedside monitor to identify and quantify clot formation and platelets function precisely and in real time.

In the past 10 years, several microfluidic devices were produced to study different biological reactions like enzymatic reaction kinetics and fluid viscosity [30]. Schoeman et al. designed a microfluidic chip to measure clot formation evoked by blood flow. Blood samples flow from a high-pressure flow channel into a lower-pressure receiver channel until a hemostatic clot formed (Fig. 21.17). The channels were coated with procoagulants: collagen and tissue factor. This allowed him to measure normal physiological blood clot to form within a clotting time of 7.5 min.

Schoeman designed another microfluidic chip with defects in reagents to mimic hemophilia A with anti-Factor VIII antibody, and he identifies an unstable clot formation as would be expected in vivo. His team also demonstrated that treatment of blood with antiplatelet P2Y12 receptor inhibitor substantially delayed the clotting time [31].

Microfluidics cell can be designed in different complex geometries that mimic stenosed arteries to study various pathological events and aim to evaluate an individual patient's coagulopathy or compliance with treatment.

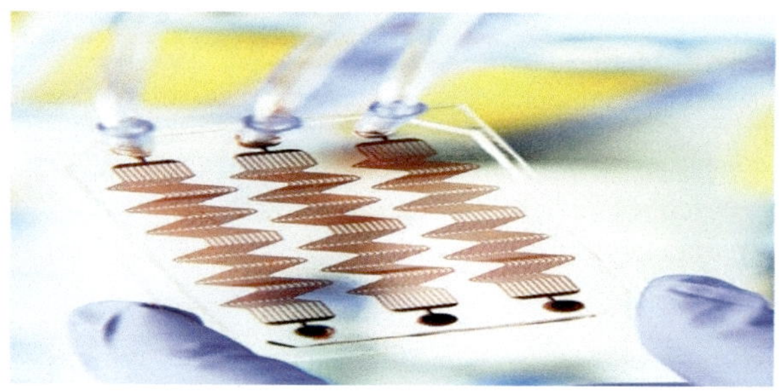

Fig. 21.17 Microfluidic 3 channels cartridge. (Courtesy of Wyss Institute at Harvard University)

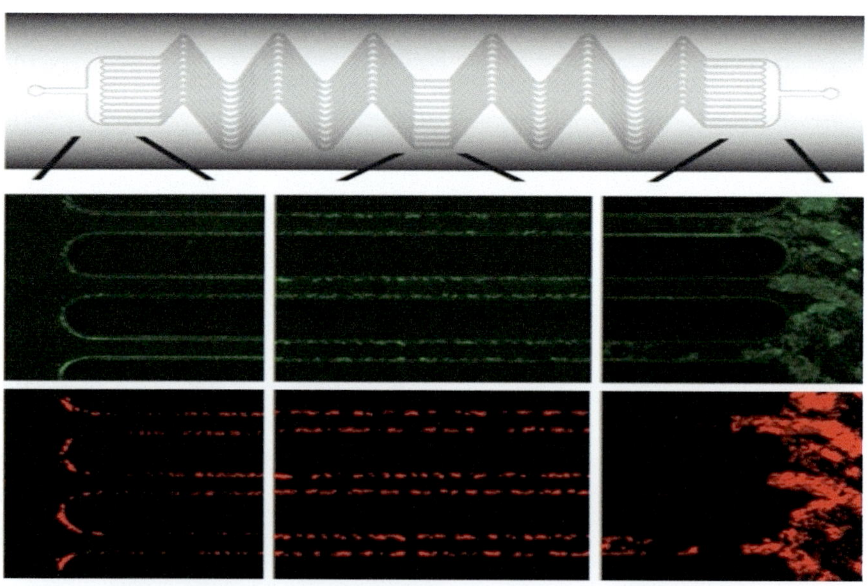

Fig. 21.16 Schematic microfluidic channels. (Courtesy of Wyss Institute at Harvard University)

Recently, the incorporation of endothelium into the operation of these devices remails a future possibility to be readily available at bedside in order to assist in clinical decision making [32–34].

In summary, microfluidic device measures patient clotting abilities under any specific physical flow pattern and, as a result, can be an invaluable tool for clinical diagnostics.

Quartz Crystal Microbalance

The basis of QCM operation relates to quartz's physical property of piezoelectricity, and as the alternating electric current passes on to the crystal, a mechanical energy generates oscillating waves with a recordable frequencies [35].

Crystal's thickness and cut is detrimental as a trade-off the generated frequency, the thinner is the crystal the higher is the resonant frequency [36].

The QCM sensor consists of a thin circular quartz that is sandwiched between a pair of electrodes and a blood sample will face the electrodes (Fig. 21.18). When sufficient AC voltage is applied to the electrodes, the crystal gets excited and generates oscillation, and a resonance will be generated with a specific frequency and will be detected and measured by a sensor. During the process of clot formation, a mass will be adsorbed on the electrodes causing change in frequency and resonance [37]. When a mass is attached to the sensor, the frequency decreases. If the mass is rigid, the decrease in frequency is proportional to the size of the mass. This linear relationship between changing in mass adsorbed on the surface of quartz crystal electrodes and proportional reduction in frequency was discovered by Sauerbrey in 1959 and established CQM algorithm foundation [33].

However, Sauerbrey equation is linear for rigid mass formation due to its even distribution with sufficiently thin adsorbed layers [34]. Therefore implementing a dissipation parameter will allow analysis of soft films that do not obey the linear relation between change in frequency and change in mass. The soft or viscoelastic will be underestimated as it is not fully coupled to the oscillating crystal. By adding and measuring the dissipation to the QCM, one can determine the adsorbed viscoelastic (soft) mass on the plate [38, 39].

Dissipation done by shutting off the driving voltage to the crystal and the energy from the oscillating crystal dissipates from the system [40]. This procedure can be repeated over 200 times per second, which gives QCM-D great sensitivity and high resolution. QCM-D measures both frequency and dissipation of the quartz crystal [41].

Laser Speckle Rheology

Laser speckle rheology (LSR) is a novel approach to evaluate the frequency-dependent process of viscoelastic blood clot formation using non-contact optical approach. A laser beam will illuminate the blood sample during the process of clot formation; light rays will be scattered by the multiple particles in the blood sample. The scattered speckles created will be captured on a high-speed camera (CMOS) (Fig. 21.19). The scale of time-varying speckle images correlated with a time-real viscoelastic clot formation and will be captured and recorded by the CMOS and analyzed by a computer software.

The Brownian motion phenomenon is one of the elements in the process of LSR evaluation, and it is defined as a random motion of particles suspended in a fluid resulting from their collision with the fast-moving particle in the

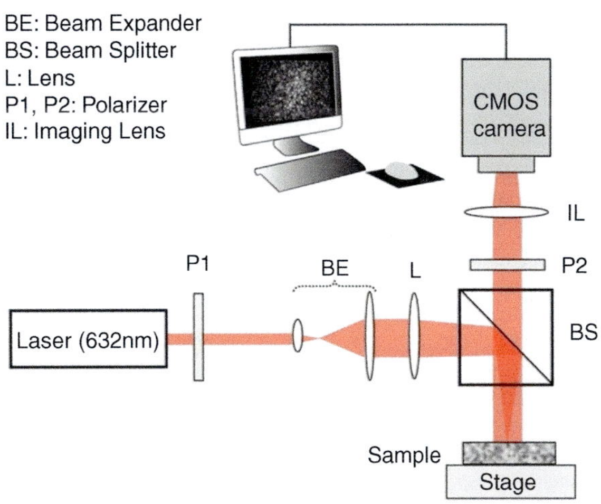

Fig. 21.19 Technology of laser speckle

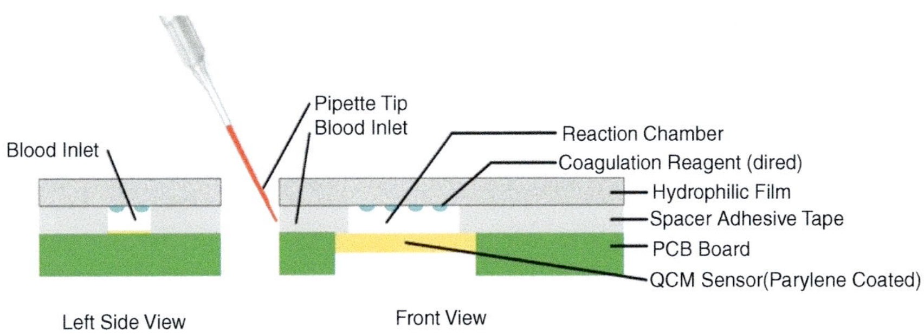

Fig. 21.18 QCM-D transducer consisting of a piezoelectric quartz sensor with two differently sized gold electrodes

fluid. The Brownian motion of blood clot has less restrictions on the scale of scattered particles reflecting wider range of speckle [42]. During the progress of clot formation with more fibrin-formation and platelets aggregation, the clot gets stiffer and restricts the scatter displacements. The camera will register lesser area of speckle fluctuations during the course of clot stiffness.

Blood coagulation status has been measured by relating the time scale of speckle intensity fluctuations with the clinically relevant coagulations parameters, including clotting time and fibrinogen content.

Markandey et al. demonstrated a close correlation between coagulation metrics measured using LSR and conventional coagulation results of activated partial thromboplastin time, prothrombin time, and functional fibrinogen levels [43].

References

1. Ganter MT, Hofer CK. Coagulation monitoring: current techniques and clinical use of viscoelastic point- of- care coagulation devices. Anesth Analg. 2008;106:1366–75.
2. Schmidt A, Israel AK, Refaai MA. The utility of thromboelastography to guide blood product transfusion. An ACLPS critical review. Am J Clin Pathol. 2019;152:407–22.
3. Nielson VG. A comparison of the thromboelastograph and the Rotem. Blood Coagul Fibrinolysis. 2007;18:247–52.
4. Wikkelso A, Wetterslev J, Møller AM, Afshari A. Thromboelastography(TEG) or thromboelastometry (ROTEM) to monitor hemostatic treatment versus usual care in adults or children with bleeding. Cochrane Database Syst Rev. 2016;(8):CD007871. https://doi.org/10.1002/14651858.pub3.
5. Gurbel PA, Bliden K, Tantry US, et al. First report of the point-of-care TEG: a technical validation study of the TEG-6S system. Platelets. 2016;27(7):642–9.
6. Lloyd-Donald P, Churilov L, Cheong B, et al. Assessing TEG6S reliability between devices and across multiple time points: a prospective thromboelastography validation study. Sci Rep. 2020;10(1):7045.
7. Theusinger OM, Schroder CM, Eismon J, Emmert Y, Seifert B, Spahn RD, Baulig W. The influence of laboratory coagulation factor levels on rotational thromboelastometry (ROTEM) during major surgery with hemorrhage. Anes Analg. 2013;117(2):314–21. Ghossh K, Shetty S., Kulkarni B. Correlation of thromboelastographic patterns and clinical presentation and rational for the use of anti-fibrinolytics in severe hemophilia patients. Haemophilia. 2007;13:734–79.
8. Juffermans NP, Wirtz MR, Balvers K, Baksaas-Aasen K, van Dieren S, Gaarder C, et al. Towards patient-specific management of trauma hemorrhage: the effect of resuscitation therapy on parameters of thromboelastometry. J Thromb Haemost. 2019;17(3):441–8.
9. Martini W, Cortez D, Dubick M, Park M, Holcomb J. Thromboelastography is better than PT, aPTT, and activated clotting time in detecting clinically relevant clotting abnormalities after hypothermia, hemorrhagic shock and resuscitation in pigs. J Trauma. 2008;65(3):53543.
10. Holcomb JB, Minei KM, Scerbo ML, Radwan ZA, Wade CE, Kozar RA, et al. Admission rapid thromboelastography can replace conventional coagulation tests in the emergency department: experience with 1974 consecutive trauma patients. Ann Surg. 2012;256(3):476–86.
11. Stensballe J. Hemostatic resuscitation for massive bleeding: the paradigm of plasma and platelets—a review of the literature. Transfusion. 2010;50(3):701–10.
12. Tapia NM, Chang A, Norman M, Welsh F, Scott B, Wall MJ Jr, Mattox KL, Suliburk J. TEG-guided resuscitation is superior to standardized MTP resuscitation in massively transfused penetrating trauma patients. J Trauma Acute Care Surg. 2013;74(2):378–85.
13. Gonzalez E, Moore EE, Moore HB, Chapman MP, Chin TL, Ghasabyan A, et al. Goal-directed hemostatic resuscitation of trauma-induced coagulopathy: a pragmatic randomized clinical trial comparing a viscoelastic assay to conventional coagulation assays. Ann Surg. 2016;263(6):1051–9.
14. Annecke T, Geisenberger T, Kurzl R, Penning R, Heindl B. Algorithm-based coagulation management of catastrophic amniotic fluid embolism. Blood Coagul Fibrinolysis. 2010;21:95–100.
15. Lang T, von Depka M. Possibilities and limitations of thrombelastometry/-graphy. Hamostaseologie. 2006;26:S20–9.
16. Karlsson O, Sporrong T, Hillarp A, Jeppsson A, Hellgren M. Prospective longitudinal study of thromboelastography and standard hemostatic laboratory tests in healthy women during normal pregnancy. Anesth Analg. 2012;115:890–8.
17. Karlsson O, Jeppsson A, Hellgren M. Major obstetric haemorrhage: monitoring with thromboelastography, laboratory analyses or both? Int J Obstet Anesth. 2014;23:10–7.
18. Collins PW, Lilley G, Bruynseels D, Laurent DB, Cannings-John R, Precious E, Hamlyn V, Sanders J, Alikhan R, Rayment R, et al. Fibrin-based clot formation as an early and rapid biomarker for progression of postpartum hemorrhage a prospective study. Blood. 2014;124(11):1727–36.
19. Ondondo BO. Management of major obstetric haemorrhage using ROTEM point-of-care haemostasis analysers can reduce blood product usage without increasing fibrinogen replacement therapy. Biomed Pharmacol J. 2018;11(3):1167–76.
20. Collins PW, Canninghs-John R, Bruynseels D, Malliah S, Dick J, Weeks AD, Sander J, Aawar N, Townson J, Hood K, Hall JE, Collis RE. Viscoelastometric-guided early fibrinogen concentrate replacement during postpartum haemorrhage: OBS2, a double-blind controlled trial. Br J Anaesth. 2017;119(3);411–21.
21. Corey FS, Walker WF. Sonic estimation of elasticity via resonance: a new method of assessing hemostasis. Ann Biomed Eng. 2015;44:1405–24.
22. Ferrante EA, Blasier KR, Givens T, Lioyd CA, Fischer TJ, Viola F. A novel device for the evaluation of hemostatic function in critical care settings. Anesth Analg. 2016;123(6):1372–9.
23. Nelb GW, Kamykowski GW, Ferry JD. Rheology of fibrin clots. V. Shear modulus, creep, and creep recovery of fine unligated clots. Biophys Chem. 1981;13:15–23.
24. Evans PA, Hawkins K, Lawrence M, Williams RL, Barrow MS, Thirumalai N, Williams PR. Rheometry and associated techniques for blood coagulation studies. Med Eng Phys. 2008;30:671–9.
25. Huffmyer JL, Fernandez LG, Haghigian C, et al. Comparison of SEER sonorheometry with rotational thromboelastometry and laboratory parameters in cardiac surgery. Anesth Analg. 2016;123:1390–9.
26. Allen TW, Viola F. A novel point-of-care approach for improving acute bleeding management. Med Lab Obser. 2018;50(9):30.
27. Fogelson AL, Neeves KB. Fluid mechanics of blood clot formation. Annu Rev Fluid Mech. 2015;47(Fogelson):377–403.
28. Ong S-E, Du H. Fundamental principles and applications of microfluidic systems. Front Biosci. 2008;13(7):2757–73.
29. Haeberle M, von Setten Z. Microfluidic lab-on-a-chip platforms, characteristics and applications. Chem Soc Rev. 2010;39(3):1153–82.
30. Zhang C, Neelamegham S. Application of microfluidic device in studies of thrombosis and hemostasis. J Platelets. 2017;28(5):434–40. Published online 2017 Jun 5. https://doi.org/10.1080/09537104.2017.1319047.

31. Diamond SL. New microfluidic paths to test for bleeding or clotting. J Cell Mol Bioeng. 2017;10(1):1–2.
32. Dixon MC. Quartz crystal microbalance with dissipation monitoring: enabling real-time characterization of biological materials and their interactions. J Biomol Tech. 2008;19(3):151–8.
33. Rodahl M, Kasemo B. A simple setup to simultaneously measure the resonant frequency and the absolute dissipation factor of a quartz crystal microbalance. Rev Sci Instr. 1996;67:3238–41.
34. Hook F, et al. Variations in coupled water, viscoelastic properties, and film thickness of a Mefp-1 protein film during adsorption and cross-linking: a quartz crystal microbalance with dissipation monitoring, ellipsometry, and surface Plasmon resonance study. Anal Chem. 2001;73:5796–804.
35. Huang X, Bai Q, Hu J, Hou D. A practical model of quartz crystal microbalance in actual applications. Sensors. 2017;17:1785. (1-9)
36. Irwin EF, Ho JE, Kane SR, Healy KE. Analysis of interpenetrating polymer networks via quartz crystal microbalance with dissipation monitoring. Langmuir. 2005;21(12):5529–36.
37. Rodahl M, Höök F, et al. Simultaneous frequency and dissipation factor QCM measurements of biomolecular adsorption and cell adhesion. Faraday Discuss. 1997;107:229–46.
38. Irwin EF, et al. Analysis of interpenetrating polymer networks via quartz crystal microbalance with dissipation monitoring. Langmuir. 2005 Jun 7;21(12):5529–36.
39. Lakshmanan RS, Efremov V, Cullen SM, Killard AJ. Blood plasma coagulation and fibrinogen concentration were studied with QCM-D. Dev Sens Actuators B Chem. 2014;192(1):23–8.
40. Tripathi MM, Hajiarian Z, Van Cott EM, Nadkarni SK. Assessing blood coagulation status with laser speckle rheology. Biomed Opt Express. 2014;5(3):817–31.
41. Weitz DA, Pine DJ. Diffusing-wave spectroscopy. In: Brown W, editor. Dynamic light scattering. New York: Oxford University Press; 1993.
42. Hayashi Y, Brun M-A, Machida K, Nagasawa M. Principles of dielectric blood coagulometry as a comprehensive coagulation test. Anal Chem. 2015;87(19).
43. Wang Z, Meng X, Li X, Wang C, Shi L, Gong P, Chen Q. Yu Y. Non-contact electromagnetic induction coagulation detection device. Australas Phys ENG Sci MED. March 2018;41(1):105–15.

Vascular Endothelial Dysfunction and Inflammatory States

22

Samuel Chijioke Onyewu, Alice Tolbert Coombs, and Fatoumata Kromah

Overview of Endothelial Cell and Function

Embryologically, EC arises from the mesoderm which is located on the ventral floor of the dorsal aorta within the aorto-gonado-mesonephros region [1, 2]. Mesenchymal cells, which arise from the mesoderm, differentiate into hemangioblasts and angioblasts. Hemangioblasts further differentiate into EC and other hematopoietic cell lines [1, 2] (Fig. 22.1).

Endothelial cells (ECs) form the endothelium as a single layer of cells lining blood vessels and lymphatics (Fig. 22.2). The endothelium forms a semi-permeable membrane barrier that limits fluid, solute, and large molecule access to the interstitium of various organs [3].

Description of Endothelial Cell and Function

Morphologically, the EC surface in an adult is composed of approximately 20–60 trillion cells and covers 3–7 m^2 surface area. EC are generally flat; however, the thickness of ECs is determined by the dynamic structure lying on its luminal surface [4]. The thickness of EC varies from less than 0.1 to 1 micrometer in capillaries, veins, and aorta, respectively [5, 6]. Depending on which organ it is located, ECs can be fenestrated or un-fenestrated [5]. ECs are covered by a "thick" endothelial glycocalyx layer which prevents capillary leakage and activation by the coagulation system. The glycocalyx covering is vital as it also acts as a barrier to regulate fluid and molecule movement and balance [3]. When ECs are fenestrated, they have pores and openings between cells that promote increased permeability and allow large molecules to pass through capillaries. Fenestrated ECs are present in the capillaries of small intestine, endocrine glands, kidney (glomeruli and renal tubules), and the choroid plexus. In contrast, ECs that are un-fenestrated are found in arteries, veins, and capillaries of the brain, skin, heart, and lung. The EC surface is cohesive, adhesive, and luminal thus allowing EC to play an integral role in the binding of transport and regulatory proteins circulating with blood cells [7]. ECs are involved in the expression of inflammatory and growth factors such as endothelial cell selectin (E-selectin) and vascular endothelial growth factor (VEGF). E-Selectin plays a key role in leukocytes adhesion. VEGF is important for the generation of ECs and maintenance of endothelial fenestrae [7]. ECs synthesize other metabolically active substances which are summarized in Table 22.1 [8–10].

ECs perform other metabolic functions and possess contractile proteins – actin, myosin, and tropomyosin. These contractile proteins generate the shape and elasticity of ECs and are integral in the vasoactive function of blood vessels [7]. One of the most important functions in the vasomotor balance is that ECs produce nitric oxide (NO) [4, 11]. NO is a principal substrate required for the maintenance of vascular tone and reactivity of blood vessels. NO inhibits the action of angiotensin II (AG II) and endothelin 1 (ET 1). ET 1 is a cellular substance produced in ECs and is a potent vasoconstrictor. In addition to inhibiting platelet and white blood cell activation, NO also maintains vascular smooth muscle cells in a non-proliferative state [12] (Fig. 22.3).

Definition of Endothelial Dysfunction

Endothelial cell structure, property, and function are quite diverse resulting in a heterogeneous endothelial environment in which organ systems vary greatly in their capacity to accomplish different functions [3]. Of note this heterogeneity in regulation of vascular tone, molecule transportation, coagulation, and hormone metabolism can be observed between organ systems and within endothelial cells of the same organ. Therefore, endothelial dysfunction is defined as an aberration in the physical integrity and/or functional processes of ECs. EC dysfunction

S. C. Onyewu · A. T. Coombs · F. Kromah (✉)
Virginia Commonwealth University Health System, Department of Anesthesiology, Richmond, VA, USA
e-mail: Alice.coomb@vcuhealth.org; Fatoumata.kromah@vcuhealth.org

© Springer Nature Switzerland AG 2021
C. S. Scher et al. (eds.), *Essentials of Blood Product Management in Anesthesia Practice*, https://doi.org/10.1007/978-3-030-59295-0_22

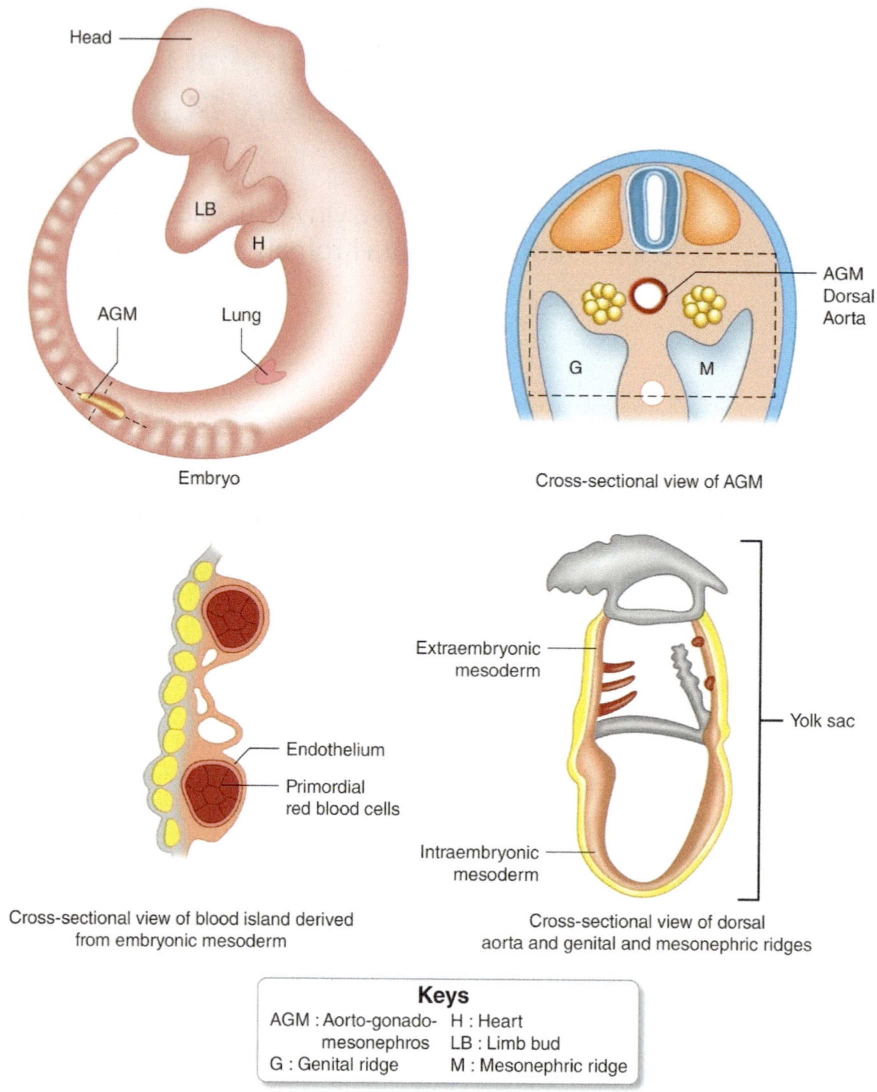

Fig. 22.1 Schematic diagram of endothelial cell embryogenesis. (Modified from image from Dr. Samuel Onyewu)

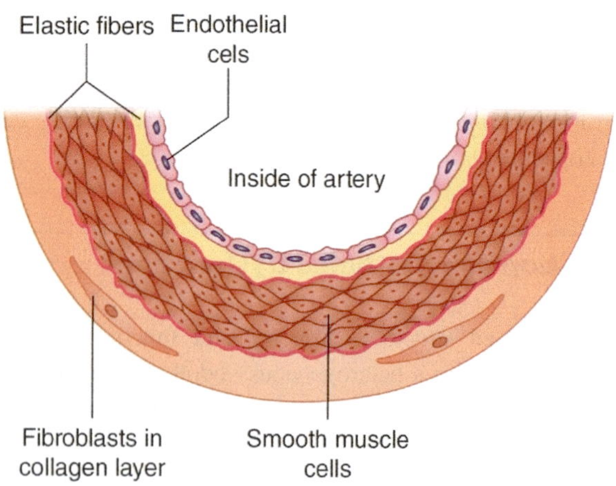

Fig. 22.2 Endothelial cell lining a vessel lumen. (Modified from Stijn AI. Ghesquiere. University of Maastricht. Nov 2005)

often results in alterations in vasoreactivity, increased propensity to thrombus and plaque formation, and leukocyte adhesion along with inflammatory changes [8–10]. EC dysfunction occurs either as a principal determinant of the pathophysiologic mechanism of a disease or as a vestige of collateral damage [1, 5]. EC activation and/or dysfunction may arise from otherwise adaptive responses which may be excessive, sustained, spatial, or temporally misplaced [13] (Fig. 22.4). ECs may be in an activated state yet not dysfunctional [8].

In summary, EC dysfunction affects multiple organ systems and is involved in many disease processes [1, 5]. Hence, ECs will serve as a reliable conduit in the understanding and possible management of different pathologic conditions. In the subsequent parts of this chapter, we will be discussing the various disease processes associated with EC dysfunction and its anesthetic implications and management.

Table 22.1 Endothelial cell characteristics and physiologic functions

Maintenance of cell membrane integrity
Fibronectin
Laminin
Collagen
Proteoglycans
Proteases
Lipid metabolism
Lipoprotein lipase receptor
Anticoagulant molecules elaboration and regulator
Heparin
Prostacyclin
Thrombomodulin
Plasminogen activator
Procoagulant molecules elaboration
Von Willebrand factor
Plasminogen activator inhibitor
Thromboxane A2
Factor V
Thromboplastin
Platelet activator factor
Vasoconstrictor factors
Angiotensin-converting enzyme
Thromboxane A2
Leukotrienes
Endothelin
Vasodilator factors
Nitric oxide
Prostacyclin
Immunity and inflammatory regulators
Interleukins 1, 6, 8
Major histocompatibility complex II
Adhesion molecules: E-selectin, P-selectin
Regulation of growth factors
Insulin growth factor
Transforming growth factor
Colony stimulating factor

Table created by Dr. Samuel Onyewu

Pathophysiology of Endothelial Dysfunction

Endothelial dysfunction is known to be associated with multiple pathologic conditions [14]. It is directly implicated in the pathogenesis and clinical course of cardiovascular conditions, diabetes mellitus, renal dysfunction, Alzheimer's disease, erectile dysfunction, and osteoporosis [15–23]. Endothelial dysfunction may result from various etiologies such as direct injury to the endothelium, infections, reactive or immunologic causes, aging, and disease states.

Etiologies of Endothelial Dysfunction

Iatrogenic

Direct injury alters the morphological architecture of the vascular ECs increasing the likelihood of thrombosis and concentric intimal thickening. Direct injury may occur following iatrogenic procedures performed to correct an underlying pathology. These include angioplasty and stent placement to improve the patency of stenosed vessels [24] (Fig. 22.5).

Infectious

Viruses and bacteria have also been implicated to EC activation [25]. Other inducers of the endothelium include lipid products, complement components, advanced glycosylation end products, hypoxia, laminar blood flow, and growth factors. See Fig. 22.4. Activated ECs secrete cytokines, chemokines, growth factors, procoagulants, and anticoagulant molecules.

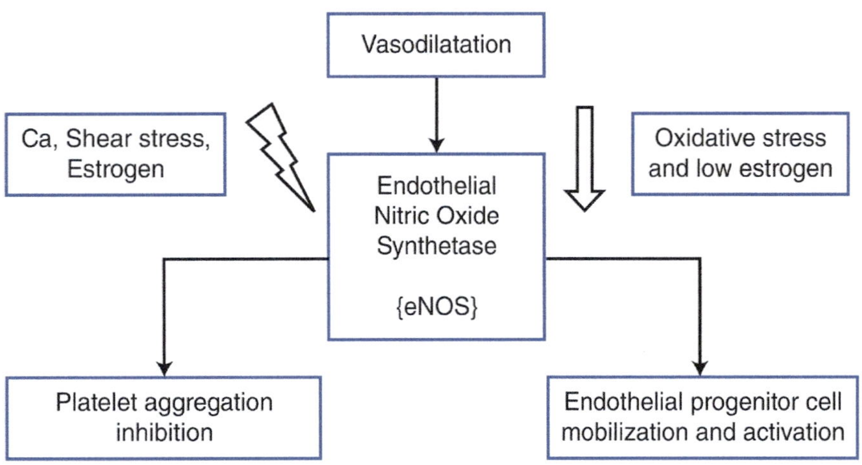

Fig. 22.3 Schematic diagram showing the functions of endothelial nitric oxide synthetase (eNOS) function, its inducers and inhibitors

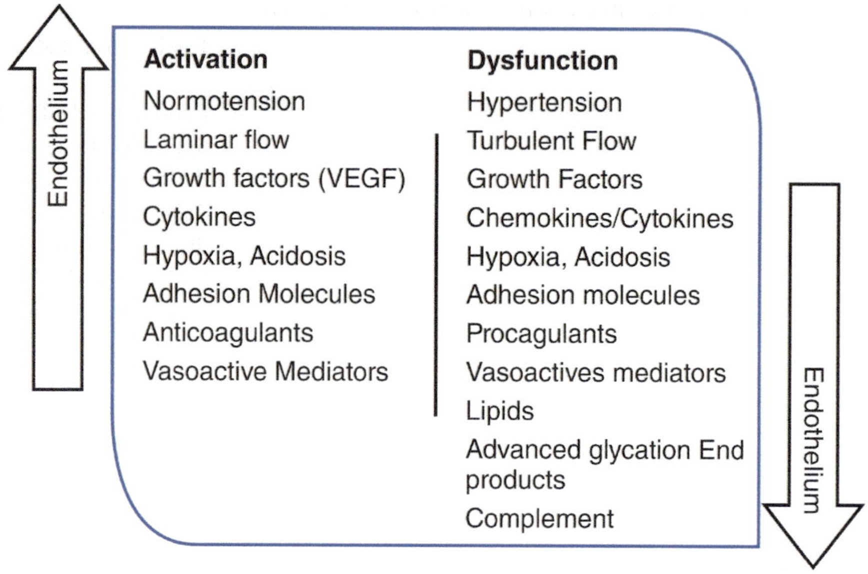

Fig. 22.4 Schematic representation of factors associated with endothelial cell activation and dysfunction. (Modified from image from Dr. Samuel Onyewu)

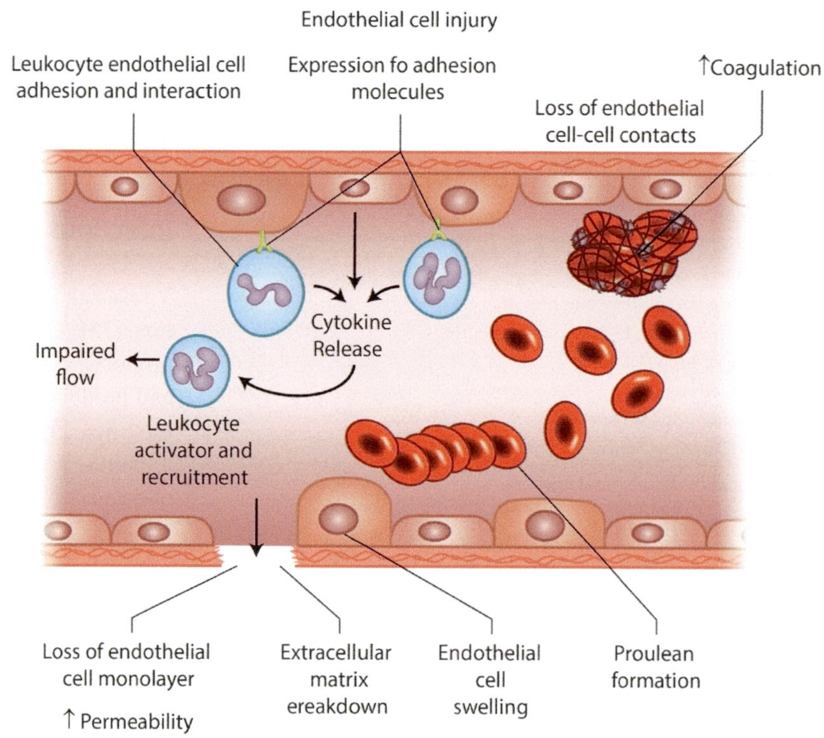

Fig. 22.5 Schematic diagram of endothelial cell injury. (Modified from: Sharfuddin A, Molitoris BA. Endothelial injury. In: Vincent JL, Hall JB, editors; 2012)

Reactive Substrates

Nicotine from chronic cigarette smoking is a burgeoning etiology for cardiovascular diseases, which accounts for a third of the deaths in cigarette smokers [26–29]. Nicotine causes morphological alterations of ECs and vascular smooth muscles inducing functional changes associated with the pathogenesis of cardiovascular diseases [30–33]. A proposed mechanism of action of nicotine-associated endothelial dysfunction is an imbalance in vascular tone, increased expression of ET-1, inducible NOS, and reduced expression of eNOS [34, 35] (Fig. 22.6).

Nicotine reduces the production and bioavailability of nitric oxide (NO), by decreasing the expression of endothelial nitric oxide synthetase (eNOS). Nicotine also causes alteration in the functional integrity of the endothelium resulting in vasospasm, stimulation of leukocytes and platelet adhesion, and thus thrombus formation [36].

Aging

Aging is an integral factor in the development of atherosclerosis, vasculopathies, and cardiovascular disease. Age-

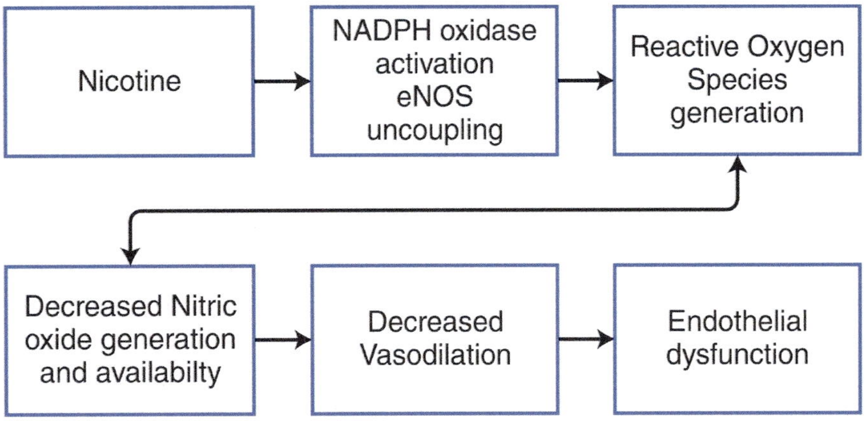

Fig. 22.6 Schematic diagram of nicotine-related endothelial dysfunction. (Modified from image from Dr. Samuel Onyewu)

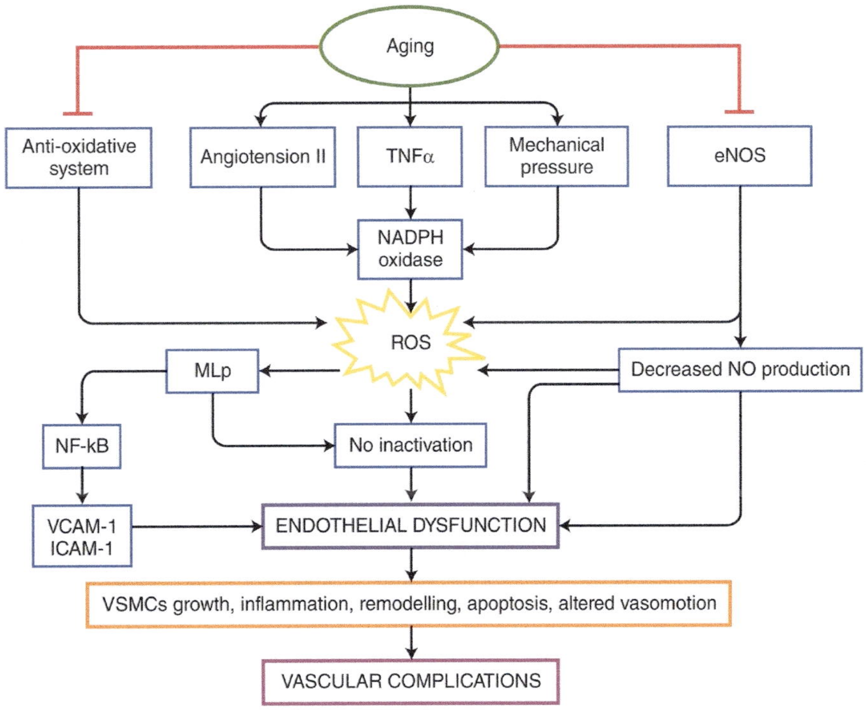

Fig. 22.7 Schematic diagram showing endothelial dysfunction related to aging. (Modified from Rodella LF, Rezzani R. Endothelial and vascular smooth cell dysfunction: a comprehensive appraisal; 2012)

related dysfunction of both endothelial and vascular smooth muscle cells has been attributed to vasospasm, thrombosis, cellular growth, oxidative stress, and inflammation [20]. Some report that aging deteriorates the balance between vasodilator and vasoconstrictor substances produced by the endothelium [20, 37–40]. Senescent ECs have attenuated angiogenic and regenerative capacity, hence limited ability to form new vascular structures [20]. Furthermore, EC senescence may alter the physiologic functions of the endothelium by altering secretion of cytokines, growth factors, and proteases in the vascular wall [41] (Fig. 22.7).

Clinical Presentation of Endothelial Dysfunction and Inflammatory States

Atherosclerosis

Atherosclerosis is a chronic inflammatory response triggered in attempt to mitigate vascular endothelial cell dysfunction, lipid accumulation and oxidation, and thrombosis [42]. Endothelial cell dysfunction along with formation of a fatty streak in which proliferation of intima vascular smooth muscle cells and extracellular matrix (ECM) deposition occurs creates an atherosclerotic atheroma (Fig. 22.8). The atheroma is an intima layer lesion that protrude into vascular lumen.

Atherosclerosis is responsible for hypertension, cardiovascular, cerebrovascular, coronary artery, and peripheral

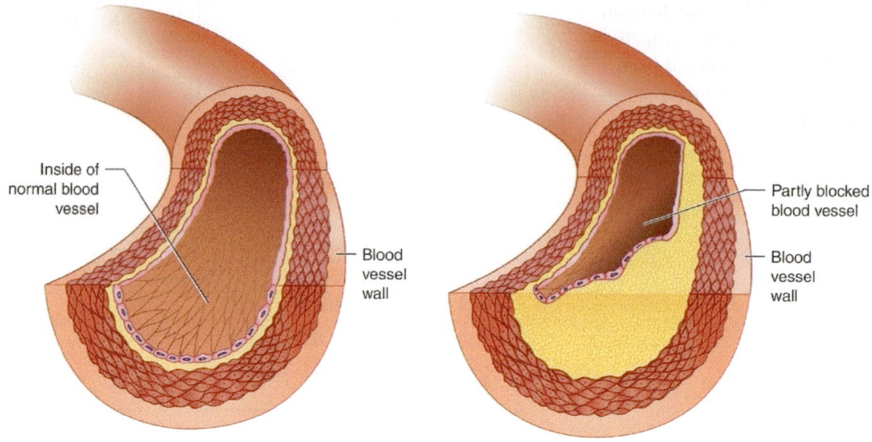

Fig. 22.8 Schematic diagram showing a well-developed atheroma constricting blood vessel lumen. (Modified from Glagov et al. [43])

Table 22.2 Risk factors for atherosclerosis

Modifiable	Non-modifiable
Hypertension	Age
Diabetes mellitus	Gender
Hyperlipidemia	Family history
Cigarette smoking	Genetics
C-reactive protein	

Table created by Dr. Samuel Onyewu

vascular diseases. In combination these diseases have been attributed to half of all deaths in the western world [16, 24]. The prevalence and severity of atherosclerosis are related to several risk factors which can be divided into modifiable and non-modifiable risk factors (Table 22.2).

Risk factors have a multiplicative effect. The presence of two risk factors result in a fourfold likelihood of having an ischemic heart event. Meanwhile, the presence of three risk factors result in a seven fold likelihood of having an ischemic heart event [24].

Non-modifiable risk factors – Age, gender, and genetics. Age greater than 45 years have been shown to have a higher likelihood of the presence of atherosclerotic lesions [42]. Men are more likely than pre-menopausal women to have atherosclerotic disease. This protective effect has been attributed to estrogen. However, the protective effect has not been shown in post-menopausal women on hormonal therapy [44]. Genetics play a significant role and has been implicated in atherosclerosis and ischemic heart disease (IHD). A few genetic disorders like familial hypercholesterolemia have a higher propensity of causing atherosclerosis. However, the association is likely multifactorial in nature and related to inherited genetic polymorphism and other established risk factors of familial clustering such as hypertension or diabetes [45].

Modifiable risk factors – Hyperlipidemia, hypertension, cigarette smoking, and diabetes (Table 22.2). Hyperlipidemia mostly hypercholesterolemia is responsible for the formation of atherosclerosis. Low-density lipoprotein (LDL) transports cholesterol to peripheral vascular tissues, while high-density lipoprotein (HDL) transports cholesterol from tissues into the liver where the cholesterol is excreted in the bile. High intake of cholesterol and saturated fat from egg yolks, animal fat, and butter increase plasma level of cholesterol. Trans-unsaturated fat used in confectionery and margarine adversely affect cholesterol profile. On the other hand, omega-3 fatty acid, found in fish oil, exercise, and moderate alcohol intake improve cholesterol profile. Hypertension both systolic and diastolic levels are important in atherosclerosis. Hypertension on its own increases the risk for IHD by 60% [16, 24]. Prolonged cigarette smoking of a pack or more a day doubles the rate of death from IHD, while smoking cessation significantly reduces the risk [24]. The nicotine released from cigarette smoking increases release of platelet-derived growth factors, ICAM-1 and VCAM-1 expression inducing EC dysfunction and atherosclerotic lesion formation [46, 47]. Diabetes mellitus induces hypercholesterolemia and markedly increases the risk of atherosclerosis. Diabetics compared to non-diabetics have a hundred-fold increase in peripheral vessel disease, and two fold increase in myocardial infarction along with increased risk of cerebral vascular accidents.

Twenty percent of cardiovascular events happen in the absence of hyperlipidemia, hypertension, cigarette smoking, and diabetes [42]. Therefore, inflammation, hyperhomocysteinemia, metabolic syndrome, dyslipidemia, lipoprotein a, and hemostatic factors increase the risk for atherosclerosis. Inflammation is present in all stages of atherogenesis, and it is closely linked to atherosclerotic plaque formation and rupture. Multiple inflammatory markers have been associated with IHD. C-reactive protein (CRP) has emerged as the most sensitive inflammatory markers [48]. CRP is an acute phase reactant produced in the liver that opsonizes bacteria and activates complements. When CRP is secreted from cells within the atherosclerotic intima, CRP activates local endothelial cells inducing a prothrombotic state and increases adhesiveness of EC to leukocytes. CRP is an independent predictor of myocardial infarction, cerebral vascular accident, peripheral arterial disease, and sudden cardiac death among healthy individuals [42]. Smoking cessation, exercise, weight loss and statins reduce CRP levels, although reduction in CRP level has not been proven to reduce cardiovascular risk [24]. Hyperhomocysteinemia is associated with coronary artery disease, peripheral vascular disease, stroke, and venous thrombosis [49]. Elevated homocysteine can be found in low intake of folate and vitamin B12; however, vitamin supplementation has not shown to preclude cardiovascular disease. Metabolic syndrome is characterized by conditions associated with insulin resistance [50]. The syndrome is also associated with hypertension, dyslipidemia, and central obesity. Dyslipidemia leads to endothelial cell dysfunction secondary to increased oxidative stress and a systemic pro-inflammatory state that leads to vascular thrombosis. Lipoprotein (a) is an altered form of LDL. Lipoprotein (a) contains apolipoprotein B-100 portion of LDL linked to apolipoprotein A. Lipoprotein (a) levels are associated with an elevated risk of coronary and cerebrovascular disease, independent of total cholesterol and LDL levels [44]. Plasminogen activator inhibitor 1 and thrombin both have procoagulant and pro-inflammatory effect. Plasminogen activator inhibitor 1, thrombin, and platelet-derived growth factors are major predictors of vascular pathology in atherosclerosis [42].

The pathogenesis of atherosclerosis is based on a composite of two theories known as the intimal cell proliferation or repetitive formation and organization of thrombi [51, 52], which is summarized as the response to injury hypothesis [53]. According to the model, atherosclerosis is produced by the following pathologic events: endothelial injury which causes increased vascular permeability, leukocyte adhesion, and thrombosis. This leads to accumulation of lipoproteins especially oxidized LDL in the vessel walls; monocytes adhere to the endothelium, followed by its migration to the intima and finally its transformation to macrophages and foam cells. Foam cells are composed of platelet adhesion, factors released from activated platelets, macrophages, and vascular wall cells. These induce smooth muscle wall cells of blood vessel wall media which lead to smooth muscle cell proliferation and ECM production. Lipids accumulate both extracellularly and within the cells (macrophages and smooth muscle cells) (Fig. 22.9).

The clinical presentation of atherosclerosis depends on the organ system affected and the severity of the atherosclerotic lesion. Its manifestation includes coronary artery disease, stroke, peripheral artery disease, hypertension, or renal failure. Sequelae of an atheromatous plaque include hemorrhage, rupture, and thrombus formation and migration with possible microemboli. The more detrimental sequelae are ischemia and aneurysm formation.

Hypertension

Hypertension is a major risk factor for atherosclerosis and other conditions such as multi-infarct dementia, aortic dissection, renal failure, and hypertensive heart disease [54] (Table 22.3).

Idiopathic (essential) hypertension accounts for 95% of the cases, while the remaining 5% are associated with secondary diseases of the renal or endocrine systems. Idiopathic hypertension is associated with short-term problems and is compatible with longevity especially when blood pressure is adequately controlled. However, uncontrolled

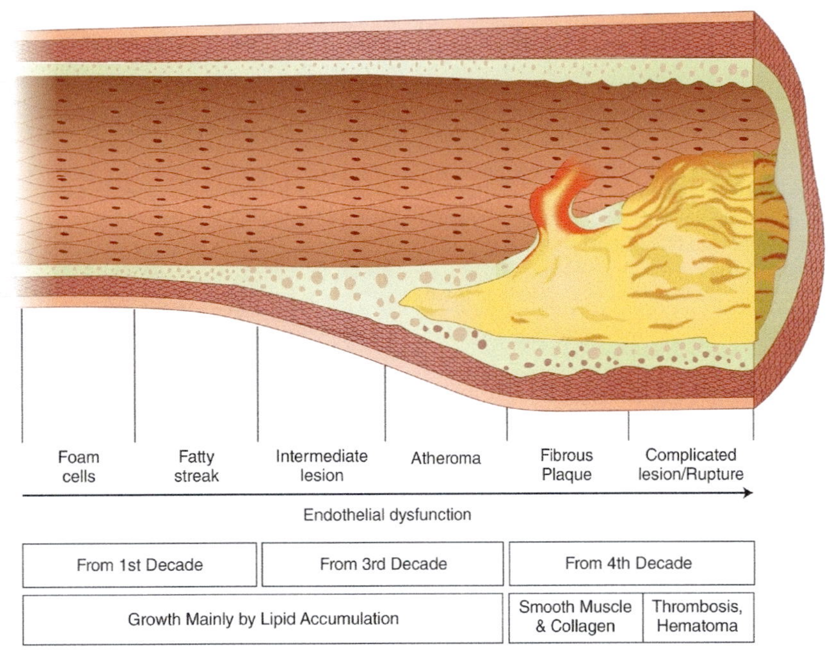

Fig. 22.9 Evolution of atheromatous plaque formation. (Modified from Story HC et al. *Circulation*. 92:1355–1379; 1995)

hypertension causes death within 1–2 years if not treated promptly. Systolic BP of 200 mmHg and diastolic pressures >120 mmHg is associated with end-organ damage such as retinal damage and exudates with or without papilledema, renal failure, and cerebral hemorrhage. Recent BP criteria developed by the American Heart association are intended to decrease the related complications [54].

Table 22.3 Types and major causes of hypertension (systolic and diastolic)

Essential hypertension (idiopathic accounts for 90–95% of cases)
Secondary hypertension is primarily due to renal or endocrine disorders
Renal
Glomerulonephritis
Chronic kidney disease
Renal artery stenosis
Polycystic kidney disease
Renal vasculitis
Renin producing tumors
Endocrine
Adrenocortical hyper function: Cushing's syndrome, primary hyperaldosteronism, congenital adrenal hyperplasia, licorice ingestion
Exogenous hormones: Glucocorticoid therapy, estrogen, sympathomimetic, tyramine containing food, monoamine oxidase inhibitors
Pheochromocytoma
Acromegaly
Hypothyroidism (myxedema)
Hyperthyroidism (thyrotoxicosis)
Pregnancy induced
Neurologic
Raised intracranial pressure
Sleep deprivation
Surgical stress from pain
Cardiovascular
Coarctation of the aorta
Polyarteritis nodosa
Volume overload

Table created by Dr. Samuel Onyewu

Regulation of blood pressure is dependent on renal autoregulation through glomerular ultrafiltration, renin angiotensin aldosterone system, sodium intake, fluid homeostasis, exercise, stress, obesity, and smoking. Adequate blood pressure monitoring is imperative in preventing atherosclerosis and other cardiovascular risk factors.

Vascular Aneurysm and Dissection

An aneurysm is a localized abnormal dilation of a blood vessel or the heart [54]. The aneurysms are either congenital or acquired, true or false. A true aneurysm is one that has all the layers of the blood vessel or the heart intact. Examples of true aneurysms are atherosclerotic, syphilitic, and congenital or ventricular aneurysm that occur following a transmural myocardial infarction. A false aneurysm is an aneurysm that has a defect in the vessel wall causing an extravascular hematoma which freely communicates with an intravascular space (pulsating hematoma). An example of a false aneurysm is a ventricular rupture contained in a pericardial adhesion or an arterial leak at the anastomosis site of a synthetic graft with a native artery. Aneurysms are also classified by shape and size. A fusiform aneurysm is a diffuse circumferential dilation of a long (up to 20 cm) vascular segment. A saccular aneurysm is a spherical outpouching that is between 5 and 20 cm, and they often contain a thrombus. A dissection on the other hand is a hematoma or hemorrhage within the walls of a blood vessel. Dissections are often but not always aneurysmal (Fig. 22.10).

The pathogenesis of an aneurysm is related to the alteration in the structure and/or function of the vessel wall connective tissue. Risk factors include intrinsic deficiency of the connective tissue wall commonly seen in Marfan's and Loeys-Dietz syndromes, Ehlers-Danlos, and vitamin C deficiencies. In Marfan's there is defect in the synthesis of fibrillin which leads to abnormal transforming growth factor

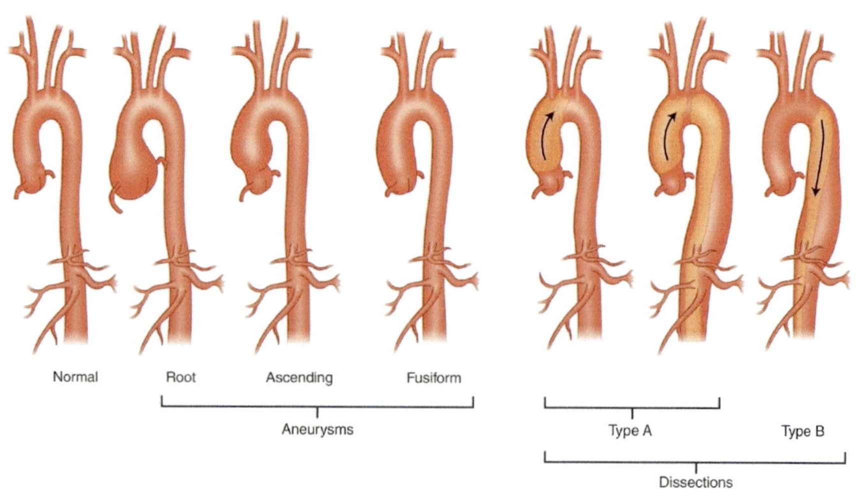

Fig. 22.10 Diagram of Aortic aneurysm and dissection. (Modified from Pinard [55])

beta (TGF-B) activity, resulting in progressive weakness of elastic tissue in the aorta. In Loeys-Dietz syndrome, mutation in TGF-B receptors leads to abnormal elastin and collagen I and III. Aneurysms in individuals with Loeys-Dietz syndrome rupture easily even at small sizes [56]. Ehlers-Danlos is also associated with defective collagen III synthesis. Vitamin C deficiency is associated with altered collagen cross-link.

Another etiology leading to aneurysm formation is the imbalance between collagen synthesis and degradation secondary to local inflammatory infiltrates and proteolytic enzymes. Metalloproteinases (MMP) from macrophages in atherosclerotic plaques and vasculitis have been implicated in aneurysm development [57]. MMP has the ability to degrade all the components (collagens, elastin, proteoglycans, laminin, fibronectin) of ECM in arterial walls. Also, there may be loss of smooth muscle cells or synthesis of non-collagenous or non-elastic ECM. This can occur due to ischemia in the media layer secondary to atherosclerotic thickening in the intima. Demand ischemia occurs due to the increased distance of oxygen and nutrients travel to supply the smooth muscles. Systemic hypertension can also occur due to narrowing of the vasa vasorum. Histologically this change is described as cystic medial degeneration. The two most important disorders that predispose to aortic aneurysms are atherosclerosis and hypertension. The symptoms of an aortic aneurysm depend on the location. It ranges from chest or abdominal pain secondary to obstruction, compression or ischemia, pulsating mass, hemorrhage with shock, and death following exsanguination.

Vascular dissection occurs when blood finds its way through the walls of an aorta. Dissection commonly occurs in middle aged (40–60-year-old) men with an underlying history of hypertension. In younger individuals the history of Marfan's disease is usually present. Dissection can also occur following aortic cannulation during cardiopulmonary bypass and cardiac catheterization. The major pathogenesis of dissection is hypertension. Hypertensive patients have medial hypertrophy of the vasa vasorum. Medial hypertrophy is associated with degenerative changes of the aortic media and variable loss of medial smooth muscle cells. Vascular dissections are also associated with inherited or acquired connective tissue disorder (Marfan's, Ehlers-Danlos, vitamin C deficiency, and copper deficiency). Types of dissection depends on the involvement of the ascending aorta. Type A and B or DeBakey I/II or III (Fig. 22.11). The presentation of vascular dissection depends on the area of involvement. Therefore, symptoms may include chest pain radiating between the scapulae, and back pain from transverse myelitis if the spinal arteries are affected. Prognosis has improved over the years, and the main goal of treatment is blood pressure control.

Vasculitis

Vasculitis is defined as inflammation of the vascular wall of arteries, veins, and capillaries. The presence of these vessels in various organ systems allows vasculitis to occur in all organs resulting in an overall general clinical presenta-

Classification of aortic dissection

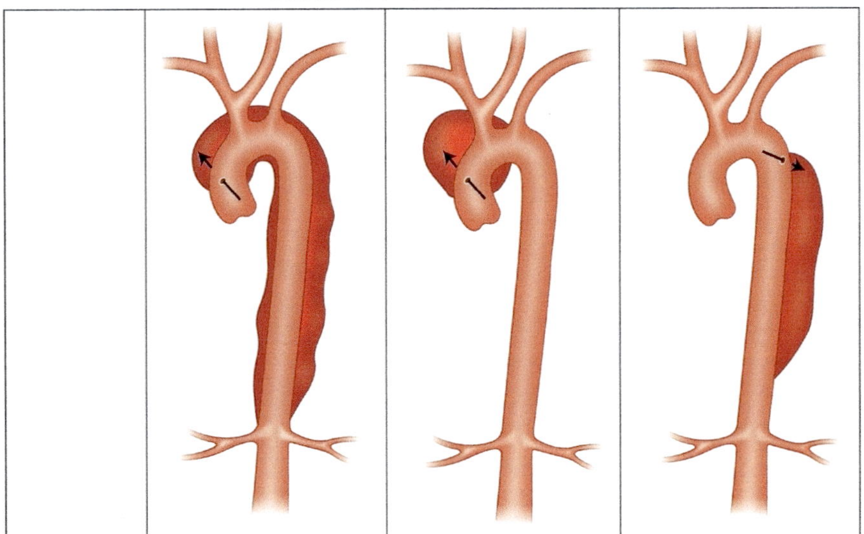

Percentage	60%	10-15%	25-30%
Type	DeBakey I	DeBakey II	DeBakey III
	Stanford A (Proximal)		Stanford B (Distal)

Fig. 22.11 Diagrammatic representations of the types of dissection. (Modified from Matthews JP, Swaminathan M, Ayoub CM. *Clinical manual and review of transesophageal echocardiography*. 2nd ed. www.accessanesthesiology.com)

tion. Approximately 20 primary types of vasculitis are recognized. Efforts have been made to classify them based on the vasculature involved, the size of the vessel they affect, associated organs implicated, pathologic mechanism, morphologic characteristic at presentation, and even patient demographics [58]. Although, this is still an evolving process, the Chapel-Hill nomenclature remains the most widely accepted classification approach [59] (Fig. 22.12).

Vasculitis is often immune mediated or caused by infection. Infectious etiologies can also lead to non-infectious vasculitis by indirectly inducing immune complexes and causing cross-reactivity. Treatment modality may be counterproductive if the etiology is not identified. Other causes of vasculitis include radiation, mechanical trauma, and biochemical toxins. Non-infectious vasculitis is initiated by immune complex deposition, antineutrophil cytoplasmic antibodies (ANCA), and anti-endothelial cell antibodies. Immune complex associated vasculitis has many similarities of other immune complex conditions such as Arthus reaction and serum sickness [60]. Examples of immune complex vasculitis include systemic lupus erythematosus (SLE), polyarteritis nodosa (PAN), and drug hypersensitivity vasculitis (penicillin and streptokinase). For patients with SLE, there is a DNA-anti-DNA complex which bind to vascular walls. About 30% of PAN patients have circulating HBsAg-anti HBsAg antibody complex [61]. Drug hypersensitivity vasculitis occurs when a drug (penicillin) binds to serum proteins. Drug hypersensitivity vasculitis can also occur when foreign protein (streptokinase) binds to antibodies and form circulating immune complexes (See Fig. 22.12). The temporal sequence of antigen-antibody complex formation is yet to be fully understood. Antineutrophil cytoplasmic antibodies (ANCAs) are described as antibodies that react against constituents (mainly enzymes) of neutrophil. Reactivity is primarily to granules, monocytes, lysosomes, and endothelial cells. ANCA can be divided into anti-myeloperoxidase (MPO-ANCA) formerly known as perinuclear ANCA (p-ANCA) and anti-proteinase- 3 (PR-3 ANCA), formerly known as cytoplasmic ANCA (c-ANCA). MPO is a lysosomal granule that produces free oxygen radicals and is induced by agents, such as propylthiouracil. PR-3 is a neutrophil azurophilic granule constituent [61, 62]. PR-3 ANCA are seen in Wegener granulomatosis, while MPO-ANCA are common with microscopic polyangiitis and Churg-Strauss syndrome. ANCAs are useful markers for diagnosis of ANCA vasculitis. The mechanism of action is activation of neutrophils which synthesize free radicals and proteolytic enzymes. The ensuing neutrophil-endothelial interaction leads to endothelial cell damage. Anti-endothelial cell antibodies are antibodies to endothelial and smooth muscle cells predisposing patients to Kawasaki disease [63, 64]. Infectious vasculitis occurs following localized invasion of bacteria and fungi. Hematogenous spread from distant infectious site following septicemia or embolization from infective endocarditis can also cause vasculitis. Organisms commonly involved are *Aspergillus* and *Mucor*. These fungi can lead to aneurysm, thrombosis, or infarction.

Diabetes Mellitus

Diabetes mellitus is a condition that is associated with impaired glucose utilization by cells. EC dysfunction associated with type 1 diabetes aka insulin-dependent diabetes is predominantly caused by the metabolic changes seen with hyperglycemia and microvascular complications prominently in retinal and renal vessels [65]. Non-insulin-dependent (type 2) diabetes is associated with obesity and metabolic

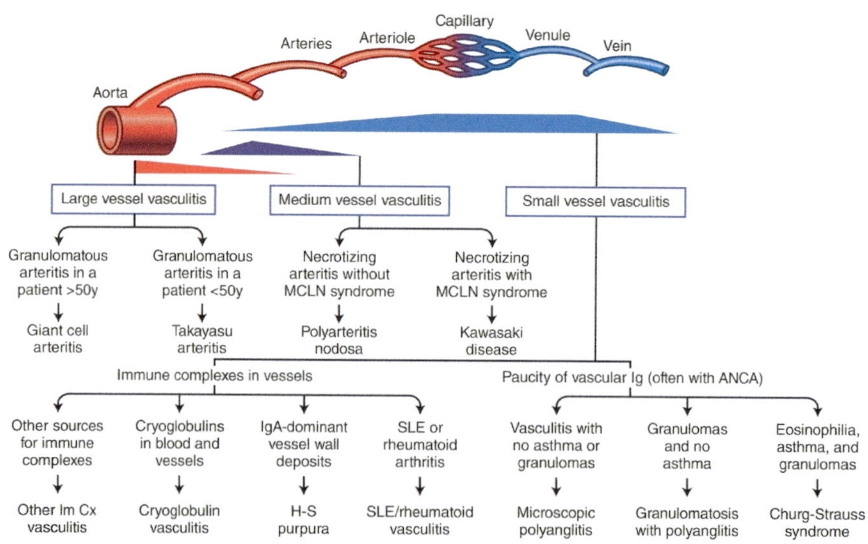

Fig. 22.12 Diagrammatic schema of the various types of vasculitis and vasculature affected. (Modified from Imboden JB, Hellmann DB, Stone JH. *Current diagnosis and treatment*; Rheumatology. 3rd ed. www.accessmedicine.com)

syndrome. In type 2 diabetes, EC dysfunction begins before the clinical onset of diabetes [66–68]. Patients with insulin-deficient diabetes (type 1) have multiple EC dysfunctions. EC dysfunction resulting in dysregulation of vascular tone, organ perfusion derangement, inhibition of inflammation/trans-endothelial transport of blood solutes, prevention of coagulation, and initiation of angiogenesis [68–75]. High fat diet has been shown to impair delivery of insulin to the interstitial space causing a dysfunction in endothelial insulin signaling [73]. Hyperglycemia causes mitochondrial fragmentation, and dysfunction leading to increased mitochondrial reactive oxygen species (ROS) production and vascular tone dysregulation, which is secondary to rapid breakdown of nitric oxide (NO) [73, 76, 77]. This has been suggested as the etiology of EC dysfunction in patients with diabetes. However, various studies have shown it is multifactorial and not just hyperglycemia (Fig. 22.13).

Perivascular adipose tissue (PVAT) found in the abdomen and blood vessels, have been described to control insulin sensitivity and endothelial function. They have shown to be critically involved in the regulation of local vascular tone and inflammation [68, 79–81]. PVAT is reported to be impaired in obesity and type 2 diabetes [70, 77, 82]. PVAT inflammation has been associated with hypoperfusion of adipose tissue, leading to concomitant hypoxia, which may alter adipocyte secretion, thus causing dysfunction in vascular tone.

Neoplasm

There are multiple tumors of endothelial origin; some are benign while others malignant. Examples of benign tumors are hemangioma and lymphangioma, while angiosarcoma is a malignant tumor. Benign tumors are lined with a layer of normal endothelial cells, filled with blood cells or lymph. Malignant tumors do not have well-organized conduits and are composed of more disorganized cells, that are constantly proliferating with no distinct morphology. CD-31 and von Willebrand's factor are endothelial markers used to identify malignant cells with poor atypia immunohistochemically [83]. Hemangiomas are very common tumors which are characterized by normal and abnormal blood vessels filled with blood. They are common in infancy and early childhood and are usually localized even though they are quite ubiquitous. Capillary hemangiomas spontaneously regress and rarely undergo malignant transformation. Cavernous hemangiomas are associated with abnormal blood vessel formation in deep tissues and are likely to cause pressure symptoms or rupture. Lymphangiomas are analogous to blood vessel hemangiomas but devoid of erythrocytes. There are two types, simple (capillary) and cavernous lymphangioma (cystic hygroma). They are quite common in the head, neck, and axilla of children. Angiosarcomas are malignant endothelial cell tumors common in adults. Angiosarcomas are associated with carcinogen exposure: arsenics, thorotrast,

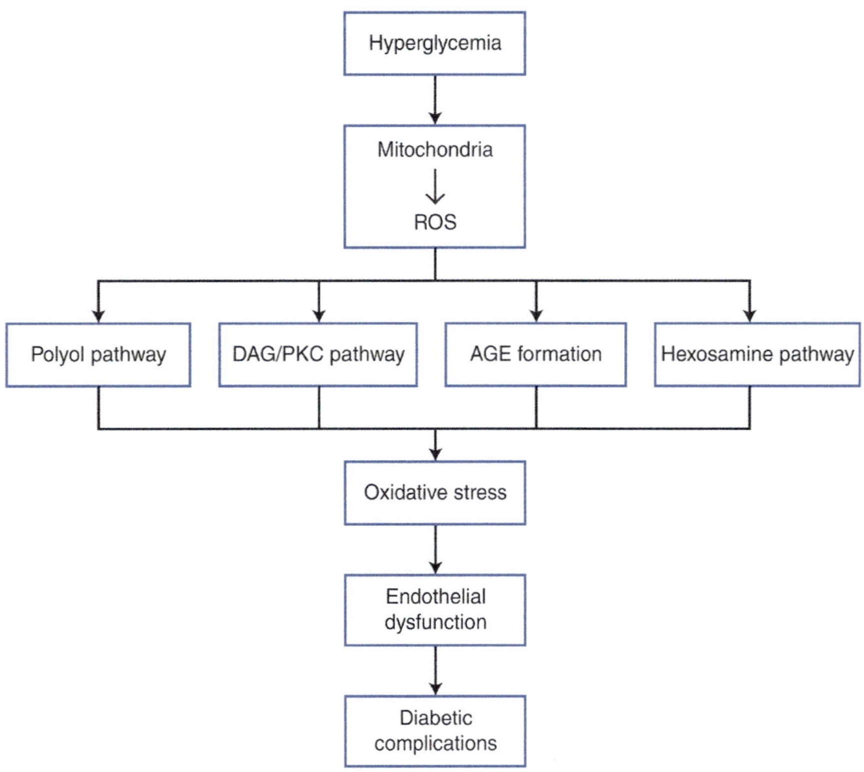

Fig. 22.13 Schematic diagram showing the effect of hyperglycemia on endothelial function. (Modified from Van den Oever et al. [78])

polyvinyl chloride, and tumors such as lymphangiosarcoma and are poorly differentiated. In contrast to angiosarcomas, hemangiomas are well differentiated.

Anesthetic Considerations

Acute Critical Illness and Endotheliopathy

Acute critically ill patients scheduled for operative intervention may have multisystem organ dysfunction that emanates from endotheliopathy [84]. The endothelium and glycocalyx are normally naturally anticoagulated by heparinoids, tissue factor pathway inhibitor, thrombomodulin system, and tissue plasminogen activator (tPA). These factors interact with other mediators to dissolve forming clots [84]. In acute severe trauma, sepsis, post cardiac arrest and MI, endothelial inflammation, and dysfunction in the anticoagulation system causes hypocoagulation [85]. In addition, there is shock-induced sympatho-adrenal hyperactivation which leads to endotheliopathy. This endothelial injury induces a severe imbalance between the quiescent and activated state, leading to hypoperfusion and increased mortality (Fig. 22.14). One in four patients admitted to and from the emergency room have some form of coagulopathy [85]. While many patients have other causes such as drug reaction or side effect, the coagulopathy that is associated with acute trauma, septic shock, bacteremia, myocardial infarction, and post cardiac arrest syndrome has a mortality rate that is three to four times higher (mortality rate of 50%) than patients with these same diagnosis without coagulopathy [86].

Preoperative Consideration

The widespread presence of EC throughout the body means that EC dysfunction may lead to generalized organ derangements and various associated conditions. Preoperatively, it is necessary to perform a thorough evaluation. Prior medical conditions such as a cerebral vascular accident, cardiovascular changes, pulmonary disease, diabetes mellitus, and medication history need to be reviewed. The planned surgical procedure and acuity of the surgery needs to be ascertained. The risks and benefits should be discussed with the patient, surgeon, and anesthesiologist. Appropriate preoperative workup, anesthetic planning, and postoperative course must be carefully addressed. Patient presenting to the operating room with severe trauma, sepsis, acute MI, and post cardiac arrest syndrome has coagulopathy and adrenal-catecholamine hyperstimulation. While the approach has been supportive and addressing matters as they evolve in the past, recent reports suggest that beta blockers and ACE inhibitors may help to optimize microcirculation through reduction or reversal of endothelial injury. This is accomplished through their impact on inhibiting the catecholamine surge associated with endotheliopathy [84].

Intraoperative Consideration

On arrival to the operating room, the standard monitors and other monitoring modalities needed should be applied based on the patient's comorbidities. Invasive versus non-invasive blood pressure management, echocardiogram, glucose, and temperature monitoring should all be considered on a case-by-case basis. It is imperative in each case to preclude potential intraoperative sequelae following induction and the possible effect of the anesthetic administered. Intraoperative bleeding can be decreased through efforts to reduce glycocalyx and endothelial injury [87]. In a recent randomized study in patients undergoing emergent thoracic aortic dissection surgery, and required transfusion, patients who received Octaplast LG (solvent/detergent-treated pooled plasma) when compared to standard FFP, the former patients (Octaplas LG) had reduced glycocalyx and endothelial injury, reduced bleeding, less transfusion requirements, use of prohemostatics, and ventilator days post operatively [88]. The concern raised is routine transfusion with glycocalyx, leading to barrier erosion which may cause coagulation dysfunction, endothelium inflammation, and injury due to contaminants or substances in the blood [87,

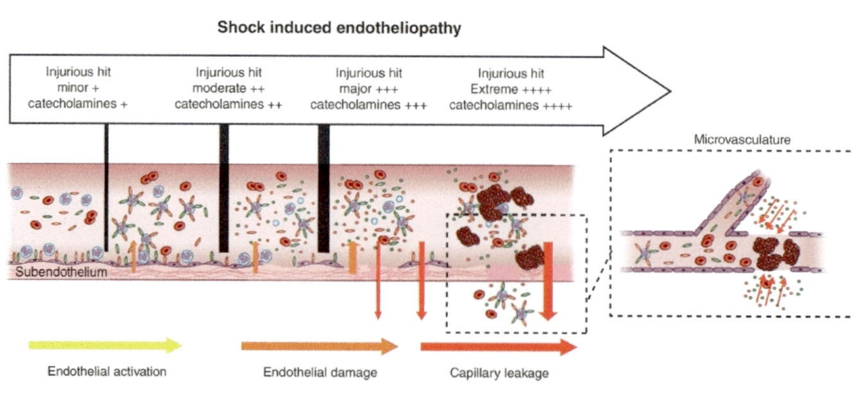

Fig. 22.14 Shock-induced endotheliopathy (SHINE). Schematic illustration of the changes in the vascular compartment with increasing disease severity and increasing sympatho-adrenal activation. (Modified from: Johansson et al. [84])

89]. Furthermore, in animal models with hemorrhagic shock, it has been shown that plasma administration when compared to crystalloid is associated with improved endothelial integrity and restoration of the glycocalyx layer [89].

Postoperative Consideration

Patients with EC dysfunction may be at risk for bleeding, hyper-hypoglycemia, and cardiovascular or cerebrovascular event. Depending on the severity of the clinical presentation, postoperative care of patients with endotheliopathy and diseases associated vascular endothelial dysfunction needs to be carefully planned before the end of the intraoperative course. Transition of care for patients with conditions involving EC dysfunction should be closely monitored. Appropriate care assessment, discussion, and planning may preclude potential complications.

Prevention/Management

The Western diet is high in unsaturated fats, and the lifestyle has become more sedentary compared to Mediterranean and Oriental diet [14]. Hence, there is a significant progression of adverse cardiovascular risk factors in western population. Pharmacological, physical activity, and lifestyle modification often may not treat or prevent EC dysfunction.

Pharmacological

The ubiquitous nature of ECs allow ECs to be plastic and amendable to therapeutic intervention [14]. Hence, ECs are reliable conduits for therapeutic interventions of various pathologic conditions. Multiple medications for hypertension, hyperlipidemia, diabetes, thrombosis, and cancers have been synthesized and prescribed to patients to prevent or treat the associated clinical sequelae of endothelial dysfunction. These medications have not shown to be curative for the various disorders associated with vascular endothelial dysfunction. There is a significant need for physical activity and lifestyle modification adjuncts.

Physical Activity

A few studies have shown that moderate-intensity aerobic exercise improves endothelial function in animals and humans with and without cardiovascular risk factors [90–93]. Exercise training has been shown to ameliorate inflammation [14]. Patients with chronic heart failure (CHF) have increased markers (tumor necrosis factor a, ICAM-1, and E selectin) for endothelial damage. However, these markers were absent in CHF patients who exercised regularly [91, 92]. It was also interesting to note that diet and exercise have synergistic effects as opposed to modification from either modality diet or exercise.

Lifestyle Modification

It has been established that various types of fats, saturated, monounsaturated, and trans-fatty acids [94–96], have been implicated in endothelial dysfunction. These specific fats have been found in partial hydrogenation of vegetable oils commonly found in margarine, pastry products, and frozen foods. A Mediterranean diet low in saturated fats, high in vegetables content, and olive oil (which contains oleic and linoleic acids) reduces endothelial dysfunction, insulin resistance, and markers of vascular inflammation [97–100]. In addition, polyphenols found in fruits, cereals, olive, vegetables, legumes, chocolate, tea, coffees and wine [101, 102] have antioxidant properties and are known to prevent endothelial dysfunction [103]. Melatonin and red wine also have antioxidant properties.

Conclusion

ECs play an important role in the homeostasis of the body, but dysfunction of EC is implicated in various inflammatory states and multiple organ system pathology. The goal of this chapter is to highlight the various pathologies associated with EC dysfunction and how it impacts anesthetic care. An overview of the potential complications and conditions associated with EC dysfunction is useful for the anesthesiologist and other anesthesia care providers to prevent or decrease perioperative morbidity and mortality. Knowledge of vascular endothelial dysfunction and inflammatory states can help guide anesthetic assessment, plan, and management. The different pathologic states associated with endothelial dysfunction have significant socioeconomic and public health impact. Adequate knowledge and modalities to address these various pathologies will ultimately improve the global and public health burden associated with diabetes and other cardiovascular diseases.

References

1. Aird WC. Endothelium in health and disease. Pharmacol Rep. 2008;60(1):139–43.
2. Galley HF, Webster NR. Physiology of the endothelium. Br J Anaesth. 2004;93(1):105–13.
3. Pries AR, Secomb TW, Gaehtgens P. The endothelial surface layer. Pflugers Arch. 2000;440:653–66.

4. Minami T, Aird WC. Endothelial cell gene regulation. Trends Cardiovasc Med. 2005;15(5):174–84.
5. Aird WC. Phenotypic heterogeneity of endothelium: I. structure, function, and mechanisms. Circ Res. 2007;100(2):158–73.
6. Florey F. The endothelial cell. Br Med J. 1966;2(5512):487–90.
7. Pasyk KA, Jakobczak BA. Vascular endothelium: recent advances. Eur J Dermatol. 2004;14(4):209–13.
8. Esper RJ, Nordaby RA, Vilarino JO, Paragano A, Caccharon JL, Machado RA. Endothelial dysfunction: a comprehensive appraisal. Cardiovasc Diabetol. 2006;5, article 4.
9. Rubanyi GM. The role of endothelium in cardiovascular homeostasis and diseases. J Cardiovasc Pharmacol. 1993;23(supplement 4):S1–S14.
10. Vanhoutte PM. Regeneration of the endothelium in vascular injury. Cardiovasc Drugs Ther. 2010;24(4):299–303.
11. Uematsu M, Ohara Y, Navas JP, Nishida K, Murphy TJ, Alexander RW, Nerem RM, et al. Regulation of endothelial cell nitric oxide synthase mRNA expression by shear stress. Am J Physiol. 1995;269(6 part 1):C1371–8.
12. Verma S, Buchanan MR, Anderson TJ. Endothelial function testing as a biomarker of vascular disease. Circulation. 2003;108(17):2054–9.
13. Aird WC. Spatial and temporal dynamics of the endothelium. J Thromb Haemost. 2005;3(7):1392–406.
14. Favero G, Paganelli C, Buffoli B, Rodella LF, Rezzani R. Endothelium and its alterations in cardiovascular diseases: life style intervention. Biomed Res Int. 2014;2014:801896.
15. Suwaidi JA, Hamasaki S, Higano ST, Nishimura RA, Holmes DR Jr, Lerman A. Long-term follow-up of patients with mild coronary artery disease and endothelial dysfunction. Circulation. 2000;101(9):948–54.
16. Schachinger V, Britten MB, Zeiher AM. Prognostic impact of coronary vasodilator dysfunction on adverse long-term outcome of coronary heart disease. Circulation. 2000;101(16):1899–906.
17. Kolka CM, Bergman RN. The endothelium in diabetes: its role in insulin access and diabetic complications. Rev Endocr Metab Disord. 2013;14(1):13–9.
18. Giacco F, Brownlee M. Oxidative stress and diabetic complications. Circ Res. 2010;107(9):1058–70.
19. Csiszar A, Toth J, Peti-Peterdi J, Ungvari Z. The aging kidney: role of endothelial oxidative stress and inflammation. Acta Physiol Hung. 2007;94(1–2):107–15.
20. Herrera MD, Mingorance C, Rodriguez-Rodriguez R, de Sotomayor MA. Endothelial dysfunction and aging: an update. Ageing Res Rev. 2010;9(2):142–52.
21. Price JM, Hellermann A, Hellermann G, Sutton ET. Aging enhances vascular dysfunction induced by the alzheimer's peptide B-amyloid. Neurol Res. 2004;26(3):305–11.
22. Burnett AL. The role of nitric oxide in erectile dysfunction: implications for medical therapy. J Clin Hypertens. 2006;8(12, supplement 4):53–62.
23. Sanada M, Taguchi A, Higashi Y, Tsuda M, Kodama I, Yoshizuma M, Ohama K. Forearm endothelial function and bone mineral loss in post-menopausal women. Atherosclerosis. 2004;176(2):387–92.
24. Mitchell RN, Schoen FJ. Blood vessels. In: Kumar V, Abbas AK, Fausto N, Aster JC, editors. Robbins and Cotran pathologic basis of diseases. 8th ed. Philadelphia: Elsevier Saunders; 2016. p. 525.
25. Kumar V, Abbas AK, Fausto N, Aster JC. Acute and chronic inflammation. In: Kumar V, Abbas AK, Fausto N, Aster JC, editors. Robbins and Cotran pathologic basis of diseases. 8th ed. Philadelphia: Elsevier Saunders; 2016. p. 47.
26. Argacha JF, Fontaine D, Adamopoulos D, Ajose A, van de Bome P, Fontaine J, et al. Acute effect of sidestream cigarette smoke extract on vascular endothelial function. J Cardiovasc Pharmacol. 2008;52(3):262–7.
27. Balakumar P, Sharma R, Singh M. Benfotiamine attenuates nicotine and uric acid-induced vascular endothelial dysfunction in the rat. Pharmacol Res. 2008;58(5–6):356–63.
28. Campbell SC, Moffatt RJ, Stamford BA. Smoking and smoking cessation- the relationship between cardiovascular disease and lipoprotein metabolism: a review. Atherosclerosis. 2008;201(2):225–35.
29. Balakumar P, Kaur J. Is nicotine a key player or spectator in the induction and progression of cardiovascular diseases? Pharmacol Res. 2009;60(5):361–8.
30. Pittilo RM. Cigarette smoking and endothelial injury: a review. Adv Exp Med Biol. 1990;273:61–78.
31. Bernhard D, Rossmann A, Wick G. Metals in cigarette smoke. IUBMB Life. 2005;57(12):805–9.
32. Rahman MM, Laher I. Structural and functional alteration of blood vessels caused by cigarette smoking: an overview of molecular mechanisms. Curr Vasc Pharmacol. 2007;5(4):276–92.
33. Luo H-L, Zang W-J, Lu J, Yu X-J, Lin Y-X, Cao Y-X. The protective effect of captopril on nicotine-induced endothelial dysfunction in rat. Basic Clin Pharmacol Toxicol. 2006;99(3):237–45.
34. Rodella LF, Rossini C, Favero G, Foglio E, Loreto C, Rezzani R. Nicotine-induced morphological changes in rat aorta: the protective role of melatonin. Cells Tissues Organs. 2012;195(3):252–9.
35. Rodella LF, Favero G, Rossini C, Foglio E, Reiter RJ, Rezzani R. Endothelin-1 as a potential marker of melatonin's therapeutic effects in smoking-induced vasculopathy. Life Sci. 2010;87(17–18):558–64.
36. Erhardt L. Cigarette smoking: an undertreated risk factor for cardiovascular disease. Atherosclerosis. 2009;205(1):23–32.
37. Ferrari AU, Radaelli A, Centola M. Invited review: aging and the cardiovascular system. J Appl Physiol. 2003;95(6):2591–7.
38. Matz RL, Andriantsitohaina R. Age-related endothelial dysfunction: potential implications for pharmacotherapy. Drugs Aging. 2003;20(7):527–50.
39. Brandes RP, Fleming I, Busse R. Endothelial aging. Cardiovasc Res. 2005;66(2):286–94.
40. Puca AA, Carrizzo A, Villa F, Ferrario A, Casaburo M, Maciag A, et al. Vascular ageing: the role of oxidative stress. Int J Biochem Cell Biol. 2003;45(3):556–9.
41. Dia D-F, Rabinovitch PS, Ungvari Z. Mitochondria and cardiovascular aging. Circ Res. 2012;110(8):1109–24.
42. Mitchell RN, Schoen FJ. Blood Vessels. In: Kumar V, Abbas AK, Fausto N, Aster JC, editors. Robbins and Cotran pathologic basis of diseases. 8th ed. Philadelphia: Elsevier Saunders; 2016. p. 498–505.
43. Glagov S, Weisenberg E, Zavins CK, Stankunavicius R, Kolettis GJ. Compensatory enlargement of human atherosclerotic coronary arteries. New Eng J Med. 1987;316(22):1371–5.
44. Kumar V, Abbas AK, Fausto N, Aster JC. Environmental and nutritional diseases. In: Kumar V, Abbas AK, Fausto N, Aster JC, editors. Robbins and Cotran pathologic basis of diseases. 8th ed. Philadelphia: Elsevier Saunders; 2016. p. 415.
45. Miller DT, Ridker PM, Libby P, Kwiatkowski DJ. Atherosclerosis: the path from genomics to therapeutics. J Am Coll Cardiol. 2007;49:1589.
46. Rodella LF, Filippini F, Bonomini F, Bresciani R, Reiter RJ, Rezzani R. Beneficial effects of melatonin on nicotine induced vasculopathy. J Pineal Res. 2010;48(2):126–32.
47. Wang XL, Raveendran M, Wang J. Genetic influence on cigarette induced cardiovascular disease. Prog Cardiovasc Dis. 2003;45(5):361–82.
48. Ridker P. C-reactive protein and the prediction of cardiovascular events among those at intermediate risk: moving an inflammatory hypothesis toward consensus. J Am Coll Cardiol. 2007;49:2129.
49. Guthikonda S, Haynes W. Homocysteine: role and implications in atherosclerosis. Curr Atheroscler Rep. 2006;8:100.

50. Meerarani P, Badimon JJ, Zias E, Fuster V, Moreno PR. Metabolic syndrome and diabetic atherothrombosis: implications in vascular complications. Curr Mol Med. 2006;6:501.
51. Libby P. The vascular biology of atherosclerosis. In: Mann D, Zipes D, Libby P, Bonow R, editors. Braunwald's heart disease. 7th ed. Philadelphia: Elsevier Saunders; 2005. p. 921.
52. Hansson G, Robertson AK, Soderber-Naucler C. Inflammation and atherosclerosis. Annu Rev Pathol. 2006;1:297.
53. Ross R. Atherosclerosis—an inflammatory disease. N Engl J Med. 1999;340(2):115–26.
54. Mitchell RN, Schoen FJ. Blood Vessels. In: Kumar V, Abbas AK, Fausto N, Aster JC, editors. Robbins and Cotran pathologic basis of diseases. 8th ed. Philadelphia: Elsevier Saunders; 2016. p. 492, 506.
55. Pinard A, Jones GT, Milewicz DM. Genetics of thoracic and abdominal aortic disease. Circ Res. 2019;124:588–606.
56. Hobeika M, Thompson RW, Muhs BE, Brooks PC, Gagne PJ. Matrix metalloproteinases in peripheral vascular disease. J Vasc Surg. 2007;45(4):849.
57. Shimizu K, Mitchell RN, Libby P. Inflammation and cellular immune responses in abdominal aortic aneurysms. Arterioscler Thromb Vasc Biol. 2006;26(5):987–94.
58. Jennette J, Falk R. Nosology of primary vasculitis. Curr Opin Rheumatol. 2007;19:10.
59. Jennette J, et al. Nomenclature of systemic vasculitides. Proposal of an international consensus conference. Arthritis Rheum. 1994;37:187.
60. Kumar V, Abbas AK, Fausto N, Aster JC. Diseases of immune system. In: Kumar V, Abbas AK, Fausto N, Aster JC, editors. Robbins and Cotran pathologic basis of diseases. 8th ed. Philadelphia: Elsevier Saunders; 2016. p. 198.
61. Mitchell RN, Schoen FJ. Blood Vessels. In: Kumar V, Abbas AK, Fausto N, Aster JC, editors. Robbins and Cotran pathologic basis of diseases. 8th ed. Philadelphia: Elsevier Saunders; 2016. p. 511.
62. Kumar V, Abbas AK, Fausto N, Aster JC. Acute and chronic inflammation. In: Kumar V, Abbas AK, Fausto N, Aster JC, editors. Robbins and Cotran pathologic basis of diseases. 8th ed. Philadelphia: Elsevier Saunders; 2016. p. 53.
63. Falcini F. Kawasaki disease. Curr Opin Rheumatol. 2006;18:33.
64. Gedalia A. Kawasaki disease: 40 years after the original report. Curr Rheumatol Rep. 2007;9:336.
65. Giacco F, Brownlee M. Oxidative stress and diabetic complications. Circ Res. 2010;107(9):1058–70.
66. De Jongh RT, Serné EH, Ijzerman RG, de Vries G, Stehouwer CDA. Impaired microvascular function in obesity: implications for obesity-associated microangiopathy, hypertension, and insulin resistance. Circulation. 2004;109(21):2529–35.
67. Caballero AE, Arora S, Saouaf R, Lim SC, Smakowski P, Park JY, et al. Microvascular and macrovascular reactivity is reduced in subjects at risk for type 2 diabetes. Diabetes. 1999;48(9):1856–62.
68. Eringa EC, Stehouwer CDA, Roos MH, Westerhof N, Sipkema P. Selective resistance to vasoactive effects of insulin in muscle resistance arteries of obese Zucker (fa/fa) rats. Am J Physiol. 2007;293(5):E1134–9.
69. Okon EB, Chung AWY, Rauniyar P, Padilla E, Tejerina T, McManus BM, et al. Compromised arterial function in human type 2 diabetic patients. Diabetes. 2005;54(8):2415–23.
70. Meijer RI, de Boer MP, Groen MR, et al. Insulin-induced microvascular recruitment in skin and muscle are related and both are associated with whole-body glucose uptake. Microcirculation. 2012;19(6):494–500.
71. Kostromina E, Gustavsson N, Wang X, Lim CY, Radda GK, Li C, et al. Glucose intolerance and impaired insulin secretion in pancreas-specific signal transducer and activator of transcription-3 knockout mice are associated with microvascular alterations in the pancreas. Endocrinology. 2010;151(5):2050–9.
72. Yudkin JS, Stehouwer CDA, Emeis JJ, Coppack SW. C-reactive protein in healthy subjects: associations with obesity, insulin resistance, and endothelial dysfunction: a potential role for cytokines originating from adipose tissue? Arterioscler Thromb Vasc Biol. 1999;19(4):972–8.
73. Kolka CM, Bergman RN. The endothelium in diabetes: its role in insulin access and diabetic complications. Rev Endocr Metab Disord. 2013;14(1):13–9.
74. Prakash R, Somanath PR, El-Remessy AB, Kelly-Cobbs A, Stern JE, Dore-Duffy P, et al. Enhanced cerebral but not peripheral angiogenesis in the Goto-Kakizaki model of type 2 diabetes involves VEGF and peroxynitrite signaling. Diabetes. 2012;61(6):1533–42.
75. Chang SC, Yang WCV. Hyperglycemia induces altered expressions of angiogenesis associated molecules in the trophoblast. Evid Based Complement Alternat Med. 2013;2013. 11 pages. 457971.
76. Shenouda SM, Widlansky ME, Chen K, Xu G, Holbrook M, Tabit CE, et al. Altered mitochondrial dynamics contributes to endothelial dysfunction in diabetes mellitus. Circulation. 2011;124(4):444–5.
77. Sharma A, Bernatchez PN, de Haan JB. Targeting endothelial dysfunction in vascular complications associated with diabetes. J Vasc Med. 2012;2012. 12 pages.750126.
78. Van den Oever AM, Raterman HG et al. Endothelial dysfunction, Inflammation, and apoptosis in diabetes mellitus. Med Inflam. 2017;7.
79. Greenstein AS, Khavandi K, Withers SB, Sonoyama K, Clancy O, Jeziorska M, et al. Local inflammation and hypoxia abolish the protective anticontractile properties of perivascular fat in obese patients. Circulation. 2009;119(12):1661–70.
80. Chatterjee TK, Stoll LL, Denning GM, Harrelson A, Blomkalns AL, Idelman G, et al. Proinflammatory phenotype of perivascular adipocytes: influence of high-fat feeding. Circ Res. 2009;104(4):541–9.
81. Henrichot E, Juge-Aubry CE, Pernin A, Pache JC, Velebit V, Dayer JM, et al. Production of chemokines by perivascular adipose tissue: a role in the pathogenesis of atherosclerosis? Arterioscler Thromb Vasc Biol. 2005;25(12):2594–9.
82. Withers SB, Agabiti-Rosei C, Livingstone DM, Little MC, Aslam R, Malik RA, et al. Macrophage activation is responsible for loss of anticontractile function in inflamed perivascular fat. Arterioscler Thromb Vasc Biol. 2011;31(4):908–13.
83. Mitchell RN, Schoen FJ. Blood vessels. In: Kumar V, Abbas AK, Fausto N, Aster JC, editors. Robbins and Cotran pathologic basis of diseases. 8th ed. Philadelphia: Elsevier Saunders; 2016. p. 520.
84. Johansson P, Stensballe, J, Ostrowski SR. Shock induced endotheliopathy (SHINE) in acute critical illness - a unifying pathophysiologic mechanism. Crit Care. 2017;21(1):25.
85. Kim J, Kim K, Lee JH, Jo YH, Kim T, Rhee JE, Kang KW. Prognostic implication of initial coagulopathy in out-of-hospital cardiac arrest. Resuscitation. 2013;84(1):48–53.
86. Holcomb JB, Minei KM, Scerbo ML, Radwan ZA, Wade CE, Kozar RA, Gill BS, Albarado R, McNutt MK, Khan S, et al. Admission rapid thrombelastography can replace conventional coagulation tests in the emergency department: experience with 1974 consecutive trauma patients. Ann Surg. 2012;256(3):476–86.
87. Kozar RA, Peng Z, Zhang R, Holcomb JB, Pati S, Park P, et al. Plasma restoration of endothelial glycocalyx in a rodent model of hemorrhagic shock. Anesth Analg. 2011;112:1289–95.
88. Stensballe J, Ulrich AG, Nilsson JC, Henriksen HH, Olsen PS, Ostrowski SR, et al. Resuscitation of endotheliopathy and bleeding in thoracic aortic dissection: the viper-Octa randomized clinical pilot trial. Anesth Analg. 2018;127(4):920–7.

89. Pati S, Potter DR, Baimukanova G, Farrel DH, Holcomb JB, Schreiber MA. Modulating the endotheliopathy of trauma: factor concentrate versus fresh frozen plasma. J Trauma Acute Care Surg. 2016;80:576–84.
90. Brown MD, Feairheller DL. Are there race-dependent endothelial cell responses to exercise? Exerc Sport Sci Rev. 2013;41(1):44–54. [PMC free article] [PubMed] [Google Scholar]
91. Flynn KE, Piña IL, Whellan DJ, Lin L, Blumenthal JA, Ellis JA, et al. Effects of exercise training on health status in patients with chronic heart failure HF-ACTION randomized controlled trial. J Am Med Assoc. 2009;301(14):1451–9. [PMC free article] [PubMed] [Google Scholar]
92. Downing J, Balady GJ. The role of exercise training in heart failure. J Am Coll Cardiol. 2011;58(6):561–9. [PubMed] [Google Scholar]
93. Niebauer J. Effects of exercise training on inflammatory markers in patients with heart failure. Heart Fail Rev. 2008;13(1):39–49. [PubMed] [Google Scholar]
94. Cuevas AM, Germain AM. Diet and endothelial function. Biol Res. 2004;37(2):225–30.
95. Vogel RA. The Mediterranean diet and endothelial function: why some dietary fats may be healthy. Cleve Clin J Med. 2000;67(4, article 232):235–6. Erratum in Cleveland Clinic Journal of Medicine, vol. 67, no. 7, article 467, 2000
96. Lopez-Garcia E, Schulze MB, Meigs JB, Manson JE, Rifai N, Stampfer MJ, et al. Consumption of trans fatty acids is related to plasma biomarkers of inflammation and endothelial dysfunction. J Nutr. 2005;135(3):562–6.
97. Silva JM, Saldanha C. Diet, atherosclerosis and atherothrombotic events. Rev Port Cardiol. 2007;26(3):277–94.
98. Esposito K, Marfella R, Ciotola M, Di Palo C, Giugliano G, D'Armiento M, et al. Effect of a Mediterranean-style diet on endothelial dysfunction and markers of vascular inflammation in the metabolic syndrome: a randomized trial. J Am Med Assoc. 2004;292(12):1440–6.
99. Estruch R, Martínez-González MA, Corella D, Salas-Salvado J, Ruiz-Gutierrez V, Covas MI, et al. Effects of a Mediterranean-style diet on cardiovascular risk factors a randomized trial. Ann Intern Med. 2006;145(1):1–11.
100. Ryan M, Mcinerney D, Owens D, Collins P, Johnson A, Tomkin GH. Diabetes and the Mediterranean diet: a beneficial effect of oleic acid on insulin sensitivity, adipocyte glucose transport and endothelium-dependent vaso-reactivity. Month J Assoc Phys. 2000;93(2):85–91.
101. Grassi D, Desideri G, Ferri C. Flavonoids: antioxidants against atherosclerosis. Nutrients. 2010;2(8):889–902.
102. Rezzani R, Rodella LF, Tengattini S, Bonomini F, Pechanova O, Kojsova S, et al. Protective role of polyphenols in cyclosporine A-induced nephrotoxicity during rat pregnancy. J Histochem Cytochem. 2006;54(8):923–32.
103. Landberg R, Naidoo N, van Dam RM. Diet and endothelial function: from individual components to dietary patterns. Curr Opin Lipidol. 2012;23(2):147–55.

23 Obstetrical Blood Management

Colleen B. Yen, Monica M. DiLorenzo, and Daniel Katz

Overview and Introduction

Transfusion in obstetrics presents unique challenges and considerations. The most common indication for transfusion in this population is post partum hemorrhage (PPH). Obstetrical blood management goes hand in hand with PPH. One cannot become proficient in obstetrical blood management without intimate knowledge of PPH. Likewise, properly managing PPH should lead to a decreased need for blood products, which is the best strategy when it can be attained. Therefore, this chapter will begin with the critical management steps for PPH that should lead to a decreased need for transfusion and will end with specific transfusion management strategies.

Epidemiology and Definition

Post partum hemorrhage affects approximately 2% of parturients [1, 2] and is one of the leading causes of maternal deaths worldwide, accounting for over 27% of maternal deaths [3].

Post partum hemorrhage was classically defined as estimated blood loss (EBL) >500 mL for a vaginal delivery and EBL >1000 mL for a cesarean delivery and was divided into primary PPH, occurring within 24 hours of birth, and secondary PPH, occurring more than 24 hours and up to 12 weeks post partum. However, these definitions are overly simplistic, and current definitions vary by society and expert opinion [4–10]. Further, since blood loss is difficult to estimate and is often underestimated, societies including ACOG [4] have created programs such as the reVITALize program to standardize definitions in obstetrics and have included other metrics in addition to blood loss such as vital sign changes as supplemental criteria regardless of the estimated blood loss (EBL). Additionally, although some define PPH as EBL >1000 mL, which would decrease the number of patients labeled with PPH, blood loss greater than 500 mL for a normal spontaneous vaginal delivery (NSVD) is still considered to be abnormal [4] and should prompt an escalation of care.

Risk Factors for Obstetric Hemorrhage

Several studies have identified risk factors for postpartum hemorrhage and are presented in Table 23.1.

While identifying patients at risk for PPH is an important step in hemorrhage planning and management, probably the most important take away is that there is a very high incidence

Table 23.1 Risk factors for postpartum hemorrhage [4, 11–14]

Risk factors involving a highly or overly distended uterus	Other risk factors
Macrosomia	Prolonged labor
Twin or multiple gestation	Augmented labor
Polyhydramnios	Rapid labor
	History of PPH
	Episiotomy
	Pre eclampsia
	BMI >40
	Operative delivery
	Coagulopathy
	Anticoagulant or antithrombotic medication use
	Thrombocytopenia
	Morbidly adherent placenta
	Asian or Hispanic ethnicity
	Chorioamonitis

C. B. Yen (✉) · M. M. DiLorenzo
The Mount Sinai Hospital, Department of Anesthesiology, Perioperative and Pain Medicine, New York, NY, USA
e-mail: colleen.yen@mountsinai.org; Monica.dilorenzo@mountsinai.org

D. Katz
Icahn School of Medicine at Mount Sinai, Department of Anesthesiology, New York, NY, USA
e-mail: Daniel.katz@mountsinai.org

© Springer Nature Switzerland AG 2021
C. S. Scher et al. (eds.), *Essentials of Blood Product Management in Anesthesia Practice*,
https://doi.org/10.1007/978-3-030-59295-0_23

of PPH in patients with no known risk factors. Risk stratification tools have not proven to be specific. In fact, Bateman et al. in a population study of almost 900,000 deliveries with more than 25,000 episodes of PPH found that in patients aged 20–40 years who had a normal spontaneous vaginal delivery (NSVD) complicated by atony that required transfusion, only 38% of patients had one of the risk factors tested [13]. The conclusion is that even though we can identify high risk patients with scoring systems, every patient on the labor floor is at risk for PPH. This highlights the importance of labor and delivery units being prepared with plans and resources to rapidly respond to unexpected hemorrhage events. Specific management strategies will be discussed later in this chapter.

Preventing PPH and Blood Transfusion

The most important step in obstetrical transfusion management is preventing obstetrical hemorrhage. It is important to recognize that PPH is frequently preventable and represents an area for improvement in obstetric care and outcomes. Several major obstetric and anesthesiology societies recommend the use of uterotonic medications as first-line prevention of PPH. An active type and screen should also be obtained and confirmed at the first sign of hemorrhage, if not in all obstetric patients at the time of presentation in labor [4, 15], as discussed above, unanticipated hemorrhage in patients with few or no risk factors is not uncommon.

When thinking about preventing PPH, it is important to recall that the vast majority of PPH cases (60–80%) are due to uterine atony, followed by retained placenta, defects in coagulation, uterine inversion, and genital tract trauma [13, 14], which are summarized as the 4 Ts in Table 23.2.

Active management of the third stage of labor (delivery of the placenta) reduces the risk of PPH and is defined as administration of a prophylactic uterotonic [16], early umbilical cord clamping, and controlled cord traction to facilitate placental delivery. Active management of the third stage of labor is recommended for every delivery, and oxytocin or its analogue carbetocin, which causes uterine contraction and prostaglandin production, is considered to be the drug of choice for first-line treatment. Per a Cochrane meta-analysis, oxytocin was found to probably reduce blood loss and the need for additional uterotonics, though optimal dose and timing have yet to be determined [6, 16–19]. When necessary, additional uterotonics such as misoprostol, methylergonovine, and carboprost have been shown to be effective when used with or immediately following oxytocin [20–26]. It is important to keep in mind that each uterotonic comes with potential side effects and may be contraindicated in patients with certain conditions, summarized in Table 23.3.

Table 23.2 Common causes of PPH [13, 14]

Tone	Uterine atony
Tissue	Placental retention/morbidly adherent placenta
Trauma	Tears and lacerations
Thrombin	Coagulopathy

Occasionally, in cases where severe hemorrhage is anticipated and would be challenging to control, such as in placenta percreta, surgical strategies to prevent bleeding may be employed. Arterial balloon catheters may be placed in a preemptive manner and are most commonly placed in the uterine arteries; however more proximal balloons in the iliac arteries and the aorta have also been used [29]. Uterine artery embolization has been used in such a manner for both prophylactic control of bleeding [30] or as a rescue measure as part of a uterine conservation strategy [31]. A significant number of patients, however, will continue to bleed in spite of uterine artery embolization given the redundancy of blood flow to the uterus [32], and in these cases emergent uterine artery embolization or hysterectomy may be required.

Recognition and Quantification of PPH

One of the largest challenges in obstetrical blood management is estimating how much blood has been lost and determining how much blood to replace. Physiologic perturbations are often late signs of hypovolemia in young, healthy parturient [33]. Peripheral and splanchnic vasoconstriction facilitates the relocation of blood from venous capacitance vessels to the central circulation, allowing blood pressure and heart rate to remain near normal until blood loss exceeds 1500 mL in most parturient [33].

Other indicators of blood loss, such as hematocrit and lactate levels, also present challenging limitations. Changes in hematocrit and hemoglobin often take hours to manifest, and

Table 23.3 Second-line uterotonics [26–28]

Uterotonic	Mechanism of action	Common side effects	Possible contraindications
Misoprostol	Prostaglandin E1 causes uterine contraction	Nausea, vomiting, maternal pyrexia	Concern for aspiration or increased oxygen demand
Methylergonovine	Semi-synthetic ergot alkaloid increases tone, rate, and amplitude of rhythmic contractions	Hypertension	Hypertension, coronary artery disease, preeclampsia
Carboprost	Analogue of prostaglandin F2 alpha causes smooth muscle contractions	Bronchospasm, hypertension, nausea, vomiting, diarrhea	Asthma, hypertension, concern for aspiration

a nadir may not be reached until post partum day 2 or 3 [34] and are further confounded by crystalloid administration as well as clinical states such as pre eclampsia where vascular permeability is altered [35, 36]. Arterial lactate levels have been successfully used as a surrogate marker for tissue perfusion in trauma [37, 38], sepsis [39], and gastrointestinal bleeding [40], and the lactate level trend and absolute value have been used in obstetrics to assess oxygen delivery and the need for transfusion or to assess for the efficacy of interventions aimed at facilitating tissue perfusion, though data supporting their use in PPH is limited. However, the utility of both hematocrit and lactate testing may be limited by the availability of point-of-care testing and laboratory turn around times. In fact, they may result so late as to provide no clinical value to a provider managing an acute or rapid hemorrhage.

Patient Blood Management and PPH

Current guidelines for transfusion are based on evidence specific to the non-pregnant adult major trauma and military medicine patient and recommend the use of formulaic transfusion of packed red blood cells (PRBC), fresh frozen plasma (FFP), and cryoprecipitate in fixed ratios [41, 42]. However, the baseline coagulation profile of a pregnant patient and a non-pregnant patient is very different, and there is no data to extrapolate the formulaic transfusion used in trauma and military medicine to obstetric hemorrhage [41–43]. This is especially true in regard to components such as fibrinogen (discussed below) in which transfusion of plasma-based products can incite a dilutional coagulopathy.

First, we will discuss the change in coagulation status in the term parturient and subsequently the impact of the coagulopathy of PPH on this coagulation status, with emphasis on fibrinogen level as a therapeutic target. Next, we will discuss steps in anticipation for PPH including blood product availability and triggers for transfusion of PRBC specifically. Further, we will discuss massive transfusion protocols in obstetric anesthesia, transfusion of incompatible blood in a patient with multiple antibodies, and cell salvage. Importantly, we will stress the ability of viscoelastic testing to overcome many of the shortfalls of traditional coagulation testing in the management of PPH. Finally, we will discuss pharmacologic adjuncts including antifibrinolytics, fibrinogen concentrates, prothrombin complex concentrates, recombinant activated factor VIIa, and calcium in obstetrical blood management.

Change in Coagulation Factors in the Pregnant Patient

Pregnancy is a hypercoagulable state [43, 44]. In the pregnant patient, there is an increase in procoagulant activity (characterized by increases in factors V, VII, VIII, IX, X, XII, von Willebrand factor, and fibrinogen) and a decrease in endogenous anticoagulant activity (characterized by increases in heparin cofactor I1 antitrypsin, protein S activity, and activated protein C resistance) [43, 44]. Platelet count may decrease during pregnancy (gestational thrombocytopenia) but rarely occurs to a level that contributes to risk of bleeding [45].

The change in fibrinogen in a term pregnancy is important and significant; fibrinogen level in a pregnant patient at term ranges from 350 to 650 mg/dL, which is nearly double in the fibrinogen level in a non-pregnant patient [43]. The change in fibrinogen may not be reflected in a facility's reference range, which may cause the under-recognition of hypofibrinogenemia. Other laboratory markers of coagulation such as the prothrombin time (PT) and partial thromboplastin time (PTT) do not usually become abnormal during obstetric hemorrhage until large volumes of blood have already been lost [43].

Coagulopathy in Postpartum Hemorrhage

Coagulopathy associated with PPH is likely a complex interaction between dilution, local consumption, disseminated consumption, and increased fibrinolysis [46, 47]. Although an increase in procoagulant activity is seen in the pregnant patient, these protective mechanisms may be quickly overcome in the setting of massive blood loss [47]. The rapid consumption of clotting factors and platelets in massive hemorrhage can quickly exceed the normal surplus of coagulation factors [47]. Furthermore, critical levels of prothrombin, factor V, factor VII, and platelets are reached after a loss of greater than 200% of calculated blood volume, whereas life-threatening levels of fibrinogen are reached after a loss of only 140% [47].

Fibrinogen

Although factor repletion is an important component of preventing coagulopathy, fibrinogen deserves special consideration as a biomarker in the diagnosis of hemorrhage and as a potential therapeutic target for the management of hemorrhage. Fibrinogen is one of the main building blocks in coagulation, and a low fibrinogen level has been identified as an early predictor of severe PPH [44, 48]. Charbit et al. assessed coagulation profiles of 128 patients with atonic PPH (after administration of a second-line uterotonic) for 24 hours after onset of bleeding. Maternal fibrinogen level was independently associated with severe PPH; for every 1 g/L decrease in fibrinogen, there was a 2.6-fold increased odds of severe PPH. A baseline fibrinogen level ≤2 g/L taken at the time of bleeding onset had a positive predictive value of 100% [42, 44, 49]. These results demonstrate that a low fibrinogen level during the early phase of postpartum bleeding can predict the later development of severe PPH [44].

Blood Product Availability

One of the earliest steps in patient blood management is to have blood products available when needed. Practices in routine laboratory testing of the obstetric patient vary by institution and can vary from no routine testing to a universal type and screen. Although hemorrhage bundles encourage use of preemptive type and screen for moderate-risk patients and type and cross-match for high-risk patients, less guidance is given as to what should be done in the low-risk population who still contribute to a significant portion of patients with PPH [50]. The ASA Task Force on Obstetric Anesthesia practice guidelines state that the literature is insufficient to determine whether type and screen leads to fewer maternal anesthetic complications and whether type and cross-match is necessary for healthy and uncomplicated parturients [51]. From a cost analysis perspective, universal type and screen for all patients is not cost-effective and only marginally reduces the need to transfuse uncrossed blood [52]. Each institution must determine their own approach based on local guidelines, patient mix, and cost-effectiveness while maximizing the degree of clinical impact [44].

Massive Transfusion Protocol

When the maternal rate of bleeding is rapid, several units of blood products will not suffice to ensure avoidance of maternal morbidity and mortality. In the event of massive hemorrhage, large volumes of blood products are needed expeditiously, and massive transfusion protocols (MTPs) were developed for this purpose. The criteria to meet massive transfusion is discussed elsewhere.

As discussed, there is no consensus on the optimal RBC-to-plasma ratio in the management of obstetric hemorrhage. Popular ratios for transfusion include PRBC/FFP/platelet ratio of 6:4:1 or 4:4:1. While some societies such as ACOG recommend fixed product ratios for obstetric hemorrhage MTPs, others such as the Royal College of Obstetricians and Gynecologists (RCOG) recommend set volumes of plasma following RBC transfusion [43]. The CMQCC recommends that transfusion be based on vital signs and should not be delayed while awaiting laboratory results [43]. In the obstetric patient, many transfusion protocols include cryoprecipitate, in anticipation of a rapid decrease in fibrinogen during severe hemorrhage.

Implementation of a massive transfusion protocol has been shown to improve the timeline of blood transfusion and to be cost-effective due to a lower overall usage of blood products [44]. Additionally, utilization of the MTP not only improves the line of communication for ordering and transporting blood products from the blood bank to the labor and delivery unit but also ensures that blood products continue to be available until surgical and hemostatic control of hemorrhage has occurred [44].

A survey of 60 directors of academic obstetric anesthesia units across the United States reported that 95% of labor and delivery units had an MTP protocol [44, 53]. However, most centers lacked a standardized initiation cut off which caused variability in use. Most institutions with an initiation standard used a cut-off of 1500 mL with uncontrolled bleeding [53].

Multiple Antibodies and Transfusion of Incompatible Blood

Specific patient populations including patients with sickle cell disease, thalassemia, and hemophilia have higher rates of blood antibodies [53]. These patients are still at risk for obstetric hemorrhage and may require transfusion. Usually, every effort is made to avoid the transfusion of incompatible blood, through efforts including prophylactic preparation of cross-matched blood products 48 hours prior to induction of labor, use of cell salvage, and early intervention for obstetric hemorrhage such as uterine artery embolization and hysterectomy to obtain surgical control [53]. If the transfusion of incompatible units becomes necessary, the clinician should transfuse in ascending order of clinical hemolytic severity of the antibody of concern. The blood bank, hematology, and maternal fetal medicine should be involved if transfusion of known incompatible blood is to take place [53].

Transfusion Triggers for PRBC Transfusion in Non-MTP Circumstances

There is no optimal Hob/Hot goal that must be met during obstetric hemorrhage; however the common threshold of a Hob of 7 g/ld. or a Hot of 21% is commonly cited [50, 54]. Although a Hot of 18–25% may be tolerated in an otherwise healthy parturient, most experts agree that PRBC transfusion is warranted with a Hot of less than 25% in the setting of active bleeding [47]. A higher Hot during ongoing hemorrhage both maintains tissue and organ perfusion and improves overall coagulation status [47]. Clinical markers including serum pH, lactate, base deficit, and bicarbonate have been extensively studied as markers of resuscitation success in shock [53]. As a patient's volume status may change rapidly during hemorrhage resuscitation, it is recommended to repeat testing every 30–45 minutes until the hemorrhage is controlled [43]. However, during an acute event, there can be significant fluctuations and variability in measurements, and therefore laboratory tests should not be used as the sole criteria to transfuse packed red blood cells (PRBCs). Anesthesiologists often use these values in conjunction with evidence of hypovolemia and oxygen debt such as oliguria, refractory hypotension/tachycardia, and arterial lactate to guide PRBC transfusions. Other clinical endpoints of successful resuscitation include a maintained mean arterial pressure ≥65 mmHg, sustained mental status, and acid-based status [53]. It would make sense that institutions that perform QBL would integrate these values into transfusion algorithms. As it stands current transfusion practice is a delicate balance between under- and over-resuscitation, with negative consequences for both.

Cell Salvage

For a long time, the use of cell salvage during obstetric hemorrhage was considered controversial due to the possibility of amniotic fluid embolism (AFE) and maternal alloimmunization to fetal RBC antigens [43, 47, 48]. Newer data suggests that the risk of AFE and maternal-fetal alloimmunization can be decreased by use of leukocyte depletion filters (LDF) and separation of suction for blood and amniotic fluid prior to placental delivery [48]. Newer generation LDF are effective in decreasing the number of amniotic fluid proteins, bacterial contamination, free hemoglobin, and potassium [48]. With these new separate filters, large case series have demonstrated a lower risk profile for salvaged blood, with no cases of AFE reported, and are now supported in current guidelines.

However, obstetric hemorrhage is unpredictable, and a major challenge is the inability to set up cell salvage for every delivery [43]. As such, emphasis has been put on identification of those at high risk for obstetric hemorrhage, including multiple gestation, placenta previa, and invasive placentation [43]. The ACOG and ASA support cell salvage in parturients in whom large blood loss is expected (>20% of blood volume) [43, 48, 55]. Cell salvage may be especially useful in settings with limited blood product availability or in specific obstetric populations including rare blood types and Jehovah's Witnesses [43, 47]. Any patient receiving salvaged blood should undergo testing for fetal RBC exposure and administered Rh immunoglobulin if clinically indicated [43].

Goal-Directed Therapy and Viscoelastic Testing

An obstacle to avoiding coagulopathy in PPH lies in the limitations of traditional coagulation testing. Traditional coagulation tests such as prothrombin time (PT), partial thromboplastin time (PTT), and clauss fibrinogen assays do not give the full picture of hemostasis during obstetric hemorrhage and only provide guidance on initial clot formation [56, 57]. It is well-recognized that these traditional coagulation tests are poor predictors of bleeding [42]. During obstetric hemorrhage, PT and PTT often remain within normal range even until blood loss reaches 4000–5000 ml [42]. Further, these tests may have long turnaround times (60–90 minutes); thus results are less relevant in an acutely changing situation, and many clinicians may decide to transfuse based on a protocol-based approach or upon clinical judgment [42]. The issue with formulaic transfusion is that not all obstetric hemorrhage is the same, and patients may present with a variety of bleeding phenotypes. In many cases administering FFP may cause a dilutional coagulopathy, especially in the case of hypofibrinogenemia. Plasma transfusion must occur in large volumes to be effective, which may lead to volume overload or other transfusion reactions [58, 59].

Viscoelastic testing via thromboelasography (TEG) or thromboelastometry (ROTEM) overcome many of the shortfalls of traditional coagulation tests. TEG and ROTEM assess and graphically display the viscoelastic properties from clot formation to clot lysis, provide actionable information within minutes, and allow for specific goal-directed therapy. An important advantage of these assays is the quick turnaround time, with an evaluation of clot kinetics generated in 5–10 minutes [42]. Studies in the obstetric population have shown both agreement and correlation between viscoelastic testing parameters and traditional coagulation assays, with a decreased time for data acquisition [60, 61]. This is especially true for measurements of fibrinogen, which has been shown to be a prognostic indicator and therapeutic target in obstetric hemorrhage. A FibTEM A5, which is the amplitude of the FibTEM trace at 5 minutes after the start of clot formation, measures the effect of fibrinogen by eliminating the contribution of platelets to clot strength by way of the addition of cytochalasin D and has been shown to correlate with plasma fibrinogen level [62]. A FibTEM A5 of 12 mm correlates approximately with a plasma fibrinogen level of 2.2 g/L [62]. In 2019, McNamara et al. presented 4 years of data on a ROTEM-guided algorithm for obstetric hemorrhage. The data compared the use of shock packs, which included four units of PRBC, four units of FFP, and one dose of platelets, and a ROTEM-guided algorithm with administration of fibrinogen concentrates. The data showed a significant reduction in morbidity, specifically transfusion-associated circulatory overload (TACO) likely secondary to a decrease in the transfusion of FFP, and a decrease in the number of units and total volume of blood products transfused per patient [62]. Comparator studies are ongoing, with early results demonstrating that viscoelastic testing driven algorithms can decrease the amount of products given

[49, 63, 64], ICU admission [49, 63], hysterectomy [49], and length of stay with decreased cost [49].

Pharmacologic Adjuncts in Postpartum Hemorrhage

Maternal death from postpartum hemorrhage may occur within hours of onset, especially in clinical settings without robust blood banks or with the ability to collaborate with a nearby blood bank [53]. Pharmacologic adjuncts including antifibrinolytics, fibrinogen concentrates, prothrombin complex concentrate (PCC), recombinant factor VIIa (rFVIIa), and calcium may aid in both high and low blood bank resource settings as adjuncts to massive transfusion protocols.

Antifibrinolytics

TXA is a potent antifibrinolytic that binds to lysine residues in plasminogen and plasmin, preventing plasmin activation and clot breakdown. It is used widely in the management of hemorrhage in the cardiac surgery and trauma patient [43, 53] and is shown to significantly reduce perioperative blood loss and RBC transfusion without an increase in thrombotic events [47]. The utility of TXA in postpartum hemorrhage has been recognized since the release of data from the World Maternal Antifibrinolytic Trial (WOMAN Trial) in 2017 [65]. Including over 20,000 parturients across almost 200 hospitals in 21 countries, women randomized to receive 1 g IV TXA after losing 500 mL of blood had a decreased incidence of death from bleeding (RR 0.64 [95%CI: 0.49–0.85 $p = 0.045$]) when compared to placebo. If the TXA was administered within 3 hours of delivery, maternal death was decreased by over 30%. Importantly, the WOMAN trial found no increase in thromboembolic events or renal dysfunction in patients who received TXA. The recommended treatment dose of TXA is 1 g intravenously, with a second gram administered if bleeding continues after 30 minutes, or if hemorrhage recurs within 24 hours of delivery [48]. The WHO, ACOG, and CMQCC now include TXA recommendations in their obstetric hemorrhage guidelines [43]. Several small RCTs and meta-analyses studying antifibrinolytic therapy in the postpartum period demonstrate that TXA use is associated with a reduction in blood loss, decreased need for additional uterotonic agents, and higher hemoglobin levels after 24 hours [47]. Another unanswered questioned is whether one should wait for hemorrhage to start as was the study design in the WOMAN trial or if it should be given prophylactically for high-risk situations such as placenta percreta.

Fibrinogen Concentrates

While fibrinogen has been identified as a biomarker for severe PPH, the optimal fibrinogen concentration to prevent coagulopathy is not known. However, the threshold of 200 mg/dl has been shown to be predictive of progression to further hemorrhage, has been used as a cut off value for repletion, and is the currently recommended threshold for repletion by the American Society of Anesthesiologists [51]. With regard to repletion strategy, it is important to note that prophylactic treatment prior to the onset of hypofibrinogenemia is an ineffective strategy [66, 67]. Therefore, to optimize transfusion management, firstly the measurement of fibrinogen levels should occur rapidly, and, secondly, fibrinogen-containing products must be readily available. The first issue can be overcome with rapid lab protocols or viscoelastic testing if available. The second issue is that due to high levels of fibrinogen present in term parturients, products such as FFP can dilute fibrinogen levels until the extremes of blood loss.

Two therapeutic options are available for fibrinogen replacement: cryoprecipitate and fibrinogen concentrate [42]. The fibrinogen concentration in cryoprecipitate ranges from 3 to 30 g/L, leading to a potentially inconsistent effect, and requires two to three freeze-thaw cycles prior to administration, which can potentially cause a delay in administration [42]. Also, cryoprecipitate is not virally inactivated and is not available in all locations [68]. Fibrinogen concentrate has been used as a rapid alternative for fibrinogen repletion in obstetric hemorrhage [49, 63, 67]. Fibrinogen concentrates are a manufactured concentrated form of fibrinogen produced from human plasma. It comes as a powder to be reconstituted, does not require refrigeration, and therefore may easily be stored near the patient in a controlled release compartment system such as Pyxis [42]. Unlike cryoprecipitate, fibrinogen concentrates do not require cross-match [45, 48] and have decreased risk of infectious complications since viral activation and the removal of antigens and antibodies occurs during the manufacturing process [42, 48]. Appropriate fibrinogen concentrate therapy can prevent unnecessary product transfusion and complications of transfusion such as volume overload and allergic reactions [45]. The cost of fibrinogen concentrate varies by location; however studies looking at the cost of utilizing fibrinogen concentrate instead of traditional MTP or shock packs have found it to be either cost saving or cost neutral when taking into account the complications from transfusion reactions and the cost of wasted blood products [49, 63]. The cost-effectiveness of fibrinogen concentrate and cryoprecipitate in the management of severe obstetric hemorrhage should be further explored [49]. A final and important limitation of fibrinogen concentrate is that unlike cryoprecipitate, fibrinogen concentrate contains no fibrin stabilizing factors or factor XIII, which in very large hemorrhages can cause coagulopathy if not repleted.

Prothrombin Complex Concentrates and Recombinant Activated Factor VIIa

The data for proper dosing and safety of PCCs in PPH is limited [48]. They carry a major risk of thrombosis with their usage, and clinical experience in the obstetric population are limited to case reports in women who have extreme coagulation derangements or refractory hemorrhage [69–71]. The advantages of PCCs lie in that they are standardized in their composition and activity, unlike FFP in which factor composition and efficacy are highly variable. They are also stored at room temperature and can have shelf-lives of over 36 months, which make them highly advantageous in areas with limited blood bank resources. More data in the obstetric population are needed before they can be considered for anything other than severe life-threatening hemorrhage that is refractory to all other therapies, as indicated in the ACOG hemorrhage bundle [50].

In the setting of intractable obstetric hemorrhage, recombinant activated factor VIIa (rFVIIa) may be considered. Like PCC, rFVIIa is associated with arterial and venous thrombosis [47], continues to be recommended only as a last ditch effort to stop life-threatening bleeding when all other efforts have failed, and has no proven survival benefit [48]. Although there is no optimal dose range for the parturient, 60–90 μg/kg IV is mentioned in guidelines [47]; however lower doses including 40 μg/kg and 20 μg/kg have been attempted and may carry less risk of thrombosis [72]. It should be noted that women who receive rFVIIa during management of amniotic fluid embolism may have worse outcomes compared to those who did not [73]. A novel topical application of rFVIIa has been described in a five patient case series in patients with placenta previa [74]. Bleeding was well-controlled in all cases; however, more data is needed to determine both safety and efficacy of this technique.

Calcium

Vigilance of maternal calcium levels is of paramount importance during obstetric hemorrhage. Calcium is needed for adequate myocardial contractility as well as vascular tone. Additionally, it is a co-factor in almost every step of coagulation and is necessary for hemostasis [75]. Calcium levels can drop precipitously during obstetric hemorrhage due to hemodilution from non-calcium containing IV fluids and from the administration of citrated blood products that chelate calcium. Citrate from blood products can be cleared relatively quickly by the liver; however, any hepatic impairment from underlying or acute disease including hypotension or hypothermia can delay clearance and cause hypocalcemia. As such, ionized calcium should be checked frequently and kept in the normal physiologic range during any major obstetric hemorrhage. In any case where calcium levels cannot be monitored, pre-emptive repletion should be considered. Lastly, both acidosis and hypothermia can have profound negative impacts on hemostasis and coagulation. Coagulation function diminishes once pH drops below 7.2, with prolongation of PT and PTT as well as diminished platelet function [76, 77]. Interestingly, coagulation function remains impaired upon pH neutralization with sodium bicarbonate administration which may have other deleterious effects on physiology [78, 79]. It would seem based on this evidence that the best way to ameliorate dysfunction by acidosis is to prevent its onset through oxygen delivery optimization when possible. Hypothermia, which can be associated with fluid administration, insensible loss, and redistribution with induction of anesthesia, can impair coagulation with a 10% drop in factor activity level per 1 °C drop in temperature [80]. Although clinically significant coagulopathy does not seem to appear until core temperature drops below 33 °C, efforts to warm patients during resuscitation should begin early [81]. Maintaining core temperature through monitoring and warming efforts such as forced air warming and administering warmed fluids and blood products is well within the expertise of the anesthesiologist. Rapid infusion devices that deliver large volumes of warm fluid are often employed in major surgical procedures and ought to be used in PPH when indicated and should be readily available on the labor floor.

Conclusion

PPH management is a complex process requiring constant vigilance and support from every discipline. The goals of the anesthesiologist in these cases are to place invasive monitors and lines, coordinate the administration of uterotonic agents, direct transfusion practices including interpretation of POC coagulation and lab tests, manage patient hemodynamics, as well as optimize non-transfusion based therapies such that the obstetrician can focus on surgical modalities to manage the uterus and achieve hemostasis.

References

1. Callaghan WM, Kuklina EVBC. Trends in postpartum hemorrhage: United States, 1994-2006. Am J Obs Gynecol. 2010;202(4):353, e1-6.
2. Tuncalp O, Souza JP, GMI. New WHO recommendations on prevention and treatment of postpartum hemorrhage. Int J Gynaecol Obstet. 2013;123(3):254–6.

3. Say L, Chou D, Gemmill A, et al. Global causes of maternal death: A WHO systemic analysis. Lancet Glob Heal. 2014;2(6):e323.
4. Committee on Practice Bulletins-Obstetrics. Practice bulletin no. 183: postpartum hemorrhage. Obstet Gynecol. 2017;130(4):e168–86.
5. Prevention and management of postpartum haemorrhage: green-top guideline no. 52. BJOG 2017;124(5):e106–49.
6. Lyndon A, Lagrew D. CMQCC OB Hemorrhage Tootkit V 2.0.
7. Leduc D, Senikas V, Lalonde A, et al. Active management of the third stage of labour: Prevention and treatment of postpartum hemorrhage. J Obs Gynaecol Canada [J D'obstétrique Gynécologie du Canada]. 2009;31(10):980–93.
8. WHO recommendations for the prevention and treatment of postpartum haemorrhage. 2012.
9. Abdul-Kadir R, McLintock C, Ducloy A-S, et al. Evaluation and management of postpartum hemorrhage: consensus from an international expert panel. Transfusion. 2014;54(7):1756–68.
10. Sentilhes L, Vayssière C, Deneux-Tharaux C, et al. Postpartum hemorrhage: guidelines for clinical practice from the French College of Gynaecologists and Obstetricians (CNGOF): In collaboration with the French Society of Anesthesiology and Intensive Care (SFAR). Eur J Obs Gynecol Reprod Biol. 2016;198:12–21. http://www.ncbi.nlm.nih.gov/pubmed/26773243
11. Mhyre JM, Shilkrut A, Kuklina EV, et al. Massive blood transfusion during hospitalization for delivery in New York State, 1998–2007. Obstet Gynecol. 2013;122(6):1288–94. https://doi.org/10.1097/AOG.0000000000000021.
12. Sheiner E, Sarid L, Levy A, Seidman DS, Hallak M. Obstetric risk factors and outcome of pregnancies complicated with early postpartum hemorrhage: A population-based study. J Matern Fetal Neonatal Med. 2005;18(3):149–54. https://doi.org/10.1080/14767050500170088.
13. Bateman BT, Berman MF, Riley LE, Leffert LR. The epidemiology of postpartum hemorrhage in a large, nationwide sample of deliveries. Anesth Analg. 2010;110(5):1368–73. https://doi.org/10.1213/ANE.0b013e3181d74898.
14. Ring L, Landau R. Postpartum hemorrhage: anesthesia management. Semin Perinatol. 2019;43(1):35–43.
15. SOAP Postpartum Hemorrhage Protocol. 2019.
16. Salati J, Leathersich S, Williams M, Cuthbert A, Tolosa J. Prophylactic oxytocin for the third stage of labour to prevent postpartum haemorrhage. Cochrane Database Syst Rev. 2019 April; 29(4):CD001808. PMID: 31032882
17. Goffman D, Ananth CV, Fleischer A, D'Alton M, Lavery JA, et al. The New York State Safe Motherhood Initiative: EarlyImpact of Obstetric Haemorrhage Bundle Implementation. Am J. Perinatol. 2019 Nov; 36(13):1344–50. PMID:30609429
18. WHO Recommendations for the prevention and treatment of postpartum hemorrhage. WHO Recomm Prev Treat Postpartum Haemorrhage. 2012.
19. Westhoff G, Cotter AM, Tolosa JE. Prophylactic oxytocin for the third stage of labour to prevent postpartum haemorrhage. Cochrane Database Syst Rev. 2013;10:CD001808. https://doi.org/10.1002/14651858.CD001808.pub2.
20. Gallos ID, Williams HM, Price MJ, et al. Uterotonic agents for preventing postpartum haemorrhage: a network meta-analysis. Cochrane Database Syst Rev. 2018;4:CD011689. https://doi.org/10.1002/14651858.CD011689.pub2.
21. Roth JV. Some unanswered questions about temperature management. Anesth Analg. 2009;109(5):1695–9. https://doi.org/10.1213/ANE.0b013e3181b763ae.
22. Harber CR, Levy DM, Chidambaram S, Macpherson MB. Life-threatening bronchospasm after intramuscular carboprost for postpartum haemorrhage. BJOG. 2007;114(3):366–8. https://doi.org/10.1111/j.1471-0528.2006.01227.x.
23. Butwick AJ, Carvalho B, Blumenfeld YJ, El-Sayed YY, Nelson LM, Bateman BT. Second-line uterotonics and the risk of hemorrhage-related morbidity. Am J Obstet Gynecol. 2015;212(5):642.e1-7. https://doi.org/10.1016/j.ajog.2015.01.008.
24. Magee LA, Namouz-Haddard S, Cao V, Koren G, von Dadelazen P. Labetolol for hypertension in pregnancy. Expert Opin Drug Saf. 2015;14(3):453–61. PMID:25692529.
25. Sumikura H, Inada E. Uterotonics and tocolytics for anesthesiologists. Curr Opin Anaesthesiol. 2016;29(3)282–7. PMID 26974052.
26. Allen R, O'Brien BM. Uses of misoprostol in obstetrics and gynecology. Rev Obstet Gynecol. 2009;2(3):159–68. https://www.ncbi.nlm.nih.gov/pubmed/19826573.
27. Novartis Pharmaceuticals Corporation. Methylergonovine drug label. https://www.accessdata.fda.gov/drugsatfda_docs/label/2012/006035s078lbl.pdf. Accessed 22 Aug 2019.
28. Carboprost tromethamine. National Center for Biotechnology Information PubChem Database. pubchem.ncbi.nlm.nih.gov/compound/Carboprost-tromethamine. Accessed 22 Aug 2019.
29. Shahin Y, Pang CL. Endovascular interventional modalities for haemorrhage control in abnormal placental implantation deliveries: a systematic review and meta-analysis. Eur Radiol. 2018. https://doi.org/10.1007/s00330-017-5222-0.
30. Pan Y, Zhou X, Yang Z, Cui S, De W, Sun L. Retrospective cohort study of prophylactic intraoperative uterine artery embolization for abnormally invasive placenta. Int J Gynaecol Obstet. 2017;137(1):45–50. https://doi.org/10.1002/ijgo.12090.
31. Aoki M, Tokue H, Miyazaki M, Shibuya K, Hirasawa S, Oshima K. Primary postpartum hemorrhage: outcome of uterine artery embolization. Br J Radiol. 2018:20180132. https://doi.org/10.1259/bjr.20180132.
32. Kim J-E, So YH, Kim BJ, Kim SM, Choi YH, Sung CK. Postpartum hemorrhage from non-uterine arteries: clinical importance of their detection and the results of selective embolization. Acta Radiol. 2017: https://doi.org/10.1177/0284185117738547.
33. Baird E. Identification and management of obstetric hemorrhage. Anesth Clin. 2017;35(1):15–34.
34. Kodkany B, Derman R. Pitfalls in assessing blood loss and decision to transfer. In: Lynch C, Keith L, Lalonde A, Karoshi M, editors. A Textbook of Postpartum Hemorrhage. Dumfries: Sapiens Publishing; 2006. p. 35–3.
35. Bills VL, Salmon AH, Harper SJ, et al. Impaired vascular permeability regulation caused by the $VEGF_{165}b$ splice variant in pre-eclampsia. BJOG. 2011;118(10):1253–61. https://doi.org/10.1111/j.1471-0528.2011.02925.x.
36. Dai D-M, Cao J, Yang H-M, et al. Hematocrit and plasma albumin levels difference may be a potential biomarker to discriminate preeclampsia and eclampsia in patients with hypertensive disorders of pregnancy. Clin Chim Acta. 2017;464:218–22. https://doi.org/10.1016/j.cca.2016.12.001.
37. Hamada SR, Rosa A, Gauss T, et al. Development and validation of a pre-hospital "Red Flag" alert for activation of intra-hospital haemorrhage control response in blunt trauma. Crit Care. 2018;22(1):113. https://doi.org/10.1186/s13054-018-2026-9.
38. Javali RH, Ravindra P, Patil A, et al. A clinical study on the initial assessment of arterial lactate and base deficit as predictors of outcome in trauma patients. Indian J Crit Care Med. 2017;21(11):719–25. https://doi.org/10.4103/ijccm.IJCCM_218_17.
39. Ryoo SM, Lee J, Lee Y-S, et al. Lactate level versus lactate clearance for predicting mortality in patients with septic shock defined by sepsis-3. Crit Care Med. 2018;46(6):e489–95. https://doi.org/10.1097/CCM.0000000000003030.
40. Shah A, Chisolm-Straker M, Alexander A, Rattu M, Dikdan S, Manini AF. Prognostic use of lactate to predict inpatient mortality in acute gastrointestinal hemorrhage. Am J Emerg Med. 2014;32(7):752–5. https://doi.org/10.1016/j.ajem.2014.02.010.

41. Collins PW, Bell SF, de Lloyd L, Collis RE. Management of postpartum haemorrhage: from research into practice, a narrative review of the literature and the Cardiff experience. Int J Obstet Anesth. 2019;37:106–17. https://doi.org/10.1016/j.ijoa.2018.08.008.
42. Shah A, Collis RE. Managing obstetric haemorrhage: is it time for a more personalised approach? Anaesthesia. 2019;74(8):961–4. https://doi.org/10.1111/anae.14661. PMID:30950513.
43. O'Brien KL, Shainker SA, Lockhart EL. Transfusion management of obstetric hemorrhage. Transfus Med Rev. 2018;32(4):249–55. https://doi.org/10.1016/j.tmrv.2018.05.003.
44. Butwick AJ, Goodnough LT. Transfusion and coagulation management in major obstetric hemorrhage. Curr Opin Anaesthesiol. 2015;28(3):275–84. https://doi.org/10.1097/ACO.0000000000000180.
45. Sahin AS, Ozkan S. Treatment of obstetric hemorrhage with fibrinogen concentrate. Med Sci Monit. 2019;25:1814–21. https://doi.org/10.12659/msm.914234.
46. Collis RE, Collins PW. Haemostatic management of obstetric haemorrhage. Anaesthesia. 2015;70:78–86. https://doi.org/10.1111/anae.12913.
47. Baird EJ. Identification and management of obstetric hemorrhage. Anesthesiol Clin. 2017;35(1):15–34. https://doi.org/10.1016/j.anclin.2016.09.004.
48. Higgins N, Patel SK, Toledo P. Postpartum hemorrhage revisited: new challenges and solutions. Curr Opin Anaesthesiol. 2019;32(3):278–84. https://doi.org/10.1097/aco.0000000000000717.
49. Snegovskikh D, Souza D, Walton Z, et al. Point-of-care viscoelastic testing improves the outcome of pregnancies complicated by severe postpartum hemorrhage. J Clin Anesth. 2018;44:50–6. https://doi.org/10.1016/j.jclinane.2017.10.003.
50. American College of Obstetricians and Gynecologists. Maternal safety bundle for obstetric hemorrhage. 2015;(November):1–29. https://www.acog.org/-/media/Districts/District-II/Public/SMI/v2/HEMSlideSetNov2015.pdf?dmc=1&ts=20190625T1556366928.
51. Practice guidelines for perioperative blood management. Anesthesiology. 2015;122(2):241–75. https://doi.org/10.1097/aln.0000000000000463.
52. Einerson BD, Stehlikova Z, Nelson RE, Bellows BK, Kawamoto K, Clark EAS. Transfusion preparedness strategies for obstetric hemorrhage: a cost-effectiveness analysis. Obstet Gynecol. 2017;130(6):1347–55. https://doi.org/10.1097/AOG.0000000000002359.
53. Kogutt BK, Vaught AJ. Postpartum hemorrhage: blood product management and massive transfusion. Semin Perinatol. 2019;43(1):44–50. https://doi.org/10.1053/j.semperi.2018.11.008.
54. Lyndon A, Lagrew D, Main E, Cape V. A California toolkit to transform maternity care improving ealth care response to obstetric hemorrhage version 2. 0 a California quality improvement toolkit THE OBSTETRIC HEMORRHAGE TASK FORCE improving health care response to obstetric hemorrhage Versi. 2015.
55. Wong CA, Toledo P. To salvage (routinely) or not to salvage: that is the question. Anaesthesia. 2019;74(8):957–60. https://doi.org/10.1111/anae.14667. PMIAD:30963553.
56. De Lloyd L, Bovington R, Kaye A, et al. Standard haemostatic tests following major obstetric haemorrhage. Int J Obstet Anesth. 2011;20(2):135–41. https://doi.org/10.1016/j.ijoa.2010.12.002.
57. Larsen JB, Hvas AM. Predictive value of whole blood and plasma coagulation tests for intra- and postoperative bleeding risk: a systematic review. Semin Thromb Hemost. 2017;43(7):772–805. https://doi.org/10.1055/s-0037-1602665.
58. Solomon C, Collis RE, Collins PW. Haemostatic monitoring during postpartum haemorrhage and implications for management. Br J Anaesth. 2012;109(6):851–63. https://doi.org/10.1093/bja/aes361.
59. Hendrickson JE, Roubinian NH, Chowdhury D, Brambilla D, Murphy EL, Wu Y, Ness PM, Gehrle EA, Snyder EL, Hauser RG, Gottschall JL, Kleinman S, Kakaiya R, Strauss R. Incidence of transfusion reactions: a multi-center study utilizing systematic active surveillance and expert adjudication. Transfusion. 2016;56(10):2587–96. https://doi.org/10.1097/CCM.0b013e31823da96d.Hydrogen.
60. Katz D, Hamburger J, Batt D, Zahn J, Beilin Y. Point-of-care fibrinogen testing in pregnancy. Anesth Analg. 2018;XXX(Xxx):1–3. https://doi.org/10.1213/ane.0000000000003301.
61. Girard T, Mörtl M, Schlembach D. New approaches to obstetric hemorrhage: the postpartum hemorrhage consensus algorithm. Curr Opin Anaesthesiol. 2014;27(3):267–74. https://doi.org/10.1097/ACO.0000000000000081.
62. McNamara H, Kenyon C, Smith R, Mallaiah S, Barclay P. Four years' experience of a ROTEM ® -guided algorithm for treatment of coagulopathy in obstetric haemorrhage. Anaesthesia. 2019;74(8):984–91. https://doi.org/10.1111/anae.14628. PMID:30950521.
63. Mallaiah S, Barclay P, Harrod I, Chevannes C, Bhalla A. Introduction of an algorithm for ROTEM-guided fibrinogen concentrate administration in major obstetric haemorrhage. Anaesthesia. 2015;70(2):166–75. https://doi.org/10.1111/anae.12859.
64. Mallaiah S, Chevannes C, McNamara H. Use of ROTEM® in major obstetric haemorrhage. Anaesthesia. 2015;70(6):759–60. https://doi.org/10.1111/anae.13103.
65. Shakur H, Roberts I, Fawole B, et al. Effect of early tranexamic acid administration on mortality, hysterectomy, and other morbidities in women with post-partum haemorrhage (WOMAN): an international, randomised, double-blind, placebo-controlled trial. Lancet. 2017;389(10084):2105–16. https://doi.org/10.1016/S0140-6736(17)30638-4.
66. Wikkelsø AJ, Edwards HM, Afshari A, et al. Pre-emptive treatment with fibrinogen concentrate for postpartum haemorrhage: randomized controlled trial. Br J Anaesth. 2015;114(4):623–33. https://doi.org/10.1093/bja/aeu444.
67. Collins PW, Cannings-John R, Bruynseels D, et al. Viscoelastometric-guided early fibrinogen concentrate replacement during postpartum haemorrhage: OBS2, a double-blind randomized controlled trial. Br J Anaesth. 2017;119(3):411–21. https://doi.org/10.1093/bja/aex181.
68. McDonnell NJ, Browning R. How to replace fibrinogen in postpartum haemorrhage situations? (Hint: Don't use FFP!). Int J Obstet Anesth. 2018;33:4–7. https://doi.org/10.1016/j.ijoa.2017.08.008.
69. Nakauchi-Tanaka T, Sohda S, Someya K, Kono K, Hamada H, Yoshikawa H. Acquired haemophilia due to factor VIII inhibitors in ovarian hyperstimulation syndrome: case report. Hum Reprod. 2003;18(3):506–8. https://doi.org/10.1093/humrep/deg112.
70. Matsuoka A, Sasaki H, Sugimori C, Hirabuki S, Hoshiba T, Fujiwara H. Acquired hemophilia A manifesting as plasma transfusion-uncontrolled severe bleeding 2 weeks after chorioamnionitis-induced abortion. J Obstet Gynaecol Res. 2017;43(4):763–7. https://doi.org/10.1111/jog.13270.
71. Glynn JC. Prothrombin complex for massive obstetric haemorrhage. Anaesthesia. 2007;62:202–3.
72. Shaylor R, Weiniger CF, Austin N, et al. National and international guidelines for patient blood management in obstetrics: a qualitative review. Anesth Analg. 2017;124(1):216–32. https://doi.org/10.1213/ANE.0000000000001473.
73. Leighton Barbara L, Wall Michael H, Lockhart Ellen M, Phillips Louise E, Zatta AJ. Use of recombinant factor VIIa in patients with warfarin-associated intracranial hemorrhage. Anesthesiology. 2011;115(6):1201–8. http://ovidsp.ovid.com/ovidweb.cgi?T=JS&PAGE=reference&D=emed7&NEWS=N&AN=2005358465.
74. Schjoldager BTBG, Mikkelsen E, Lykke MR, et al. Topical application of recombinant activated factor VII during cesarean delivery

for placenta previa. Am J Obstet Gynecol. 2017;216(6):608.e1–5. https://doi.org/10.1016/j.ajog.2017.02.024.

75. Palta S, Saroa R, Palta A. Overview of the coagulation system. Indian J Anaesth. 2014;58(5):515–23. https://doi.org/10.4103/0019-5049.144643.
76. Ganter MT, Pittet JF. New insights into acute coagulopathy in trauma patients. Best Pract Res Clin Anaesthesiol. 2010;24(1):15–25. https://doi.org/10.1016/j.bpa.2009.09.010.
77. Meng ZH, Wolberg AS, Monroe DM, Hoffman M. The effect of temperature and pH on the activity of factor VIIa: implications for the efficacy of high-dose factor VIIa in hypothermic and acidotic patients. J Trauma. 2003;55(5):886–91. https://doi.org/10.1097/01.TA.0000066184.20808.A5.
78. Graf H, Leach W, Arieff AI. Evidence for a detrimental effect of bicarbonate therapy on hypoxic lactic acidosis. Science (80-). 1984;227(4688):754–5.
79. Martini WZ, Dubick MA, Pusateri AE, Park MS, Ryan KL, Holcomb JB. Does bicarbonate correct coagulation function impaired by acidosis in swine? J Trauma – Inj Infect Crit Care. 2006;61(1):99–106. https://doi.org/10.1097/01.ta.0000215574.99093.22.
80. Elmer J, Wilcox SR, Raja AS. Massive transfusion in traumatic shock. J Emerg Med. 2013;44(4):829–38. https://doi.org/10.1016/j.jemermed.2012.11.025.
81. De Robertis E, Kozek-Langenecker SA, Tufano R, Romano GM, Piazza O, Zito Marinosci G. Coagulopathy induced by acidosis, hypothermia and hypocalcaemia in severe bleeding. Minerva Anestesiol. 2015;81(1):65–75.

Pediatric Blood Management

24

Michelle M. Sheth, Meera Gangadharan, Destiny F. Chau, Norma J. Klein, and Renira Rugnath

Introduction

Pediatric patient blood management (PBM) is an interdisciplinary, evidence-based approach to improving patient outcomes through anemia prevention and treatment, optimization of hemostasis, and minimization of perioperative blood loss. These practices are well established in the adult literature and are supported by various health organizations including the World Health Organization, the American Society of Anesthesiology, the Australian National Blood Authority, and the European Society of Anesthesiology. However, while these practices have been well established for the adult patient population, pediatric PBM lags behind [1–5].

In general, the anesthesiology literature reaffirms that children are not little adults and that unique differences must be recognized for successful outcomes. Adult PBM strategies may not be directly extrapolated to pediatric patients, so guidelines addressing patient physiology and disease processes are necessary. Pediatric patients must always be treated with attention to unique features of each growth phase. For instance, neonates and children have higher average hemoglobin concentrations and oxygen requirements than adults [6]. Additionally, transfusion practices may differ significantly between children's hospitals [7]. In response, recent steps have been taken to standardize methodology. Comprehensive standards were released in 2010 by the Society of Advancement of Blood Management (a Pediatric section was added in 2016), who define PBM as, "the timely application of evidence-based medical and surgical concepts designed to maintain hemoglobin concentration, optimize hemostasis, and minimize blood loss as to improve patient outcome" [1]. Blood transfusions are not without risk, so the decision to transfuse must involve a consideration of the risks and benefits [8]. Thus, this chapter will describe pediatric physiology from the premature neonate through adolescence, the preoperative evaluation, blood conservation strategies, surgical discipline-specific considerations, and evidence-based transfusion guidelines.

History of Pediatric Blood Transfusion

Among the early documented experiments with blood transfusions is the transfusion to a 15-year-old with fever who became weak and pale after leeching proved unsuccessful. He was transfused with blood from a lamb donor. He survived, but the donor succumbed. This sacrificial act was repeated a few more times with only one recipient surviving the procedure. These transfusions were provided by Jean-Baptiste Denys, the personal physician to King Louis XIV in the seventeenth century. Subsequently, Jean-Baptiste was charged with murder, and the procedure was banned [9]. Centuries passed before blood transfusions were conducted in the pediatric patient population. The first neonatal blood transfusion occurred on March 4, 1908, at a New York children's hospital. The newborn was delivered with forceps; however, within 12 hours, the neonate developed a tongue hematoma and facial swelling. She became febrile,

M. M. Sheth (✉)
UMMC, Department of Anesthesiology, Jackson, MS, USA
e-mail: Msheth2@umc.edu

M. Gangadharan
Department of Anesthesiology, UAMS, Little Rock, AR, USA

D. F. Chau
Department of Anesthesiology and Pain Medicine, Arkansas Children's Hospital, University of Arkansas for Medical Sciences, Little Rock, AR, USA

N. J. Klein
University of California Medical Center Davis (UCDMC), University of California, Davis, Department of Anesthesiology & Pain Medicine, Sacramento, CA, USA

R. Rugnath
University of Mississippi Medical Center, School of Medicine, Jackson, MS, USA

© Springer Nature Switzerland AG 2021
C. S. Scher et al. (eds.), *Essentials of Blood Product Management in Anesthesia Practice*,
https://doi.org/10.1007/978-3-030-59295-0_24

restless, and pale, and it became evident a transfusion was required. Her father was the donor for the transfusion, and both the neonate and the father survived. With that, the foundation for the practice of pediatric blood transfusion was established [10].

Anatomical and Physiological Characteristics of Blood in Premature Neonates, Infants, and Children

Many anatomic, physiologic, and hematologic differences between children and adults, even between different age groups, have been identified. The following sections will discuss current standards in pediatric PBM and transfusion guidelines in light of these differences.

Fetal Blood Development

To understand physiological characteristics of blood, one must first review fetal blood development. A fetus attains viability between the 23rd and 26th weeks of gestation. The hematologic system of these fragile patients differs considerably from that of an older child. In utero, erythrocyte production begins in the yolk sac (at 3–6 weeks of gestation), then it migrates to the liver (6–22 weeks of gestation) and finally to the bone marrow. Erythrocyte production and maturation in the fetus is controlled by growth factors produced by the fetus, rather than maternally transferred factors. Erythropoietin is produced by the liver in utero. After birth, the kidneys become the site of erythropoietin synthesis [11]. The quantity of iron in the fetus increases throughout gestation. Preterm infants have less iron than full-term infant [12]. In extremely premature infants, the hematologic system is frequently supported with blood component transfusions and nutritional support.

Blood Volume

Estimation of a child's blood volume and blood loss may be difficult, as children have an increased blood volume: body mass ratio compared to adults. The increased blood volume varies with age, such that the blood volume of a child may be as high as 90, 80, and 70 mL/kg at birth, 1 month, and 5 years, respectively. During active bleeding, the hemoglobin and hematocrit values may not accurately predict blood cell mass. Therefore, a child may maintain a normal blood pressure value in spite of a 15–20% blood volume loss [13]. Mottling, altered consciousness, and delayed capillary refill >3 seconds are likely to precede evident hypotension, but a narrowed pulse pressure and loss of arterial pulse contour may be more indicative of significant blood loss than hypotension and tachycardia. In the case of premature infants and neonates, significant anemia may be reflected in nonspecific signs such as poor feeding, slow weight gain, apnea, bradycardia, and decreased activity. Furthermore, the neonatal heart contains proportionally less contractile tissue and has a limited ability to increase cardiac output in the face of a hemorrhage-induced reduction in oxygen carrying capacity [14, 15].

Normal Red Blood Cell Parameters in Preterm and Term Neonates

The normal red blood cell parameters listed in Table 24.1 were obtained by analyzing a very large database (17,634 tests performed on 12,016 neonates in western USA) who had blood tests during their routine care [11]. Only tests from neonates who were expected to have normal values were included. Mean corpuscular volume (MCV) and mean corpuscular hemoglobin (MCH) decreased in a linear fashion with increasing gestational age. Mean corpuscular hemoglobin concentration (MCHC) does not change based on gestational age. The hemoglobin and hematocrit increase from 22 weeks to 40 weeks gestation. The hemoglobin increases by 0.21 g/dl and the hematocrit by 0.64% for every week increase in gestational age. In neonates 35 weeks to 42 weeks of gestation, the hematocrit levels increase by 3.6 +/− 0.5% in the first 4 hours after birth, secondary to fluid shifting out of the intravascular space. Hematocrit levels remained unchanged in the same time period for neonates 29 to 34 weeks of gestation but are reduced by 6 +/− 0.3% in neonates less than 29 weeks of gestation [16].

Neonatal Hemoglobin Levels and Oxygen Dissociation

At birth, a term neonate's hemoglobin is ~70% hemoglobin F (HgbF) and ~ 30 hemoglobin A (HgbA) [15]. The *p50* of HgbF is 18 mmHg, but the *p50* in HgbA is 25 mmHg. Thus, HgbF is associated with a leftward shift in the oxyhemoglobin dissociation curve, or an increased oxygen affinity. This increased oxygen affinity results from HgbF's decreased affinity for 2,3 diphosphoglycerate (2,3-DPG),

Table 24.1 Normal red cell parameters in preterm and term neonates

Parameter	<25 weeks	40 weeks
MCV	119 +/− 7 fl	106 +/− 4 fl
MCH	40 +/− 2 pg	36 +/− 2 pg
MCHC	34 +/− 1 g/dl	34 +/− 1 g/d

Table information from: Christensen et al. [72]

the stabilizer of the deoxyhemoglobin state. Although this is associated with an increased ability of the fetus to extract oxygen from the maternal placental circulation, it is a theoretical disadvantage in the extrauterine environment under conditions of hypoxic stress. During the first several months of life, an infant's hemoglobin levels fall from 14 to 20 g/dL to a mean ~ 11 g/dL in term infants and as low as ~7 g/dL in preterm infants. This "physiologic anemia" is the result of decreased erythropoietin production and the shorter life span of HgbF (e.g., 90 vs. 120 days for HgbA) [14]. This transient but functional anemia tends to occur earlier and to a more notable degree in preterm infants. In preterm infants, the switch from fetal hemoglobin production to predominantly HgbA production occurs at the post-conceptional age of 37 weeks. It is unaffected by the duration of time that the infant spends in the extrauterine environment [17]. Also, neonatal erythropoietin is produced in monocytes, the adrenal cortex, and the kidney, but postnatally, it is produced in the peritubular renal cells. A confounding issue for sick neonates is that they often undergo repeated blood testing, amounting to 0.8–3.1 mL/kg/day blood loss [18]. For example, a 0.5 mL blood sample in a 1 kg neonate, if extrapolated to a 70 kg patient, is a 35 mL blood sample, something rarely removed at one time in an adult patient [19].

Coagulation System Development

The coagulation system undergoes developmental changes as the fetus grows in utero and changes continue after birth. Coagulation factors do not cross the placenta; instead, they are synthesized by the fetus and can be detected as early as 10 weeks of gestation. Challenges to studying developmental hemostasis in the newborn include small sample sizes in studies, the need for small volumes of blood for assays, and the different physiological states of test subjects especially the premature neonatal population. Diagnosis of bleeding disorders in newborns requires an understanding of normal values of coagulation factor levels in these patients. Table 24.2 shows how various levels of coagulation proteins in newborn infants differ from adult values. Although newborns have lower levels of coagulation factors than adults, their hemostatic system appears to function without spontaneous hemorrhage. Extremely low birth weight infants, at a corrected age of 6 months, achieve the same levels of factor II, V, VII, and X as healthy full-term infants of the same age. Antithrombin III, protein C, and protein S showed the same pattern of development as that of term infants [20]. These findings have clinical implications. Newborns are fairly resistant to heparin probably because of low levels of AT III. Since APTT is prolonged in infants, one should monitor factor Xa activity to titrate unfractionated heparin in this age group [21]. Homozygous deficiency of factor II, X, and XI can be difficult to diagnose because the lower limits of normal coincide with the levels found in these deficient states. Homozygous factor V, VII, IX, XIII and fibrinogen deficiency can be diagnosed at birth, because the levels in the disease state are much lower than the lower limit of normal in this age group. Moderate and severe forms of factor VIII deficiency (hemophilia A) can also be diagnosed in the newborn period. Von Willebrand factor levels are high in the neonate, and there is a greater percentage of the efficacious high molecular weight multimers. Hence only severe forms of von Willebrand's disease are likely to be diagnosed in the newborn period. Neonatal fibrinogen is different from the adult form. Thromboelastography (TEG) studies indicate that a dysfunctional state of fibrinogen exists in infancy [22]. Neonatal plasminogen function is also less effective than its adult counterpart. However, tissue plasminogen activator inhibitor levels are high. This indicates that fibrinolytic activity is attenuated in the neonate compared to the adult [23].

Table 24.2 Various tests of coagulation and levels of coagulation proteins in premature vs term newborns

Various tests of coagulation and levels of coagulation proteins in newborn infants		
Test	30–36 weeks	Term
Fibrinogen	=	=
II	↓	↓
VII	=	= by day 5
IX	↓	↓
X	↓	↓
XI	↓	↓
XII	↓	↓
Prekallikrein	↓	↓
HMWK	↓	= by 1 month
V	= by day 5 of life	= by day 5 of life
VIII	↑	↑
VwF	↑	↑
XIII	= by day 5 of life	= by day 5 of life
Plasminogen	↓	↓
Antithrombin III	↓	↓, = by 3 months
Heparin cofactor II	↓	↓
Protein S	↓	↓
Protein C	↓	↓
α_2 Macroglobulin	↑	↑
C1 INH	↓	↓
α_2 Antiplasmin	↓	= by day 5
α_1 Antitrypsin	=	=

Table information from: Andrew M 1987 [73], and Andrew M 1988 [74]

HMWK high molecular weight kininogen, *VwF* von Willebrand factor, *C1 INH* C1 esterase inhibitor

Table 24.3 Diseases that require special consideration

Disease process	Abnormality	Recommendation
Sickle cell disease	Low hematocrit, iron overload	Threshold of Hb 10 g/dL prior to surgery requiring general anesthesia if at risk of critical illness [25]
Anemia of prematurity	Low hematocrit, low iron stores	Limit preoperative blood draws; add iron supplementation [19]
Liver failure	Coagulation abnormalities. Anemia of chronic disease	Coagulation lab tests prior to surgery to assess baseline [26]
Cirrhosis	Thrombocytopenia, low serum albumin, clotting factors II, VII, IX, X abnormalities	Platelet and FFP +/− cryoprecipitate administration preoperatively if indicated by test results or clinical coagulopathy [26]
Renal failure	Anemia of chronic disease	Erythropoiesis-stimulating agents [4]
Congenital heart disease (cyanotic)	Decreased oxygen delivery	Threshold of Hb 9 g/dL if adequate oxygenation and normal end organ perfusion [25, 27]
Noncyanotic heart disease	Intracardiac shunting, cardiac failure	Threshold of Hb 7 g/dL if stable [19, 27]; 8 g/dL if clinical signs of symptomatic anemia [27]
Pediatric oncology	Pancytopenia, thrombocytopenia, aplastic anemia	Preoperative labs and appropriate transfusion [28]

Preoperative Assessment

Preoperative assessment to stratify hemorrhage risk is important. Neonates and infants are less tolerant of blood loss compared to older children and adults, and significant blood loss may go unrecognized. Poor hematopoiesis with reduced erythropoietin levels and production, repeat blood draws, and poor iron availability contribute to the high rate of anemia seen in critically ill children [24]. Specific disease processes that require special preoperative consideration are detailed in Table 24.3. The impact of each of these conditions on the requirement for an allogeneic blood transfusion may vary depending on the patient's age and disease severity.

Estimating Allowable Blood Loss

Prior to all surgeries, it is important to assess the child's tolerance for and likelihood of requiring a blood transfusion. A restrictive red blood cell (PRBC) transfusion threshold in the adult patient population is associated with unchanged, if not improved, morbidity and mortality [29]. Application of similar thresholds in the pediatric patient population, along with nutrition and anemia support, is thought to produce similar outcomes [30–34].

Table 24.4 Calculation technique for estimated blood volume (EBV)

Estimated blood volume calculation	
Age	Estimated blood volume (EBV)
Preemies	90–100 *mL/kg*
Term neonate to 3 months	80–90 *mL/kg*
>3 months of age to 3 years	70–80 *mL/kg*
>3 years of age	70 *mL/kg*

Estimating the maximum allowable blood loss requires calculation of the child's estimated blood volume (EBV), which is a product of both age and weight. This is described in Table 24.4 and Eq. 24.1.

Equation 24.1 The maximum allowable blood loss (MABL) is a function of the EBV, the patient's initial hematocrit (H_0), and the minimal or target hematocrit (H_1)

$$\text{MABL} = \frac{\text{EBV} \times (H_0 - H_1)}{H_0} \quad (24.1)$$

Perioperative Conservation Strategies in Pediatric Patients

PBM Standards and Goals

Due to these anatomical, physiological, and hematological variances, special considerations and strategies should be employed during the use of PBM tactics. Recent data highlighting the serious hazards of allogeneic blood transfusions have contributed to the development of perioperative patient blood management (PBM) and conservation strategies. Patient blood management is most useful for procedures with expected severe blood loss, as it focuses on blood conservation and preventative measures and has been shown to reduce blood product transfusions, mortality, and costs [35, 36]. However, defining PBM standards for infants and children is much more challenging than for adults, as transfusion practices vary considerably by patient categories, conditions, and settings. Therefore, in order to develop and implement an institutional pediatric PBM program as supported as its adult-centered counterpart, multidisciplinary health professionals and administrative support system involvement is critical, with proper education for the involved team members an essential factor for its success. The team should include the Anesthesiology, Surgery, Pharmacy, Transfusion Services, ICU, and administrative support. PBM goals involve optimizing and maintaining hemoglobin levels, optimizing hemostasis, minimizing blood loss, and improving patient outcomes.

Updated clinical and administrative standards for pediatric PBM were recently published by The Society for Advancement of Blood Management [1]. It is urged that a comprehensive PBM program must include age- and weight-appropriate clinical protocols and policies for the management of preoperative anemia, perioperative bleeding, and massive transfusion; these principles are expanded upon in Fig. 24.1. Goal-directed transfusion guidelines using restrictive transfusion strategies as supported by evidence are also fundamental components [1, 37, 38].

Preoperative Blood Management and Conservation

Patients at risk for intraoperative, allogeneic blood transfusions must be evaluated for preoperative anemia and bleeding abnormalities as indicated by history and examination. Preoperative anemia is widespread, as it is found in about 40% of children worldwide and 15–20% of children in industrialized countries [39, 40]. The main etiology is iron deficiency, which has a fairly simple treatment plan: iron supplementation [41]. Iron supplementation has been demonstrated to increase hemoglobin levels and decrease blood transfusions, and there is evidence that intravenous iron may result in improved responses as compared to oral iron supplementation [5]. Preoperative anemia, however, is an independent risk factor and is associated with worsened postoperative outcomes in pediatric surgical patients [5, 41–43]. Although not routinely used, recombinant erythropoietin for stimulation of erythropoiesis has been used successfully in neonates and infants for increasing the hemoglobin concentration prior to surgery. However, recombinant erythropoietin is associated with an increased burden of treatment, as it involves regular subcutaneous injections with

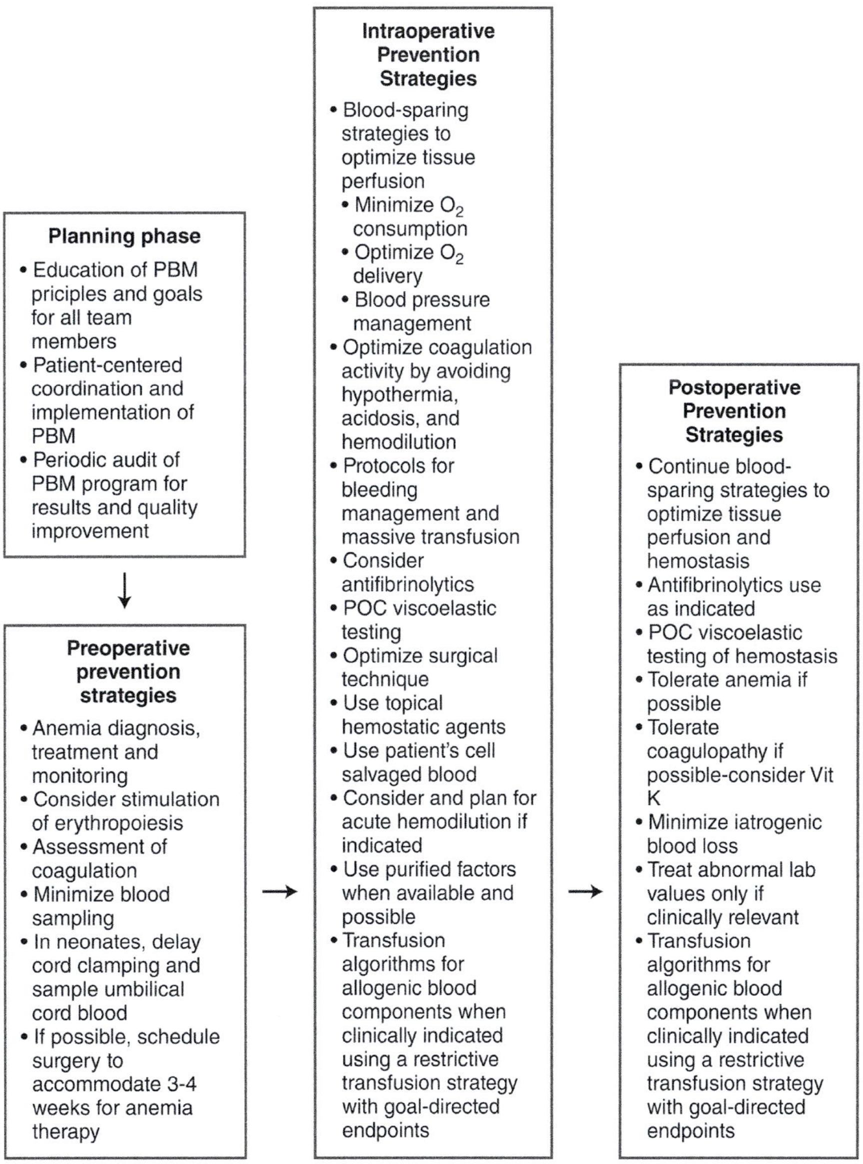

Fig. 24.1 Illustration of a comprehensive pediatric patient blood management program with general principles for perioperative blood conservation strategies. PBM patient blood management, ICU intensive care unit, POC point of care

frequent monitoring of response and iron levels. Nevertheless, it is an additional resource for patients whose parents refuse blood transfusions, whom other causes of anemia have been excluded, or who are poor responders to iron supplementation [5, 27, 41]. In the neonate, important blood conservation strategies also include the delay in umbilical cord clamping and use of umbilical cord blood for initial laboratory sampling upon delivery [38, 44].

Additional blood conservation measures include the following:

- Standardized guidelines for phlebotomy procedure.
- Obtain blood samples only when necessary.
- Optimize logistics of laboratory blood sampling, for example, bundling of tests.
- Use the smallest collection tube and the minimum acceptable volumes allowable for laboratory testing.
- Remove sampling lines early.
- Return, rather than discard, excess sample volumes to the patient.
- Use point-of-care testing devices.
- Use laboratory equipment needing only small volumes for analysis.
- Use transcutaneous instruments for hemoglobin assessment.

Intraoperative Blood Management and Conservation

If possible, surgery should be scheduled for at least 3 weeks after the initial patient evaluation to allow sufficient time for the medical evaluation and treatment of anemia [5]. Intraoperatively, the conduct of the anesthetic and surgery should favor the minimization of bleeding, promotion of hemostasis, and basic non-transfusion techniques for optimization of cardiac output and tissue perfusion (e.g., rhythm, heart rate, preload, contractility, afterload, acid/base status, electrolytes, and temperature). Appropriate surgical techniques and meticulous use of hemostatic topical agents are significant factors in decreasing surgical bleeding. Recommended multimodal blood-sparing approaches include the avoidance of non-purposeful hemodilution; optimization of acid/base status; focused blood pressure management to avoid hypotension with the judicious use of inotropic support if necessary; avoidance of hypertension to decrease the rate of bleeding; and the concurrent use of antifibrinolytics. If significant bleeding ensues, standardized bleeding management protocols and transfusion algorithms must be in place to guide management. Restrictive transfusion thresholds and goal-directed therapy guided by clinical status and by point-of-care viscoelastic testing are the current standards for most pediatric patients, but further research is needed to ascertain the best transfusion strategies for patients with life-threatening bleeding, hemodynamic instability, and cardiopulmonary disease [25]. In select cases (mostly in cardiac surgery when the parents refuse blood transfusions), acute normovolemic hemodilution (ANH) at the beginning of surgery, with return of the autologous blood towards the end of surgery, has been associated with reduction in allogeneic blood transfusions [45]. Currently, there is insufficient evidence to recommend its routine use, although if implemented, institutional protocols should be in place to ensure patient safety [4]. The first consensus for recommendations for ANH standards and best practices in cardiac surgery, sponsored by the Society for the Advancement of Blood Management and published in 2020, do not address ANH in the pediatric population [46]. A recent statement by the Transfusion and Anemia Expertise Initiative (TAXI) made recommendations for restrictive transfusion practices for the pediatric critically ill patient in the intensive care setting. However, in neonates and premature infants, the evidence supporting restrictive transfusion strategies is unclear [4, 25]. Cell salvage and reinfusion are also techniques shown to effectively reduce allogeneic blood transfusions; evidence suggests that bowel and cancer surgery are not absolute contraindications for its use. The use of factor concentrates and recombinant coagulation products should be considered as indicated for certain patients [5].

Postoperative Blood Management and Conservation

Postoperatively, PBM should continue with blood-sparing methods for optimization of tissue perfusion, minimization of bleeding and iatrogenic blood losses, treatment of coagulopathy, and utilization of antifibrinolytics as appropriate. Adding vitamin K can help if coagulopathy is present but does not require immediate treatment. If the anemia is not tolerated by the patient, the use of transfusion algorithms with restrictive strategy is recommended as guided by point-of–care viscoelastic testing [1, 43, 76].

Blood Management Recommendations for Specific Surgeries

The aforementioned recommendations are expanded upon in the next section with a focus on specific surgery types. See Tables 24.5, 24.6, and 24.7 for recommendations from major international guidelines, which specifically address pediatric PBM for cardiac and other major non-cardiac surgeries as well as special patient conditions. The level of evidence is provided for each recommendation. Published guidelines for pediatric PBM are based on systematic reviews of the pediat-

Table 24.5 Patient blood management recommendations for pediatric cardiac surgery

Pediatric cardiac surgery					
Challenges Unique cardiac physiology with often reduced reserve margins, e.g., cyanotic disease and parallel circulations Cardiopulmonary bypass (CPB) with associated hemostatic and physiologic derangements Cardiac lesions with varying surgical repair techniques, CPB approaches, and perioperative management methods					
Interventions	**Recommendations**	**Grade**			
		NATA [27]	BCSH [19]	NBA [4]	ESA [5]
Preoperative					
Anemia	Treat iron deficiency anemia with oral or IV iron	1C			1B – PO iron 1C – IV iron
	Erythropoietin in specific cases	2C			
Intraoperative					
Antifibrinolytics	Administer lysine analogs	1B	1B	R	
CPB circuit	Use miniaturized CPB for neonates and infants	1C			
Ultrafiltration	Conventional ultrafiltration or modified ultrafiltration for neonates and infants	1B			
Cell salvage	Use of cell salvage	1C	1B	PP	1B
POC testing for heparin response	Whole blood ACT or heparin concentration	1B			
AT deficiency	FFP (10 mL/kg) or antithrombin supplementation in the presence of heparin resistance secondary to antithrombin deficiency	1C			
Protamine dose	Protamine dose should be calculated based on heparin concentration	1C			
	Use direct thrombin inhibitors when heparin is contraindicated	1C			
Hemostasis monitoring	Monitoring of hemostasis to guide the administration of blood products	1B	Evidence is insufficient to make a specific recommendation	PP-viscoelastic testing	
	Blood used for cardiac surgery in neonates and infants should be used before the end of storage day 5		1C		
Postoperative					
Restrictive Hb threshold	Hemoglobin threshold for transfusion in stable, acyanotic heart disease	1B – Hb 7 g/dL asymptomatic 1B – Hb 8 g/dL with clinical signs suggesting symptomatic anemia	2B – Hb 7 g/dL asymptomatic 2C – In neonates or actively bleeding or unstable children following CPB, a higher Hb threshold may be appropriate		
	Hemoglobin threshold stable, cyanotic heart disease	1C – with clinical signs suggestive of symptomatic anemia, Hb 9 g/dL	2C – there is insufficient evidence to make a recommendation for children with cyanotic heart disease		

CPB cardiopulmonary bypass, *R* recommendation, *PP* practice point, *PO* per os, *IV* intravenous, *ACT* activated clotting time, *AT* antithrombin, *POC* point-of-care testing, *FFP* fresh frozen plasma, *Hb* hemoglobin, *PRBC* red blood cell

ric PBM literature, which are mostly observational with a paucity of high-grade evidence. Most recommendations were created from evidence where available and expert-based consensus when the evidence is weak or insufficient. Across sets of guidelines, most recommendations are generally concordant with variations from group to group due to different methodology and reviewers. Procedures usually associated with major blood loss or blood transfusions are cardiac, craniofacial, scoliosis and other major orthopedic surgeries, liver transplantation, and major trauma. Main PBM recommendations rest on preoperative screening for anemia with diagnosis and proper treatment prior to elective surgery, the administra-

Table 24.6 Patient blood management recommendations for pediatric major non-cardiac surgeries

Major non-cardiac surgeries				
Interventions	**Grade**			
	SABM [1]	NBA [4]	ESA [5]	BSCH [19]
Preoperative				
Anemia: treat iron deficiency anemia with iron		R	1B – PO iron 1C – IV iron	1C
Intraoperative				
Hb transfusion threshold		R In pediatric patients, including those who are critically ill, a restrictive transfusion strategy is suggested in hemodynamically stable pediatric patients (excluding neonates): Hb concentration < 7 g/dL, PRBC transfusion is often appropriate. Hb concentration of 7–9 g/dL, PRBC transfusion may be appropriate, based on the need to relieve clinical signs and symptoms of anemia. Hb concentration > 9 g/dL, PRBC transfusion is often unnecessary and may be inappropriate		1C With the exception of children with sickle cell disease, there is no evidence to suggest that children undergoing elective non-cardiac surgery require a higher Hb transfusion threshold than those in PICU (7 g/dl, stable patients without major comorbidity or bleeding. Excludes cyanotic children)
Antifibrinolytic – administer lysine analogs	The use of antifibrinolytics and intraoperative cell salvage collection and re-administration should be considered for all pediatric patients undergoing high blood loss surgery including, but not limited to, cardiac surgery with CPB, craniofacial surgery, and scoliosis/orthopedic surgery	R Antifibrinolytics may be considered in large blood loss cases such as scoliosis and craniofacial surgery PP Tranexamic acid should be given within 3 hours of traumatic injury		2C Tranexamic acid should be given if major blood loss associated with traumatic injury is anticipated 1B Tranexamic acid should be given when there is high risk of significant bleeding during surgery
Cell salvage			1B We recommend the use of red cell salvage, which is helpful for blood conservation in major cardiac and orthopedic surgery	2C Red cell salvage should be considered in all children at risk of significant bleeding undergoing surgery and where transfusion may be required, providing appropriately trained staff are available
Postoperative				
Hb transfusion threshold		PP In stable pediatric patients (excluding neonates) Hb <7 g/dL, PRBC transfusion is often appropriate PP Hb >9 g/dL, PRBC transfusion is often unnecessary and may be inappropriate In preterm infants requiring transfusion, there is insufficient evidence to support or refute the use of either a restrictive or liberal PRBC transfusion strategy	1C Except for premature babies and cyanotic newborns, hemoglobin targets in bleeding children are 7–9 g dL We recommend a target hemoglobin concentration of 7–9 g/dL during active bleeding	1C Hb transfusion threshold of 7 g/dL in stable patients without major comorbidity or bleeding

CPB cardiopulmonary bypass, *R* recommendation, *PP* practice point, *PO* per os, *IV* intravenous, *POC* point-of-care testing, *FFP* fresh frozen, plasma, *Hb* hemoglobin, *PRBC* red blood cell

Table 24.7 Patient blood-management recommendations for pediatric patients with special situations

Special patients and situations	
	Grade
	TAXI [25]
The patient with sickle cell disease	1B "In children with sickle cell disease who are critically ill or those at risk of critical illness, we recommend RBC transfusion to achieve a target hemoglobin concentration of 10 g/dL (rather than a hemoglobin S [HbS] of <30%) prior to a surgical procedure requiring general anesthesia"

tion of antifibrinolytics, the use of cell salvage, and restrictive transfusion strategies as guided by viscoelastic testing. Recommendations are mostly stratified by the GRADE scale with the exception of the Australian National Blood Authority which uses R (recommendation) if sufficiently high quality of data and PP (practice point) if the quality of data is weak [4]. Note that these guidelines often exclude the preterm and neonatal patient populations unless specified, as the evidence is largely inconclusive in these populations.

Blood Management Guidelines: Pediatric Considerations

A significant number of hospitalized children receive at least one blood transfusion. In fact, more than one-half of extremely low birth weight preterm infants undergo a transfusion during their initial hospitalization [19]. Therefore, the administration of blood products to children requires special consideration. Children and particularly infants have a unique physiology that requires weight-based product dosing, heightened vigilance during large volume transfusions, and special blood banking processes related to a developing immune system. Evidence supporting transfusion thresholds in children stem from a limited number of studies but, in general, evolving standards follow trends adopted in adult blood management. Our understanding of the infant's coagulation system or potential advantages of clotting factor administration is particularly lacking. Much research needs to be done to more clearly define rational and evidence-based administration in children, particularly with respect to the long-term effects of restrictive transfusion thresholds.

Adverse Reactions in Children

Recent reports suggest that children may suffer more adverse transfusion reactions (ATRs) than adults [37, 47, 48]. In particular, febrile nonhemolytic transfusion reactions (FNHTRs) have been reported to occur at a rate five times that seen in adults [48]. Because of their relatively small blood volume, children are at particular risk of deleterious effects of rapid transfusions. Cardiac arrest secondary to hyperkalemia, particularly in infants, is now established as a known hazard of rapid blood infusion rates [49, 50]. The average potassium concentration of a stored packed PRBC unit is 30–80 mEq/L, which may lead to hyperkalemic cardiac arrest when relatively high blood volumes are administered at a rapid rate [15, 18, 19]. It is recommended that transfusions in small patients be initiated at volumes less than 15–20 mL/kg at of less than 1 mL/kg/min under close monitoring, with a gradual increase in rate as tolerated [13, 19, 51]. Washed packed red blood cells (PRBCs), which have a reduced potassium content, or younger PRBCs (e.g., less than 7 days post-storage) may be requested for small patients requiring large volume transfusions, although existing evidence suggests that if administered at a moderate rate, neonatal outcomes following older versus fresh PRBCs are not significantly different [18]. Other ATRs associated with rapid transfusion in children, particularly small infants, include ionized hypocalcemia, hypothermia, and volume overload.

Stored blood products contain citrate preservative (citrate-phosphate-dextrose-adenine; CPDA) as an anticoagulant, which may bind the recipient's plasma calcium and hinder contraction and relaxation phases of the neonatal cardiac sarcoplasmic reticulum, leading to clinical hypotension [14]. Although this "citrate toxicity" can be seen in patients of all ages, the immature neonatal liver is unable to rapidly metabolize citrate contained in large volume or rapid transfusions. Whole blood, plasma, and irradiated PRBCs contain the highest concentrations of citrate anticoagulant [52, 53]. Because of their relatively large blood volume to weight ratio, children are particularly susceptible to the deleterious effects of transfusion-related hypothermia. A hypothermic child may exhibit decreased drug metabolism, apnea, and a coagulopathic state. When rapid infusion is necessary, PRBC and plasma transfusions should be run through a warming device [13, 15, 51]. Volume overload is also a risk that may not be readily appreciated in the small patient [47]. Transfusion-associated circulatory overload (TACO) is a well-defined ATR that is also seen but not readily recognized during anesthesia and surgery in the adult patient population [54]. There are no specific criteria for TACO in the pediatric population, but a typical presentation intraoperatively may include hypotension, hypoxemia, and bradycardia, nonspecific signs difficult to distinguish from transfusion-related hypocalcemia or hypothermia [47]. A dilutional coagulopathy, either from crystalloid administration or the administration of fractionated blood products absent coagulation factors or platelets, may develop after loss of 1.5–2 blood volumes [15]. A neonate's ability to regenerate coagulation factors is limited due to hepatic immaturity. Under normal conditions, however, tests of hemostasis in the preterm newborn are longer, and in the term newborn, may be are shorter than adult values; the clinical significance of this is unknown [51].

Pediatric Considerations for Pretransfusion Testing and Blood Processing

Children, particularly infants, may require special considerations with respect to pretransfusion testing and blood processing. For example, infants in the first several months of life have a reduced ability to produce alloantibodies against the major blood group antigens (e.g., A, B, AB, and D) due to an immature immunologic system; alloantibodies in a neonate's serum are of maternal origin. Therefore, prior to transfusing a young infant, the infant's pretransfusion testing should be accompanied by a test for maternal blood type and antibodies [13]. As a matter of caution, many transfusion services administer type O, Rhesus(D)-negative (Rh-neg) PRBCs to all infants under 3–6 months of age until both infant and maternal blood screening is performed [15]. When performed as a matter of routine, this safety policy may strain a hospital's O-negative blood supply. Rh-neg cellular blood products (e.g., PRBCs and platelets) and CMV-antibody negative products in general may be distributed in emergency situations for infants and young children for whom pretransfusion testing is unavailable. One concern is that the administration of Rh(D)-positive cellular blood products to a Rh-neg infant, or any female of potential childbearing age, may lead to alloantigen sensitization. Rh-neg sensitization may set the stage for Rh-incompatibility that may complicate a subsequent pregnancy or transfusion. Furthermore, Rh-neg sensitization may also lead to extravascular (i.e., delayed) hemolysis that, although typically mild, may lead to significant morbidity in younger or very small patients. CMV is transported through white blood cells and can have a devastating outcome in susceptible and immunocompromised patients.

Many blood centers only administer blood that is CMV-antibody negative to preterm and young infants. Leukoreduction (LCR), under standardized procedure and quality control, removes a substantial quantity of white blood cells from donor products. The majority, but not all, of US blood centers perform pretransfusion leukoreduction of donated cellular blood products. LCR is associated with a substantial reduction in ATRs, including FNHTRs and graft-versus-host disease (GVHD). Administration of blood that is both leukocyte-reduced and CMV-antibody negative has been shown to effectively eliminate the risk of transfusion-related CMV infection in very low birth weight preterm infants. There is some evidence that leukocyte reduction of blood products prevents or significantly reduces the risk of CMV in stem cell transplant patients and therefore arguably eliminates the need for CMV-negative blood products in susceptible populations [18].

Blood Preservatives

In an effort to reduce donor exposure, blood banks often release small aliquots of blood from a single donor unit held in preservative. The two main preservatives are AS (adenine-glucose-mannitol) and CPDA, and both contain additives that serve as nutrients to the stored PRBCs [13]. Adenine, mannitol, citrate, and dextrose in high concentrations have been associated with renal toxicity (adenine, mannitol), intraventricular hemorrhage (mannitol), hypocalcemia (citrate), and hyperglycemia (dextrose) [13, 55]. Thus, blood stored for neonatal use is often preferentially reconstituted with AS because it extends the shelf life of a PRBC from 35 in CPDA to 42 days, supporting continued use of a single donor unit [13]. As with the precautionary measures that may be used to prevent hyperkalemia, small volume (e.g., <20 mL/kg), slow-rate infusions have not been shown to be a preservative-related problem in preterm infants [13, 18, 55].

Packed Red Blood Cell (PRBC) Transfusion Guidelines

A decision to transfuse must be based on a consideration of the patient's full clinical profile, including cardiorespiratory disease, pending interventions, rate of blood loss, and comorbidities that may impact systemic oxygen delivery, rather than a single laboratory value at one point in time [3]. Furthermore, anemia should always be addressed and managed prior to making a decision to administer blood [43]. As in the adult patient population, a restrictive PRBC transfusion threshold may reduce the number of PRBC units transfused in stable, hospitalized children without an increase in untoward outcomes [30–34]. The World Health Organization (WHO) and several African societies set a transfusion threshold at 5 g/dL for symptomatic children, suggesting that this degree of anemia in asymptomatic children may be a new cutoff for transfusion avoidance in resource-poor environments [56]. A recent consensus group of international experts, the TAXI Initiative, also recommended a transfusion threshold of 5 g/dL in critically ill children without certain comorbidities when considering the hemoglobin value alone [25]. In 2019, a consensus statement was developed to guide PRBC transfusions in children undergoing cardiac surgery [27]. Further studies in both cyanotic and acyanotic children undergoing cardiac surgery have lent support to the short-term safety of lower PRBC transfusion thresholds in the pediatric cardiac patient population [57, 58].

Transfusion thresholds for preterm infants, a unique patient population with rapidly changing physiological needs, are currently based on gestational age and cardiorespiratory status [19]. Neonates are typically transfused at a higher hemoglobin value than older infants and children

[14]. Several randomized controlled trials have examined restrictive versus liberal transfusion thresholds in very low birth weight premature infants, with conflicting short-term outcome results [59–61, 67]. Systematic reviews conclude that despite a decrease in donor exposure and lower hemoglobin values, treatment endpoints and long-term outcomes remain unclear in the restrictive strategy [32, 33]. A recent multicenter trial (the ETTNO Randomized Clinical Trial) examined long-term outcomes in infants at 2 years corrected age who had birth weights less than 1 kg and concluded that the rate of disability and death were unaffected using a restrictive red blood cell transfusion threshold versus a more liberal one [62]. The thresholds for transfusion were based on individual patient factors such as postnatal age and illness acuity. A pending multicenter study, The Transfusion in Prematures (TOP) Trial will further examine longer term outcomes associated with a liberal versus a restrictive red blood cell transfusion threshold in extremely low birth weight infants. Tables 24.8 and 24.9 contain suggested PRBC transfusion guidelines based on hemoglobin value in infants.

Children tend to be managed according to adult PRBC guidelines and expert opinion [55]. Anemic children with a chronic medical condition may be physiologically compensated and are often transfused at lower hemoglobin values. As Table 24.10 demonstrates, current international PRBC trigger guidelines are similar, with slight variation during the first weeks of life.

Table 24.8 PRBC transfusion guidelines for premature[a] and young infants (<4 months PNA)

Postnatal age[b] (PNA; days)	Hemoglobin (g/dL)	
	Requiring [c]respiratory support	No respiratory support
0–7	11.5	10
8–14	10	8.5
> 14	8.5	7.5
Acute blood loss, symptomatic	10% of total blood volume	
Congenital heart disease	Cyanotic: 9 g/dL if symptomatic anemia	
	Acyanotic: 7 g/dL; symptomatic anemia: 8 g/dL	
CNS bleeding	<7–10 g/dL	
[d]Symptomatic anemia	<8 g/dL	

[a]Premature indicates an infant less than 37 weeks corrected gestational age
[b]Postnatal age (PNA) indicates the chronological age, or time elapsed birth
[c]Respiratory support is defined as a need for mechanical support ventilation or $FiO_2 > 25\%$
[d]An otherwise stable infant with bradycardia/tachycardia, poor weight gain, or apnea

Plasma Transfusion Guidelines

Plasma may be the most overly administered blood product available and is often administered based on laboratory values alone [19, 63]. In general, coagulation factor levels in infants tend to be lower than those of older children and adults, but the clinical significance of this difference is unknown [19, 64] (Table 24.11). Despite differences in coagulation factor levels, conventional test results of coagulation are often treated similarly between infants and older children [51]. As a result, routine coagulation screening may lead to inappropriate transfusions, particularly in the neonate where there is heightened anxiety over bleeding potential including intraventricular hemorrhage (IVH) [51, 65, 66]. In the absence of confounding variables that may increase bleeding risk, only 10–40% of coagulation factor activity levels are needed to achieve hemostasis. Furthermore, there is no evi-

Table 24.9 PRBC transfusion guidelines for older infants (≥4 months PNA)

Symptomatic anemia: Hgb < 7 g/dL	
Perioperative anemia with anticipated blood loss: Hgb < 8 g/dL	
Congenital heart disease	Cyanotic: 9 g/dL if symptomatic anemia
	Acyanotic: 7 g/dL; Symptomatic anemia: 8 g/dL
Acute blood loss with hemodynamic instability	8 g/dL
Acute traumatic brain injury	<10 g/dL
Chronic transfusion regimen (e.g., sickle cell anemia, thalassemia, leukemias) Hgb < 7 g/dL	

Table 24.10 RBC transfusion practices

Overview of international guidelines for red blood cell transfusions								
	British Committee for Standards in Haematology 2016 [19]		Australian National Blood Authority 2016 [4]		Canadian Blood Services 2017 [64]		Dutch Guidelines Quality Council (Concept) 2018 [74]	
Postnatal week	Respiratory support[a]	No respiratory support	Respiratory support	No respiratory support	Respiratory support	No respiratory support	Respiratory support	No respiratory support
Week 1	10–12 g/dL	<10 g/dL	11–13 g/dL	10–12 g/dL	<11.5 g/dL	<10 g/dL	<11.5 g/dL	<10 g/dL
Week 2	9.5–10 g/dL	<7.5 g/dL	10–12.5 g/dL	8.5–11 g/dL	<10 g/dL	<8.5 g/dL	<10 g/dL	<8.5 g/dL
Week ≥3	8.5–10 g/dL	<7.5 g/dL	8.5–11 g/dL	7–10 g/dL	<8.5 g/dL	<7.5 g/dL	<8.5 g/dL	<7.5 g/dL

Modified from Ree and Lopriore [75]
[a]For example, supplemental oxygen, high-flow nasal cannula, CPAP (continuous positive airway pressure), positive-pressure ventilation

Table 24.11 Screening laboratory tests for hemostasis: neonates versus adults[a]

	Preterm neonates vs. full-term neonates	Neonates vs. older children/ adults	Approximate age adult values are reached[b]
aPTT	Longer	Longer	16 years
Prothrombin time	Longer	Same or longer	16 years
Thrombin time	Longer	Same or longer	5 years
Bleeding time	Longer[c]	Shorter	1 month
PFA-100	Longer[c]	Shorter	1 month
ROTERM/TEG			
Clotting time	Same	Shorter	3 months
Clot formation time	Same	Shorter	3 months
Maximal clot firmness	Stronger	Stronger	3 months

Modified from AABB Technical Manual, 19th ed, originally from Revel-Vilk
aModified with permission from Revel-Vilk
bMaximum age reported
cIn samples drawn in the first 7 to 10 days of life
aPTT activated partial thromboplastin time, *PFA* platelet function analyzer, *ROTEM* rotating tromboelastometry, *TEG* thromboelastography

dence that an international normalized ratio (INR) value between 1.6 and 2.0 is indicative of future bleeding risk in either the adult or pediatric patient populations [13, 51]. When available, the specific coagulation product should be utilized to replace inherited or acquired coagulation deficiency, rather than plasma. Recombinant coagulation products available include factors VIII, IX, VIIa, XI, and XIII, prothrombin complex concentrate (factors II, VII, IX, X), antithrombin III, protein C, and C1 esterase inhibitor. Absolute contraindications to plasma transfusion in all age groups include volume expansion and nutritional replacement therapy. A suggested plasma transfusion volume is 10–20 mL/kg at an initial rate of 1 mL/kg/min that is gradually increased as the patient is evaluated for signs of citrate toxicity (e.g., hypocalcemia and hypotension). This dose of plasma may result in an increase in coagulation factor levels by approximately 15%, with a clinical effect lasting less than 12 hours [13]. Recommended indications for plasma therapy in children and neonates include the following.

Neonates

1. Treatment of clinically significant bleeding in the face of abnormal coagulation parameters
2. Prior to an invasive procedure in the face of abnormal coagulation parameters
3. Treatment of severe hereditary protein S deficiency
4. Treatment of protein C deficiency if recombinant factor is unavailable

Children

1. Coagulation factor consumption including disseminated intravascular coagulation (DIC)
2. Prolonged PT/aPTT >2 times midpoint normal range for age prior to an invasive procedure
3. Urgent warfarin reversal when prothrombin complex concentrate is unavailable or contraindicated (e.g., HIT (heparin-induced thrombocytopenia))
4. Treatment of idiopathic thrombotic thrombocytopenic purpura (ITP)
5. Treatment of bleeding for acquired or inherited factor deficiencies when specific factor concentrates are unavailable
6. Plasma exchange

Platelet Transfusion Guidelines

Sepsis, maternal disorders such as preeclampsia, the presence of intravenous catheters, and low blood levels of endogenous erythropoietin contribute to a high incidence (20–70%) of thrombocytopenia in preterm neonates, resulting in a high rate of platelet transfusions [18]. Platelet transfusions in children are associated with more ATRs than other fractionated blood products [47]. The threshold for a platelet transfusion usually hinges on whether the goal is to prevent future bleeding (e.g., prophylaxis) or to stop active bleeding in the face of thrombocytopenia. The definition of thrombocytopenia has been defined as 150×10^9/L in both children and adults [13]. From the neonatal period through adulthood, platelet counts are similar. Neonatal platelets may be larger and exhibit greater adhesion and faster clot initiation, although the clinical significance of this finding is unknown [19]. Taken as an isolated finding, a platelet count alone does not always predict a patient's risk of bleeding. Patients with a platelet count as low as 50×10^9/L may have normal coagulation in the absence of confounding variables such as cardiopulmonary bypass circuitry, drug administration, or an alloimmune process.

In general, platelet transfusion trigger guidelines for infants and older children tend to reflect adult guidelines [68]. A platelet count of 100×10^9/L was once the standard for surgical hemostasis; however, with ongoing clinical experience (including the high rate of ATRs associated with platelets), the suggested transfusion threshold for major non-neuraxial surgery has decreased to 50×10^9/L. Recent adult studies support a count of 20×10^9/L for central venous catheter placement [68, 69]. Although controversial, the minimum acceptable count for diagnostic lumbar puncture, a procedure frequently performed in children with a defect in platelet production, has been 10×10^9/L for many years. Following a systematic review and expert consensus, this newly recommended threshold is 50 × 10^9/L, despite supporting evidence that is of very low quality [69]. In a recent retrospective study of 900 propensity-matched, critically ill adult patients, there was no benefit following prophylactic platelet transfusions in nonbleeding patients with platelet counts as low as 20 × 10^9/L, putting into question all current guidelines [70]. Presumably because of a perceived risk of IVH, sick preterm infants and neonates often receive platelets at a higher threshold (e.g., 20–50 × 10^9/L), when a stable, nonbleeding infant or older child is unlikely to have significant bleeding at platelet counts as low as 10 × 10^9/L [13]. A recent multicenter trial (PLANET-2) examined 660 premature infants and found less 28-day mortality or episodes of major bleeding when applying a prophylactic transfusion threshold of 25 rather than 50 × 10^9/L [71].

Platelet transfusion triggers suggested in a variety of clinical situations are listed in Table 24.12. Ideally, platelets should be ABO-compatible with the recipient's blood type, because if not ABO-identical, the response as measured by platelet count may be decreased [13]. Furthermore, because all platelet preparations contain a small number of PRBCs (possibly 0.5 ml/unit), ideal donor platelets are Rh(D)-identical to prevent anti-D alloimmunization. A dose of ~5–10 mL/kg should increase a patient's platelet count by ~50–100 × 10^9/L. In the absence of life-threatening bleeding, platelet transfusions should not be given in the face of idiopathic thrombocytopenic purpura (ITP), thrombotic thrombocytopenic purpura (TTP), heparin-induced thrombocytopenia (HIT), or hemolytic uremic syndrome (HUS), either because of a risk of continued consumption (such as in ITP), or an increased risk of thrombosis [13, 64]. For children undergoing cardiopulmonary bypass or extracorporeal life support (ECLS), platelet transfusions are recommended in the face of excessive bleeding unresponsive to other measures such as heparin reversal, although a threshold of 100 × 10^9/L has traditionally been chosen [27].

Table 24.12 Platelet transfusion triggers

Platelet transfusion triggers by count (10^9/L)	
Prophylactic transfusion	
Prematurity (<37 weeks PCA)	<25
Term infants (>37 weeks PCA)	
<4 months old	<20
>4 months old	<10
Prior to lumbar puncture	<50
Patient scheduled for major invasive procedure	<50
Qualitative platelet defect (congenital or acquired)	*Any platelet count if bleeding*
CNS procedure	<100
Central venous catheter placement	*Tunneled:* <50 *Non-tunneled:* <20
Fetal and neonatal alloimmune thrombocytopenia (FNAIT)	Stable patient: <20–30 Unstable patient: <50
Patient has an FNAIT-affected sibling	<20–30
Bleeding patients	
Active bleeding	<50
Intracranial bleeding	<100
Diffuse microvascular bleeding, ECLS, cardiopulmonary bypass	<100
Qualitative platelet defect	*Any platelet count if bleeding*

Cryoprecipitate Transfusion Guidelines

Cryoprecipitate is a precipitant of fresh frozen plasma. The pediatric literature lacks clinical trials comparing differing cryoprecipitate dosing regimens or indications. There is no evidence supporting the benefit of prophylactic use of cryoprecipitate, including prior to invasive surgery. Typically administered to replace fibrinogen, a single cryoprecipitate unit contains factor VIII (80 mg), fibrinogen (150 mg), factor XIII (up to 30% that is contained in original plasma), and von Willebrand factor (up to 70% that is contained in original plasma) in a total volume of 10–15 ml [13]. It does not have to be ABO-compatible when used for non-neonates, and its small volume comparatively reduces the risk of fluid overload often seen when plasma is used to treat clotting factor deficiencies. ABO-compatibility is recommended for use in neonates secondary to their small size and concerns over hemolysis due to the alloantibodies that may be contained in the precipitate [13]. Specific virus-inactivated factor concentrates such as recombinant factor VIII, von Willebrand factor complex, or fibrinogen concentrate should be administered in lieu of cryoprecipitate when these products are available. A "pooled" unit of cryoprecipitate is the product of 5–6 donors (~100–130 ml) and, although heat-treated, may theoretically present an infectious and alloimmunization risk. Recombinant fibrinogen concentrate is not yet FDA-approved in the United States for the treatment of acquired hypofibrinogenemia.

The recommended dose for cryoprecipitate is 1 unit [e.g., 10–15 ml] per 10 kg body weight, which can be expected to increase the child's fibrinogen level by 50–100 mg/dL [13]. A generally accepted threshold for cryoprecipitate transfusion in the setting of clinically significant bleeding is 100 mg/dL. Other indications include the following:

1. Disease states with evidence of fibrinogen consumption including DIC with bleeding.
2. Hypofibrinogenemia and a pending invasive procedure.
3. Bleeding following cardiac or other major surgery with evidence of low fibrinogen level.
4. Inherited defects of fibrinogen, either quantitative (e.g., afibrinogenemia, congenital hypofibrinogenemia, Kasabach-Merritt syndrome, or hemangioma with thrombocytopenia) or qualitative (e.g., fibrinogen Cleveland, fibrinogen Marburg, etc.).

5. As treatment for hemophilia A or vWF disease in the absence of a response to desmopressin or availability of specific recombinant factor concentrates.
6. Platelet dysfunction in the face of uremia and hemodialysis is not available.
7. Fibrin sealant.

Conclusion

In conclusion, pediatric PBM consists of a customized blood conservation strategy, individualized to each patient according to their age and clinical condition. Fundamental considerations include attention to anemia, maintenance of hemoglobin concentration, optimization of hemostasis, and minimization of blood loss. Although the medical literature does not contain an abundance of evidence supporting blanket application of pediatric PBM principles, transfusion trigger thresholds have decreased as supported by an increasing number of trials. An interdisciplinary approach to patient blood management along with a dedication to education, quality control, and monitoring of institutional behavior is essential to sustained PBM practices. Education with a focus on the unique physiology of blood loss and replacement in children is imperative for patient safety. Most importantly, pediatric PBM is confirmation that we always act in the best interest of our patients.

References

1. Goobie SM, Gallagher T, Gross I, Shander A. Society for the advancement of blood management administrative and clinical standards for patient blood management programs. 4th edition (pediatric version). Paediatr Anaesth. 2019;29(3):231–6.
2. World Health Organization (WHO). Global Forum for Blood Safety: Patient Blood Management 14—15 March 2011. Found at https://www.who.int/bloodsafety/events/gfbs_01_pbm_concept_paper.pdf. Accessed Dec 20 2020.
3. American Society of Anesthesiologists Task Force on Perioperative Blood Management. Practice guidelines for perioperative blood management: an updated report by the American Society of Anesthesiologists Task Force on Perioperative Blood Management. Anesthesiology. 2015;122(2):241–75.
4. National Blood Authority (NBA) (2016). Patient blood management guidelines: module 6 – neonatal and paediatrics. Found at https://www.blood.gov.au/pbm-module-6. Accessed Dec 20 2020.
5. Kozek-Langenecker SA, Afshari A, Albaladejo P, Santullano CA, De Robertis E, Filipescu DC, Fries D, Görlinger K, Haas T, Imberger G, Jacob M, Lancé M, Llau J, Mallett S, Meier J, Rahe-Meyer N, Samama CM, Smith A, Solomon C, Van der Linden P, Wikkelsø AJ, Wouters P, Wyffels P. Management of severe perioperative bleeding: guidelines from the European Society of Anaesthesiology. Eur J Anaesthesiol. 2013;30(6):270–382. Erratum in: Eur J Anaesthesiol. 2014 Apr;31(4):247.
6. Secher EL, Stensballe J, Afshari A. Transfusion in critically ill children: an ongoing dilemma. Acta Anaesthesiol Scand. 2013;57(6):684–91. Epub 2013 May 21
7. Willems A, Harrington K, Lacroix J, Biarent D, Joffe AR, Wensley D, et al. Comparison of two red-cell transfusion strategies after pediatric cardiac surgery: a subgroup analysis. Crit Care Med. 2010;38(2):649–56.
8. Stainsby D, Jones H, Wells AW, Gibson B, Cohen H. SHOT Steering Group. Adverse outcomes of blood transfusion in children: analysis of UK reports to the serious hazards of transfusion scheme 1996–2005. Br J Haematol. 2008;141(1):73–9.
9. Lawler SD, Berkman EM. Blood Group. Encyclopædia Britannica. 2019 Jul. Found at https://www.britannica.com/science/blood-group#ref192399. Accessed Dec 20 2020.
10. Raju TNK. Historical Perspectives: Cured by the Blood: The Story of the First Neonatal Blood Transfusion. NeoReviews. 2006;7(2):e67–8.
11. Fernández KS, de Alarcón PA. Development of the hematopoietic system and disorders of hematopoiesis that present during infancy and early childhood. Pediatr Clin North Am. 2013;60(6):1273–89.
12. Widdowson EM, Spray CM. Chemical development in utero. Arch Dis Child. 1951;26(127):205–14. https://doi.org/10.1136/adc.26.127.205. PMID: 14857788; PMCID: PMC1988372.
13. Wong ECC, Roseff SD, King KE, editors. Pediatric transfusion: a physician's handbook. 4th ed. Bethesda: American Association of Blood Banks (AABB).; 2015.
14. Barcelona SL, Thompson AA, Coté CJ. Intraoperative pediatric blood transfusion therapy: a review of common issues. Part II: transfusion therapy, special considerations, and reduction of allogenic blood transfusions. Paediatr Anaesth. 2005;15(10):814–30.
15. Barcelona SL, Thompson AA, Coté CJ. Intraoperative pediatric blood transfusion therapy: a review of common issues. Part I: hematologic and physiologic differences from adults; metabolic and infectious risks. Paediatr Anaesth. 2005;15(9):716–26.
16. Jopling J, Henry E, Wiedmeier SE, Christensen RD. Reference ranges for hematocrit and blood hemoglobin concentration during the neonatal period: data from a multihospital health care system. Pediatrics. 2009;123(2):e333–7.
17. Bard H. Postnatal fetal and adult hemoglobin synthesis in early preterm newborn infants. J Clin Invest. 1973;52(8):1789–95. PMID: 4719660; PMCID: PMC302458
18. Simon TL, McCullough J, Snyder EL, Solheim BG, Strauss RG, editors. Fetal and neonatal hematopoiesis; Red blood cell transfusions for neonates and infants. In Rossi's Principles of transfusion medicine. 5th ed. West Sussex: Wiley; 2016. pp. 516–27; 535–41.
19. New HV, Berryman J, Bolton-Maggs PH, Cantwell C, Chalmers EA, Davies T, Gottstein R, Kelleher A, Kumar S, Morley SL, Stanworth SJ. British Committee for Standards in Haematology. Guidelines on transfusion for fetuses, neonates and older children. Br J Haematol. 2016;175(5):784–828. Epub 2016 Nov 11
20. Salonvaara M, Riikonen P, Vahtera E, Mahlamäki E, Heinonen K, Kekomäki R. Development of selected coagulation factors and anticoagulants in preterm infants by the age of six months. Thromb Haemost. 2004;92(4):688–96.
21. Toulon P. Developmental hemostasis: laboratory and clinical implications. Int J Lab Hematol. 2016;38(Suppl 1):66–77.
22. Brown AC, Hannan RT, Timmins LH, Fernandez JD, Barker TH, Guzzetta NA. Fibrin Network Changes in Neonates after Cardiopulmonary Bypass. Anesthesiology. 2016 May;124(5):1021–31. https://doi.org/10.1097/ALN.0000000000001058. Erratum in: Anesthesiology. 2016 Sep;125(3):610. PMID: 26914227; PMCID: PMC4837010.
23. Andrew M. The relevance of developmental hemostasis to hemorrhagic disorders of newborns. Semin Perinatol. 1997;21(1):70–85. Review
24. Sloniewsky D. Anemia and transfusion in critically ill pediatric patients: a review of etiology, management, and outcomes. Crit Care Clin. 2013;29(2):301–17. https://doi.org/10.1016/j.ccc.2012.11.005. Epub 2013 Jan 3

25. Valentine SL, Bembea MM, Muszynski JA, Cholette JM, Doctor A, Spinella PC, Steiner ME, Tucci M, Hassan NE, Parker RI, Lacroix J, Argent A, Carson JL, Remy KE, Demaret P, Emeriaud G, Kneyber MCJ, Guzzetta N, Hall MW, Macrae D, Karam O, Russell RT, Stricker PA, Vogel AM, Tasker RC, Turgeon AF, Schwartz SM, Willems A, Josephson CD, Luban NLC, Lehmann LE, Stanworth SJ, Zantek ND, Bunchman TE, Cheifetz IM, Fortenberry JD, Delaney M, van de Watering L, Robinson KA, Malone S, Steffen KM, Bateman ST, Pediatric Critical Care Transfusion and Anemia Expertise Initiative (TAXI); Pediatric Critical Care Blood Research Network (BloodNet), and the Pediatric Acute Lung Injury and Sepsis Investigators (PALISI) Network. Consensus Recommendations for RBC Transfusion Practice in Critically Ill Children From the Pediatric Critical Care Transfusion and Anemia Expertise Initiative. Pediatr Crit Care Med. 2018;19(9):884–98. PMID: 30180125; PMCID: PMC6126913
26. Northup PG, Friedman LS, Kamath PS. AGA clinical practice update on surgical risk assessment and perioperative management in cirrhosis: expert review. Clin Gastroenterol Hepatol. 2019;17(4):595–606. https://doi.org/10.1016/j.cgh.2018.09.043. Epub 2018 Sep 28
27. Faraoni D, Meier J, New HV, Van der Linden PJ, Hunt BJ. Patient blood management for neonates and children undergoing cardiac surgery: 2019 NATA guidelines. J Cardiothorac Vasc Anesth. 2019;33(12):3249–63. Epub 2019 Mar 20
28. Nellis ME, Goel R, Karam O. Transfusion management in pediatric oncology patients. Hematol Oncol Clin North Am. 2019;33(5):903–13. Epub 2019 Jul 5
29. Australian National Blood Authority, Patient Blood Management Guidelines Companion 24: Restrictive Transfusion Strategy. Found at https://www.blood.gov.au/patient-blood-management-guidelines-companions. Accessed Dec 20 2020.
30. Hébert PC, Wells G, Blajchman MA, Marshall J, Martin C, Pagliarello G, Tweeddale M, Schweitzer I, Yetisir E. A multicenter, randomized, controlled clinical trial of transfusion requirements in critical care. Transfusion Requirements in Critical Care Investigators, Canadian Critical Care Trials Group. N Engl J Med. 1999;340(6):409–17. https://doi.org/10.1056/NEJM199902113400601. Erratum in: N Engl J Med 1999 Apr 1;340(13):1056.
31. Lacroix J, Hébert PC, Hutchison JS, Hume HA, Tucci M, Ducruet T, Gauvin F, Collet JP, Toledano BJ, Robillard P, Joffe A, Biarent D, Meert K, Peters MJ. TRIPICU Investigators; Canadian Critical Care Trials Group; Pediatric Acute Lung Injury and Sepsis Investigators Network. Transfusion strategies for patients in pediatric intensive care units. N Engl J Med. 2007;356(16):1609–19.
32. Whyte R, Kirpalani H. Low versus high haemoglobin concentration threshold for blood transfusion for preventing morbidity and mortality in very low birth weight infants. Cochrane Database Syst Rev. 2011;(11):CD000512.
33. Venkatesh V, Khan R, Curley A, New H, Stanworth S. How we decide when a neonate needs a transfusion. Br J Haematol. 2013;160(4):421–33. Epub 2012 Oct 24
34. Lacroix J, Demaret P, Tucci M. Red blood cell transfusion: decision making in pediatric intensive care units. Semin Perinatol. 2012;36(4):225–31.
35. Anthes E. Evidence-based medicine: save blood, save lives. Nature. 2015;520(7545):24–6.
36. Goodnough LT, Shieh L, Hadhazy E, Cheng N, Khari P, Maggio P. Improved blood utilization using real-time clinical decision support. Transfusion. 2014;54(5):1358–65. Epub 2013 Oct 10
37. Goel R, Cushing MM, Tobian AA. Pediatric patient blood management programs: not just transfusing little adults. Transfus Med Rev. 2016;30(4):235–41. Epub 2016 Aug 1
38. Crighton GL, New HV, Liley HG, Stanworth SJ. Patient blood management, what does this actually mean for neonates and infants? Transfus Med. 2018;28(2):117–31. Epub 2018 Apr 17
39. World Health Organization- The Global Prevalence of Anaemia, 2011. Found at https://apps.who.int/iris/bitstream/10665/177094/1/9789241564960_eng.pdf. Accessed Dec 20 2020.
40. Pasricha SR. Anemia: a comprehensive global estimate. Blood. 2014;123(5):611–2.
41. Mills RJ, Davies MW. Enteral iron supplementation in preterm and low birth weight infants. Cochrane Database Syst Rev. 2012;(3):CD005095.
42. Rajasekaran S, Kort E, Hackbarth R, Davis AT, Sanfilippo D, Fitzgerald R, Zuiderveen S, Ndika AN, Beauchamp H, Olivero A, Hassan N. Red cell transfusions as an independent risk for mortality in critically ill children. J Intensive Care. 2016;4(2). PMID: 26744626; PMCID: PMC4704419
43. Goobie SM, Faraoni D, Zurakowski D, DiNardo JA. Association of preoperative anemia with postoperative mortality in neonates. JAMA Pediatr. 2016;170(9):855–62.
44. von Lindern JS, Lopriore E. Management and prevention of neonatal anemia: current evidence and guidelines. Expert Rev Hematol. 2014;7(2):195–202. Epub 2014 Feb 13
45. Crescini WM, Muralidaran A, Shen I, LeBlan A, You J, Giacomuzzi C, Treggiari MM. The use of acute normovolemic hemodilution in paediatric cardiac surgery. Acta Anaesthesiol Scand. 2018;62(6):756–64. Epub 2018 Mar 4
46. Shander A, Brown J, Licker M, Mazer DC, Meier J, Ozawa S, Tibi PR, Van der Linden P, Perelman S. Standards and best practice for acute normovolemic hemodilution: evidence-based consensus recommendations. J Cardiothorac Vasc Anesth. 2020;34(7):1755–60. Epub 2020 Jan 17
47. Narayan S. The 2019 Annual SHOT Report. Serious Hazards of Transfusion (SHOT) Working Group. Found at https://www.shotuk.org/wp-content/uploads/myimages/SHOT-REPORT-2019-Final-Bookmarked-v2.pdf. Accessed Dec 20 2020.
48. Oakley FD, Woods M, Arnold S, Young PP. Transfusion reactions in pediatric compared with adult patients: a look at rate, reaction type, and associated products. Transfusion. 2015;55(3):563–70. Epub 2014 Aug 22
49. Christensen RE, Lee AC, Gowen MS, Rettiganti MR, Deshpande JK, Morray JP. Pediatric perioperative cardiac arrest, death in the off hours: a report from wake up safe, the pediatric quality improvement initiative. Anesth Analg. 2018;127(2):472–7.
50. Morray JP. Cardiac arrest in anesthetized children: recent advances and challenges for the future. Paediatr Anaesth. 2011;21(7):722–9. Epub 2010 Nov 21
51. Fung MK, Eder AF, Spitalnik SL, Westhoff CM, editors. Chapters 22 and 24: Noninfectious complications of blood transfusions; neonatal and pediatric transfusion practice. In Technical manual. 19th ed. Bethesda: Amer Assn of Blood Banks; 2017. pp. 56–58; 61–62
52. Vraets A, Lin Y, Callum JL. Transfusion-associated hyperkalemia. Transfus Med Rev. 2011;25(3):184–96. Epub 2011 Apr 17
53. Coté CJ, Lerman J, Anderson BJ. Strategies for blood product management, reducing transfusions, and massive blood transfusion. In: A practice of anesthesia for infants and children. 6th ed. Philadelphia: Elsevier; 2018. p. 257–80.
54. Clifford L, Jia Q, Subramanian A, Yadav H, Schroeder DR, Kor DJ. Risk factors and clinical outcomes associated with perioperative transfusion-associated circulatory overload. Anesthesiology. 2017;126(3):409–18. PMID: 28072601; PMCID: PMC5309147
55. Roseff SD, Luban NL, Manno CS. Guidelines for assessing appropriateness of pediatric transfusion. Transfusion. 2002;42(11):1398–413.
56. Roberts DJ, Field S, Delaney M, Bates I. Problems and approaches for blood transfusion in the developing countries. Hematol Oncol Clin North Am. 2016;30(2):477–95.
57. Cholette JM, Rubenstein JS, Alfieris GM, Powers KS, Eaton M, Lerner NB. Children with single-ventricle physiology do not benefit from higher hemoglobin levels post cavopulmonary connection:

results of a prospective, randomized, controlled trial of a restrictive versus liberal red-cell transfusion strategy. Pediatr Crit Care Med. 2011;12(1):39–45.

58. de Gast-Bakker DH, de Wilde RB, Hazekamp MG, Sojak V, Zwaginga JJ, Wolterbeek R, de Jonge E, Gesink-van der Veer BJ. Safety and effects of two red blood cell transfusion strategies in pediatric cardiac surgery patients: a randomized controlled trial. Intensive Care Med. 2013;39(11):2011–9. Epub 2013 Aug 31.
59. Whyte RK. Neurodevelopmental outcome of extremely low-birth-weight infants randomly assigned to restrictive or liberal hemoglobin thresholds for blood transfusion. Semin Perinatol. 2012;36(4):290–3.
60. Bell EF, Strauss RG, Widness JA, Mahoney LT, Mock DM, Seward VJ, Cress GA, Johnson KJ, Kromer IJ, Zimmerman MB. Randomized trial of liberal versus restrictive guidelines for red blood cell transfusion in preterm infants. Pediatrics. 2005;115(6):1685–91. PMID: 15930233; PMCID: PMC2866196.
61. Chen HL, Tseng HI, Lu CC, Yang SN, Fan HC, Yang RC. Effect of blood transfusions on the outcome of very low body weight preterm infants under two different transfusion criteria. Pediatr Neonatol. 2009;50(3):110–6.
62. Franz AR, Engel C, Bassler D, Rüdiger M, Thome UH, Maier RF, Krägeloh-Mann I, Kron M, Essers J, Bührer C, Rellensmann G, Rossi R, Bittrich HJ, Roll C, Höhn T, Ehrhardt H, Avenarius S, Körner HT, Stein A, Buxmann H, Vochem M, Poets CF, Investigators ETTNO. Effects of liberal vs restrictive transfusion thresholds on survival and neurocognitive outcomes in extremely low-birth-weight infants: the ETTNO Randomized Clinical Trial. JAMA. 2020;324(6):560–70. PMID: 32780138; PMCID: PMC7420159
63. Puetz J, Witmer C, Huang YS, Raffini L. Widespread use of fresh frozen plasma in US children's hospitals despite limited evidence demonstrating a beneficial effect. J Pediatr. 2012;160(2):210–215.e1. https://doi.org/10.1016/j.jpeds.2011.08.013. Epub 2011 Sep 14.
64. Canadian Blood Services: Clinical Guide to Transfusion. Chapter 13: Neonatal and Pediatric Transfusion. Lau W. Found at https://professionaleducation.blood.ca/en/node/174/pdf. Accessed Dec 20 2020.
65. Girelli G, Antoncecchi S, Casadei AM, Del Vecchio A, Isernia P, Motta M, Regoli D, Romagnoli C, Tripodi G, Velati C. Recommendations for transfusion therapy in neonatology. Blood Transfus. 2015;13(3):484–97. PMID: 26445308; PMCID: PMC4607607
66. Tripodi A, Ramenghi LA, Chantarangkul V, De Carli A, Clerici M, Groppo M, Mosca F, Mannucci PM. Normal thrombin generation in neonates in spite of prolonged conventional coagulation tests. Haematologica. 2008;93(8):1256–9. Epub 2008 Apr 9
67. Kirpalani H, Whyte RK, Andersen C, Asztalos EV, Heddle N, Blajchman MA, Peliowski A, Rios A, LaCorte M, Connelly R, Barrington K, Roberts RS. The Premature Infants in Need of Transfusion (PINT) study: a randomized, controlled trial of a restrictive (low) versus liberal (high) transfusion threshold for extremely low birth weight infants. J Pediatr. 2006;149(3):301–7.
68. Sloan SR, Parker RI. Current status of platelet transfusion in pediatric patients. Transfus Med Rev. 2016;30(4):230–4. Epub 2016 Aug 4
69. Kaufman RM, Djulbegovic B, Gernsheimer T, Kleinman S, Tinmouth AT, Capocelli KE, Cipolle MD, Cohn CS, Fung MK, Grossman BJ, Mintz PD, O'Malley BA, Sesok-Pizzini DA, Shander A, Stack GE, Webert KE, Weinstein R, Welch BG, Whitman GJ, Wong EC, Tobian AA. AABB. Platelet transfusion: a clinical practice guideline from the AABB. Ann Intern Med. 2015;162(3):205–13.
70. Warner MA, Chandran A, Frank RD, Kor DJ. Prophylactic platelet transfusions for critically ill patients with thrombocytopenia: a single-institution propensity-matched cohort study. Anesth Analg. 2019;128(2):288–95. PMID: 29293185; PMCID: PMC6026075
71. Curley A, Stanworth SJ, Willoughby K, Fustolo-Gunnink SF, Venkatesh V, Hudson C, Deary A, Hodge R, Hopkins V, Lopez Santamaria B, Mora A, Llewelyn C, D'Amore A, Khan R, Onland W, Lopriore E, Fijnvandraat K, New H, Clarke P, Watts T, PlaNeT2 MATISSE Collaborators. Randomized trial of platelet-transfusion thresholds in neonates. N Engl J Med. 2019;380(3):242–51. Epub 2018 Nov 2
72. Christensen RD, Del Vecchio A, Henry E. Expected erythrocyte, platelet and neutrophil values for term and preterm neonates. J Matern Fetal Neonatal Med. 2012;25(Suppl 5):77–9. Review. PubMed PMID: 23025775
73. Andrew M, Paes B, Milner R, Johnston M, Mitchell L, Tollefsen DM, Powers P. Development of the human coagulation system in the full-term infant. Blood. 1987;70(1):165–72.
74. Andrew M, Paes B, Milner R, Johnston M, Mitchell L, Tollefsen DM, Castle V, Powers P. Development of the human coagulation system in the healthy premature infant. Blood. 1988;72(5):1651–7. PMID: 3179444
75. Ree IMC, Lopriore E. Updates in neonatal hematology: causes, 1083 risk factors, and management of anemia and thrombocytopenia. Hematol Oncol Clin North Am. 2019;33(3):521–32. https://doi.org/10.1016/j.hoc.2019.01.013. Epub 2019 Mar 23. Review. PubMed PMID: 31030817
76. Goobie SM, Haas T. Perioperative bleeding management in pediatric patients. Curr Opin Anaesthesiol. 2016;29(3):352–8. https://doi.org/10.1097/ACO.0000000000000308. PMID: 26844864.

Blood Management in the Liver Transplant Patient

25

Diana Romano, Jeron Zerillo, and Natalie Smith

Introduction

During liver transplantation, management of blood and blood component transfusion is complex given the pathophysiologic derangements of hemostasis in cirrhosis. Patients with end-stage liver disease are at higher risk for both bleeding and thrombosis compared to healthy volunteers. Patients with end-stage liver disease (ESLD) often demonstrate perturbations in the coagulation system from decreased production of coagulation factors. These alterations often result in abnormal results for standard laboratory assessment including prothrombin time (PT), activated partial thromboplastin time (PTT), international normalized ratio (INR) and platelet count. Abnormalities in these tests, like elevated INR and thrombocytopenia have traditionally been regarded as indicative of higher bleeding risk, especially in those with ESLD. However, decision-making based on these abnormal laboratory tests alone may actually be hazardous to the ESLD patient, and evaluation of hemostasis is often more complex. In this chapter, we will discuss the hemostatic alterations in ESLD, the evaluation of coagulation status in ESLD, and management of coagulopathy during liver transplantation including blood and other product transfusion as a means to treat coagulopathy and bleeding.

Coagulopathy in Cirrhosis

Cirrhosis has a profound impact on the hemostatic system as the liver is the major synthesizer of coagulation factors as well as proteins involved in fibrinolysis and thrombopoietin for platelet production. The liver synthesizes procoagulant factors II, V, VII, IX, X, XI, XII, and XIII, and a reduction of the activity in these factors is frequently observed in ESLD patients [1]. On the other hand, most inhibitors of coagulation (anti-thrombin, heparin cofactor II, protein C, protein S, and tissue factor pathway inhibitor) and components of the fibrinolytic system (plasminogen, α2-antiplasmin, plasmin inhibitor) are also synthesized in the liver and are similarly decreased [1]. As such, a balanced decrease in synthesis of pro- and anti-coagulation factors in ESLD can result in a relative homeostasis in ESLD. However, with such a fragile balance, ESLD patients are at risk of developing either hypo- or hypercoagulable states. In fact, tissue factor is produced in hepatocytes and believed to be a principal physiological activator of coagulation. It is released by damaged hepatocytes and may play a role in the hypercoagulable aspects of liver diseases [2].

Platelets play an important role in coagulation, and their quantity and quality are often profoundly decreased in ESLD. This is largely driven by portal hypertension and subsequent platelet sequestration and destruction by the spleen (hypersplenism). Reduced synthesis of thrombopoetin, the growth factor required for platelet production, also leads to a reduction in circulating platelets. Platelets may additionally be consumed in coagulopathy, and bone marrow suppression may further exacerbate thrombocytopenia [2].

Von Willebrand Factor (vWF) is synthesized in endothelial cells and is increased in liver disease causing increased platelet aggregation. The vWF which inactivates metalloproteinase ADAMTS13, also synthesized in the liver, is often decreased [2]. As a result, vWF breakdown is slowed, and vWF exhibits increased activity. This supports platelet adhesion despite reduced platelet functional capacity [3, 4]. Of the factors listed above, factor VIII and vWF can be viewed as the only factors which are typically increased in concentration compared to the majority that are typically reduced due to overall impaired protein synthesis [1].

D. Romano (✉) · N. Smith · J. Zerillo
The Icahn School of Medicine at Mount Sinai Hospital, Department of Anesthesiology, Perioperative and Pain Management, New York, NY, USA
e-mail: Diana.Romano@mountsinai.org; Natalie.smith@mountsinai.org; jeron.zerillo@mountsinai.org

© Springer Nature Switzerland AG 2021
C. S. Scher et al. (eds.), *Essentials of Blood Product Management in Anesthesia Practice*,
https://doi.org/10.1007/978-3-030-59295-0_25

Rebalanced Hemostasis

The current view is that the majority of patients with ESLD exist in a precarious balance between these pro- and anticoagulation systems, in what has been termed a state of "re-balanced hemostasis." [5] This rebalance, however, is less stable than the hemostatic balance in healthy patients [5] and is easily disturbed by complications of liver disease including infections, renal failure, and surgical stress leading to rapid shifts to a hypo- or hypercoagulable state, explaining why both bleeding and thrombotic episodes occur in these patients [5]. Importantly, traditional laboratory testing can be misleading resulting in unnecessary transfusion of factors [6].

Evaluating Coagulation Defects in ESLD

The bleeding risk in ESLD patients is typically first assessed using interview and physical examination. Medical history should focus on history of bleeding including epistaxis, spontaneous bleeding (e.g., gingival bleeding while brushing teeth), esophageal variceal bleed, history of easy bruising, history of deep vein thrombosis (DVT), pulmonary embolism (PE), or portal vein thrombosis (PVT), and history of cancer, particularly hepatocellular carcinoma (HCC). Physical exam findings suggestive of increased bleeding risk may include bruises, petechiae, or spontaneous bleeding from vascular insertion sites.

The next step to evaluate a cirrhotic patient's coagulation status is using standard laboratory tests of prothrombin time (PT), activated partial thrombin time (aPTT), and international normalized ratio (INR). Routine coagulation tests including PT/INR and PTT are in vitro tests and only measure the levels of specific individual procoagulants produced by the liver.

Historically, practitioners would prophylactically correct a prolonged PT and elevated INR prior to surgery by administering plasma, due to concerns for excessive bleeding risk. However, this assumption is likely incorrect. Clinical and laboratory studies have shown that INR does not correlate to bleeding risk in cirrhotic patients [6]. Routine correction of hemostasis abnormalities by plasma or platelet transfusion in patients with liver disease is not indicated and may even do more harm than good by disrupting the patients' so-called rebalanced hemostasis discussed above [5]. In addition, when plasma is given to correct an elevated INR, it is commonly under-dosed. The dose of plasma to correct an elevated INR is 10–15 ml/kg. However, providers give an average of 1–2 units which exposes the patient to all the risks of transfusion, including transfusion-associated acute lung injury (TRALI), transfusion-associated circulatory overload (TACO), and portal venous congestion without adequately correcting the INR. Warner et al. showed that in nearly 7000 patients receiving plasma with a median pretransfusion INR of 1.9 and a median transfusion volume of two units, (20% of which were administered prophylactically before a procedure), the median decrease in INR was 0.4 with complete INR normalization in only 12% of the patients. Reductions in INR were modest with pretransfusion INR values <3 [7].

More sophisticated point-of-care tests of coagulation such as viscoelastic testing including thromboelastography (TEG) and rotational thromboelastometry (ROTEM) represent a helpful technique for evaluating whole blood clotting. Use of viscoelastic testing is likely superior to traditional PT/INR and PTT for evaluating cirrhotic patient's underlying hemostatic abnormalities due to the tests' ability to quantify clot initiation, propagation, and breakdown in real time to identify specific abnormalities. The ROTEM test contains several component tests: EXTEM which analyzes the extrinsic coagulation pathway, INTEM which analyzes the intrinsic pathway, FIBTEM which analyzes the contribution of fibrinogen to coagulation, and APTEM which detects fibrinolysis. An additional test, HEPTEM, can be used to detect heparin effects [8]. The most relevant ROTEM tests for liver transplantation are the EXTEM, FIBTEM, and APTEM. Commonly used thromboelastometry parameters include the clotting time (CT) representing clotting factor activation, clot formation time (CFT) and α-angle which correlate with factor amplification and fibrin cross-linkage, Amplitude at 5 and 10 minutes (A5 and A10) and maximum clot firmness (MCF), represent clot strength and correlate to platelets and fibrinogen activity on the EXTEM, and fibrinogen on the FIBTEM. Maximum lysis (ML) indicates the maximum amount of clot breakdown [9]. One distinct advantage of ROTEM over standard laboratory assessment is the speed; results (including CT, CFT, A5, A10) can be obtained within 5–10 minutes of starting the assay. A5/A10 have been shown to have an excellent correlation with thrombocytopenia and hypofibrinogenemia and may potentially guide early transfusion of relevant blood products during liver transplantation [10]. Evidence supports the use of these tests to guide transfusion in actively bleeding patients without liver disease and has shown a reduction in the amount of transfusion and decreased risk of postoperative thrombosis [8, 11, 12]. In liver transplant surgery, utilization of ROTEM to guide transfusion may decrease blood loss and plasma transfusion [13–15]. ROTEM-guided hemorrhage prediction in ESLD is an area of ongoing research with promising results thus far [16, 17]. Evidence as to any long-term benefits in morbidity and mortality with of the use of thromboelastometry in liver transplantation is limited. One case control study of ROTEM in 303 liver transplant patients showed that use of ROTEM reduced blood product administration in patients with MELD >21, reduced surgical complications and postoperative renal failure, and was associated with better preservation of the liver graft with lower rates of graft dysfunction and re-transplant as well as lower early mortality [18]. However, a randomized controlled trial of 28 patients undergoing liver transplantation using thromboelastography-guided transfusion versus standard laboratory coagulation testing showed significantly less plasma transfusion in the thromboelastography group, but no difference in 3-year survival.

Another major advantage of ROTEM is its high negative predictive value—during ongoing bleeding a normal ROTEM may indicate a surgical source of bleeding rather than coagulopathy [11]. We recommend baseline ROTEM at the start of the procedure and then again at least after reperfusion or more frequently if abnormal or continued diffuse bleeding occurs.

Liver Transplant and Intraoperative Changes in Coagulation Status

The main causes of bleeding during liver transplantation include inadequate surgical hemostasis, coagulopathy (dilutional or consumptive), hyperfibrinolysis, transmural hydrostatic pressure such as portal hypertension, hypothermia, release of inflammatory mediators, and heparin/TPA infusion from the graft itself. There are three distinct phases in liver transplantation each with specific potential complications.

Pre-anhepatic Stage

The pre-anhepatic stage begins at surgical incision and ends when blood flow to the patient's liver is stopped. The hallmark of this phase is dissection and exposure of the hilum. Careful observation of the surgical field is key as surgical bleeding is most likely to occur during this phase. Vascular access should be adequately placed and blood products prepared accordingly due to the potential for sudden acute bleeding during the pre-anhepatic phase. Rapid infusing capability is a baseline requirement. Bleeding is most likely to be encountered in patients with portal hypertension, where fragile venous structures may rupture and be difficult to control surgically. In patients with severe portal hypertension, including those who have undergone previous transjugular intrahepatic portosystemic shunt (TIPS) procedures, disruption of porto-systemic shunts into the abdominal wall and peritoneum may be unavoidable for surgical exposure.

Risk of bleeding is increased in patients with previous upper abdominal surgeries (including previous transplants) and/or history of spontaneous bacterial peritonitis due to adhesions. Patients presenting with alcoholic hepatitis or alcoholic cirrhosis may have increased bleeding risk due to the direct toxic effect of alcohol on the bone marrow, as well as suppression of megakaryocyte function causing thrombocytopenia and impaired platelet function [19]. In contrast, patients with HCC are at increased risk of developing venous thromboembolic complications including both PVT and non-splanchnic venous thromboembolism such as DVT and PE [20]. In addition, non-neoplastic PVT is more frequent in cirrhotic patients than in the general population and has been reported to be associated with a thrombophilic genotype in up to 69.5% of cirrhotic patients with PVT [21, 22]. Additionally, in patients requiring continuous renal replacement therapy (CVVH) during liver transplantation, thrombosis of the CVVH circuit was more rapid and more common than in control subjects [23]. It has been reported that patients with primary biliary cirrhosis exhibit less fibrinolysis and preserved capacity for thrombin generation compared with other etiologies for cirrhosis [24, 25].

The primary goal of anesthetic management during the pre-anhepatic phase is to maintain normovolemia using directed colloid/crystalloid/transfusion therapy when required based on a combination of observation of the surgical field and baseline viscoelastic testing obtained early in the case. Patients with ESLD are at increased risk of dilutional coagulopathy compared to the general population due to baseline low levels of coagulation factors, thus judicious use of fluids is not only important for the patient's cardiopulmonary and volume status but also to their potential for coagulation.

Large fluid and blood product resuscitation may increase central venous pressure (CVP) which theoretically may increase bleeding secondary to increased portal hypertension. However, maintaining low CVP during the pre-anhepatic phase with the intention of reducing blood loss is controversial, with some reports showing maintenance of lower CVP (<5 mmHg) by forced diuresis, fluid restriction, nitroglycerin, and morphine to be associated with increased rates of postoperative renal failure and 30-day mortality [26] and others showing no difference in perioperative renal function and postoperative complications between normal and low CVP groups [27].

Anhepatic Stage

The second phase of liver transplantation is the anhepatic stage which begins with clamping of the porta hepatis and ends at reperfusion of the new liver graft. There are three main surgical techniques for the anhepatic phase [28]. Total vascular isolation with inferior vena cava (IVC) replacement involves placing clamps across the porta hepatis, infrahepatic IVC, and suprahepatic IVC followed by removal of the liver and associated vasculature and replacement with the donor graft and vessels. IVC clamping may result in major hemodynamic instability due to sudden decrease in preload and thus cardiac output with requisite volume resuscitation and vasopressor support to tolerate this technique. A second technique, called the piggy back technique, involves clamping the porta-hepatis and the hepatic veins; this involves a side clamp at the junction of the hepatic veins and the IVC. The piggy back technique preserves partial IVC flow and maintains partial preload and cardiac output compared to total caval replacement. Additionally, a temporary portocaval shunt can be placed to better preserve preload during the anhepatic phase. The piggy back technique is associated with a more complicated surgical anastomosis compared with total caval replacement. A third method for maintaining cardiac output during the anhepatic phase is veno-venous bypass (VVB). For this method, a femoral vein canula (and sometimes a portal vein cannula) and an upper body venous cannula (such as internal jugular or subclavian vein) are placed and blood from the lower body is returned to the right atrium via a bypass circuit prior to total vascular isolation. Once the patient is anhepatic, vasopressor and inotropic support may be preferable to support blood pressure rather than fluid therapy, as excessive resuscitation during this phase could lead to volume overload at reperfusion causing acute right heart failure or congestion of the liver graft, impairing its function.

Once the recipient hepatectomy is performed, any preexisting function of the patient's own liver is lost. This includes metabolizing anesthetic drugs and citrate from transfused blood products leading to potential citrate toxicity. Coagulopathy may be observed due to accumulation of endogenous tPA and other endogenous anticoagulants which are normally metabolized by the liver. As tPA increases the conversion of plasminogen to plasmin, which then aids in the breakdown of fibrin to fibrin split products, the end result is that fibrinogen production is slowed and fibrin is consumed leading to increased blood loss [24, 29].

Neohepatic Stage

The final stage of liver transplantation, the neohepatic phase, starts at reperfusion and ends at the completion of surgery. Reperfusion may result in significant hemodynamic lability. At this point reperfusion of the new graft occurs by restoring venous blood flow through portal venous inflow and the inferior vena cava outflow. During this time, the stagnant venous blood in the portal system and lower body systemic circulation, in addition to the preservative solution and endogenous metabolites within the liver graft itself, are released into the systemic circulation. Reperfusion can be complicated by right ventricular distension and dysfunction, pulmonary vascular constriction, systemic hypotension, arrhythmias, and cardiac arrest. Management of this critical period involves improving cardiac dysfunction using vasopressors, antiarrhythmics, and membrane stabilization but rarely involves acute changes in blood management. In the neohepatic phase, new coagulopathy can occur due to hyperfibrinolysis. In addition to the tPA effect seen during the anhepatic phase, in the neohepatic phase, fibrinolysis is enhanced by the release of tPA from the donor endothelium secondary to injury by ischemia and reperfusion [30]. Heparin-like activity may also be seen after graft reperfusion either from release of exogenous heparin from the donor liver used in the preservation process or from release of endogenous heparin-like substances from the ischemic graft endothelium [30, 31]. Although it is typically short-lived, patients with higher sensitivity to heparin may not clear it rapidly and develop coagulopathy; the use of protamine in this special case has been shown to improve blood loss [32]. Lastly, decreased blood temperature (from cold preservation solution), metabolic acidosis, and reduced cardiovascular function may all play some roles in coagulopathy in the neohepatic stage [30], many of which will reverse with time once the liver graft begins functioning. Graft quality plays an important role in the neohepatic period as delayed or primary non-function of the graft will cause worsening coagulopathy. Select risk factors for graft failure include marginal grafts, poor preservation, and prolonged cold and/or warm ischemia times [33].

Red Blood Cell Transfusion in Liver Transplantation

There is no current standard transfusion pattern followed during liver transplantation. One Canadian study reported that practice patterns differed significantly among eight major liver transplantation centers for RBC, plasma, and platelets [34]. Identifying a uniform transfusion strategy is difficult due to differences in the availability of point of care coagulation testing and difficulty in predicting intraoperative blood transfusion requirements from preoperative variables [35, 36].

Strategies for Blood Conservation

Frequent hematologic complications such as anemia, thrombocytopenia, and coagulopathy found in liver transplant patients present a significant barrier when trying to avoid/minimize allogeneic blood product transfusion. This being said, in order to reduce the incidence of exposure-related complications, several strategies could be employed [28]. Acute normovolemic hemodilution (ANH) is one strategy entailing removal of blood, typically via central access, during the pre-anhepatic stage with maintenance of normovolemia with crystalloid or colloid replacement. Lowering of the patient's hemoglobin concentration using ANH minimizes the effect of surgical blood loss (hemorrhaged blood has a lower hematocrit) and preserves platelets and coagulation factors found in the autologous blood for autotransfusion in a later stage of the surgery. This technique can only be used in patients with high starting hemoglobin concentration and hemodynamic stability. Similarly, phlebotomy without replacement with crystalloid or colloid has been proposed by other groups [37].

RBC salvage using a cell salvage device is a well-established technique in liver transplant allowing large volumes of shed blood to be returned to the patient without the potential for alloimmunization or other allogeneic blood transfusion complications [28]. Contraindications to the technique include infected material in the surgical field and malignancy. Several small studies, however, have evaluated the oncological safety of cell salvage in liver transplant patients with HCC and have not found negative effects on mortality or recurrence rate associated with its use [38–41]. Additional studies are warranted to confirm or refute these findings. Using techniques such as ANH and cell salvage, some institutions have achieved non-RBC transfusion liver transplantation [42].

Factor Concentrates for Liver Transplant

In the absence of bleeding, correction of cirrhotic coagulopathy is not recommended. Replacement of factors with plasma and correction of thrombocytopenia by platelet transfusion requires significant volume administration; the resultant increase in central venous pressure and portal pressures may in fact increase the risk of vascular hemorrhage [43]. Large volumes of plasma (10–15 ml/kg) are required to increase factor levels by 15–30%; each unit of plasma increases the risk of TRALI and TACO and furthermore may lead to hypocalcemia and hypothermia and may increase coagulopathy [44]. Patients undergoing liver transplant are at higher risk for TRALI than the general surgical population [45–48]. Transfusion in liver transplant is associated with longer length of stay, decreased survival, kidney injury, reoperation, and infection [33]. Prophylactic platelet transfusion in liver transplant exposes patients to the risks of transfusion, specifically TRALI and ARDS, and is associated with decreased patient and graft survival [44, 49, 50].

However, when clinical bleeding does occur, patients with end-stage liver disease are at increased risk of dilutional coagulopathy and hypofibrinogenemia compared to other patients. During liver transplant, endothelial glycocalyx injury acts as an anticoagulant and may lead to autoheparinization [51]. Surgical bleeding may be further complicated by increased fibrinolysis secondary to decreased clearance of tPA during the anhepatic phase and increased release of tPA from the graft liver at reperfusions [51]. In fact, the liver graft may worsen coagulopathy if graft function is delayed secondary to prolonged ischemic times, marginal quality graft, or extended criteria donor [33]. As such, in the presence of bleeding during liver transplant, transfusion to correct coagulopathy can be complex and a variety of hemostatic products should be considered.

Fibrinogen

Fibrinogen is the first clotting factor to decrease by a clinically significant degree via dilution. While fibrinogen is present in plasma, a large volume of plasma would be required to effectively replace fibrinogen and paradoxically may lead to further dilution. Fibrinogen is available in several forms including cryoprecipitate and fibrinogen concentrates. Cryoprecipitate is the product of partially thawed plasma and yields 15 mL per unit of plasma. It contains a range from 120 to 800 mg of fibrinogen per unit. It also contains factor VIII, factor XIII, vWF and fibronectin [44]. One single donor unit of cryoprecipitate (15 mL) can increase fibrinogen by approximately 10 mg/dL in a 60 kg person [44]. In North America two forms of fibrinogen concentrate are available including Fibryga (Octapharma, Austria) and RiaSTAP (CSL Behring, Germany). Each dose contains 1 g of fibrinogen which is reconstituted in sterile water. Compared to cryoprecipitate, fibrinogen concentrates are available without delays because they are stored at room temperature and do not require thawing or blood typing [44]. Additionally, the manufacturing process is designed to decrease the risk of transfusion reaction and pathogen transmission [44].

In trauma, massive hemorrhage is associated with a fibrinogen level less than 1.5 g/L. As such, trauma guidelines recommend maintaining fibrinogen between 1.5 and 2 g/L using an initial dose of 3–4 g of fibrinogen concentrate or 50 mL/kg of cryoprecipitate [52]. A ROTEM FIBTEM MCF of 7 in trauma was associated with a fibrinogen level of 2 g/L and may help guide transfusion [52].

A systematic review comparing the effect of plasma transfusion, to fibrinogen concentrate for the management of bleeding in all-comers, revealed equivocal results in controlling bleeding with plasma transfusion, with only 28% of studies showing positive outcomes (decreased bleeding or mortality) [53]. On the other hand, 70% of the 21 fibrinogen studies showed positive outcomes. Three studies directly compared plasma to fibrinogen concentrate and found that fibrinogen transfusion was associated with reduced blood loss, decreased total transfusion, decreased ICU and hospital stay, and increased plasma fibrinogen level [53].

Studies evaluating the efficacy and safety of fibrinogen concentrates and cryoprecipitate in liver transplant patients also utilized prothrombin complex concentrates and are discussed in the following section.

Prothrombin Complex Concentrates

Prothrombin complex concentrates (PCC) are the factors purified from the supernatant from slowly thawing plasma [44, 54]. Most available PCCs contain four factors (4F PCC) (factor II, VII, IX, and X), and early versions contained three factors (Factor II, IX, and X). Early preparations of PCC were associated with thrombosis (venous thromboembolism, myocardial infarction, disseminated intravascular coagulation), but newer products are considered safer because they maintain factors in inactivated states and contain anticoagulant proteins [55]. In the United States, 4F PCC is available as KCentra (CSL Behring, Germany) and contains heparin, protein C, protein S, and antithrombin anticoagulants as well [56]. PCC dosing is based on the factor IX content which is approximately 500 IU per vial. PCC is reconstituted with 20 mL of sterile fluid for a factor IX concentration of 25 IU/mL [44]. Compared to plasma, PCC may restore factor levels without the risk of volume overload and decreased risk of transfusion reaction due to viral inactivation and nanofiltration [55].

Most safety and dosing for 4F PCC comes from studies on warfarin-treated patients. In a multicenter clinical trial, PCC was noninferior compared to plasma for reduction in INR and hemostasis in major bleeding related to warfarin and was associated with a similar adverse event rate [57]. Another study evaluating the thromboembolic complications associated with PCC for emergent warfarin reversal (due to bleeding or need for surgical procedure) found a 3.8% incidence of thromboembolism (1 MI, 3 CVA, 1 DVT, 1 splenic infarct) related to PCC (24 IU/kg) [58]. Given that the patients in the study were on warfarin as secondary prophylaxis to prevent stroke and had a preexisting thrombogenic condition, the authors concluded that the potentially increased risk of thromboembolism from PCC administration was only mildly increased compared to baseline [58].

Data on PCC in liver disease is limited. Pereira and colleagues evaluated the utility of four different doses of 4F PCC (ranging from 12.5–50 IU/kg) with vitamin K, in patients with liver disease experiencing life-threatening bleeding and noted an improvement in hemostasis after PCC administration [59]. Another group used an in vitro thrombin generation assay to evaluate the efficacy of PCC in liver transplant [60]. PCC restored thrombin generation in the liver transplant patients using low-dose PCC (0.2 IU/mL – equivalent to 10 IU/kg) compared to plasma (dose equivalent to 2–3 units of plasma) which was not able to restore thrombin generation. Additionally, low-dose PCC was not able to restore thrombin generation in patients treated with warfarin. The authors concluded that a lower dose of PCC was adequate for restoration of thrombin generation in transplant patients compared to those requiring warfarin reversal [60].

The PROTON trial, a multicenter randomized, double-blinded study evaluating efficacy and safety 4F PCC in liver transplant is ongoing; end points include transfusion totals, estimated blood loss, rescue medications, and safety endpoints including serious adverse events focusing on thromboembolic events [61].

Several studies in liver transplant have evaluated ROTEM-based algorithms for fibrinogen replacement and PCC transfusion using a range of ROTEM based protocols. Krichner and colleagues used a FIBTEM MCF of 6 mm and an EXTEM MCF of 35 mm to guide fibrinogen with a goal fibrinogen level of 1.5–2 g/L [62]. Of the 153 patients who received fibrinogen, the average dose was 6.3 grams. An EXTEM CT >80s was used to trigger PCC administration (25 IU/Kg). Patients who required fibrinogen concentrate or PCC also received more RBC, plasma, and platelets and were more likely to require reoperation [62]. There was no difference in thrombotic complications between the conventional group and the group who received Fibrinogen concentrate and/or 4F PCC ($p = 0.31$). Hepatic artery thrombosis did not differ between groups with an overall incidence of 4.1%, PE occurred in 3/266 patients (1.1% incidence), and PVT and myocardial infarction each had an overall incidence of 0.4% [62].

A different group compared conventional transfusion practices to a ROTEM-guided algorithm which included fibrinogen concentrate and 4F PCC using different parameters [63]. ROTEM was performed at baseline, at reperfusion and after transplant. EXTEM A5 < 25 mm and FIBTEM A10 < 10 mm triggered fibrinogen transfusion by either cryoprecipitate or fibrinogen concentrate. PCC was administered when EXTEM CT >80s. Using propensity score matching, the group found decreased transfusion of RBC and plasma in the ROTEM group compared to the conventional group, there was no difference in transfusion of cryoprecipitate or platelets, complications, length of stay, or mortality [63].

More studies and standardized dosing algorithms are necessary to further evaluate fibrinogen concentrates and PCC in liver transplant recipients; these preliminary studies suggest that these products are safe to use and do not increase the risk of thrombosis and potentially decrease transfusion requirements.

Recombinant Activated Factor VII (rFVIIa)

Recombinant activated factor VII is a serine protease that converts inactive factor IX and X to active forms. rFVIIa was first used clinically in hemophilia patients who lacked factor VIII or IX, and high doses are required for hemophilia (90 mcg/kg) [44]. In the setting of perioperative bleeding, rFVIIa administration will restore activated FXa, restoring activity of the Xase complex which leads to thrombin generation; therefore rFVIIa can only work to restore hemostasis if adequate prothrombin is present for FXa to act on, as such prior repletion of prothrombin by plasma or PCC administration is necessary for rFVIIa to work [54]. Similarly, thrombin generation will not restore hemostasis in the absence of fibrinogen; thus fibrinogen levels must be replete before administration of rFVIIa for it to be effective [54].

Recombinant factor VIIa is associated with a risk for thromboembolic complications. Administration of rFVIIa in intracranial hemorrhage and cardiac surgical patients is associated with increased risk of thromboembolic events [64]. A systematic review and meta-analysis of 35 randomized controlled trials evaluated the frequency of thromboembolic events related to administration of rFVIIa, thromboembolic events occurred in 9% (401/4468) of patients, and specifically the incidence of arterial thrombus was higher in the rFVIIa group (5.5% vs. 3.2% $p = 0.003$) and coronary thrombosis (2.9% vs. 1.1%, $p = 0.002$) compared to placebo [65]. The risk of arterial thrombosis increased with patient age with an incidence of 10.8% in patients over 75 years old compared to a 4.1% incidence with placebo ($p = 0.02$). The dose ranges in the studies reviewed were wide—ranging from less than 80 mcg/kg to greater than 120 mcg/kg; the authors conclude that rFVIIa is associated with increased risk of arterial thromboembolism especially in older patients [65].

rFVIIa in Liver Disease

Several studies, including randomized controlled trials, have evaluated the utility of rFVIIa in the liver transplant population. Two small studies (less than 10 patients each) suggest that rFVIIa administration decreases transfusion requirements in liver disease patients [66, 67]; others have failed to find a difference in transfusion and long-term outcomes [68–71]. In fact, several studies suggest increased transfusion requirement and decreased patient and graft survival in patients who receive rFVIIa [72, 73]. To date, there is no evidence for increased thromboembolic events in liver transplant patients who receive rFVIIa [64, 67–69, 72, 73]. There is insufficient evidence to conclude benefit or harm for rFVIIa in this population.

Antifibrinolytics

Antifibrinolytic agents currently available include aminocaproic acid and tranexamic acid. Aprotinin, a trypsin inhibitor, was available prior to 2008 when it was withdrawn after evidence suggested increase in postoperative mortality after coronary artery bypass surgery [74]. Several studies in liver transplant compared outcomes before and after the removal of aprotinin from the market. Retrospective reviews comparing blood loss before and after aprotinin withdrawal have shown mixed results with some reporting more bleeding since the withdrawal of aprotinin and others showing no difference in transfusions [75, 76]. Currently available antifibrinolytics like tranexamic acid have been shown to reduce transfusion requirements without increased risk of hepatic artery thrombosis, venous thromboembolism, or mortality [77, 78]. Antifibrinolytic agents are typically only administered if there is viscoelastic testing evidence of hyperfibrinolysis, rather than prophylactically [62, 63].

Conclusion

In conclusion, hemostatic alterations in ESLD require careful evaluation. Care providers must set aside pre-conceived biases regarding abnormal standard laboratory results, as the majority of ESLD patients live in a state of "rebalanced hemostasis," and viscoelastic testing of whole blood clotting may aid in elucidating a patient's coagulation status. These tools are especially useful in diagnosing and managing evolving coagulopathies during liver transplant. Special consideration should be paid to patient anatomical and physiological challenges such as portal hypertension which may cause increased surgical bleeding. Strategies for blood management include conservation techniques, replacement of whole blood or its components, replacement of specific factor concentrates, and potentially antifibrinolytics when necessary. Although many options are available, tailoring to the individual patient's clinical picture is the key to good clinical outcomes.

References

1. Wada H, Usui M, Sakuragawa N. Hemostatic abnormalities and liver diseases. Semin Thromb Hemost. 2008;34(8):772–8. https://doi.org/10.1055/s-0029-1145259.
2. Hartmann M, Szalai C, Saner FH. Hemostasis in liver transplantation: pathophysiology, monitoring, and treatment. World J Gastroenterol. 2016;22(4):1541–50. https://doi.org/10.3748/wjg.v22.i4.1541.
3. Hugenholtz GCG, Adelmeijer J, Meijers JCM, Porte RJ, Stravitz RT, Lisman T. An unbalance between von Willebrand factor and ADAMTS13 in acute liver failure: implications for hemostasis and clinical outcome. Hepatology. 2013;58(2):752–61. https://doi.org/10.1002/hep.26372.
4. Lisman T, Bongers TN, Adelmeijer J, et al. Elevated levels of von Willebrand factor in cirrhosis support platelet adhesion despite reduced functional capacity. Hepatology. 2006;44(1):53–61. https://doi.org/10.1002/hep.21231.
5. Lisman T, Porte RJ. Rebalanced hemostasis in patients with liver disease: evidence and clinical consequences. Blood. 2010;116(6):878–85. https://doi.org/10.1182/blood-2010-02-261891.

6. Saner FH, Kirchner C. Monitoring and treatment of coagulation disorders in end-stage liver disease. Visc Med. 2016;32(4):241–8. https://doi.org/10.1159/000446304.
7. Warner MA, Hanson AC, Weister TJ, et al. Changes in international normalized ratios after plasma transfusion of varying doses in unique clinical environments. Anesth Analg. 2018;127(2):349–57. https://doi.org/10.1213/ANE.0000000000003336.
8. Williams B, McNeil J, Crabbe A, Tanaka KA. Practical use of thromboelastometry in the management of perioperative coagulopathy and bleeding. Transfus Med Rev. 2017;31(1):11–25. https://doi.org/10.1016/j.tmrv.2016.08.005.
9. Katz D, Beilin Y. Disorders of coagulation in pregnancy. Br J Anaesth. 2015;115 Suppl 2:ii75-88. doi: 10.1093/bja/aev374
10. Hashir A, Singh S, Krishnan G, Subramanian RGS. Correlation of early ROTEM parameters with conventional coagulation tests in patients with chronic liver disease undergoing liver transplant. Indian J Anesth. 2017;61(18):622–8. https://doi.org/10.4103/ija.IJA.
11. Pierce A, Pittet J-F. Practical understanding of hemostasis and approach to the bleeding patient in the OR. Adv Anesth. 2014;32(1):1–21. https://doi.org/10.1002/ana.22528.Toll-like.
12. Wikkelsø A, Wetterslev J, Møller AM, Afshari A. Thromboelastography (TEG) or rotational thromboelastometry (ROTEM) to monitor haemostatic treatment in bleeding patients: A systematic review with meta-analysis and trial sequential analysis. Anaesthesia. 2017;72(4):519–31. https://doi.org/10.1111/anae.13765.
13. Smart L, Mumtaz K, Scharpf D, et al. Rotational thromboelastometry or conventional coagulation tests in liver transplantation: comparing blood loss, transfusions, and cost. Ann Hepatol. 2017;16(6):916–23. https://doi.org/10.5604/01.3001.0010.5283.
14. Roullet S, Freyburger G, Cruc M, et al. Management of bleeding and transfusion during liver transplantation before and after the introduction of a rotational thromboelastometry-based algorithm. Liver Transplant. 2015;21(2):169–79. https://doi.org/10.1002/lt.24030.
15. Northup P, Reutemann B. Management of coagulation and anticoagulation in liver transplantation candidates. Liver Transplant. 2018;24(8):1119–32. https://doi.org/10.1002/lt.25198.
16. Tafur LA, Taura P, Blasi A, et al. Rotation thromboelastometry velocity curve predicts blood loss during liver transplantation. Br J Anaesth. 2016;117(6):741–8. https://doi.org/10.1093/bja/aew344.
17. Dötsch TM, Dirkmann D, Bezinover D, et al. Assessment of standard laboratory tests and rotational thromboelastometry for the prediction of postoperative bleeding in liver transplantation. Br J Anaesth. 2017;119(3):402–10. https://doi.org/10.1093/bja/aex122.
18. Álamo JM, León A, Mellado P, et al. Is "intra-operating room" thromboelastometry useful in liver transplantation? A case-control study in 303 patients. Transplant Proc. 2013;45(10):3637–9. https://doi.org/10.1016/j.transproceed.2013.11.008.
19. Marroni CA, De Medeiros FA, Fernandes SA, et al. Liver transplantation and alcoholic liver disease: history, controversies, and considerations. World J Gastroenterol. 2018;24(26):2785–805. https://doi.org/10.3748/wjg.v24.i26.2785.
20. Zanetto A, Campello E, Spiezia L, Burra P, Simioni P, Russo FP. Cancer-associated thrombosis in cirrhotic patients with hepatocellular carcinoma. Cancers (Basel). 2018;10(11):1–19. https://doi.org/10.3390/cancers10110450.
21. Rodríguez-Castro KI, Porte RJ, Nadal E, Germani G, Burra P, Senzolo M. Management of nonneoplastic portal vein thrombosis in the setting of liver transplantation: a systematic review. Transplantation. 2012;94(11):1145–53. https://doi.org/10.1097/TP.0b013e31826e8e53.
22. Amitrano L, Guardascione MA, Ames PRJ. Coagulation abnormalities in cirrhotic patients with portal vein thrombosis. Clin Lab. 2007;53(11–12):583–9.
23. Agarwal B, Shaw S, Hari MS, Burroughs AK, Davenport A. Continuous renal replacement therapy (CRRT) in patients with liver disease: is circuit life different? J Hepatol. 2009;51(3):504–9. https://doi.org/10.1016/j.jhep.2009.05.028.
24. Cleland S, Corredor C, Ye JJ, Srinivas C, McCluskey SA. Massive haemorrhage in liver transplantation: consequences, prediction and management. World J Transplant. 2016;6(2):291. https://doi.org/10.5500/wjt.v6.i2.291.
25. Segal H, Cottam S, Potter D, Hunt BJ. Coagulation and fibrinolysis in primary biliary cirrhosis compared with other liver disease and during orthotopic liver transplantation. Hepatology. 1997;25(3):683–8. https://doi.org/10.1002/hep.510250332.
26. Schroeder RA, Collins BH, Tuttle-Newhall E, et al. Intraoperative fluid management during orthotopic liver transplantation. J Cardiothorac Vasc Anesth. 2004;18(4):438–41. https://doi.org/10.1053/j.jvca.2004.05.020.
27. Feng ZY, Xu X, Zhu SM, Bein B, Zheng S. Sen. Effects of low central venous pressure during preanhepatic phase on blood loss and liver and renal function in liver transplantation. World J Surg. 2010;34(8):1864–73. https://doi.org/10.1007/s00268-010-0544-y.
28. Sakai T. Liver Transplantation Anesthesiology. In: KST S, editor. Anesthesia and Perioperative Care for Organ Transplantation. New York: Springer Science+Business Media; 2017. p. 353–64. https://doi.org/10.1213/ane.0000000000002483.
29. Kong HY, Huang SQ, Zhu SM, Wen XH. Role of anhepatic time in endothelial-related coagulation in liver transplantation. Minerva Anestesiol. 2013;79(4):391–7.
30. De Boer MT, Molenaar IQ, Hendriks HGD, Slooff MJH, Porte RJ. Minimizing blood loss in liver transplantation: progress through research and evolution of techniques. Dig Surg. 2005;22(4):265–75. https://doi.org/10.1159/000088056.
31. Kettner SC, Gonano C, Seebach F, et al. Endogenous heparin-like substances significantly impair coagulation in undergoing orthotopic liver transplantation. Anesth Analg. 1998;86(4):691–5. https://doi.org/10.1097/00000539-199804000-00002.
32. Bayly PJM, Thick M. Reversal of post-reperfusion coagulopathy by protamine sulphate in orthotopic liver transplantation. Br J Anaesth. 1994;73(6):840–2. https://doi.org/10.1093/bja/73.6.840.
33. Donohue CI. Reducing transfusion requirements in liver transplantation. World J Transplant. 2015;5(4):165. https://doi.org/10.5500/wjt.v5.i4.165.
34. Ozier Y, Pessione F, Samain E, et al. Institutional variability in transfusion practice for liver transplantation. Anesth Analg. 2003;97(3):671–9. https://doi.org/10.1213/01.ANE.0000073354.38695.7C.
35. Findlay JY, Rettke SR. Poor prediction of blood transfusion requirements in adult liver transplantations from preoperative variables. J Clin Anesth. 2000;12(4):319–23. https://doi.org/10.1016/S0952-8180(00)00162-8.
36. Steib A, Freys G, Lehmann C, Meyer C, Mahoudeau G. Intraoperative blood losses and transfusion requirements during adult liver transplantation remain difficult to predict. Can J Anesth. 2001;48(11):1075–9. https://doi.org/10.1007/BF03020372.
37. Massicotte L, Lenis S, Thibeault L, Sassine M, Seal RRA. Effect of low central venous pressure and phlebotomy on blood product transfusion requirements during liver transplantations. Liver Transplant. 2006;12:117–23. https://doi.org/10.1002/lt.20559.
38. Araujo RL, Pantanali CA, Haddad L, Filho JAR, D'Albuquerque LAC, Andraus W. Does autologous blood transfusion during liver transplantation for hepatocellular carcinoma increase risk of recurrence? World J Gastrointest Surg. 2016;8(2):161. https://doi.org/10.4240/wjgs.v8.i2.161.
39. Foltys D, Zimmermann T, Heise M, et al. Liver transplantation for hepatocellular carcinoma-is there a risk of recurrence caused by intraoperative blood salvage autotransfusion? Eur Surg Res. 2011;47(3):182–7. https://doi.org/10.1159/000330746.

40. Liang TB, Li DL, Liang L, et al. Intraoperative blood salvage during liver transplantation in patients with hepatocellular carcinoma: efficiency of leukocyte depletion filters in the removal of tumor cells. Transplantation. 2008;85(6):863–9. https://doi.org/10.1097/TP.0b013e3181671f2e.
41. Muscari F, Suc B, Vigouroux D, et al. Blood salvage autotransfusion during transplantation for hepatocarcinoma: does it increase the risk of neoplastic recurrence? Transpl Int. 2005;18(11):1236–9. https://doi.org/10.1111/j.1432-2277.2005.00207.x.
42. Massicotte L, Denault AY, Beaulieu D, Thibeault L, Hevesi Z, Nozza A, Lapointe RAR. Transfusion rate for 500 consecutive living donor liver transplantations: experience of one liver transplantation center. Transplantation. 2012;94(11):e66–7. https://doi.org/10.1097/TP.0b013e318274ab4a.
43. Lisman T, Porte RJ. Pathogenesis, prevention, and management of bleeding and thrombosis in patients with liver diseases. Res Pract Thromb Haemost. 2017;1(2):150–61. https://doi.org/10.1002/rth2.12028.
44. Chow JH, Lee K, Abuelkasem E, Udekwu OR, Tanaka KA. Coagulation management during liver transplantation: use of fibrinogen concentrate, recombinant activated factor vii, prothrombin complex concentrate, and antifibrinolytics. Semin Cardiothorac Vasc Anesth. 2018;22(2):164–73. https://doi.org/10.1177/1089253217739689.
45. Toy P, Gajic O, Bacchetti P, et al. Transfusion-related acute lung injury: incidence and risk factors. Clin Trials Obs. 2012;119(7):1757–68. https://doi.org/10.1182/blood-2011-08-370932.An.
46. Clifford L, Jia Q, Subramanian A, et al. Characterizing the epidemiology of postoperative transfusion-related acute lung injury. Anesthesiology. 2015;122:12–20.
47. Benson AB, Austin GL, Berg M, et al. Transfusion-related acute lung injury in ICU patients admitted with gastrointestinal bleeding. Intensive Care Med. 2010;36(10):1710–7. https://doi.org/10.1007/s00134-010-1954-x.
48. Smith NK, Kim S, Hill B, Goldberg A, DeMaria S, Zerillo J. Transfusion-Related Acute Lung Injury (TRALI) and Transfusion-Associated Circulatory Overload (TACO) in liver transplantation: a case report and focused review. Semin Cardiothorac Vasc Anesth. 2018;22(2). https://doi.org/10.1177/1089253217736298.
49. De Boer MT, Christensen MC, Asmussen M, et al. The impact of intraoperative transfusion of platelets and red blood cells on survival after liver transplantation. Anesth Analg. 2008;106(1):32–44. https://doi.org/10.1213/01.ane.0000289638.26666.ed.
50. Pereboom ITA, De Boer MT, Haagsma EB, Hendriks HGD, Lisman T, Porte RJ. Platelet transfusion during liver transplantation is associated with increased postoperative mortality due to acute lung injury. Anesth Analg. 2009;108(4):1083–91. https://doi.org/10.1213/ane.0b013e3181948a59.
51. Schiefer J, Lebherz-Eichinger D, Erdoes G, et al. Alterations of endothelial glycocalyx during orthotopic liver transplantation in patients with end-stage liver disease. Transplantation. 2015;99(10):2118–23. https://doi.org/10.1097/TP.0000000000000680.
52. Spahn DR, Bouillon B, Cerny V, et al. Managment of bleeding and coagulopathy following major trauma: an updated European guideline. Crit Care. 2013;17:R76.
53. Kozek-Langenecker S, Sørensen B, Hess JR, Spahn DR. Clinical effectiveness of fresh frozen plasma compared with fibrinogen concentrate: a systematic review. Crit Care. 2011;15(5):R239. https://doi.org/10.1186/cc10488.
54. Ghadimi K, Levy JH, Welsby IJ. Prothrombin Complex Concentrates for Bleeding in the Perioperative Setting. Anesth Analg. 2016;122(5):1287–300. https://doi.org/10.1016/j.physbeh.2017.03.040.
55. Sørensen B, Spahn DR, Innerhofer P, Spannagl M, Rossaint R. Clinical review: prothrombin complex concentrates – evaluation of safety and thrombogenicity. Crit Care. 2011;15(1):1–9. https://doi.org/10.1186/cc9311.
56. CSL Behring. [Package insert] Kcentra Prothrombin Complex Concentrate (Human). 2013.
57. Sarode R, Milling TJ, Refaai MA, et al. Efficacy and safety of a 4-factor prothrombin complex concentrate in patients on vitamin K antagonists presenting with major bleeding: a randomized, plasma-controlled, phase IIIb study. Circulation. 2013;128(11):1234–43. https://doi.org/10.1161/CIRCULATIONAHA.113.002283.
58. Majeed A, Eelde A, Ågren A, Schulman S, Holmström M. Thromboembolic safety and efficacy of prothrombin complex concentrates in the emergency reversal of warfarin coagulopathy. Thromb Res. 2012;129(2):146–51. https://doi.org/10.1016/j.thromres.2011.07.024.
59. Pereira D, Liotta E, Mahmoud AA. The use of Kcentra® in the reversal of coagulopathy of chronic liver disease. J Pharm Pract. 2018;31(1):120–5. https://doi.org/10.1177/0897190017696952.
60. Abuelkasem E, Hasan S, Mazzeffi MA, Planinsic RM, Sakai T, Tanaka KA. Reduced requirement for prothrombin complex concentrate for the restoration of thrombin generation in plasma from liver transplant recipients. Anesth Analg. 2017;125(2):609–15. https://doi.org/10.1213/ANE.0000000000002106.
61. Arshad F, Ickx B, Van Beem RT, et al. Prothrombin complex concentrate in the reduction of blood loss during orthotopic liver transplantation: PROTON-trial. BMC Surg. 2013;13(1):1. https://doi.org/10.1186/1471-2482-13-22.
62. Kirchner C, Dirkmann D, Treckmann JW, et al. Coagulation management with factor concentrates in liver transplantation: a single-center experience. Transfusion. 2014;54(1):2760–8. https://doi.org/10.1111/trf.12707.
63. Zamper RPC, Amorim TC, Queiroz VNF, et al. Association between viscoelastic tests-guided therapy with synthetic factor concentrates and allogenic blood transfusion in liver transplantation: a before-after study. BMC Anesthesiol. 2018;18(1):1–12. https://doi.org/10.1186/s12871-018-0664-8.
64. Yank V, Tuohy CV, Logan AC, et al. Systematic review: benefits and harms of in-hospital use of recombinant factor VIIa for off-label indications. Ann Intern Med. 2011;154(8)529–40.
65. Levi M, Levy JH, Andersen HF, Truloff D. Safety of recombinant activated factor VII in randomized clinical trials. N Engl J Med. 2010;363(19):1791–800.
66. Hendriks HGD, Meijer K, De Wolf JTM, et al. Reduced transfusion requirements by recombinant factor VIIa in orthotopic liver transplantation. Transplantation. 2001;71(3):402–5. https://doi.org/10.1097/00007890-200102150-00011.
67. Busani S, Semeraro G, Cantaroni C, Masetti M, Marietta M, Girardis M. Recombinant activated factor VII in critical bleeding after orthotopic liver transplantation. Transplant Proc. 2008;40(6):1989–90. https://doi.org/10.1016/j.transproceed.2008.05.021.
68. Planinsic RM, van der Meer J, Testa G, et al. Safety and efficacy of a single bolus administration of recombinant factor VIIa in liver transplantation due to chronic liver disease. Liver Transplant. 2005;11(8):895–900. https://doi.org/10.1002/lt.20458.
69. Lodge JPA, Jonas S, Jones RM, et al. Efficacy and safety of repeated perioperative doses of recombinant factor VIIa in liver transplantation. Liver Transplant. 2005;11(8):973–9. https://doi.org/10.1002/lt.20470.
70. Bosch J, Thabut D, Bendtsen F, et al. Recombinant factor VIIa for upper gastrointestinal bleeding in patients with cirrhosis: a randomized, double-blind trial. Gastroenterology. 2004;127(4):1123–30. https://doi.org/10.1053/j.gastro.2004.07.015.
71. Lodge JPA, Jonas S, Oussoultzglou E, et al. Recombinant coagulation factor VIIa in major liver resection. Anesthesiology. 2005;102(4):269–75. https://doi.org/10.1097/01.sa.0000172532.43755.3b.

72. Pham HP, Hsu SX, Parker-Jones S, Samstein B, Diuguid D, Schwartz J. Recombinant activated factor VII in patients with acute liver failure with UNOS Status 1A: a single tertiary academic centre experience. Vox Sang. 2014;106(1):75–82. https://doi.org/10.1111/vox.12067.
73. Scheffert JL, Taber DJ, Pilch NA, McGillicuddy JW, Baliga PK, Chavin KD. Timing of factor VIIa in liver transplantation impacts cost and clinical outcomes. Pharmacotherapy. 2013;33(5):483–8. https://doi.org/10.1002/phar.1230.
74. Fergusson DA, Hebert PC, Mazer CD, et al. A comparison of aprotinin and llysine analogues in high risk cardiac surgery. N Engl J Med. 2008;358(22):2319–31. https://doi.org/10.1056/NEJMoa1602001.
75. Trzebicki J, Kosieradzki M, Flakiewicz E, et al. Detrimental effect of aprotinin ban on amount of blood loss during liver transplantation: single-center experience. Transplant Proc. 2011;43(5):1725–7. https://doi.org/10.1016/j.transproceed.2011.01.182.
76. Schofield N, Sugavanam A, Thompson K, Mallet SV. No increase in blood transfusions during liver transplantation since the withdrawal of aprotinin. Liver Transplant. 2014;20:584–90. https://doi.org/10.1002/lt.23839.
77. Molenaar IQ, Warnaar N, Groen H, TenVergert EM, Slooff MJH, Porte RJ. Efficacy and safety of antifibrinolytic drugs in liver transplantation: a systematic review and meta-analysis. Am J Transplant. 2007;7(1):185–94. https://doi.org/10.1111/j.1600-6143.2006.01591.x.
78. Badenoch A, Sharma A, Gower S, et al. The effectiveness and safety of tranexamic acid in orthotopic liver transplantation clinical practice: a propensity score matched cohort study. Transplantation. 2017;101(7):1658–65. https://doi.org/10.1097/TP.0000000000001682.

Liberal vs. Conservative Blood Strategies

26

Lisa Farmer, Deepinder S. Mann, and Donald S. Prough

Abbreviations

AABB	American Association of Blood Banks
ASA	American Society of Anesthesiologists
ATLS	Advanced Trauma Life Support
DO_2	Delivery oxygen
ECG	Electrocardiogram
ESA	Erythropoietic-stimulating agents
FDA	Food and Drug Administration
FOCUS	Functional Outcomes in Cardiovascular patients Undergoing Surgical Repair
Hgb	Hemoglobin
ICP	Intracranial pressure
NISHOT	Noninfectious serious hazards of transfusions
O_2	Oxygen
PPH	Postpartum hemorrhage
RBC	Red blood cell
SCA	Society of Cardiovascular Anesthesiologists
STS	Society of Thoracic Surgeons
TAXI	Transfusion and Anemia Expertise Initiative
TBI	Traumatic brain injury
TIPS	Transjugular intrahepatic portosystemic shunt
TXA	Tranexamic acid
TITR	Transfusion Indication Threshold Reduction
TRACS	Transfusion Requirements After Cardiac Surgery
TRiCS	Transfusion Requirements in Cardiac Surgery
VO_2	Oxygen consumption

L. Farmer (✉) · D. S. Mann · D. S. Prough
Department of Anesthesiology, The University of Texas Medical Branch at Galveston, Galveston, TX, USA
e-mail: lrfarmer@utmb.edu; dsmann@utmb.edu; dsprough@utmb.edu

Introduction

Historically, the standard approach to anemia in a hospitalized patient was to treat liberally with allogenic blood transfusions to maintain a hemoglobin ([Hgb]) exceeding 10 g/dL, i.e., the customary transfusion trigger was 10 g/dL. The safety of a more conservative approach was suggested by normovolemic hemodilution studies of the late 1990s which established that healthy, elderly, and stable cardiac patients compensated for severe anemia without increases in serum lactate, suggesting that tissue oxygenation remained adequate as long as intravascular volume was maintained [1]. Multiple studies report that allogenic blood transfusions are both risky to patients and costly to hospitals [2, 3]. In fact, mortality increases in a dose-dependent manner with each intraoperative red blood cell (RBC) unit transfused [4]. Thus, if outcomes are similar, a conservative strategy with a more restrictive transfusion trigger is recommended for most patient populations.

Reducing unnecessary blood transfusions through application of appropriate restrictive transfusion strategies has become the standard of care [5]. Numerous randomized controlled trials have shown that restrictive transfusion triggers are safe for most hemodynamically stable, nonbleeding patients [6]. Over the last 20 years, transfusion guidelines from multiple international societies, including the Society of Cardiovascular Anesthesiologists (SCA) and the Society of Thoracic Surgeons (STS), recommend restrictive transfusion strategies with a [Hgb] threshold of 7 g/dL in asymptomatic patients [6–10]. A higher [Hgb] threshold of 8 g/dL is suggested for postoperative patients, hospitalized patients with preexisting cardiovascular disease, and symptomatic patients with chest pain, congestive heart failure, orthostatic hypotension, or tachycardia unresponsive to fluid resuscitation [1]. For patients with acute coronary syndrome, recommendations differ, although most guidelines support a restrictive transfusion trigger between 7 g/dL and 9 g/dL [8, 10–12].

© Springer Nature Switzerland AG 2021
C. S. Scher et al. (eds.), *Essentials of Blood Product Management in Anesthesia Practice*,
https://doi.org/10.1007/978-3-030-59295-0_26

It is important to note that guidelines from most societies target hemodynamically stable patients without significant ongoing bleeding [6]. There is not enough evidence to support either restrictive or liberal transfusion strategies in unstable patients or in patients with active bleeding, although patients with active gastrointestinal bleeding and those with hemorrhagic shock have been studied most extensively [13]. Patients with hemorrhagic shock should be transfused empirically with RBCs, plasma, and platelets in fixed ratios until life-threatening bleeding is controlled.

As frontline administrators of blood products, anesthesiologists are thought to be involved in almost half of the decisions to transfuse the 21 million blood components used annually [14]. The American Society of Anesthesiologists (ASA) generally support restrictive transfusion practices, defined as a [Hgb] threshold of less than 8 g/dL, and report that the decision to transfuse should be based on a patient's generalized risk of developing complications from inadequate tissue oxygenation as opposed to a single [Hgb] trigger [15, 16]. Since initial guidelines were published in 1996, the ASA has agreed that transfusions are rarely indicated when [Hgb] is greater than 10 g/dL and is usually indicated when [Hgb] <6 g/dL [17]. Unfortunately, the ASA and other international societies are unable to give clear [Hgb] thresholds for patients at risk for tissue hypoxia and end-organ dysfunction in the acute care setting [18].

Anemia is common, affecting 20–40% of surgical patients and is a strong predictor of perioperative transfusions [19]. Perioperative anemia is an independent predictor of worsened patient outcomes, including increased length of hospital and ICU stay, and is associated with increased risk of postoperative complications and mortality [3, 20]. The combination of perioperative anemia and intraoperative blood transfusions further increases morbidity and mortality. It is unclear which factors cause the risks of acute anemia to exceed the risks associated with allogenic blood transfusions, especially for high-risk patients with ongoing blood loss. The challenge is to differentiate patients who will benefit from conservative transfusion strategies from those that will be compromised by them, and thus not benefit from the procedure.

Under normal physiologic conditions, systemic oxygen (O_2) delivery (DO_2) exceeds O_2 consumption (VO_2) in a 5:1 ratio creating a positive O_2 reserve [18, 21]. In anemic patients, compensatory mechanisms allow for increased cardiac output, right shifting of the oxyhemoglobin dissociation curve, and altered regional blood flow to increase O_2 extraction and maintain tissue DO_2 [3]. Surgical stressors and anesthetic medications lead to multiple factors that disrupt normal O_2 supply-demand, which influence patients' tolerance to and compensation for anemia. For example, hypoventilatory hypoxia, common perioperatively, compromises DO_2 at the same time that surgical trauma and pain increases VO_2. Anesthetic drugs can reduce cardiac contractility and cause widespread vasodilation, limiting the patient's ability to increase DO_2 via increased cardiac output and altered regional blood flow. Hypotension, intravascular volume changes, and increased catecholamines, all of which are common perioperatively, further limit blood flow to vital organs. Clinicians must incorporate available indicators of DO_2 into the decision to transfuse [22].

Traditional neurologic, cardiovascular, and respiratory features of tissue hypoxia are masked during general anesthesia. Unstable vital signs can result from anesthetic side effects or surgical manipulation, making it difficult to determine the primary driver of changes in heart rate, blood pressure, and electrocardiogram. Furthermore, inadequate tissue perfusion is possible despite normal blood pressure and heart rate [23]. Hypovolemia can result from ongoing perioperative losses or from relative changes in systemic vasodilation associated with anesthesia. Tissue hypoxia secondary to hypovolemia is readily reversed by restoration of intravascular volume. Assessing the heart rate, blood pressure, urinary output, and laboratory response to fluid challenges provide partial information. Intermittent boluses of vasopressors can temporize severe hypotension during ongoing volume resuscitation, but careful evaluation of intravascular volume is necessary to assure end-organ perfusion is maintained.

Intraoperative Transfusion Strategies

When choosing between conservative and liberal transfusion strategies, it is important to consider the clinical context including both surgical type and patient comorbidities. In 2016, Hovaguiman and Myles [18] performed a meta-analysis on 31 randomized controlled trials in which they grouped patients into five context-specific strata. In patients with cardiovascular disease undergoing cardiac or vascular procedures and in elderly patients undergoing orthopedic procedures, application of restrictive transfusion strategies resulted in increased "inadequate O_2 supply" events and/or mortality. Application of restrictive transfusion triggers in acute care, medical-surgical patients and in younger patients with subarachnoid bleeding or traumatic brain injury showed similar outcomes to the liberal transfusion group. This suggests an approach to perioperative transfusions that "one size may not fit all" [24]. More research is needed to identify which high-risk patients will do better with a less conservative approach.

During anesthesia a primary goal is to maintain adequate tissue perfusion and DO_2. DO_2 is dependent on multiple physiologic parameters other than [Hgb]. Clinicians should strive to reduce O_2 demand and optimize heart rate, rhythm, contractility, preload, and afterload before deciding to transfuse except in the case of hemorrhagic shock [25].

Intravascular deficits should be treated with crystalloid administration and anesthesia-related vasodilation with vasopressors. The decision to transfuse must be based on multiple factors including the potential for or actual ongoing bleeding, intravascular volume status, signs of organ ischemia, and the adequacy of cardiopulmonary reserve [15]. Each of these factors is challenging to measure, requires astute clinical judgment to interpret, and is more subjective than an arbitrary [Hgb]. Integration of patient data through vigilance and meticulous monitoring is key in determining when transfusions are necessary during surgery.

Estimating blood loss is a critical step in transfusion decisions but better techniques are necessary to improve accuracy with its measure. Multiple reports show that estimation of blood loss is difficult, frequently inaccurate, and inconsistent among nurses, surgeons, and anesthesiologists [26, 27]. The rate, magnitude, and potential for ongoing bleeding must also be considered. The definition of massive hemorrhage varies but generally includes one of the following criteria: need for >10 units of red blood cells, loss of ≥one blood volume in 24 hours, loss of ≥50% of blood volume in 3 hours, or blood loss ≥150 mL/min.

The Advanced Trauma Life Support (ATLS) identifies four classes of hemorrhage based on estimated blood loss, as shown in Table 26.1 [28, 29]. Class I hemorrhage involves loss of 15% of blood volume and results in minimal hemodynamic changes. Class II involves loss of 15–30% of blood volume and results in tachycardia without a change in systolic blood pressure. It is important to note that pulse pressure will begin to narrow with loss of 15–30% of blood volume as diastolic blood pressure increases to maintain tissue perfusion [28]. Increased diastolic blood pressure and a base deficit of −2 to −6 mEq/L may be the first marker of ongoing blood loss and ensuing metabolic acidosis [29]. Class II hemorrhage is usually effectively corrected with fluid administration although transfusion maybe indicated if the patient has preexisting anemia or cardiovascular disease. Class III hemorrhage involves loss of 30–40% of blood volume resulting in significant tachycardia (HR 120–140 bpm), hypotension, base deficit of −6 to −10 mEq/L, and oliguria. Blood loss of >40% of estimated blood volume defines Class IV hemorrhage and results in marked tachycardia (HR >140), severe hypotension, base deficit greater than −10 mEq/L, and anuria. Immediate transfusion of blood and blood products is indicated for Class III or IV hemorrhage to restore intravascular volume, maintain DO_2, and prevent development of coagulopathy [29].

Table 26.1 Advanced trauma life support classes of hemorrhage [29, 30]

	Class I	Class II	Class III	Class IV
Blood loss %	<15	15–30	30–40	>40
Pulse rate	<100	100–120	120–140	>140
Blood pressure	No change	No change	Decreased	Greatly decreased
Pulse pressure	Normal to increased	Decreased	Decreased	Decreased
Urinary output (ml/hr)	>30	20–30	5–15	Minimal
Base deficit (mEq/L)	0 to −2	−2 to −6	−6 to −10	−10 or less
Blood products needed	Unlikely	Possible	Yes	Activate massive transfusion protocol

Estimating intravascular blood volume is challenging due to inaccuracies of intraoperative blood loss measurements, intercompartmental fluid shifts, and the dilutional effects of crystalloid administration [17]. Meticulous monitoring for vital organ perfusion and clinical indications of tissue hypoxia is key in assessing the intravascular volume status of surgical patients. Preoperative evaluation of volume status with careful attention to conditions associated with increased volume losses, diuretic use, and duration of preoperative fasting is important in pre-surgical patients. The blood pressure and heart rate response to anesthesia induction, blood loss, and fluid administration are common metrics used to estimate volume status. Urinary output of at least 0.5 mL/kg/h is a sign of adequate intravascular volume and adequate renal perfusion. Non-invasive cardiac output monitors and assessment of cardiac chamber size with echocardiography provide a more objective measure of fluid responsiveness. Invasive pressure measures such as stroke volume or pulse pressure variation or trends in central venous pressure or pulmonary arterial occlusion pressure should be used as needed to respond to the dynamic volume changes associated with surgery and anesthesia [23].

Hypovolemia is associated with labile blood pressure during anesthesia and exaggerated changes in [Hgb] with fluid administration. After transfusion and without ongoing blood loss, euvolemic adults should have a 1 g/dL rise in [Hgb] for every unit of RBCs given. Of note, 10 ml/kg of RBCs will produce similar effects in children. Hypovolemic patients will have larger than expected increases in [Hgb] with each unit of RBCs transfused and conversely will have greater dilution of [Hgb] with fluid administration.

The critical [Hgb] required for each patient varies inversely with cardiovascular reserve [30]. Clinicians must consider a patient's comorbidities, response to fluid administration, and need for vasoactive medications to determine cardiopulmonary reserve. Transfusion is usually not necessary when a patient is able to compensate for acute anemia without signs of tissue hypoxia. High-risk patients with low cardiopulmonary reserve do not tolerate the combination of acute anemia and impaired compensatory response. The increase in cardiac output and heart rate required to compensate for anemia in these patients cause increased myocardial O_2 demands.

Transfusions may be necessary before laboratory measurements of [Hgb] during acute intraoperative bleeding. During acute blood loss, [Hgb] will be normal or misleadingly high unless substantial volumes of asanguineous fluids have been administered, making [Hgb] a less accurate trigger for transfusion. To guide transfusions, the clinician must continuously assess the operative field, hemodynamic response to volume administration, and laboratory values. Meticulous monitoring for signs of tissue hypoxia, such as unstable vital signs, ECG changes, echocardiographic wall motion abnormalities, cerebral oximetry, new onset of oliguria, metabolic acidosis, elevated base excess, or increased serum lactate, is key to optimize end-organ perfusion. The best intraoperative monitoring technique and optimal physiologic metrics and biomarkers needed to establish individual transfusion thresholds have not been identified in adult or pediatric patients [15, 25].

Comprehensive Conservative Strategies

Conservative transfusion strategies are preferred if tissue perfusion and DO_2 can be maintained. This is only possible with a more comprehensive approach to anemia and perioperative bleeding. After implementing broad-based restrictive transfusion strategies, multiple institutions have reported a significant decrease in blood utilization and have shown similar to improved outcomes for patients in restrictive transfusion groups compared to those in liberal groups [31–34].

Careful preoperative assessment is necessary to identify potential for organ ischemia and risk factors for bleeding [15, 19]. Cardiopulmonary reserve should be optimized to improve tolerance to acute anemia and anesthesia. Whenever possible, anticoagulant and antiplatelet drugs should be stopped early enough to allow their effects to dissipate. If identified early, preoperative anemia is a modifiable risk, but effective management requires screening 4–8 weeks preoperatively to allow time to regenerate RBC mass. Treatment of preoperative anemia should be considered for all high-risk patients undergoing major elective procedures, especially if the procedure is associated with a >10% likelihood of needing a blood transfusion [13, 35].

Intraoperatively, every attempt should be made to minimize blood loss and improve the patient's tolerance to anemia, such that restrictive transfusion triggers can be utilized and transfusions avoided. Goal-directed fluid therapy and appropriate use of inotropic and vasoactive drugs is important to assure adequate DO_2 during surgery. Meticulous attention to hemostasis is the job of both the surgeon and the anesthesiologist. Surgical technique and appropriate use of hemostatic agents are key determinants of perioperative blood loss [19]. ASA practice guidelines for perioperative blood management recommend using multimodal protocols and algorithms to decrease bleeding whenever possible [15]. Aggressively treating hypothermia, acidosis, and hypocalcemia is critical to facilitate clot formation; otherwise this triad creates a vicious cycle, prolonging surgery and increasing blood loss. Additional techniques to minimize blood loss may include maintaining the blood pressure at the lowest safe level, lowering of central venous pressure, and careful positioning [19].

Prophylactic use of cell saver and antifibrinolytics for patients at risk for excessive bleeding is advocated. Hemostasis requires adequate presence of coagulation factors, platelets, and fibrinogen to produce a stable clot. Use of point-of-care testing such as viscoelastic monitoring to guide fresh frozen plasma, platelets, cryoprecipitate, factor concentrates, and antifibrinolytic drugs is recommended and has been shown to significantly reduce transfusion requirements [15].

Application of conservative transfusion strategies are also advocated in the postoperative period. Use of iron to treat postoperative iron deficiency will improve the patient's tolerance to anemia, as symptoms frequently resolve prior to regeneration of RBC mass once iron stores have been replaced [5]. Post-operative blood loss can be significantly reduced by minimizing laboratory tests and using low-volume collection tubes. A comprehensive approach to anemia and meticulous control of blood loss are required to minimize transfusion and improve patient outcomes.

The remainder of this chapter will focus on outcomes of liberal versus conservative transfusion strategies in specific high-risk patient populations.

Transfusion Strategies in Cardiac Surgery

Cardiac surgery is frequently associated with significant blood loss, and patients undergoing cardiac surgery have limited cardiopulmonary reserve due to common high-risk comorbidities. The STS Adult Cardiac Surgery Database notes that 50% of patients undergoing cardiac procedures receive blood transfusions [12]. The 2010 Transfusion Requirements After Cardiac Surgery (TRACS) study found that transfusions were an independent risk factor for morbidity and mortality in this patient population [36]. These finding are supported by several other retrospective studies and systematic reviews. For example, patients undergoing coronary artery bypass grafting experienced an increase risk of death and pneumonia after high amounts of RBC transfusions [37, 38]. Of course, during acute hemorrhage associated with cardiac surgery, RBC transfusions can be lifesaving by providing increased O_2-carrying capacity and improved microcirculation [39].

TRACS documented the safety of restrictive transfusion strategies after cardiopulmonary bypass, showing no difference in the 30-day mortality between patients transfused to a restrictive goal ([Hgb] >8 g/dL, hematocrit >24%) versus liberal ([Hgb] >10 g/dL, hematocrit >30%). In 2015, the safety of restrictive strategies in cardiac surgery was questioned when the Transfusion Indication Threshold Reduction (TITRe2) clinical trial reported a significantly increased 90-day mortality in the restrictive group compared to the liberal group [40]. In 2017 the Transfusion Requirements in Cardiac Surgery III (TRiCS III) trial concluded that for patients at moderate to high risk of death, application of a restrictive strategy ([Hgb] threshold <7.5 g/dL) was non-inferior to a liberal strategy for outcomes including death and major disability (myocardial infarction, stroke, or new-onset renal failure with dialysis). These outcomes were achieved with less blood being transfused [41]. The current international consensus on evidence-based patient blood management strongly recommend a restrictive transfusion trigger of [Hgb] <7.5 g/dL for patients undergoing cardiac surgery [13].

[Hgb] is not the only indication for blood transfusion in this population. All cardiac surgery patients are at risk for both tissue hypoxia from anemia and worsened outcomes secondary to blood transfusions. Current STS and SCA guidelines for patients with [Hgb] between 7 and 10 g/dL undergoing cardiac surgery recommend transfusion in patients with "critical noncardiac end-organ ischemia," active blood loss, or clinical indication of tissue hypoxia [7]. Low mixed venous O_2 saturation or electrocardiographic or echocardiographic evidence of myocardial ischemia is defined as an indication of tissue hypoxia.

Treatment of preoperative anemia can be challenging in cardiac surgery patients due to the urgency of the procedure and US Food and Drug Administration (FDA) restrictions against use of erythropoietic-stimulating agents (ESAs) in cardiac and vascular surgery [31]. Implementing a variety of other conservative strategies including meticulous surgical hemostasis, use of antifibrinolytic agents, thromboelastographic guided coagulation algorithms, postoperative use of intravenous iron, and application of restrictive transfusion thresholds result in decreased number of transfusions, less kidney injury, shorter length of hospital stays, and lower costs [31].

Transfusion Strategies in Orthopedic Surgery

Although a [Hgb] threshold of 7 g/dL appears safe for most asymptomatic orthopedic patients, the current American Association of Blood Banks (AABB) guidelines for RBC transfusions recommend a restrictive [Hgb] trigger of 8 g/dL for this population [6, 32]. Hip fracture patients represent a vulnerable orthopedic population as most are elderly and have cardiovascular disease or other comorbidities associated with decreased cardiovascular reserve. In 2011, the Functional Outcomes in Cardiovascular patients Undergoing Surgical repair (FOCUS) trial assessed hip fracture patients who were over 50 years of age and had a history of either cardiovascular disease, diabetes, peripheral vascular disease, or smoking. Restrictive strategies were found non-inferior to liberal strategies regarding 30-and-60 day mortality and morbidity [42]. The current international consensus on evidence-based patient blood management concludes that high-risk hip fracture patients who are treated with restrictive transfusion triggers have similar critical outcomes to patients transfused liberally [13]. Another benefit of restrictive strategies in this population is that 42% fewer patients receive transfusions in the restrictive transfusion group ([Hgb] trigger <8 g/dL) compared to the liberal threshold groups [13]. Symptomatic anemia, defined as chest pain, congestive heart failure, tachycardia, or hypotension unresponsive to fluid, should be used as criteria for transfusion even when [Hgb] >8 g/dL [32, 42].

A variety of conservative transfusion strategies have been studied in orthopedic surgery. Use of tranexamic acid in hip and knee arthroplasty is instrumental at reducing overall blood loss and transfusion requirements, especially if given prior to tourniquet deflation [15]. Identification and effective management of preoperative anemia is advocated for elective major orthopedic procedures [13]. Anesthetic techniques such as maintenance of normothermia and controlled hypotension can decrease blood loss. Regional anesthesia, especially in major joint surgery, can significantly reduce perioperative blood loss [43]. Reducing perioperative blood loss in total knee arthroplasty has additional benefits, such as decreased intra-articular hemorrhage, limb swelling, postoperative pain, and increased range of motion leading to improved rehabilitation and patient satisfaction [44].

Transfusion Strategies in the Pediatric Population

Pediatric anemia is common, occurring in up to 75% of critically ill children, resulting in almost half of PICU patients receiving a blood transfusion if admitted for more than 48 hours [45]. The risks of anemia and transfusions differ in pediatric patients. Children appear to tolerate anemia better than adult populations as they typically do not have flow limiting lesions that jeopardize DO_2 to vital organs. However, noninfectious serious hazards of transfusions (NISHOT), in particular transfusion-associated lung injury and transfusion-associated circulatory overload, are much more prevalent in critically ill children for unclear reasons [25]. In fact, RBC transfusion is an independent risk factor for mortality in critically ill children [46].

In critically ill, hemodynamically stable children, a restrictive transfusion strategy is non-inferior to a liberal transfusion strategy and reduces exposure to blood products, making restrictive strategies preferred during periods of hemodynamic stability [25]. The 2007 Transfusion Requirements in the Pediatric Intensive Care Unit (TRIPICU) study was a multicenter, randomized controlled trial that compared restrictive ([Hgb] ≤ 7 g/dL) to liberal ([Hgb] ≤ 9.5 g/dL) transfusion thresholds in critically ill children. TRIPICU reported similar rates of multi-organ dysfunction in both groups, although restrictive practices reduced transfusion frequency by half [47]. A study of acute pediatric burn patients found that a restrictive transfusion group ([Hgb] <7 g/dL) had significantly lower mortality than a liberal transfusion group ([Hgb] <10 g/dL) [48].

Despite the benefits of reduced RBC transfusions in children, pediatric intensivists have been slow to adopt restrictive practices [25]. There is limited evidence to guide transfusion decisions in critically ill hemodynamically unstable patients, defined as mean arterial pressure greater than 2 standard deviations below normal mean for age or an increase in cardiovascular support (vasoactive drugs or fluids) over the last 2 hours [47]. Likewise, there is lack of evidence to guide transfusion strategies for critically ill children undergoing surgical procedures, especially for medically fragile patients with complicated physiology [45].

The 2018 Pediatric Critical Care Transfusion and Anemia Expertise Initiative (TAXI) brought together international, multidisciplinary experts to address different types of critically ill children, including those with non-hemorrhagic and hemorrhagic shock, non-life-threatening bleeding, and traumatic brain injury [25]. Consensus of >80% was reached for each recommendation, including the need to consider the overall clinical context (symptoms, signs, physiologic markers, laboratory results) and the risks, benefits, and alternatives when deciding to transfuse. The use of physiologic-based metrics and biomarkers of DO_2 are recommended, but the experts could not give guidance on thresholds or priorities of these measures to inform transfusion decisions. More research is needed to identify biomarkers and/or physiologic measures that suggest intolerance to anemia and indicate a patient-specific likelihood of transfusion benefit.

Figure 26.1 represents an RBC transfusion clinical decision support tree that summarizes the TAXI recommendations for critically ill children [25]. [Hgb] should be measured before transfusion unless a patient has life-threatening bleeding. Transfusion is recommended for [Hgb] <5 g/dL and should be considered if [Hgb] is between 5 and 7 g/dL in general or during periods of non-life-threatening bleeding. For acute brain injury patients, transfusion should be considered for [Hgb] between 7 and 10 g/dL. Due to inadequate evidence, TAXI could not recommend for or against the use of brain O_2 monitoring to guide transfusion decisions. During non-hemorrhagic shock, all strategies to augment DO_2 and decrease O_2 demands should be considered before transfusion. TAXI recommended not transfusing patients who are hemodynamically stable with a [Hgb] >7 g/dL. The post transfusion goal should be to relieve the indication for transfusion as opposed to achievement of a certain [Hgb]. During hemorrhagic shock, empiric ratios of RBCs, plasma, and platelets should be given until bleeding is controlled as children with life-threatening hemorrhage have >50% mortality [45].

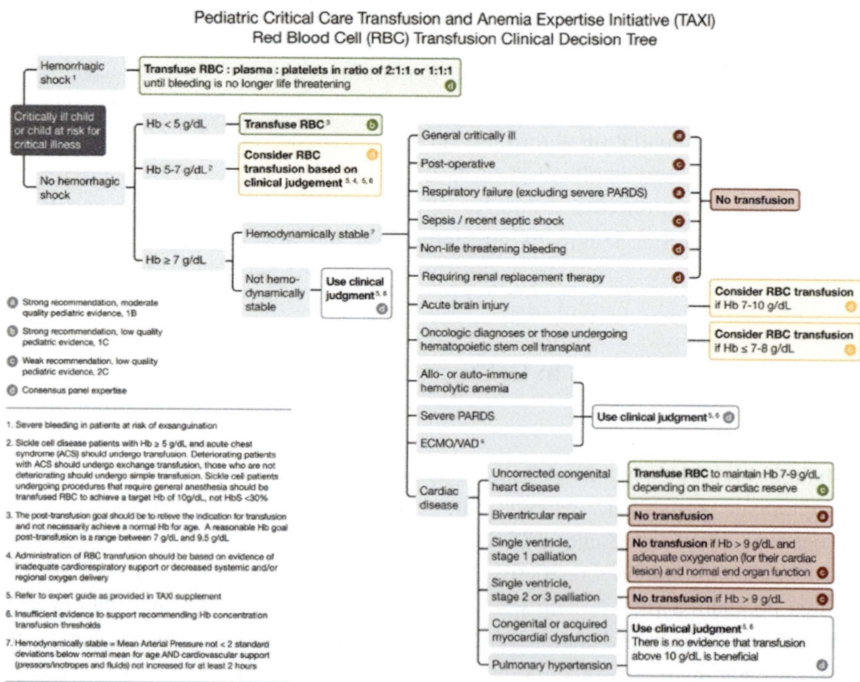

Fig. 26.1 Pediatric critical care Transfusion and Anemia Expertise Initiative (TAXI). Red Blood Cell (RBC) Transfusion Clinical Decision Tree. Transfusion and Anemia Expertise Initiative (TAXI) RBC transfusion decision tree for critically ill children. ACS acute chest syndrome, ECMO extracorporeal membrane oxygenation, Hb hemoglobin, HbS Hb S, PARDS pediatric acute respiratory distress syndrome, VAD ventricular assist device. (With permission from Valentine et al. [25])

Transfusion Strategies in the Obstetric Population

Maternal anemia is common and is associated with increased premature delivery and worsened child morality [49]. Multiple physiologic changes occur during pregnancy to assure adequate DO_2 to the parturient and developing fetus. These include increased maternal 2, 3-diphosphoglycerate, plasma volume, red cells, and cardiac output. Dilutional anemia develops as the increase in plasma volume exceeds that of red cell mass. Oral iron and folic acid supplementation, both of which are part of routine antenatal care, help the parturient tolerate anemia and avoid the associated adverse outcomes.

Physiologic changes provide a compensatory reserve that allows the parturient to tolerate the acute blood loss commonly associated with delivery [50]. Post-delivery changes of increased peripheral resistance and hemoconcentration help maintain blood pressure and further reduce the need for transfusion [50]. Despite this compensatory reserve, approximately 1% of women receive a blood transfusion after spontaneous vaginal delivery and 5–6% after instrumental deliveries or cesarean sections [51]. Pregnancy, especially when accompanied by preeclampsia, is associated with increased risk of transfusion reactions [52].

There is considerable variability in transfusion guidelines among international obstetric societies, likely due to the lack of clear evidence specific for obstetric patients regarding safety of conservative transfusion strategies. Most societies recommend transfusing based on the degree of blood loss even though there are well-known inaccuracies in peripartum blood loss measurements especially at higher volumes [49]. Hancock et al. [53] found that improved accuracy of blood loss measurement did not result in earlier identification of postpartum hemorrhage (PPH). Clinicians must assess vital signs and severity of bleeding to determine when transfusion is indicated. A high suspicion for PPH as well as a standardized approach to patients at risk for hemorrhage is needed. These may include preemptive blood ordering, emergency release of blood products, and massive transfusion protocols.

PPH is a leading cause of maternal death after childbirth. At term, uterine blood flow is approximately 5 liters per minute, which can result in a high rate of blood loss. Clinicians must maintain a high index of suspicion for PPH in order to recognize and treat it quickly. A 2017 Cochrane review of the efficacy of antifibrinolytic drugs for treating primary PPH found that intravenous tranexamic acid (TXA) reduces risk of maternal death from bleeding if given early, ideally 1–3 hours after childbirth, although it did not reduce the risk of serious bleeding or need for blood transfusion. The use of TXA was not associated with increased risk of thromboembolic events in this population [54].

Strategies to reduce unnecessary transfusions in the obstetric population include treatment of preoperative anemia, decreasing iatrogenic blood loss, optimization of hemostasis, and establishment of transfusion thresholds [49]. Anemia and iron deficiency, common in the postpartum period, are associated with decreased exercise tolerance, impaired lactation, reduced cognitive performance, emotional instability, and depression all of which can interfere with maternal baby bonding. Treatment with iron may protect against these negative effects [49]. Adequate fibrinogen necessary to optimize hemostasis during obstetric hemorrhage varies between 100 and 200 mg/dL depending on the obstetric society guideline [49]. Additional research focused on context-specific indicators of volume status and tissue O_2 delivery in obstetric patients, especially as it applies to maternal hemorrhage, is needed to determine the safety of restrictive versus liberal transfusion practices in the obstetric population.

Transfusion Strategies in GI Bleeding

Upper gastrointestinal bleeding is a very common cause of acute blood loss and therefore a very common cause for transfusion. For patients who are not experiencing massive exsanguination, a [Hgb] transfusion trigger <7 g/dL has been shown to be superior to a liberal threshold <9 g/dL. A key trial from 2013 found most patients in the restrictive group had lower 45-day mortality, fewer rebleeding events, fewer cardiac complications, and shorter hospital stays compared to a liberal group. Importantly, patients with Child-Pugh class C cirrhosis did not see the mortality benefit [55]. Currently, for bleeding varices, the American Association for the Study of Liver Disease recommends transfusing when [Hgb] approaches 7 g/dL with a goal of maintaining between 7 and 9 g/dL [56]. Additional strategies to reduce bleeding and keep patients above transfusion triggers include early use of vasoactive drugs (e.g., octreotide or vasopressin), early esophagogastroduodenectomy, and the use of transjugular intrahepatic portosystemic shunt (TIPS) in selected patients [57].

Geriatrics

In the general geriatric population, the prevalence of anemia may be as high as 25%. The elderly are the most common group to receive transfusions for anemia treatment. There is some evidence that the presence of anemia, independent of other comorbidities, can be a risk factor for the development of dementia and rapid cognitive decline [58]. The mechanism for this is unknown. Chronic hypoxia and systemic effects from micronutrient deficiency are two possible explanations for this association [59]. Other researchers have not found a link between anemia and delirium [60]. Currently, it is unknown whether simply being a geriatric patient necessitates either liberal or conservative transfusion thresholds.

Neurologic Injury

For many acute neurological injuries, patients presenting with anemia is an independent and significant predictor of poor outcomes [61, 62]. Adequate O_2 delivery is key during the early phases of brain injury. However, during these events normal brain auto-regulation is suspected to be altered. For many common injuries (including acute stroke, intracerebral hemorrhage, and subarachnoid hemorrhage), several studies have found harm or no benefit to liberal transfusion goals compared to restrictive [61, 63–66].

Traumatic brain injury (TBI) is the most common cause of death in the first half of life, and many survivors are left with permanent impairment. More than 1/3 of patients with TBIs are transfused. Extra-cerebral injuries are the most common precipitator of transfusion. Not only is auto-regulation affected, but there is also concern that even mild anemia may cause vasodilation and thereby increase intracranial pressure in these patients [67].

Many trials have included small numbers of TBI patients; however, there is not enough information for a clear consensus whether liberal or restrictive transfusions strategies are superior. A clinician survey found most medical providers felt a threshold between 7 and 8 g/dL was best for acute brain injury in general. When it came to TBIs, however, there were nearly an equal number of responders in all groups between 7 and 10 g/dL [68]. There is also disagreement if those presenting with high ICPs might have different thresholds. A multicenter, randomized controlled trial (HEMOTION trial) may shed light on this area in the future (results expected in 2021) [69].

Patients who develop intracerebral hemorrhage while treated with antiplatelet drugs can have worse outcomes compared to patients with normal platelet function. The role of platelet transfusion has been investigated in this population. In a recent trial, platelet transfusion was associated with greater disability at 3 months than in those who did not receive platelets [70]. This study excluded patients with platelet counts <100,000/L, and there was a relatively low rate of acute strokes in the trial. The role of platelet function tests to selectively choose who might benefit from transfusion is ongoing [71]. Some experts suggest avoiding platelet administration unless a surgical intervention is planned regardless of what antiplatelet agent the patient has taken [72].

References

1. Auron M, Duran Castillo MY, Kumar A. Parsimonious blood use and lower transfusion triggers: what is the evidence? Cleve Clin J Med. 2017;84(1):43–51. Epub 2017/01/14.
2. Shander A, Hofmann A, Ozawa S, Theusinger OM, Gombotz H, Spahn DR. Activity-based costs of blood transfusions in surgical patients at four hospitals. Transfusion. 2010;50(4):753–65. Epub 2009/12/17.
3. Shander A, Javidroozi M, Ozawa S, Hare GM. What is really dangerous: Anaemia or transfusion? Br J Anaesth. 2011;107(Suppl 1):i41–59. Epub 2011/12/22.
4. Johnson DJ, Scott AV, Barodka VM, Park S, Wasey JO, Ness PM, et al. Morbidity and mortality after high-dose transfusion. Anesthesiology. 2016;124(2):387–95. Epub 2015/11/17.
5. Shander A, Bracey AW Jr, Goodnough LT, Gross I, Hassan NE, Ozawa S, et al. Patient blood management as standard of care. Anesth Analg. 2016;123(4):1051–3. Epub 2016/09/20.
6. Carson JL, Guyatt G, Heddle NM, Grossman BJ, Cohn CS, Fung MK, et al. Clinical practice guidelines from the AABB: red blood cell transfusion thresholds and storage. JAMA. 2016;316(19):2025–35. Epub 2016/10/13.
7. Society of Thoracic Surgeons Blood Conservation Guideline Task F, Ferraris VA, Brown JR, Despotis GJ, Hammon JW, Reece TB, et al. 2011 Update to the Society of Thoracic Surgeons and the Society of Cardiovascular Anesthesiologists blood conservation clinical practice guidelines. Ann Thorac Surg. 2011;91(3):944–82. Epub 2011/03/01.
8. Retter A, Wyncoll D, Pearse R, Carson D, McKechnie S, Stanworth S, et al. Guidelines on the management of anaemia and red cell transfusion in adult critically ill patients. Br J Haematol. 2013;160(4):445–64. Epub 2013/01/03.
9. Napolitano LM, Kurek S, Luchette FA, Corwin HL, Barie PS, Tisherman SA, et al. Clinical practice guideline: red blood cell transfusion in adult trauma and critical care. Crit Care Med. 2009;37(12):3124–57. Epub 2009/09/24.
10. National Blood Authority. Patient blood management guidelines: module 3 – medical: quick reference guide. Canberra, Australia: National Blood Authority, 2012. https://www.blood.gov.au/system/files/documents/20180426-Module3-QRG.pdf.
11. Hamm CW, Bassand JP, Agewall S, Bax J, Boersma E, Bueno H, et al. ESC Guidelines for the management of acute coronary syndromes in patients presenting without persistent ST-segment elevation: The Task Force for the management of acute coronary syndromes (ACS) in patients presenting without persistent ST-segment elevation of the European Society of Cardiology (ESC). Eur Heart J. 2011;32(23):2999–3054. Epub 2011/08/30.
12. Qaseem A, Humphrey LL, Fitterman N, Starkey M, Shekelle P, Clinical Guidelines Committee of the American College of Physicians. Treatment of anemia in patients with heart disease: a clinical practice guideline from the American College of Physicians. Ann Intern Med. 2013;159(11):770–9. Epub 2013/12/04.
13. Mueller MM, Van Remoortel H, Meybohm P, Aranko K, Aubron C, Burger R, et al. Patient blood management: recommendations from the 2018 Frankfurt consensus conference. JAMA. 2019;321(10):983–97. Epub 2019/03/13.
14. Wanderer JP, Rathmell JP. Perioperative transfusion: a complicated story. Anesthesiology. 2015;122(1):A23. Epub 2015/01/23.
15. American Society of Anesthesiologists Task Force on Perioperative Blood M. Practice guidelines for perioperative blood management: an updated report by the American Society of Anesthesiologists Task Force on Perioperative Blood Management*. Anesthesiology. 2015;122(2):241–75. Epub 2014/12/30.
16. Practice guidelines for perioperative blood transfusion and adjuvant therapies: an updated report by the American Society of Anesthesiologists Task Force on Perioperative Blood Transfusion and Adjuvant Therapies. Anesthesiology. 2006;105(1):198–208.
17. Practice Guidelines for blood component therapy: a report by the American Society of Anesthesiologists Task Force on Blood Component Therapy. Anesthesiology. 1996;84(3):732–47. Epub 1996/03/01.
18. Hovaguimian F, Myles PS. Restrictive versus liberal transfusion strategy in the perioperative and acute care settings: a context-specific systematic review and meta-analysis of randomized controlled trials. Anesthesiology. 2016;125(1):46–61. Epub 2016/05/12.

19. Thakrar SV, Clevenger B, Mallett S. Patient blood management and perioperative anaemia. BJA Education. 2017;17(1):28–34. Epub 2017.
20. Musallam KM, Tamim HM, Richards T, Spahn DR, Rosendaal FR, Habbal A, et al. Preoperative anaemia and postoperative outcomes in non-cardiac surgery: a retrospective cohort study. Lancet. 2011;378(9800):1396–407. Epub 2011/10/11.
21. Englesbe MJ, Pelletier SJ, Diehl KM, Sung RS, Wahl WL, Punch J, et al. Transfusions in surgical patients. J Am Coll Surg. 2005;200(2):249–54. Epub 2005/01/25.
22. Yazer MH, Triulzi DJ. AABB red blood cell transfusion guidelines: something for almost everyone. JAMA. 2016;316(19):1984–5. Epub 2016/10/13.
23. Teirney P, Ahmed B, Nichol A. Shock: causes, initial assessment and investigations. Anaesth Intensive Care Med. 2017;18(3):118–21.
24. Wanderer JPR, J.P. Perioperative and acute care transfusion strategies: one size may not fit all. Anesthesiology. 2016;125(1):A21.
25. Valentine SL, Bembea MM, Muszynski JA, Cholette JM, Doctor A, Spinella PC, et al. Consensus recommendations for rbc transfusion practice in critically ill children from the pediatric critical care transfusion and anemia expertise initiative. Pediatr Crit Care Med. 2018;19(9):884–98. Epub 2018/09/05.
26. Lopez-Picado A, Albinarrate A, Barrachina B. Determination of perioperative blood loss: accuracy or approximation? Anesth Analg. 2017;125(1):280–6. Epub 2017/04/04.
27. Rothermel LD, Lipman JM. Estimation of blood loss is inaccurate and unreliable. Surgery. 2016;160(4):946–53. Epub 2016/08/22.
28. Mutschler M, Paffrath T, Wolfl C, Probst C, Nienaber U, Schipper IB, et al. The ATLS((R)) classification of hypovolaemic shock: a well established teaching tool on the edge? Injury. 2014;45(Suppl 3):S35–8. Epub 2014/10/07.
29. Galvagno SM, Nahmias JT, Young DA. Adtvanced trauma life support Update 2019 Management and Applications for adults and special populations. Anesthesiology Clin. 2019;37:13–32.
30. Robertie PG, Gravlee GP. Safe limits of isovolemic hemodilution and recommendations for erythrocyte transfusion. Int Anesthesiol Clin. 1990;28:197–204.
31. Gross I, Seifert B, Hofmann A, Spahn DR. Patient blood management in cardiac surgery results in fewer transfusions and better outcome. Transfusion. 2015;55(5):1075–81. Epub 2015/01/08.
32. Gupta PB, DeMario VM, Amin RM, Gehrie EA, Goel R, Lee KHK, et al. Patient blood management program improves blood use and clinical outcomes in orthopedic surgery. Anesthesiology. 2018;129(6):1082–91. Epub 2018/08/21.
33. Leahy MF, Hofmann A, Towler S, Trentino KM, Burrows SA, Swain SG, et al. Improved outcomes and reduced costs associated with a health-system-wide patient blood management program: a retrospective observational study in four major adult tertiary-care hospitals. Transfusion. 2017;57(6):1347–58. Epub 2017/02/06.
34. Goodnough LT, Maggio P, Hadhazy E, Shieh L, Hernandez-Boussard T, Khari P, et al. Restrictive blood transfusion practices are associated with improved patient outcomes. Transfusion. 2014;54(10 Pt 2):2753–9. Epub 2014/07/06.
35. Chandra S, Kulkarni H, Westphal M. The bloody mess of red blood cell transfusion. Crit Care. 2017;21(Suppl 3):310. Epub 2018/01/04.
36. Hajjar LA, Vincent JL, Galas FR, Nakamura RE, Silva CM, Santos MH, et al. Transfusion requirements after cardiac surgery: the TRACS randomized controlled trial. JAMA. 2010;304(14):1559–67. Epub 2010/10/14.
37. Weightman WM, Gibbs NM, Sheminant MR, Newman MA, Grey DE. Moderate exposure to allogeneic blood products is not associated with reduced long-term survival after surgery for coronary artery disease. Anesthesiology. 2009;111(2):327–33. Epub 2009/07/25.
38. Likosky DS, Paone G, Zhang M, Rogers MA, Harrington SD, Theurer PF, et al. Red blood cell transfusions impact pneumonia rates after coronary artery bypass grafting. Ann Thorac Surg. 2015;100(3):794–800; discussion 1. Epub 2015/07/26.
39. Yuruk K, Almac E, Bezemer R, Goedhart P, de Mol B, Ince C. Blood transfusions recruit the microcirculation during cardiac surgery. Transfusion. 2011;51(5):961–7. Epub 2010/12/08.
40. Murphy GJ, Pike K, Rogers CA, Wordsworth S, Stokes EA, Angelini GD, et al. Liberal or restrictive transfusion after cardiac surgery. N Engl J Med. 2015;372(11):997–1008. Epub 2015/03/12.
41. Mazer CD, Whitlock RP, Fergusson DA, Hall J, Belley-Cote E, Connolly K, et al. Restrictive or liberal red-cell transfusion for cardiac surgery. N Engl J Med. 2017;377(22):2133–44. Epub 2017/11/14.
42. Carson JL, Terrin ML, Noveck H, Sanders DW, Chaitman BR, Rhoads GG, et al. Liberal or restrictive transfusion in high-risk patients after hip surgery. N Engl J Med. 2011;365(26):2453–62. Epub 2011/12/16.
43. Richman JM, Rowlingson AJ, Maine DN, Courpas GE, Weller JF, Wu CL. Does neuraxial anesthesia reduce intraoperative blood loss? A meta-analysis. J Clin Anesth. 2006;18(6):427–35. Epub 2006/09/19.
44. Lu Q, Peng H, Zhou GJ, Yin D. Perioperative blood management strategies for total knee arthroplasty. Orthop Surg. 2018;10(1):8–16. Epub 2018/02/10.
45. Cure P, Bembea M, Chou S, Doctor A, Eder A, Hendrickson J, et al. 2016 Proceedings of the National Heart, Lung, and Blood Institute's scientific priorities in pediatric transfusion medicine. Transfusion. 2017;57(6):1568–81. Epub 2017/04/04.
46. Rajasekaran S, Kort E, Hackbarth R, Davis AT, Sanfilippo D, Fitzgerald R, et al. Red cell transfusions as an independent risk for mortality in critically ill children. J Intensive Care. 2016;4:2. Epub 2016/01/09.
47. Lacroix J, Hebert PC, Hutchison JS, Hume HA, Tucci M, Ducruet T, et al. Transfusion strategies for patients in pediatric intensive care units. N Engl J Med. 2007;356(16):1609–19. Epub 2007/04/20.
48. Voigt CD, Hundeshagen G, Malagaris I, Watson K, Obiarinze RN, Hasanpour H, et al. Effects of a restrictive blood transfusion protocol on acute pediatric burn care: transfusion threshold in pediatric burns. J Trauma Acute Care Surg. 2018;85(6):1048–54. Epub 2018/09/27.
49. Shaylor R, Weiniger CF, Austin N, Tzabazis A, Shander A, Goodnough LT, et al. National and international guidelines for patient blood management in obstetrics: a qualitative review. Anesth Analg. 2017;124(1):216–32. Epub 2016/08/25.
50. Ekeroma AJ, Ansari A, Stirrat GM. Blood transfusion in obstetrics and gynaecology. Br J Obstet Gynaecol. 1997;104(3):278–84. Epub 1997/03/01.
51. Shakur H, Elbourne D, Gulmezoglu M, Alfirevic Z, Ronsmans C, Allen E, et al. The WOMAN Trial (World Maternal Antifibrinolytic Trial): tranexamic acid for the treatment of postpartum haemorrhage: an international randomised, double blind placebo controlled trial. Trials. 2010;11(40):40. Epub 2010/04/20.
52. Thurn L, Wikman A, Westgren M, Lindqvist PG. Incidence and risk factors of transfusion reactions in postpartum blood transfusions. Blood Adv. 2019;3(15):2298–306. Epub 2019/08/02.
53. Hancock A, Weeks AD, Lavender DT. Is accurate and reliable blood loss estimation the 'crucial step' in early detection of postpartum haemorrhage: an integrative review of the literature. BioMed Central. 2015;15:230.
54. Shakur H, Beaumont D, Pavord S, Gayet-Ageron A, Ker K, Mousa HA. Antifibrinolytic drugs for treating primary postpartum haemorrhage. Cochrane Database Syst Rev. 2018;2:CD012964. Epub 2018/02/21.
55. Villanueva C, Colomo A, Bosch A, Concepcion M, Hernandez-Gea V, Aracil C, et al. Transfusion strategies for acute upper gas-

trointestinal bleeding. N Engl J Med. 2013;368(1):11–21. Epub 2013/01/04.
56. Garcia-Tsao G, Abraldes JG, Berzigotti A, Bosch J. Portal hypertensive bleeding in cirrhosis: risk stratification, diagnosis, and management: 2016 practice guidance by the American Association for the study of liver diseases. Hepatology. 2017;65(1):310–35. Epub 2016/10/28.
57. Wells M, Chande N, Adams P, Beaton M, Levstik M, Boyce E, et al. Meta-analysis: vasoactive medications for the management of acute variceal bleeds. Aliment Pharmacol Ther. 2012;35(11):1267–78. Epub 2012/04/11.
58. Atti AR, Palmer K, Volpato S, Zuliani G, Winblad B, Fratiglioni L. Anaemia increases the risk of dementia in cognitively intact elderly. Neurobiol Aging. 2006;27(2):278–84. Epub 2005/05/17.
59. Hong CH, Falvey C, Harris TB, Simonsick EM, Satterfield S, Ferrucci L, et al. Anemia and risk of dementia in older adults: findings from the Health ABC study. Neurology. 2013;81(6):528–33. Epub 2013/08/02.
60. Myint PK, Owen S, McCarthy K, Pearce L, Moug SJ, Stechman MJ, et al. Is anemia associated with cognitive impairment and delirium among older acute surgical patients? Geriatr Gerontol Int. 2018;18(7):1025–30. Epub 2018/03/03.
61. Le Roux PD. Participants in the international multi-disciplinary consensus conference on the critical care management of subarachnoid h. Anemia and transfusion after subarachnoid hemorrhage. Neurocrit Care. 2011;15(2):342–53. Epub 2011/07/20.
62. Milionis H, Papavasileiou V, Eskandari A, D'Ambrogio-Remillard S, Ntaios G, Michel P. Anemia on admission predicts short- and long-term outcomes in patients with acute ischemic stroke. Int J Stroke. 2015;10(2):224–30. Epub 2014/11/27.
63. Salim A, Hadjizacharia P, DuBose J, Brown C, Inaba K, Chan L, et al. Role of anemia in traumatic brain injury. J Am Coll Surg. 2008;207(3):398–406. Epub 2008/08/30.
64. Festic E, Rabinstein AA, Freeman WD, Mauricio EA, Robinson MT, Mandrekar J, et al. Blood transfusion is an important predictor of hospital mortality among patients with aneurysmal subarachnoid hemorrhage. Neurocrit Care. 2013;18(2):209–15. Epub 2012/09/12.
65. Lelubre C, Bouzat P, Crippa IA, Taccone FS. Anemia management after acute brain injury. Crit Care. 2016;20(1):152. Epub 2016/06/18.
66. Hebert PC, Wells G, Blajchman MA, Marshall J, Martin C, Pagliarello G, et al. A multicenter, randomized, controlled clinical trial of transfusion requirements in critical care. Transfusion requirements in critical care investigators, Canadian Critical Care Trials Group. N Engl J Med. 1999;340(6):409–17. Epub 1999/02/11.
67. Tango HK, Schmidt AP, Mizumoto N, Lacava M, Cruz RJ Jr, Auler JO Jr. Low hematocrit levels increase intracranial pressure in an animal model of cryogenic brain injury. J Trauma. 2009;66(3):720–6. Epub 2009/03/12.
68. Badenes R, Oddo M, Suarez JI, Antonelli M, Lipman J, Citerio G, et al. Hemoglobin concentrations and RBC transfusion thresholds in patients with acute brain injury: an international survey. Crit Care. 2017;21(1):159. Epub 2017/06/19.
69. Turgeon AF, Lauzier F, Fergusson DA (2018) Blood transfusion in critically ill patients with traumatic brain injury. In: Vincent JL. (eds) Annual Update in Intensive Care and Emergency Medicine 2018. Cham. https://doi.org/10.1007/978-3-319-73670-9_3.
70. Baharoglu MI, Cordonnier C, Salman RA, de Gans K, Koopman MM, Brand A, et al. Platelet transfusion versus standard care after acute stroke due to spontaneous cerebral haemorrhage associated with antiplatelet therapy (PATCH): a randomised, open-label, phase 3 trial. Lancet. 2016;387(10038):2605–13. Epub 2016/05/15.
71. Cheng KY, Tsang CP, Leung GKK, Lui WM. The application of point-of-care platelet function assay in guiding platelet transfusion in aspirin-users with intracranial haemorrhages. J Clin Neurosci. 2018;55:52–6. Epub 2018/07/26.
72. Dastur CK, Yu W. Current management of spontaneous intracerebral haemorrhage. Stroke Vasc Neurol. 2017;2(1):21–9. Epub 2017/09/30.

Hereditary Coagulation Disorders

27

Sanjana A. Malviya, Yi Deng, and Melissa Nikolaidis

Introduction

Inherited bleeding disorders are uncommon and exist in <1% of the general population [1–3]. These disorders range from abnormalities involving platelets (primary hemostasis), coagulation factors (secondary hemostasis), clot lysis (tertiary hemostasis), and blood vessels. The vast majority (>95%) of inherited bleeding disorders are predominated by hemophilias and von Willebrand disease (vWD) [3]. They, along with other common inherited and acquired bleeding disorders, are discussed in detail elsewhere in this book. The aim of this chapter is to highlight the rarer congenital disorders that result in defects in hemostasis. In some of these syndromes, a bleeding diathesis is the predominate feature, while in others the bleeding is self-limiting and clinically mild. In the following section, we will categorize them according to disorders in primary, secondary, and tertiary hemostasis, before concluding the chapter with a concise overview on anesthetic concerns and management of this patient population.

Hereditary Disorders Affecting Primary Hemostasis

Primary hemostasis is the process of platelets attaching to damaged endothelium and forming an initial plug. Classically, disorders of primary hemostasis manifest in excessive bleeding from skin and mucus membranes after minor trauma. They are typically divided into *functional* versus *quantitative* platelets defects. In a large case series involving surgical patients with inherited platelet disorders, Orsini et al. showed excessive bleeding occurred in 19.7% of cases in the perioperative period, with a higher incidence in those with functional (24.8%) versus quantitative platelet disorders (13.4%) [4].

Functional Platelet Disorders

Functional disorders indicate deficient platelet activity within the clotting cascade, with or without accompanying thrombocytopenia. These can be further classified according to the mechanism of defect affecting adhesion, activation, or aggregation.

Bernard-Soulier Syndrome (BSS) BSS results from a group of autosomal recessive (AR) mutations encoding the glycoprotein complex GPIb/IX/V, which forms the platelet receptor for von Willebrand factor (vWF) [5]. Platelets with this defect are unable to adhere and aggregate at the site of vascular injury. In addition, this glycoprotein complex is involved in megakaryocytosis and platelet turnover, so BSS patients develop both thrombocytopenia and abnormally large platelets (macrothrombocytopenia) [6]. Diagnostically, patients exhibit prolonged bleeding time and abnormal riscocetin-induced agglutination not corrected by addition of normal plasma (distinguishing it from vWD). However, platelet aggregation time and clot retraction time are normal. Treatment involves donor platelet transfusion and/or tranexamic acid to control bleeding events [7].

Storage Pool Disorders This set of diverse, yet rare inherited, disorder affects platelet granule (alpha and dense granule) biogenesis and release, leading to deficiency in platelet activation and aggregation [5]. Examples include gray platelet syndrome, Paris Trousseau syndrome, and Quebec platelet disorder [6]. Gray platelet syndrome is best characterized here, exhibiting macrothrombocytopenia, reduced aggregation, and abnormal thrombus formation. Patients

S. A. Malviya · Y. Deng · M. Nikolaidis (✉)
Baylor College of Medicine, Department of Anesthesiology, Houston, TX, USA
e-mail: malviya@bcm.edu; Sanjana.Malviya@bcm.edu; yd1@bcm.edu; nikolaid@bcm.edu

© Springer Nature Switzerland AG 2021
C. S. Scher et al. (eds.), *Essentials of Blood Product Management in Anesthesia Practice*,
https://doi.org/10.1007/978-3-030-59295-0_27

usually see mild-to-moderate clinical bleeding [6]. Dense granule disorders include Hermansky-Pudlak and Wiskott-Aldrich syndromes (WAS, see below). Hermansky-Pudlask patients have normal platelet counts and morphology but defective aggregation [8]. In addition, they can be associated with oculocutaneous albinism and granulomatous colitis. Typical management includes platelet transfusion and desmopressin to enhance platelet activity [5].

Glanzmann Thrombasthenia (GT) GT is an AR defect in glycoprotein complex GPIIb/IIIa resulting in the inability of fibrinogen to crosslink platelets. As such, platelet aggregation is greatly diminished [5, 8]. Patients with this disease may be refractory to platelet transfusions because of alloantibodies to the GPIIb/IIIa complex [9]. In these cases, the use of recombinant factor VIIa may be necessary for both hemostasis and prophylaxis [7, 10].

Quantitative Platelet Disorders

Quantitative platelet disorders frequently manifest in the newborn or adolescent period. In addition to low platelet count, they can be further sub-classified by platelet size, into small (i.e., WAS and X-linked thrombocytopenia), normal (i.e., familial platelet disorder, congenital amegakaryocytic thrombocytopenia, and thrombocytopenia absent radius (TAR) syndrome), or large platelets (i.e., MHY9-related thrombocytopenia, X-linked macrothrombocytopenia) [11].

Wiskott-Aldrich Syndrome WAS is characterized by X-linked defect in the WAS gene, leading to a triad of recurrent sinopulmonary infections, eczema, and thrombocytopenia [12, 13]. Platelet dysfunction arises from abnormal dense granules production and increased splenic turnover [14]. X-linked microthrombocytopenia (XLT) is a milder form of this condition, characterized by only microthrombocytopenia without other systemic symptoms. Together these conditions occur in 1:250,000 live births [13]. Patients present in the first year of life with petechiae, easy bruising, and spontaneous or prolonged bleeding. Life-threatening episodes of gastrointestinal (GI) and/or intracranial hemorrhages (ICH) occur in 10–30% of patients [14].

Congenital Amegakaryocytic Thrombocytopenia (CAMT) CAMT is an AR mutation of the *MPL* gene responsible for the thrombopoietin receptor and megakaryocyte production. Patients with CAMT present with severe thrombocytopenia and mucocutaneous hemorrhage at birth which may worsen throughout life. Diagnosis is confirmed by severe thrombocytopenia, absent megakaryocytes in bone marrow, and genetic testing. Treatments include platelet transfusion and stem cell transplant [11].

Thrombocytopenia Absent Radius (TAR) Syndrome TAR syndrome is an AR deletion of the 1q21.1 chromosome, a segment that includes 11 genes and occurs in 1:100,000–1:200,000 live births [15]. Patients have hypomegakaryocytic thrombocytopenia and bilateral radial aplasia. Thrombocytopenia is most severe at birth but usually resolves by school age [11]. It is estimated that 15% of children with TAR syndrome may have congenital heart disease, most commonly tetralogy of Fallot and atrial septal defects. In addition, renal anomalies can occur in 20% of patients [15].

MHY9-related Thrombocytopenia This is a family of autosomal dominant (AD) disorders involving mutations in the myosin heavy-chain gene MYH9. These conditions are also known as May-Hegglin anomaly, Fechtner syndrome, Sebastian syndrome, and Ebstein syndrome [11]. Symptoms include thrombocytopenia, hearing loss, renal failure, and cataracts [11]. Diagnosis is made by visualization of cytoplasmic inclusions in neutrophils and giant platelets on peripheral blood smear [16]. These patients may require cataract surgery and renal transplant at an early age.

X-linked macrothrombocytopenia is characterized by a mutation in the GATA binding protein, leading to defective maturation of megakaryocytes, deficient alpha granules, and hemolytic anemia [11]. Patients tend to have frequent bleeding diathesis with low hemoglobin reserve.

Other Congenital Syndromes Associated with Disorders of Platelet Function

In addition to the aforementioned disorders, there are a number of hereditary, systemic syndromes with platelet dysfunctions, albeit in a more ancillary fashion.

Down's Syndrome (DS) Trisomy 21, or DS, is a well-known syndrome associated with several hematologic derangements. The neonatal period can present with neutrophilia, polycythemia, and thrombocytopenia [17]. Thrombocytopenia is usually mild to moderate and quickly abates with age [18]. The postulated mechanism is dysfunctional megakaryopoiesis as well as prolonged megakaryocyte progenitor lifespan during gestation. DS is also associated with an increased risk of myeloproliferative disease and leukemia at an early age. Hepatosplenomegaly, petechiae, and/or frank bleeding are not uncommon [19]. Current recommendations include obtaining a preoperative complete blood count (CBC) to evaluate for anemia, thrombocytopenia, and hyperleukocytosis [19]. In addition, the American Academy of Pediatrics (AAP) recommends a screening CBC at birth and an annual hemoglobin level check thereafter [19].

Trisomy 13, 18 with modern medical expertise, 50% of patients with Trisomy 13 and 18 have an expected survival beyond the first week of life [20]. Eighty-three percent of Trisomy 18 patients are born with mild thrombocytopenia [20]. Given these patients' frequent need for corrective or palliative surgeries, a preoperative CBC is essential [13].

DiGeorge Syndrome the 22 q11.2 deletion syndrome is the most prevalent chromosomal microdeletion syndrome, occurring in 1:4000 births [13]. It presents as a triad of congenital heart disease, thymic hypoplasia, and hypoparathyroidism [21]. Hemostatic defects in DiGeorge syndrome come from a defective GPIb platelet receptor and abnormal platelet adhesion. In addition, these patients face a 200X increased risk of idiopathic thrombocytopenic purpura (ITP) [13, 21, 22]. Studies have shown that DiGeorge patients have 4X increase in excessive bleeding and 3X increase in transfusion rates during cardiac surgery [23, 24].

Noonan Syndrome Noonan syndrome is a heterogenetic AD disorder occurring in 1:1000–1:2500 live births [25]. Patients have a myriad of abnormalities including facial dysmorphism, cardiac anomalies, genital defects, and short stature. Ninety percent have laboratory abnormalities in platelet function (aggregation and release) and coagulation tests (factor deficiencies), causing bleeding diathesis in 40% of those affected [25]. Prior to surgery, it may be prudent to refer to hematology for further assessment of coagulopathy and management recommendations [26, 27].

Cornelia de Lange Syndrome (CdLS) CdLS is a rare AD disorder precipitated by a mutation in the NIBPL gene [28]. Patients have multi-organ abnormalities including growth retardation, characteristic facies, limb abnormalities, and severe cognitive impairment [28]. Thrombocytopenia is present in 35% of patients, which may be transient or can progress to chronic ITP in 16% [13]. Current screening protocols recommend assessing platelet level at diagnosis and every 5 years after [13].

Jacobsen Syndrome partial deletion of chromosome 11 with characteristic multi-organ deformities including abnormal facies, cognitive impairment, GI tract and cardiac malformation, and dysmorphogenesis of hands and feet [29]. Interestingly, patients have pancytopenia including macrothrombocytopenia at birth as well as functional platelet defect, which may persist despite transfusions [13, 29]. As a result, it may be important to obtain hematology referral and platelet function testing prior to surgery.

Ehlers-Danlos Syndrome (EDS) EDS is an AD family of inherited collagen disorders occurring in 1:5000 people. There are five subtypes, with most exhibiting skin hyperextensibility, joint hypermobility, delayed wound healing, and atrophic scarring. In addition, capillary and platelet fragility is observed due to defective collagen in membrane scaffolding [13]. Although most patients have normal prothrombin time (PT) and activated partial thromboplastin time (aPTT), coagulation factor deficiencies have been reported in all subtypes [30]. Vascular type EDS, or type IV, is associated with a mutation in Col3A1 gene causing defects in medium-to large-sized blood vessels. These patients are at high risk of spontaneous vessel rupture in the GI tract, uterus, lungs, spleen, and liver [31]. Furthermore, 26–50% of these patients have defective platelet aggregation [31, 32]. Special surgical considerations exist for all EDS patients as they are predisposed to joint dislocation, skin damage, aneurysm formation, and vascular dissection.

Hereditary Disorders Affecting Secondary Hemostasis

Secondary hemostasis is the process of crosslinked fibrin reinforcing the platelet plug to generate a stable clot. Patients with disorders affecting secondary hemostasis typically present with soft-tissue and retroperitoneal bleeding, hematomas, or hemarthroses. Fibrin formation represents the final step in the coagulation cascade and is dependent on many coagulation factors synthesized by the liver. Deficiencies at any step within the cascade may lead to clinical coagulopathy, with the most researched conditions being hemophilia A and B (deficiencies in factors (F) VIII and IX, respectively). These are discussed in detail elsewhere.

The rare inherited coagulation disorders (RICD) are a heterogenous collection of AR conditions affecting other coagulation factors, including FII, V, VII, X, XI, and XIII, which affect $\leq$1 in 500,000 individuals each [2, 33]. In addition, combined FV/VIII deficiency due to mutation in the LMAN1 gene and variable combined factor deficiency with congenital deficiencies in vitamin K-dependent factors (FII, VII, IX, X) have also been described [2, 34, 35].

Clinical symptoms vary significantly between each disorder and even between patients afflicted with the same disorder [36]. Unlike hemophilia, factor levels do not always correlate with bleeding tendency. Patients tend to display prolonged PT or aPTT, and diagnosis is confirmed by testing for specific factor activity levels [36]. The therapeutic goals is to restore factor levels by infusing recombinant factor concentrates (available for FVII and XIII), plasma-derived concentrates (FX and XIII), prothrombin complex concentrate (PCC), fresh frozen plasma (FFP), and/or cryoprecipitate. Therapeutic plasma exchange is an excellent option if minimizing volume overload is paramount [2]. The British Committee for Standards in Haematology (BCSH) guidelines recommend avoiding high bleeding risk activities, selecting invasive procedures with minimum bleeding risk, and ensuring adequate communication between a hemophilia center and the treating physician. Antifibrinolytic and topical hemostatic agents should be used whenever possible, and intraoperative thromboelastography may prove invaluable in guiding factor replacement [2, 37].

Hereditary Disorders Affecting Tertiary Hemostasis

Tertiary hemostasis involves fibrinogen formation and lysis. There are two types of hereditary fibrinogen disorders which directly affect this process. Type I is an AR quantitative defect, in which fibrinogen levels are either low (hypofibrinogenemia) or absent (afibrinogenemia) [38]. These patients typically present with mild spontaneous bleeding events in the neonatal period, but symptoms can significantly worsen later in life. In addition, patients may experience severe obstetric hemorrhage, excessive bleeding post-provocation or intervention, and even delayed wound healing. Intriguingly, they are also at risk for paradoxical thromboembolic complications in both the arterial and venous vasculature, occurring up to 30.1% of patients [2, 38–40]. Type II, or dysfibrinogenemia, is an AD qualitative defect in which there is fibrinogen dysfunction as well as abnormal fibrinolysis. These patients predictably present with bleeding and/or thromboembolic complications as well [41].

Hereditary fibrinogen disorders are characterized by prolonged PT and aPTT, thrombin time, low fibrinogen levels, and abnormal fibrinogen function test. Management options include raising the functional levels to above 1–1.5 g/L using fibrinogen concentrate or cryoprecipitate [41]. Tranexamic acid may be used for bleeding prophylaxis before surgical procedures [41]. Fibrinogen replacement therapy is complicated by thrombosis in up to 30% of patients, so clinicians must exercise caution and hematology referral is often prudent [41].

Other Hereditary Disorders with Defects in Coagulation System

Inherited Thrombophilias

Besides genetic conditions which increase bleeding propensities, several hereditary coagulation disorders exist in which the risk of thrombosis is conversely increased. The most common ones include factor V Leiden, prothrombin G20210A, protein C/S deficiency, and antithrombin deficiency. These conditions are described in the chapter detailing hypercoagulable states.

Vasculitis and Autoimmune Conditions

Hereditary Hemorrhagic Telangiectasias (HHT) also known as Osler-Weber-Rendu syndrome, HHT is an AD inherited defect occurring in 1:5000–1:8000 individuals [42, 43]. It is associated with elevated levels of vascular transforming growth factor, which is expressed on vascular endothelial cells and promotes cell proliferation [42]. As a result, telangiectasias and arteriovenous malformations (AVMs) are a hallmark of this disease [44]. Early in the disease course, recurrent epistaxis is the most common presenting feature, while in latter stages visceral AVMs predominate in the pulmonary, hepatic, and cerebral circulations [42]. AVMs may enlarge during pregnancy due to increased circulating blood volume, cardiac output, and venous congestion due to the gravid uterus [42, 45]. In addition to hemorrhagic risk, AVMs can also promote circulatory dysfunction by inducing right to left shunting, paradoxical emboli, pulmonary hypertension, and high-output heart failure [42]. Spinal AVMs are rare but may hamper neuraxial anesthesia [44]. Finally, patients often have debilitating anemia due to recurrent hemorrhagic episodes [42].

Antiphospholipid Antibody Syndrome (APS) APS is an autoimmune (AI) disease characterized by the presence of antiphospholipid antibodies in serum, mainly lupus anticoagulant, anticardiolipin antibodies, and anti-B2 glycoprotein antibodies. These antibodies are purported to affect multiple components of coagulation pathway including protein C, platelets, fibrinolysis, annexin V, and blood vessels [46]. APS exists either in isolation (primary APS) or in association with preexisting AI conditions like systemic lupus erythematosus (SLE) (secondary APS) [47]. A separate and often life-threatening form termed catastrophic APS (CAPS) is associated with thrombotic microangiopathy and multiple organ thromboses. APS is diagnosed by the presence of autoantibodies and at least one clinical feature (i.e., vascular thrombosis, recurrent fetal loss, etc.) [48]. Deep vein thrombosis (DVT) and cerebral vascular events predominate most presentations of APS, although cardiac valve disease and coronary atherosclerosis can manifest as well [47, 49–51]. In terms of coagulation defects, 20% of patients are also at risk for a mild-moderate thrombocytopenia [48]. This is postulated to result from increased platelet destruction by APS antibodies; therefore platelet supplementation does not reduce the risk of bleeding [52].

APS patients are very difficult to manage perioperatively. They alternatingly can be at risk of thrombosis due to withdrawal from anticoagulation and the hypercoagulable state of surgery or at risk for bleeding from excessive anticoagulation and thrombocytopenia [48]. No consensus guidelines exist; however several studies recommend the reduction of perioperative risk via the following methods: (1) minimize periods without anticoagulation, (2) restart postoperative anticoagulation as early as possible, (3) use mechanical thromboprophylaxis methods to reduce the risk of DVTs, and (4) encourage early mobilization after surgery [47, 52]. If the patients are therapeutic on coumadin, they will need extended bridging protocols with heparin as the International Normalized Ratio (INR) goals are typically higher in this population (INR >3) [47, 48, 52]. Lastly, heparin monitoring should be performed with anti-FXa levels instead of aPTT, as circulating lupus anticoagulant may falsely elevate baseline aPTT [48].

Systemic Vasculitis several types of systemic vasculitis such as Behchet's syndrome (BS) and ANCA-associated vasculitis have manifestations of venous and arterial thrombosis. BS is characterized by oral and genital ulcerations, uveitis, skin lesions, and vasculitis involving cerebral and GI systems [53]. These patients exhibit an abnormally high production of procoagulant factors and thrombin, which along with impaired fibrinolysis leads to increased risk of DVTs and superficial vein thrombophlebitis. Less commonly, arterial thrombosis and aneurysms may present as well [53]. Similarly, patients with ANCA-associated vasculitis often have antibodies to plasminogen, causing impaired fibrinolysis and arterial/venous thromboembolism [53].

Hereditary Liver Disease

Liver dysfunction and cirrhosis are associated with major disruptions in the coagulation system, including disturbances in primary, secondary, and tertiary hemostasis. Thrombocytopenia develops from portal hypertension causing congestive splenomegaly, while platelet dysfunction arises from increased endothelial production of nitric oxide and prostacyclin which inhibit platelet activation [54–56]. The liver produces both procoagulant and anticoagulant factors, which may be reduced unpredictably during disease states. Similarly, pro-fibrinolytic and antifibrinolytic forces fall into disequilibrium in cirrhosis and unpredictably manifest in periods of hyper or hypofibrinolysis [54–56]. Cirrhotic patients often have conventional laboratory abnormalities in coagulation that do not reflect clinical risk of bleeding [54]. Therefore, viscoelastic coagulation tests such as rotational thromboelastometry (ROTEM) and thromboelastography (TEG) may serve as better tools in assessing functional coagulation status in these patients [55, 56].

There are many inherited metabolic and genetic defects that can cause premature liver dysfunction. Bleeding risk is thought to be more pronounced in patients with hepatocellular rather than cholestatic liver injury [56]. As it is impossible to list all hereditary conditions that can induce liver dysfunction, instead we will focus on the three most prevalent genetic disorders that impact hepatic function in the surgical population.

Hereditary Hemochromatosis (HH) HH, occurring in 1:250 individuals, is an AR mutation of the HFE gene, leading to increased iron absorption, iron overload, and tissue damage. In HH, iron accumulates in hepatocytes, causing oxidative stress leading to hepatocyte injury and cirrhosis [57]. Laboratory markers assessing liver function are abnormal in 75% of patients [58]. Those afflicted with HH are also predisposed to develop hepatocellular carcinoma, with prevalence ranging from 12.4% to 45% [59]. Lastly, patients may develop cardiomyopathy, diabetes, arthritis, and abnormal skin pigmentation [57].

Alpha-1-Antitrypsin (AAT) Deficiency AAT deficiency is characterized by an AR mutation of the AAT gene which encodes a serine protease inhibitor produced by the liver [57]. Mutant AAT accumulates within hepatocytes, causing apoptosis and resulting hepatocellular injury. In the lung, functional AAT normally protects against the degradation of elastin, which is responsible for maintaining lung parenchyma. Loss of function leads to early-onset emphysema, which is gravely exacerbated by smoking [60, 61]. Overall, hepatic dysfunction is estimated to be present in 10–15% of children and 43% of adults with AAT deficiency, with prevalence increasing with age [62].

Wilson's Disease also known as hepatolenticular degeneration, Wilson's disease is caused by AR mutation of the ATP7B gene that occurs in 1:30,000 live births [57]. This gene encodes the ATPase which transports copper into bile and then incorporates it into ceruloplasmin for excretion. In Wilson's disease, defective ATPase leads to elevated levels of free copper, which damages hepatocytes and induces oxidative injury and apoptosis. Clinically, liver dysfunction prevails in 40–73% of patients and has a variety of manifestations including acute hepatitis, acute fulminant liver failure, chronic hepatitis, and cirrhosis [63, 64]. Aside from liver disease, patients may also have neurologic, psychiatric, ocular, and cardiac ailments due to deposition of copper in basal ganglia, eyes, and heart, respectively [65].

General Considerations for Anesthetic Management

Hereditary coagulation disorders are varied in scope and presentation, so there cannot be one uniform approach to management. In general, many scenarios of unexpected perioperative hemorrhage can be avoided by maintaining a high index of suspicion for bleeding diathesis. The American Society of Anesthesiologists (ASA) clinical practice guidelines recommend a thorough "preoperative evaluation of a patient to identify risk factors for requiring a blood transfusion, including reviewing previous medical records, conducting a patient or family interview, reviewing existing laboratory test results and ordering additional laboratory tests when indicated" [66]. The BCSH states that a bleeding history should be sought including "family history, evidence of excessive post-traumatic or post-surgical bleeding, and the use of antithrombotic drugs" [67]. In addition, physical exam specifically focused on often neglected aspects such as petechiae, ecchymosis, pallor, telangiectasias, joint deformities, and hyper-elasticity of skin, which when present should raise suspicion of a possible systemic disorder (Table 27.1).

Table 27.1 History and physical exam features of hereditary coagulation disorders

Pediatrics
Umbilical stump bleeding
Bleeding post circumcision
Intracranial hemorrhage in neonatal period
Prolonged bleeding after heel-stick
General
Easy bruising or bleeding with minor trauma or in absence of trauma
Mucocutaneus bleeding with tooth brushing, prolonged nose bleeds
Excessive or prolonged bleeding after trauma, surgery, dental procedures
Menorrhagia
Prolonged bleeding during childbirth
Hemarthroses, retroperitoneal bleeding
History of liver disease
Family history
Recurrent bleeding symptoms
Excessive post-procedural bleeding
Liver disease
Physical exam findings
Petechiae, jaundice, telangiectasias, hypermobility of joints, musculoskeletal abnormalities, anemia, hepatosplenomegaly

Routine laboratory testing may be normal and cannot exclude a coagulation disorder [66] (Table 27.2). If suspicion is high for an underlying bleeding diathesis, hematology should be consulted early to seek further testing and offer guidance on perioperative management [33, 67].

Obstetric Anesthesia

Hematologic State During Pregnancy obstetric (OB) patients undergo several physiologic changes that alter the patient's coagulation profile. The plasma volume increase outstrips red blood cell (RBC) production increase so physiological anemia of pregnancy develops [68]. Mild thrombocytopenia is typically seen, and the coagulation factor activity doubles at term [68, 69].

Neuraxial Anesthesia in the general OB population, the risk of an epidural or spinal hematoma after neuraxial anesthesia is 1:168,000 [68]. Any patients presenting with hemostatic defects will likely be at greater risk of neuraxial complications. In those with thrombocytopenia, there is currently no specific platelet nadir that is predictive of future hematoma formation, although a 2015 survey suggests most OB anesthesiologist would not attempt neuraxial technique if the platelet level is <50,000 per μL [70, 71]. Other hereditary coagulation disorders are so rare that literature guidance on individual patient management is mostly lacking. In hemophiliacs, neuraxial anesthesia has been documented successfully if factor deficiencies were corrected beforehand [7]. Because factor levels decrease significantly in the postpartum period, some authors suggest checking it prior to the removal of epidural catheter [69]. Disorders like HHT, EDS, and certain vasculitides can have spinal vasculature involvement and caution must be exercised when performing neuraxial techniques.

Mode of Delivery while there are no specific contraindications, Cesarean delivery in neonates with known

Table 27.2 Common laboratory studies in inherited coagulopathies

	Primary hemostasis		Secondary hemostasis								Tertiary hemostasis		
	Quantitative platelet disorders	Functional platelet disorders	FVIII	FII	FV	FV/VIII	FVII	FX	FXI	FXIII	Afibrinogenemia	Hypo-fibrinogenemia	Dys-fibrinogemeia
Platelet count	↓	↔	↔	↔	↔	↔	↔	↔	↔	↔	↔	↔	↔
Bleeding time	↑	↑	↑/↔	↔	↔	↔	↔	↔	↔	↔	↔	↔	↔
PT	↔	↔	↔	↑	↑	↑	↑	↑	↔	↔	↑/↔	↑/↔	↑/↔
aPTT	↔	↔	↑	↔	↑	↑	↔	↑	↑	↔	↑/↔	↑/↔	↑/↔
TT	↔	↔	↔	↔	↔	↔	↔	↔	↔	↔	↑	↑	↑
Fibrinogen	↔	↔	↔	↔	↔	↔	↔	↔	↔	↔	↓/0	↓	Normal

PT prothrombin time, *aPTT* activated partial thrombin time, *TT* thrombin time, *F* factor inherited coagulation disorders is associated with the lowest risk of ICH, while assisted vaginal delivery carries the highest risk [68]. If vaginal delivery is sought, care must be taken to reduce the risk of ICH via avoidance of invasive fetal monitoring and delivery instrumentation [68]. For patients with known coagulation factor disorders, factor levels should be checked at regular intervals throughout pregnancy and maintained at near-normal levels during the peripartum period. Treatment of intrapartum hemorrhage can be aided with the addition of tranexamic acid, desmopressin, recombinant factors, and blood components [68, 69]. Finally, point-of-care testing modalities like ROTEM and TEG as well as rapid platelet function test (i.e., PFA-100, Plateletworks, etc.) may gain wider adoption in the future [69].

Regional Anesthesia

Currently there are no guidelines regarding the use of regional anesthesia in patients with hereditary coagulation disorders. Peripheral nerve blocks have been performed safely in patients with moderate to severe hemophilia A and FXI deficiency, provided that the deficient factor levels had been corrected prior to the procedure [72, 73]. Nevertheless, given the lack of comprehensive research, patients must be evaluated on an individual basis for the risk versus benefit of undergoing regional anesthesia [74].

Cardiac Anesthesia

Cardiac surgery and cardiopulmonary bypass (CPB) inflict multiple insults to the hemostatic profile. Blood contact with the CPB circuit induces an intense inflammatory response leading to activation of both pro-and anticoagulation pathways. These derangements are further exacerbated by hypothermia, acidosis, hemodilution, and systemic heparinization. Clearly, patients with hereditary coagulation disturbances are particularly tricky to manage in this scenario. Literature is again scarce here, with most being case reports of patients with hemophilia or vWD [75]. In an Australian case series of hemophiliac and vWD patients undergoing CPB, 12% developed bleeding requiring re-operation, compared to 1.9% in the general population [76]. However, these patients did not have increased hospital length of stay nor worsened mortality [76]. Other case reports suggest that patients deficient in coagulation factors may benefit from perioperative measurement of factor and inhibitor levels, as well as repletion of those factors either with concentrates or plasma [75]. Intraoperatively, factors are supplemented immediately after coming off bypass, and then continued daily for 7–10 days, postoperatively. Again, a multidisciplinary approach with cardiac anesthesiologist, hematologist, and cardiac surgeon involvement is key [2, 75, 76].

Orthopedic Surgery

All patients with disorders of secondary hemostasis are at risk for recurrent hemarthrosis and chronic joint arthropathy necessitating surgical correction. Again, much of the data regarding orthopedic surgery comes from patients with hemophilia and vWD. In patients with hemophilia undergoing elective orthopedic procedures, it is recommended to replete factor activity level to 100% perioperatively and maintain levels >60% postoperatively for 2 weeks [77]. Those patients with factor inhibiting antibodies may benefit from higher doses of factor concentrate, use of "bypassing agents" such as activated PCC or recombinant FVIIa, and/or plasmapheresis to reduce antibody burden prior to surgery [77]. Patients with vWD can be treated with desmopressin and FVIII repletion prior to surgery [77].

There are limited data regarding patients with rare bleeding disorders and undergoing orthopedic surgery. In a retrospective case series of 22 patients with rare inherited coagulation disorders, 20% had suffered significant bleeding complications after surgery (defined as requiring more than 2 units of red cell transfusion) despite the fact that most of them had received prophylactic factor replacements [36]. Patients with bleeding events were more likely to have low baseline factor levels prior to the procedure [36]. Furthermore, in a study of patients with inherited platelet disorders undergoing orthopedic surgery, 12.5% suffered excessive bleeding in the perioperative period [4]. Similar to other high-risk procedures, these patients may benefit from preoperative platelet transfusions, use of desmopressin to enhance platelet function, and antifibrinolytic agents.

Conclusion

Although overall rare, there exists a myriad of hereditary disorders that can affect hemostasis and coagulation. Each condition and each patient afflicted with the same condition can present with different degrees of coagulation defect. In addition, many of these inherited disorders are associated with comorbidities that require surgical correction. It is therefore paramount for the anesthesiologist to recognize and identify risk factors for bleeding and thrombosis through a detailed preoperative evaluation, determine the need for further diagnostic work up, and work together with other specialties to optimally manage these patients during the perioperative period.

References

1. Bhave P, McGiffin D, Shaw J, et al. Guide to performing cardiac surgery in patients with hereditary bleeding disorders. J Card Surg. 2015;30(1):61–9. https://doi.org/10.1111/jocs.12464.
2. Strauss ER, Mazzeffi MA, Williams B, Key NS, Tanaka KA. Perioperative management of rare coagulation factor deficiency states in cardiac surgery. Br J Anaesth. 2017;119(3):354–68. https://doi.org/10.1093/bja/aex198.
3. Mensah PK, Gooding R. Surgery in patients with inherited bleeding disorders. Anaesthesia. 2015;70(Suppl 1):112–20, e39–40. https://doi.org/10.1111/anae.12899.
4. Orsini S, Noris P, Bury L, et al. Bleeding risk of surgery and its prevention in patients with inherited platelet disorders. Haematologica. 2017;102(7):1192–203. https://doi.org/10.3324/haematol.2016.160754.
5. Cattaneo M. Inherited platelet-based bleeding disorders. J Thromb Haemost. 2003;1(7):1628–36. http://www.ncbi.nlm.nih.gov/pubmed/12871299.
6. Nurden AT, Nurden P. Inherited disorders of platelet function: selected updates. J Thromb Haemost. 2015;13(Suppl 1):S2–9. https://doi.org/10.1111/jth.12898.
7. Bannow BS, Konkle BA. Inherited bleeding disorders in the obstetric patient. Transfus Med Rev. 2018;32(4):237–43. https://doi.org/10.1016/j.tmrv.2018.06.003.
8. Handin RI. Inherited platelet disorders. Hematology Am Soc Hematol Educ Program. 2005:396–402. https://doi.org/10.1182/asheducation-2005.1.396.
9. Hayward CPM. Inherited platelet disorders. Curr Opin Hematol. 2003;10(5):362–8. http://www.ncbi.nlm.nih.gov/pubmed/12913791.
10. Nurden AT, Freson K, Seligsohn U. Inherited platelet disorders. Haemophilia. 2012;18(Suppl 4):154–60. https://doi.org/10.1111/j.1365-2516.2012.02856.x.
11. Drachman JG. Inherited thrombocytopenia: when a low platelet count does not mean ITP. Blood. 2004;103(2):390–8. https://doi.org/10.1182/blood-2003-05-1742.
12. Candotti F. Clinical manifestations and pathophysiological mechanisms of the Wiskott-Aldrich syndrome. J Clin Immunol. 2018;38(1):13–27. https://doi.org/10.1007/s10875-017-0453-z.
13. Sarangi SN, Acharya SS. Bleeding disorders in congenital syndromes. Pediatrics. 2017;139(2):e20154360. https://doi.org/10.1542/peds.2015-4360.
14. Rivers E, Worth A, Thrasher AJ, Burns SO. How I manage patients with Wiskott Aldrich syndrome. Br J Haematol. 2019;185(4):647–55. https://doi.org/10.1111/bjh.15831.
15. Greenhalgh KL, Howell RT, Bottani A, et al. Thrombocytopenia-absent radius syndrome: a clinical genetic study. J Med Genet. 2002;39(12):876–81. https://doi.org/10.1136/jmg.39.12.876.
16. Ruhoy SM, Yates A. Macrothrombocytopenia with Döhle body-like granulocyte inclusions: a case report of May-Hegglin anomaly in a 33-year-old white woman with an update on the molecular findings of MYH9 -related disease. Lab Med. 2016;47(3):246–50. https://doi.org/10.1093/labmed/lmw033.
17. Martínez-Macías FJ, Bobadilla-Morales L, González-Cruz J, et al. Descriptive study of the complete blood count in newborn infants with Down syndrome. Am J Med Genet. 2017;173A:897–904. https://doi.org/10.1002/ajmg.a.38097.
18. Hord JD, Gay JC, Whitlock JA. Thrombocytopenia in neonates with trisomy 21. Arch Pediatr Adolesc Med. 1995;149(7):824–5.
19. Lewanda AF, Matisoff A, Revenis M, et al. Preoperative evaluation and comprehensive risk assessment for children with Down syndrome. Paediatr Anaesth. 2016;26:356–62. https://doi.org/10.1111/pan.12841.
20. Wiedmeier S, Henry E, Christensen R. Hematological abnormalities during the first week of life among neonates with trisomy 18 and trisomy 13: data from a multi-hospital healthcare system. Am J Med Genet. 2008;146A:312–20. https://doi.org/10.1002/ajmg.a.32107.
21. Lambert MP, Arulselvan A, Schott A, et al. The 22q11.2 deletion syndrome: cancer predisposition, platelet abnormalities and cytopenias. Am J Med Genet A. 2018;176(10):2121–7. https://doi.org/10.1002/ajmg.a.38474.
22. Lawrence S, McDonald-McGinn DM, Zackai E, Sullivan KE. Thrombocytopenia in patients with chromosome 22q11.2 deletion syndrome. J Pediatr. 2003;143(2):277–8. https://doi.org/10.1067/S0022-3476(03)00248-8.
23. Brenner MK, Clarke S, Mahnke DK, et al. Effect of 22q11.2 deletion on bleeding and transfusion utilization in children with congenital heart disease undergoing cardiac surgery. Pediatr Res. 2016;79(2):318–24. https://doi.org/10.1038/pr.2015.216.
24. Yeng Yeoh T, Scavonetto F, Hamlin RJ, Burkhart HM, Sprung J, Weingarten TN. Perioperative management of patients with DiGeorge syndrome undergoing cardiac surgery. J Cardiothorac Vasc Anesth. 2014;28(4):983–9. https://doi.org/10.1053/j.jvca.2013.10.025.
25. Artoni A, Selicorni A, Passamonti SM, et al. Hemostatic abnormalities in Noonan syndrome. Pediatrics. 2014;133(5):e1299–304. https://doi.org/10.1542/peds.2013-3251.
26. Nugent DJ, Romano AA, Sabharwal S, Cooper DL. Evaluation of bleeding disorders in patients with Noonan syndrome: a systematic review. J Blood Med. 2018;9:185–92. https://doi.org/10.2147/JBM.S164474.
27. Morice A, Harroche A, Cairet P, Khonsari RH. Preoperative detailed coagulation tests are required in patients with Noonan syndrome. J Oral Maxillofac Surg. 2018;76(7):1553–8. https://doi.org/10.1016/j.joms.2017.12.012.
28. Cavalleri V, Bettini LR, Barboni C, et al. Thrombocytopenia and Cornelia de Lange syndrome: still an enigma? Am J Med Genet. 2016;170A(1):130–4. https://doi.org/10.1002/ajmg.a.37390.
29. Mattina T, Perrotta CS, Grossfeld P. Jacobsen syndrome. Orphanet J Rare Dis. 2009;4(1):9. https://doi.org/10.1186/1750-1172-4-9.
30. De Paepe A, Malfait F. Bleeding and bruising in patients with Ehlers–Danlos syndrome and other collagen vascular disorders. Br J Haematol. 2004;127:491–500.
31. Busch A, Hoffjan S, Bergmann F, et al. Vascular type Ehlers-Danlos syndrome is associated with platelet dysfunction and low vitamin D serum concentration. Orphanet J Rare Dis. 2016;11(1):1–8. https://doi.org/10.1186/s13023-016-0491-2.
32. Wiesmann T, Castori M, Malfait F, Wulf H. Recommendations for anesthesia and perioperative management in patients with Ehlers-Danlos syndrome. Orphanet J Rare Dis. 2014;9(1):109–18. https://doi.org/10.1186/s13023-014-0109-5.
33. Mensah PK, Gooding R. Surgery in patients with inherited bleeding disorders. Anaesthesia. 2015;70:112–e40. https://doi.org/10.1111/anae.12899.
34. Bolton-Maggs PHB. The rare inherited coagulation disorders. Pediatr Blood Cancer. 2013;60(S1):S37–40. https://doi.org/10.1002/pbc.24336.

35. Acharya SS. Rare bleeding disorders in children: identification and primary care management. Pediatrics. 2013;132(5):882–92. https://doi.org/10.1542/peds.2012-3662.
36. Siboni SM, Biguzzi E, Pasta G, et al. Management of orthopaedic surgery in rare bleeding disorders. Haemophilia. 2014;20(5):693–701. https://doi.org/10.1111/hae.12387.
37. Mumford AD, Ackroyd S, Alikhan R, et al. Guideline for the diagnosis and management of the rare coagulation disorders. Br J Haematol. 2014;167(3):304–26. https://doi.org/10.1111/bjh.13058.
38. Casini A, Neerman-Arbez M, Ariëns RA, de Moerloose P. Dysfibrinogenemia: from molecular anomalies to clinical manifestations and management. J Thromb Haemost. 2015;13:909–19. https://doi.org/10.1111/jth.12916.
39. Stanciakova L, Kubisz P, Dobrotova M, Stasko J. Congenital afibrinogenemia: from etiopathogenesis to challenging clinical management. Expert Rev Hematol. 2016;9(7):639–48. https://doi.org/10.1080/17474086.2016.1200967.
40. Korte W, Poon M-C, Iorio A, Makris M. Thrombosis in inherited fibrinogen disorders. Transfus Med Hemother. 2017;44(2):70–6. https://doi.org/10.1159/000452864.
41. Shapiro SE. Diagnosis and management of dysfibrinogenemia. Clin Adv Hematol Oncol. 2018;16(9):602–5.
42. Lomax S, Edgcombe H. Anesthetic implications for the parturient with hereditary hemorrhagic telangiectasia. Can J Anesth. 2009;56:374–84. https://doi.org/10.1007/s12630-009-9076-z.
43. Chieira D, Conceição L, Semedo E, Almeida V. Osler-Weber-Rendu syndrome: an anaesthetic challenge? BMJ Case Rep. 2016;2016:bcr2015213647. https://doi.org/10.1136/bcr-2015-213647.
44. Weingarten TN, Hanson JW, Anusionwu KO, et al. Management of patients with hereditary hemorrhagic telangiectasia undergoing general anesthesia: a cohort from a single academic center's experience. J Anesth. 2013;27(5):705–11. https://doi.org/10.1007/s00540-013-1601-0.
45. Crawford M, Burns R, Cooper S, Mackay T. Hereditary haemorrhagic telangiectasia in pregnancy: regional and general anaesthesia. Int J Obstet Anesth. 2018;33:84–6. https://doi.org/10.1016/j.ijoa.2017.11.002.
46. Previtali E, Bucciarelli P, Passamonti SM, Martinelli I. Risk factors for venous and arterial thrombosis. Blood Transfus. 2011;9(2):120–38. https://doi.org/10.2450/2010.0066-10.
47. Madan R, Khoursheed M, Kukla R, Al-Mazidi M, Behbehani A. The anaesthetist and the antiphospholipid syndrome. Anaesthesia. 1997;52:72–4. https://doi.org/10.1111/j.1365-2044.1997.010-az010.x.
48. Saunders KH, Erkan D, Lockshin MD. Perioperative management of antiphospholipid antibody-positive patients. Curr Rheumatol Rep. 2014;16(7):426. https://doi.org/10.1007/s11926-014-0426-7.
49. Cervera R, Piette JC, Font J, et al. Antiphospholipid syndrome: clinical and immunologic manifestations and patterns of disease expression in a cohort of 1,000 patients. Arthritis Rheum. 2002;46(4):1019–27. https://doi.org/10.1002/art.10187.
50. Zuily S, Huttin O, Mohamed S, Marie PY, Selton-Suty C, Wahl D. Valvular heart disease in antiphospholipid syndrome. Curr Rheumatol Rep. 2013;15(320–328). https://doi.org/10.1007/s11926-013-0320-8.
51. Hegde VAP, Vivas Y, Shah H, et al. Cardiovascular surgical outcomes in patients with the antiphospholipid syndrome—a case-series. Heart Lung Circ. 2007;16(6):423–7. https://doi.org/10.1016/j.hlc.2007.03.010.
52. Erkan D, Leibowitz E, Berman J, et al. Perioperative medical management of antiphospholipid syndrome: hospital for special surgery experience, review of literature, and recommendations. J Rheumatol. 2002;29(4):843–9.
53. Emmi G, Silvestri E, Squatrito D, et al. Thrombosis in vasculitis: from pathogenesis to treatment. Thromb J. 2015;13(1):15. https://doi.org/10.1186/s12959-015-0047-z.
54. Tripodi A, Mannucci PM. The coagulopathy of chronic liver disease. N Engl J Med. 2011;365(2):147–56. https://doi.org/10.1056/NEJMra1011170.
55. Kiamanesh D, Rumley J, Moitra VK. Monitoring and managing hepatic disease in anaesthesia. Br J Anaesth. 2013;111(Suppl 1):i50–61. https://doi.org/10.1093/bja/aet378.
56. Weeder PD, Porte RJ, Lisman T. Hemostasis in liver disease: implications of new concepts for perioperative management. Transfus Med Rev. 2014;28(3):107–13. https://doi.org/10.1016/j.tmrv.2014.03.002.
57. Scorza M, Elce A, Zarrilli F, Liguori R, Amato F, Castaldo G. Genetic diseases that predispose to early liver cirrhosis. Int J Hepatol. 2014;2014:1–11. https://doi.org/10.1155/2014/713754.
58. Niederau C, Strohmeyer G, Stremmel W. Epidemiology, clinical spectrum and prognosis of hemochromatosis. Adv Exp Med Biol. 1994;356:293–302. https://doi.org/10.1007/978-1-4615-2554-7_31.
59. Beaton MD, Adams PC. Prognostic factors and survival in patients with hereditary hemochromatosis and cirrhosis. Can J Gastroenterol. 2006;20(4):257–60. https://doi.org/10.1155/2006/428048.
60. Mahadeva R, Lomas DA. Genetics and respiratory disease bullet 2: alpha1-antitrypsin deficiency, cirrhosis and emphysema. Thorax. 1998;53(6):501–5. https://doi.org/10.1136/thx.53.6.501.
61. Gooptu B, Ekeowa UI, Lomas DA. Mechanisms of emphysema in 1-antitrypsin deficiency: molecular and cellular insights. Eur Respir J. 2009;34(2):475–88. https://doi.org/10.1183/09031936.00096508.
62. Clark VC. Liver transplantation in alpha-1 antitrypsin deficiency. Clin Liver Dis. 2017;21(2):355–65. https://doi.org/10.1016/j.cld.2016.12.008.
63. Capone K, Azzam RK. Wilson's disease: a review for the general pediatrician. Pediatr Ann. 2018;47(11):e440–4. https://doi.org/10.3928/19382359-20181026-01.
64. Merle U, Schaefer M, Ferenci P, Stremmel W. Clinical presentation, diagnosis and long-term outcome of Wilson's disease: a cohort study. Gut. 2007;56(1):115–20. https://doi.org/10.1136/gut.2005.087262.
65. Moores A, Fox S, Lang A, Hirschfield G. Wilson disease: Canadian perspectives on presentation and outcomes from an adult ambulatory setting. Can J Gastroenterol. 2012;26(6):333–9. https://doi.org/10.1155/2012/123431.
66. American Society of Anesthesiologists Task Force on Perioperative Blood Management. Practice guidelines for perioperative blood management. Anesthesiology. 2015;122(2):241–75. https://doi.org/10.1097/ALN.0000000000000463.
67. Chee YL, Crawford JC, Watson HG, Greaves M. Guidelines on the assessment of bleeding risk prior to surgery or invasive procedures. Br J Haematol. 2008;140(5):496–504. https://doi.org/10.1111/j.1365-2141.2007.06968.x.
68. Katz D, Beilin Y. Disorders of coagulation in pregnancy. Br J Anaesth. 2015;115:ii75–88. https://doi.org/10.1093/bja/aev374.
69. Chow L, Farber MK, Camann WR. Anesthesia in the pregnant patient with hematologic disorders. Hematol Oncol Clin North Am. 2011;25(2):425–43. https://doi.org/10.1016/j.hoc.2011.01.003.
70. Practice guidelines for obstetric anesthesia. Anesthesiology. 2016;124(2):270–300. https://doi.org/10.1097/ALN.0000000000000935.
71. Basaran A, Basaran M, Basaran B, Sen C, Martin JN. Controversial clinical practices for patients with preeclampsia or HELLP syndrome: a survey. J Perinat Med. 2015;43(1). https://doi.org/10.1515/jpm-2014-0109.
72. Sripada R, Reyes JJ, Sun R. Peripheral nerve blocks for intraoperative management in patients with hemophilia A. J Clin Anesth. 2009;21(2):120–3. https://doi.org/10.1016/j.jclinane.2008.06.030.
73. Yoshikawa S, Kumano I, Satoh Y, Yufune S. Anesthetic management using peripheral nerve block in patients with factor XI

deficiency: a case report. JA Clin Rep. 2016;2(1):17. https://doi.org/10.1186/s40981-016-0047-4.

74. Shah UJ, Narayanan M, Smith JG. Anaesthetic considerations in patients with inherited disorders of coagulation. Contin Educ Anaesth Crit Care Pain. 2015;15(1):26–31. https://doi.org/10.1093/bjaceaccp/mku007.
75. Rossi M, Jayaram R, Sayeed R. Do patients with haemophilia undergoing cardiac surgery have good surgical outcomes? Interact Cardiovasc Thorac Surg. 2011;13:320–31. https://doi.org/10.1510/icvts.2011.272401.
76. Bhave P, McGiffin D, Shaw J, et al. A guide to performing cardiac surgery in patients with hereditary bleeding disorders. J Card Surg. 2015;30:61–9.
77. Mansour J, Graf K, Lafferty P. Bleeding disorders in orthopedic surgery. Orthopedics. 2012;35(12):1053–62. https://doi.org/10.3928/01477447-20121120-09.

28 Metabolism, Pathophysiology, and Clinical Considerations of Iron Overload, a Comprehensive Review

Andrew Jesse Garcia, Chikezie N. Okeagu, Alan David Kaye, and Alaa Abd-Elsayed

Introduction

Experimentation with blood transfusion dates back to the seventeenth century when Richard Lower demonstrated the ability to keep dogs that had had their blood volume intentionally depleted alive by transfusion of blood from other dogs [1]. In 1818, Dr. James Blundell, a British obstetrician, performed the first documented transfusion of human blood, transfusing several donors' blood into a patient with gastric cancer. Despite a temporary improvement in his condition, the patient died two days later. In the ensuing years, Dr. Blundell performed several more transfusions using human blood, with little success, however, as at least five of the ten patients died. Furthermore, some of those who survived are reported to have experienced headache, backache, fever, and dark-colored urine [2]. In 1840, the first successful transfusion of whole blood was performed in 1840 by Samuel Armstrong Lane, with the aid of Dr. Blundell, to treat a patient with hemophilia [3], setting the stage for what would one day become a standard component of the treatment many medical conditions.

Since these early days, the practice of blood transfusion has drastically evolved. Initially considered a risky and dubious practice, widely rejected by the medical establishment, blood product transfusion has become a staple of medical care in America and around the world. The indications and diseases for which transfusion is indicated are vast, and thus, thousands of these procedures take place each day. Approximately 21 million blood components are transfused in the USA each year, the majority of which are units of red blood cells (RBCs), which account for roughly 36,000 units daily [4]. Transfusion of blood products peaked in 2011 when nearly 7% of hospitalized patients received red blood cell (RBC) transfusion [5].

Much of the credit for the massive expansion in the acceptance and use of blood transfusions from the days of Blundell to the modern-day is due to the tremendous strides that have been made in improving the safety of transfusion. In its nascent days, blood transfusion presented a host of potentially life-threatening risks that were mostly unknown to the recipients, and those administering the transfusions. This began to change in 1900, when Karl Landsteiner described the ABO blood grouping system [6]. Since then, several more advancements have been made in transfusion medicine, with each improving the safety and applicability of blood transfusions. Due largely to the 1982 discovery that HIV could be transmitted through transfusion of blood and the fervid stigma that surrounded the disease at the time, the risk of infection transmission associated with blood transfusion is relatively well known. However, due to the stringent screening and testing that potential donors and blood products undergo, the risk of contracting HIV, viral hepatitis, or any other of the host of potentially transmissible diseases is remarkably low [7, 8]. Nevertheless, transfusion still carries many other risks, especially in those patients who require frequent transfusion. Risks such as contamination of stored

A. J. Garcia
Department of Anesthesiology, LSUHSC New Orleans, New Orleans, LA, USA

George Washington University School of Medicine and Health Sciences, Washington, DC, USA
e-mail: garcia13@gwu.edu

C. N. Okeagu
Department of Anesthesiology, LSUHSC New Orleans, New Orleans, LA, USA
e-mail: cokeag@lsuhsc.edu

A. D. Kaye (✉)
Department of Anesthesiology and Pharmacology, Toxicology, and Neurosciences, Louisiana State University School of Medicine-Shreveport, Shreveport, LA, USA

LSU Health Shreveport School of Medicine, New Orleans, LA, USA

Tulane School of Medicine, New Orleans, LA, USA
e-mail: akaye@lsuhsc.edu

A. Abd-Elsayed
Department of Anesthesiology, University of Wisconsin School of Medicine and Public Health, Madison, WI, USA
e-mail: abdelsayed@wisc.edu

© Springer Nature Switzerland AG 2021
C. S. Scher et al. (eds.), *Essentials of Blood Product Management in Anesthesia Practice*,
https://doi.org/10.1007/978-3-030-59295-0_28

blood products, Transfusion-Related Acute Lung Injury (TRALI); Transfusion Associated Circulatory Overload (TACO); Transfusion-Mediated Immunosuppression, immune and hemolytic reactions; and Transfusion-Related Iron Overload (TRIO) represent serious and potentially fatal complications of blood transfusion [7–9]. This chapter will present a brief overview of iron metabolism, and explore the signs, symptoms, diagnosis, and treatments of TRIO.

Iron Metabolism and Homeostasis

Iron is essential to a wide array of biological processes. It serves as a vital component in proteins required for oxygen transport, mitochondrial respiration, nucleic acid replication and repair, host defense, cell signaling, and various other fundamental processes [10]. In excess, however, iron poses potential risks of harmful effects on the human body. Under normal physiological conditions, the level and locations of iron within the body are tightly regulated [11, 12]. Iron is efficiently stored and recycled by the body; any iron that is lost must be replenished through diet (~1–2 mg daily) [12, 13].

Although dietary iron is found in a variety of forms, the absorption of non-heme iron has been the best characterized. After ingestion and enzymatic breakdown of iron -containing food, the iron is maintained in a soluble and readily absorbable form by the stomach's low pH. The GI tract then takes up iron. The proximal parts of the small intestine, namely, the duodenum and first part of the jejunum, are responsible for the bulk of absorption. Iron traverses across the apical membrane of the enterocyte via the Divalent Metal Transporter 1 (DMT1); It is then transported across the basolateral membrane of the cell by Ferroportin 1 (FPN1) and into the bloodstream where it circulates bound to transferrin. Iron that does not enter the bloodstream remains in the enterocyte and is stored as ferritin [11]. The majority of absorbed iron is delivered to the bone marrow for incorporation into RBCs and erythroid precursors. Smaller amounts are found within myoglobin in muscles and proteins and enzymes of other cells. Excess iron is stored as ferritin in the liver. The primary mode of maintaining iron hemostasis is through the recycling of senescent erythrocytes by reticuloendothelial macrophages; These macrophages also store iron s ferritin after RBC breakdown until it is incorporated into new erythrocytes [11, 12].

A sophisticated signaling network helps to regulate iron levels in the body. Hepcidin, a protein made in the liver, helps mediate this process. When sufficient iron levels are perceived by the liver, more hepcidin is produced, which binds to FPN1 on hepatocytes, absorptive enterocytes, and iron recycling macrophages and inhibits iron absorption and release from stores. Contrarily, when iron levels are low, hepcidin levels remain low, allowing for more dietary iron absorption and release from stores. In healthy humans, this process helps to maintain total body iron levels between 3 and 5 g [10, 11]. Disruption of this delicate process can lead to abnormally high or low iron levels, both of which can have pathologic effects on the body.

Pathophysiology of Iron Overload

Iron overload disorders are subdivided into primary, or those that result from a genetic defect in the hepcidin-ferropotin axis, and secondary, which are usually the result of ineffective erythropoiesis, liver disease, or excess exogenous iron. Hereditary hemochromatosis, of which there are several subtypes, is an example of a primary iron overload disorder [11, 13, 14]. Primary iron overload will not be covered in-depth in this chapter; However, many of the clinical manifestations and some of the management approaches that will be discussed can also be applied to primary iron overload disorders.

TRIO, a type of secondary iron overload results from the accumulation of iron that is a byproduct of frequent blood transfusion. Several conditions require frequent blood transfusions as a component of treatment, thereby increasing the risk of developing TRIO. Patients with diseases such as thalassemia, sickle cell, cancers such as leukemia, myelodysplastic syndromes, and aplastic anemia are often dependent on frequent blood transfusions to maintain adequate hemoglobin levels [12, 15]. Low hemoglobin, or anemia, is problematic as hemoglobin is responsible for delivering oxygen throughout the body. When a person becomes anemic rapidly, such as in the setting of massive blood loss, or when they have an inborn defect in hemoglobin synthesis that results in defective or low levels of hemoglobin, RBC transfusion is often required to restore the oxygen-carrying capacity of the blood [16]. While RBC transfusion delivers much needed hemoglobin to patients, it also invariably administers an iron load as each unit of RBCs contains 200–250 mg of iron. That amount of iron would cause most people to develop iron overload after the transfusion of 10–20 units of blood [15]. This can be especially problematic given the fact that many of the conditions being treated with RBC transfusion, though they result in inadequate or defective hemoglobin production, do not have a depleting effect on iron levels; that is, iron levels can be normal or even high at baseline before the additional iron received from transfusion [17]. The body does not have an effective mechanism by which excess iron is actively excreted and only loses about 1–2 mg daily through the sloughing of skin and mucosal cells, menstruation, and other minor bleeding [10, 12, 15]. Iron levels are usually controlled through the regulation of absorption and mobilization of stores described previously, but this mechanism is not equipped to deal with the large influx of iron from multiple transfusions.

Iron normally circulates in the plasma bound to transferrin. In non-diseased states, only about 30% of transferrin is saturated with iron [11, 13]. Iron overload occurs when the binding capacity of transferrin is surpassed, leaving unbound iron to circulate freely and subsequently deposit in tissues [11, 13, 15]. This process of iron deposition is called hemosiderosis. It is thought that certain tissues such as those of myocardial muscle, endocrine tissue, and hepatocytes are more susceptible to hemosiderosis due to a mechanism mediated by calcium channels [18]. The deposited iron contributes to oxidant mediated injury to the cells as iron catalyzes the conversion of hydrogen peroxide to free radical ions that attack cellular membranes, proteins, and DNA [12, 13].

Signs, Symptoms, and Diagnosis of Iron Overload

The signs and symptoms of iron overload are nonspecific and dependent on the location and extent of damage caused by iron deposition. Iron most commonly deposits in the liver, heart, and glands of the endocrine system [12]. As a consequence of the resultant oxidative damage, patients can develop cirrhosis and hepatocellular carcinoma (liver), cardiomyopathies and heart failure (heart), and endocrinopathies such as diabetes (islet cells of pancreas), and gonadal dysfunction (pituitary). Iron deposition in the skin can result in a bronze appearance [10]. Iron deposition in joints can lead to arthropathy [15]. Excess iron deposition has also been associated with neurodegenerative disorders such as Alzheimer's and Parkinson's, kidney disease, cancer, and mineral and bone disorders [10]. Furthermore, some evidence suggests that high iron levels increase the risk of infection as excess iron can promote the growth and virulence of bacteria [19].

Early diagnosis of iron overload is critical to avoid the potential complications of excess iron. Several serum markers are available for use in screening for iron overload including, ferritin, iron, transferrin saturation, total iron binding capacity (TIBC), and nontransferrin-bound iron (NTBI). Ferritin is used most frequently as it is widely available, is inexpensive, and is generally a good reflection of body iron stores [13, 18, 20]. Ferritin levels above 200 ng/ml (449 pmol/l) in women or 300 ng/ml in men are suggestive of iron overload [13]. However, since ferritin can also be increased in the setting of inflammatory processes, autoimmune disease, and other chronic illness, elevated ferritin alone cannot diagnose iron overload. TSAT can also be a useful indicator of total body iron. Saturation above 45% in women and 50% in men should raise suspicion for overload [13]. TSAT is a very dynamic measure that is influenced by a wide range of physiological and temporal factors, which limits its clinical utility [13, 20, 21].

If serum assays suggest iron overload, evaluation of liver iron is warranted. The liver is the primary iron storage organ, and as such, liver iron levels reflect total body iron stores [18, 20]. Liver biopsy is the only direct way to assess liver iron concentration and remains the most precise method. Biopsy also allows for evaluation of liver histology, which can provide valuable information regarding the presence and progression of liver disease. The drawbacks of biopsy include expense, and the risks (bleeding, infection) and discomfort associated with the procedure. Other noninvasive mechanisms of measuring liver iron concentration exist. These include computed tomography (CT), magnetic resonance imaging (MRI), and superconducting quantum interference device (SQUID). These imagining modalities are largely limited by accessibility, affordability, and need for further validation [18, 20]. Furthermore, CT scan carries with it the risks of radiation exposure. Aside from tests intended to directly assess iron, it is also prudent to regularly monitor susceptible organs for signs of end organ damage (i.e., echocardiography, regular blood work).

Treatments

Chelating agents are the mainstay of treatment for iron overload. These agents work by forming complexes with plasma non-transferrin bound iron (NTBI) and intracellular iron, promoting excretion. There are currently three iron chelating agents available, deferoxamine (DFO), deferasirox (DFX), and deferiprone (DFP). They preferentially act on plasma iron pools since this source is more readily available than iron stored as ferritin or hemosiderin, which are turned over less frequently (every few days in the case of hepatocytes). In the liver, the chelated iron is excreted through the biliary system into the feces. The extent by which elimination in the feces or urine occurs depends on the chelating agent.

Deferoxamine (DFO)

Deferoxamine (DFO) is an iron-binding compound produced by a bacteria *Streptomyces pilosus* and was the first iron-chelating agent developed over 50 years ago [22, 23]. A single molecule of the agent binds iron atoms in a 1:1 fashion, forming a feroxamine complex that is metabolically inert. DFO has poor oral absorption and thus requires either subcutaneous or IV administration. Vitamin C is often administered at the time of DFO infusion to enhance excretion of chelatable iron, but this typically is only done if patients are vitamin C deficient [24, 25]. Furthermore, DFO has a short half-life, necessitating continuous infusion of the drug over a period of 8 hours or more [22]. DFO is taken up efficiently by hepatocytes, where it chelates hepatocellular iron and is excreted in bile. In cells, it induces autophagy of cytosolic ferritin after localization to lysosomes. This iron is then bound to DFO and cleared from the cell, where it is eliminated primarily by the kidneys [25, 26].

Major adverse events to DFO therapy include local infusion site reactions such as erythema and pruritis; ocular toxicities such as decreased visual acuity and night blindness; audiologic toxicities sensorineural hearing loss and tinnitus; bone abnormalities and growth retardation; hypersensitivity reactions; and increased infection risk to the bacteria *Yersinia* and *Klebsiella* [22]. Additionally, high-dose therapy has been associated with pulmonary toxicity, neurotoxicity, and decreased plasma zinc in limited case series, particularly in children [27]. Contraindications to DFO consist of renal impairment necessitating dose adjustment (25–50% of normal dose) at creatinine clearance of 10–50 ml/minute [28]. Treatment should be avoided in patients with a creatinine clearance ≤10 ml/minute or during dialysis [28]. Adherence has also been listed as a challenge with DFO, with compliance rates reported around 59–78% in patients with beta-thalassemia, particularly in the elderly patients and those with coexisting psychiatric disorders [29]. Monitoring of DFO therapy consists of serum creatinine at baseline and every month thereafter, serum electrolytes at baseline and every 1–3 months, ophthalmic and auditory exam at baseline and annually, and growth, height, and body weight measurements in children at baseline and every 3 months thereafter. Aluminum and zinc levels should also be monitored as needed [30].

Management of adverse events of DFO can be managed both for local reactions and for systemic reactions. For local site reactions, clinicians should rotate infusion sites, apply local anesthetic or corticosteroid cream, and infuse hydrocortisone along with DFO as needed [28]. Auditory effects can be managed by limiting exposure to loud noises, avoiding high doses in children if they have a low iron burden, holding chelator doses as needed, and monitoring via audiometry [26]. Ocular abnormalities can be managed via holding doses as needed and monitoring via visual acuity tests, slit-lamp exam, and annual fundoscopy [26]. Osteologic complications can be managed by limiting doses to <30 mg/kg/day in growing children, holding or reducing chelator doses, and monitoring growth charts every 3 months [25, 26]. Due to the risk of infection, chelation should be held in the setting of acute febrile illness or unexplained fever [27].

DFO is currently approved by the FDA for chronic iron overload due to transfusion-dependent anemias [31]. Of the three chelators, it is the most established agent for reduction of serum ferritin and cardiac and hepatic iron and improvement of iron-induced cardiac complications. It has been linked to prolonged survival in patients with thalassemia since its use starting in the 1970s [25, 26, 32, 33].

Deferasirox (DFX)

Deferasirox (DFX) binds iron atoms in a 2:1 fashion (2 DFX: 1 iron atom). Like DFO, it forms a complex with plasma iron. Unlike DFO, DFX also has good oral bioavailability and has the longest half-life of the three chelators [23, 29, 32, 34]. DFX is readily taken up by hepatocytes, where it can bind hepatocellular iron and get eliminated in the bile [25]. In cells, however, DFX chelates cytosolic iron, leading to ferritin degradation. Lastly, DFX-iron complexes are eliminated primarily via the hepatobiliary route rather than through urine [25].

Major adverse events to DFX therapy occur most commonly with higher doses (≥25–35 mg/kg/day for dispersible tablets) [25, 26]. These include gastrointestinal (GI) effects such as abdominal pain, nausea, and vomiting; GI bleeding (rarely); skin reactions (pruritis and rash); hepatic impairment including elevation of transaminases and fulminant hepatic failure (rarely); cytopenias including leukopenia and thrombocytopenia; auditory and ophthalmic toxicity-and renal impairment [28]. Among the three available iron chelators, DFX, in particular, has been associated with an increased risk of acute renal failure in patients with iron overload [35]. Absolute contraindications to DFX include pregnancy and thrombocytopenia, with dose reductions for renal impairment (eGFR <40 mL/minute/1.73 m^2) and hepatic impairment (Child-Pugh stage B or worse) [36]. DFX dose should be reduced by 50% if eGFR is between 40 and 60 mL/minute/1.73 m^2 and in patients with moderate hepatic impairment (Child-Pugh stage B). It should be avoided in patients with eGFR <40 mL/minute/1.73 m^2 and Child-Pugh stage C or worse hepatic impairment [35, 36]. Monitoring for DFX includes CBC with differential at baseline and monthly thereafter, renal function at baseline and monthly, serum electrolytes at baseline and monthly, urinalysis at baseline and every 1–3 months thereafter, LFTs at baseline and monthly thereafter, and ophthalmic and auditory exam at baseline and annually [26, 28, 30].

Management of adverse effects for DFX are based on resolving cutaneous, GI, renal, and hepatic sequalae [25, 26]. For mild to moderate cutaneous reactions such as skin rash, doses should be continued, as these reactions tend to resolve spontaneously. For more severe skin rashes, DFX should be held and patients treated with low-dose oral steroids. DFX may be reinitiated at 50% of last dose after resolution of symptoms. For GI side effects such as diarrhea, antidiarrheal medicines should be considered for up to 2 days along with hydration. Adjusting DFX dosing schedule to the evening rather than the morning, and switching liquid used to reconstitute medication may also help. For abdominal pain, avoiding medications that irritate the GI tract and sipping water or other clear fluids while avoiding solid food for a few hours following dose can also help resolve pain. This, along with antiemetics, may also help for nausea and vomiting. For renal impairment, consider dose reductions in serum creatinine >33% above baseline, with halting of therapy until resolution. In cases of stress including sepsis, dehydration, and acute kidney injury, doses should be held, and if patient develops Fanconi syndrome as a result of treatment [28].

DFX is currently approved by the FDA for iron overload due to chronic transfusions in patients 2 years and older, and non-transfusion-dependent thalassemia syndromes in patients ≥10 years of age, with liver iron concentrations (LIC) ≥5 mg iron/g dry weight and with serum ferritin >300 ng/mL [36]. While not as efficacious as DFO for preventing sequalae of transfusion iron overload, DFX has been reported to reduce hepatic iron and ferritin levels similar to DFO with doses ≥20–30 mg/kg/day and to reduce cardiac iron overload and preserve cardiac function [37].

Deferiprone (DFP)

Deferiprone (DFP) binds iron in a 3:1 fashion that chelates iron from lysosomes and mitochondria, in addition to both parenchymal and reticuloendothelial cells [26, 38]. It is rapidly absorbed orally, with a peak blood level after 45 minutes of ingestion. It is cleared rapidly from the plasma through conversion to a glucuronide derivative in the urine. Like DFO, it is primarily excreted through the urine. DFP has been associated with better rates of adherence than DFO in patients with thalassemia major [24].

Major adverse events to DFP therapy include chromaturia; GI effects such as abdominal pain, nausea, vomiting, diarrhea, and dyspepsia that typically resolve within weeks; agranulocytosis (ANC <0.5 × 10^9/L); neutropenia (ANC <1.5 × 10^9/L); liver enzyme elevations; neurologic toxicity including gait abnormalities, ataxia, and nystagmus; arthropathies; and zinc deficiency [25, 26]. Adverse effects are reversible upon discontinuation of the drug. Contraindications to DFP therapy include agranulocytosis or neutropenia, pregnancy, and previous hypersensitivity reactions including Henoch-Schonlein purpura, urticaria, or periorbital edema with skin rash [39]. Monitoring for DFP includes CBC with differential at baseline and weekly during the first year of therapy and bimonthly after that so long as no neutropenia occurs, weight and BMI, zinc levels every 3 months and as needed, and liver function tests at baseline and monthly [28, 30].

Management of adverse effects to DFP include adjustments for neutropenia and agranulocytosis, GI distress, arthropathy, liver enzyme elevations, and zinc deficiency. For neutropenia, chelator should be held for a few weeks with possibility for rechallenge once ANC >1.5 × 10^9. If agranulocytosis develops, chelator should be discontinued without expectation for rechallenge, and IV antibiotics should be initiated if patient becomes febrile. Granulocyte colony-stimulating factor (G-CSF) may be initiated if low ANC persists. For GI distress, therapy should be held and rechallenged with food or as liquid formulation. Antiemetics may be initiated if nausea/vomiting is present. For arthropathy, NSAID analgesics may be used for mild symptoms, with rechallenge possible at lower dose upon resolution of arthropathy. Liver enzyme elevations often are asymptomatic, but in the setting that elevated transaminases persist >2 times the normal limit, DFP should be discontinued. For zinc deficiency, a zinc supplement can be administered [27, 28].

DFP is FDA-approved for the treatment of transfusional iron overload due to thalassemia syndromes resistant to first-line treatments with DFO or DFX [39]. Efficacy for DFP is increased in the setting of cardiac iron overload, particularly when used in combination with DFO compared to DFO alone. Efficacy is reduced, however, for reduction of hepatic iron and serum ferritin [26, 28].

Combinations

Combination of the chelators DFO and DFP have been shown to act synergistically to remove iron. This is due to a shuttle mechanism in which DFP removes iron from cells and passes it onto DFO, which allows DFP to reenter cells and extract more iron [25]. The drug can also rapidly access NTBI fractions in plasma and shuttle this to DFO, creating a more efficient system of iron removal. Efficacy for such combination therapy has resulted in reductions in hepatic and myocardial iron, improvement in cardiac function, and reductions of total iron burden in patients with beta-thalassemia [40, 41]. Several dosing regimens are effective such as, simultaneous administration of chelators, alternating chelators daily, and sequential administration of chelators in the morning and evening. Combination therapy with DFO and DFP has shown superior efficacy for the management of cardiac iron overload in both overt and non-overt cardiac dysfunction [42]. Overt cardiac dysfunction can be managed via continuous IV DFO therapy 50 mg/kg/day and DFO 25 mg orally three times daily as soon as possible [40, 41]. Table 28.1 comparing these three agents and details of their use is listed below.

Table 28.1 Comparison of iron chelators [43]

	DFO	DFX	DFP
Usual dose	25–60 mg/kg/day 5–7 days/week over 8–12 hours/day [25]	20–40 mg/kg once daily for dispersible tablet; 14–28 mg/kg once daily for film coated table and sprinkles [25]	75 mg/kg/day in three divided doses (up to 99 mg/kg/day) [25]
Route of administration	IV or subcutaneous	Dispersible tablet, film coated tablet, sprinkles	Oral solution or tablets
Half-life	20 minutes	8–18 hours	1–3 hours
Excretion	Urine + fecal	Fecal	Urine
Major adverse effects	Local infusion reactions Auditory and ophthalmologic effects Growth and bone defects Hypersensitivity reactions and systemic allergic reactions increased susceptibility to *Yersinia enterocolitica* and *Klebsiella pneumoniae* infections	Gastrointestinal symptoms (15%) Diarrhea (8.8%) Abdominal pain (5%) Nausea and vomiting (14.3%) Skin rash (5–11%) Elevations of creatinine (36%) Rise in hepatic enzymes (2%)	Gastrointestinal symptoms (33% in first year) Neutropenia (including agranulocytosis) (9.5%) Rise in transaminases (7%) Arthropathy (3.9–41%)
Contraindications	Severe renal impairment or dialysis Hypersensitivity Pregnancy (but has been used in third trimester)	Moderate-to-severe renal impairment (creatinine clearance <60 mL/minute) Hepatic impairment Pregnancy	History of or high risk of neutropenias or agranulocytosis Hypersensitivity (including Henoch Schonlein purpura (urticaria and periorbital edema with skin rash)) Pregnancy
Advantages	Most long-term evidence for use Relatively fewer adverse effects if used at normal doses Only chelating drug that can be used in pregnancy	Once daily oral administration Large adverse effect profile but lower probability of serious adverse effects	Most evidence for cardiac iron removal
Disadvantages	Inconvenience of parenteral administration Poor compliance Increased toxicity when ferritin falls <1000 ng/mL, requiring reduction of dose	Cost	Weekly blood count monitoring Weaker efficacy for hepatic iron removal
Monitoring	Growth in children every 3 months Serum creatinine monthly Ophthalmologic/audiologic exams periodically	Liver function tests and renal function tests (serum creatinine and urinalysis) monthly	Complete blood count weekly Liver function tests monthly

Abbreviations: *DFO* deferoxamine, *DFX* deferasirox, *DFP* deferiprone

General Considerations for Chelation Therapy

The aim of iron chelation therapy is to reduce levels of reactive NTBI as quickly as possible to remove all excess iron from the body [25, 26, 44]. Iron chelation is an effective means of improving survival in iron overload states by decreasing the risk of heart failure and morbidities from transfusion iron overload [37]. Almost all patients who require long-term blood transfusions will require iron chelation therapy during management of their conditions. Chelation strategies fall into the following categories: prevention therapy (balancing iron intake and excretion from transfusion), rescue therapy (removal of iron once it has accumulated), intensive therapy (before pregnancy or bone marrow transplant), and emergency therapy (if heart failure develops) [25].

The Goals of iron chelation therapy are based on the presence of specific clinical signs and symptoms. If cardiac iron overload is present, the main goal is to reduce excess iron from the heart. If no cardiac iron overload is present, then the goal is to maintain appropriate body iron storage levels while avoiding chelation toxicity [29]. During treatment, patients should also be monitored for chelator-associated toxicity and efficacy of therapy [25]. The response to chelation depends on the dose applied, duration of exposure, and rate of blood transfusion. Follow-up consists of continuous monitoring for changes in total body iron, changes in cardiac, hepatic, and endocrine organ function, and adverse events from chelation therapy.

Iron chelation should be performed prophylactically, before clinically significant iron accumulation [25, 33]. Specialized management is required in patients with severe renal impairment or anuria [28]. Furthermore, chelation agents should be avoided (preferentially) or used with great caution in patients who are pregnant or breast-feeding [25, 33, 45].

Pretreatment Investigations

Before treatment with iron chelators, patients should be evaluated for appropriate use [30]. This is accomplished by assessment of iron studies, including serum ferritin, transferrin saturation, liver iron concentration (LIC) by magnetic resonance imaging (MRI), and cardiac iron concentration by cardiac magnetic resonance (CMR). Furthermore, evaluation of organ function should be accomplished, including complete blood count (CBC), aspartate aminotransferase (AST), alanine aminotransferase (ALT), serum creatinine and creatinine clearance, urinalysis for proteinuria, electrocardiogram (ECG), echocardiogram for left ventricular ejection fraction (LVEF), follicle-stimulating hormone (FSH), luteinizing hormone (LH), and testosterone (in boys) or estradiol (in girls) in peripubertal or pubertal patients, growth assessment in children, and hearing and ophthalmologic tests [30].

Recommendations for Use of Iron Chelation

Transfusion-Dependent Thalassemia (TDT)

Guideline recommendations for patients with transfusion-dependent thalassemia (TDT) are based on recommendations from the Thalassemia International Federation (TIF) [25]. The mainstay treatment consists of chelation therapy with the goal of balancing iron excretion with iron accumulation. This is associated with improved survival and a decreased risk of heart failure [25]. The prevention of iron overload is preferable to rescue therapy, consisting of DFO after occurrence of >10–20 transfusions, serum ferritin >1000 ng/mL, or both. Second-line agents include DFP and DFX. Vitamin C administration at a rate of 2–3 mg/kg/day should be used as a supplement at the time of DFO infusion to increase availability of chelatable iron in patients who may be vitamin C deficient. If total body iron has already reached harmful levels by the initiation of chelation therapy, then the duration, dose, and frequency of therapy should be raised to achieve a negative iron balance, guided by the rate of transfusion. Given individual variations in transfusion rate, the optimal chelation regimen should be tailored for each individual. In patients who are noncompliant with DFO therapy or have suffered an adverse event, oral iron can be used as an alternative. DFX is preferred to DFP due to a better safety profile [25].

If patients have developed severe iron overload (defined as serum ferritin >3000 ng/mL for at least 3 months) or overt iron-induced cardiotoxicity (defined as LVEF <55%), intensive or combined iron chelation therapy should be employed [26, 40]. Preference is for DFX and DFP in this particular situation. Monitoring for chelation therapy in TDT includes regular ferritin (until below 1000 ng/mL), LIC yearly, and T2* MRI to measure heart iron content yearly [25, 26].

Non-transfusion-Dependent Thalassemia (NTDT)

Iron chelation in NTDT should be initiated with DFX in patients >10 years of age when >1 of the following are present: liver iron concentration >5 mg iron/g dry weight; serum ferritin >800 ng/mL; or serum ferritin >300 to <800 ng/mL when clinical picture or laboratory results suggest iron overload [26, 34, 46]. DFX is recommended due to the absence of data from larger randomized studies with other agents [46]. Monitoring for iron overload status should be done via LIC 6 months after start of therapy and every 6–12 months thereafter, and via serum ferritin every 3 months [46].

Sickle Cell Disease (SCD)

Iron chelation for SCD should be done in consultation with a hematologist and after documentation of transfusional iron overload. Per NIH guidelines, individuals with SCD should receive iron chelation based on the following indications: (1) liver iron stores >5–7 mg/g dry weight; (2) cumulative transfusions of 120 mL pure red blood cells/kg body weight; or (3) serum ferritin >1000 ng/mL (steady state) [47]. Preferred therapy is DFO subcutaneously, supplemented with vitamin C to help increase iron excretion in those who are vitamin C deficient [48].

Myelodysplastic Syndrome (MDS)

Indications for iron chelation in those with MDS is based on major recommendations of the MDS Foundation Working Group for Transfusional Iron Overload and the National Comprehensive Cancer Network. Iron chelation should be initiated when >1 of the following are present: (1) serum ferritin >1000 ng/mL varies based on transfusion rate; (2) patient transfusion need is consistently >2 units/month for >1 year; or (3) patient becomes unresponsive to or ineligible for primary therapy. Chelation therapy should be done with the goal of preserving organ function and monitored based on transfusion frequency. Treatment should continue so long as the patient requires transfusion therapy and iron overload remains clinically relevant. There is no clear consensus on the agent of choice, with some guidelines suggesting discretion of the treating physician and others suggesting DFO or DFX [49, 50].

NCCN guidelines suggest initiating therapy after >20–30 RBC transfusions, especially in patients with lower risk

MDS or who are transplant candidates. These guidelines recommend daily chelation with DFO subcutaneously or DFX orally. It should be mentioned that some guidelines such as the British Society of Haematology (BSH) recommend DFO as first-line therapy due to a longer record of safety and efficacy [51]. Chelation should be monitored with the goal of reducing serum ferritin from >2500 to <1000 ng/mL [49].

Other Iron Overload Conditions

Iron chelation can also treat aplastic anemia. Guidelines for therapy come from the BSH and are performed on an individual patient basis. Guidelines suggest using DFX as the chelator of choice only when DFO is inadequate or contraindicated but should be done with caution in patients taking nephrotoxic drugs due to cumulative renal toxicity [52]. DFP does have evidence for success but is not recommended in neutropenic patients [52].

Other Treatment Modalities

Additional treatment options also exist for specific patients. Phlebotomy can be used for iron removal in HSCT and SCD patients. Exchange transfusion can prevent iron overload in SCD patients, which can reduce the need for iron chelation later on. Splenectomy has been used in thalassemia patients and those with high transfusion requirements. Calcium channel blockers have been used in thalassemia patients to reduce cardiac iron uptake. HSCT itself has been used in thalassemia and SCD patients, and those with congenital and acquired aplastic anemias.

Phlebotomy

The purpose of phlebotomy is to remove units of RBC as a means of depleting total body iron. Each unit of RBC removed (about 420 mL) depletes the body of around 200 mg of iron [53]. Phlebotomy has been reported in case series to reduce serum ferritin levels to <300 ng/mL in nearly half the patients who undergo such procedure [54]. Phlebotomy is a useful treatment option for TDT, however contraindicated in diseases already complicated by anemia such as NTDT. TIF guidelines recommend against phlebotomy for patients with NTDT due to anemia [46]. BSH guidelines further recommend phlebotomy for aplastic anemia and iron overload in the setting of immunosuppression and in post-transplant patients [52]. Major adverse effects of phlebotomy, often during or immediately following procedure, include headaches, nausea, and dizziness [54].

Exchange Transfusion for Sickle Cell Disease

Exchange transfusion is a means of preventing iron overload and the need for chelation therapy in SCD patients, and providing stability of iron levels in patients who are already iron overloaded at beginning of exchange transfusion [55]. Additionally, combination therapy of exchange transfusion with DFX and DFO has been shown to be effective in reducing iron stores to target levels [47, 53].

Splenectomy for Thalassemia

Splenectomy in the setting of thalassemia is primarily done to decrease consumption of blood and transfusion requirement, with the goal of reducing iron overload [25]. The procedure is performed more as an adjunct or alternative to transfusion therapy, rather as first-line therapy. It is rarely performed, however, due to risks of procedure, including infection pulmonary hypertension, and thrombosis, and improved access and safety of standard blood transfusion. Additionally, splenectomy is usually avoided in children <5 years of age due to greater risk of infection following the procedure [25]. Adverse events associated with splenectomy include, infection and sepsis, increased risk of thrombosis, and possible increased organ damage as a result of removing the spleen, since this organ acts as a reservoir for iron scavengers, which can result in an acute decrease of iron removal [56].

Guideline-Directed Therapy for Splenectomy in TDT

For patients with TDT, splenectomy should be considered in patients >5 years of age with increased transfusion requirements that exceed the ability to control with iron chelation therapy. Increased blood requirement defined as annual transfusion volume (75% hematocrit or higher; 200–220 ml/kg/year) after ruling out alloimmunization, concurrent infection, and suboptimal transfusion therapy [25].

Guideline-Directed Therapy for Splenectomy in NTDT

In general, splenectomy should be avoided in children <5 years of age due to greater infection risk. Splenectomy can be considered in the following settings: (1) poor growth/development due to worsening anemia and both transfusion and iron chelation not available or possible; (2) hypersplenism leading to worsening anemia, leucopenia, or thrombocytopenia; (3) symptomatic splenomegaly such as LUQ pain or early satiety or massive splenomegaly with possible splenic rupture [46].

Laparoscopic splenectomy is performed over open procedures unless otherwise directed [46]. The gallbladder should be evaluated if gallstones are present. Febrile patients undergoing splenectomy should be evaluated and treated immediately due to risks of post-splenectomy sepsis. Vaccination with pneumococcal 23-valent polysaccharide vaccine, HIB, meningococcal, and influenza vaccine should be given based on recommended schedule per CDC special populations schedule if indicated. Prophylactic antibiotic therapy should be given for >2 years after splenectomy or longer at discretion of treating clinician. Given an increased risk of thrombosis or cerebrovascular disease, splenectomized patients should receive standard guideline-directed treatment if thrombotic or cerebrovascular complications arise, including transfusion therapy and anticoagulant/antiplatelet treatment for prevention. Lastly, aspirin should be considered in patients with elevated platelet counts (>500 × 10^9/L) [46].

Hematopoietic Stem Cell Transplant (HSCT)

HSCT is unique among treatments for iron overload in that it is the only existing curative therapy for thalassemia [56]. It also allows phlebotomy to become an effective option for reducing iron overload. Recommendations for use come from the European Blood and Marrow Transplantation Inborn Error Working Party and Pediatric Diseases Working Party. Per recommendations, young patients with thalassemia major with HLA identical siblings should be offered HSCT immediately, before the development of iron overload and subsequent organ damage. HSCT with a well-matched unrelated donor is also an option in children with history of lifelong control of iron overload without complications [36]. Lastly, patients with Diamond-Blackfan anemia (DBA) may be considered for transplant if <10 years of age if an HLA-matched donor is available, especially if the patient is transfusion-dependent [57].

Calcium Channel Blockers for Thalassemia

L-type calcium-channel channels (LTCC) and T-type calcium channels (TTCC) have a role in cardiac iron uptake during iron overload conditions, particularly thalassemia. Calcium channel blockers that improve cardiac function in preclinical studies include LTCC blockers verapamil, nifedipine, and amlodipine, and the TTCC blocker efonidipine. Only amlodipine has been tested in human studies and has shown benefit with concomitant iron chelation therapy [58].

Evidence for use of amlodipine comes from RCTs evaluating amlodipine with iron chelation in patients with beta-thalassemia major. The combination was found to reduce myocardial iron concentrations at 6 and 12 months but did not result in significant differences in T2* measured CMR, LVEF, serum ferritin, LIC, or adverse events [59].

Management of Specific Patient Populations

Children

Management of iron overload for children, regardless of disease, may require higher transfusion rates to maintain normal growth and development [60]. Those who develop transfusion-dependent anemias may be at risk of severe hepatic iron burden as early as two years of age in addition to cardiac iron overload. Although this tends to occur later than hepatic iron burden [60]. In general, children should be monitored for iron overload via serum ferritin every three months or earlier based on therapy failure or poor compliance. Additional monitoring via MRI for LIC yearly and myocardial T2* MRI. Myocardial monitoring frequency is dependent on baseline T2* with the following recommendations: (1) yearly in children with significant iron overload even if baseline T2* is normal (>20 ms); (2) every two years in children with well-controlled iron levels based on serum ferritin, LIC, and T2*; and (3) every six months in children with severe iron overload (T2* <10 ms) [60].

Iron chelation in children, like adults, tends to first consider DFO therapy, mainly due to a better side effect profile and compliance compared to DFX. Children should be monitored for adverse effects on bone growth, particularly defects like rickets-like bone lesions, metaphyseal changes, and spinal damage with loss of sitting height. Auditory adverse events should also be done, particularly in children with a low iron burden, as they tend to be more prone to adverse auditory effects from chelation therapy. DFX can be used as second-line therapy as it is FDA approved as first-line therapy for chronic iron overload due to blood transfusions. DFX, in comparison to DFO, has seen less reported adverse events on growth or development in patients with SCD or thalassemia. Renal function, however, should be monitored closely, as it has been associated with decreases in GFR in case series [41]. DFP is approved as second-line therapy for transfusional iron overload due to thalassemia syndromes by the FDA. However, it should be avoided in children with a history of unexplained neutropenia or bone marrow failure syndromes [6]. Adverse bone growth effects, such as bony dysplasia and deformation have also been reported [42]. (Lastly, children with neoplastic blood disorders and those having received bone marrow transplant should be treated for iron overload via periodic phlebotomy or iron chelation in the setting of severe iron overload [6].

Pregnancy

To date, no guidelines have been developed regarding iron chelation therapy in pregnancy. Recommendations for iron chelation in pregnant patients, regardless of disease, are to consider DFO as the safest option during pregnancy and breastfeeding. DFO should be discontinued during the first trimester, with consideration for reinstatement during the second and third trimesters [31]. DFX and DFP are not recommended during pregnancy and should be discontinued during pregnancy and breastfeeding [36, 39]. Female patients who are taking DFX should consider using contraception with two forms, as DFX may decrease effectiveness of hormone contraceptives via induction of CYP3A4 [36].

Future Directions

While transfusion therapy confers many vital benefits, it also puts patients at risk of the harmful complications of iron overload. Iron chelation therapy remains the standard of care for managing transfusion-related iron overload, and investigations into refining these therapies to make them more effective, convenient, and tolerable are ongoing [61, 62]. Research into developing agents to modify previously untargeted aspects of iron metabolism is also underway. Evidence suggests that exogenous transferrin may help normalize NTBI levels and curb the toxic effects of iron overload [63]. Targeting hepcidin to influence iron absorption and mobilization is also being studied [64–67]. Further refinement of these treatments will hopefully one day provide useful adjuncts and alternatives to existing options.

References

1. Fastag E, Varon J, Sternbach G. Richard Lower: the origins of blood transfusion. J Emerg Med. 2013;44(6):1146–50.
2. Learoyd P. The history of blood transfusion prior to the 20th century-part 2. Transfus Med. 2012;22(6):372–6.
3. Passerini HM. Contemporary transfusion science and challenges. AACN Adv Crit Care. 2019;30(2):139–50.
4. Blood Needs & Blood Supply [Internet]. 2019. Available from: https://www.redcrossblood.org/donate-blood/how-to-donate/how-blood-donations-help/blood-needs-blood-supply.html.
5. Goel R, Chappidi MR, Patel EU, Ness PM, Cushing MM, Frank SM, et al. Trends in red blood cell, plasma, and platelet transfusions in the United States, 1993–2014. JAMA J Am Med Assoc. 2018;319(8):825–7.
6. Tan SY, Graham C. Karl Landsteiner (1868–1943): originator of ABO blood classification. Singap Med J. 2013;54(5):243–4.
7. Goodnough LT. Risks of blood transfusion. Anesthesiol Clin North Am. 2005;23(2):241–52, v.
8. Goodnough LT, Brecher ME, Kantner MH, AuBochon JP. Transfusion medicine. First of two parts. Blood transfusion. N Engl J Med. 1999;340(6):438–47. https://doi.org/10.1056/NEJM199902113400606.
9. Barty R, Jamula E, Wang G, Liu Y, Leber B, Heddle N; UHA. Transfusion-related iron overload: a covert risk of supportive cancer care. Blood. 2013;122(21):3656. https://doi.org/10.1182/blood.V122.21.3656.3656.
10. Dev S, Babitt JL. Overview of iron metabolism in health and disease. Hemodial Int. 2017;21:S6–S20.
11. Anderson GJ, Frazer DM. Current understanding of iron homeostasis. Am J Clin Nutr. 2017;106(Suppl 6):1559S–66S.
12. Andrews NC. Disorders of iron metabolism. N Engl J Med. 1999;341(26):1986–95.
13. Fleming RE, Ponka P. Iron overload in human disease. N Engl J Med. 2012;366(4):348–59.
14. Milic S, Mikolasevic I, Orlic L, Devcic E, Starcevic-Cizmarevic N, Stimac D, et al. The role of iron and iron overload in chronic liver disease. Med Sci Monit. 2016;22:2144–51.
15. Gao C, Li L, Chen B, Song H, Cheng J, Zhang X, et al. Clinical outcomes of transfusion-associated iron overload in patients with refractory chronic anemia. Patient Prefer Adherence. 2014;8:513–7.
16. Cascio MJ, DeLoughery TG. Anemia: evaluation and diagnostic tests. Med Clin N Am. 2017;101(2):263–84.
17. Camaschella C, Nai A. Ineffective erythropoiesis and regulation of iron status in iron loading anaemias. Br J Haematol. 2016;172(4):512–23.
18. Porter J, Viprakasit V. Iron overload and chelation. In: Guidelines for the management of transfusion dependent thalassemia. 3rd ed. Nicosia: Thalassaemia International Federation; 2014. p. 42–97.
19. Cross JH, Bradbury RS, Fulford AJ, Jallow AT, Wegmüller R, Prentice AM, et al. Oral iron acutely elevates bacterial growth in human serum. Sci Rep. 2015;5:16670.
20. Wood JC. Diagnosis and management of transfusion iron overload: the role of imaging. Am J Hematol. 2007;82(12 Suppl):1132–5.
21. Elsayed ME, Sharif MU, Stack AG. Transferrin saturation: a body iron biomarker. Adv Clin Chem. 2016;75:71–97.
22. Fisher S, Brunskill S, Doree C, Gooding S, Chowdhury O, Roberts D. Desferrioxamine mesylate for managing transfusional iron overload in people with thalassaemia. Cochrane Database Syst Rev. 2013;(8).
23. Xia S, Zhang W, Huang L, Jiang H. Comparative efficacy and safety of deferoxamine, deferiprone and deferasirox on severe thalassemia: a meta-analysis of 16 randomized controlled trials. PLoS One. 2013;8(12):1–9.
24. Kwiatkowski JL. Management of transfusional iron overload – differential properties and efficacy of iron chelating agents. J Blood Med. 2011;2:135–49.
25. Cappellini MD, Cohen A, Porter J, Taher A, Viprakasit V. Guidelines for the management of transfusion dependent thalassemia (TDT). Thalass Int Fed. 2014;20(20):42–98.
26. Marsella M, Borgna-Pignatti C. Transfusional iron overload and iron chelation therapy in thalassemia major and sickle cell disease. Hematol Oncol Clin North Am, Elsevier Inc. 2014;28(4):703–27.
27. Ware HM, Kwiatkowski JL. Evaluation and treatment of transfusional iron overload in children. Pediatr Clin North Am, Elsevier Inc. 2013;60(6):1393–406.
28. Saliba AN, El Rassi FTA. Clinical monitoring and management of complications related to chelation therapy in patients with β-thalassemia. Expert Rev Hematol. 2016;9(2):151–68.
29. Kwiatkowski JL. Current recommendations for chelation for transfusion-dependent thalassemia. Ann N Y Acad Sci. 2016;1368(1):107–14.
30. Remacha Á, Sanz C, Contreras E, De Heredia CD, Grifols JR, Lozano M, et al. Guidelines on haemovigilance of post-transfusional iron overload. Blood Transfus. 2013;11(1):128–39.
31. DailyMed – DEFEROXAMINE – deferoxamine mesylate injection, powder, lyophilized, for solution.
32. Hoffbrand AV, Taher A, Cappellini MD. How I treat transfusional iron overload. Blood. 2012;120(18):3657–69.
33. Brittenham GM. Iron-chelating therapy for transfusional iron overload. N Engl J Med. 2011;364(2):146–56.

34. Bollig C, Schell L, Rucker G, Allert R, Motschall E, Niemeyer C, et al. Deferasirox for managing iron overload in people with thalassaemia (Review). 2014;(2).
35. Huang W-F, Chou H-C, Tsai Y-W, Hsiao F-Y. Safety of deferasirox: a retrospective cohort study on the risks ofgastrointestinal, liver and renal events. Pharmacoepidemiol Drug Saf. 2014;23:1176–82.
36. DailyMed – EXJADE- deferasirox tablet, for suspension.
37. Pennell DJ, Porter JB, Piga A, Lai Y, El-beshlawy A, Belhoul KM, et al. Clinical trials and observations myocardial iron removal in b -thalassemia major (CORDELIA). 2018;123(10):1447–55.
38. Fisher SA, Brunskill SJ, Doree C, Chowdhury O, Gooding S, Roberts DJ. Oral deferiprone for iron chelation in people with thalassaemia. [Update of Cochrane Database Syst Rev. 2007;(3):CD004839; PMID: 17636775]. Cochrane Database Syst Rev. 2013;8:CD004839.
39. DailyMed – FERRIPROX- deferiprone tablet, film coated.
40. Hammond J, Thompson AA, Fogel MA, Hammond K, Kokroko J, Kwiatkowski JL. Combination oral chelation in adult patients with transfusion-dependent thalassemia and high iron burden. J Pediatr Hematol Oncol. 2019;41(1):E47–50.
41. Gomber S, Jain P, Sharma S, Narang M. Comparative efficacy and safety of oral iron chelators and their novel combination in children with thalassemia. Indian Pediatr. 2016;53(3):207–10.
42. Pennell DJ, Udelson JE, Arai AE, Bozkurt B, Cohen AR, Galanello R, et al. Cardiovascular function and treatment in β-thalassemia major. Circulation. 2013;128(3):281–308.
43. Kwiatkowski J, Fedorowicz Z, Aird W. Transfusional iron overload. Dynamed. 2019:1–107. https://www.dynamed.com/condition/transfusional-iron-overload.
44. Coates TD, Wood JC. How we manage iron overload in sickle cell patients. Br J Haematol. 2017;177(5):703–16.
45. Fisher SA, Trivella M, Doree C, Fortin PM, Madgwick KV, Estcourt LJ, et al. Interventions for improving adherence to iron chelation therapy in people with sickle cell disease or thalassaemia. Cochrane Database Syst Rev. 2018;5(5):CD012349.
46. Taher A, Vichinsky E, Khaled M, Cappellini MD, Viprakasit V. Guidelines for the management of non transfusion dependent thalassemia (NTDT). Thalass Int Fed. 2017;22(22):1–117.
47. Evidence-based management of sickle cell disease: expert panel, 2014. National Heart, Lung and Blood Institute. 2014. https://www.nhlbi.nih.gov/health-topics/evidence-based-management-sickle-cell-disease.
48. National Heart Lung and Blood Institute. The management of sickle cell disease. 2002. https://www.nhlbi.nih.gov/files/docs/guidelines/sc_mngt.pdf?
49. Al-Kali A, Bejar R, Bennett JM, Hetty Carraway C; Clinic Cancer Center Stefan Barta MK; Þ Fox Chase Cancer Center M, et al. Myelodysplastic syndromes NCCN guidelines ® NCCN myelodysplastic syndromes panel members. 2017;15(1):60–87.
50. Bennett JM. Consensus statement on iron overload in myelodysplastic syndromes. Am J Hematol. 2008;83(11):858–61.
51. Killick SB, Carter C, Culligan D, Dalley C, Das-Gupta E, Drummond M, et al. Guidelines for the diagnosis and management of adult myelodysplastic syndromes. Br J Haematol. 2014;164(4):503–25.
52. Killick SB, Bown N, Cavenagh J, Dokal I, Foukaneli T, Hill A, et al. Guidelines for the diagnosis and management of adult aplastic anaemia. Br J Haematol. 2016;172(2):187–207.
53. Porter J, Garbowski M. Consequences and management of iron overload in sickle cell disease. Hematology Am Soc Hematol Educ Program. 2013;2013:447–56.
54. Panch SR, Yau YY, West K, Diggs K, Sweigart T, Leitman SF. Initial serum ferritin predicts number of therapeutic phlebotomies to iron depletion in secondary iron overload. Transfusion. 2015;55(3):611–22.
55. Kelly S, Quirolo K, Marsh A, Neumayr L, Garcia A, Custer B. Erythrocytapheresis for chronic transfusion therapy in sickle cell disease: survey of current practices and review of the literature. Transfusion. 2016;56(11):2877–88.
56. Taher AT, Weatherall DJ, Cappellini MD. Thalassaemia. Lancet. 2018;391(10116):155–67.
57. Vlachos A, Ball S, Dahl N, Alter BP, Sheth S, Ramenghi U, et al. Diagnosing and treating Diamond Blackfan anaemia: results of an international clinical consensus conference. Br J Haematol. 2008;142(6):859–76.
58. Kumfu S, Chattipakorn S, Chattipakorn N. T-type and L-type calcium channel blockers for the treatment of cardiac iron overload: an update. J Cardiovasc Pharmacol. 2017;70(5):277–83.
59. Sadaf A, Hasan B, Das JK, Colan S, Alvi N. Calcium channel blockers for preventing cardiomyopathy due to iron overload in people with transfusion-dependent beta thalassaemia. Cochrane Database Syst Rev. 2018;7(7):CD011626.
60. Aydinok Y, Kattamis A, Viprakasit V. Current approach to iron chelation in children. Br J Haematol. 2014;165(6):745–55.
61. Yassin MA, Soliman AT, De Sanctis V, Hussein RM, Al-Okka R, Kassem N, et al. Jadenu ® substituting Exjade ® in iron overloaded β-thalassemia major (BTM) patients: a preliminary report of the effects on the tolerability, serum ferritin level, liver iron concentration and biochemical profiles. Mediterr J Hematol Infect Dis. 2018;10(1):e2018064.
62. Shah NR. Advances in Iron chelation therapy: transitioning to a new oral formulation. Drugs Context. 2017;6:212502.
63. Li H, Rybicki AC, Suzuka SM, Von Bonsdorff L, Breuer W, Hall CB, et al. Transferrin therapy ameliorates disease in B-thalassemic mice. Nat Med. 2010;16(2):177–82.
64. Liu J, Sun B, Yin H, Liu S. Hepcidin: a promising therapeutic target for iron disorders. Medicine (United States). 2016;95(14):e3150.
65. Parrow NL, Gardenghi S, Rivella S. Prospects for a hepcidin mimic to treat β-thalassemia and hemochromatosis. Expert Rev Hematol. 2011;4(3):233–5.
66. Breda L, Gardenghi S, Guy E, Rachmilewitz EA, Weizer-Stern O, Adamsky K, et al. Exploring the role of hepcidin, an antimicrobial and iron regulatory peptide, in increased iron absorption in β-thalassemia. Ann N Y Acad Sci. 2005;1054:417–22.
67. Pietrangelo A. Hepcidin in human iron disorders: therapeutic implications. J Hepatol. 2011;54(1):173–81.

Blood Transfusion Pitfalls

29

Patrick O. McConville, Jason M. Buehler, and Blake A. Moore

Febrile Non-hemolytic Reactions

Incidence

The occurrence of febrile non-hemolytic transfusion reactions FNHTRs is estimated between 0.1% and 1% of transfusions. Such reactions are much more common in children with 0.2% versus 0.05% in adults [52].

Mechanism

There are two main causes of FNHTRs Cytokines present in the donor blood product and recipient antibodies against antigens present on donor granulocytes or leukocytes. Cytokines including interleukins and tumor necrosis factor are produced and released from leukocytes from blood products during storage [30]. The duration of blood storage may increase the amount of cytokines present, thereby increasing the incidence of a reaction in the product recipient [31, 67]. Additionally, recipient antibodies against various leukocyte or granulocyte antigens in the donor blood may form complexes which subsequently result in endotoxin release and fever [3, 15].

Any type of blood product may cause FNHTRs although the most common sources are packed red blood cells (PRBCs) and platelets.

Presentation

An increase in temperature of 1–2 °C approximately 1–6 hours after blood transfusion in the absence of other more significant symptoms such as hemolysis or hypotension is the most common presentation.

Prevention

Leukocyte reduction is used to reduce the incidence of FNHTRs. This may occur either prior to the storage of blood or prior to transfusion in the recipient. Leukocyte reduction (leukoreduction) prior to storage results in a greater degree of prevention of FNHTRs. Leukoreduction prior to blood storage is effective in removing leukocytes in addition to the cytokines that they may release during storage. Leukoreduction just prior to transfusion may still allow accumulated cytokine sources of FNHTRs.

Management

As with any suspected transfusion reaction, cessation of the transfusion is the first step in management. Clinical monitoring for more severe transfusion reaction symptoms including hemolysis, hypotension, hypoxia, dyspnea, rash, and anaphylaxis is critical. Supportive care should be provided until more life-threatening reactions can be excluded. Immediate clerical blood product verification should ensue. Additional laboratory analysis may be required for more severe symptoms.

P. O. McConville
The University of Tennessee Medical Center, Department of Anesthesiology, Knoxville, TN, USA
e-mail: PMcConvi@utmck.edu

J. M. Buehler (✉)
University of Tennessee at Knoxville Medical Center, Department of Anesthesiology, Knoxville, TN, USA
e-mail: jbuehler@utkmc.edu

B. A. Moore
Section on Cardiothoracic Anesthesia, University of Tennessee Graduate School of Medicine, Knoxville, TN, USA
e-mail: Bamoore@utmck.edu

© Springer Nature Switzerland AG 2021
C. S. Scher et al. (eds.), *Essentials of Blood Product Management in Anesthesia Practice*,
https://doi.org/10.1007/978-3-030-59295-0_29

Urticarial Transfusion Reaction

Incidence

The reported incidence of urticaria in response to transfusions is highest with platelets at around 2% [21, 29]. Red blood cell transfusions are associated with urticaria in 0.1–0.5% of patients [59].

Mechanism

Representing approximately 90% of allergic transfusion reactions [17, 61], urticaria may be associated with other more severe reactions to transfusions such as hypotension or bronchospasm. Immunologically mediated release of histamine by mast cells or basophils occurs via an IgE antibody response to donor plasma antigens and culminates in the cutaneous symptoms of pruritus and characteristic rash.

Presentation

The appearance of a skin rash during or shortly after the transfusion of blood products in the absence of more severe symptoms. The hives appear as pale red dots or plaques and are often accompanied by itching.

Prevention

The removal or reduction of plasma from blood products may decrease the incidence of transfusion-induced urticaria [5, 66, 70].

Management

As with any potential sign of allergic reaction, monitoring for other symptoms is warranted. Urticarial reactions, while potentially uncomfortable, do not necessarily require cessation of the transfusion. The administration of antihistamines may reduce symptoms.

Post-transfusion Purpura

Incidence

The incidence of post-transfusion purpura (PTP) is a rare complication that is difficult to quantify due to the frequency of confounding sources of thrombocytopenia in critically ill patients. Studies have found the incidence to be 1:24,000 units transfused [63]. Females represent the vast majority of cases reported [47, 50].

Mechanism

Post-transfusion purpura occurs when antibodies destroy platelets that contain the HPA-1 antigen following a blood transfusion. HPA-1 antigens are found in the majority of the population and therefore the majority of blood donors. Exposure to these antigens by a previously sensitized blood transfusion recipient results in thrombocytopenia in the days following a blood transfusion. Most patients with PTP are multiparous women who were exposed to the HPA-1 antigen during pregnancy and develop thrombocytopenia after a subsequent transfusion.

Presentation

Patients experiencing PTP have a falling platelet count 4–14 days after a transfusion of platelet containing packed red blood cells. Red blood cell transfusion contains microparticles of platelets, and exposure results in destruction of platelets that can concomitantly result in bleeding [60]. Diagnosis is confirmed with the presence of antibodies to HPA-1 in the recipient.

Prevention

Patients known to have antibodies to the HPA-1 antigen may be transfused HPA-1 antigen negative blood, although such knowledge would be rare and only anticipated in patients who previously had PTP.

Management

Since PTP is only evident in the days following transfusion of packed red blood cells (PRBCs), treatment is often delayed. IV immunoglobulin, plasmapheresis, or corticosteroids are recommended [1, 51]. Subsequent transfusions of blood products should be HPA-1 antigen negative.

Altered Oxygen Affinity

Mechanism

2,3-Diphosphoglycerate binds to hemoglobin and reduces oxygen affinity, thereby allowing oxygen to be released from hemoglobin and delivered to tissues in vivo. Packed red blood cells placed into cold storage begin to lose their 2,3 2,3-diphosphoglycerate (2,3-DPG) levels within days and can be completely depleted before transfusion [25, 74]. Blood stored for multiple days therefore theoretically may have a reduced ability to deliver oxygen to tissues in transfusion recipients due to reduced 2,3-DPG. Efforts to maintain 2,3-DPG in stored blood have been made to produce the oxygen delivery achieved in fresh PRBCs [14, 32–34, 78]. In clinical studies however, the absence of 2,3-DPG does not fully explain the reduced oxygen delivery of aged red blood cells in the transfusion recipient [13]. It is also known that 2,3-DPG levels are restored to >95% of pre-transfusion levels within 72 hours of transfusion [27]. A 2015 study in China shows that the movement of oxygen from hemoglobin, not just the affinity, is negatively impacted over the duration of storage. Oxygen release ability, however, was found to be reduced in the last 2 weeks of storage [42]. There is no evidence to demonstrate increased risk related to duration of blood storage prior to transfusion. Four recent large randomized trials, ABLE [41], TRANSFUSE [12], INFORM [28], and RECESS [68], fail to link length of storage with adverse or beneficial outcomes. But the debate over the duration of storage and risk profile continues due to issues with regard to methodology and statistical evaluation of studies of this nature [73].

Delayed Hemolytic Transfusion Reaction

Incidence

The incidence of delayed hemolytic transfusion reaction is variable, with a range from 1:40 to 1:11,000. The symptoms of DHTR are often subtle and confounded with other variables in transfusion recipients such as ongoing blood loss. Likewise, the patient population has a widely variable range of susceptibility to DHTRs which results in an unknown overall incidence.

Mechanism

Upon exposure to foreign red blood cell antigens during transfusion or pregnancy, patients develop antibodies to such antigens. Implicated antigens such as Kidd, Duffy, and Kell have been identified. Antibody formation can take weeks or months, and in the absence of further exposure to foreign antigens, antibody levels can drop to undetectable levels over time. Further exposure to the foreign antigen in subsequent transfusions may result in an increase in antibody production, resulting in hemolysis over days to weeks. A study in sickle cell disease patients found that those patients having regular transfusions were much less likely to have a DHTR than those only occasionally receiving blood transfusions [57].

Presentation

Since hemolysis takes place in the spleen and liver extravascularly, patient symptoms are often minimal. Antibodies attack only transfused red blood cells containing the antigen, which results in a slow decline in hematocrit. Depending on the rate of hemolysis, patients may rarely experience hematuria, jaundice, or acute kidney injury.

Prevention

Screening for antibodies in blood transfusion recipients, along with crossmatching may reduce the incidence of delayed hemolytic transfusion reactions. Effective prevention of DHTRs is limited in scope. Screening for antibody formation after blood transfusion or pregnancy in order to detect such antibodies prior to their decrease has been suggested as a possible preventative measure.

Management

When a delayed hemolytic transfusion reaction is suspected, hydration to prevent renal damage and monitoring of hemoglobin levels are suggested. Confirmatory testing can be obtained with direct antibody testing but may be undetectable if antibody titers fall. Automated red blood cell exchange, where incompatible red blood cells are removed and replaced with compatible red blood cells, has been used to limit the sequelae after DHTRs are suspected [71].

Infections

Incidence

Bacteria, viruses, and more rarely parasites and prions may result in infections in blood product recipients. Platelets, which are stored at room temperature, have the highest incidence of bacterial contamination and results in infectious complications in approximately 1 in 2000–3000 according to the CDC. Other blood products such as PRBCs are stored cold which reduces bacterial growth, and therefore infectious transmission is significantly less common. *Treponema pallidum, Klebsiella, Pseudomonas*, and Syphilis represent a few of the bacterial pathogens transmittable from bacteremic patients who are asymptomatic or from improper aseptic blood collection or administration technique.

Donated blood is tested for HIV, hepatitis B and C, West Nile virus, and HTLV. Testing for Zika virus is now mandated in the United States by the FDA. Screening questions including world travel, medical history, IV drug use, and sexual behavior are used to reduce the transmission of viruses to extremely rare levels. Cytomegalovirus (CMV) and human parvovirus B19 (HPV B19) are clinically silent in most patients and therefore may be transmitted commonly to transfusion recipients. Most patients experience no adverse sequelae, however with the exception of immunocompromised patients who can experience significant complications including pneumonia, hepatitis, and encephalitis.

- HIV 1:1.5–2 million
- HBV 1:200,000
- HCV 1: 1–2 million

Dengue fever has been transmitted through blood products, and donors who have travelled to areas endemic to such diseases are rejected.

West Nile, hepatitis A and E, and babesiosis have rarely been transmitted through blood transfusions.

Malaria and, less commonly, Chagas disease represent parasitic infections transmissible through blood donation.

Prions are misfolded proteins that are rarely transmitted to blood product recipients which cause several rapidly progressive neurological diseases that results in dementia and death. Creutzfeldt-Jakob disease and chronic wasting disease are examples of Prion disorders.

Prevention

Blood donation patients are screened for risk factors including symptoms of current or recent infections, risky behavior including IV drug use and sexual practices, and travel to areas of the world known to have high rates of infection. Donated blood products are tested for HCV, HBV, HIV, HTLV, and West Nile and Zika viruses. Aseptic technique is mandatory to reduce contamination of bacterial infection both in the collection and administration of blood products. Additionally, the need for blood or blood product transfusion is increasingly scrutinized. Transfusions should be limited to patients who have a clearly positive benefit to risk ratio.

Management

Blood product recipients suspected of having a transfusion-related infection should undergo confirmatory testing and be treated with antibiotics, antivirals or otherwise depending on the causative pathogen. The blood bank should be notified immediately to reduce the chance that additional patients are exposed to contaminated products.

Acute Hypotensive Transfusion Reactions

Incidence

Due to the usually brief and reversible nature of acute hypotensive transfusion reactions, the reported incidence is low and likely underreported. The reported incidence to the CDC from 2010 to 12 was between 0.05% and 2.6% based on voluntary submissions [26, 49].

Mechanism

The introduction of leukoreductive filters in the 1990s was intended to reduce febrile transfusion reactions and infections. Additionally, ACE inhibitors were expanding in use throughout the United States to manage hypertension. Patients taking ACE inhibitors who required blood products while negatively charged leukocyte reduction filters were being used experienced increased bradykinin-mediated hypotension. Bradykinin is generated from factor XII (Hageman factor) interaction with negatively charged surfaces. Bradykinin stimulates B2 receptors which increase nitric oxide and prostaglandins, which results in hypotension. Angiotensin-converting enzyme is normally responsible with inhibiting bradykinin, which explains why ACE inhibitors are associated with hypotension in such patients [4].

Presentation

A decrease of systolic, diastolic, or mean arterial pressure by 30 mmHg with transfusion of blood products, in the absence of other symptoms of anaphylaxis such as bronchospasm or hemolysis and resolution of symptoms after cessation of transfusion.

Prevention

Cessation of angiotensin-converting enzyme (ACE) inhibitors preoperatively or prior to blood transfusion for 24–48 hours.

Management

Cessation of transfusion along with supportive therapy and exclusion of other etiologies of transfusion-related hypotension resulting from transfusion are necessary.

Air Embolism

Incidence

The incidence of air embolism during the transfusion of blood products is unknown, as the majority of cases do not result in clinical manifestations. Air introduction into the venous system can result in clinical symptoms ranging from mild tachypnea to cardiac or respiratory failure.

Mechanism

Venous air embolism requires a gradient between the source of air and the pressure inside the vessel. Normal venous pressure will prevent the flow of air bubbles from intravenous tubing provided that such air bubbles are not under increased pressure. Blood products hung from above the level of entry into the vein favor infusion of desired blood products. Air bubbles at atmospheric pressure in IV tubing are not under enough pressure in most transfusions to result in movement through tubing into the venous system. Pressurized products from rapid infusers or compression bags however can exceed venous pressure resulting in embolism. Air entry of 20 cc/second may result in symptoms in patients, and rates of 70–500 cc/second can be fatal [36, 37, 54].

Small quantities of air can dissolve in the bloodstream or diffuse across the alveolar membranes in the pulmonary vasculature. Larger volumes of air can obstruct cardiac output mechanically or travel into the pulmonary arteries and overwhelm the ability of the pulmonary alveoli filtration system. Additionally, massive cytokine release may trigger ARDS and coagulopathy.

Presentation

Depending on the volume of entrained air and the pressure at which it enters the vasculature, embolic air can be dissolved in the blood or filtered in the pulmonary alveoli and result in no clinical signs or symptoms. Significant air embolism can result in complications common to other types of pulmonary embolism including dysrhythmias, ST changes, pulmonary vasoconstriction, ventilation and perfusion mismatching, and right heart failure. Massive air emboli can fail to exit the right ventricular outflow tract and result in air lock and total cardiovascular collapse. Classically a "mill-wheel" murmur may be present. Trans-esophageal echocardiogram is diagnostic in intraventricular embolic scenarios and may detect as little as 0.02 ml/kg of air [69].

Prevention

VAE, while not a transfusion reaction, is a consequence of the route of administration of blood products. Given the substantial risks associated with VAE, it is worth mentioning with transfusion reactions. As with any complication of blood transfusion, the first step in prevention is limiting the use of blood products to necessary recipients. Blood transmission should occur through approved and effective filtration devices. Pressure application of products should be limited to patients requiring rapid transfusion. Rapid infusion systems utilized for massive transfusion, such as the Smiths Medical Level 1® Fast Flow Fluid Warmer or the Belmont® Rapid Infuser, incorporate air detection systems to alert clinicians to air in the delivery circuit. These systems can help reduce the risk of lethal air embolism, but vigilance is essential to avoid inadvertent air embolism.

Management

Immediate cessation of blood transfusion is mandatory for any acute changes in cardiac, respiratory, or neurological symptoms. Supportive care including fluid administration, oxygenation, and hemodynamic assistance should be provided. Cardiopulmonary resuscitation with chest compressions and pharmacologic intervention should be considered per ACLS guidelines. Forcing the obstructive air through the vasculature with inotropic support and chest compressions may be required in significant events of air embolism. Additionally, manual aspiration of air from the right ventricle from a central venous line can be effective if positioned correctly.

Acute Hemolytic Reactions

Incidence

The incidence of acute hemolytic reaction has reduced significantly with the introduction of systems designed to prevent human and machine error. Current estimates range from 2.5 to 7.9 per 100,000 units transfused [16]. The incidence in underdeveloped health systems, however, may be closer to 1 in 100 units [2].

Mechanism

The development of acute hemolytic reactions can occur due to both immune- and non-immune-mediated processes. Immune-mediated acute hemolysis is due to transfusion of red blood cells with antigens that are incompatible with the recipient's immune system, usually due to anti-A or anti-B antibodies. Less commonly, antibodies may be formed to other antigens including Kell and Duffy. Interaction of these antibodies with recipient antigens leads to complement activation and intravascular hemolysis. Extravascular hemolysis, however, occurs when the antibodies bind to RBC antigens and result in sequestration within the reticuloendothelial system where phagocytosis occurs. Activation of macrophages leads to a systemic response which is manifest as fever and chills as well as back and abdominal flank pain.

Non-immune-mediated acute hemolysis is commonly a result of co-administration with incompatible crystalloid, thermal injury, or mechanical disruption of the cell membranes causing hemolysis. Exposure of red blood cells to hypo-osmolar crystalloid results in free water entering the cells, which leads to cellular swelling and hemolysis. Thermal injury to red blood cells can occur through both excessive heat and freezing. Cell membrane injury can result both directly from heat and from ice crystal formation during red blood cell freezing in the absence of cryoprotective agents such as glycerol. Mechanical disruption can occur through exposure to external forces during transfusion through small-gauge intravenous catheters or through cardiopulmonary bypass pumps.

Presentation

The most common symptoms seen with acute hemolytic reactions are not the classically described triad of flank pain, fever, and red or brown urine. The clinical presentation can include a myriad of symptoms including fever, chills, flank or abdominal pain, hypotension, dyspnea, hemoglobinuria, diffuse intravascular coagulopathy, acute renal failure, shock, and death.

Prevention

The introduction of pretransfusion compatibility screening has significantly reduced the incidence of acute hemolytic reactions. System-based practices to ensure proper patient identification throughout the screening and transfusion process should be strictly followed to prevent acute hemolytic reactions due to clerical error.

Management

If an acute hemolytic reaction is suspected, the transfusion should be immediately stopped. Additionally, supportive management should be instituted to prevent complications including cardiovascular instability, renal failure, respiratory failure, and the development of coagulation disorders.

Transfusion-Associated Graft Versus Host Disease

Incidence

The development of transfusion-associated graft versus host disease (TA-GVHD) is extremely rare with radiation of transfused products or through pathogen reduction techniques [16] with only 348 confirmed and reported cases in the last 50 years [46]. While radiation or pathogen reduction is typically performed prior to transfusing immunocompromised patients, it is important to note that over half of all documented TA-GVHD cases have occurred in immunocompetent patients.

Mechanism

The development of TA-GVHD starts with transfusion of blood components that contain viable T-lymphocytes. The T-lymphocytes are normally recognized as foreign by the recipient's immune system and cleared quickly. The engraftment of donor T-lymphocytes into the transfusion recipient may occur when the recipient immune system either cannot mount a proper response or does not recognize the donor T-lymphocytes as foreign [1]. While immunosuppression may play a role, there is also evidence to suggest that matching of donor and recipient HLA haplotypes may allow engraftment of donor T cells into the immunocompetent recipient. Immunocompetent patients are at increased risk when they receive donations from close family members or from a donor with homozygous HLA haplotypes that match at least one allele on the recipient. Once donor T cells have engrafted, they can initiate an immune response by recipient natural killer cells, macrophages, and other T cells against recipient tissues [39]. Once symptoms initially manifest, mortality occurs within weeks in 80–90% of patients.

Presentation

The presenting symptoms of TA-GVHD typically manifest within 2–30 days following transfusion [40] and may affect the cutaneous, gastrointestinal, and hematologic systems. The most common symptoms are the development of a rash, fever, elevated transaminase, pancytopenia, diarrhea, bone marrow hypoplasia, and hepatomegaly. The accompanying rash is typically a diffuse maculopapular rash which may develop and progress to generalized erythroderma and desquamation. Mortality is typically the result of severe neutropenia which leads to untreatable infections [62].

Prevention

Leukoreductive techniques which aim at reducing T cells from transfused products have been proposed to reduce this risk of TA-GVHD [40]. In high-risk patients, the transfusion of fresh blood units should be avoided. Units that have been stored for less than 72–96 hours are more likely to contain T-lymphocytes that retain the ability to proliferate in the recipient. T-lymphocytes have diminishing capacity for protein synthesis and proliferation as storage time increases [8].

Irradiation of PRBCs has also been proposed to be partially protective. Irradiation with at least 2500 cGy of gamma rays has been shown to render the donor's T cells incapable of proliferation within the recipient [22, 44, 55]. Preclinical data suggests that pathogen inactivation processes may be more protective of a leukoreduction technique than irradiation [7, 18, 23]. The addition of intercalating agents, such as amotosalen or riboflavin, to transfused products allows the molecule to dock between nucleic acid pairs in leukocyte DNA. Ultraviolet illumination of the blood product then activates the intercalating agent, which permanently crosslinks the helical strands. This crosslinking prevents further cellular replication and inactivates the T cell [35] while also reducing the risk of bacterial and viral transmission through the same process [45]. Regardless of which method is employed, attempts to reduce transfusion of active T-lymphocytes should be employed in patients at risk for TA-GVHD.

Management

Mortality remains high in TA-GVHD despite aggressive supportive therapies. Care should be made to maintain euvolemia and avoid electrolyte disturbances that accompany severe diarrhea. A slight survival advantage has been shown in patients treated with hematopoietic cell transplantation, although there is often not enough time to find a suitable donor. Immunosuppression has also been described to help control symptoms [40].

Transfusion-Associated Circulatory Overload

Incidence

The general incidence of transfusion-associated circulatory overload (TACO) has been estimated at 0.7%, or 10.0 per 100,000 units transfused [16, 56]. In the perioperative period, the incidence appears to be higher at around 3–11%. The highest rates appear in vascular (12.1%), transplant (8.8%), and thoracic (7.2%) surgeries, while lower rates are observed in obstetric and gynecologic patients (1.4%). There does not appear to be a difference between genders with an incidence of 4.8% in men and 3.8% in women [10]. Increased risk correlates with an increase in the number of transfused units, while other risk factors appear to include Caucasian race and pre-existing cardiac and pulmonary diseases [48].

Mechanism

The development of TACO can be influenced by volume- and non-volume-associated mediators. Volume mediators include hypervolemia from transfusion as well as increased hydrostatic pressure which leads to the development of pulmonary edema. Non-volume mediators include erythrocyte-derived microparticles, cell-free hemoglobin, and nitric oxide scavenging which may also promote fluid shifting into the lung.

Presentation

The clinical presentation of TACO consists of a myriad of symptoms associated with volume overload. The diagnostic criteria for TACO are variably described in the literature but typically includes a set of signs and symptoms that develop within 12 hours of transfusion. The International Society for Blood Transfusion criteria include the development of acute respiratory distress or pulmonary edema and two or more of the following symptoms: alterations in the cardiovascular system suggesting volume overload and/or a rise in B-type natriuretic peptide. A separate set of diagnostic criteria has also been proposed for the perioperative period and includes new onset of three of the following within 6 hours of a perioperative transfusion: acute respiratory distress, evidence of positive fluid balance, elevated brain natriuretic peptide, radiographic evidence of pulmonary edema, evidence of left heart failure, and/or elevated central venous pressure [10, 24].

Prevention

In patients at risk for the development of TACO, clinicians should reduce transfusion rate and, if possible, transfuse one unit at a time while assessing the patient's response. Risk factors for TACO include chronic kidney disease, left ventricular dysfunction, baseline beta-blockers, emergency surgery, increased colloid or crystalloid use, and use of plasma products or mixed blood products [9].

Management

That management of TACO is primarily supportive. Clinicians may consider the use of diuretic medications to assist with volume overload [1].

Transfusion-Related Acute Lung Injury

Incidence

The incidence of TRALI has decreased significantly since the introduction of mitigating strategies in the early 2000s. Prior to mitigation, the incidence of TRALI was estimated to be 0.04–0.1%. With the addition of mitigation, the incidence has decreased significantly to an estimated 0.0081% [58, 65, 72]. The incidence of TRALI remains relatively high in the surgical population with an overall incidence of 1.3–1.4%, with the highest rates seen in thoracic (3%), vascular (2.7%), and transplant (2.2%) cases [9].

Mechanism

Two separate mechanisms for the development of TRALI have been described. In the first, antibodies present in the donor product react with anti-human leukocyte or anti-human neutrophil antigens in the recipient. This results in an inflammatory cascade which results in the development of pulmonary edema. Pre-existing inflammatory states, recent surgery, and concurrent infections may increase the risk. A second separate mechanism has been described as a two-hit model. In this model, neutrophils are believed to be sequestered into the lung parenchyma prior to the transfusion where they are primed through cytokine release. The second hit occurs when the recipient neutrophils are activated by a factor in the donor blood product. The resulting inflammatory cascade within the lung parenchyma results in pulmonary edema [6, 19, 64].

Presentation

The clinical presentation of TRALI is characterized by acute onset of respiratory distress that occurs during the transfusion or up to 6 hours afterward. Classically, the clinical characteristics include hypoxemia with a PaO2/FiO2 <300 or SPO2 <90% on room air, bilateral infiltrates on frontal chest x-ray, no evidence of circulatory overload, and no pre-existing acute lung injury or acute respiratory distress syndrome before the transfusion [43]. Less commonly, patients may also exhibit pink frothy airway secretions, fever, hypotension, or cyanosis [75].

Prevention

Several strategies have been developed to prevent the occurrence of TRALI with blood transfusions: exclusion of donors implicated in TRALI cases, exclusive use of FFP from un-transfused males or FFP treated with solvent/detergent, and leukodepletion of cellular blood components prior to giving to patients with anti-leukocyte antibodies [43]. These strategies have been shown to significantly reduce the risk of TRALI [20] but have been variably implemented across the blood banking centers [38].

Management

Patients who are suspected to have TRALI are treated primarily through discontinuation of the transfusion and supportive care. Hypoxemia is a significant risk with TRALI which often times requires ventilatory support [76]. Patients can also develop hypovolemia and require significant volume and vasopressor support. In rare circumstances, extracorporeal membrane oxygenation and plasmapheresis have been successfully employed [77].

Transfusion-Related Immune Modulation (TRIM)

TRIM describes the observation of immune modulation, both proinflammatory and suppression effects, which occurs to the recipient following transfusion. The phenomenon was first described in the 1970s when it was demonstrated that solid organ transplant recipients who also were transfused had improved graft survival [53]. In oncologic processes, however, transfusion has been repeatedly associated with worse outcomes. The presence of donor leukocytes in transfused blood has been linked with the phenomenon of TRIM and appears to be at least partially responsible for the negative effects in outcomes for transfusion recipients, as evidenced by the reduction, albeit sustained presence, of TRIM in leukoreduced donor products [11]. An extensive discussion of this topic is beyond the scope of this chapter, but its inclusion reemphasizes the importance of adhering to transfusion guidelines in order to avoid unnecessary transfusion to keep patients safe.

References

1. Aubron C, Aries P, Le Niger C, Sparrow RL, Ozier Y. How clinicians can minimize transfusion-related adverse events? Transfus Clin Biol. 2018;25(4):257–61. https://doi.org/10.1016/j.tracli.2018.08.158.
2. Bassi R, Aggarwal S, Bhardwaj K, Thakur KK. Patterns of adverse transfusion reactions in a tertiary care centre of North India: a step towards hemovigilance. Indian J Hematol Blood Transfus. 2017;33(2):248–53. https://doi.org/10.1007/s12288-016-0684-9.
3. Brittingham TE, Chaplin H Jr. Febrile transfusion reactions caused by sensitivity to donor leukocytes and platelets. J Am Med Assoc. 1957;165(7):819–25. https://doi.org/10.1001/jama.1957.02980250053013.
4. Bruno DS, Herman JH. Acute hypotensive transfusion reactions. Lab Med. 2006;37(9):542–5.
5. Buck SA, Kickler TS, McGuire M, Braine HG, Ness PM. The utility of platelet washing using an automated procedure for severe platelet allergic reactions. Transfusion. 1987;27(5):391–3. https://doi.org/10.1046/j.1537-2995.1987.27587320530.x.

6. Bux J, Sachs UJ. The pathogenesis of transfusion-related acute lung injury (TRALI). Br J Haematol. 2007;136(6):788–99. https://doi.org/10.1111/j.1365-2141.2007.06492.x.
7. Castro G, Merkel PA, Giclas HE, Gibula A, Andersen GE, Corash LM, Lin JS, Green J, Knight V, Stassinopoulos A. Amotosalen/UVA treatment inactivates T cells more effectively than the recommended gamma dose for prevention of transfusion-associated graft-versus-host disease. Transfusion. 2018;58(6):1506–15. https://doi.org/10.1111/trf.14589.
8. Chang H, Voralia M, Bali M, Sher GD, Branch DR. Irreversible loss of donor blood leucocyte activation may explain a paucity of transfusion-associated graft-versus-host disease from stored blood. Br J Haematol. 2000;111(1):146–56. https://doi.org/10.1046/j.1365-2141.2000.02330.x.
9. Clifford L, Jia Q, Subramanian A, Yadav H, Schroeder DR, Kor DJ. Risk factors and clinical outcomes associated with perioperative transfusion-associated circulatory overload. Anesthesiology. 2017;126(3):409–18. https://doi.org/10.1097/ALN.0000000000001506.
10. Clifford L, Jia Q, Yadav H, Subramanian A, Wilson GA, Murphy SP, Pathak J, Schroeder DR, Ereth MH, Kor DJ. Characterizing the epidemiology of perioperative transfusion-associated circulatory overload. Anesthesiology. 2015;122(1):21–8. https://doi.org/10.1097/ALN.0000000000000513.
11. Connor JP, O'Shea A, McCool K, Sampene E, Barroilhet LM. Peri-operative allogeneic blood transfusion is associated with poor overall survival in advanced epithelial ovarian cancer; potential impact of patient blood management on cancer outcomes. Gynecol Oncol. 2018;151(2):294–8. https://doi.org/10.1016/j.ygyno.2018.08.040.
12. Cooper DJ, McQuilten ZK, Nichol A, Ady B, Aubron C, Bailey M, Bellomo R, Gantner D, Irving DO, Kaukonen K-M, McArthur C, Murray L, Pettilä V, French C, TRANSFUSE Investigators and the Australian and New Zealand Intensive Care Society Clinical Trials, G. Age of red cells for transfusion and outcomes in critically ill adults. N Engl J Med. 2017;377(19):1858–67. https://doi.org/10.1056/NEJMoa1707572.
13. d'Almeida MS, Gray D, Martin C, Ellis CG, Chin-Yee IH. Effect of prophylactic transfusion of stored RBCs on oxygen reserve in response to acute isovolemic hemorrhage in a rodent model. Transfusion. 2001;41(7):950–6. https://doi.org/10.1046/j.1537-2995.2001.41070950.x.
14. de Korte D, Kleine M, Korsten HG, Verhoeven AJ. Prolonged maintenance of 2,3-diphosphoglycerate acid and adenosine triphosphate in red blood cells during storage. Transfusion. 2008;48(6):1081–9. https://doi.org/10.1111/j.1537-2995.2008.01689.x.
15. de Rie MA, van der Plas-van Dalen CM, Engelfriet CP, von dem Borne AE. The serology of febrile transfusion reactions. Vox Sang. 1985;49(2):126–34. https://doi.org/10.1111/j.1423-0410.1985.tb00780.x.
16. Delaney M, Wendel S, Bercovitz RS, Cid J, Cohn C, Dunbar NM, Apelseth TO, Popovsky M, Stanworth SJ, Tinmouth A, Van De Watering L, Waters JH, Yazer M, Ziman A, Biomedical Excellence for Safer Transfusion, C. Transfusion reactions: prevention, diagnosis, and treatment. Lancet. 2016;388(10061):2825–36. https://doi.org/10.1016/S0140-6736(15)01313-6.
17. Domen RE, Hoeltge GA. Allergic transfusion reactions: an evaluation of 273 consecutive reactions. Arch Pathol Lab Med. 2003;127(3):316–20. https://doi.org/10.1043/0003-9985(2003)127<0316:ATR>2.0.CO;2.
18. Fast LD, DiLeone G, Marschner S. Inactivation of human white blood cells in platelet products after pathogen reduction technology treatment in comparison to gamma irradiation. Transfusion. 2011;51(7):1397–404. https://doi.org/10.1111/j.1537-2995.2010.02984.x.
19. Fung YL, Silliman CC. The role of neutrophils in the pathogenesis of transfusion-related acute lung injury. Transfus Med Rev. 2009;23(4):266–83. https://doi.org/10.1016/j.tmrv.2009.06.001.
20. Funk MB, Heiden M, Volkers P, Lohmann A, Keller-Stanislawski B. Evaluation of risk minimisation measures for blood components – based on reporting rates of transfusion-transmitted reactions (1997–2013). Transfus Med Hemother. 2015;42(4):240–6. https://doi.org/10.1159/000381996.
21. Geiger TL, Howard SC. Acetaminophen and diphenhydramine premedication for allergic and febrile nonhemolytic transfusion reactions: good prophylaxis or bad practice? Transfus Med Rev. 2007;21(1):1–12. https://doi.org/10.1016/j.tmrv.2006.09.001.
22. Goes EG, Borges JC, Covas DT, Orellana MD, Palma PV, Morais FR, Pela CA. Quality control of blood irradiation: determination T cells radiosensitivity to cobalt-60 gamma rays. Transfusion. 2006;46(1):34–40. https://doi.org/10.1111/j.1537-2995.2005.00669.x.
23. Grass JA, Wafa T, Reames A, Wages D, Corash L, Ferrara JL, Lin L. Prevention of transfusion-associated graft-versus-host disease by photochemical treatment. Blood. 1999;93(9):3140–7. Retrieved from https://www.ncbi.nlm.nih.gov/pubmed/10216113.
24. International Society of Blood Transfusion Working Party on Haemovigilance. Transfusion-Associated circulatory overload (TACO) definition. 2018. Retrieved from http://www.isbtweb.org/fileadmin/user_upload/TACO_2018_definition_March_2019.pdf.
25. Hamasaki N, Rose ZB. The binding of phosphorylated red cell metabolites to human hemoglobin A. J Biol Chem. 1974;249(24):7896–901. Retrieved from https://www.ncbi.nlm.nih.gov/pubmed/4430678.
26. Harvey AR, Basavaraju SV, Chung KW, Kuehnert MJ. Transfusion-related adverse reactions reported to the National Healthcare Safety Network Hemovigilance Module, United States, 2010 to 2012. Transfusion. 2015;55(4):709–18. https://doi.org/10.1111/trf.12918.
27. Heaton A, Keegan T, Holme S. In vivo regeneration of red cell 2,3-diphosphoglycerate following transfusion of DPG-depleted AS-1, AS-3 and CPDA-1 red cells. Br J Haematol. 1989;71(1):131–6. https://doi.org/10.1111/j.1365-2141.1989.tb06286.x.
28. Heddle NM, Cook RJ, Arnold DM, Liu Y, Barty R, Crowther MA, Devereaux PJ, Hirsh J, Warkentin TE, Webert KE, Roxby D, Sobieraj-Teague M, Kurz A, Sessler DI, Figueroa P, Ellis M, Eikelboom JW. Effect of short-term vs. long-term blood storage on mortality after transfusion. N Engl J Med. 2016;375(20):1937–45. https://doi.org/10.1056/NEJMoa1609014.
29. Heddle NM, Klama L, Meyer R, Walker I, Boshkov L, Roberts R, Chambers S, Podlosky L, O'Hoski P, Levine M. A randomized controlled trial comparing plasma removal with white cell reduction to prevent reactions to platelets. Transfusion. 1999;39(3):231–8. https://doi.org/10.1046/j.1537-2995.1999.39399219278.x.
30. Heddle NM, Klama L, Singer J, Richards C, Fedak P, Walker I, Kelton JG. The role of the plasma from platelet concentrates in transfusion reactions. N Engl J Med. 1994;331(10):625–8. https://doi.org/10.1056/NEJM199409083311001.
31. Heddle NM, Klama LN, Griffith L, Roberts R, Shukla G, Kelton JG. A prospective study to identify the risk factors associated with acute reactions to platelet and red cell transfusions. Transfusion. 1993;33(10):794–7. https://doi.org/10.1046/j.1537-2995.1993.331094054613.x.
32. Hess JR, Hill HR, Oliver CK, Lippert LE, Greenwalt TJ. Alkaline CPD and the preservation of RBC 2,3-DPG. Transfusion. 2002;42(6):747–52. https://doi.org/10.1046/j.1537-2995.2002.00115.x.
33. Hogman CF, Knutson F, Loof H, Payrat JM. Improved maintenance of 2,3 DPG and ATP in RBCs stored in a modified additive solution. Transfusion. 2002;42(7):824–9. https://doi.org/10.1046/j.1537-2995.2002.00148.x.

34. Hogman CF, Lof H, Meryman HT. Storage of red blood cells with improved maintenance of 2,3-bisphosphoglycerate. Transfusion. 2006;46(9):1543–52. https://doi.org/10.1111/j.1537-2995.2006.00893.x.
35. Irsch J, Lin L. Pathogen inactivation of platelet and plasma blood components for transfusion using the INTERCEPT blood system. Transfus Med Hemother. 2011;38(1):19–31. https://doi.org/10.1159/000323937.
36. Kashuk JL, Penn I. Air embolism after central venous catheterization. Surg Gynecol Obstet. 1984;159(3):249–52. Retrieved from https://www.ncbi.nlm.nih.gov/pubmed/6433496.
37. King MB, Harmon KR. Unusual forms of pulmonary embolism. Clin Chest Med. 1994;15(3):561–80. Retrieved from https://www.ncbi.nlm.nih.gov/pubmed/7982347.
38. Kleinman S, Grossman B, Kopko P. A national survey of transfusion-related acute lung injury risk reduction policies for platelets and plasma in the United States. Transfusion. 2010;50(6):1312–21. https://doi.org/10.1111/j.1537-2995.2010.02659.x.
39. Kleinman S, Stassinopoulos A. Transfusion-associated graft-versus-host disease reexamined: potential for improved prevention using a universally applied intervention. Transfusion. 2018;58(11):2545–63. https://doi.org/10.1111/trf.14930.
40. Kopolovic I, Ostro J, Tsubota H, Lin Y, Cserti-Gazdewich CM, Messner HA, Keir AK, DenHollander N, Dzik WS, Callum J. A systematic review of transfusion-associated graft-versus-host disease. Blood. 2015;126(3):406–14. https://doi.org/10.1182/blood-2015-01-620872.
41. Lacroix J, Hebert PC, Fergusson DA, Tinmouth A, Cook DJ, Marshall JC, Clayton L, McIntyre L, Callum J, Turgeon AF, Blajchman MA, Walsh TS, Stanworth SJ, Campbell H, Capellier G, Tiberghien P, Bardiaux L, van de Watering L, van der Meer NJ, Sabri E, Vo D, ABLE Investigators, Canadian Critical Care Trials, G. Age of transfused blood in critically ill adults. N Engl J Med. 2015;372(15):1410–8. https://doi.org/10.1056/NEJMoa1500704.
42. Li Y, Xiong Y, Wang R, Tang F, Wang X. Blood banking-induced alteration of red blood cell oxygen release ability. Blood Transfus. 2016;14(2):238–44. https://doi.org/10.2450/2015.0055-15.
43. Liumbruno GM, Sodini ML, Grazzini G, Tuscan Transfusion S. Recommendations from the Tuscan Transfusion System on the appropriate use of solvent/detergent-inactivated fresh-frozen plasma. Blood Transfus. 2008;6(1):25–36. Retrieved from https://www.ncbi.nlm.nih.gov/pubmed/18661921.
44. Luban NL, Drothler D, Moroff G, Quinones R. Irradiation of platelet components: inhibition of lymphocyte proliferation assessed by limiting-dilution analysis. Transfusion. 2000;40(3):348–52. https://doi.org/10.1046/j.1537-2995.2000.40030348.x.
45. Makroo RN, Sardana R, Mediratta L, Butta H, Thakur UK, Agrawal S, Chowdhry M, Kumar S, Chokroborty S. Evaluation of bacterial inactivation in random donor platelets and single-donor apheresis platelets by the INTERCEPT blood system. Asian J Transfus Sci. 2018;12(2):146–53. https://doi.org/10.4103/ajts.AJTS_87_17.
46. Manduzio P. Transfusion-associated graft-versus-host disease: a concise review. Hematol Rep. 2018;10(4):7724. https://doi.org/10.4081/hr.2018.7724.
47. McCrae KR, Herman JH. Posttransfusion purpura: two unusual cases and a literature review. Am J Hematol. 1996;52(3):205–11. https://doi.org/10.1002/(SICI)1096-8652(199607)52:3<205::AID-AJH13>3.0.CO;2-E.
48. Menis M, Anderson SA, Forshee RA, McKean S, Johnson C, Holness L, Warnock R, Gondalia R, Worrall CM, Kelman JA, Ball R, Izurieta HS. Transfusion-associated circulatory overload (TACO) and potential risk factors among the inpatient US elderly as recorded in Medicare administrative databases during 2011. Vox Sang. 2014;106(2):144–52. https://doi.org/10.1111/vox.12070.
49. Metcalf RA, Bakhtary S, Goodnough LT, Andrews J. Clinical pattern in hypotensive transfusion reactions. Anesth Analg. 2016;123(2):268–73. https://doi.org/10.1213/ANE.0000000000001387.
50. Mueller-Eckhardt C. Post-transfusion purpura. Br J Haematol. 1986;64(3):419–24. https://doi.org/10.1111/j.1365-2141.1986.tb02198.x.
51. Mueller-Eckhardt C, Kiefel V. High-dose IgG for post-transfusion purpura-revisited. Blut. 1988;57(4):163–7. https://doi.org/10.1007/bf00319544.
52. Oakley FD, Woods M, Arnold S, Young PP. Transfusion reactions in pediatric compared with adult patients: a look at rate, reaction type, and associated products. Transfusion. 2015;55(3):563–70. https://doi.org/10.1111/trf.12827.
53. Opelz G, Sengar DP, Mickey MR, Terasaki PI. Effect of blood transfusions on subsequent kidney transplants. Transplant Proc. 1973;5(1):253–9. Retrieved from https://www.ncbi.nlm.nih.gov/pubmed/4572098.
54. Orebaugh SL. Venous air embolism: clinical and experimental considerations. Crit Care Med. 1992;20(8):1169–77. https://doi.org/10.1097/00003246-199208000-00017.
55. Pelszynski MM, Moroff G, Luban NL, Taylor BJ, Quinones RR. Effect of gamma irradiation of red blood cell units on T-cell inactivation as assessed by limiting dilution analysis: implications for preventing transfusion-associated graft-versus-host disease. Blood. 1994;83(6):1683–9. Retrieved from https://www.ncbi.nlm.nih.gov/pubmed/8123860.
56. Philip J, Pawar A, Chatterjee T, Mallhi RS, Biswas AK, Dimri U. Non infectious complications related to blood transfusion: an 11 year retrospective analysis in a tertiary care hospital. Indian J Hematol Blood Transfus. 2016;32(3):292–8. https://doi.org/10.1007/s12288-015-0565-7.
57. Pirenne F, Narbey D, Chadebech P, Mekontso-Dessap A, Bartolucci P, Rieux C, Michel M, Pakdaman S, Djoudi R, Galacteros F, Habibi A. Incidence and risk of delayed hemolytic transfusion reaction in sickle cell disease patients based on a prospective study. Blood. 2016;128(22). Retrieved from http://www.bloodjournal.org/content/128/22/95.
58. Rana R, Fernandez-Perez ER, Khan SA, Rana S, Winters JL, Lesnick TG, Breanndan Moore S, Gajic O. Transfusion-related acute lung injury and pulmonary edema in critically ill patients: a retrospective study. Transfusion. 2006;46(9):1478–83. https://doi.org/10.1111/j.1537-2995.2006.00930.x.
59. Sarkodee-Adoo CB, Kendall JM, Sridhara R, Lee EJ, Schiffer CA. The relationship between the duration of platelet storage and the development of transfusion reactions. Transfusion. 1998;38(3):229–35. https://doi.org/10.1046/j.1537-2995.1998.38398222865.x.
60. Sarode R. Complications of transfusion. (Merck Manual). Retrieved from https://www.merckmanuals.com/professional/hematology-and-oncology/transfusion-medicine/complications-of-transfusion.
61. Savage WJ, Tobian AA, Savage JH, Hamilton RG, Ness PM. Atopic predisposition of recipients in allergic transfusion reactions to apheresis platelets. Transfusion. 2011;51(11):2337–42. https://doi.org/10.1111/j.1537-2995.2011.03160.x.
62. Schroeder ML. Transfusion-associated graft-versus-host disease. Br J Haematol. 2002;117(2):275–87. https://doi.org/10.1046/j.1365-2141.2002.03450.x.
63. Shtalrid M, Shvidel L, Vorst E, Weinmann EE, Berrebi A, Sigler E. Post-transfusion purpura: a challenging diagnosis. Isr Med Assoc J. 2006;8(10):672–4. Retrieved from https://www.ncbi.nlm.nih.gov/pubmed/17125110.

64. Silliman CC. The two-event model of transfusion-related acute lung injury. Crit Care Med. 2006;34(5 Suppl):S124–31. https://doi.org/10.1097/01.CCM.0000214292.62276.8E.
65. Silliman CC, Boshkov LK, Mehdizadehkashi Z, Elzi DJ, Dickey WO, Podlosky L, Clarke G, Ambruso DR. Transfusion-related acute lung injury: epidemiology and a prospective analysis of etiologic factors. Blood. 2003;101(2):454–62. https://doi.org/10.1182/blood-2002-03-0958.
66. Silvergleid AJ, Hafleigh EB, Harabin MA, Wolf RM, Grumet FC. Clinical value of washed-platelet concentrates in patients with non-hemolytic transfusion reactions. Transfusion. 1977;17(1):33–7. https://doi.org/10.1046/j.1537-2995.1977.17177128881.x.
67. Stack G, Snyder EL. Cytokine generation in stored platelet concentrates. Transfusion. 1994;34(1):20–5. https://doi.org/10.1046/j.1537-2995.1994.34194098597.x.
68. Steiner ME, Ness PM, Assmann SF, Triulzi DJ, Sloan SR, Delaney M, Granger S, Bennett-Guerrero E, Blajchman MA, Scavo V, Carson JL, Levy JH, Whitman G, D'Andrea P, Pulkrabek S, Ortel TL, Bornikova L, Raife T, Puca KE, Kaufman RM, Nuttall GA, Young PP, Youssef S, Engelman R, Greilich PE, Miles R, Josephson CD, Bracey A, Cooke R, McCullough J, Hunsaker R, Uhl L, McFarland JG, Park Y, Cushing MM, Klodell CT, Karanam R, Roberts PR, Dyke C, Hod EA, Stowell CP. Effects of red-cell storage duration on patients undergoing cardiac surgery. N Engl J Med. 2015;372(15):1419–29. https://doi.org/10.1056/NEJMoa1414219.
69. Sviri S, Woods WP, van Heerden PV. Air embolism--a case series and review. Crit Care Resusc. 2004;6(4):271–6. Retrieved from https://www.ncbi.nlm.nih.gov/pubmed/16556106.
70. Tobian AA, Savage WJ, Tisch DJ, Thoman S, King KE, Ness PM. Prevention of allergic transfusion reactions to platelets and red blood cells through plasma reduction. Transfusion. 2011;51(8):1676–83. https://doi.org/10.1111/j.1537-2995.2010.03008.x.
71. Tormey CA, Stack G. Limiting the extent of a delayed hemolytic transfusion reaction with automated red blood cell exchange. Arch Pathol Lab Med. 2013;137(6):861–4. https://doi.org/10.5858/arpa.2012-0154-CR.
72. Toy P, Gajic O, Bacchetti P, Looney MR, Gropper MA, Hubmayr R, Lowell CA, Norris PJ, Murphy EL, Weiskopf RB, Wilson G, Koenigsberg M, Lee D, Schuller R, Wu P, Grimes B, Gandhi MJ, Winters JL, Mair D, Hirschler N, Rosen RS, Matthay MA, Group, T. S. Transfusion-related acute lung injury: incidence and risk factors. Blood. 2012;119(7):1757–67. https://doi.org/10.1182/blood-2011-08-370932.
73. Trivella M, Stanworth SJ, Brunskill S, Dutton P, Altman DG. Can we be certain that storage duration of transfused red blood cells does not affect patient outcomes? BMJ. 2019;365:l2320. https://doi.org/10.1136/bmj.l2320.
74. Valtis DJ. Defective gas-transport function of stored red bloodcells. Lancet. 1954;266(6803):119–24. https://doi.org/10.1016/s0140-6736(54)90978-2.
75. van Stein D, Beckers EA, Sintnicolaas K, Porcelijn L, Danovic F, Wollersheim JA, Brand A, van Rhenen DJ. Transfusion-related acute lung injury reports in the Netherlands: an observational study. Transfusion. 2010;50(1):213–20. https://doi.org/10.1111/j.1537-2995.2009.02345.x.
76. Vlaar AP, Binnekade JM, Prins D, van Stein D, Hofstra JJ, Schultz MJ, Juffermans NP. Risk factors and outcome of transfusion-related acute lung injury in the critically ill: a nested case-control study. Crit Care Med. 2010;38(3):771–8. https://doi.org/10.1097/CCM.0b013e3181cc4d4b.
77. Wallis JP. Transfusion-related acute lung injury (TRALI): presentation, epidemiology and treatment. Intensive Care Med. 2007;33(Suppl 1):S12–6. https://doi.org/10.1007/s00134-007-2874-2.
78. Yoshida T, AuBuchon JP, Dumont LJ, Gorham JD, Gifford SC, Foster KY, Bitensky MW. The effects of additive solution pH and metabolic rejuvenation on anaerobic storage of red cells. Transfusion. 2008;48(10):2096–105. https://doi.org/10.1111/j.1537-2995.2008.01812.x.

30 Blood Transfusion and Traumatic Brain Injury

Jose V. Montoya-Gacharna and Samir Kendale

Traumatic Brain Injury Definition and Epidemiology

Traumatic brain injury (TBI) is an acquired sudden injury secondary to blunt or penetrating mechanisms to the brain that disrupts its normal functioning. TBI can cause serious physical, cognitive, and psychosocial disabilities for the patient and cost for families and the healthcare system; the Centers for Disease Control and Prevention (CDC) estimated that in 2010, 2.5 million suffered from TBI and accounted for 87% of visits to the emergency department, 11% of hospitalizations, and 2% of deaths. Estimates show that 3.2–5.3 million persons have a TBI-related disability in the United States [1]. TBI is such complex health public issue that the US government has created the constitutional tools to be confronted. The Traumatic Brain Injury Act of 2008 authorized research and public health activities associated with TBI [2]. Studies performed in the United States before 2006 showed an incidence of TBI around 140/100,000 persons [3]. In 2003, Rutland-Brown et al. reported a mortality of 17.5/100,000 per year secondary to TBI [4]. During the period 1997–2007, approximately 580,000 persons died due to TBI in the United States [5]. All age groups are affected. TBI is a major cause of disability and death especially in the young adult population [6]. Mortality is higher in patients older than 65 years, in whom TBI is mostly related to falls [7, 8]. Men are more frequently affected than women. The majority of deaths are caused by motor vehicle accidents, suicides, and falls [5]. TBI can occur as an isolated injury or be associated with trauma to other areas of the body. It is classified as mild, moderate, and severe depending on the mechanism of injury and clinical signs and symptoms. The clinical assessment of TBI patients includes the Glasgow coma score and radiographic data. The scale assigns values 1–5 according to clinical responses including eye opening, motor response, and verbal response. Scores of 13–15 points correlate to mild, 9–12 points moderate, and <8 points severe brain injury [9].

Pathophysiology of TBI

A primary direct mechanical injury is followed by a delayed secondary injury after TBI [9, 10]. Injury to the brain impairs cerebral autoregulation of cerebral blood flow and causes metabolic derangements and the activation of a cascade of molecular signals. Several pathologic stages have been identified after TBI. Initially, a similar process to ischemia produces an increase in lactic acid, cell membrane permeability, and edema. The disruption of the blood-brain barrier also occurs. Depletion of ATP produces failure of ATP-dependent pumps. In the second stage, there is a sustained membrane depolarization with release of excitatory neurotransmitters such as glutamate and aspartate as well as activation of voltage-dependent calcium and sodium channels. Massive release of K+ associated with the release of excitatory neurotransmitters and calcium accumulation has also been identified [11]. Calcium overload in the mitochondria induces oxidative stress and mitochondrial dysfunction. A rapid increase in glucose followed by glucose metabolic depression can also be detected. Activation of lipid peroxidases, proteases, and phospholipases triggers apoptosis and cell death. In addition to all the mechanisms described, the damage to the blood-brain barrier causes the leakage of molecules (plasma derived factors) and cells involved in neuroinflammation (macrophages, lymphocytes, and neutrophils) and microglia activation [10].

J. V. Montoya-Gacharna (✉)
NYU Langone Medical Center, Department of Anesthesiology, New York, NY, USA
e-mail: jose.montoya-gacharna@nyumc.org

S. Kendale
Beth Israel Deaconess Medical Center, Department of Anesthesia, Perioperative Care & Pain Medicine, Boston, MA, USA
e-mail: skendale@bidmc.harvard.edu

© Springer Nature Switzerland AG 2021
C. S. Scher et al. (eds.), *Essentials of Blood Product Management in Anesthesia Practice*,
https://doi.org/10.1007/978-3-030-59295-0_30

When a mechanism of rapid acceleration and deceleration occurs, axonal breakdown follows. This injury is known as diffuse axonal injury [12]. Systemic inflammation and catecholamine increases can cause organ dysfunction in other areas. For example, neurogenic pulmonary edema can occur after TBI [13]. More detailed information regarding the mechanisms involved in TBI are described in several reviews [10, 11, 14].

Early neurosurgical assessment and therapy are crucial after TBI. Prevention of increase in intracranial pressure (ICP) or decrease in cerebral perfusion pressure (CPP) has been the most important clinical goal in the management of TBI; however more complex mechanisms of injury should be also taken into account [11]. Several molecular targets are being investigated for the treatment of secondary injury following TBI [10]. Improving the energy at the cellular level, decreasing the production of free radicals, maintaining the homeostasis of ions and glucose, and reducing cell death could be important targets involved in the management of TBI. Recent guidelines were developed by the Brain Trauma Foundation regarding severe TBI and include recommendations regarding the type of decompressive craniotomy, prophylactic hypothermia, hyperosmolar therapy, CSF drainage, ventilation therapy; the use of anesthetics, analgesics, sedatives, and steroids; nutrition; infection prophylaxis; DVT thrombosis prophylaxis; and seizure prophylaxis [15]. Updated recommendations include intracranial pressure monitoring, CPP monitoring, and advanced cerebral monitoring including jugular bulbar monitoring of AVDO2 [15].

Traumatic Brain Injury and Coagulopathy

Patients that have suffered severe TBI can present with abnormalities in their standard coagulation tests (INR, PT, and PTT) at hospital admission. Although isolated TBI occurs with minimal blood loss, coagulopathy could also be present. Coagulopathy may manifest initially as a hypocoagulable state that follows to a hypercoagulable state associated with a tendency for thrombosis [16]. Within minutes after TBI, fibrin degradation products and D-dimer are detectable followed by depletion of fibrinogen [8]. The prevalence of coagulopathy after TBI has a wide range from 7% [17] to 63% [18]. It is also more prevalent in severe TBI (60%) [19, 20]. Coagulopathy is less common in mild head injury [21]. There are more patients with coagulopathy with severe (76.7%) versus moderate (52.7%) head injury [22]. A meta-analysis of 22 studies showed that 35.2% of isolated TBIs had acute traumatic coagulopathy. Those patients had worse outcomes and a mortality between 17% and 86% [23]. Trauma-induced coagulopathy is a predictor of unfavorable neurological outcome in the pediatric population [24]. The PROPP trial demonstrated that patients that suffered TBI and hemorrhagic shock had also more pronounced coagulopathy [25]. In a prospective longitudinal study of moderate and severe head injury, there were 67% of patients with coagulopathy [22]. Several factors are involved with the development of coagulopathy including blood transfusion, surgical intervention, polytrauma, and severity of head injury [22]. The mechanism of injury also could be involved in the development of coagulopathy; in a retrospective study of 534 patients that evaluated blunt versus penetrating injury, patients with penetrating trauma were more coagulopathic and received more units of blood than the blunt cohort [26]. In a prospective study with 120 patients, trauma-induced coagulopathy was present in 46.6% of patients and was associated with acidosis in 60%; there was a decline in coagulation activation, increased thrombin formation, and fibrinolysis. Tissue factor, tissue factor pathway inhibitor, protein C, and protein S were low. As previously mentioned, patients have abnormalities in standard coagulation tests at admission to the emergency department [27]. In a prospective study of 572 patients, severe isolated TBI was independently associated with delayed clot formation [28]. Abnormalities in the coagulation process increase morbidity and mortality. Multiple mechanisms are associated with the activation of the coagulopathy. For instance, brain-derived cellular microvesicles (BDMV) are produced by injured glial cells and neurons and induce a hypercoagulable state in animal models [25]. Maegele et al. identified several risk factors related to the development of coagulopathy after blunt force trauma [29]. They include age >75 years [30, 31], >2L IVF at admission [31], GCS <8 at scene of injury [31, 32], injury severity score >16 [32], abbreviate injury scale (AIS) head = 5 [31, 33], subarachnoid hemorrhage, brain edema, midline shift on CT [32], abnormal pupils [30], SBP <90 [31, 32], Hb <12.4 mg/dL [34], serum glucose >151 mg/dL [34], arterial base deficit >6 mmol/L [33], and presence of at least two factors, of age >50 years, shock index (SI) >1, or abnormal pupils [30]. Moreover, INR has been identified as a hematological prognostic indicator in severe TBI requiring decompressive craniectomy [35]. Interestingly, normalization of INR through specific management of coagulopathy is independently associated with lower mortality in acute traumatic coagulopathy in isolated TBI in a retrospective study of 157 patients [36]. It is not clear whether the management of hypocoagulable state after TBI is similar as the presence after other types of traumas in the body.

Traumatic Brain Injury and Red Blood Cell Transfusion

Anemia and TBI Outcome

Anemia reduces the oxygen-carrying capacity of blood. Additionally, cerebral autoregulation may be impaired in patients with TBI. This combination of factors, in which oxygen delivery to brain tissue may be substantially diminished, may confer further injury than the effect of either alone [37]. Nonetheless, the relationship between anemia and outcomes after TBI remains elusive. Some studies have found associations between low hemoglobin concentrations and mortality or poorer neurologic outcome [38–40], as well as the converse that higher hemoglobin levels were associated with improved neurologic outcome [41]. There is some evidence, however, that suggests no link between anemia alone and worse outcomes in TBI patients [42–44]. The lack of consensus is not surprising considering the nature of these retrospective explorations, which are limited by variations in sample size and study population, differing definitions of anemia, differing outcome definitions, and the potential for unidentified confounding variables.

Transfusion and TBI Outcome

Although anemia is potentially associated with poor outcomes, transfusion of red blood cells with the goal of correcting anemia in TBI patients may not be a benign intervention. Transfusion of red blood cells in TBI patients is fairly common, with anywhere between 8.5% and 55% of TBI patients receiving RBC transfusion, depending on inclusion criteria and study design [40, 44–48]. RBC transfusion has been associated with a number of adverse outcomes, including increased ICU length of stay [46, 49], mortality [40, 44, 45, 49, 50], and other composite measures including ARDS, acute renal failure, and sepsis [44, 50]. Additionally, there may also be a relationship between RBC transfusion and long-term outcomes, specifically worse Glasgow outcome scale scores, Rancho Los Amigos Levels of Cognitive Functioning Scale scores, Disability Rating Scale scores, and Functional Status Examination scores assessed at either 6 months or 1 year [47, 48]. Many of these adverse outcomes, both short-term and long-term, however, may be as well contingent upon patient population and characteristics. One study, for example, suggested that the associations between transfusion and mortality may be dependent on the Glasgow coma score upon presentation or limited to patients in whom there was no evidence of shock [50].

For this reason, there has been significant interest in ascertaining thresholds for RBC transfusion, namely, whether there is a hemoglobin threshold at which harm of transfusion surpasses benefit. International clinician attitudes vary with regard to decisions to transfuse. Most physicians use a threshold of around 8 g/dl, though this may vary based on a variety of factors [51]. For example, neurosurgeons tend to transfuse at higher threshold than trauma surgeons or critical care physicians, and many physicians consider factors other than solely the hemoglobin threshold when deciding whether to transfuse RBCs, such as multiple trauma, presence of shock, and planned surgery [52, 53].

The literature on transfusion thresholds remains nebulous, and not only for patients with TBI. A Cochrane review suggested no difference in mortality between liberal and restrictive transfusion strategies [54]. In TBI patients, there has been evidence that a more liberal transfusion strategy (transfusing at a hemoglobin level of 10 g/dl) was associated with increased risk of progressive hemorrhagic injury and thromboembolic events [55, 56], but there has been little evidence of a difference in mortality, clinical improvement, or length of stay related to varying transfusion threshold [57, 58].

Finally, while limited clinical equipoise exists with regard to transfusion threshold, there is some consensus that the age of transfused blood is not associated with worse outcomes in patients with TBI [59, 60].

Traumatic Brain Injury and Plasma Transfusion

A standard practice to guide the transfusion of plasma during bleeding has been the use of coagulation times (PT, aPTT, and INR). However, a retrospective study of 4310 neurosurgical patients showed that preoperative elevated PT was not associated with an increased risk of perioperative hemorrhagic complications [61]. In the preoperative period, it is not recommended to correct a mildly prolonged INR in a stable hemodynamically patient [62]. The American Society for Anesthesiology Task Force recommends to transfuse plasma in four clinical settings: (1) for correction of excessive microvascular bleeding with INR >2 in the absence of heparin; (2) when standard coagulopathy tests are not available and there is excessive bleeding secondary to coagulation factor deficiencies; (3) when more than one volume of blood has been given; and (4) when reversal of warfarin is necessary and there is no available PCC or when factor deficiency is present but the specific factor is not available [63]. The European Society of Anesthesiology guideline recommends against the use of plasma transfusion for pre-procedural correction of mildly to moderately elevated INR, but recommends early targeted correction of coagulation factor deficiencies [64].

Several retrospective studies do not support the transfusion of plasma to reverse TBI-induced coagulopathy. A study of patients with TBI and moderate coagulopathy (INR 1.4–2.0) showed that FFP transfusion alone or in combination with packed RBCs resulted in poor long-term functional outcome [65]. Zhang et al. showed that patients with TBI who received plasma transfusion had significant higher mortality regardless of the severity of TBI in a prospective study of

618 patients [66]. According to Leeper et al., plasma transfusions and TBI were two independent predictors for fibrinolysis shutdown and were associated with a poor prognosis in pediatric patients with TBI. This author recommends that plasma transfusions should not be targeted to INR but to rTEG, ACT, and clinical bleeding [67].

Traumatic Brain Injury and Platelet Transfusion

Platelet function may be abnormal after TBI; for instance, platelets derived from TBI patients respond poorly to adenosine diphosphate (ADP) and arachidonic acid [68–70]. A prospective study of 153 patients showed that ADP inhibition of platelet function was increased in moderate-to-severe TBI vs mild TBI. This ADP inhibition at admission was not associated with in-hospital mortality or CT scan lesion expansion, and there were no differences in mean reduction of ADP inhibition from platelet transfusion vs no platelet transfusion [71]. Platelet dysfunction (ADP inhibition >60% on TEG) is an independent predictor of increased mortality in patients with severe TBI [72]. A platelet count higher than 100 k/L has been used for patients undergoing a neurosurgical procedure [73] and has been endorsed by the British Committee for Standards in Haematology (BCHS) Blood Transfusion Task Force [74]. A similar recommendation was found in the pediatric population. BCHS guidelines recommend a value higher than 100 k/L for neonates and 75–100 k/L for children. A threshold of 50 k/L in pediatric craniotomies has also been suggested [75]. A case series showed an association with postoperative intracranial bleeding in neurosurgical patients with platelets less than 100 K/L [76]. A goal-directed platelet transfusion to correct platelet dysfunction could be a better approach. Furay compared 35 patients who suffered TBI and had platelet dysfunction with 51 historic controls. Patients who received platelet transfusion had lower mortality (9% vs 35%) [72]. The role of platelet assay for guiding platelet transfusion in neurosurgical patients has not been validated.

Patients who suffered TBI and are on antiplatelet therapy are a challenge for the anesthesiologist. Unfortunately, there are no recommendations regarding this issue. A retrospective study of 328 patients with TBI and on antiplatelet therapy with aspirin or clopidogrel showed that platelet transfusion did not reduce mortality in patients >50 years old [77]. A cohort analysis of TBI patients treated with aspirin before trauma detected a higher mortality after platelet transfusion and failed to improved platelet function [78]. Platelet transfusion is able to reverse ASA-induced platelet inhibition but not the inhibition of platelet function produced by TBI [79]. An observational study of six US trauma centers of adults on antiplatelet therapy who suffered TBI blunt injury showed that transfused patients had higher injury severity scores and admission CT scores. Interestingly platelet transfusion reduced platelet inhibition to aspirin but not to clopidogrel. Platelet transfusion was associated with longer length of stay but no differences in mortality [80]. A prospective study of 243 patients with isolated intracranial hemorrhage and preinjury P2Y12 inhibitors showed a lower rate of bleeding progression and a decrease of neurosurgical intervention with platelet transfusion [81]. On the other hand, the ratio of platelet to plasma and RBCT could affect outcomes of TBI patients. A retrospective observational study of 385 patients with isolated blunt TBI who received a plasma-to-red cell ratio >1 was an independent predictor for reduced hospital mortality but not the same for platelet-to-red cell ratio >1. A systematic review of seven retrospective cohort studies found that platelet transfusion was associated with elevated odds ratio for in-hospital mortality [82]. However, another retrospective study of TBI patients who received RBCT, plasma, and platelets in a 1:1:1 ratio compared with non-ratio-based transfusion patients showed improve survival among those patients with ratio-based transfusions [83].

Transfusion of Cryoprecipitate

Acquired hypofibrinogenemia can occur in TBI with multiple trauma. The decrease in fibrinogen associated with the dilution of coagulation factors favors TBI-induced coagulopathy. Cryoprecipitate is used in the treatment of hypofibrinogenemia and hemophilia. Cryoprecipitate is a source of fibrinogen, factor VIII, VWF, and factor XIII [84]. The replenishment of fibrinogen with cryoprecipitate, in theory, should decrease the coagulopathy that occurs after trauma. Decrease in plasma fibrinogen increases red blood cell transfusion and mortality. A recent cohort study of 33 patients who suffered severe TBI showed that the rate of coagulopathy at 24 hours was lower but not significantly different than the control group; however, the in-hospital mortality was significantly lower in those patients treated with cryoprecipitate [85]. A retrospective cohort study of patients with severe multiple trauma and TBI and infusion of cryoprecipitate within 90 minutes of admission showed a decrease in mortality at 24 hours of 8% vs 13%. It also reduced the amount of blood transfusion products (RBCT 7 ± 1 unit vs 17 ± 3 units; FFP 9 ± 1 units vs 16 ± 3 units; platelets 3 ± 1 units vs 15 ± 4 units). The European Society of Anesthesiology guidelines recommend the use of cryoprecipitate as an alternative when fibrinogen is not available [86]. The BCHS guideline recommends prophylactic administration of cryoprecipitate to pediatric patients with a fibrinogen <1 g/L and significant risk of bleeding at a critical anatomical area [87].

Antifibrinolytic Medications and Traumatic Brain Injury

Antifibrinolytic agents prevent the destruction of the blood clot and are able to reduce bleeding. They have been shown to reduce mortality during postpartum hemorrhage and perioperative blood transfusion without increasing the risk of thromboembolic events [88] and possibly TBI [89]. Tranexamic acid (TXA) is also able to reduce blood transfusion in total hip arthroplasty [90], traumatic femur surgery [91], and cesarean section [92].

Several trials are ongoing to determine whether antifibrinolytic therapy could be effective after TBI. The CRASH-2 study showed that adult trauma patients with significant bleeding would benefit from the use of TXA. The risk of death due to bleeding significantly was reduced in the TXA group compared to placebo group (4.9% vs 5.7%, RR 0.85, 95% CI 0.76–0.96). There were no increases in thrombotic complications compared with the control group and fewer focal ischemic lesions [93]. The CRASH-2 intracranial bleeding study was a prospective randomized controlled trial within the CRASH-2 trial to evaluate the effect of TXA on intracranial hemorrhage growth after TBI. TXA use reduced hematoma expansion and resulted in fewer deaths compared to placebo. A post hoc evaluation of 270 patients from the CRASH-2 trial with intracranial bleeding was not able to exclude side effects after TXA but suggested further research [94]. The CRASH-3 trial is currently in course and is evaluating the effect of early treatment with TXA on death and disability in TBI patients [95].

A recent trial evaluation of TXA at a 1 g loading dose followed by an 8-hour infusion reduced intracerebral hematoma expansion and improved clinical outcomes after acute stroke secondary to intracerebral hemorrhage. The study showed no differences in the functional status or death of patients at 90 days from injury between TXA or placebo groups [96]. A sub-study of the CRASH-3 trial is evaluating the mechanistic effects of TXA on TBI. The study will determine the intracranial bleeding volume after injury by computed tomography [97].

A retrospective review of 4476 patients who suffered all adult trauma showed that in patients with lower GCS, TXA was used significantly more in patients with higher injury severity score (ISS), penetrating injuries, and higher incidence of severe head injury or transfusion requirements. Patient who received TXA had lower mortality rate (0% vs 10.1%) and increase of GCS to 14–15. There were no differences on thromboembolic events [98].

A recent randomized double-blind, placebo-controlled clinical trial of 80 patients showed that TXA after TBI was able to reduce intraoperative intracranial bleeding [99]. A meta-analysis found five randomized controlled trials of patients with TBI treated with TXA. There was a decrease in hematoma expansion. After exclusion of one of the studies after a sensitivity analysis, there were significant differences in mortality and neurologic outcomes between TXA and placebo groups without difference in thrombotic events [89].

It is important to indicate that recently it has been reported that isolated TBI has a characteristic coagulopathy with delayed clot formation that is not associated with fibrinolysis abnormalities. The authors suggest that these findings may indicate that early coagulation factor replacement should be done over antifibrinolytic therapy in severe isolated TBI [28]. However, a recent study showed that rFVII in early treatment did not decrease mortality or improve clinical outcomes after TBI [100].

Conclusions

Traumatic brain injury is a serious public health concern that generates thousands of TBI-related deaths and disabilities. TBI induces a specific type of coagulopathy that is more complex with associated injuries. An adequate management of TBI-induced coagulopathy is critical for patient outcome. Most of the current medical evidence for the transfusion of blood products and its derivatives comes from retrospective and prospective studies. More double-blinded trials are necessary to effectively improve the management of coagulopathy during TBI.

References

1. Selassie AW, et al. Incidence of long-term disability following traumatic brain injury hospitalization, United States, 2003. J Head Trauma Rehabil. 2008;23(2):123–31.
2. Zaloshnja E, et al. Prevalence of long-term disability from traumatic brain injury in the civilian population of the United States, 2005. J Head Trauma Rehabil. 2008;23(6):394–400.
3. George W. Rutherford, MD et. al. Epidemiology of adult traumatic brain injury. Institute of Medicine Committee on Gulf, W., V. Health: brain injury in, and O. long-term health. In: Gulf war and health: long-term consequences of traumatic brain injury. Vol. 7. Washington, DC: National Academies Press (US); 2008.
4. Rutland-Brown W, et al. Incidence of traumatic brain injury in the United States, 2003. J Head Trauma Rehabil. 2006;21(6):544–8.
5. Coronado VG, et al. Surveillance for traumatic brain injury-related deaths--United States, 1997–2007. MMWR Surveill Summ. 2011;60(5):1–32.
6. Faul MC, V. Handbook of clinical neurology. Vol. 127. 2015. Elsevier. Amsterdam, Netherlands.
7. Mak CHK, et al. Traumatic brain injury in the elderly: is it as bad as we think? Curr Transl Geriatr Exp Gerontol Rep. 2012;1(3):171–8.

8. Thompson HJ, McCormick WC, Kagan SH. Traumatic brain injury in older adults: epidemiology, outcomes, and future implications. J Am Geriatr Soc. 2006;54(10):1590–5.
9. Moppett IK. Traumatic brain injury: assessment, resuscitation and early management. Br J Anaesth. 2007;99(1):18–31.
10. Sulhan S, et al. Neuroinflammation and blood-brain barrier disruption following traumatic brain injury: pathophysiology and potential therapeutic targets. J Neurosci Res. 2020;98(1):19–28.
11. Prins M, et al. The pathophysiology of traumatic brain injury at a glance. Dis Model Mech. 2013;6(6):1307–15.
12. Tang-Schomer MD, et al. Mechanical breaking of microtubules in axons during dynamic stretch injury underlies delayed elasticity, microtubule disassembly, and axon degeneration. FASEB J. 2010;24(5):1401–10.
13. Kinoshita K. Traumatic brain injury: pathophysiology for neurocritical care. J Intensive Care. 2016;4:29.
14. Ladak AA, Enam SA, Ibrahim MT. A review of the molecular mechanisms of traumatic brain injury. World Neurosurg. 2019;131:126–32.
15. Carney N, et al. Guidelines for the management of severe traumatic brain injury, fourth edition. Neurosurgery. 2017;80(1):6–15.
16. Laroche M, et al. Coagulopathy after traumatic brain injury. Neurosurgery. 2012;70(6):1334–45.
17. Chhabra G, et al. Hypofibrinogenemia in isolated traumatic brain injury in Indian patients. Neurol India. 2010;58(5):756–7.
18. Shehata M, Afify MI, El-Shafie M, Khaled M. Prevalence and clinical implications of coagulopathy in patients with isolated head trauma. Med J Cairo Univ. 2011;79:131–7.
19. Hoyt DB. A clinical review of bleeding dilemmas in trauma. Semin Hematol. 2004;41(1 Suppl 1):40–3.
20. Harhangi BS, et al. Coagulation disorders after traumatic brain injury. Acta Neurochir. 2008;150(2):165–75; discussion 175.
21. Gomez PA, et al. Mild head injury: differences in prognosis among patients with a Glasgow Coma Scale score of 13 to 15 and analysis of factors associated with abnormal CT findings. Br J Neurosurg. 1996;10(5):453–60.
22. Shrestha A, Joshi RM, Devkota UP. Contributing factors for coagulopathy in traumatic brain injury. Asian J Neurosurg. 2017;12(4):648–52.
23. Epstein DS, et al. Acute traumatic coagulopathy in the setting of isolated traumatic brain injury: a systematic review and meta-analysis. Injury. 2014;45(5):819–24.
24. Podolsky-Gondim GG, et al. The role of coagulopathy on clinical outcome following traumatic brain injury in children: analysis of 66 consecutive cases in a single center institution. Childs Nerv Syst. 2018;34(12):2455–61.
25. Stolla M, et al. Current state of transfusion in traumatic brain injury and associated coagulopathy. Transfusion. 2019;59(S2):1522–8.
26. Martin G, et al. Relationship of coagulopathy and platelet dysfunction to transfusion needs after traumatic brain injury. Neurocrit Care. 2018;28(3):330–7.
27. Albert V, et al. Early posttraumatic changes in coagulation and fibrinolysis systems in isolated severe traumatic brain injury patients and its influence on immediate outcome. Hematol Oncol Stem Cell Ther. 2019;12(1):32–43.
28. Samuels JM, et al. Severe traumatic brain injury is associated with a unique coagulopathy phenotype. J Trauma Acute Care Surg. 2019;86(4):686–93.
29. Maegele M, et al. Coagulopathy and haemorrhagic progression in traumatic brain injury: advances in mechanisms, diagnosis, and management. Lancet Neurol. 2017;16(8):630–47.
30. Epstein DS, et al. Acute traumatic coagulopathy in the setting of isolated traumatic brain injury: definition, incidence and outcomes. Br J Neurosurg. 2015;29(1):118–22.
31. Wafaisade A, et al. Acute coagulopathy in isolated blunt traumatic brain injury. Neurocrit Care. 2010;12(2):211–9.
32. Talving P, et al. Coagulopathy in severe traumatic brain injury: a prospective study. J Trauma. 2009;66(1):55–61; discussion 61–2.
33. Lustenberger T, et al. Early coagulopathy after isolated severe traumatic brain injury: relationship with hypoperfusion challenged. J Trauma. 2010;69(6):1410–4.
34. Alexiou GA, et al. Admission glucose and coagulopathy occurrence in patients with traumatic brain injury. Brain Inj. 2014;28(4):438–41.
35. Corbett JM, Ho KM, Honeybul S. Prognostic significance of abnormal hematological parameters in severe traumatic brain injury requiring decompressive craniectomy. J Neurosurg. 2019:1–7.
36. Epstein DS, et al. Normalization of coagulopathy is associated with improved outcome after isolated traumatic brain injury. J Clin Neurosci. 2016;29:64–9.
37. Xia ZY, et al. Effects of hemoglobin level on the early postsurgical cerebral metabolism in patients with severe traumatic brain injury. Brain Inj. 2017;31(5):697–701.
38. Sekhon MS, et al. Association of hemoglobin concentration and mortality in critically ill patients with severe traumatic brain injury. Crit Care. 2012;16(4):R128.
39. Litofsky NS, et al. The negative impact of anemia in outcome from traumatic brain injury. World Neurosurg. 2016;90:82–90.
40. Duane TM, et al. The effect of anemia and blood transfusions on mortality in closed head injury patients. J Surg Res. 2008;147(2):163–7.
41. Griesdale DE, et al. Hemoglobin area and time index above 90 g/L are associated with improved 6-month functional outcomes in patients with severe traumatic brain injury. Neurocrit Care. 2015;23(1):78–84.
42. Yang CJ, et al. The association between anemia and the mortality of severe traumatic brain injury in emergency department. J Trauma. 2011;71(6):E132–5.
43. Oddo M, et al. Anemia and brain oxygen after severe traumatic brain injury. Intensive Care Med. 2012;38(9):1497–504.
44. Salim A, et al. Role of anemia in traumatic brain injury. J Am Coll Surg. 2008;207(3):398–406.
45. Boutin A, et al. Transfusion of red blood cells in patients with traumatic brain injuries admitted to Canadian trauma health centres: a multicentre cohort study. BMJ Open. 2017;7(3):e014472.
46. Moman RN, et al. Red blood cell transfusion in acute brain injury subtypes: an observational cohort study. J Crit Care. 2019;50:44–9.
47. Leal-Noval SR, et al. Effects of red blood cell transfusion on long-term disability of patients with traumatic brain injury. Neurocrit Care. 2016;24(3):371–80.
48. Warner MA, et al. Transfusions and long-term functional outcomes in traumatic brain injury. J Neurosurg. 2010;113(3):539–46.
49. Boutin A, et al. Hemoglobin thresholds and red blood cell transfusion in adult patients with moderate or severe traumatic brain injuries: a retrospective cohort study. J Crit Care. 2018;45:133–9.
50. Elterman J, et al. Transfusion of red blood cells in patients with a prehospital Glasgow Coma Scale score of 8 or less and no evidence of shock is associated with worse outcomes. J Trauma Acute Care Surg. 2013;75(1):8–14; discussion 14.
51. Badenes R, et al. Hemoglobin concentrations and RBC transfusion thresholds in patients with acute brain injury: an international survey. Crit Care. 2017;21(1):159.
52. Lessard Bonaventure P, et al. Red blood cell transfusion in critically ill patients with traumatic brain injury: an international survey of physicians' attitudes. Can J Anaesth. 2019;66(9):1038–48.
53. Sena MJ, et al. Transfusion practices for acute traumatic brain injury: a survey of physicians at US trauma centers. Intensive Care Med. 2009;35(3):480–8.

54. Carson JL, et al. Transfusion thresholds and other strategies for guiding allogeneic red blood cell transfusion. Cochrane Database Syst Rev. 2016;10:Cd002042.
55. Robertson CS, et al. Effect of erythropoietin and transfusion threshold on neurological recovery after traumatic brain injury: a randomized clinical trial. JAMA. 2014;312(1):36–47.
56. Vedantam A, et al. Progressive hemorrhagic injury after severe traumatic brain injury: effect of hemoglobin transfusion thresholds. J Neurosurg. 2016;125(5):1229–34.
57. McIntyre LA, et al. Effect of a liberal versus restrictive transfusion strategy on mortality in patients with moderate to severe head injury. Neurocrit Care. 2006;5(1):4–9.
58. Carr KR, et al. Association between relative anemia and early functional recovery after severe traumatic brain injury (TBI). Neurocrit Care. 2016;25(2):185–92.
59. Yamal JM, et al. Association of transfusion red blood cell storage age and blood oxygenation, long-term neurologic outcome, and mortality in traumatic brain injury. J Trauma Acute Care Surg. 2015;79(5):843–9.
60. Ruel-Laliberte J, et al. Effect of age of transfused red blood cells on neurologic outcome following traumatic brain injury (ABLE-tbi Study): a nested study of the Age of Blood Evaluation (ABLE) trial. Can J Anaesth. 2019;66(6):696–705.
61. Dutzmann S, et al. On the value of routine prothrombin time screening in elective neurosurgical procedures. Neurosurg Focus. 2012;33(5):E9.
62. West KL, Adamson C, Hoffman M. Prophylactic correction of the international normalized ratio in neurosurgery: a brief review of a brief literature. J Neurosurg. 2011;114(1):9–18.
63. American Society of Anesthesiologists Task Force on Perioperative Blood, M. Practice guidelines for perioperative blood management: an updated report by the American Society of Anesthesiologists Task Force on Perioperative Blood Management*. Anesthesiology. 2015;122(2):241–75.
64. Kozek-Langenecker SA, et al. Management of severe perioperative bleeding: guidelines from the European Society of Anaesthesiology. Eur J Anaesthesiol. 2013;30(6):270–382.
65. Anglin CO, et al. Effects of platelet and plasma transfusion on outcome in traumatic brain injury patients with moderate bleeding diatheses. J Neurosurg. 2013;118(3):676–86.
66. Zhang LM, et al. Increased transfusion of fresh frozen plasma is associated with mortality or worse functional outcomes after severe traumatic brain injury: a retrospective study. World Neurosurg. 2017;104:381–9.
67. Leeper CM, et al. Overresuscitation with plasma is associated with sustained fibrinolysis shutdown and death in pediatric traumatic brain injury. J Trauma Acute Care Surg. 2018;85(1):12–7.
68. Wohlauer MV, et al. Early platelet dysfunction: an unrecognized role in the acute coagulopathy of trauma. J Am Coll Surg. 2012;214(5):739–46.
69. Davis PK, et al. Platelet dysfunction is an early marker for traumatic brain injury-induced coagulopathy. Neurocrit Care. 2013;18(2):201–8.
70. Castellino FJ, et al. Traumatic brain injury causes platelet adenosine diphosphate and arachidonic acid receptor inhibition independent of hemorrhagic shock in humans and rats. J Trauma Acute Care Surg. 2014;76(5):1169–76.
71. Guillotte AR, et al. Effects of platelet dysfunction and platelet transfusion on outcomes in traumatic brain injury patients. Brain Inj. 2018;32(13–14):1849–57.
72. Furay E, et al. Goal-directed platelet transfusions correct platelet dysfunction and may improve survival in patients with severe traumatic brain injury. J Trauma Acute Care Surg. 2018;85(5):881–7.
73. Practice parameter for the use of fresh-frozen plasma, cryoprecipitate, and platelets. Fresh-Frozen Plasma, Cryoprecipitate, and Platelets Administration Practice Guidelines Development Task Force of the College of American Pathologists. JAMA. 1994;271(10):777–81.
74. Estcourt LJ, et al. Guidelines for the use of platelet transfusions. Br J Haematol. 2017;176(3):365–94.
75. Goobie SM, Haas T. Bleeding management for pediatric craniotomies and craniofacial surgery. Paediatr Anaesth. 2014;24(7):678–89.
76. Chan KH, Mann KS, Chan TK. The significance of thrombocytopenia in the development of postoperative intracranial hematoma. J Neurosurg. 1989;71(1):38–41.
77. Downey DM, et al. Does platelet administration affect mortality in elderly head-injured patients taking antiplatelet medications? Am Surg. 2009;75(11):1100–3.
78. Bachelani AM, et al. Assessment of platelet transfusion for reversal of aspirin after traumatic brain injury. Surgery. 2011;150(4):836–43.
79. Briggs A, et al. Platelet dysfunction and platelet transfusion in traumatic brain injury. J Surg Res. 2015;193(2):802–6.
80. Holzmacher JL, et al. Platelet transfusion does not improve outcomes in patients with brain injury on antiplatelet therapy. Brain Inj. 2018;32(3):325–30.
81. Jehan F, et al. Is there a need for platelet transfusion after traumatic brain injury in patients on P2Y12 inhibitors? J Surg Res. 2019;236:224–9.
82. Leong LB, David TK. Is platelet transfusion effective in patients taking antiplatelet agents who suffer an intracranial hemorrhage? J Emerg Med. 2015;49(4):561–72.
83. Jokar TO, et al. Ratio-based resuscitation in trauma patients with traumatic brain injury: is there a similar effect? Am Surg. 2016;82(3):271–7.
84. Wong H, Curry N, Stanworth SJ. Blood products and procoagulants in traumatic bleeding: use and evidence. Curr Opin Crit Care. 2016;22(6):598–606.
85. Shibahashi K, et al. Initial results of empirical cryoprecipitate transfusion in the treatment of isolated severe traumatic brain injury: use of in-house-produced cryoprecipitate. Neurol Med Chir (Tokyo). 2019;59(10):371–8.
86. Kozek-Langenecker SA, et al. Management of severe perioperative bleeding: guidelines from the European Society of Anaesthesiology: first update 2016. Eur J Anaesthesiol. 2017;34(6):332–95.
87. New HV, et al. Guidelines on transfusion for fetuses, neonates and older children. Br J Haematol. 2016;175(5):784–828.
88. Shakur H, et al. Antifibrinolytic drugs for treating primary postpartum haemorrhage. Cochrane Database Syst Rev. 2018;2:Cd012964.
89. Weng S, et al. Effect of tranexamic acid in patients with traumatic brain injury: a systematic review and meta-analysis. World Neurosurg. 2019;123:128–35.
90. Sandri A, et al. Perioperative intravenous tranexamic acid reduces blood transfusion in primary cementless total hip arthroplasty. Acta Biomed. 2019;90(1-s):81–6.
91. Haghighi M, et al. Does tranexamic acid reduce bleeding during femoral fracture operation? Arch Bone Jt Surg. 2017;5(2):103–8.
92. Wang Y, Liu S, He L. Prophylactic use of tranexamic acid reduces blood loss and transfusion requirements in patients undergoing cesarean section: a meta-analysis. J Obstet Gynaecol Res. 2019;45(8):1562–75.
93. Roberts I, et al. The CRASH-2 trial: a randomised controlled trial and economic evaluation of the effects of tranexamic acid on death, vascular occlusive events and transfusion requirement in bleeding trauma patients. Health Technol Assess. 2013;17(10):1–79.
94. Perel P, et al. CRASH-2 (Clinical Randomisation of an Antifibrinolytic in Significant Haemorrhage) intracranial bleeding study: the effect of tranexamic acid in traumatic brain injury-

-a nested randomised, placebo-controlled trial. Health Technol Assess. 2012;16(13):iii–xii, 1–54.
95. Roberts I, et al. Tranexamic acid for significant traumatic brain injury (The CRASH-3 trial): statistical analysis plan for an international, randomised, double-blind, placebo-controlled trial. Wellcome Open Res. 2018;3:86.
96. Sprigg N, et al. Tranexamic acid for hyperacute primary IntraCerebral Haemorrhage (TICH-2): an international randomised, placebo-controlled, phase 3 superiority trial. Lancet. 2018;391(10135):2107–15.
97. Mahmood A, Roberts I, Shakur H. A nested mechanistic sub-study into the effect of tranexamic acid versus placebo on intracranial haemorrhage and cerebral ischaemia in isolated traumatic brain injury: study protocol for a randomised controlled trial (CRASH-3 Trial Intracranial Bleeding Mechanistic Sub-Study [CRASH-3 IBMS]). Trials. 2017;18(1):330.
98. Morte D, et al. Tranexamic acid administration following head trauma in a combat setting: does tranexamic acid result in improved neurologic outcomes? J Trauma Acute Care Surg. 2019;87(1):125–9.
99. Ebrahimi P, et al. Intravenous tranexamic acid for subdural and epidural intracranial hemorrhage: randomized, double-blind, placebo-controlled trial. Rev Recent Clin Trials. 2019;14(4):286–91.
100. Lombardo S, et al. Factor VIIa administration in traumatic brain injury: an AAST-MITC propensity score analysis. Trauma Surg Acute Care Open. 2018;3(1):e000134.

Transfusion-Related Immunomodulation in Relation to Perioperative Infection/Cancer: Biology, Evidence, and Controversy in Transfusion

31

Atish Patel and Bruce D. Spiess

Background

Red blood cell (RBC) transfusions have evolved to be one of the most common medical interventionsa in the United States and are given to approximately three to four million patients each year (14+ million units per year) [1, 2]. The number of RBC transfusions peaked in 2012–2013 with subsequent years demonstrating some decrease. Causes put forth by blood bankers for this decrease include the 2008–2009 economic downturn, but it has persisted and expanded since the economy has recovered. Far more realistic is the appreciation by medicine that transfusion is associated with (causes) adverse outcomes. RBC transfusion has long been known to carry significant risks. However, the transfusion decision is rarely an in-depth risk-benefit analysis.

Historically, focus has been on ABO-Rh compatibility, virus, pathogen avoidance, and whether blood banking was able to meet the demands created by expanding, evermore complex medical/surgical care in an aging population. The first reports of serious hepatitis transmission occurred in 1947, yet the use of transfusion grew until the human immunodeficiency virus transfusion crisis [3]. The viral risks exceeded 10–40% seroconversion in some places, but it was not until the late 1980s that critical steps were taken to reduce the risks to below 1/1–4,000,000 units infused [3, 4].

Today, blood transfusion still has many serious side effects, which are often under-appreciated by physicians. A contemporary list of transfusion risks includes (in order of frequency): non-hemolytic febrile reactions (higher in non-leukoreduced blood products), allergic reactions (not including anaphylaxis), transfusion-associated circulatory overload, metabolic toxicities and derangements, transfusion-related immunomodulation (TRIM), transfusion-associated lung injury (TRALI), post-transfusion purpura, graft-versus-host disease, transfusion-transmitted viruses, parasites and bacteria, and anaphylaxis, among others [5–7]. It can be argued that TRIM is present to some degree in all patients who have received an allogeneic transfusion and therefore should be listed as the number one complication of transfusion. TRALI, allergic reactions, non-hemolytic febrile reactions, graft-versus-host disease, and anaphylaxis are ultimately immune-mediated, therefore all are TRIM. TRIM has also become synonymous with increased nosocomial infection and/or cancer recurrence.

TRALI is widely noted to be the most frequent cause of death after transfusion [8]. The contribution of TRIM to the morbidity and mortality of hospitalized critically ill patients may well outdistance the effects of TRALI in leading to bad outcomes. TRALI is itself a result of TRIM, and TRIM happens near universally. The decision to transfuse a patient is most often made based upon a perceived risk (fear) of decreased oxygen-carrying capacity imputed by not transfusing. Many academic surgical and medical societies have guidelines regarding appropriate RBC transfusion triggers (usually a range of hemoglobin or hematocrit). Medicine has underdeveloped monitoring capabilities for tissue oxygen delivery/utilization; thus the anxiety leading to transfusion behavior is based on perceived risk often with little data. We believe that few who make the transfusion decision fully appreciate the literature regarding TRIM and that such knowledge, if acquired, could well promote caution when ordering an RBC transfusion. This review will examine controversial/contradictory literature as well as the biologic mechanisms of TRIM. In the end, the review will question

The work contained within is solely the author's own and each has contributed from conception through writing and reviewing.

A. Patel (✉)
Vanderbilt University Medical Center, Department of Anesthesiology, Nashville, TN, USA
e-mail: atish.patel@vumc.org

B. D. Spiess
University of Florida Health, Gainesville, FL, USA
e-mail: bspiess@anest.ufl.edu

© Springer Nature Switzerland AG 2021
C. S. Scher et al. (eds.), *Essentials of Blood Product Management in Anesthesia Practice*,
https://doi.org/10.1007/978-3-030-59295-0_31

the ethical/quality control point: Is unnecessary RBC transfusion an avoidable human error in medicine?

History of TRIM

There is strong evidence of TRIM-related effects on transfusion recipients. Increased rates of tumor recurrence are noted in transfusion versus non-transfusion patients, as are nosocomial infections. Because a patient does not manifest a nosocomial infection does not in itself mean that he/she has not experienced some level of TRIM. Nosocomial infections kill and cost billions of dollars with per patient cost of over $50–75,000 USD in complications [9]. Because over 60% of ICU-treated patients receive a blood transfusion, the relationship between transfusion and the current ICU bacteria may be related.

TRIM was first embraced as a concept in the 1970s with orthotropic renal transplantation. Opelz et al. [10] conducted a prospective, multicenter study that found kidney organ survival rates to be higher in patients who received allogeneic blood transfusions (ABTs; 90% vs 82%, P = 0.02). The results pointed to a dose-dependent relationship between RBC transfusion and immunosuppression. Improved overall survival rate at a 5-year follow-up, in addition to animal and observational studies, showed similar results, which led to widespread and liberal use of ABTs, especially with transplantation in order to decrease graft-versus-host complications [10–14]. At times, patients were transfused when their hemoglobin was in excess of 10gm/dL solely for the purpose of creating immunosuppression. In the late 1980s, in addition to organ transplants, transfusions were liberally administered to women experiencing recurrent spontaneous abortion (thought to be an immune-related maternal attack on the fetus) [15]. Today, those who argue against TRIM and transfusion dismiss or ignore these historical facts. Some explain the renal allograft data as due to a time when allogeneic blood was not leukoreduced. The effect of leukoreduction will be discussed later. Notably, leukoreduction may lessen but does not eliminate TRIM.

The practice of using transfusion as a way to intentionally immune inhibit a recipient ended with two events: with the onset of the AIDS and hepatitis C epidemics along with the advent of cyclosporine immunosuppressives and other modern immunosuppressive agents. Transfusion as a medical technique to intentionally immunosuppress came to a halt.

Cancer Recurrence

After the beneficial immunosuppressive effect of transfusion was recognized, Gantt, in 1981 [16], suggested an association between transfusion and increased cancer recurrence, raising concern that the outcome for patients undergoing curative surgery for a malignancy might be worsened. The reasoning was, if transfusion downregulated the recipient's immune system, it might also enhance tumor growth and the implantation/growth of metastases. Since then, multiple observational studies, randomized controlled trials (RCTs), and meta-analyses have been published pointing toward higher rates of cancer recurrence, especially colorectal, bladder, and most recently hematopoietic/leukemic cancers [17, 18, 37–43].

The focus of transfusion then shifted in the late 1980s when several researchers began to suggest that some of the adverse patient outcomes that had been attributed to intractable disease and comorbid conditions were in fact complications of transfusion therapy. This led to retrospective and prospective observational studies, in addition to animal studies in the following decade, which implicated TRIM as causing higher postoperative infection rates. Neil Blumberg compiled data from these studies and found that patients receiving perioperative transfusion (compared with those not receiving transfusion) had a higher risk of developing postoperative bacterial infection (as much as 200–1000% higher).

Much needed RCTs to verify this surprising evidence soon followed. Several small- to medium-sized RCTs in the early 1990s containing between 50 and 500 patients were conducted that showed higher postoperative infections in orthopedic, colorectal, and cardiac surgeries [17, 18]. In 1998, an association between non-leukoreduced ABTs and short-term overall mortality (up to 3 months post-transfusion) was described by van de Watering et al. [19] That study compared cardiac surgery patients receiving non-white blood cell (WBC)-reduced versus WBC-reduced allogeneic RBCs [19]. The study had been designed to investigate an association between ABT and the risk of postoperative infection, but instead of conclusively showing increased infection, the investigators observed an increase in mortality. This evidence linking ABTs to increased postoperative infections and mortality led to the creation of several larger RCTs, which then showed mixed evidence.

Mechanism

The current understanding is that ABTs create both immunomodulatory and pro-inflammatory effects predominantly through the following mechanisms: [20] (1) infusion of allogeneic mononuclear cells; (2) soluble biologic response modifiers released in a time-dependent manner from WBC granules or membranes into the supernatant fluid of RBC or platelet concentrates during storage; and/or (3) soluble human leukocyte antigen (HLA) class I peptides that circulate in allogeneic plasma.

Multiple studies support the mechanism that allogeneic WBCs bearing class II HLA antigens are directly involved in immunosuppressing hosts receiving ABTs. The initial studies in the 1970s surrounding renal transplants found that patients who had pre-transplant, WBC-reduced blood transfusions showed less immunological benefit. This led to further animal studies by Kao [21] and Bordin [22] that demonstrated immune suppression in recipient mice receiving allogeneic WBCs. Other animal studies [23, 24] looked at the tumor growth-promoting effects of ABTs and noticed that naive animals infused with cells from a donor (given an ABT), or directly given an ABT, had higher rates of pulmonary nodules. When the donor animal's cells or blood were WBC reduced, malignancy rates were restored back to normal in the naive host animals. There was actually a dose-response relationship between the volume of ABT and the number of pulmonary tumor nodules. Because the negative effect of blood transfusion could be eliminated with leukoreduction, it was fair to implicate WBCs (or their products) as causing the noted immunomodulatory effects. In addition to increased pulmonary nodules, these animal studies also hinted at a proliferation of transforming growth factor (TGF)-β-positive suppressor T-cells. Reed et al. [25] discovered that donor CD200 molecules (specifically on dendritic antigen-presenting cells [APCs]) interact with host $\gamma\delta$-suppressor T-cells, thereby releasing TGF-β and suppressing host immune defenses.

These revelations led to further studies by Beko [26] and Dizik [27] that looked at HLA compatibility between donors and recipients. They concluded that the long-term persistence of a small amount of allogeneic donor WBCs, including dendritic APCs, in the recipient (microchimerism) may account for the downregulation of the recipient's immune system. In addition to TGF-β, as mentioned above, microchimerism may also result in the release of interleukin-4 and interleukin-10 from T-helper type 2 (Th-2) lymphocytes [28]. These cytokines inhibit T-helper type 1 (Th-1) cells, and impairment of Th-1 cytokine secretion results in impairment of various functions of cellular immunity (including antigen processing, macrophage activation, the T-cell cytotoxic function, and neutrophil and monocyte cytocidal activity) [29].

A retrospective study by Utter [30] evaluated 163 American combat veterans who received transfusion in theater of operation. He found that 10% of veterans (as much as 20% in Korean War veterans) had evidence of transfusion-associated microchimerism (TA-MC) that, in some instances, lasted upward of 60 years. This was in comparison to the control group who did not receive transfusion and showed a TA-MC rate of 0.7%. Further work by Nelson [31] supported that TA-MC is involved in the pathogenesis of several chronic graft-versus-host-type diseases. More importantly, a more recent study by Reed [32] revealed that TA-MC is present in approximately one-half of transfusion and severely injured patients at hospital discharge and is *not* affected by leukoreduction. So, the issue regarding whether leukoreduction is a cure or prevention of TRIM is based on controversial data.

In addition to allogeneic mononuclear cells, a number of bioactive soluble molecules and factors have been shown to detach from these WBCs during storage and have also been implicated in the pathogenesis of TRIM. Nielsen et al. [33] reported that the concentration of histamine, eosinophil cationic protein and protein X, myeloperoxidase, and plasminogen activator inhibitor-1 can increase up to 3- to-25-fold in the supernatant fluid of RBC components during storage. These cytokines/protein messengers are known to inhibit neutrophil function. Other authors [34, 35] also discovered HLA class 1 antigen and Fas ligand to be among these bioactive soluble molecules released during storage – and both of these have been shown to inhibit the natural killer and cytotoxic T-cells of the recipient, which impairs the destruction of virus-infected cells. The supernatant of stored RBCs with and without leukoreduction is immunosuppressive.

Lastly, it has also been suggested that soluble HLA proteins and immune-reactive HLA peptides are involved in the effects of TRIM. Non-polymorphic peptides derived from HLA class I molecules induce antigen-nonspecific immunosuppression, while polymorphic HLA class I peptides have antigen-specific immunomodulatory effects [36]. During transfusion, allogeneic plasma introduces soluble HLA antigens to the recipient's thymic circulation. According to Roelen [37], a partial or fully matched HLA-DR (HLA with the DR isotope) between host and recipient will lead to tolerance and immunosuppression, whereas a fully mismatched HLA-DR will lead to alloimmunization. The mechanism also relies on the viability of donor dendritic APCs (presenting HLA antigens) along with co-stimulatory signals. Non-viable dendritic APCs and a lack of co-stimulatory signals (presumed to be provoked by long refrigerated blood storage times), despite HLA compatibility, can result in T-cell inactivation and anergy [33]. Experiments in laboratory animals have shown that when two antigens are introduced, the host's response to one antigen is almost always decreased. In humans, a wide variety of different antigens are introduced during ABT, and a similar decreased host response as seen in mice could be occurring.

Despite the numerous postulated mechanisms above, it is worth mentioning that Bruson et al. [38] have conclusively shown that ABTs definitely lead to impaired natural killer cell function, alteration in T lymphocyte ratios, defective antigen presentation, suppression of lymphocyte blastogenesis, decreased macrophage phagocytic function, and inhibited neutrophil function [38].

Microparticles of the cell membrane are budded and lost from intact erythrocytes during storage. These microparticles are composed of phosphatidyl serine along with certain proteins. CD-40L is expressed on the surface of platelets as well as, to a lesser degree, erythrocytes. CD-40L is immunosuppressive in itself and has been implicated as a protein that sets up the pulmonary vasculature to react, leak, and develop TRALI. CD-40L increases in concentration in the plasma the longer blood is stored, as are the microparticles of budded cell membranes. Macrophages phagocytize these particles, which makes a great deal of sense in that macrophages are programmed to recognize dead or dying cells, clear the circulation of these, and recognize cell membranes as potential invaders. When macrophages are exposed to a great deal of these lipids, they become lipid laden, swollen, and dysfunctional as they are "full" and satiated from ingesting particles. The longer blood is stored, the larger the number of microparticles that get infused. Inflammation and oxidative stress can further worsen these immunomodulatory effects, as oxidated lipids are particularly inflammatory. We do not know whether oxidized phosphatidyl serine versus non-oxidized is more or less inflammatory/immunosuppressive. Some of the latest thinking on preserving RBCs during blood banking involves efforts to make the stored RBCs anoxic thereby decreasing oxidative stress. By reducing oxygen free radical generation, the budding of microparticles is reduced. That technology is not yet in use, but it makes an interesting future research question to examine. We have previously been working on ways to increase oxygen delivery to stored blood during blood banking…which might well be exactly the wrong thing to do (Table 31.1).

Postoperative Infection Rates

As mentioned above, the concept of TRIM, although initially embraced as a therapeutic advantage for renal transplantation in the 1970s and 80s, never drew questioning by the medical care community as to why or when we should transfuse patients. A "belief" persisted, with a particular paternalism, that (1) blood transfusion was good and that the risks were minimal and (2) "your doctor knows what is best for you!" Such paternalism continued even in the face of huge numbers of people infected and dying of hepatitis C due to transfusion.

Table 31.1 Postulated mechanisms of the transfusion-related immunomodulation effect [20]

Clonal deletion of specific lines of immune cells
Induction of suppressor T-cells
Production of anti-idiotypic antibodies
Suppression of natural killer cell activity
Polarization of the immune system to the T-helper type 2 responses, with suppression of T-helper type 1 responses
Selection of non-responder-type immune cells
Mixed microchimerism
Induction of apoptosis, resulting in the death of specific types of immune-competent cells
Accumulation in the supernatant of stored components of soluble molecules (e.g., histamine, eosinophil cationic protein, eosinophil protein X) that inhibit neutrophil function
Accumulation in the supernatant of stored components of soluble molecules (i.e., soluble Fas ligand or soluble human leukocyte antigen class I molecules) that inhibit the immune response
Others

Even today, with a very large supportive literature, the issue of TRIM is still debated. Skeptics of TRIM have put dismissive comments in the literature [39]. Some of this represents doubts about a controversial subject wherein proponents of TRIM are seen to represent a threat to mainstream beliefs about the "goodness" of transfusion and the standard of practice (10 g/dL as a transfusion trigger). However, early proponents of TRIM like Tartter and Blumberg may have also been victims of bad timing. Their work came during and just after the catastrophic transfusion-transmitted AIDS epidemic of 1981–1987. Few clinicians and investigators in transfusion medicine had any enthusiasm for adding further layers of potential negativity to the already catastrophic news headlines regarding HIV contamination of the blood supply. New data demonstrating that transfusion was even more dangerous to patients than originally believed in the early 1980s might represent a "piling on" and a further attack upon the much-revered medical teaching.

With some animal studies suggesting that TRIM is mediated by donor allogeneic WBCs that either directly downregulate the recipient's immune function or indirectly mediate the alleged TRIM effects by releasing soluble mediators into the supernatant fluid of RBCs during storage, nine RCTs were conducted to determine if leukoreduction of blood led to lower postoperative infection rates.

Six of the nine studies showed lower postoperative infection rates with leukoreduction, and the other three did not: the three not showing a reduction in TRIM by leukoreduction have been criticized for their design, whereas the others were simply accepted as fact. Perhaps the paternalism and belief system of transfusion again overcame science.

The study by van der Watering et al. [19] randomized 871 eligible patients with colorectal cancer receiving blood to get leukocyte-depleted RBCs or packed cells without a buffy coat. They reported "no statistically significant differences" in overall infection or cancer rates between the two groups. A potential flaw in this study is that buffy coat-depleted cells are inherently leukoreduced. Therefore, when the control arm of an RCT consists of already-leukoreduced blood, especially considering it was buffy coat-depleted and not just buffy coat-reduced (leading to greater leukoreduction), one would expect little if any difference in immunosuppression between the control and treatment arms.

Wallis randomized 597 patients undergoing elective coronary artery or heart valve surgery to receive either plasma-reduced, buffy coat-depleted, or WBC-filtered RBC [40].

The authors concluded that there was no difference in infection rates between the three arms ***after they* excluded urinary tract infections (UTIs)**, which were significantly elevated in the plasma-reduced arm [40]. UTIs are most definitely a significant nosocomial infection of major importance to postoperative adverse outcomes, length of hospital stay, and even mortality. When including UTIs and comparing all postoperative infections among the three arms (plasma-reduced 33%, buffy coat-depleted 19%, WBC-filtered 22%; P = 0.03 adjusted for other variables), there is at least an 11% increase in infections between fully (WBC-filtered) and partially (buffy coat-depleted) leukoreduced cells. Additionally, the authors claimed to have higher infection rates in the WBC-filtered arm at the 3-month follow-up [40]. However, the majority of these were self-reported infections that were proven by bacterial culture, radiologic findings, or documented fever while the study participant was as inpatient. Self-reporting of infection is a notoriously ineffective and unscientific way to follow this potentially devastating outcome.

Titlestad randomized 112 patients to receive leukocyte-depleted erythrocyte suspensions or non-leukocyte-depleted erythrocyte suspensions to patients undergoing colorectal surgery [41]. Despite claiming that "no significant difference between the transfusion groups was seen on any single infectious event," the infection rate in the leukoreduced arm was still 7% lower (38% vs. 45%; P = 0.52). Additionally, with a P-value as a high as 0.52 and small patient population (compared to the other studies exceeding 500+ patients), the validity of the result is questionable [41].

A meta-analysis of the nine studies by Neil Blumberg [42], limiting patients who actually received transfusions (n = 3093) and applying the intention to treat principle, demonstrated that leukoreduced transfusions significantly reduced the odds of postoperative infection (odds ratio = 0.522; 95% CI, 0.332–0.821; P = 0.005). Another meta-analysis by Fergusson et al. [43], including only transfused patients as well, found a statistically and clinically significant reduction in postoperative infection following leukoreduction (relative risk [RR] = 0.60; 95% CI, 0.38–0.93). Today, therefore, it is generally accepted that leukoreduction itself decreases the effects of TRIM, yet it still exists and is a problem [44].

A meta-analysis by Vamvakas et al. [39] reached contrary conclusions. However, their meta-analysis included hundreds of non-transfused patients that were intentionally excluded from the original RCTs, as well as from two meta-analyses that showed higher postoperative infections. Non-transfused patients are not relevant when it comes to the question of whether transfusion-related immunomodulation has clinically significant effects or whether leukoreduction can reduce such effects [42]. The reasoning for this is that one must compare leukoreduced versus non-leukoreduced blood transfusions to determine the true effect of immunomodulation. The use of the intention-to-treat analysis (compared to the as-treated analysis) in this instance included patients that did not receive transfusions, accounting for more than 10% of the analyzed patients in most cases, therefore diluting any potential beneficial effect of leukoreduction.

For rigorous statistical analyses, inclusion of any patient that was randomized is usually critical. However, exclusion of these patients provides a more scientifically valid examination of the outcomes between patients who received non-leukoreduced or leukoreduced transfusions, excluding patients who received no transfusions at all. Fergusson [43] has argued this point successfully and shown that trial investigators can exclude patients' data from analysis, without risking bias, when ineligible patients are mistakenly randomized into a trial.

Most problematically, this study does not in all instances correspond to the actual data from the original studies. Rather, for some of the clinical trials, the meta-analyses included "imputed" outcomes. This effort was an attempt to retrospectively create an "intention-to-treat analysis." The authors took non-transfused patients from several studies and the number of postoperative infections and divided them in half. They then added these non-transfused patients and infections back to the actual published data from the transfused patients. However, as mentioned, data from non-transfused patients, and certainly data not derived from experimental results, have little to no scientific validity in assessing either transfusion immunomodulation or the effects of leukoreduction [42].

The British Isles have essentially done a large human experiment. They intentionally went to universal leukoreduction which was a misdirected attempt to avoid the transfusion of prions (potential mad cow disease) among their population. The thinking at the time was that the vector for "mad cow" disease must be neutrophil transmitted, and thus by universal leukoreduction, they would eliminate/reduce that potential catastrophic aspect for blood transfusion. We now know that prions are carried in the plasma and have nothing to do with leukocytes. The incidence of perioperative infection did not change across Britain from before leukoreduction to after it was established, and those patients not transfused do far better. Even with that data, the "belief" that leukoreduction reduces TRIM persists. Perhaps we really do not have a scientific answer – only "beliefs" and desires to find things better persist with regard to transfusion.

Most recently, a meta-analysis by Kwon [45] in 2016 investigated the impact of allogeneic versus autologous leukocyte-filtered blood transfusions on the incidence of postoperative infections in adult surgical patients. They evaluated 16 randomized controlled trials involving 6586 randomized (ITT) patients (4615 APP patients) in various clinical settings. The results demonstrated an overall 26% risk reduction among the leukocyte-filtered blood group in postoperative infections when analyzed by APP (RR = 0.74; 95% CI, 0.60–0.92; P = 0.007) and a 22% risk reduction when analyzed by ITT (RR = 0.78; 95% CI, 0.65–0.94; P = 0.009). Leukocyte-filtered blood was also associated with a significant reduction in length of stay (standardized difference of mean = −0.74; 95% CI, −1.32 to −0.15; P = 0.014) and all-cause mortality (RR = 0.74; 95% CI, 0.57–0.95; P = 0.018) [45]. We can safely conclude that leukocyte-filtered (reduced) blood transfusions are associated with significantly lower postoperative infection rates in both the APP and ITT populations. This lends support to the argument that non-leukocyte-reduced whole blood has deleterious immunosuppressive effects.

Additionally, an argument made by many of the skeptics that doubted or underestimated the effects TRIM over the past two decades was that transfusion is a surrogate marker for the severity of the patient's condition or other confounding factors. And while it is true that confounded associations can sometimes lead to adverse outcomes, sometimes even at high as a 100%, outcomes beyond the point begin to point toward cause and effect. According to A.B. Hill's "rules of causality" (the basis of evidence-based medicine), a positively strong dose-response relationship is a good indicator for causality and not simply correlation. Therefore, an increasing dose of blood should in theory lead to a larger response of immunosuppression and/or postoperative infection. Blumberg et al. eloquently expounded on this theory in a 2007 TRANSFUSION publication in which he drew parallels with smoking and lung cancer in which a cause and effect is taken as proven [45]. The risk of lung cancer in patients that smoke is so far above what confounders could cause, that without RCT's medicine has assigned it causality. Similarly, the rate of perioperative immunosuppression is so high, up to sevenfold increased, after transfusion that confounders cannot be responsible [45].

Furthermore, transfusion practices vary almost an order of magnitude in the clinical setting, from patient to patient, physician to physician, and hospital to hospital. The contention that transfusion could act as a precise and reliable indicator of clinical tumor staging or severity of illness is, in retrospect, implausible.

Conclusion

In 2010, President Bill Clinton made the statement that unnecessary RBC transfusion was the third largest killer by human error of Americans. He may well have been correct, and the problem now is how to define a "necessary transfusion." Clearly, we do not have an answer to that, but the data on TRIM should be sobering to the medical care community. Perioperative infection prolongs hospital stay and is linked to any number of other adverse outcomes, and a great deal of money is spent on giving prophylactic antibiotics as well as the appropriate timing of these antibiotics before surgery. The risks of TRIM and the outcome data are of the same magnitude of effect when one looks at transfusion and perioperative infection as that seen with proper use of antibiotics. Yet few physicians, hospital administrators, or regulators see the connection or are willing to expend the same resources to educate medical personnel on patient blood management or reducing unnecessary transfusion. Few if any hospital epidemiologists know of the effect of transfusion and TRIM on infection in their hospital. There still appears to exist the same bias and teaching that blood transfusion is good. Those places that have implemented comprehensive blood management programs have seen reductions in perioperative infection rates. Perhaps persons of influence in The Joint Commission and the Centers for Medicare & Medicaid Services should examine President Clinton's words and reflect on how we should change our practice to understand the importance of TRIM.

Future research need not spend time and effort proving that TRIM exists. It does. What needs to be researched are more methods to reduce RBC storage defects and efforts to educate the medical community regarding proper/best practices in transfusion medicine. Patient blood management is leading efforts to use focused methods to reduce anemia and salvage the patient's own blood, and with these interventions, perhaps nosocomial infection and cancer recurrence can be reduced.

Conflict of Interest None.

References

1. Ellingson KD, Sapiano MRP, Haass KA, et al. Continued decline of blood collection and transfusion in the United States-2015. Transfusion. 2017;57:1588–98.
2. Edens C, Haass KA, Cumming M, et al. Evaluation of the National Healthcare Safety Network Hemovigilance Module for transfusion-related adverse reactions in the United States. Transfusion. 2019;59:524–33.
3. Block TM, Alter HJ, London WT, Bray M. A historical prospective on the discovery and elucidation of the hepatitis B virus. Antivir Res. 2016;131:109–23.
4. Stramer SL. Current perspectives in transfusion-transmitted infectious diseases: emerging and re-emerging infections. ISBT Sci Ser. 2014;9:30–6.
5. Perrotta PL, Snyder EL. Non- infectious complications of transfusion therapy. Blood Rev. 2001;15:69–83.
6. Hendrickson JE, Hillyer CD. Noninfectious serious hazards of transfusion. Anesth Analg. 2009;108:759–69.
7. Gilliss BM, Looney MR, Gropper MA. Reducing non-infectious risks of blood transfusion. Anesthesiology. 2011;115:635–49.
8. Harvey AR, Basavaraju S, Chung KW, Kuehnert M. Transfusion-related adverse reactions reported to the National Healthcare

Safety network Hemovigilance Module, United States 2010–2012. Transfusion. 2015;55:709–18.
9. Manoukian S, Stewart S, Dancer S, et al. Estimating excess length of stay due to healthcare-associated infections: a systemic review and meta-analysis of statistical methodology- Review. J Hosp Acquir Infect. 2018;100:222–35.
10. Opelz G, Sengar DP, Mickey MR, Terasaki PI. Effect of blood transfusions on subsequent kidney transplants. Transplant Proc. 1973;5:253–9.
11. Morris PJ, Ting A, Stocker J. Leukocyte antigens in renal transplantation. 1. The paradox of blood transfusions in renal transplantation. Med J Aust. 1968;24:1088–90.
12. Fabre JW, Morris PJ. The mechanism of specific immunosuppression of renal allograft rejection by donor strain blood. Transplantation. 1972;14:634–40.
13. Thoenes GH, Pielsticker K, Schreiber MA. Blood transfusion-induced facilitation of kidney graft survival in rats (congenic-resistant strains). Clin Nephrol. 1980;13:133–41.
14. Keowan PA, Descamps B. Improved renal allograft survival after blood transfusion: a non-specific, erythrocyte-mediated immunoregulatory process? Lancet. 1979;8106:20–2.
15. Gatenby PA, Cameron K, Simes RJ, Adelstein S, Bennett MJ, Jansen RP, Shearman RP, Stewart GJ, Whittle M, Doran TJ. Treatment of recurrent spontaneous abortion by immunization with paternal lymphocytes: results of a controlled trial. Am J Reprod Immunol. 1993;29:88–94.
16. Gantt CL. Red blood cells for cancer patients. Lancet. 1981;2:363.
17. Murphy P, Heal JM, Blumberg N. Infection or suspected infection after hip replacement surgery with autologous or homologous blood transfusions. Transfusion. 1991;31:212–7.
18. Jensen LS, Kissmeyer-Nielsen P, Wolff B, Qvist N. Randomised comparison of leucocyte-depleted versus buffy-coat-poor blood transfusion and complications after colorectal surgery. Lancet. 1996;348:841–5.
19. van de Watering LMG, Hermans J, Houbiers JGA, van den Broek PJ, Bouter H, Boer F, Harvey MS, Huysmans HA, Brand A. Beneficial effect of leukocyte depletion of transfused blood on post-operative complications in patients undergoing cardiac surgery: a randomized clinical trial. Circulation. 1998;97:562–8.
20. Vamvakas EC, Blajchman MA. Transfusion-related immunomodulation (TRIM): an update. Blood Rev. 2007;21:327–48.
21. Kao KJ. Induction of humoral immune tolerance to major histocompatibility complex antigens by transfusions of UV-B irradiated leukocytes. Blood. 1996;88:4375–82.
22. Bordin JO, Heddle NM, Blajchman MA. Biologic effects of leukocytes present in transfused cellular blood products. Blood. 1994;84:1705–21.
23. Blajchman MA, Bardossy I, Carmen R, Sastry A, Singal DP. Allogeneic blood transfusion-induced enhancement of tumor growth: two animal models showing amelioration by leukodepletion and passive transfer using spleen cells. Blood. 1993;81:1880–2.
24. Clark DA, Gorczynski RM, Blajchman MA. Transfusion-related immunomodulation due to peripheral blood dendritic cells expressing the CD200 tolerance signaling molecule and alloantigen. Transfusion. 2008;48:814–21.
25. Reed SG. TGF-β in infections and infectious disease. Microbes Infect. 1999;1:1313–25.
26. Beko KR, Tran HO, Hewitt CW, Black KS, Patel MP, Ramsamooj R, Martin DC. Mechanisms of prior blood transfusion-cyclosporine-induced tolerance: a potential role for immune-cellular chimerism. Transplant Proc. 1991;23:147–8.
27. Dzik WH. Mononuclear cell microchimerism and the immunomodulatory effect of transfusion. Transfusion. 1994;34:1007–12.
28. Kirkley SA, Cowles J, LPelligrini Jr VD, Harris CM, Boyd AD, Blumberg N. Blood transfusion and total joint replacement surgery: T-helper 2 cytokine secretion and clinical outcome. Transf Med. 1998;8:195–204.
29. Gafter U, Kalechman Y, Sredni B. Blood transfusion enhances production of T-helper-2 cytokines and transforming growth factor beta in humans. Clin Sci (Lond). 1996;91:519–23.
30. Utter GH, Lee TH, Rivers RM, Montalvo L, Wen L, Chafets DM, Reed WF, Busch MP. Microchimerism decades after transfusion among combat-injured US veterans from the Vietnam, Korean, and World War II conflicts. Transfusion. 2008;48:1609–15.
31. Nelson JL. HLA relationships of pregnancy, microchimerism and autoimmune disease. J Reprod Immunol. 2001;52:77–84.
32. Reed W, Lee TH, Norris PJ, Utter GH, Busch MP. Transfusion-associated microchimerism: a new complication of blood transfusions in severely ill patients. Semin Hematol. 2007;44:24–31.
33. Nielsen HJ, Reimert CM, Pedersen AN, Brünner N, Edvardsen L, Dybkjaer E, Kehlet H, Skov PS. Time-dependent, spontaneous release of white cell- and platelet-derived bioactive substances from stored human blood. Transfusion. 1996;36:960–5.
34. Ghio M, Contini P, Mazzei C, Brenci S, Barberis G, Filaci G, Indiveri F, Puppo F. Soluble HLA class I, HLA class II, and Fas ligand in blood components: a possible key to explain the immunomodulatory effects of allogeneic blood transfusion. Blood. 1999;93:1770–7.
35. Puppo F, Contini P, Ghio M, Brenci S, Scudeletti M, Filaci G, Ferrone S, Indiveri F. Soluble human MHC class I molecules induce soluble Fas-ligand secretion and trigger apoptosis in activated CD8+ Fas (CD95)+ T lymphocytes. Int Immunol. 2000;12:195–203.
36. Magee CC, Sayegh MH. Peptide-mediated immunosuppression. Curr Opin Immunol. 1997;9:669–75.
37. Roelen DL, van Rood JJ, Brand A, Claas FH. Immunomodulation by blood transfusions. Vox Sang. 2000;78:273–5.
38. Brunson ME, Alexander JW. Mechanisms of transfusion-induced immunosuppression. Transfusion. 1990;30:651–8.
39. Vamvakas EC, Blajchman MA. Deleterious clinical effects of transfusion-associated immunomodulation: fact or fiction? [review]. Blood. 2001;97:1180–95.
40. Wallis JP, Chapman CE, Orr KE, Clark SC, Forty JR. Effect of WBC reduction of transfused RBCs on postoperative infection rates in cardiac surgery. Transfusion. 2002;42:1127–34.
41. Titlestad IL, Ebbesen LS, Ainsworth AP, Lillevang ST, Qvist N, Georgsen J. Leukocyte-depletion of blood components does not significantly reduce the risk of infectious complications. Results of a double-blinded, randomized study. Int J Color Dis. 2001;16:147–53.
42. Blumberg N. Deleterious clinical effects of transfusion immunomodulation: proven beyond a reasonable doubt. Transfusion. 2005;45:33S–9; discussion 39S–40.
43. Fergusson D, Aaron SD, Guyatt G, Hebert P. Post-randomization exclusions: the intention to treat principle and excluding patients from analysis. BMJ. 2002;325:652–4.
44. Blumberg N, Zhao H, Wang H, Messing S, Heal JM, Lyman GH. The intention to treat principle in clinic trials and meta-analysis of leukoreduced blood transfusion in surgical patients. Transfusion. 2007;47:573–81.
45. Kwon S, Lew S, Chamberlain RS. Leukocyte filtration and postoperative infections. J Surg Res. 2016;205:499–509.

Origins of Blood Products

32

Elyse M. Cornett, Matthew B. Novitch, Cody Koress, Mitchell C. Fuller, Samuel Carlson, Jennifer Kaiser, Natalia Okon, and Alan David Kaye

Introduction

The first recorded transfusion occurred in 1628 by British physician William Harvey who also discovered the circulation of blood [1]. The first successful transfusion occurred in 1665 and involved transferring blood from one dog to another dog, and in 1667 blood was successfully transferred from sheep to humans. In 1900, Karl Landsteiner discovered blood groups A, B, and O when he mixed the red cells and serum of each of his staff, ultimately revealing why some blood transfusions are deadly [2]. The ABO blood typing system is still relevant today in transfusion and transplantation.

Technological development facilitated the elaboration of the cardiovascular system, which is fundamentally defined by the transportation of blood to tissue. Blood is a living tissue composed of three types of blood cells: *red blood cells* (erythrocytes), *white blood cells* (leukocytes), and *platelets* (thrombocytes). This cellular component comprises 40% of the total blood volume [3]. The function of red blood cells (RBC) is to transport oxygen to peripheral tissues and carry carbon dioxide away from tissues. The function of white blood cells (WBC) is to defend the body against infectious disease and foreign materials by orchestrating the human immune response. Thrombocyte's assist in blood clotting and coagulation homeostasis [4]. *Plasma* comprises 60% of blood by volume and functions as the liquid component of blood, which carries the cellular components (RBC, WBC, and platelets) to peripheral tissues [5].

Blood transfusion has been used by clinicians since the twentieth century to treat pathophysiologic conditions such as anemia and hemorrhage. Transfusion of blood products, (which are collected, tested, prepared, stored, and transported in concordance with FDA regulations from a donor to a patient), are needed to sustain life or improve conditions. While whole blood can provide improved oxygen-carrying capacity, volume expansion, and replacement of clotting factors, specific component therapy is equally effective and a more efficient use of donated blood [6]. Packed red blood cells (RBCs), washed RBCs, WBC-depleted RBCs, fresh frozen plasma (FFP), cryoprecipitate, platelets, and white blood cells are commercially made and can also be processed from bone marrow [7].

There are guidelines to ensure the safety of blood transfusions and to ensure that blood products are safe. Efforts to ensure safety include increased staff trainings on the blood

E. M. Cornett
LSU Health Shreveport, Department of Anesthesiology, Shreveport, LA, USA
e-mail: ecorne@lsuhsc.edu

M. B. Novitch (✉)
University of Washington Medical Center, Department of Anesthesiology, Seattle, WA, USA
e-mail: mnovitch@uw.edu

C. Koress
LSU Health Sciences Center, Department of Anesthesiology, New Orleans, LA, USA
e-mail: ckores@lsuhsc.edu

M. C. Fuller
Froedtert Hospital, Medical College of Wisconsin, Milwaukee, WI, USA
e-mail: mfuller@mcw.edu

S. Carlson · J. Kaiser
Medical College of Wisconsin, Department of Anesthesiology, Wauwatosa, WI, USA
e-mail: Sacarlson@mcw.edu; jkaiser@mcw.edu

N. Okon
Department of Anesthesiology, Wauwatosa, WI, USA
e-mail: nokon@mcw.edu

A. D. Kaye
Department of Anesthesiology and Pharmacology, Toxicology, and Neurosciences, Louisiana State University School of Medicine-Shreveport, Shreveport, LA, USA

LSU Health Shreveport School of Medicine, New Orleans, LA, USA

Tulane School of Medicine, New Orleans, LA, USA
e-mail: akaye@lsuhsc.edu

© Springer Nature Switzerland AG 2021
C. S. Scher et al. (eds.), *Essentials of Blood Product Management in Anesthesia Practice*,
https://doi.org/10.1007/978-3-030-59295-0_32

transfusion process, and more detailed blood donor recruitment processes. Research has demonstrated that screening questions for blood donors are the single most important factor in reducing transfusion-transmitted infections [8]. These questions help identify important risk factors for transfusion-associated adverse events including, testing positive for HIV or other infections, drug use, travel history, and sexual history.

This chapter will elucidate the high-yield anatomy and physiology of blood product origins for clinical anesthesiologists, and the products themselves. Emphasis will be placed on bone marrow structure, hematopoietic components, stromal components, mesenchymal stem cells, and specific blood products.

Bone Marrow Structure

The bone is a porous structure comprised of mineralized calcium compounds, cells, and vessels. The mature human skeleton is divided into the axial skeleton and the appendicular skeleton. The axial skeleton includes the ossicles of the middle ear, the hyoid bone, the rib cage, sternum, and vertebral column. The appendicular includes the limb bones, pectoral, and pelvic girdle. Bone marrow is protected by cortical bone in the trabecular or cancellous portion of bone. At birth, bone marrow is hematopoietically active throughout the skeleton and classified as red marrow. However, by puberty, hematopoietic activity becomes restricted to the bone marrow found in the axial skeleton. The red marrow in long bones transitions to yellow marrow comprised of adipose cells [9].

Bone marrow functions as the major hematopoietic organ in the body and a primary lymphoid tissue. Bone marrow provides the essential microenvironment support for the proliferation, differentiation, and release of blood cells. Erythrocytes, granulocytes, monocytes, lymphocytes, and platelets all primarily arise from bone marrow. Bone marrow resides within a meshwork of trabecular bone embedded within hematopoietic tissue islands and adipose cells.

Overall, the structure of bone is arranged into cylindrical subunits called osteons. The cortex is the external structure consisting of compact bone composed from hydroxyapatite and type one collagen. Trabeculae are the internal portions of the bone arranged into networks of spicules that enclose the thin-walled sinusoids of bone marrow. The inner surface of the trabeculae bone spicules is covered by an endosteal lining of endosteal cells. This lining is a single layer of flat, elongated cells that form a continuous membrane over the trabeculae surface. Underlying the endosteal cells is a discontinuous basement membrane. Adventitial reticular cells support the endosteal lining and contain progenitors of osteoblasts, adipocytes, and chondrocytes. Within the interstitial space of the endothelial lined sinusoids are organized clusters of hematopoietic cells and fat cells. The ratio of fat cells to hematopoietic cells is 1:1 in a healthy adult [10].

Nutrient supply of the bone marrow cavity is organized in a circular pattern with blood flowing from the center, out to the periphery, and back into the center of the cavity. Entry of these nutrient canals differs among those and flat bones. In long bones, the nutrient canal enters the cavity obliquely comprised of one artery and one or two veins. In flat bones, numerous vessels enter as large or small nutrient canals into the marrow cavity. A central longitudinal vein serves as the primary venous the marrow channel. Arteries that enter the cavity split into ascending or descending branches and run coiling around the longitudinal vein. The ascending and descending branches give rise to thin-walled arterioles that extend out toward the cortical bone. Plexuses of venous sinuses near the cortical bone anastomose with the arterioles and drain into collecting venules that extend backward toward the central longitudinal vein. Blood vessels of the bone marrow are composed of a layer of flat endothelial cells lacking a basement membrane. This bone marrow barrier prevents immature blood cells from leaving the marrow. Myelinated and non-myelinated nerve bundles enter through the nutrient canal as part of the periarterial sheath to provide innervation to the smooth muscle of the vessels. Bone marrow does not have a lymphatic drainage system [11].

Hematopoetic Components

Pioneering research by Alexander Friedenstein in the 1960s characterized bone as the sum of two cellular components, *hematopoietic* tissue and *supportive stroma* tissue [12]. Hematopoietic tissue is defined as tissue able to give rise to blood cells, cumulatively comprising the blood system. The blood system has more than ten cell types that perform many physiologic functions that are necessary for life. All blood cell types arise from a common hematopoietic stem cell (HSC), which is majorly found in bone marrow, the major site of adult hematopoiesis. HSC first activates in late embryogenesis when the fetus outgrows its transplacental diffusive capacity. The earliest intra-embryo site for HSC generation is the aorta-gonad-mesonephros (AGM), later becoming the liver, kidney, and finally bone marrow, close to the time of gestation. At this point HSC is responsible for producing over 10^{10}–10^{12} blood cells each day for the entire lifespan of the infant [13]. Hematopoiesis is a constantly active and highly plastic process, which regenerates blood cells of all lineages that can be described in three distinct stages: *polypotent* with lifelong self-renewal potential, *multipotent* with limited self-renewal potential, and lineage-specific tissue progenitor [14]. The first stage of hematopoiesis is represented by the uncommitted (pluripotent) HSC, which maintains three primary roles, to self-renew, to become quiescent, and to differentiate into a tissue-specific progenitor. In order for the human body to maintain the ability to make new blood for an entire lifespan, HSC self-renewal assures a continued source of pluripotent bone marrow stem cells. The polypotent stage has been recently subtyped as alpha, beta, and gamma families with specification bias for myeloid fate and lymphoid fate, respectively, shedding insight into age-related immune depression [15]. The second stage of hematopoiesis is characterized by a multipotent stem cell with less self-renewal capacity and a stronger ability to differentiate into a lineage-specific cell. The third stage of hematopoiesis includes all myeloid and lymphoid tissues including, lymphocytes, granulocytes, erythrocytes, megakaryocytes, and monocytes.

The list of regulation factors that dictate hematopoietic stem cell differentiation, called hematopoiesis, is both intrinsic and extrinsic and incorporates a vast spectrum of molecular signaling networks. Hematopoiesis is central to both normal and pathological clinical medicine, which explains why the elderly have decreased immune system protection and an increased likelihood of prevalent hematologic cancers such as leukemias and lymphomas [16]. Intrinsic regulation of hematopoiesis includes genetic and epigenetic elements. Epigenetic methylation can drive the expressional activation of genes responsible for differentiation [17]. Genetic expressivity is robustly regulated via transcription factors and can select for the tissue fate of the HSC. For example, the pluripotent HSC differentiates to a multipotent form via IL6 and stem cell factor, whereas the second step of HSC differentiation to a particular blood organ is molecularly programmed by GM-CSF, M-CSF, IL-1 to IL-5, INF, TNF, and a myriad of endocrine growth factors [18]. Additionally, homeostatic extrinsic regulation factors in the bone marrow microenvironment provide extracellular signaling that supply direct and indirect control of hematopoietic component differentiation. Bone marrow stroma in the long bone of adult bone marrow is the major regulatory entity, but other regulatory contributions are made by endothelial cells, non-myelinating Schwann cells, megakaryocytes, macrophages, and osteoblasts [19]. Signaling from sympathetic nerves, oxygen conditions, and numerous circulating factors all supply direct and indirect control of HSC.

There are five fates of the HSC that together represent the hematopoietic components: lymphopoiesis, granulocytopoiesis, erythropoiesis, megakaryocytopoiesis, and monocytopoiesis. Understanding the physiological function of these components guides clinical decision-making when deciding when to use a whole blood product or specific blood products [20]. *Lymphopoiesis* results in pro-NK cells, pro-T cells, and pro-B cells that further differentiate to their mature forms at distal sites, such as the thymus and spleen. NK cells are key players in eliminating tumorigenic tissue and intracellular viral infections by targeted cell lysis and activation of the adaptive immune system [21]. Adaptive immunity has B cell and T cell arms, which generate antibodies and perform target cell lysis/proliferation of the adaptive response. Additionally, B and T cell immunity orchestrates a long-lived protective response to immunization. *Granulocytopoiesis* generates neutrophils, basophils, and eosinophils and minorly contributes to the monocyte differentiation pathway– with the major monocyte pathway being *monocytopoiesis* [14]. Monocytes can then further divide into polymorphonuclear cells, dendritic cells, and macrophages. Combined, granulocytopoiesis and monocytopoiesis comprise an innate immunity, which utilizes pattern recognition receptors (PRRs) to bind pathogen-associated molecular patterns (PAMPs) and elicit an exquisite immune response [22]. Innate immunity can clear infection by phagocytosis of foreign particles or by a pantheon of alternative mechanisms (i.e., NETosis). Megakaryocytopoiesis is a fourth pathway that generates platelets. The final pathway, *erythropoiesis*, is the process where over two million red blood cells per second are generated from myeloid precursor cells. In homeostasis, red blood cells transport oxygen for tissue perfusion. Dysregulation of erythropoiesis results in common blood disorders like anemia, sickle cell disease, paroxysmal nocturnal hemoglobinuria, and β-thalassemia [23]. Major technological advances in cell sorting and diagnostic efficacy have enabled hematopoietic component usage, decreasing wasteful administration of whole blood cell products when specific products are adequate.

Stroma

Beyond hematopoietic tissue, Friedenstein also identified supportive stroma. The stroma is defined as a heterogeneous population of cells within a tissue or organ, which provide structural and connective roles. While not directly implicated in hematopoiesis, stroma cells of the bone marrow contribute to the microenvironment, which influences hematopoietic cell function and differentiation [24]. Anatomically, stromal cells are found between outer surfaces of the blood vessel and bone surfaces but are not cells with direct hematopoietic lineage. Stroma cells of the bone marrow provide both structural and physiological functions for hematopoietic cells and include into a broad array of cell types including bone, cartilage, adipocyte, and supportive hematopoietic tissue [25]. A specific subset of stromal cells called *mesenchymal stem cells* are hypothesized to possess stem cell characteristics with potential for multiple lineage differentiation.

There are a variety of cells within bone marrow stroma, each of which assists with a unique function. *Endothelial cells* are derivatives of the endothelial stem cells and function to form sinusoids, or small blood vessel within organs. *Osteoclasts and osteoblasts* function in bone resorption and creation, respectively. *Adipocytes* are fat cells that store energy in the form of triacylglycerols and cholesterol. *Macrophages* help provide iron for hemoglobin and the subsequent production of red blood cells. *Fibroblasts* are true structural cells, which provide reticular connective tissue and stability to the niche [26]. Bone marrow has characteristic and substantial blood flow mediated via the sinusoidal vessels, which provide a nutrient-rich environment that supports extravascular hematopoiesis. Stromal fibroblasts are known for their supportive role in hematopoiesis and bone development. While understood to be integrally involved in hematopoiesis, much is still unknown concerning their exact morphology. Stromal fibroblasts coat the sinusoid wall and express collagen type I and II, populate the marrow before hematopoietic cells appear, and appear to be functionally involved in developmental coupling of osteogenesis and vascularity [25]. Bone disease in humans is linked with increases in these stromal fibroblasts, potentially leading to osteosclerosis [25].

Proliferation, differentiation, and maturation of hematopoietic cells depend on the stroma of the bone marrow due to the role it plays in niche development, and function in cytokine signal production. These niches also play a significant role in the development of tumor cell metastasis within the bone marrow, leading to the tumor cell propensity for metastasizing to bone [27]. Multiple factors contribute to this propensity for a tumor to metastasize including substantial blood flow, adhesive molecules, which provide recognition and interaction between stromal cells, extracellular matrix, and endothelial cells, and growth factors critical to ensuring remodeling. Growth and physical factors, hypothesized to play a significant role in tumor cell development within the bone marrow stroma, include platelet-derived growth factor, transforming growth factor-β, fibroblast growth factor, insulin growth factor, acidic pH, low oxygen levels, and high extracellular calcium concentration [25–27]. In vitro studies suggest that the significant potential for proliferation may be associated with capacity for self-renewal and support the hypothesis that stem cells within the stromal cell lines are capable of giving rise to multiple lineages and potentially contributing to osteogenic cancers [27, 28].

Mesenchymal Stem Cells

Mesenchymal stem cells (MSCs) are a subset of stromal supportive tissue that are also known as mesenchymal stromal cells, multipotent adult progenitor cells, and marrow-isolated multilineage inducible cells [29, 30]. These alternative names are controversial, however, as no in vivo self-renewal potential has ever been clearly demonstrated with isolated MSCs.

MSCs are non-hematopoietic adult stem cells that can differentiate into endodermal, mesodermal, and ectodermal lineages (i.e., multipotency). MSCs were first discovered as a component of the bone marrow stroma that demonstrated classic tri-lineage potential for adipogenesis, chondrogenesis, and osteogenesis. MSC's also reside in the spleen, liver, and other B-cell lymphopoiesis progenitor tissues [31] Histologically, MSCs are identified by their unique cell surface marker expression [32] and can be identified by several markers (CD)44, CD73, CD90, and CD105 and by a lack of expression of hematopoetic antigens, CD11b, CD14, CD19 CD34, CD45, CD79, and HLA (human leucocyte antigen)-DR. There is controversy as to how to properly define a cell population that shares stem cell marker expression but may be more biologically divergent, depending on location.

The clinical utility of MSCs have potential for considerable in vitro expansion, proliferation, and differentiation. Mesenchymal stem cells can be harvested from donor amniotic fluid, adipose tissue, dental tissue, bone marrow, and Wharton's jelly in the umbilical cord [33, 34]. As such, the therapeutic applications of MSCs are extensive. Ex vivo expansion of MSCs for in vivo transplantation can regenerate bone and stromal structures while supporting hematopoiesis. Additionally, bone marrow stromal cell transplantation is beneficial compared to total marrow transplantation because a significant population of cells can be generated from a small marrow aspirate, avoiding unnecessary surgery.

Stromal cells assist in fast bone formation, faster and more fully than a total marrow transplant [25]. Underscoring the importance of a viable MSC population in clinical transplants, damage to the MSCs due to pre-transplant radiation therapy can prevent effective maintenance and lineage preservation. The use of MSC transplant in conjunction with hematopoietic stem cell transplant may limit the required dose of hematopoietic stem cells to be translated and improve the overall outcome of transplant therapy [27, 28].

In recent years, the applications for MSCs have grown to include immunomodulation of refractory acute graft-versus-host disease in bone marrow transplant patients, drug resistant epilepsy in children, multiple sclerosis, and diabetes [35–38]. There is a clinically indicated role for MSCs as native support to the growth and prosperity of hematopoietic tissue in vivo, adjunctive to hematopoietic stem cell transplantation, and as the primary transplantation tissue.

Specific Products

Whole blood can be divided into different products: packed red blood cells (PRBCs), cryoprecipitate, platelets, and fresh frozen plasma (FFP). Isolated components of whole blood are each indicated for unique circumstances, rendering the division, separate storage, and administration more efficacious than that of complete whole blood [39]. In the context of the predominant shortage of blood products, this separation becomes espcially practical [40].

Packed Red Blood Cells

Packed red blood cells (PRBCs) are indicated for preventing or improving hypoxia. Pragmatically, the presence and degree of hypoxia is estimated with hemoglobin or hematocrit markers serving as substitutes for intracellular pO_2. These measures alone do not account for physiologic compensation and must be evaluated in a clinical context. If hypoxia is threatened in a non-urgent context, especially with asymptomatic patients, measures apart from transfusion– such as iron supplementation or B_{12} tablets– are preferred. Tissue oxygenation depends not only on the concentration of hemoglobin but also on the hemoglobin saturation and oxygen requirement factors, which are influenced by the physiologic state of the patient. While a hemoglobin of 7 g/L may indicate sufficient perfusion in a young, healthy patient, the same hemoglobin concentration may be inadequate in an elderly patient, or someone with ongoing bleeding. Hemoglobin levels above 10 g/L rarely require transfusion, while those less than 6 g/L very frequently require transfusion. As an estimate, a single unit of PRBCs increases an adult's hemoglobin by 1 g/dL [41]. Other substrates may be preferable to replete volume, though a volume loss of at least 40% often requires additional PRBC transfusion. Red blood cells may also be leukodepleted, irradiated, washed, or frozen, with each preparation specifically indicated for the prevention of certain infectious conditions or immunologic reactions to PRBCs. For example, washed red blood cells are indicated in IgA deficiency, prevention of certain allergic reactions, and prevention of febrile reactions from transfusion [41].

Fresh Frozen Plasma

Fresh frozen plasma (FFP) is prepared from whole blood or derived from such via apheresis (in which red blood cells are immediately reintroduced to the donor while the plasma is retained). It is frozen at −18 °C or less and is used immediately upon thawing or is stored for no more than 24 hours. It comprises the liquid, acellular, component of blood, roughly 50% by volume. Plasma contains all protein factor and antibody components of blood but does not contain platelets. It is transfused to replace deficient or defective plasma proteins. Indications for FFP include replacement of multiple plasma proteins (as in disseminated intravascular coagulation or liver failure), massive transfusion in patients with relevant coagulation deficiencies, immediate warfarin reversal, thrombotic thrombocytopenic purpura patient transfusion, and replacement of proteins for which specific concentrates are unavailable. Fresh frozen plasma should not be used if a more specific factor concentrate is available, or if a more effective therapy reversal agent (i.e., vitamin K) can be used instead. It should not be employed for volume expansion when other volume expanders are considered more safe and effective [42].

Cryoprecipitate

Cryoprecipitate is collected by thawing fresh frozen plasma from whole blood at 0–6 °C and collecting the solid component. It provides fibrinogen, fibronectin, ADAMTS13, von Willebrand factor, and factors VIII and XIII. When isolated recombinant proteins are unavailable and the use of fresh frozen plasma (FFP) is undesirable from a volume-status standpoint, cryoprecipitate may be used to replenish fibrinogen or factor XIII in respective deficiencies. Use in bleeding uremic patients may be considered, but not as a first-line replenishing agent. Similarly, it may be used in factor VIII deficiency (hemophilia A) or von Willebrand's disease after efforts fail to obtain isolated factor concentrates [42].

Platelets

Platelets are white blood cell remnants, which are crucial to clot formation and hemostasis. They're collected from either whole blood or apheresis techniques (plasma and platelets are removed from the blood before reintroduction into the donor). Variable levels of red and white blood cells may remain with the platelets, depending upon the collection technique. The platelets are then stored in plasma. The primary hemostatic platelet plug is an initial response of the body to vascular injury, which prevents bleeding. This temporary "plug" is formed by an intricate interaction between platelets, coagulation factors, von Willebrand Factor, damaged vessel wall protein, and phospholipids. It is later replaced by a more stable fibrin clot, in secondary hemostasis. The goal of platelet transfusion is to supply the body with sufficient numbers of functional platelets to maintain hemostasis. Indications include serious risk of bleeding, active bleeding from thrombocytopenia, or dysfunctional platelets. Patients with cancer, aplastic anemia, central nervous system trauma, or who require cardiopulmonary bypass are at risk of requiring platelet transfusion [42].

Because platelet transfusion carries risk, the clinical context of the patient must be accounted for when evaluating the risks and benefits. Infectious and immunogenic risks may be minimized by transfusing platelets from a single donor, especially with HLA matching. When platelet levels remain above 50,000, bleeding from thrombocytopenia is unlikely, even in a surgical context. Spontaneous bleeding is unlikely to occur from platelet deficit until the number drops below 10,000 platelets. This is maybe used as a transfusion cutoff even in asymptomatic patients. Simultaneous clinical factors, like fever and coagulopathy, may increase the bleeding risk, and justify a less restrictive transfusion threshold [43]. In cases of mucous membrane bleeding that is hemodynamically significant, platelet transfusion should be initiated regardless of laboratory values. In surgical patients or those with active bleeding, a threshold of 50,000 is justifiable [43]. For autoimmune disorders like immune thrombocytopenic purpura, platelet transfusion may be of limited benefit, as the issue is related to platelet destruction. Concentrate transfusion may still provide benefit to alleviate active bleeding. Often, intravenous immunoglobulin may augment the patient reaction to platelets and provide direct therapeutic benefit. In heparin-induced thrombocytopenia type II, or thrombotic thrombocytopenic purpura, platelet transfusions are contraindicated due to the increased risk of thrombosis. Leukoreduction of platelet transfusion product is indicated to decrease the frequency of transfused CMV infection, HLA allo-immunization, and recurrent febrile nonhemolytic reactions [42, 43].

Conclusion

A thorough understanding of blood product anatomy and physiology is an asset to the modern practicing physician. Ordering the correct blood products can significantly limit wasteful use of blood, thereby reducing the risk to patients and avoiding inflated healthcare costs.

References

1. History of blood transfusions 1628 to now. Red Cross Blood Services [Internet]. Cited 25 Oct 2019. Available from: https://www.redcrossblood.org/donate-blood/blood-donation-process/what-happens-to-donated-blood/blood-transfusions/history-blood-transfusion.html.
2. Farhud DD, Yeganeh MZ. A brief history of human blood groups. Iran J Public Health. 2013;42(1):1–6.
3. Sharma R, Sharma S. Physiology, blood volume. StatPearls. 2018.
4. Prinyakupt J, Pluempitiwiriyawej C. Segmentation of white blood cells and comparison of cell morphology by linear and naïve Bayes classifiers. Biomed Eng Online. 2015:30;14:63. https://doi.org/10.1186/s12938-015-0037-1. PMID: 26123131; PMCID: PMC4485641.
5. Mathew J, Bhimji SS. Physiology, blood plasma. StatPearls. 2018.
6. Yaddanapudi S, Yaddanapudi LN. Indications for blood and blood product transfusion. Indian J Anaesth, Indian Society of Anaesthetists. 2014;58:538–42.
7. Haldiman L, Zia H, Singh G. Improving appropriateness of blood utilization through prospective review of requests for blood products: the role of pathology residents as consultants. Lab Med. 2014;45(3):264–71.
8. Harris JC, Crookston KP. Blood product safety. Nat Clim Chang. 2013;3:606–7.
9. Dave U, Koury MJ. Chapter 5: structure of the marrow and the hematopoietic microenvironment. In: Kaushansky K, Lichtman MA, Prchal JT, Levi MM, Press OW, Burns LJ, Caligiuri M, editors. Williams hematology. 9th ed. New York: McGraw-Hill; 2016.
10. Kumar V, Abbas AK, Aster JC, Perkins JA. Robbins and Cotran pathologic basis of disease. Philadelphia : Saunders/Elsevie: 2010 p. 1391.
11. Islam A, Glomski C, Henderson ES. Bone lining (endosteal) cells and hematopoiesis: a light microscopic study of normal and pathologic human bone marrow in plastic-embedded sections. Anat Rec [Internet]. 1990 [Cited 17 Oct 2019];227(3):300–6. Available from: http://www.ncbi.nlm.nih.gov/pubmed/2372137.
12. Grayson WL, Bunnell BA, Martin E, Frazier T, Hung BP, Gimble JM. Stromal cells and stem cells in clinical bone regeneration. Nat Rev Endocrinol, Nature Publishing Group. 2015;11:140–50.
13. Levine MN, Raskob G, Beyth RJ, Kearon C, Schulman S. Hemorrhagic complications of anticoagulant treatment. Chest [Internet]. 2004 [Cited 14 Dec 2016];126(3):287S–310 S. Available from: http://linkinghub.elsevier.com/retrieve/pii/S0012369215314951.
14. Michael A. Rieger TS. Hematopoiesis. Cold Spring Harb Lab Press [Internet]. 2012 [Cited 17 Oct 2019]. Available from: https://www.ncbi.nlm.nih.gov/pmc/articles/PMC3504436/pdf/cshperspect-MDV-a008250.pdf.
15. Beerman I, Bhattacharya D, Zandi S, Sigvardsson M, Weissman IL, Bryder D, et al. Functionally distinct hematopoietic stem cells modulate hematopoietic lineage potential during aging by a mechanism of clonal expansion. Proc Natl Acad Sci [Internet]. 2010 [Cited 17 Oct 2019];107(12):5465–70. Available from: http://www.ncbi.nlm.nih.gov/pubmed/20304793.
16. Xie M, Lu C, Wang J, McLellan MD, Johnson KJ, Wendl MC, et al. Age-related mutations associated with clonal hematopoietic expansion and malignancies. Nat Med [Internet]. 2014 [Cited 17 Oct 2019];20(12):1472–8. Available from: http://www.nature.com/articles/nm.3733.
17. Farlik M, Halbritter F, Müller F, Choudry FA, Ebert P, Klughammer J, et al. DNA methylation dynamics of human hematopoietic stem cell differentiation. Cell Stem Cell [Internet]. 2016 [Cited 17 Oct 2019];19(6):808–22. Available from: https://www.sciencedirect.com/science/article/pii/S1934590916303605.
18. Travlos GS. Normal structure, function, and histology of the bone marrow. Toxicol Pathol [Internet]. 2006 [Cited 17 Oct 2019];34(5):548–65. Available from: http://www.ncbi.nlm.nih.gov/pubmed/17067943.
19. Decker MN. The extrinsic regulation of hematopoietic stem cells in health and disease [Internet]. 2018 [Cited 17 Oct 2019]. Available from: https://search.proquest.com/docview/2130899557?pq-origsite=gscholar.
20. Gaur DS, Negi G, Chauhan N, Kusum A, Khan S, Pathak VP. Utilization of blood and components in a tertiary care hospital. Indian J Hematol Blood Transfus [Internet]. 2009 [Cited 17 Oct 2019];25(3):91–5. Available from: http://link.springer.com/10.1007/s12288-009-0027-1.
21. Vivier E, Raulet DH, Moretta A, Caligiuri MA, Zitvogel L, Lanier LL, et al. Innate or adaptive immunity? The example of natural killer cells. Science [Internet]. 2011 [Cited 17 Oct 2019];331(6013):44–9. Available from: http://www.ncbi.nlm.nih.gov/pubmed/21212348.
22. Iwasaki A, Medzhitov R. Control of adaptive immunity by the innate immune system. Nat Immunol [Internet]. 2015 [Cited 17 Oct

2019];16(4):343–53. Available from: http://www.ncbi.nlm.nih.gov/pubmed/25789684.
23. Liang R, Ghaffari S. Advances in understanding the mechanisms of erythropoiesis in homeostasis and disease. Br J Haematol [Internet]. 2016 [Cited 17 Oct 2019];174(5):661–73. Available from: http://www.ncbi.nlm.nih.gov/pubmed/27442953.
24. Bernardo ME, Fibbe WE. Mesenchymal stromal cells and hematopoietic stem cell transplantation. Immunol Lett. 2015;168(2):215–21.
25. Krebsbach PH, Kuznetsov SA, Bianco P, Robey PG. Bone marrow stromal cells: characterization and clinical application. Crit Rev Oral Biol Med. 1999;10(2):165–81.
26. Moschetta M, Kawano Y, Sacco A, Belotti A, Ribolla R, Chiarini M, et al. Bone marrow stroma and vascular contributions to myeloma bone homing. Curr Osteoporos Rep. 2017;15(5):499–506.
27. Beresford JN. Osteogenic stem cells and the stromal system of bone and marrow. Clin Orthop Relat Res. 1989;240:270–80.
28. Abbuehl J-P, Tatarova Z, Held W, Huelsken J. Long-term engraftment of primary bone marrow stromal cells repairs niche damage and improves hematopoietic stem cell transplantation. Cell Stem Cell. 2017;21(2):241–255.e6.
29. D'Ippolito G, Diabira S, Howard GA, Menei P, Roos BA, Schiller PC. Marrow-isolated adult multilineage inducible (MIAMI) cells, a unique population of postnatal young and old human cells with extensive expansion and differentiation potential. J Cell Sci. 2004;117(Pt 14):2971–81.
30. Jiang Y, Jahagirdar BN, Reinhardt RL, Schwartz RE, Keene CD, Ortiz-Gonzalez XR, Reyes M, Lenvik T, Lund T, Blackstad M, Du J, Aldrich S, Lisberg A, Low WC, Largaespada DA, Verfaillie CM. Pluripotency of mesenchymal stem cells derived from adult marrow. Nature. 2002:4;418(6893):41–9. https://doi.org/10.1038/nature00870. Epub 2002 Jun 20. Erratum in: Nature. 2007 Jun 14;447(7146):879–80. PMID: 12077603.
31. Lindner U, Kramer J, Rohwedel J, Schlenke P. Mesenchymal stem or stromal cells: toward a better understanding of their biology? Transfus Med Hemother. 2010;37:75–83.
32. Ding DC, Chang YH, Shyu WC, Lin SZ. Human umbilical cord mesenchymal stem cells: a new era for stem cell therapy. Cell Transplant, Cognizant Communication Corporation. 2015;24:339–47.
33. Ullah I, Subbarao RB, Rho GJ. Human mesenchymal stem cells – current trends and future prospective. Biosci Rep. 2015;35(2):1–18.
34. Kobolak J, Dinnyes A, Memic A, Khademhosseini A, Mobasheri A. Mesenchymal stem cells: identification, phenotypic characterization, biological properties and potential for regenerative medicine through biomaterial micro-engineering of their niche. Methods. 2016;99:62–8.
35. Cohen JA, Imrey PB, Planchon SM, Bermel RA, Fisher E, Fox RJ, et al. Pilot trial of intravenous autologous culture-expanded mesenchymal stem cell transplantation in multiple sclerosis. Mult Scler J. 2018;24(4):501–11.
36. Squillaro T, Peluso G, Galderisi U. Clinical trials with mesenchymal stem cells: an update. Cell Transplant, Cognizant Communication Corporation. 2016;25:829–48.
37. Krasowska-Kwiecien A, Gozdzik J, Jarocha D, Wozniak M, Czogala W, Wiecha O, et al. Mesenchymal stem cells as a salvage treatment for severe refractory graft-vs-host disease in children after bone marrow transplantation. Transplant Proc. 2019;51(3):880–9.
38. Milczarek O, Jarocha D, Starowicz-Filip A, Kwiatkowski S, Badyra B, Majka M. Multiple autologous bone marrow-derived CD271+ mesenchymal stem cell transplantation overcomes drug-resistant epilepsy in children. Stem Cells Transl Med. 2018;7(1):20–33.
39. Basu D, Kulkarni R. Overview of blood components and their preparation. Indian J Anaesth. 2014;58(5):529–37.
40. Kim HO. In-vitro stem cell derived red blood cells for transfusion: are we there yet? Yonsei Med J. 2014;55:304–9.
41. Liumbruno G, Bennardello F, Lattanzio A, Piccoli P, Rossetti G. Recommendations for the transfusion of red blood cells. Blood Transfus. 2009;7:49–64.
42. Circular of information for the use of human blood and blood components.
43. Drews RE, Weinberger SE. Thrombocytopenic disorders in critically ill patients. Am J Respir Crit Care Med, American Lung Association. 2000;162:347–51.

Blood Conservation and Management in Cardiac Surgery

33

Blake A. Moore and Patrick O. McConville

Cardiac surgical procedures requiring cardiopulmonary bypass necessitate systemic anticoagulation and exposure to the pro-inflammatory extracorporeal circuit. Surgical procedures already account for 50% of all allogeneic blood product administration. Cardiac surgical procedures are at high risk for bleeding and allogeneic transfusion. Transfusion rates in cardiac surgery vary widely, with rates of 40–90% of cardiac surgical patients will receive a transfusion; cardiac surgical procedures consist of 10–20% of total blood product administration in the United States [1–4].

Perioperative transfusion of any product in CABG has been associated with worse outcomes in a dose-dependent manner, including increased mortality, renal failure, prolonged mechanical ventilation, and serious infection [5]. Even long-term survival is negatively impacted by perioperative transfusion in CABG surgery [6].

Patients undergoing cardiac surgery are also likely to be anemic by the WHO (World Health Organization) definition. The WHO defines anemia as <130 g/L for males and <120 g/L in females. By this metric 20–30% of cardiac surgical patients are anemic prior to surgery [7].

Blood products are a finite resource that also introduce risk, but they are also critical in modern cardiac surgery. Allogeneic blood products and commercially produced blood products should be preserved and given in accordance with guidelines to avoid unnecessary transfusion and risks of allogeneic transfusion and to limit the risks of administering pharmacological agents to augment hemostasis. Newer pharmacological agents that are derived from human proteins can serve to replace or reduce fresh frozen plasma and cryoprecipitate administration through coagulation factor replacement (four-factor prothrombin complex concentrates such as *Beriplex®*, *Kcentra®*) and lyophilized human fibrinogen administration (*RiaSTAP®*, *fibryga®*). Understanding the basics of the broad mechanisms of the hemostatic system, specifically, platelet function, the endothelium, fibrinolysis, and coagulation factors, is essential to improving outcomes in cardiac surgery while also preserving precious blood resources and containing costs.

The Society of Thoracic Surgeons and the Society of Cardiovascular Anesthesiologists have released guidelines on blood conservation with a most recent update in 2011. Highlights of the 2011 Guidelines Recommendations are included below and included the following [4]:

- There is good evidence in support of lysine analogs to reduce blood loss (I,[A]).
- P2Y12 inhibitors should be discontinued prior to cardiac surgery (I,[B]), while point-of-care testing for ADP responsiveness may be a reasonable measure to plan earlier interventions (IIb, [C]).
- Cell salvage is a reasonable means of conserving blood and limiting use of allogeneic blood transfusion (IIb,[B]).

In 2017, the European Association for Cardiothoracic Surgery (EACTS) and the European Association of Cardiothoracic Anaesthesiology (EACTA) have given further guidance on blood conservation and management in cardiac surgical patients. Highlights from the 2017 guidelines will be discussed later in this chapter.

B. A. Moore
Section on Cardiothoracic Anesthesia, University of Tennessee Graduate School of Medicine, Knoxville, TN, USA
e-mail: Bamoore@utmck.edu

P. O. McConville (✉)
The University of Tennessee Medical Center, Department of Anesthesiology, Knoxville, TN, USA
e-mail: PMcConvi@utmck.edu

© Springer Nature Switzerland AG 2021
C. S. Scher et al. (eds.), *Essentials of Blood Product Management in Anesthesia Practice*,
https://doi.org/10.1007/978-3-030-59295-0_33

The Cardiopulmonary Bypass Circuit and the Hematologic Inflammatory Response

The hemostatic system normally is a balance between the complex interactions of injured endothelium, platelets, and the serial interactions of circulating hemostatic proteins resulting in clot formation and the subsequent interactions between regulatory proteins that culminate in fibrinolysis. Many of the reactions that result in thrombin's terminal cleavage of fibrinogen to form a fibrin clotting matrix occur in the presence of both calcium and platelet phospholipid that is present in activated, prothrombotic platelet surfaces or endothelium.

Exposure of blood to the cardiopulmonary bypass *circuit* results in a profound inflammatory response mediated by complement, neutrophils, endothelium, monocytes, and platelet-activating response with release of PF4 by alpha granules [8, 9]. The inflammatory response is, therefore, systemic and multifactorial. As a consequence of localized ischemia with associated ischemia-reperfusion injury, microemboli, exogenous heparin, *and even hypothermia*, cardiopulmonary bypass can result in marked coagulopathy [10]. The surface activation mechanisms of hemostasis are related to endothelial injury which leads to extrinsic pathway tissue factor production and activation. This mechanism of coagulation ignition is the accepted primary mechanism of cardiac surgery-induced coagulopathy. The coagulation cascade is traditionally presented in a simplistic but organized manner that allows for an overview of the components of the biochemical reactions that occur with hemostasis while failing to demonstrate the complex interconnected nature of the pathway that allows for the appropriate balance between hemostasis and clot lysis that prevents intravascular thrombosis from a runaway reaction or uncontrolled bleeding from inadequate activation. The culmination of the reactions of the intrinsic pathway, extrinsic pathway, and common pathways results in the terminal reaction where thrombin cleaves fibrinogen to produce soluble fibrin, which subsequently forms insoluble clot when factor XIII crosslinks strands of fibrin. Thrombin accelerates the hemostatic pathway reactions by amplification of hemostatic reactions, it promotes inflammatory mediators' activation and chemotactic mechanisms, and it also serves to activate protein C, which serves to temper the hemostatic reactions through negative feedback mechanisms. As a most important component of the hemostatic system, it is believed that cardiopulmonary bypass may affect the thrombin burst, resulting in coagulopathy by thrombocytopenia (platelet consumption), diminished platelet interactions, and the concentration of protein substrates present [10].

Preoperative Anemia

Elective cases should be postponed in anemic patients. The management of anemia will likely include iron supplementation. While the exact time and benefits of iron administration have not been determined, it is a reasonable intervention to provide for elective cardiac surgical procedures. There is evidence to support the use of IV iron to treat IDA (iron deficiency anemia) (Meta-analysis PLoS One 2019). Preoperative anemia is a modifiable risk factor for postoperative morbidity and mortality in cardiac surgery (Ann Thorac Surg 2013). Erythropoietin has demonstrated to reduce red cell transfusion in some studies of non-anemic patients undergoing cardiac surgery. The expert consensus is that erythropoietin with or without iron supplementation should be considered in patients undergoing cardiac surgery in an elective setting [11].

Management of Anticoagulants and Antiplatelet Drugs

Prior to cardiac surgery, many surgical patients will have been receiving anticoagulants or antiplatelet drugs for both coronary disease or related medical problems. Aspirin should be routinely continued for CABG, despite increased blood loss, due to reduced thrombotic events, including acute kidney injury [12–14]. The EACTS/EACTA 2017 Guidelines also recommend continuing aspirin in low-risk patients for CABG or to restart as soon as safely possible if bleeding risk is excessive or the patient refuses blood transfusions [11]. Aspirin should otherwise be held for 5 days before cardiac surgery. Resumption of aspirin within 48 hours of CABG has demonstrated a significantly significant reduction in mortality [15].

Many patients with coronary disease may be on dual antiplatelet therapy (DAPT) prior to cardiac surgery. For non-emergent cases, the P2Y12-receptor antagonist should be held in accordance with their respective pharmacologic profile. Aspirin therapy should be continued during this period according to the EACTS/EACTA 2017 Guidelines. Figure 33.1 outlines the management of aspirin and P2Y12 antagonists for cardiac surgery.

The EACTS/EACTA 2017 Guidelines also have recommendations for perioperative management of GpIIb/IIIa inhibitors, vitamin K antagonists (VKA), LMWH (enoxaparin), and direct oral anticoagulants (DOAC). The direct oral anticoagulants include the direct thrombin inhibitor dabigatran and the factor Xa inhibitors (rivaroxaban, apixaban, edoxaban). The drugs in these various classes are commonly prescribed to patients undergoing cardiac surgery for related disease processes and must be managed appropriately in the perioperative period to limit post-cardiopulmonary bypass bleeding. With regard to LMWH or unfractionated heparin (UFH), which may be utilized as a bridge treatment for those on anticoagulation for prevention of thrombotic events, anticoagulant bridge therapy should only be considered in those who are at high risk for thrombotic events [11]. GpIIb/IIIa inhibitors should be discontinued 4 hours prior to surgery, VKA should be discontinued 3–5 days prior to surgery to achieve an INR <1.5, LMWH should be held >24 hours prior to surgery, and DOAC should be held >48 hours prior to surgery [11, 16]. Only those patients at high risk for thrombotic events should receive LMWH or UFH bridges from oral anticoagulation. These patients include those with recent acute pulmonary embolism (<4 weeks from surgery), atrial fibrillation with CHA_2DS_2-VASc score >4, and patients with a mechanical heart valve [16]. Figure 33.2 gives a perioperative timeline of the management of these agents in elective cardiac surgery.

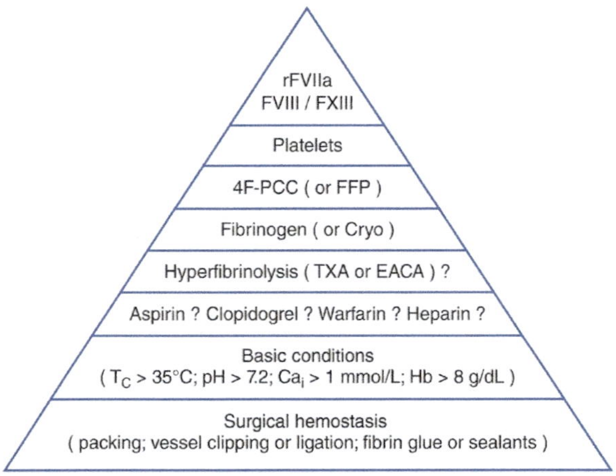

Fig. 33.1 Management of antiplatelet therapy in patients having coronary artery bypass grafting surgery. [a]Complex and redo operations, severe renal insufficiency, hematological diseases, and hereditary deficiencies in platelet function. [b]Recent stent implantation, recent thromboembolic event, and alarming angiographic results. [c]Until the recommended DAPT period is completed. ASA, acetylsalicylic acid; DAPT, dual antiplatelet therapy; GPIIb/IIIa, glycoprotein IIb/IIIa. (Modified from Task Force on Patient Blood Management for Adult Cardiac Surgery of the European Association for Cardio-Thoracic S et al. [11])

Retrograde and Antegrade Autologous Priming

Retrograde autologous priming involves replacement of the crystalloid in the CPB cannulas with blood prior to initiation of CPB to limit hemodilution. This technique is currently recommended for consideration as part of blood conservation efforts in cardiac surgery. Several studies have demonstrated that RAP reduces hemodilution and transfusion in cardiac surgery, although no large randomized trials have demonstrated its benefit [17, 18].

Off-Pump Cardiac Surgery

Two recent large studies have shown reduced transfusion rates in off-pump CABG procedures. The CORONARY Investigators and GOPCABE study found reduced transfusion rates in off-pump CABG procedures [19, 20]. Based on these studies and despite the limitations, including lack of blinding to treatment, exclusion after randomization, and an unspecified transfusion protocol, it is reasonable to consider off-pump CABG procedures in certain patients.

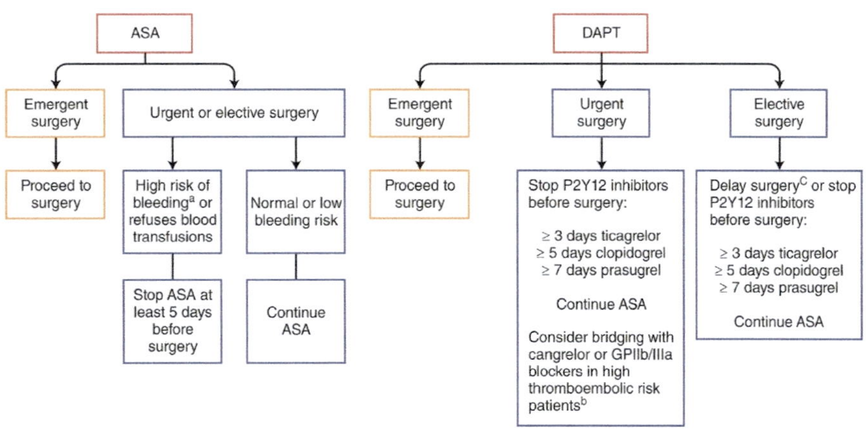

Fig. 33.2 Management of oral anticoagulation in patients with an indication for pre- and/or postoperative bridging. [a]Bridging with UFH/LMWH should start when INR values are below specific therapeutic ranges. [b]Discontinuation should be prolonged to 472 h if creatinine clearance is 50–79 ml/min/1.73 m^2 or Z96 h if creatinine clearance is o50 ml/min/1.73 m^2. DOACs, direct oral anticoagulants; INR, international normalized ratio; LMWH, low-molecular-weight heparin; UFH, unfractionated heparin; VKAs, vitamin K antagonists. (Modified from Task Force on Patient Blood Management for Adult Cardiac Surgery of the European Association for Cardio-Thoracic S et al. [11])

Acute Normovolemic Hemodilution

Acute normovolemic hemodilution (ANH) has been used for patients undergoing surgical procedures with high risk of bleeding in order to attempt to limit allogeneic transfusion of red blood cells, platelets, and clotting factors. It was first described in the 1970s [21, 22]. ANH is a blood conservation technique that sequesters the patient's whole blood prior to surgical intervention in order to administer at the conclusion of the case when surgical bleeding has been controlled and to treat coagulopathy. The blood is stored during the procedure until such time it is needed to transfuse back to the patient. Following withdrawal of whole blood, the blood volume is replaced with crystalloid or colloid to maintain intravascular volume. In some more recently published studies, it has demonstrated a statistically significant reduction in the reduction of allogeneic transfusions for high-risk surgical cases [23].

While the potential benefits of ANH are still being investigated, recent retrospective analysis, meta-analysis, and prospective trials have demonstrated reduced transfusion requirements in cardiac surgical patients who receive ANH [24, 25]. ANH has also demonstrated a myocardial protective effect during cardiac surgery, with less inotropic support, reduced incidence of dysrhythmias, and lower levels of circulating biomarkers indicative of myocardial injury [26]. Future studies may provide further insight into whether a specific subset of patients would benefit from ANH during cardiac surgery. The technique is not widely utilized because of the challenges of both blood acquisition and storage. Should the autologous blood be compromised or otherwise prevented from transfusing back to the patient, there is additional risk of necessary allogeneic blood transfusion.

Platelet-Rich Plasma

Originally reported to reduce bleeding in cardiac surgery in 1977 by Harke et al., the use of platelet-rich plasma in cardiac surgery has yielded mixed results in subsequent studies [27]. A recent randomized controlled trial in aortic surgery with deep hypothermic circulatory arrest demonstrated reduced allogeneic transfusion in patients who received autologous platelet-rich plasma [28]. It is reasonable to consider the use of autologous platelet-rich plasma as part of a blood conservation plan in cardiac surgery, but there are remaining questions as to the utility of platelet-rich plasma in cardiac surgery. Questions that require additional investigation include improvement in clinical outcomes, indications for its use, and cost-effectiveness, among others [29].

Management of Bleeding Cardiac Surgical Patients

It is recommended in both the STS/SCA 2011 guidelines and the more recent EACTA/EACTS 2017 guidelines that a multidisciplinary team should be involved in managing the post-cardiopulmonary bypass patient with coagulopathy by formulating a plan to treat bleeding patients using evidence to guide therapy (Class I, Level of Evidence C) [11]. Antifibrinolytic agents, tranexamic acid or epsilon-aminocaproic acid, have Class I, Level A evidence of efficacy for limiting coagulopathy and bleeding in cardiac surgery and should be utilized to reduce allogeneic blood transfusion. Using targeted products with evidence of coagulopathy, including TEG, ROTEM, or POC testing, is preferable to subjectively treating coagulopathy in non-life-threatening bleeding in cardiac surgical patients (Class IIa, Level of Evidence B) [11]. In patients with appropriate oxygen delivery undergoing cardiopulmonary bypass, a hematocrit of 21–24% during cardiopulmonary bypass to limit allogeneic transfusion is sufficient [30]. Massive transfusion protocols should be utilized when life-threatening bleeding occurs. A general approach would be to address post-cardiopulmonary bypass in the manner presented in Fig. 33.3.

The patient's preoperative medication profile should be considered when treating coagulopathy. Additionally, surgical hemostasis should be secured while the anesthesiologist should be vigilant in physiological management, including active warming and pH management of acidosis, and treatment of hypocalcemia and anemia.

With regard to specific targeting of bleeding with products of the coagulation cascade, it should be further emphasized that fibrinogen is an important component of clot formation. Fibrinogen makes up the largest component of the coagulation factors by weight and is found only in the vascular space, with no reserves [32]. Indeed, perioperative fibrinogen level has been shown to correlate with bleeding in cardiac surgery in multiple studies [33, 34]. Hypofibrinogenemia in the setting of coagulopathy and evidence of bleeding should be treated (cryoprecipitate or fibrinogen concentrate), but a recent meta-analysis failed to show benefit of routine use of fibrinogen concentrate for hypofibrinogenemia in cardiac surgical patients [35]. More

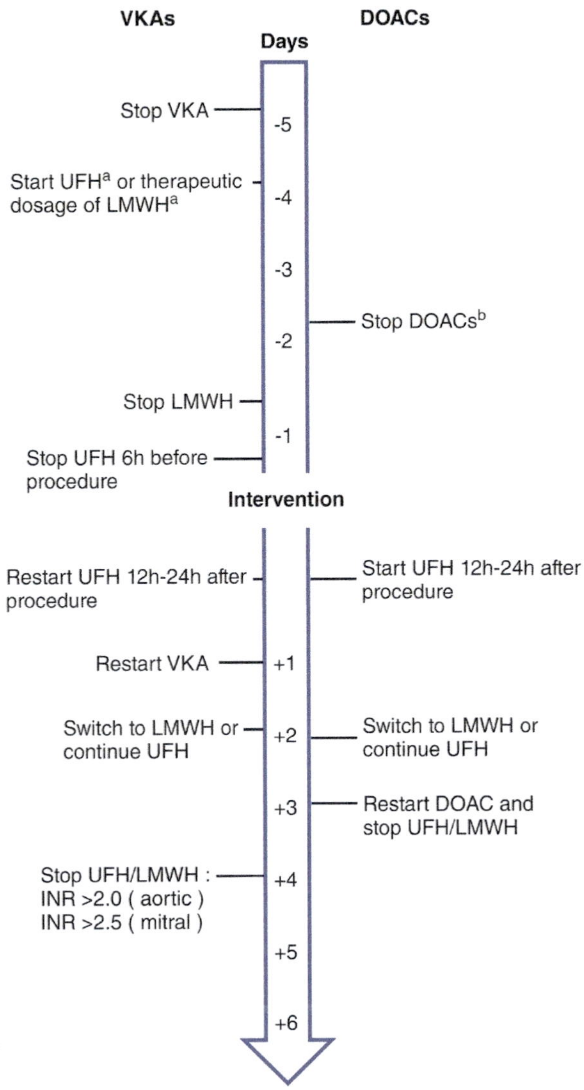

Fig. 33.3 Pyramid of therapy in coagulopathic patients. (Modified from Görlinger [31]). The sequence of hemostatic therapeutic interventions starts from the bottom of the pyramid and then continues to the top until hemostasis is achieved. Cai, ionized calcium; FFP, fresh frozen plasma; FVIII, coagulation factor VIII/von Willebrand factor concentrate; FXIII, coagulation factor XIII concentrate; Hb, hemoglobin; PCC, prothrombin complex concentrate; rFVIIa, activated recombinant factor VII; Tc, core temperature [31, 32]

recently, the role of fibrinogen therapy has been assessed by consensus in a subcommittee of the European Association of Cardiothoracic Anesthesiology. The recommendations include testing and correction of hypofibrinogenemia but also recognize the paucity of data to endorse the routine use of fibrinogen concentrate [36]. A recent noninferiority study (FIBRES) of fibrinogen concentrate versus cryoprecipitate for the management of symptomatic hypofibrinogenemia (defined as <150–200 mg/dL) demonstrated that concentrates are noninferior to cryoprecipitate administration [37]. Fibrinogen levels necessary to counter coagulopathy have yet to be determined, but hypofibrinogenemia as defined by <150–200 mg/dL in the setting of coagulopathic bleeding should be considered as a corrective measure to minimize other allogeneic blood products or riskier prothrombotic concentrates, such as PCCs or rVIIa [38].

The use of platelets in cardiac surgery should be limited to severe thrombocytopenia (<50 × 10^9/L) or in the setting of concomitant antiplatelet drug use with evidence of bleeding [11]. The prothrombin complex concentrate (PCCs) are three- or four-factor preparations that include vitamin K-dependent coagulation factors (II, IX, X, VII) and varying concentrations of protein C, protein S, and antithrombin. The evidence for administration of these agents or fresh frozen plasma (FFP) involve bleeding with deficiency of vitamin K-dependent coagulation factors. There is no evidence to support the use of recombinant factor seven (rFVIIa) in cardiac surgery at this time. Its use should be used in uncontrolled bleeding refractory to other measures only.

Cardiac surgical patients are at high risk for the complications of allogeneic transfusion given the massive assault on the coagulation cascade as a result of systemic heparinization, preoperative comorbidities (anemia, kidney disease), perioperative medical therapy targeting platelet function or the coagulation system, hypothermia, ischemia, and the proinflammatory response that occurs in response to a surgical stress. While much work is needed to determine optimal management of these patients, there is consensus on a framework of management that involves a large, multidisciplinary team. The perioperative physician should be apprised of the recommendations to provide optimal care for these patients. Figure 33.4 provides an overview of the entire perioperative period, wherein monitoring, interrogation, and intervention are needed to limit unnecessary transfusion and provide evidence-based care.

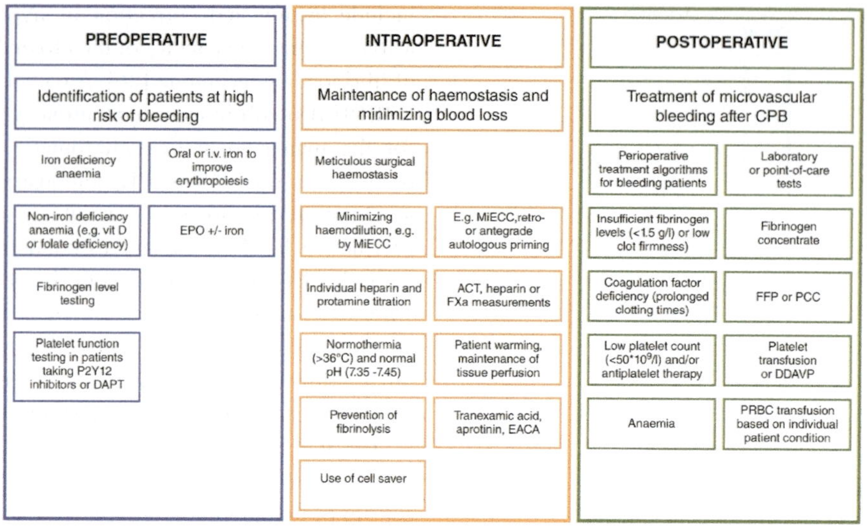

Fig. 33.4 Hemostatic monitoring throughout the perioperative period and possible treatment modalities. ACT, activated clotting time; CPB, cardiopulmonary bypass; DAPT, dual antiplatelet therapy; DDAVP, desmopressin; EACA, e-aminocaproic acid; EPO, erythropoietin; FFP, fresh frozen plasma; i.v., intravenous; MiECC, minimally invasive extracorporeal circulation circuit; PCC, prothrombin complex concentrate; PRBC, packed red blood cells. (Modified from Task Force on Patient Blood Management for Adult Cardiac Surgery of the European Association for Cardio-Thoracic S et al. [11])

References

1. Wells AW, Mounter PJ, Chapman CE, Stainsby D, Wallis JP. Where does blood go? Prospective observational study of red cell transfusion in North England. BMJ. 2002;325(7368):803.
2. Stover EP, Siegel LC, Parks R, Levin J, Body SC, Maddi R, et al. Variability in transfusion practice for coronary artery bypass surgery persists despite national consensus guidelines: a 24-institution study. Institutions of the Multicenter Study of Perioperative Ischemia Research Group. Anesthesiology. 1998;88(2):327–33.
3. Hajjar LA, Vincent JL, Galas FR, Nakamura RE, Silva CM, Santos MH, et al. Transfusion requirements after cardiac surgery: the TRACS randomized controlled trial. JAMA. 2010;304(14):1559–67.
4. Society of Thoracic Surgeons Blood Conservation Guideline Task F, Ferraris VA, Brown JR, Despotis GJ, Hammon JW, Reece TB, et al. 2011 update to the Society of Thoracic Surgeons and the Society of Cardiovascular Anesthesiologists blood conservation clinical practice guidelines. Ann Thorac Surg. 2011;91(3):944–82.
5. Koch CG, Li L, Duncan AI, Mihaljevic T, Cosgrove DM, Loop FD, et al. Morbidity and mortality risk associated with red blood cell and blood-component transfusion in isolated coronary artery bypass grafting. Crit Care Med. 2006;34(6):1608–16.
6. Koch CG, Li L, Duncan AI, Mihaljevic T, Loop FD, Starr NJ, et al. Transfusion in coronary artery bypass grafting is associated with reduced long-term survival. Ann Thorac Surg. 2006;81(5):1650–7.
7. Hogan M, Klein AA, Richards T. The impact of anaemia and intravenous iron replacement therapy on outcomes in cardiac surgery. Eur J Cardiothorac Surg. 2015;47(2):218–26.
8. Harker LA, Malpass TW, Branson HE, Hessel EA 2nd, Slichter SJ. Mechanism of abnormal bleeding in patients undergoing cardiopulmonary bypass: acquired transient platelet dysfunction associated with selective alpha-granule release. Blood. 1980;56(5):824–34.
9. Edmunds LH Jr. Inflammatory response to cardiopulmonary bypass. Ann Thorac Surg. 1998;66(5 Suppl):S12–6; discussion S25-8.
10. Kaplan JA, Augoustides JGT, Manecke GR, Maus T, Reich DL. Kaplan's cardiac anesthesia: for cardiac and noncardiac surgery 7th Edition. Elsevier 2017.
11. Task Force on Patient Blood Management for Adult Cardiac Surgery of the European Association for Cardio-Thoracic S, the European Association of Cardiothoracic A, Boer C, Meesters MI, Milojevic M, Benedetto U, et al. 2017 EACTS/EACTA Guidelines on patient blood management for adult cardiac surgery. J Cardiothorac Vasc Anesth. 2018;32(1):88–120.
12. Lazar HL. The use of preoperative aspirin in cardiac surgery: the ruling on the field stands. J Card Surg. 2017;32(12):775–6.
13. Hillis LD, Smith PK, Anderson JL, Bittl JA, Bridges CR, Byrne JG, et al. 2011 ACCF/AHA guideline for coronary artery bypass graft surgery. A report of the American College of Cardiology Foundation/American Heart Association Task Force on Practice Guidelines. Developed in collaboration with the American Association for Thoracic Surgery, Society of Cardiovascular Anesthesiologists, and Society of Thoracic Surgeons. J Am Coll Cardiol. 2011;58(24):e123–210.
14. Liu H, Li J, Chen M, Yang T, Ruan Z, Su J, et al. A meta-analysis of randomized and observational studies: aspirin protects from cardiac surgery-associated acute kidney injury. Heart Surg Forum. 2019;22(4):E301–E7.
15. Mangano DT, Multicenter Study of Perioperative Ischemia Research G. Aspirin and mortality from coronary bypass surgery. N Engl J Med. 2002;347(17):1309–17.
16. Terwindt LE, Karlas AA, Eberl S, Wijnberge M, Driessen AHG, Veelo DP, et al. Patient blood management in the cardiac surgical setting: an updated overview. Transfus Apher Sci. 2019;58(4):397–407.
17. Hofmann B, Kaufmann C, Stiller M, Neitzel T, Wienke A, Silber RE, et al. Positive impact of retrograde autologous priming in adult patients undergoing cardiac surgery: a randomized clinical trial. J Cardiothorac Surg. 2018;13(1):50.
18. Rosengart TK, DeBois W, O'Hara M, Helm R, Gomez M, Lang SJ, et al. Retrograde autologous priming for cardiopulmonary bypass: a safe and effective means of decreasing hemodilution and transfu-

sion requirements. J Thorac Cardiovasc Surg. 1998;115(2):426–38; discussion 38–9.
19. Lamy A, Devereaux PJ, Prabhakaran D, Taggart DP, Hu S, Paolasso E, et al. Off-pump or on-pump coronary-artery bypass grafting at 30 days. N Engl J Med. 2012;366(16):1489–97.
20. Diegeler A, Borgermann J, Kappert U, Breuer M, Boning A, Ursulescu A, et al. Off-pump versus on-pump coronary-artery bypass grafting in elderly patients. N Engl J Med. 2013;368(13):1189–98.
21. Hallowell P, Bland JH, Buckley MJ, Lowenstein E. Transfusion of fresh autologous blood in open-heart surgery. A method for reducing bank blood requirements. J Thorac Cardiovasc Surg. 1972;64(6):941–8.
22. Lawson NW, Ochsner JL, Mills NL, Leonard GL. The use of hemodilution and fresh autologous blood in open-heart surgery. Anesth Analg. 1974;53(5):672–83.
23. Jarnagin WR, Gonen M, Maithel SK, Fong Y, D'Angelica MI, Dematteo RP, et al. A prospective randomized trial of acute normovolemic hemodilution compared to standard intraoperative management in patients undergoing major hepatic resection. Ann Surg. 2008;248(3):360–9.
24. Henderson RA, Mazzeffi MA, Strauss ER, Williams B, Wipfli C, Dawood M, et al. Impact of intraoperative high-volume autologous blood collection on allogeneic transfusion during and after cardiac surgery: a propensity score matched analysis. Transfusion. 2019;59(6):2023–9.
25. Barile L, Fominskiy E, Di Tomasso N, Alpizar Castro LE, Landoni G, De Luca M, et al. Acute normovolemic hemodilution reduces allogeneic red blood cell transfusion in cardiac surgery: a systematic review and meta-analysis of randomized trials. Anesth Analg. 2017;124(3):743–52.
26. Licker M, Sierra J, Kalangos A, Panos A, Diaper J, Ellenberger C. Cardioprotective effects of acute normovolemic hemodilution in patients with severe aortic stenosis undergoing valve replacement. Transfusion. 2007;47(2):341–50.
27. Harke H, Tanger D, Furst-Denzer S, Paoachrysanthou C, Bernhard A. Effect of a preoperative separation of platelets on the postoperative blood loss subsequent to extracorporeal circulation in open heart surgery (author's transl). Anaesthesist. 1977;26(2):64–71.
28. Zhou SF, Estrera AL, Loubser P, Ignacio C, Panthayi S, Miller C 3rd, et al. Autologous platelet-rich plasma reduces transfusions during ascending aortic arch repair: a prospective, randomized, controlled trial. Ann Thorac Surg. 2015;99(4):1282–90.
29. Bai SJ, Zeng B, Zhang L, Huang Z. Autologous platelet-rich plasmapheresis in cardiovascular surgery: a narrative review. J Cardiothorac Vasc Anesth. 2020;34(6):1614–21.
30. von Heymann C, Sander M, Foer A, Heinemann A, Spiess B, Braun J, et al. The impact of an hematocrit of 20% during normothermic cardiopulmonary bypass for elective low risk coronary artery bypass graft surgery on oxygen delivery and clinical outcome--a randomized controlled study [ISRCTN35655335]. Crit Care. 2006;10(2):R58.
31. Görlinger K. Coagulation management during liver transplantation. Hamostaseologie. 2006;26(3 Suppl 1):S64–76.
32. Görlinger K, Shore-Lesserson L, Dirkmann D, Hanke AA, Rahe-Meyer N, Tanaka KA. Management of hemorrhage in cardiothoracic surgery. J Cardiothorac Vasc Anesth. 2013;27(4 Suppl):S20–34.
33. Karlsson M, Ternstrom L, Hyllner M, Baghaei F, Nilsson S, Jeppsson A. Plasma fibrinogen level, bleeding, and transfusion after on-pump coronary artery bypass grafting surgery: a prospective observational study. Transfusion. 2008;48(10):2152–8.
34. Karkouti K, McCluskey SA, Syed S, Pazaratz C, Poonawala H, Crowther MA. The influence of perioperative coagulation status on postoperative blood loss in complex cardiac surgery: a prospective observational study. Anesth Analg. 2010;110(6):1533–40.
35. Li JY, Gong J, Zhu F, Moodie J, Newitt A, Uruthiramoorthy L, et al. Fibrinogen concentrate in cardiovascular surgery: a meta-analysis of randomized controlled trials. Anesth Analg. 2018;127(3):612–21.
36. Erdoes G, Koster A, Meesters MI, Ortmann E, Bolliger D, Baryshnikova E, et al. The role of fibrinogen and fibrinogen concentrate in cardiac surgery: an international consensus statement from the Haemostasis and Transfusion Scientific Subcommittee of the European Association of Cardiothoracic Anaesthesiology. Anaesthesia. 2019;74(12):1589–600.
37. Callum J, Farkouh ME, Scales DC, Heddle NM, Crowther M, Rao V, et al. Effect of fibrinogen concentrate vs cryoprecipitate on blood component transfusion after cardiac surgery: the fibres randomized clinical trial. JAMA. 2019;322:1–11.
38. Ranucci M, Pistuddi V, Baryshnikova E, Colella D, Bianchi P. Fibrinogen levels after cardiac surgical procedures: association with postoperative bleeding, trigger values, and target values. Ann Thorac Surg. 2016;102(1):78–85.

34 Platelet-Rich Plasma: Not for Athletes Only

Ryan T. Gualtier, Luis Chabla-Penafiel, and Anuragh Trikha

Platelet Rich Plasma (PRP) is increased concentration of autologous platelet suspended in small amount of plasma produced by centrifugation of patient's own blood. Use of PRP has been widely studied in bone and tendon tissue healing and reconstruction [1]. Platelets contains alpha granules which are important source of anabolic growth factors including fibroblast growth factors (FGF), bone morphogenic proteins (BMP), transformation growth factor beta-1 (TGF-β1), platelet-derived grown factor (PDGF), basic fibroblast grown factor (BFGF), vascular endothelial grown factor (VEGF), epidermal grown factor, insulin-like growth factor, and several others [2]. In fact, PRP is known to contain more than 1,500 bioactive proteins [1]. These factors are important for biological processes including wound healing, inhibiting inflammation and pain, chemotaxis, neovascularization, synthesis of extracellular matrix, and scar formation which aides in improvement in soft tissue healing, vascularization of grafts and bone [3]. Normal platelet ranges between 150,000 and 350,000 μ/L. PRP contains four to six times concentration greater than whole blood. Improvement in bone and soft tissue healing properties have been demonstrated with concentration of platelets of 1,000,000 μ/L, which is the concentration of platelets in commercial platelet systems [2].

There are four different types of PRP variations which give each commercial system its unique properties, including leukocyte-rich PRP (LR-PRP), pure PRP, or leukocyte-poor PRP (LP-PRP), platelet-rich fibrin, and leukocyte-and-platelet-rich fibrin. LP-PRP increases anti-inflammatory mediators including IL-4 and IL-10, whereas LR-PRP significantly increases proinflammatory markers including TNF-alpha, IL-6, INF-gamma, and IL-1-beta and metalloproteinases which antagonize the anabolic cytokines within platelets [2].

Commercial PRP systems use different methods to collect platelets concentrate layer. Generally, whole blood is mixed with anticoagulation factors and centrifuged to obtain platelets. The centrifugation process separates whole blood to RBC layer, platelet-poor plasma layer, and "buffy coat" layer containing platelets with or without leukocytes. The platelet concentrate layer is isolated using various processing techniques. These platelets can then be either directly injected into the patient or activated via different compounds that leads to degranulation and release of growth factors [2].

The current clinical review shows abundant high-quality evidence of use of LP-PRP for osteoarthritis (OA) of the knee and LR-PRP for lateral epicondylitis. Moderate high-quality evidence supports the use of LR-PRP injection for patellar tendinopathy and LP-PRP for donor site pain in patellar tendon graft BTB (bone-tendon-bone) ACL reconstruction and plantar fasciitis [1]. At this time, the following diagnoses do not have high-quality evidence available; however, small clinical trials have shown promising results. These include rotator cuff tendinopathy, osteoarthritis of the hip, donor site pain in ACL reconstruction with patellar tendon autograft, and high ankle sprains.

Osteoarthritis of the Knee

Osteoarthritis is a disease of synovial joints caused by failure in repair of joint damage resulting in alteration of joint structures. It is the most common musculoskeletal disorder leading to functional decline, mobility limitations, and disability of aging population. The most common clinical manifestation of osteoarthritis is joint pain. 240 million people suffer from osteoarthritis globally. Current nonsurgical treatment modalities include physiotherapy, analgesia, nonsteroidal anti-inflammatory drugs, and intra-articular injections, such as hyaluronic acid, corticosteroids, or ozone, with the purpose of reducing symptoms and improving joint function [4]. In vitro and ex vivo studies have provided the foundation for

R. T. Gualtier (✉) · L. Chabla-Penafiel · A. Trikha
New York University School of Medicine, Department of Anesthesiology, Perioperative Care, and Pain Medicine, New York, NY, USA
e-mail: Ryan.gualtier@nyulangone.org

© Springer Nature Switzerland AG 2021
C. S. Scher et al. (eds.), *Essentials of Blood Product Management in Anesthesia Practice*,
https://doi.org/10.1007/978-3-030-59295-0_34

this interest, and positive effects of PRP have been observed, including chondrogenic differentiation of pluripotent mesenchymal cells with expression of cartilage specific genes, chondrocyte proliferation, increased extracellular matrix production, and inhibition of catabolic pathways [5]. Despite the prevalence, no FDA-approved disease-modifying osteoarthritis drugs currently exist to prevent, slow, or halt knee osteoarthritis [6].

Abundant high-quality evidence supports the use of LP-PRP intra-articular injection for osteoarthritis of the knee. Shen et al. [4] performed a meta-analysis of 14 randomized clinical trials comprising 1423 individuals between 2011 and 2016 to compare intra-articular PRP injections to various controls including saline placebo, hyaluronic acid, ozone, and corticosteroids. Compared with control, PRP injections significantly reduced WOMAC (Western Ontario and McMaster Universities Osteoarthritis Index) pain subscores at 3, 6, and 12 months follow-up ($p = 0.02$, 0.004, <0.001, respectively); PRP significantly improved WOMAC physical function sub-scores at 3, 6, and 12 months ($p = 0.002$, 0.01, <0.001, respectively); PRP also significantly improved total WOMAC scores at 3, 6, and 12 months (all $p < 0.001$). PRP did not significantly increase the risk of post-injection adverse events (RR, 1.40 [95% CI, 0.80–2.45], $I^2 = 59\%$, $p = 0.24$). Subgroup analysis further showed that PRP is more efficacious in patients with mild-to-moderate osteoarthritis [2].

Lucia et al. [7] performed a narrative review of the meta-analysis and systemic reviews in 2019, and according to the narrators, at present, results from RCTs seem to favor PRP use over other intra-articular treatments to improve pain scales in the short and medium term (6–12 months), but the overall level of evidence is low. They concluded that this is likely the result of a lack of standardization of PRP products, scarceness of high-quality RCTs not showing high risks of bias, and poor patient stratification for inclusion in the RCTs.

A meta-analysis by Riboh et al. [5] included six randomized controlled trials and three prospective comparative studies with a total of 1055 patients. Injection of LP-PRP resulted in significantly better WOMAC scores than did injection of hyaluronic acid (mean difference, −21.14; 95% CI, −39.63 to −2.65) or placebo (mean difference, −17.84; 95% CI, −34.95 to −0.73). No difference was observed in LR-PRP. SUCRA (surface under the cumulative ranking) analysis showed that LP-PRP was the highest ranked treatment for both measures of clinical efficacy using the International Knee Documentation Committee (IKDC) subjective score and WOMAC score. This is likely due to the biological basis of LP-PRP and LR-PRP as mentioned in the Introduction section. Thus, intra-articular LP-PRP may be the preferred preparation for the treatment of knee osteoarthritis symptoms [2].

Lateral Epicondylitis

Lateral epicondylitis, also known as tennis elbow, affects 1–3% of adults each year. It often affects the dominant arm in patients with high demand of gripping or repetitive wrist movements. Individuals between the ages of 35 and 50 years are at high risk. Elbow tenderness and pain with resisted wrist extension are common manifestations of lateral epicondylar tendinopathy. Overuse and repetitive microtraumas of wrist extensor tendons are believed to be the mechanism of injury of lateral epicondylitis. The lesion starts as a tear in the extensor tendon leading to abnormal microvascular response. It is commonly associated with functional disorder and pain of the elbow joint. Initial interventions include rest, activity or equipment modification, nonsteroidal anti-inflammatory medication, bracing, and physical therapy. If these treatments fail to improve the pain and tenderness, second-line treatments such as cortisone injections, prolotherapy, autologous blood injections, PRP injections, and needling of the extensor tendon origin have been recommended. If patients continue to report pain and dysfunction despite these measures, surgery is then considered [8]. Abundant high-quality evidence supports the use of LR-PRP injection for lateral epicondylitis who have failed to respond to conservative treatments [2].

Mishra et al. [8] evaluated 230 patients in a large multicenter double-blinded prospective randomized controlled trial. All the patients had at least 3 months of symptoms and failed conservative therapy. The patients were randomly divided into PRP treatment and active control, and all patients had their extensor tendon needled with and without PRP, respectively. No statically significant difference was found at 12 weeks in this study. However, at 24 weeks, the PRP-treated patients reported an improvement of 71.5% in their pain scores compared with 56.1% in the control group ($P = 0.019$). 29.1% of the PRP-treated patients reported significant elbow tenderness versus 54.0% in the control group ($P = 0.009$). Success rates for patients with 24 weeks of follow-up were 83.9% in the PRP group compared with 68.3% in the control group ($P = 0.037$).

Gosens et al. [9, 10] conducted a double-blind randomized controlled trial with a 2-year follow-up to determine effectiveness of LR-PRP compared with corticosteroid injection in patients with chronic lateral epicondylitis. The primary analysis included visual analog scale (VAS) pain scores and disabilities of the arm, shoulder, and hand (DASH) outcome scores. When baseline VAS and DASH scores were compared with the scores at 1 year follow-up, VAS was successful and statistically significant in PRP as compared to corticosteroid (73% vs. 49%, $P < 0.001$), as well as DASH when compared to corticosteroid (73% vs. 51%, $p = 0.005$). When baseline VAS and DASH scores were compared with the scores at a 2-year follow-up, both groups significantly improved over time. However, the DASH scores of the corticosteroid group returned to baseline levels, while those of the PRP group significantly improved.

Rotator Cuff Tendinopathies

Rotator cuff tendinopathies are one of the most common reasons why patients present with shoulder pain and disability. In fact, it's not only athletes who suffer from rotator cuff tears, but they can happen to anyone with routine daily activities or with overuse. An estimated 50% of patients presenting with shoulder pain may be diagnosed with rotator cuff tendinopathy, including supraspinatus partial thickness tears and tendonosis [11]. The goal of the treating physician is to reduce patients' pain and, by doing so, hopefully improve function. Unfortunately, many patients are refractory to these conservative therapies, which include rest, multimodal pain regimen, physical therapy, and corticosteroid injections, and surgery becomes the only viable option. Due to the relative avascular nature of tendons, their regenerative potential is limited; however, there is some clinical evidence that PRP may help revascularize the area of injury and promote healing. Several RCTs have investigated whether PRP can be utilized for improving pain and functional outcomes in rotator cuff pathology.

In a placebo-controlled double-blind randomized clinical trial by Kesikburun et al. [12], a total of 40 patients were enrolled, with [12] history of shoulder pain for >3 months during overhead-throwing activities [1], MRI findings of rotator cuff tear, and [11] minimum of 50% reduction in shoulder pain with administration of anesthetic injection. Patients received 5 ml of PRP or 5 ml of saline via ultrasound-guided injection into the subacromial space. In addition, all patients underwent a 6-week standard exercise program. Outcomes were measured via the Western Ontario Rotator Cuff (WORC) Index, Shoulder Pain and Disability Index (SPADI), VAS, and shoulder pain with Neer Test at 3, 6, 12, and 24 weeks, as well as 1 year after injection. At the 1-year follow-up, PRP was found to be no more effective in improving quality of life, pain, disability, and shoulder ROM than placebo patients who were treated with physical therapy.

Rha et al. [2] went on to compare the effects of PRP with those of dry needling on shoulder pain and function in patients with rotator cuff disease. 39 patients with supraspinatus tendon lesions less than 1.0 cm, but not a complete tear, were included. Half of the group received two dry-needling procedures, and the other half received two PRP injections to the affected shoulder at 4-week intervals utilizing ultrasound guidance. SPADI, passive ROM, and a physician rating scale at 6 months follow-up were used to measure outcomes. The clinical effect of PRP was found to be superior to dry needling at 6 months.

In another study by Shams et al. [11], a similar outcome was reached in regard to PRP vs corticosteroid for the treatment of symptomatic rotator cuff tears. 40 patients with symptomatic rotator cuff tears were assessed pre-injection, 6 weeks, and 3 and 6 months after injection utilizing the American Shoulder and Elbow Surgeons Standardized Shoulder Assessment Form (ASES), Constant-Murley Score (CMS), Simple Shoulder Test (SST), and Visual Analog Scale (VAS) for pain. Both injection groups showed statistical significance with outcomes over time compared to those pre-injection. At 12 weeks, there was also a statistically significant difference between the PRP and corticosteroid group, in favor of PRP, although there was no significance after 6 months. Therefore, the group summarized that subacromial PRP may be considered a good alternative to corticosteroid injections in those with a contraindication to corticosteroid administration.

Osteoarthritis of the Hip

Osteoarthritis (OA) of the hip has not been studied as extensively as OA of the knee; however, little evidence of its efficacy does exist. OA is a slowly evolving process, which typically is characterized by pain, stiffness, and decreased range of motion. Overall, roughly 40% of those over 65 years old may suffer from OA of the hip or knee [13]. The prevalence of hip OA alone may account for 7–25% in white patients over 55 years [11]. OA is brought on by biomechanical and biochemical factors which leads to cartilage disruption and bone hypertrophy. Within the knee or hip joint, proinflammatory cytokines and proteinases interfere with the normal production of hyaluronic acid (HA), which results in a significantly reduced molecular weight and viscoelasticity leading to degradation of articular cartilage and joint function [14]. As the joints affected by OA have a lower than normal concentration of HA, any exogenous administration of HA should increase the synovial fluid viscosity, leading to improved shock absorption and lubricating capabilities. In addition, HA is known to stimulate the body's own endogenous HA synthesis via CD44 receptor binding [15].

The current non-operative treatment modalities for OA of the hip include both non-pharmacologic and pharmacological therapies aimed at reducing pain, stiffness, and disability. Intra-articular corticosteroid injections tend to temporarily reduce pain and improve function [16], however do not change the natural progression of the disease and may also have negative effect on hip structures [17].

There have been four major RCTs comparing PRP to hyaluronic acid for OA of the hip. Battaglia et al. [5] looked to compare clinical efficacy of PRP vs HA at 12 months of follow-up in patients with hip OA. 100 patients with chronic unilateral hip OA were enrolled and randomly assigned PRP or HA via ultrasound-guided injection. Patients were evaluated at 1, 3, 6, and 12 months using visual analog scale and Harris Hip Score (HHS). At the 1- and 3-month follow-up, both groups showed overall improvement. At 6 and 12 months, there was a slight worsening, however no statistical difference between HA and PRP. In conclusion, the study noted PRP injections to be efficacious in terms of functional improvement and pain reduction, but not superior to HA at 12 months' follow-up.

Di Sante et al. also compared the efficacy of HA vs PRP with ultrasound-guided intra-articular injection [18]. They looked at 43 patients with unilateral severe hip OA. Patients were randomly assigned to receive HA or PRP and received three injections in total (one per week). Patients were evaluated at baseline, week 4, and week 16. Primary outcomes were measured with VAS and WOMAC. Results revealed that compared to baseline, the PRP-treated VAS scores were significantly decreased at 4 weeks, but not at 16 weeks, which indicates an early effect on pain that was not sustained at a longer-term follow-up. In contrary, the HA group had a significant decrease in both VAS and WOMAC values between baseline and 16 weeks.

In an RTC performed by Dallari et al. [14], ultrasound-guided injection of PRP and hyaluronic acid was performed separately and in combination for hip osteoarthritis. The primary outcome measure was a change in pain intensity as assessed by VAS at 2, 6, and 12 months. Other measures included WOMAC and concentration of growth factors in PRP and their correlation with clinical outcomes. A total of 111 patients were randomly assigned to receive three weekly injections of either PRP (44 patients), PRP + HA (31 patients), or HA (36 patients). At all follow-ups, PRP had the lowest VAS scores. The results indicated the intra-articular PRP injections do offer significant clinical improvement in patients with hip OA without relative side effects.

Doria et al. [13] also performed a prospective controlled double-blinded RCT on 80 patients with symptomatic early hip OA. The measures included WOMAC, VAS, and Harris Hip Score, which were evaluated before and at 6 and 12 months post-treatment. Both groups showed a significant improvement from baseline at both endpoints; however, PRP did not offer significantly better results compared to HA in patients with moderate OA.

Although data is limited in regard to PRP for intra-articular injections for hip osteoarthritis, it does show some promising results with pain reduction and improved function by patient-reported scores. Several studies do show PRP with an earlier onset to pain reduction compared to HA; however there is no statistical difference as time goes on, particularly at 12 months post-injection. More high-quality studies are necessary to see whether PRP can be utilized as a modality for delaying hip surgery due to OA.

Anterior Cruciate Ligament Tears

Anterior cruciate ligament (ACL) tears are one of the most common sports medicine-related injuries, which makes ACL reconstructive surgery one of the most frequently performed procedures in the field [19]. Majority of these patients are young and athletic, with high expectations of recovering from their injury and returning to the sport. Although most of the current surgical techniques can provide satisfactory results, it's not 100% guaranteed, and not all patients are able to regain their pre-injury activity level. Clinical results may be shaped not only by the type of graft used but even factors such as pre-injury knee laxity. Due to the nature of these injuries and the expectations by the patients, most research is looking into ways to improve ACL healing, reduce failure rate, and improve on recovery times. PRP is one of these sought-after approaches that are being looked at more closely as a potential therapeutic agent.

A prospective randomized trial performed by Vogrin et al. [20] concluded that platelet gel produced from autologous platelet-rich plasma and applied locally demonstrated a significantly higher level of vascularization in the osteoligamentous interface in 4–6 weeks (0.33 ± 0.09) in PG-treated group than the control group (0.16 ± 0.09, $p < 0.001$). An observational study performed by Sanchez et al. [21] evaluated the gross morphologies of the grafts on second-look arthroscopy in 37 volunteers who underwent either conventional (control group, $n = 15$) or platelet-rich plasma preparation rich in growth factors assisted ($n = 22$) ACL reconstruction with an autogenous hamstring. Biopsy specimen was evaluated by the use of Ligament Tissue Maturity Index to assess the histologic changes during the 6- to 24-month postoperative period of graft maturation. It was found that newly formed connective tissue, resembling synovial-like tissue, enveloped the treated graft in 77.3% of the PRGF-treated grafts and 40% of the controls.

Systematic literature review by Di Matteo et al. [22] showed that the only advantage of PRP is related to a better graft maturation over time, without clear beneficial effects in terms of clinical outcome, bone-graft integration, and prevention of bony tunnel enlargement. Recent literature review by Riediger et al. [23] concluded that the research failed to show significant clinical benefit of using biologics like PRP and therefore does not support the routine use in ACLR. However, there is some evidence that use of PRP may promote graft harvest site healing, graft maturation and reduce tunnel widening in the short term. A prospective, randomized, and double-blinded clinical study by Seijas et al. [24] evaluated the donor site anterior knee pain in "patellar graft" or "bone-tendon-bone" (BTB) autograft ACL reconstruction with the application of autologous plasma rich in growth factors (PRGF). PRGF group showed decreased donor site pain in comparison to the control group, with significant differences in the first two postoperative months of follow-up. The current study does not show clinical effect of PRP on graft integration or maturation, but limited studies have shown positive results in decreasing patellar tendon donor site pain.

Patellar Tendinopathy

Patellar tendinopathy is a common cause of pain among athletes, known as "jumper's knee." It has been associated with activities involving jumping, more specifically repetitive jumping. Patellar tendinopathy is not an inflammatory disorder; it's a degenerative disorder. Tendinosis occurs with progressive degeneration of the tendinous tissue and inability for repair.

Risk factors associated with patellar tendinopathy include high body mass index, large abdominal circumference, limb-length discrepancy, flat foot arch, weak quadriceps, and low flexibility of both quadriceps and hamstring muscles. However, tendinopathy does not occur in all people with the same type of activity; therefore there must be both intrinsic and extrinsic factors.

Patellar tendinopathy can cause pain that is debilitating and impede with a patient's mobility. Patients usually present with pain over the proximal and distal part of the patella tendon. Patients will report pain of the proximal tendon when the knee is flexed and report pain of the distal tendon when the knee is extended. A provocative test is the single leg squat test, which causes increased load on the patellar tendon. Ultrasound and MRI are useful imaging for diagnosis. Common differential diagnosis includes patellofemoral pain syndrome, fat-pad syndrome, meniscal tears, cartilage lesions, and referred pain.

Common treatment modalities include eccentric exercises, extracorporeal shock wave therapy, steroid injections, sclerosing agents, and hyaluronic acid. The last resort is surgery. There is interest in PRP. PRP has a high concentration of growth factors, which can help stop the degeneration of the tendon. These growth factors work on tenocytes, cells that maintain homeostasis in tendons. Some of these growth factors include platelet-derived growth factor, vascular endothelial growth factor, epidermal growth factor, and insulin-like growth factor. They promote proliferation, cell differentiation, chemotaxis, and angiogenesis. However, there is conflicting evidence to support PRP over other modalities for patellar tendinopathy.

There have been several studies looking at PRP for patellar tendinopathy. They have looked at PRP vs saline, PRP vs dry needling, PRP vs extracorporeal shock wave therapy, and PRP vs steroids. Some studies have shown that PRP is superior over other modalities, and some studies have not. A study conducted by Scott et al. [17] showed that PRP was not more effective than saline for the improvement of patellar tendinopathy symptoms. His study looked at both LR-PRP and LP-PRP. The study occurred over 3 sites, with a sample size of 20 patients in each arm, followed over 12 weeks. There was no statistical difference, but he noted that the LR-PRP arm at both 6 weeks and 12 weeks had an increase in pain. They hypothesized that this was due to the introduction of WBC, which increased the inflammatory process. The study was limited by the sample size and the lack of standardization of physical therapy, and the patients were mostly young adults to middle-aged males.

PRP may be effective over dry needling. A study conducted by Dragoo et al. [15] showed that PRP plus dry needling was superior over dry needling alone. He showed an acceleration in recovery but that over time the effects were decreased. Notable in this study was that the PRP group reported significant decrease in pain and an improvement in symptoms and function. PRP may also be more effective over extracorporeal shock wave therapy (ESWT). Vetrano et al. [25] looked at a total of 43 patients that were comparable in age, sex, and level of sport participation. He followed the patients over 1 year. At both 6 months and 12 months, there was an improvement in pain and function. The researchers noted that the improvement of tendinopathy with PRP might be possible because they did not inject PRP with local anesthetics. However, previous investigations have shown that both ESWT and PRP increase the number of tenocytes and production of collagen type I and type III, which are needed for tendon repair.

The discrepancies in the studies can be attributed to the preparation of PRP and with the amount of PRP injected into the tendon. Amounts have ranged from 3 mL to 5 mL. Moreover, there is a lack of standardization on how PRP is prepared. Another question that has yet to be answered is the frequency of injections. Most studies have looked at single injections, with an average follow-up of 1 year. These patients may benefit from repeat injections in lieu of a single injection.

Plantar Fasciitis

Plantar fasciitis is a common cause of heel pain, affecting people of different lifestyles. It can be caused by overuse from prolonged standing and running. Risk factors include high arch, leg length discrepancy, obesity, sedentary lifestyles, and tightness of the Achilles tendon and intrinsic foot muscles. Like patellar tendinopathy, it is a chronic process of degeneration and not believed to be secondary to acute inflammation. Plantar fasciitis is diagnosed through physical exam and history. Patients will report heel pain, tightness in the morning, and improvement of pain after ambulation. However, toward the end of the day, there may be increased pain. On physical exam, it will be noted that the patient usually guards the foot that is affected. Pressure on the medial plantar calcaneal region will cause a sharp and stabbing pain. Imaging is not necessary to diagnose plantar fasciitis. But both ultrasound and MRI are the best modalities.

Plantar fasciitis is treated conservatively. This includes rest, acetaminophen, nonsteroidal anti-inflammatory drugs, massage, and modification of activity. If there is no improvement, or little improvement with physical therapy, other modalities are recommended. These include percutaneous needling, steroid injection, anterior night splint, and Botox. The use of PRP for plantar fasciitis seems appealing and is being used more.

A study by Sherpy et al. [26] showed that PRP vs steroid injection had comparable results. Patients in both groups improved clinically. Patients that received steroid injection had better outcome with ultrasound evaluation, with a decrease in thickness, and the fascia became more hyperechoic. Monto et al. [27] showed that PRP was superior to steroid injections for severe chronic plantar fasciitis. He studied patients over 24 months and showed that patient's function initially improved with steroid injections, and then there was a decline. With PRP there was a steady increase in function, the maximum function at 3 months, which stayed stable until 24 months. It should be noted that most studies looking at PRP injections usually use a volume of 3–5 mL; Monto et al. [27] used 9 mL. It is uncertain if the volume contributed to a positive effect. But it can be hypothesized that with increased volume, there are more growth factors released that aid in the repair of the damaged collagen. Research conducted by Jain et al. also showed the PRP was more beneficial over steroid injections, highlighting that the effects of PRP were longer-lasting than steroids.

A meta-analysis by Yang et al. [28] showed that PRP does not have a short-term benefit on functional status or pain, but it has a better long-term effect. The reason why PRP may not have a short-term effect is because the growth factors in PRP need time for the regenerative process. The advantage of PRP compared to steroids is that there is less risk for abscesses, osteomyelitis, fat pad atrophy, and plantar fascia tears.

In contrast to steroid injections, Kim et al. [29] looked at PRP vs dextrose prolotherapy (DP). He took 11 patients and injected them with dextrose prolotherapy, a total of 2 injections. Ten patients were injected with PRP, in a series of two injections. He found that there was an improvement in both pain and function that was sustained over 6 months, and there was no difference between DP and PRP. His study was limited by the small sample size, and there was no placebo. Therefore, there are an abundance of studies looking at PRP for PF, with conflicting efficacy. However, PRP may be more appealing with less risk of side effects when compared to steroids. Moreover, patients may need more than one injection of PRP.

Conclusion

PRP shows promise in treating several musculoskeletal diseases. PRP works by releasing factors that are important for wound healing, inhibiting inflammation and pain, chemotaxis, neovascularization, synthesis of extracellular matrix, and scar formation, which aids in soft tissue healing. There are several studies looking at PRP for osteoarthritis of the knee, lateral epicondylitis, ACL reconstruction, rotator cuff tendinopathy, osteoarthritis of the hip, patella tendinopathy, and planter fasciitis. These studies have demonstrated that PRP may be an alternative treatment and may avoid some side effects of common treatments, i.e., steroid injections. However, there is no consensus into which PRP variation is better and which preparation process is superior. Larger studies and standardization of PRP processing may be moving forward.

References

1. Han C, Na Y, Zhu Y, Kong L, Eerdun T, Yang X, Ren Y. Is platelet-rich plasma an ideal biomaterial for arthroscopic rotator cuff repair? A systematic review and meta-analysis of randomized controlled trials. J Orthop Surg Res. 2019;14(1):183. https://doi.org/10.1186/s13018-019-1207-9.
2. Le AD, Enweze L, Debaun MR, Dragoo JL. Platelet-rich plasma. Clin Sports Med. 2019;38(1):17–44. https://doi.org/10.1016/j.csm.2018.08.001.
3. Urits I, Viswanath O, Galasso AC, Sottosani ER, Mahan KM, Aiudi CM, et al. Platelet-rich plasma for the treatment of low back pain: a comprehensive review. Curr Pain Headache Rep. 2019;23(7):52. https://doi.org/10.1007/s11916-019-0797-6.
4. Shen L, Yuan T, Chen S, Xie X, Zhang C. The temporal effect of platelet-rich plasma on pain and physical function in the treatment of knee osteoarthritis: systematic review and meta-analysis of randomized controlled trials. J Orthop Surg Res. 2017;12(1):16. https://doi.org/10.1186/s13018-017-0521-3.
5. Riboh JC, Saltzman BM, Yanke AB, Fortier L, Cole BJ. Effect of leukocyte concentration on the efficacy of platelet-rich plasma in the treatment of knee osteoarthritis. Am J Sports Med. 2015;44(3):792–800. https://doi.org/10.1177/0363546515580787.
6. Rashid H, Kwoh CK. Should platelet-rich plasma or stem cell therapy be used to treat osteoarthritis? Rheum Dis Clin North Am. 2019;45(3):417–38. https://doi.org/10.1016/j.rdc.2019.04.010.
7. Gato-Calvo L, Magalhaes J, Ruiz-Romero C, Blanco FJ, Burguera EF. Platelet-rich plasma in osteoarthritis treatment: review of current evidence. Ther Adv Chronic Dis. 2019;10:2040622319825567. https://doi.org/10.1177/2040622319825567.
8. Mishra AK, Skrepnik NV, Edwards SG, Jones GL, Sampson S, Vermillion DA, Vermillion DA, Ramsey ML, Karli DC, Rettig AC. Efficacy of platelet-rich plasma for chronic ten-

nis elbow. Am J Sports Med. 2013;42(2):463–71. https://doi.org/10.1177/0363546513494359.
9. Gosens T, Peerbooms JC, Laar WV, Oudsten BLD. Ongoing positive effect of platelet-rich plasma versus corticosteroid injection in lateral epicondylitis. Am J Sports Med. 2011;39(6):1200–8. https://doi.org/10.1177/0363546510397173.
10. Peerbooms JC, Sluimer J, Bruijn DJ, Gosens T. Positive effect of an autologous platelet concentrate in lateral epicondylitis in a double-blind randomized controlled trial. Am J Sports Med. 2010;38(2):255–62. https://doi.org/10.1177/0363546509355445.
11. Shams A, El-Sayed M, Gamal O, Ewes W. Subacromial injection of autologous platelet-rich plasma versus corticosteroid for the treatment of symptomatic partial rotator cuff tears. Eur J Orthop Surg Traumatol. 2016;26(8):837–42. https://doi.org/10.1007/s00590-016-1826-3.
12. Kesikburun S, Tan AK, Yılmaz B, Yaşar E, Yazıcıoğlu K. Platelet-rich plasma injections in the treatment of chronic rotator cuff tendinopathy. Am J Sports Med. 2013;41(11):2609–16. https://doi.org/10.1177/0363546513496542.
13. Dawson J, Linsell L, Zondervan K, Rose P, Randall T, Carr A, Fitzpatrick R. Epidemiology of hip and knee pain and its impact on overall health status in older adults. Rheumatology. 2004;43:497–504. https://doi.org/10.1093/rheumatology/keh086.
14. Dallari D, Stagni C, Rani N, Sabbioni G, Pelotti P, Torricelli P, Tschon M, Giavaresi G. Ultrasound-guided injection of platelet-rich plasma and hyaluronic acid, separately and in combination, for hip osteoarthritis: a randomized controlled study. Am J Sports Med. 2016;44:664–71. https://doi.org/10.1177/0363546515620383.
15. Dragoo JL, Wasterlain AS, Braun HJ, Nead KT. Platelet-rich plasma as a treatment for patellar tendinopathy. Am J Sports Med. 2014;42(3):610–8. https://doi.org/10.1177/0363546513518416.
16. Battaglia M, Guaraldi F, Vannini F, Rossi G, Timoncini A, Buda R, Giannini S. Efficacy of ultrasound-guided intra-articular injections of platelet-rich plasma versus hyaluronic acid for hip osteoarthritis. Orthopedics. 2013;36(12):e1501–8. https://doi.org/10.3928/01477447-20131120-13.
17. Scott A, Laprade RF, Harmon KG, Filardo G, Kon E, Villa SD, et al. Platelet-rich plasma for patellar tendinopathy: a randomized controlled trial of leukocyte-rich PRP or leukocyte-poor PRP versus saline. Am J Sports Med. 2019;47(7):1654–61. https://doi.org/10.1177/0363546519837954.
18. Sante LD, Villani C, Santilli V, Valeo M, Bologna E, Imparato L, et al. Intra-articular hyaluronic acid vs platelet-rich plasma in the treatment of hip osteoarthritis. Med Ultrason. 2016;18(4):463. https://doi.org/10.11152/mu-874.
19. Anitua E, Sánchez M, Nurden AT, Nurden P, Orive G, Andía I. New insights into and novel applications for platelet-rich fibrin therapies. Trends Biotechnol. 2006;24(5):227–34. https://doi.org/10.1016/j.tibtech.2006.02.010.
20. Vogrin M, Rupreht M, Dinevski D, Hašpl M, Kuhta M, Jevsek M, et al. Effects of a platelet gel on early graft revascularization after anterior cruciate ligament reconstruction: a prospective, randomized, double-blind, clinical trial. Eur Surg Res. 2010;45(2):77–85. https://doi.org/10.1159/000318597.
21. Sánchez M, Anitua E, Azofra J, Prado R, Muruzabal F, Andia I. Ligamentization of tendon grafts treated with an endogenous preparation rich in growth factors: gross morphology and histology. Arthroscopy J Arthrosc Relat Surg. 2010;26(4):470–80. https://doi.org/10.1016/j.arthro.2009.08.019.
22. Matteo BD, Loibl M, Andriolo L, Filardo G, Zellner J, Koch M, Angele P. Biologic agents for anterior cruciate ligament healing: a systematic review. World J Orthop. 2016;7(9):592. https://doi.org/10.5312/wjo.v7.i9.592.
23. Riediger MD, Stride D, Coke SE, Kurz AZ, Duong A, Ayeni OR. ACL reconstruction with augmentation: a scoping review. Curr Rev Musculoskelet Med. 2019;12(2):166–72. https://doi.org/10.1007/s12178-019-09548-4.
24. Seijas R, Cuscó X, Sallent A, Serra I, Ares O, Cugat R. Pain in donor site after BTB-ACL reconstruction with PRGF: a randomized trial. Arch Orthop Trauma Surg. 2016;136(6):829–35. https://doi.org/10.1007/s00402-016-2458-0.
25. Vetrano M, Castorina A, Vulpiani MC, Baldini R, Pavan A, Feretti A. Platelet-rich plasma versus focused shock wave in the treatment of jumper's knee in athletes. Am J Sports Med. 2013;41(4):795–803. https://doi.org/10.1177/0363546513475345.
26. Sherpy NA, Hammad MA, Hagrass HA, Samir H, Abu-ElMaaty SE, Mortada MA. Local injection of autologous platelet rich plasma compared to corticosteroid treatment of chronic plantar fasciitis patients: a clinical and ultrasonographic follow-up study. Egypt Rheumatol. 2016;38:247–52. https://doi.org/10.1016/j.ejr.2015.09.008.
27. Monto RR. Platelet-rich plasma efficacy versus corticosteroid injection treatment for chronic severe plantar fasciitis. Foot Ankle Int. 2017;35(4):313–8. https://doi.org/10.1177/1071100713519778.
28. Yang WY, Han YH, Cao XW, Pan JK, Lin JT, Liu J. Platelet-rich plasma as a treatment for plantar fasciitis: a meta-analysis of randomized controlled trails. Medicine (Baltimore). 2017;96(44):e8475. https://doi.org/10.1097/MD.0000000000008475.
29. Kim E, Lee JH. Autologous platelet-rich plasma versus dextrose prolotherapy for the treatment of chronic recalcitrant plantar fasciitis. PMR. 2014;6(2):152–8. https://doi.org/10.1016/j.pmrj.2013.07.003.

Blood Transfusions for Burn Patients

35

Rayhan Tariq, Christopher Hoffman, Mingqiang Li, and Henry Liu

Introduction

An estimated 180,000 deaths annually are caused by burns-related injury worldwide [1]. Nearly 500,000 people receive medical treatment for burn-related events, and 3500 burn patients die annually from their burn injury in the United States alone. There were 40,000 burn patients hospitalized in the United States in 2016, including 30,000 at hospital burn centers [2]. The length of hospitalization is approximately calculated for an average of 1 day per 1% burned total body surface area (TBSA) and increases with age and the presence of inhalation or other co-existing injuries [3].

Anemia is one of the major challenging consequences after severe burn injury and often requires blood transfusion. There are two types of anemia that present in burn patients: anemia due to acute blood loss and due to critical illness. During the first 1–2 weeks after severe burn injury, acute blood loss anemia develops from thermal injury and repeated surgical procedures for the burn wounds as well as from intrinsic physiologic changes such as decreased hematopoiesis, red blood cell (RBC) sequestration, and increased RBC destruction [4, 5]. Anemia of critical illness prevails usually after week 3 and is multifactorial, and it can be caused by an imbalance between decreased production (dampened erythropoiesis, reduced erythropoietin production, nutritional deficits) and increased destruction (amplified sequestration, abnormal RBC morphology, increased metabolism and inflammatory response) of RBCs [6]. Burn patients with >20% TBSA usually need intensive care hospitalization with the probability of multiple blood transfusions over the course of hospitalization. Burn patients were transfused a mean of 14 units of packed RBCs during their hospitalization.

Massive blood transfusion is often common and substantial in burn patients as mentioned above. Blood transfusion carries its own risks which include immunosuppression, transfusion-related lung injury (TRALI), transfusion-associated circulatory overload (TACO), and infection transmission. A correlation between blood transfusions and infection in burn patients is well-documented for many years [6, 7]. One multicenter retrospective study and one retrospective single center study both reported an increased risk of blood stream infection by 11% for each unit transfused [7, 8]. An increased mortality has also been reported with increased transfusion rate.

Hypercoagulability and coagulopathy are also major challenging consequences of severe burn injury and require early detection and extensive intervention. A burn injury can potentially induce a systemic hypercoagulable state shortly after admission and during period of recovery. This hypercoagulability is usually driven by tissue injury, excessive inflammatory response, and hypoperfusion. A coagulopathic status, such as disseminated intravascular coagulopathy (DIC), is associated with severe burn injuries greater than 40% TBSA [9]. Risk of coagulopathy and excessive bleeding leads to a wide range of clinical presentation in hemostatic profiles in burn patients including anemia; normo-, hyper-, and hypocoagulability; and hyperfibrinolysis.

Epidemiology of Blood Transfusion in Burn Injury

Several studies have described the transfusion need in burn patients in relationship between percentage of TBSA burn and the transfusion rate. Birdsell et al. reported in a study with 109 pediatric burn patients that 100% of children with ≥30%

R. Tariq · C. Hoffman
Thomas Jefferson University Hospital, Department of Anesthesiology, Philadelphia, PA, USA

M. Li
Xiangyang Central Hospital, Department of Anesthesiology, Xiangyang, Hubei, China

H. Liu (✉)
Department of Anesthesiology and Perioperative Medicine, Milton S. Hershey Medical Center, Penn State College of Medicine, Hershey, PA, USA

© Springer Nature Switzerland AG 2021
C. S. Scher et al. (eds.), *Essentials of Blood Product Management in Anesthesia Practice*,
https://doi.org/10.1007/978-3-030-59295-0_35

TBSA received a blood transfusion, but no blood transfusions were given for TBSA ≤5% [8]. Yogore et al. described in a study with 1282 burn patients that 5.7% of patients with ≤10% TBSA burn, 21% patients with 11 to 20% TBSA burn, 39% patients with 21–30% TBSA burn, and 62% patients with >30% TBSA burn required blood transfusion [10]. Palmieri et al. noted that 74.7% of 620 patients with ≥20% TBSA burn from 21 medical centers needed blood transfusion(s) [6]. Posluszny et al. found that 88.7% of patients with ≥20% TBSA required a blood transfusion(s) [11]. Wu et al. described that 86.5% of 133 patients with ≥40% TBSA demanded blood transfusion(s) and 97.7% demanded a plasma transfusion(s) [12]. Lu et al. reported a necessity for blood transfusion in 71.9% of 89 patients with 15–65% TBSA and a necessity for plasma transfusion(s) in 44.9% [13].

It is noteworthy the historical rate of blood transfusion as it relates to TBSA burn percentage. The transfusion rate has been documented in several studies in earlier days. Graves et al. noted an average of 19.7 units in patients with >10% TBSA [7]. Vasko et al. found that patients with >10% TBSA received an average of 8.94 units and patients with >30% TBSA required 17 units [14]. Palmieri et al. described that patients with ≥20% TBSA were transfused on average with 13.7 ± 1.1 units and patients with burns ≥50% TBSA received >30 units of RBC transfusion. Patients with >40% TBSA required at least 11 units of RBCs [6]. Posluszny et al. showed that patients with >40% TBSA demanded on average a blood transfusion of 20 units [11]. Wu et al. reported that patients with ≥40% TBSA were given an average of 68.2 units of blood [12].

These numbers showed the liberal trend for blood transfusion in burn patients traditionally. The Transfusion Requirements in Critical Care (TRICC) trial for stable ICU patients triggered a shift from traditionally liberal transfusion strategy (hemoglobin 10–12 g/dL) toward a currently more restrictive strategy (hemoglobin 7–8 g/dL), supported by outcomes that a restrictive strategy was at least as safe as the liberal strategy and was able to decrease hospital mortality in restrictive group [15]. Burn patients were excluded in the TRICC trial and its following studies. In 2017, a large, multicenter, randomized, and prospective trial of blood transfusion investigation, entitled "Transfusion Requirement in Burn Care Evaluation (TRIBE)," compared the restrictive strategy of blood transfusion versus the liberal strategy in patients with burn injury >20% TBSA [16]. The results showed no statistically significant differences in mortality, hospital length of stay, ICU stay, or safety [16].

Burn Injury and Coagulopathy

While blood transfusion in a burn patient may reduce the adverse effect associated with anemia, blood transfusion is associated with some side effects of its own. The major side effects include pulmonary edema, volume overload, immune suppression, TRALI, and potentially coagulopathy. Transfusion-related coagulopathy is usually secondary to massive transfusion which leads to dilutional coagulopathy. Burn injury is a known disruptor of coagulation cascade displaying a wide range of presentations from sub-clinical manifestation to fulminant DIC. The underlying pathophysiology is the propagation of both thrombosis and fibrinolysis mediated by inflammatory cytokines and release of tissue factors. The natural anticoagulants are subsequently depleted. The hypothermia and hemodilution secondary to aggressive fluid resuscitation also contribute to the coagulation abnormality. These changes resemble those disturbances in major trauma or sepsis [17]. Because of previously mentioned reasons, it is very helpful to obtain a dynamic measurement of blood coagulation for an accurate assessment of the current coagulation status for the management of these burn patients. This can be achieved quickly and point-of-care basis by viscoelastic testing of blood in current medical practice. Correction of the coagulopathic defects decreases the associated morbidity and mortality. Empirical evidence suggests that viscoelastic tests such as thromboelastography can better guide transfusion when used in complement with the traditional blood coagulation tests [18]. The use of specific blood components could somewhat limit the patients' exposure to the risk associated with blood products. However, it seems like the use of viscoelastic testing or specific blood component products (cryoprecipitate, fibrinogen concentrate, and prothrombin complex concentrate) is still not widely adopted, especially in developing countries [19].

TRIBE Trial and the Optimal Blood Transfusion Threshold in Burn Patients

It is widely accepted now that restrictive blood transfusion is as effective as liberal strategy in ICU patients. This is largely the result of the 1999 Transfusion Requirements in Critical Care (TRICC) trial. However, the TRICC trial was not designed to be specific to burn patients and considered a mix of all the ICU patients. Burn patients have some unique pathophysiological alterations. A hypermetabolic state, prolonged hospitalization, and need for multiple surgeries are some of the characteristic features of severe burn injury in critical care facility. The Transfusion Requirement in Burn Care Evaluation (TRIBE) trial is one of the first major prospective, randomized, controlled clinical trials that focused particularly on transfusion-related issues in burn patients. The goal of TRIBE was to compare outcomes under a restrictive blood transfusion policy (maintaining a hemoglobin level at 7–8 g/dL) to a traditional transfusion policy (maintaining hemoglobin at 10–11 g/dL) [16]. In this TRIBE clinical trial, 345 patients across 18 medical centers were randomized to a restrictive (hemoglobin level at 7–8g/dL) or liberal (hemoglobin level at 10–11g/dL) transfusion strategy throughout hospitalization. The median blood transfusion in restrictive group was 8 units, i.e., half of the 16 units in the liberal group. Patients were studied during their entire hospital stay including any ICU stay and surgical procedures. The authors found no difference in incidence of bloodstream infections, organ dysfunction, mechanical ventilation days, time to wound healing, and 30-day mortality. This well-designed clinical trial presents high-quality evidence that a conservative blood management therapy is non-inferior to liberal approach in burn patients while reducing exposure to blood products and conserving this very valuable commodity.

Summary

In the United States, nearly 500,000 people will need certain medical treatment for burn-related injuries, and 3500 burn patients die from their burn injury annually. Risks of excessive bleeding and sepsis cause a wide range of abnormal hemostatic profiles in burn patients including anemia; normo-, hyper-, and hypocoagulability; and hyperfibrinolysis. Correction of the coagulopathic defects decreases the associated morbidity and mortality. Viscoelastic tests such as thromboelastography and other point-of-care tests can better guide transfusion practice and management of coagulation problems when used in complement with the traditional blood coagulation tests. These measured deficits of platelets, fibrinogen, and factors then be then replenished with more specific blood components. The TRIBE trial identified the optimal blood transfusion threshold in burn patients. The TRIBE trial was a well-designed prospective randomized multicenter trial that showed similar outcomes in a restrictive (hemoglobin 7–8g/dL) versus liberal (hemoglobin 10–11g/dL) transfusion strategy. A restrictive blood transfusion was well tolerated in burn patients while reducing exposure to blood products and providing economic benefits by reducing blood consumption and hospital stay.

References

1. WHO, fact sheets [Internet]. Burns; Available from: https://www.who.int/news-room/fact-sheets/detail/burns. Accessed on 28 Aug 2019.
2. National Burn Repository: Report of Data from 2017. American Burn Association. https://www.google.com/search?source=hp&ei=7BpnXcm_JdDy5gLR2b_gCw&q=national+burn+repository+report+of+data+from+2005-2015+executionexception&oq=National+Burn+Repository%3A+Report+of+Data+from+2005-2015+&gs_l=psy-ab.1.0.33i29 912.4172.4172..10004...0.0..0.324.500.0j1j0j1......0....2j1..gws-wiz.....0....10001%3A0%2C154.GAJ2PGw0Atw. Accessed on 28 Aug 2019.
3. Taylor SL, Sen S, Greenhalgh DG, Lawless M, Curri T, Palmieri TL. Real-time prediction for burn length of stay via median residual hospital length of stay methodology. J Burn Care Res. 2016;37(5):e476–82. https://doi.org/10.1097/BCR.0000000000000332. PMID: 27355650.
4. Kimber RJ, Lander H. The effect of heat on human red cell morphology, fragility, and subsequent survival in vivo. J Lab Clin Med. 64:922–33. PMID: 14239955.
5. Loebl EC, Marvin JA, Curreri W, Baxter CR. Erythrocyte survival following thermal injury. J Surg Res. 1974;16:96–101. https://doi.org/10.1016/0022-4804(74)90016-x. PMID: 4818344.
6. Palmieri TL, Caruso DM, Foster KN, Cairns BA, Peck MD, Gamelli RL, et al. Effect of blood transfusion on outcome after major burn injury: a multicenter study. Crit Care Med. 2006;34(6):1602–7. https://doi.org/10.1097/01.CCM.0000217472.97524.0E. PMID: 16607231.
7. Graves TA, Cioffi WG, Mason AD Jr, McManus WF, Pruitt BA Jr. Relationship of transfusion and infection in a burn population. J Trauma. 1989;29(7):948–52; discussion 952–4. https://doi.org/10.1097/00005373-198907000-00007. PMID: 2746705.
8. Birdsell DC, Birch JR. Anemia following thermal burns: a survey of 109 children. Can J Surg. 1971;14(5):345–50. PMID: 5315619.
9. King DR, Namias N, Andrews DM. Coagulation abnormalities following thermal injury. Blood Coagul Fibrinolysis. 2010;21(7):666–9. https://doi.org/10.1097/MBC.0b013e32833ceb08. PMID: 20689402.
10. Yogore MG 3rd, Boral L, Kowal-Vern A, Patel H, Brown S, Latenser BA. Use of blood band services in a burn unit. J Burn Care Res. 6:835–41.
11. Posluszny JAGR. Anemia of thermal injury: combined acute blood loss anemia and anemia of critical illness. J Burn Care Res. 2006;27(6):835–41. https://doi.org/10.1097/01.BCR.0000245418.73538.25. PMID: 17091079.
12. Wu G, Zhuang M, Fan X, Hong X, Wang K, Wang H, et al. Blood transfusions in severe burn patients: epidemiology and predictive factors. Burns. 2016;42(8):1721–7. https://doi.org/10.1016/j.burns.2016.06.002. PMID: 27576934.
13. Lu RP, Lin FC, Ortiz-Pujols SM, Whinna HC, Cairns BA, Key NS. Blood utilization in patients with burn injury and association with clinical outcomes (CME). Transfusion. 2013;53(10):2212–21; quiz 2211. https://doi.org/10.1111/trf.12057. PMID: 23278449.
14. Vasko SD, Burdge JJ, Ruberg RL, Verghese AS. Evaluation of erythropoietin levels in the anemia of thermal injury. J Burn Care Rehabil. 1991;12(5):437–41. PMID: 1752878.
15. Hebert PC, Wells G, Blajchman MA, Marshall J, Martin C, Pagliarello G, et al. A multicenter, randomized controlled clinical trial of transfusion requirements in critical care. N Engl J Med. 1999;340(6):409–17. https://doi.org/10.1056/NEJM199902113400601. PMID: 9971864.
16. Palmieri TL, Holmes JH, Arnoldo B, Peck M, Potenza B, Cochran A, et al. Transfusion requirement in burn care evaluation (TRIBE): a multicenter randomized prospective trial of blood transfusion in major burn injury. Ann Surg. 2017;266(4):595–602. https://doi.org/10.1097/SLA.0000000000002408. PMID: 28697050.
17. Dobson GP, Letson HL, Sharma R, Sheppard FR, Cap AP. Mechanisms of early trauma-induced coagulopathy: the clot thickens or not? J Trauma Acute Care Surg. 2015;79(2):301–9. https://doi.org/10.1097/TA.0000000000000729. PMID: 26218701.
18. Marsden NJ, Van M, Dean S, Azzopardi EA, Hemington-Gorse S, et al. Measuring coagulation in burns: an evidence-based systematic review. Scars Burn Heal. 2017;3:1–13. https://doi.org/10.1177/2059513117728201. PMID: 29799542.
19. Lavrentieva A, Depetris N, Kaimakamis E, Berardino M, Stella M. Monitoring and treatment of coagulation abnormalities in burn patients. An international survey on current practices. Ann Burns Fire Disasters. 2016;29(3):172–7. PMID: 28149244.

36 Prehospital Transfusions by First Providers

Marie-Christine Wright, Chikezie N. Okeagu, Alaina L. Broussard, Keith P. Delaune, Shukan Patel, Elyse M. Cornett, and Alan David Kaye

Introduction

In 1628, English physician William Harvey published his landmark work, *Exercitatio Anatomica de Motu Cordis et Sanguinis in Animalibus* (commonly *De motu cordis*), in which he described the circulation of blood in the body by the heart. Although it was widely accepted that blood played an essential role in the sustenance of life, little was known about how it was delivered to the tissues to serve this vital function. In fact, the prevailing belief theorized by Galen ~1500 years earlier stated that blood was continuously produced and distributed by the liver and completely absorbed by the tissues [1]. His discovery led to intense investigation into blood circulation, resulting in successful transfusion experiments in animals within a few decades of the publication of *De motu cordis*, and ultimately culminating in the successful transfusion of human blood by Dr. James Blunndell in 1818 [2, 3]. Today, blood transfusion is the most common procedure performed in US hospitals [4].

The indications for blood transfusion are vast and include a number of conditions that result in blood loss and anemia, including hemorrhage [5]. Hemorrhage is responsible for up to 40% of deaths in trauma [6]. Massive hemorrhage also presents a host of physiological derangements that jeopardize the survival of trauma patients. Recognized as the "triad of death," the combination of hypothermia, metabolic acidosis, and coagulopathy, when present, portends a poor prognosis (see Fig. 36.1). Severe hemorrhage can directly lead to hypothermia. Failure to control hemorrhage leads to increased sympathetic tone, which diverts blood away from non-vital organs in an attempt to preserve perfusion of vital organs. This eventually leads to a mismatch between oxygen demand and oxygen delivery, forcing the body to rely on anaerobic metabolism, which results in the accumulation of acidic compounds such as lactic acid and ketone bodies. It also results in a drop in pH and the development of metabolic acidosis. In an attempt to control the massive blood loss, the body activates the coagulation cascade, and clotting factors are quickly depleted leading to a consumptive coagulopathy. Furthermore, these derangements each can potentiate each other leading to worsening acidosis, coagulopathy, and hypothermia [7–10].

The recognition that promptly addressing these factors gives patients the best chance at a favorable outcome has led to the development of various damage control resuscitation (DCR) strategies [11]. Transfusion of blood products is a staple of DCR protocols and one of the first tools employed upon the arrival of the patient at a trauma center [6, 10, 11]. However, elements of the triad can present within minutes, long before patients arrive at the hospital [12, 13]. In fact, up to 56% of trauma patients die before arrival at the hospital [14]. As such, there has been much interest in resuscitation

M.-C. Wright
University of Toledo School of Medicine, Department of Pediatrics, Toledo, LA, USA
e-mail: Marie.wright@utoledo.edu

C. N. Okeagu
Department of Anesthesiology, LSU School of Medicine, New Orleans, LA, USA
e-mail: cokeag@lsuhsc.edu

A. L. Broussard · K. P. Delaune
Ochsner Clinic, Department of Anesthesiology, New Orleans, LA, USA
e-mail: Alaina.broussard@ochsner.org; keith.delaune@ochsner.org

S. Patel
Department of Anesthesiology, LSU Health Sciences Center, New Orleans, LA, USA
e-mail: spat23@lsuhsc.edu

E. M. Cornett (✉)
Department of Anesthesiology, LSU Health Shreveport, Shreveport, LA, USA
e-mail: ecorne@lsuhsc.edu

A. D. Kaye
Departments of Anesthesiology and Pharmacology, Toxicology and Neurosciences, Louisiana State University School of Medicine-Shreveport, Shreveport, LA, USA

LSU Health Shreveport School of Medicine, New Orleans, LA, USA

Tulane School of Medicine, New Orleans, LA, USA
e-mail: akaye@lsuhsc.edu

© Springer Nature Switzerland AG 2021
C. S. Scher et al. (eds.), *Essentials of Blood Product Management in Anesthesia Practice*,
https://doi.org/10.1007/978-3-030-59295-0_36

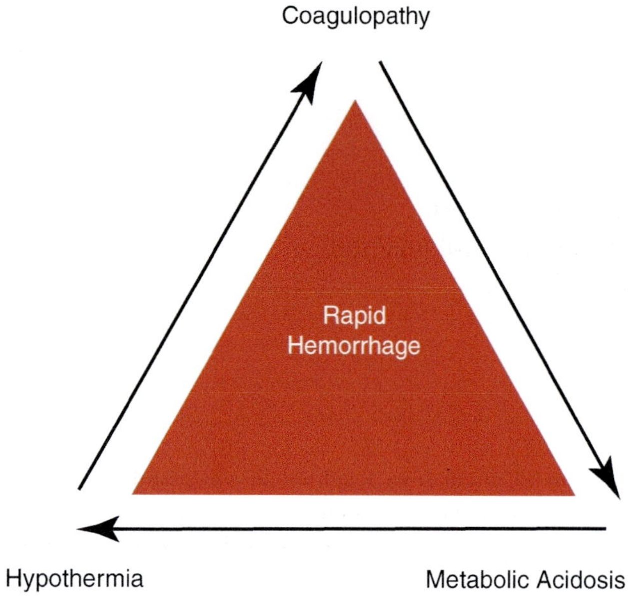

Fig. 36.1 Triad of death

measures that can be initiated prior to arrival at the hospital, and this includes the administration of prehospital blood transfusions (PHBT) [11, 14–17].

Developed with influence from treatment regimens for soldiers injured during military conflict, modern DCR aims to mitigate rapid hemorrhage, with a balanced ratio of plasma, platelets, and red blood cells to mimic reconstituted whole blood [18, 19]. Traditionally, crystalloid-based resuscitation in the prehospital setting has been common; however there has been recent interest in developing approaches that emphasize earlier transfusion of blood [11, 20]. While administering blood products should theoretically help to curb the physiological effects of hemorrhage and lead to increased survival, research into the outcomes of these protocols has yielded mixed results. A randomized trial by Sperry et al. demonstrated that prehospital administration of thawed plasma resulted in a lower 30-day mortality than standard resuscitation with crystalloid solution (23% vs 33%) [20]. Shackelford et al. also found reduced 24-hour and 30-day mortality in those that received prehospital transfusion (red cells within 30 minutes of injury) in the US military combat setting [21]. Contrarily, Moore et al. found no difference in a 28-day mortality in trauma patients receiving plasma vs saline [22]. Similarly, a recent systematic review and meta-analysis examining the effectiveness of PHBT in reducing mortality by Rijnhout et al. could not find conclusive benefit of PHBT [23].

Aside from the equivocal outcomes data, there is additional controversy surrounding prehospital transfusion. The practice of administering blood outside of the hospital setting carries with it inherent feasibility and logistical issues. For instance, there are legitimate concerns regarding the availability and storage of blood products [17]. Blood products need to be stored at acceptable temperatures and have to be utilized before expiration. Moreover, warming of blood products before administration is advised [23, 24]. Failure to do so will worsen hypothermia and exacerbate the physiologic derangements of the triad [8, 9, 13, 23]. Ensuring that these requirements are met can be expensive [23, 24]. Furthermore, as there is not time to determine the blood type of a trauma victim in the setting of life-threatening traumatic hemorrhage, universal donor types must be on hand to avoid inciting immunological rejection of the donor blood and worsening the patient's condition. Additionally, even if blood is properly cross-matched or universal donor blood is used, there can be negative reactions to blood transfusion such as anaphylaxis, circulatory overload, and lung injury that first responders administering transfusions outside of the hospital may be ill-equipped to deal with [20, 23].

Despite these potential risks, very few patients are reported to have these complications [20, 23]. A lack of standardization of PHBT protocols makes it difficult to definitively determine their contribution to mortality prevention in trauma, and the promise that has been shown by some studies suggests that PHBT may in fact provide benefit if protocols can be optimized. The prospect of being able to reduce the percentage of negative outcomes associated with traumatic hemorrhage makes further exploration into the concept a worthwhile endeavor. This chapter will explore different aspects of PHBT. It will provide an overview of the different blood products available for transfusion and discuss in more detail aspects of storage and transportation and guidelines for PHBT. Finally, we will further discuss recent clinical findings and potential considerations for the future of PHBT.

Blood Products

Blood donation is highly regulated in the United States by the Food and Drug Administration (FDA). Blood donors must be between 16 and 65 years of age, must weigh at least 110 pounds, and exclude those with certain medical conditions or other infectious etiologies [25]. Donors are also screened for recent travel exposures, new tattoos or piercings, hemoglobin concentration, blood pressure, medications, and pregnancy [25]. In addition to screening questionnaires, blood is tested for different infectious diseases after donation including HIV, hepatitis B and C, WNV, HTVL, CMV, EBV, syphilis, and Chagas [25]. Blood facilities in the United States are frequently inspected and are required to meet high-quality standards which are outlined in the Public Health Service Act 42 and enforced by the FDA to ensure the US blood supply is as safe as possible [26]. Whole blood is collected from donors and should be separated into components within 5–8 hours via refrigerated centrifugation [27]. Apheresis is an alternative blood collection method which collects specific components of blood while simultaneously returning the remaining blood back to the donor using filtration techniques [27].

Whole blood is an unprocessed blood product which contains all components of physiologic circulating blood including red blood cells (RBC), plasma, platelets, and leukocytes [27]. Since whole blood contains multiple different elements, there are many adverse reactions that can occur when foreign blood is given to a recipient [27]. Antigens on a red blood cell, such as "A" or "B," determine a person's blood type as "A," "B," "AB," or "O." Rh factor is another antigen that determines if blood type is "positive" or "negative" [25]. If ABO blood type is not correctly matched beforehand, antibodies can be formed against the foreign antigen and can cause fatal acute hemolytic transfusion reactions [25]. To avoid this type of reaction, if a blood type is unknown, the universal blood donor "O negative" should be given [25]. Whole blood can be stored at a licensed blood bank for 35 days at 1–6 °C in an anticoagulant solution, citrate phosphate dextrose adenine (CPDA-1) [27]. The US military occasionally uses "warm fresh whole blood" (WFWB) donated from "walking blood banks" (WBB) in combat-related trauma [28]. WFWB expires after storage at room temperature for 24 hours or refrigerated for 8 hours [28]. The biggest disadvantage for using WFWB in traumatic combat situations is the risk of acute hemolytic reaction. This is related to mismatched blood types and the possibility of transmitting infections [28]. The advantages for using whole blood transfusions is that whole blood contains all natural blood components in physiologic ratios without preservatives or additives and can be stored as one modality allowing easier access in emergency situations [28]. A 2009 study by Spinella et al. demonstrated that WFWB is associated with an improved 30-day survival in combat-related patients with hemorrhagic shock compared to component blood transfusion [28]. Due to the physiologic components of whole blood, easier storage, and access, whole blood may be advantageous to prevent hemorrhagic mortality before first responders reach the hospital with a critical patient.

Packed red blood cells (PRBCs) are blood products that contain 200 mL of concentrated RBCs to a hematocrit of 75% [29]. PRBCs are used to quickly increase oxygen-carrying capacity in patients who are severely anemic (hemoglobin < 7 g/dl) or have severe occult blood loss [29]. After receiving 1 unit of PRBC, a patient's hemoglobin and hematocrit are expected to rise by 1 g/dl and 3%, respectively [29]. As with whole blood, ABO compatibility is essential to avoid transfusion reactions [25]. Packed red blood cells are also available to certain populations as "washed," "leukoreduced," or "irradiated." *Washed red cells* are washed with sterile saline which removes 98% of plasma, platelets, and cellular debris and reduces leukocyte concentration [29]. Washed PRBCs are indicated in patients with a history of allergic reaction to transfusion and IgA deficiency but must be used within 24 hours of saline washing [29]. *Leukoreduced red cells* are PRBCs with 99.9% of leukocytes filtered out reducing the risk of CMV, EBV, and HTLV infections and febrile reactions [29]. *Irradiated red cells* are gamma-radiated PRBCs which kill all lymphocytes [29]. This blood product is indicated to prevent donor versus host disease in immunocompromised patients, lymphoma patients, stem cell and marrow transplant patients, and intrauterine transfusions [29]. PRBCs can be stored at 1–6 °C at a blood bank for up to 42 days. When dispensed, PRBCs can be stored in a blood bank cooler for 6 hours [27]. Transfusion with PRBCs can play an important role in prehospital treatment of patients who experience hemorrhagic shock because the highly concentrated hemoglobin allows for a rapid increase in oxygen-carrying capacity which is vital for organ function in patients who have lost severe amounts of blood.

Fresh frozen plasma (FFP) contains all clotting factors, protein C, protein S, antithrombin III, albumin, immunoglobulins, tissue factor pathway inhibitor, and fibrinogen [30]. These elements are separated from whole blood and must be frozen within 6 hours of phlebotomy to preserve clotting factors [30]. FFP is indicated in patients with significant coagulation factor deficiencies including congenital deficiencies, microvascular bleeding with elevated PT and PTT, dilutional coagulopathy related to massive blood replacement, disseminated intravascular coagulation, and coagulopathy secondary to liver pathology [29]. FFP is also used in urgent reversal of warfarin therapy and in combination with plasmapheresis to treat thrombocytopenic purpura and hemolytic uremic syndrome [29]. FFP expires after 1 year in a blood bank freezer at ≤18 °C but must be used 5 days after thawing [27].

Liquid plasma (LP) contains the same blood components as FFP, but it is immediately stored at 1–6 °C instead of freezing after phlebotomy. Liquid plasma expires 5 days after the whole blood that it was extracted from, so approximately 26–40 days depending on anticoagulation solution used [27]. Liquid plasma contains less clotting factors than FFP, for example, clotting factors V and VIII begin to decrease after 6 hours [27]. The longer shelf life of LP compared to thawed FFP is advantageous for adequate supplies of plasma. ABO compatibility is also a concern for plasma transfusions, but the matching system is opposite to that of RBC compatibility [31]. Since plasma contains only antibodies, as opposed to antigens that are located on RBCs, the universal plasma donor type is AB plasma which contains no antibodies [31]. Liquid plasma may play a larger role in prehospital transfusion in the future related to its longer shelf life as compared to thawed FFP.

Platelets are an essential component of clot formation in the blood. Platelets can be collected from single whole blood, pooled whole blood (platelets from 4–6 donors), or apheresis procedures [29]. Prophylactic platelet transfusions are indicated in thrombocytopenic patients or bleeding surgical patients when the platelet count is below 50,000 or below 100,000 if the risk of bleeding is clinically significant [29]. They are also needed in patients with microvascular bleeding with known platelet dysfunction but contraindicated in idiopathic thrombocytopenia purpura (ITP) [29]. Platelets are stored at room temperature (20–24 °C) with continuous gentle agitation to avoid clot formation, but the shelf life is only 5 days [29].

Cryoprecipitate is a blood product that contains concentrated factor VIII, factor XIII, fibrinogen, fibronectin, and von Willebrand's factor [29]. Cryoprecipitate is indicated for pro-

Table 36.1 Blood products analyzed by components, expiration date, and storage requirements

Blood product	Composition	Expiration date	Storage
Whole blood	Unprocessed RBC, plasma, platelets, clotting factors, and leukocytes in physiologic ratios	21 days in CPD or CP2D 35 days in CPDA-1	1–6 °C
Packed red blood cells (PBRCs)	RBCs only (small residual plasma and leukocytes unless radiated or filtered)	42 days	1–6 °C
Fresh frozen plasma (FFP)	All clotting factors, antithrombin III, albumin, immunoglobulin, fibrinogen protein C and S, and tissue factor pathway inhibitor	365 days 5 days after thaw	≤−18 °C 1–6 °C before transfusion
Liquid plasma (LP)	Same as FFP, but less clotting factors, never frozen	5 days after expiration of whole blood extracted from (21 + 5 or 35 + 5)	1–6 °C
Cryoprecipitate	Clotting factors VIII and XIII, von Willebrand factor, fibrinogen, and fibronectin	365 days	≤−18 °C
Platelets	Platelets only	5 days	20–24 °C with continuous gentle agitation

phylaxis in perioperative patients with congenital fibrinogen deficiencies, patients with von Willebrand's disease that is unresponsive to DDAVP or currently bleeding, and correction of microvascular bleeding in massive blood transfusions with fibronectin concentrations between 80 and 100 mg/dl [29]. Blood fibronectin concentration can be raised by 50 mg/dl with administration of one unit of cryoprecipitate per 10 kg [29]. Cryoprecipitate transfusion allows for replenishment of important end components for the formation of fibrin clots and does not require ABO matching before use [25]. For these reasons, cryoprecipitate may also play an important role in prehospital treatment when massive transfusion protocol is needed.

Currently, the massive transfusion protocol requires PRBC, FFP, and platelets transfused in a 1:1:1 ratio for "damage control resuscitation" in hemorrhaging patients with severe trauma [32]. These traumatic scenarios are seen daily throughout the United States by first responders. Massive transfusion achieves the goals of quickly enhancing oxygen-carrying capacity and correcting intravascular volume depletion and trauma-induced coagulopathies while administering in a 1:1:1 ratio to prevent dilutional coagulopathy [32]. Prehospital transfusions of hemorrhaging patients can address these fatal problems before reaching a medical facility (Table 36.1).

Transportation, Storage, and Expiration

Prehospital transfusions by first providers may improve outcomes in patients; however, implementing such protocols in Emergency Medical Services (EMS) in the United States is futile if the blood products reaching patients are of lesser quality than those received at a hospital. Intense oversight and regulation are needed to preserve blood product quality from the time of deployment until administration in the field. Unfortunately, such tight regulations can be logistical barriers to the widespread implementation of prehospital transfusion practices. Of these barriers, the regulation of temperature during transport remains the most difficult aspect of bringing blood into the field. Above ideal temperatures, the blood products may expire rapidly, making the practice of bringing blood on every emergency call (where they might not be used) extremely costly. Maintaining a lower temperature minimizes the metabolic activity of the blood, prolonging its shelf life. Freezing the blood, however, is not feasible—at temperatures below 2 °C, the red blood cells may become dehydrated and subsequently hemolyze. Additionally, ice crystal formation can cause RBC membrane damage [33]. That being said, whole blood and pRBCs are not the only products used in transfusion, and unfortunately, different products are best maintained at different temperatures.

The tight control of temperature maintains the standard of care, ensuring patients receive the same quality of blood products administered in the Emergency Room. These temperatures, in addition to preventing damage and contamination, prolong the shelf life of the products. Shelf life is generally described as the maximum time at which administered products are still effective. The American Association of Blood Banks (AABB) works closely with the FDA to produce standards for temperature targets in both the storage and transport of each blood product [34]. The following descriptions of each type of blood products' recommended storage/transportation temperatures and expiration dates are from the 2018 AABB Temperature Standards [35].

The AABB recommends the storage of pRBC preparations at a temperature between 1 and 6 °C and transportation at a temperature between 1 and 10 °C. The shelf life for pRBCs is determined by the time at which 75% of transfused red blood cells are still viable in the circulation 24 hours after administration. Depending on the specific anticoagulant used, shelf life varies from 21 to 42 days.

For platelet preparations, the AABB recommends storage at temperatures between 20 and 24 °C (room temperature) with continuous agitation. During transportation platelet preparations should be kept at the same temperature; however continuous agitation is not necessary. The continuous agitation in storage has been thought to reduce platelet hypoxia and the subsequent damaging decrease in pH due to lactic acid production [36]. The shelf life for platelet products is generally only 5 days.

The AABB recommends FFP storage at temperatures less than or equal to −18 °C. At these temperatures, the shelf life is up to 12 months from the date of collection (up to 36 months if kept at temperatures below −25 °C). However, FFP must be thawed before administration, and once thawed, the shelf life decreases to between 1 and 5 days depending on the preparation.

For cryoprecipitate, the AABB recommends storage at temperatures less than or equal to −18 °C. Similar to FFP, cryoprecipitate also has to be thawed. Once thawed it should be kept at room temperature until administration; however, it quickly expires within 6 hours.

As mentioned earlier, a major obstacle for the systematic implementation of prehospital transfusions is the transport of these products into the field at temperatures meeting the demands of regulatory laws and recommendations. Specialized containers used for transport are primarily built around their ability to keep whole blood and blood components at the target temperature for transport. Such containers are usually coolers of some sort with the ability to be remotely monitored and controlled to maintain a very specific temperature, regardless of the external environment. Coolers seem to be preferred over the use of standard blood product refrigerators due to the mobility of coolers in the field. The two main components of these storage devices are an insulated container and a coolant insert or packet. One commonly used product is Pelican BioThermal's (USA) Crēdo™ Medic Pack Series 4 EMT cooler, capable of holding 2 units of pRBCs and 2 units of plasma. The Medic Pack consists of an outer carrying shell, a middle vacuum pack container, and an internal thermal container filled with heavy water [37]. The heavy water is frozen (for at least 8 hours) prior to use and once used thaws to around 3.8 °C, the melting point of heavy water. Results of testing showed the pack could maintain blood product temperatures between 1 and 6 °C for runs up to 24 hours [38]. Similarly, companies have started production on coolers made specifically for temperature-sensitive blood/medication transport. FaraeTec's (USA) LifeBox 50 consists of a rugged outer shell (unlike the Crēdo™ Medic Pack) with a reticulated polystyrene shell beneath it, a carbon aerogel vacuum-insulated panel, a zero-permeability vapor barrier for panel protection, and an inner plastic corrugated lining [39]. The LifeBox, like the Crēdo™ Medic Pack, contains a phase change material to help maintain target temperatures. Neither box requires batteries for operation, giving them both an advantage over more expensive options. However, these containers are not cheap. Investigations into more affordable options (containers not specifically made for such extreme temperature control) found that safe storage and transport weren't possible with simpler, cheaper materials [40]. It can be postulated that as more EMS departments throughout the country adopt prehospital transfusion protocols, companies will develop more optimal storage containers perhaps at a more affordable price.

With the advent of prehospital transfusions in the field, much of what has been implemented does not follow a nationally standardized protocol. A few EMS programs throughout the country have successfully implicated protocols that make prehospital transfusions by EMS personnel effective both medically and financially. Departments must take care to maintain low wastage and misuse of an already diminished national supply of blood. To mitigate this risk, it's imperative that EMS departments engage in a partnership with a local hospital or blood bank to allow rotation of the EMS's blood supplies. Short shelf lives mean that products not used in the field may go to waste; therefore "exchanging" them for newer supplies from a local hospital or blood bank ensures that the near-expiration blood products will likely be used quickly in the hospital setting [41]. Certain EMS departments have also implemented a standard that all onboard units of blood or blood components are to be from different donations, allowing first providers to continue to administer indicated products if one of the units causes a transfusion reaction [38].

EMS stations have used other equipment in the introduction of prehospital transfusion protocols. In some instances, temperature probes were added to the specialized coolers, able to display the temperature on the dashboard of an ambulance, personnel department of an aircraft, or remotely to a supervisor. EMS stations also invested in specialized refrigeration units that allow for precise temperature control of stored blood products [38]. Such refrigerators have advanced technology including triple-redundant thermometers with software that can send texts and alert staff in cases of malfunction or rising temperatures [42]. Some programs incorporated devices including point-of-care hemoglobin meters to assist in determining if transfusion is indicated. Additionally, portable warming devices are necessary to allow first providers to rapidly heat blood products for transfusion of large amounts. In experimental trials, one of these warming devices, the Warrior Lite, was able to warm blood products from 10 °C to 35 °C at a rate of 200 mL/min [43].

The process of integrating prehospital transfusions into emergency medical services in the field is not without logistical complications. Each department must decide if implementing such protocols is cost-effective for their area. Factors to consider include the incidence of shock/trauma in the area, availability of a local hospital system and/or blood bank to establish a blood-sharing program with, cost of fitting emergency vehicles and stations with the appropriate equipment, and equipment upkeep. Equipment such as coolers are the victims of excessive wear and tear due to the demanding environment first providers operate in daily. Not only are these coolers expensive, but the process of preconditioning and installation are expensive and time-consuming [38]. Wastage of expensive blood products due to misuse, poor storage protocols, or uncontrollable factors (i.e., vehicle breakdown) may also contribute to increased costs. It is also expensive, yet exceedingly important, to train all personnel in the storage, transportation, and administration per protocol of these products [44]. Departments also must implement strict documentation protocols, which can be time-consuming for personnel. Much of the current research on prehospital transfusions by first providers understandably focuses on indication criteria for transfusion and patient outcomes. However, as more EMS departments throughout the country develop prehospital transfusion programs, more research should be directed at the cost-effectiveness of these programs to determine if the process can be financially streamlined.

All of the logistical barriers discussed above have prevented widespread implementation of such practices in EMS throughout the United States. Historically, the US military has carried blood products in medical evacuation helicopters for some time [45]. The timeline of different departments implementing similar practices is hard to delineate. The Norwegian Helicopter Emergency Medical Services has reportedly deployed aircraft with blood on board intermittently for the last 30 years before finally making it standard for every flight to carry blood products in 2013 [17]. Australia seems to be one of the first to implement prehospital transfusions in civilian air ambulances circa 2011, with the United Kingdom following soon after [46]. In 2016, a study showed that of 235 helicopter emergency medical services in the United States, only 25.3% carried blood products. Of those that did, only 60% carried blood products on every flight [47]. Since then many different emergency services such as Life Flight (USA) have implemented prehospital transfusion protocols where possible. Interestingly, since 2009, cruise lines have successfully implemented protocols for warm fresh whole blood transfusion (WFWB) using donors on-board [17]. Reportedly in 2017, Cypress Creek EMS and Harris County Emergency Services District 48 of Harris County, Texas, were the first to carry and transfuse whole blood to patients as a civilian ground EMS service in the United States [41]. In 2018, San Antonio, Texas, became the first metropolitan area to equip paramedics and seven fire departments with whole blood for prehospital transfusions [48]. As research on the results of these programs surfaces, the United States can anticipate the implementation of similar practices in EMS departments throughout the country. As the prevalence of prehospital blood transfusions further increases, more research should highlight the main logistical barriers to program incorporation and allow the healthcare community to delineate areas of improvement that increase the cost-effectiveness of these programs, standardize protocols for transfusion, and most importantly improve patient outcomes.

Guidelines for Transfusion and Risks

Guidelines for transfusions vary from hospital to hospital and from society to society; however the general purpose and backbone of various guidelines all express the same thing. During a surgical procedure, the responsibility of transfusing blood usually falls on the anesthesiologist; as such the American Society of Anesthesiologists has published its own guidelines on the subject. These guidelines are broken down into four sections: Patient Evaluation, Preadmission Patient Preparation, Preprocedure Preparation, and Intraoperative and Postoperative Management of Blood Loss (see Table 36.2).

Transfusion in critical care and trauma medicine has different guidelines than that of a preplanned surgery. However, the overall goal of both scenarios is the same which is to stabilize the patient and prevent any long-term complications, if possible. The American College of Critical Care Medicine in conjunction with the Society of Critical Care Medicine has transfusion recommendations relating to seven areas: (1) critically ill, (2) sepsis, (3) patients at risk for or with acute lung injury or ARDS, (4) neurological injury and disease, (5) RBC transfusion risks, (6) alternatives to RBC transfusion, and (7) strategies to reduce transfusions. See Table 36.3.

The American Association of Blood Banks has also put forth their own guidelines for transfusions; however in the surgical and acute setting, guidelines by the ASA and ACCCM may be more practical. The AABB sets forth its guidelines in the form of two recommendations. See Table 36.4.

In many instances, a RBC transfusion is critical to the survival of the patient; however, transfusion reactions do occasionally occur and should be accounted for any time blood products are given. Acute intravascular hemolytic transfusion reactions occur when red blood cells break down due to either a complement-mediated immune mechanism (usually secondary to ABO incompatibility) or physical damage to the cells (osmotic or temperature related). Severe complications such as shock and DIC are often related to ABO incompatibility and less so with physical damage. Signs of ABO incompatibility in the operating room include hypotension, shock, and fever. If ABO incompatibility is suspected, the transfusion should be stopped immediately, and supportive measures to maintain blood pressure should be done. Transfusion of blood products such as platelets, FFP, and cryoprecipitate will help in decreasing the consumptive coagulopathy [52]. Syndromes such as transfusion-associated circulatory overload (TACO) and transfusion-related acute lung injury (TRALI) usually occur 6 hours after transfusion which involve respiratory distress and are oftentimes life-threatening. TACO is characterized by pulmonary hydrostatic edema, while TRALI presents as pulmonary permeability edema [53]. TRALIs are caused by donor antibodies in plasma containing blood components (FFP, platelets, RBCs) interacting with antigens on the patient's granulocytes. This reaction subsequently results in granulocyte aggregation and complement activation in the lung capillaries, leading to fever, hypoxemia, acute respiratory distress, and increased peak airway pressure. The symptoms are similar to the symptoms seen in transfusion-related circulatory overload, but fever sets TRALI apart [54]. Platelet transfusion often puts the patient at risk for bacterial contamination. Platelets are stored at 20–24 degrees Celsius which facilitates growth of bacteria. There has been a large decline in the number of transfusion reaction cases related to new screening methods to detect contamination being implemented. However, contaminated products are occasionally missed by screening, as such patients who develop hyperthermia and hypotension after a transfusion should be suspected for having bacterially contaminated products given to

Table 36.2 Transfusion guidelines set forth by the American Society of Anesthesiologists [49]

Patient evaluation

1. Review of previous medical records, paying particular attention to history of previous blood transfusion and current medications (warfarin, clopidogrel, aspirin, or other NOACs)
2. History of congenital coagulopathies, thrombotic events, and risk factors for organ ischemia
3. Efforts should be made to discuss the possible need for a transfusion, and the risk and benefits of such a procedure and patient preferences toward a blood transfusion should also be elicited
4. Current labs should be checked, a physical exam performed, and any additional labs ordered

Preadmission patient preparation

1. For patients with CKD, renal insufficiency, or transfusion refusal, erythropoietin with or without iron may be used to help lower risks
2. For patients on anticoagulants, discontinuation should only be done after consulting with the proper specialist
3. For patients on antiplatelet agents, discontinuation is desired before the start of the procedure
4. For patients undergoing procedures where significant blood loss is expected, blood products should be available on short notice

Pre-procedure preparation

1. A restrictive RBC strategy should be used
   (a) Transfusion requirements for hemoglobin's ranging between 6 and 10 g/dL should be based on current or potential bleeding, intravascular volume status, signs of end-organ ischemia, and cardiopulmonary reserve
   (b) Administration of RBCs should be done unit by unit
   (c) A protocol for avoidance of transfusions may be used as a strategy to reduce blood loss for patients whom transfusion is refused or is not possible
   (d) Massive transfusion protocol may be implemented when available as a method to optimize RBC delivery in massively bleeding patients
2. Reversal of anticoagulants
   (a) For urgent reversal of warfarin, administer prothrombin complex concentrates or FFP
   (b) Admitter vitamin K for selected patients for nonurgent reversal of warfarin, except when rapid restoration of anticoagulation after surgery is required
3. Antifibrinolytics for prophylaxis of excessive blood loss
   (a) For patients undergoing cardiopulmonary bypass, the use of antifibrinolytic therapy for prophylaxis of the use of allogenic blood transfusions is recommended
   (b) Antifibrinolytic therapy for prophylaxis should be considered in certain orthopedic surgery
   (c) Antifibrinolytic therapy for prophylaxis should be considered in liver surgery and other clinical circumstances at high risk for excessive bleeding
4. Acute normovolemic hemodilution (ANH)
   (a) Consider ANH to reduce the need for allogeneic blood transfusion in patients at high risk for excessive bleeding (e.g., major cardiac, orthopedic, thoracic, or liver surgery), if possible

Table 36.2 (continued)

Intraoperative and postoperative management of blood loss

1. Allogenic RBC transfusion
   (a) Administer blood without consideration of length of storage
   (b) Leukocyte-reduced blood may be used for reducing complications with allogenic blood transfusion
2. Reinfusion of recovered RBCs
   (a) Reinfuse recovered RBCs as a blood-sparing intervention when applicable
3. Intraoperative and postoperative patient monitoring
   (a) Visual assessment of the surgical field in collaboration with the surgeon to look for any excessive bleeding should be performed periodically
   (b) Inspect suction canisters, surgical sponges, and surgical drains to access for a quantitative measurement of blood loss
   (c) Monitor perfusion of vital organs using standard ASA monitors (i.e., blood pressure, heart rate, oxygen saturation, EKG)
   (d) In patients where anemia is suspected, the monitoring of hemoglobin and hematocrit levels is vital and should account for estimated blood loss
   (e) In patients where coagulopathy is suspected, monitoring coagulations studies such as INR, aPTT, and fibrinogen concentration may be warranted
   (f) Signs and symptoms of transfusions reactions should be looked for periodically (hyperthermia, urticaria, respiratory distress, etc.). Should these symptoms occur, stop the transfusion immediately
4. Treatment of excessive bleeding
   (a) Ordering a platelet count before transfusion may be beneficial; however it is often times not possible. Anticoagulation drug status should also be assessed in patients with excessive bleeding
   (b) If at all possible, order coagulation studies such as PT, INR, and aPTT before transfusion with FFP
   (c) Fibrinogen levels should be monitored before the infusion of cryoprecipitate
   (d) In patients with excessive bleeding and platelet dysfunction, desmopressin may be considered. Topical agents such as fibrin glue or thrombin gel may be used as well
   (e) If the cause of the excessive bleeding is fibrinolysis, then agents such as Ɖ-aminocaproic acid or tranexamic acid may be used
   (f) If the coagulations studies reveal an increased INR, then PCCs may be used
   (g) After all other approaches have been exhausted, one may consider using recombinant factor VII to alleviate the bleeding
   (h) Concentrated fibrinogen may also be beneficial

Table 36.3 Transfusion guidelines from the American College of Critical Care Medicine [50]

Recommendations regarding RBC transfusion in the following patient populations
Generally, critically ill patient
1. Indications for RBC transfusions include signs of extreme blood loss such as in hemorrhagic shock, hemorrhage, hemodynamic instability, or below average oxygen delivery
2. A threshold of 7 g/dL to transfuse RBCs is as effective as using a threshold of 10 g/dL in critically ill patients with hemodynamically stable anemia, except possibly in patients with acute myocardial ischemia
3. Solely using hemoglobin as a marker for transfusion is not advised. Several factors such as intravascular volume status, shock, duration of symptoms, and hemodynamic parameters should be taken into account
4. Transfusion of RBCs should be administered as single units when possible
5. Consider transfusion if Hb is 7 g/dL in critically ill patients requiring mechanical ventilation (MV), resuscitated critically ill trauma patients, and critically ill patients with stable cardiac disease. Using a threshold of 10 g/dL is not beneficial in these instances
6. RBC transfusion should not be considered as the sole method to improve tissue oxygen consumption in critically ill patients
7. Patients with a history of acute coronary syndromes with associated anemia may benefit from an RBC transfusion
Sepsis[a]
1. The transfusion needs for septic patients must be assessed individually because optimal transfusion thresholds in septic patients are not known and there is no clear evidence that blood transfusions increase tissue oxygenation
Patients at risk for or with acute lung injury (ALI) or acute respiratory distress syndrome (ARDS)[a]
1. ALI and ARDS are common clinical complications of massive transfusions
2. In patients at risk for ALI or ARDS, every attempt should be made at avoiding RBC transfusions
3. TRALI or ARDS events following transfusions should be reported to the blood bank
4. RBC transfusion is not a viable option to help wean a patient from mechanical ventilation
Patients with neurological injury and disease[a]
1. There are no benefits in using a threshold of 10 g/dL to initiate transfusions in patients with moderate-to-severe traumatic brain injury
2. RBC transfusions in patients with neurological injury should be assessed on an individual basis as there are currently no guidelines
Transfusion risks[a]
1. RBC transfusion is associated with increased risk of nosocomial infection (wound infection, pneumonia, sepsis)
2. Multiple organ failure and systemic response syndrome are rare but often deadly risk factors that must be considered when performing a transfusion
3. The benefits of leukocyte depletion of RBC transfusions is still being studied
4. RBC transfusions are independently associated with increased ICU and hospital stays, complications, and mortality
5. Patients who undergo a RBC transfusion are at a higher risk for an increased ICU and hospital admission, complications, and death
There is a relationship between transfusion and ALI and ARDS
Alternatives to RBC transfusions[a]
1. Increased reticulocytosis via recombinant human erythropoietin can decrease transfusion requirements
2. Hemoglobin-based oxygen carriers (HBOCs) are being studied for use in critically ill patients but have not yet been approved for use in the United States
Strategies to reduce RBC transfusions[a]
1. The use of low-volume adult or pediatric blood sampling tubes and reduction of diagnostic laboratory testing are associated with a reduction in phlebotomy volumes and a reduction in blood transfusion
2. Devices that conserve waste blood for use again are connected with a reduction in phlebotomy volume

[a]There is insufficient data to support Level 1 recommendations on this topic

Table 36.4 Transfusion guidelines from the American Association of Blood Banks [51]

First recommendation
1. A hemoglobin of 7 g/dL should be used as the threshold to initiate RBC transfusion in hemodynamically stable patients, including critically ill patients
2. For patients undergoing orthopedic or cardiac surgery and those with preexisting cardiovascular disease, transfusion threshold of 8 g/dL may be used
3. The recommendations do not apply to the following conditions: acute coronary syndrome, severe thrombocytopenia, patients treated for hematological or oncological disorders at risk of bleeding, and chronic transfusion dependent anemia
Second recommendation
1. Patients, including neonates, should receive RBC units selected at any point within their dating period rather than limiting patients to RBC units stored for less than 10 days

them. In patients who develop hypocalcemia and hypomagnesemia, citrate toxicity should be considered. Citrate is commonly used as an anticoagulant in blood products; however, it also readily binds calcium and magnesium. In cases where large numbers of blood components are transfused over a short time, the metabolism of citrate is overcome. Lastly, allergic reactions due to patient IgE antibodies attacking proteins in the plasma of donated blood products do occur. Patients usually develop urticaria and other erythematous skin manifestations, which can subside spontaneously or with diphenhydramine administration. Occasionally, the reaction is so severe that it can lead to anaphylaxis [55].

Recent Clinical Findings

Hemorrhagic shock is the leading cause of preventable death among trauma patients, with risk highest in the prehospital setting [56, 57]. Rapid transport is "essential" but can be delayed by uncontrollable variables. Prehospital transfusion combined with hemorrhage control techniques can save lives of trauma patients [56–58]. The "golden hour" following a major trauma is the most decisive, and prehospital transfusion can optimize transport survival and coordination with the receiving hospital to improve patient outcome [58]. Prehospital blood transfusion does not result in increased transport times to the hospital and may shorten transport time [57, 59].

Coagulopathy, hypothermia, and acidosis comprise the lethal triad in hemorrhaging trauma patients [23, 60]. Damage control resuscitation attempts to correct or mitigate the effects of this triad using early hemorrhage control, permissive hypotension, warming the patient to reduce coagulopathy, minimizing crystalloid use, and early transfusion of RBCs, plasma, and platelets [15, 58, 61–63].

Coagulopathy begins shortly after trauma, and massive bleeding rapidly leads to hypoperfusion and shock [58]. Trauma-induced coagulopathy is the primary predictor of blood transfusion requirements and increased mortality. Over-dilution with crystalloids and RBCs, acidosis, overactivated coagulation cascade, fibrinolysis, and hypothermia are all contributing factors to trauma-induced coagulopathy [15, 58, 61].

Transfusion does not guarantee that bleeding will stop, and post-traumatic injury fibrinolysis can exacerbate bleeding. An antifibrinolytic agent like tranexamic acid (TXA) can be used with blood products [61]. Additionally, prehospital plasma transfusion quickly corrects deficiencies of critical coagulation factors and acts as an ideal volume expander by "[remaining] in the intravascular space." Plasma also reduces endothelial permeability by preventing endothelial glycocalyx degradation [60].

Hemorrhagic damage control guidelines in the United States and Europe prefer "early transfusion of warmed blood products" [56]. Whole blood is best for transfusing hemorrhaging trauma patients, as it eliminates the issue of storage lesion in both red blood cells and platelets [61]. Blood components replaced fresh whole blood related to the ability to store these longer. A minority of Helicopter Emergency Medical Services (HEMS) carry cold whole blood, while the US military uses warm fresh whole blood because each soldier is prescreened as a source [23]. While hospitals administer RBC/FFP/platelets in the optimal 1:1:1 ratio, most HEMS carry only RBCs due to storage logistics, and plasma and platelets are not necessarily available in prehospital settings [23].

Storage and transportation of blood products for prehospital transfusion are feasible [64, 65]. Refrigeration with continuous temperature monitoring and an active cooler need to be on-board the transport vehicle [23, 64]. Ideally, a fluid warmer should be on-board, as transfusing cold blood products may exacerbate hypothermia and lead to complications [23, 57]. Fresh dried plasma may provide a solution to the logistical issues involved in thawing FFP for prehospital transfusion [23]. The cost and short shelf half-life of blood products remain a concern, but supplying and storing blood products for prehospital transfusion can be done easily while minimizing wastage by consistently returning unused products before expiration [56, 63].

Prehospital transfusion is safe, with rare minor adverse events, although blood transfusion in any setting is not risk-free [15, 22, 23, 56, 57, 66]. Most prehospital emergency treatment is administered by personnel who do not commonly transfuse blood. These caregivers would need education and training/support to regularly include transfusion as an option in prehospital care. However, studies have shown similar outcomes among professions [56, 64].

The most commonly used criterion for prehospital transfusion is SBP < 90 mmHg; tachycardia (rate > 120), unquantified hypoperfusion, GCS < 8, and loss of verbal contact are also used as criteria. Other indications for transfusion included penetrating trauma, traumatic limb amputation, and suspected ongoing bleeding. Physicians clinically assess patient volume status, while paramedics use "defined parameters for blood pressure or heart rate" [56].

Many studies on prehospital transfusion exclude patients with traumatic brain injury, although traumatic brain injury continues to be a primary cause of death among trauma patients [61, 67]. Hypertonic saline is preferable to blood products, because its osmolarity—which is higher than that in blood—draws fluid away from edematous brain tissue, thus reducing ICP and secondary brain injury by ameliorating brain perfusion [61]. Among hypotensive patients with traumatic brain injury and poly-trauma patients with traumatic brain injury, patients who received plasma benefited from improved neurological outcomes. Improved outcomes associated with prehospital plasma transfusion were likely attributable to coagulation factors and fibrinogen that promote neuroprotective mechanisms that "reduce brain lesion size and swelling" [67].

While most patients requiring prehospital blood transfusions are severely injured male trauma patients, studies should also address pediatric patients receiving prehospital blood transfusions [20, 64, 65]. A sizeable subset of pediatric patients requiring transport includes non-trauma neonates with symptomatic anemia or thrombocytopenia, and pediatric prehospital transfusion protocols should be developed for such patients, including "point-of-care evaluation of Hgb and platelet counts" versus the more typical hemodynamic criteria [65]. Because the pediatric patient population includes neonates, infants, and children under 14, transport teams must carry specialized infusion equipment [65].

Recognizing the need for evidence-based guidelines on prehospital transfusion, the Department of Defense funded three controlled, randomized trials: the COMBAT (Control of Major Bleeding After Trauma) trial, the PAMPer (Prehospital Air Medical Plasma) study, and the PUPTH (Prehospital Use of Plasma in Traumatic Hemorrhage) trial

Table 36.5 Positive and negative benefits of prehospital transfusion blood products and crystalloids (*note that all can exacerbate hypothermia if products or patient are not warmed*)

	PRBCs	Plasma	Plasma/RBCs (1:1)	Whole blood	Crystalloids
Positive	Transport oxygen to tissues	(1) Quickly corrects deficiencies of critical coagulation factors (2) Ideal volume expander; remains in intravascular space (3) Reduces endothelial permeability (4) Promotes neuroprotective mechanisms in TBI patients	Provides both oxygen transport to tissues and mitigates TIC	(1) Ideal because it is physiologically closest (2) No storage lesion issues	(1) Easier to store (2) Less costly and more readily available than blood products (3) No transfusion-related adverse events
Negative	(1) Can cause overdilution with crystalloids, contributing to TIC (2) Does not stop bleeding (3) Requires refrigeration with continuous temperature monitoring (4) Small-risk adverse transfusion events	(1) FFP must be kept in cold storage and takes time to thaw; correctable by using freeze-dried plasma (2) Small-risk adverse transfusion events	(1) Logistics of air and ground transport storing two types of blood products (2) Small-risk adverse transfusion events	(1) Shorter storage time (2) Small risk of adverse transfusion events	Dilutes coagulation factors

[60]. The PUPTH trial was withdrawn related to lack of patient enrollment.

The PAMPer Study conducted a pragmatic, multicenter cluster-randomized phase 3 trial comparing patients receiving thawed plasma against patients receiving standard-of-care (crystalloid) resuscitation before RBCs during emergency air transport, using 30-day mortality as the primary outcome. The intervention group experienced significantly lower 24-hour and 30-day mortality, and a lower median prothrombin-time ratio than the standard-of-care group, regardless of subsequent prehospital RBC transfusion [20]. Survival curves showed differences beginning 3 hours after randomization and continuing through the 30 days noteworthy given most hemorrhagic deaths take place within the first 3 hours following the trauma injury [20, 56]. Moreover, the intervention group did not experience a higher rate of inflammatory-mediated complications and had a low rate of minor allergic or transfusion-related events [20]. The authors reasoned that reduced bleeding and/or coagulopathy, attenuation of inflammatory response, and decreased endothelial trauma-induced dysfunction as mechanisms by which prehospital plasma transfusion conferred these survival benefits [20].

The COMBAT study was a pragmatic, randomized, single-center trial comparing trauma patients in hemorrhagic shock receiving 2 units of plasma against patients receiving normal saline during rapid ground transport to a level 1 trauma center in an urban setting. The primary outcome was 28-day mortality. Prehospital plasma transfusion did not correlate with a significant reduction in 28-day mortality. For urban areas with short transport times, the effort to thaw and transfuse plasma may outweigh any benefits [22].

Most of the literature has failed to establish positive short- or long-term survival benefits for civilian patients [57], with some studies showing improved outcomes and others showing no difference [15, 59, 66]. Prehospital research, including randomized controlled trials, carry logistical and ethical challenges, including difficulty with "cohort matching, sample sizes, and data collection" [23, 56, 68]. Increased survival to hospital, but no difference in in-hospital survival benefits [15]. This indicates the need to reevaluate how receiving hospitals manage trauma patients in hemorrhagic shock. See Table 36.5.

Summary and Conclusion

The practice of blood transfusion has evolved. While originally considered a risky practice, transfusion of blood products has become a staple of medical care around the world. In fact, blood donation is now highly regulated in the United States by the Food and Drug Administration. There are many kinds of blood products including whole blood, packed red blood cells, fresh frozen plasma, liquid plasma, platelets, and cryoprecipitate. Guidelines for transfusions vary from hospital to hospital and from society to society; however, the general purpose and backbone of various guidelines express similar things, and during a surgical procedure, the responsibility of transfusing blood usually falls on the anesthesiologist. Since there is so much variability in guidelines for blood transfusions, the Department of Defense funded three controlled, randomized trials: the COMBAT (Control of Major Bleeding After Trauma) trial, the PAMPer (Prehospital Air Medical Plasma) study, and the PUPTH (Prehospital Use of Plasma in Traumatic Hemorrhage) trial. However, prehospital research, including randomized controlled trials, carry logistical and ethical challenges, including difficulty with cohort matching, sample sizes, and data collection. In the future, there is a need for studies that are consistent and take these concerns into consideration.

References

1. Bolli R. William Harvey and the discovery of the circulation of the blood. Circ Res. 2019;124(9):1300–2.
2. Learoyd P. The history of blood transfusion prior to the 20th century--part 1. Transfus Med. 2012;22(5):308–14.
3. Learoyd P. The history of blood transfusion prior to the 20th century-part 2. Transfus Med. 2012;22:372–6.
4. Pfuntner A, Wier LM, Stocks C. Most frequent procedures performed in U.S. Hospitals, 2011: statistical brief #165. Healthcare Cost and Utilization Project (HCUP) statistical briefs; 2006.
5. Yaddanapudi S, Yaddanapudi LN. Indications for blood and blood product transfusion. Indian J Anaesth. Indian Society of Anaesthetists. 2014;58:538–42.
6. Curry N, Hopewell S, Dorée C, Hyde C, Brohi K, Stanworth S. The acute management of trauma hemorrhage: a systematic review of randomized controlled trials. Crit Care. 2011;15:R92.
7. Mikhail J. The trauma triad of death: hypothermia, acidosis, and coagulopathy. AACN Clin Issues. 1999;10(1):85–94.
8. Gaunt C, Woolley T. Management of haemorrhage in major trauma. Contin Educ Anaesth Crit Care Pain. 2014;14:251–5.
9. Gerecht R. The lethal triad. Hypothermia, acidosis & coagulopathy create a deadly cycle for trauma patients. JEMS. 2014;39(4):56–60.
10. Kauvar DS, Lefering R, Wade CE. Impact of hemorrhage on trauma outcome: an overview of epidemiology, clinical presentations, and therapeutic considerations. J Trauma Inj Infect Crit Care. 2006;60:S3–11.
11. Rehn M, Weaver AE, Eshelby S, Røislien J, Lockey DJ. Prehospital transfusion of red blood cells in civilian trauma patients. Transfus Med. 2018;28(4):277–83.
12. Carroll RC, Craft RM, Langdon RJ, Clanton CR, Snider CC, Wellons DD, et al. Early evaluation of acute traumatic coagulopathy by thrombelastography. Transl Res. 2009;154(1):34–9.
13. Brohi K, Singh J, Heron MCT. Acute traumatic coagulopathy. J Trauma Acute Care Surg. 2003;54(6):1127–30.
14. Geeraedts LMG, Pothof LAH, Caldwell E, De Lange-De Klerk ESM, D'Amours SK. Prehospital fluid resuscitation in hypotensive trauma patients: do we need a tailored approach? Injury. 2015;46:4–9.
15. Rehn M, Weaver A, Brohi K, Eshelby S, Green L, Røislien J, et al. Effect of prehospital red blood cell transfusion on mortality and time of death in civilian trauma patients. Shock. 2019;51(3):284–8.
16. Holcomb JB, Donathan DP, Cotton BA, Del Junco DJ, Brown G, von Wenckstern T, et al. Prehospital transfusion of plasma and red blood cells in trauma patients. Prehosp Emerg Care. 2015;19(1):1–9.
17. Zielinski MD, Stubbs JR, Berns KS, Glassberg E, Murdock AD, Shinar E, et al. Prehospital blood transfusion programs: capabilities and lessons learned. J Trauma Acute Care Surg. 2017;82:S70–8.
18. Borgman MA, Spinella PC, Perkins JG, Grathwohl KW, Repine T, Beekley AC, et al. The ratio of blood products transfused affects mortality in patients receiving massive transfusions at a combat support hospital. J Trauma Inj Infect Crit Care. 2007;63:805–13.
19. Holcomb JB, Tilley BC, Baraniuk S, Fox EE, Wade CE, Podbielski JM, et al. Transfusion of plasma, platelets, and red blood cells in a 1:1:1 vs a 1:1:2 ratio and mortality in patients with severe trauma: the PROPPR randomized clinical trial. JAMA. 2015;313:471–82.
20. Sperry JL, Guyette FX, Brown JB, Yazer MH, Triulzi DJ, Early-Young BJ, et al. Prehospital plasma during air medical transport in trauma patients at risk for hemorrhagic shock. N Engl J Med. 2018;379:315–26.
21. Shackelford SA, Del Junco DJ, Powell-Dunford N, Mazuchowski EL, Howard JT, Kotwal RS, et al. Association of prehospital blood product transfusion during medical evacuation of combat casualties in Afghanistan with acute and 30-day survival. JAMA. 2017;318:1581–91.
22. Moore HB, Moore EE, Chapman MP, McVaney K, Bryskiewicz G, Blechar R, et al. Plasma-first resuscitation to treat haemorrhagic shock during emergency ground transportation in an urban area: a randomised trial. Lancet. 2018;392(10144):283–91.
23. Rijnhout TWH, Wever KE, Marinus RHAR, Hoogerwerf N, Geeraedts LMG, Tan ECTH. Is prehospital blood transfusion effective and safe in haemorrhagic trauma patients? A systematic review and meta-analysis. Injury. 2019;50(5):1017–27.
24. Adams PW, Warren KA, Guyette FX, Yazer MH, Brown JB, Daily BJ, et al. Implementation of a prehospital air medical thawed plasma program. J Trauma Acute Care Surg. 2019;87:1077–81.
25. Org® WR, Lockwood W. Blood transfusions.
26. Howard PR. Basic and applied concepts of blood banking and transfusion practices.
27. Basu D, Kulkarni R. Overview of blood components and their preparation. Indian J Anaesth. 2014;58(5):529–37.
28. Cap AP, Beckett A, Benov A, Borgman M, Chen J, Corley JB, et al. Whole blood transfusion. Mil Med. 2018;183(suppl_2):44–51.
29. Arya RC, Wander G, Gupta P. Blood component therapy: which, when and how much. J Anaesthesiol Clin Pharmacol. 2011;27(2):278.
30. Kelley W, Guzman N. Fresh frozen plasma (FFP). In: StatPearls. Treasure Island: StatPearls Publishing; 2019.
31. Liumbruno G, Bennardello F, Lattanzio A, Piccoli P, Rossetti G, Italian Society of Transfusion Medicine and Immunohaematology (SIMTI) Work Group as IS of TM and I (SIMTI) W. Recommendations for the transfusion of plasma and platelets. Blood Transfus. 2009;7(2):132–50.
32. Holcomb JB, Tilley BC, Baraniuk S, Fox EE, Wade CE, Podbielski JM, et al. Transfusion of plasma, platelets, and red blood cells in a 1:1:1 vs a 1:1:2 ratio and mortality in patients with severe trauma. JAMA. 2015;313(5):471.
33. Orlov D, Karkouti K. The pathophysiology and consequences of red blood cell storage. Anaesthesia. 2015;70:29–e12.
34. American Association of Blood Banks. Regulatory affairs.
35. American Association of Blood Banks. AABB temperature standards 2018; 2018.
36. Hunter S, Nixon J, Murphy S. The effect of the interruption of agitation on plateletquality during storage for transfusion. Transfusion. 2001;41(6):809–14.
37. Pelican BioThermal Technologies. Crēdo™ Medic Pack Series 4 248 EMT.
38. Louzon MJ, Hess JR, Metcalf RA, Pagano MB. Establishing prehospital transfusion with Airlift Northwest and Harborview Medical Center; 2017.
39. Faretec Incorporated responder products. LifeBox 50 transport container.
40. Stein C, Caetano E. Transportation of blood in a helicopter emergency medical service: the importance of specialised equipment. SAJCC. 2016;32(2):62–3.
41. Dogde M, Thompson D, Bank EA, Nealy W, Fisher AD. Whole blood in EMS may save lives. J Emerg Med Serv. 2018;43(2):50–4.
42. Levon Vartanian M. Blood on the ground | EMS World.

43. Lehavi A, Yitzhak A, Jarassy R, Heizler R, Katz YS, Raz A. Comparison of the performance of battery-operated fluid warmers. Emerg Med J. 2018;35(9):564–70.
44. McGinity AC, Zhu CS, Greebon L, Xenakis E, Waltman E, Epley E, et al. Prehospital low-titer cold-stored whole blood. J Trauma Acute Care Surg. 2018;84:S115–9.
45. Malsby RF, Quesada J, Powell-Dunford N, Kinoshita R, Kurtz J, Gehlen W, et al. Prehospital blood product transfusion by U.S. Army MEDEVAC during combat operations in Afghanistan: a process improvement initiative. Mil Med. 2013;178(7):785–91.
46. Bodnar D, Rashford S, Hurn C, Quinn J, Parker L, Isoardi K, et al. Characteristics and outcomes of patients administered blood in the prehospital environment by a road based trauma response team. Emerg Med J. 2014;31(7):583–8.
47. Karl A, Pham T, Yanosky JD, Lubin J. Variability of uncrossmatched blood use by helicopter EMS programs in the United States. Prehosp Emerg Care. 2016;20(6):688–94.
48. Zhu CS, Pokorny DM, Eastridge BJ, Nicholson SE, Epley E, Forcum J, et al. Give the trauma patient what they bleed when and where they need it: establishing a comprehensive regional system of resuscitation based on patient need utilizing cold-stored, low-titer O+ whole blood. Transfusion. 2019;59:1429–38.
49. Apfelbaum JL, Nuttall GA, Connis RT, Harrison CR, Miller RD, Nickinovich DG. Practice guidelines for perioperative blood management. Anesthesiology. 2015;122(2):241–75.
50. Napolitano LM, Kurek S, Luchette FA, Corwin HL, Barie PS, Tisherman SA, et al. Clinical practice guideline: red blood cell transfusion in adult trauma and critical care*. Crit Care Med. 2009;37(12):3124–57.
51. Carson JL, Guyatt G, Heddle NM, Grossman BJ, Cohn CS, Fung MK, et al. Clinical practice guidelines from the AABB. JAMA. 2016;316(19):2025.
52. Sahu S, Hemlata AV. Adverse events related to blood transfusion. Indian J Anaesth. 2014;58(5):543–51.
53. Semple JW, Rebetz J, Kapur R. Transfusion-associated circulatory overload and transfusion-related acute lung injury. Blood. 2019;133(17):1840–53.
54. Roubinian N. TACO and TRALI: biology, risk factors, and prevention strategies. Hematology Am Soc Hematol Educ Program. 2018;2018(1):585–94.
55. Yasuda H, Ohto H, Yamaguchi O, Sakuma S, Suzuki T, Mita M, et al. Three episodes of delayed hemolytic transfusion reactions due to multiple red cell antibodies, anti-Di, anti-Jk and anti-E. Transfus Sci. 2000;23(2):107–12.
56. Shand S, Curtis K, Dinh M, Burns B. What is the impact of prehospital blood product administration for patients with catastrophic haemorrhage: an integrative review. Injury. 2019;50:226–34.
57. Peters JH, Smulders PSH, Moors XRJ, Bouman SJM, Meijs CMEM, Hoogerwerf N, et al. Are on-scene blood transfusions by a helicopter emergency medical service useful and safe? A multicentre case-control study. Eur J Emerg Med. 2019;26(2):128–32.
58. Tonglet ML, Greiffenstein P, Pitance F, Degesves S. Massive bleeding following severe blunt trauma: the first minutes that can change everything. Acta Chir Belg. 2016;116(1):11–5.
59. Holcomb JB, Swartz MD, DeSantis SM, Greene TJ, Fox EE, Stein DM, et al. Multicenter observational prehospital resuscitation on helicopter study (PROHS). J Trauma Acute Care Surg. 2017;83:S83.
60. Brown JB, Guyette FX, Neal MD, Claridge JA, Daley BJ, Harbrecht BG, et al. Taking the blood bank to the field: the design and rationale of the prehospital air medical plasma (PAMPer) trial HHS public access. Prehosp Emerg Care. 2015;19(3):343–50.
61. Eick BG, Denke NJ. Resuscitative strategies in the trauma patient: the past, the present, and the future. J Trauma Nurs. 2018;25(4):254–63.
62. Heuer M, Hussmann B, Lefering R, Kaiser GM, Eicker C, Guckelberger O, et al. Prehospital fluid management of abdominal organ trauma patients—a matched pair analysis. Langenbecks Arch Surg. 2015;400(3):371–9.
63. Sherren P, Burns B. Prehospital blood transfusion: 5-year experience of an Australian helicopter emergency medical service. Crit Care. 2013;17(Suppl 2):P295.
64. Heschl S, Andrew E, de Wit A, Bernard S, Kennedy M, Smith K. Prehospital transfusion of red cell concentrates in a paramedic-staffed helicopter emergency medical service. Emerg Med Australas. 2018;30(2):236–41.
65. Fahy AS, Thiels CA, Polites SF, Parker M, Ishitani MB, Moir CR, et al. Prehospital blood transfusions in pediatric trauma and non-trauma patients: a single-center review of safety and outcomes. Pediatr Surg Int. 2017;33(7):787–92.
66. Miller BT, Du L, Krzyzaniak MJ, Gunter OL, Nunez TC. Blood transfusion: in the air tonight? J Trauma Acute Care Surg. 2016;81(1):15–20.
67. Hernandez MC, Thiels CA, Aho JM, Habermann EB, Zielinski MD, Stubbs JA, et al. Prehospital plasma resuscitation associated with improved neurologic outcomes after traumatic brain injury. J Trauma Acute Care Surg. 2017;83(3):398–405.
68. Smith IM, James RH, Dretzke J, Midwinter MJ. Prehospital blood product resuscitation for trauma: a systematic review. Shock. 2016;46(1):3–16.

Whole Blood Is Back

37

Chris Murphy and Hyung Sun Choi

Abbreviations

CDP	Citrate phosphate dextrose
CPDA	Citrate phosphate dextrose adenine
EMS	Emergency medical services
FFP	Fresh frozen plasma
FST	Forward Surgical Team
FWB	Fresh whole blood
PRBCs	Packed red blood cells
PT	Prothrombin time
PTT	Partial thromboplastin time
SWB	Stored whole blood
WFWB	Warm fresh whole blood

Introduction

In the early years of transfusion therapy, whole blood was the only option available to practitioners. Over time with the emergence of blood banking technology and the fractionation of whole blood into its separate components, transfusion therapy and the treatment of hemorrhage have evolved away from the use of whole blood to component therapy. This allows for more efficient utilization of products. However, wide-scale use of warm fresh whole blood (WFWB) by the military in Iraq and Afghanistan has reignited interest in the civilian sector, with major trauma centers evaluating the use of whole blood in the treatment of hemorrhage. This chapter will examine the history of blood transfusions and the impact of trauma on coagulation and then provide the benefits of whole blood transfusions to component therapy in the treatment of traumatic hemorrhage and massive transfusion.

C. Murphy (✉)
Department of Anesthesiology, University of Mississippi Medical Center, Jackson, MS, USA
e-mail: cmurphy5@umc.edu

H. S. Choi
Department of Anesthesiology, Montefiore Medical Center, Bronx, NY, USA

The History of Blood Transfusion Therapy

The first documented blood transfusion into a human was performed in France in 1667. Dr. Jean-Baptiste Denys directly transfused blood from the femoral artery of a lamb through a silver tube inserted into the patient's vein. The transfusion was a success and prompted further experimentation with transfusion therapy. A subsequent patient received lamb to human transfusion with the goal of treating the man's psychosis, and he ended up receiving multiple transfusions due to the drastic improvement in his condition. He was later found to be suffering from neurosyphilis secondary to a *Treponema pallidum* infection, and the systemic reaction to the lamb's blood transfusion was causing a fever high enough to kill the bacteria. Due to continuing transfusion reactions in subsequent patients, the practice of blood transfusion was banned in England, France, and even by the Pope [1]. The practice of blood transfusion did not resume again until the 1800s, and in 1818, Dr. James Blundell, an obstetrician at Guy's Hospital, carried out the first documented direct transfusion when he aspirated venous blood from a donor with a syringe and injected it into a patient for the treatment of postpartum hemorrhage [2]. The practice was refined with the discovery of blood types by Karl Landsteiner in 1900, and further with the development of crossmatching techniques by Ottenberg in 1912 [1]. With the development of citrated solutions in 1910, it became possible to carry out the transfusion of stored whole blood, a practice that saw widespread use for the first time in World War I [3]. The emergence of blood banking from World War I was one of the most importance medical advances of the conflict, and it grew and refined over the course of the coming decades. With the advent of whole blood fractionation techniques following

© Springer Nature Switzerland AG 2021
C. S. Scher et al. (eds.), *Essentials of Blood Product Management in Anesthesia Practice*,
https://doi.org/10.1007/978-3-030-59295-0_37

Table 37.1 Possible indications for whole blood use

Indication		Reason
Pediatric	Neonatal exchange transfusion	Treatment of hyperbilirubinemia [6]
	Cardiac surgery	Minimize donor exposure [7]
	Craniofacial surgery	Reduced incidence of coagulopathy, minimized donor exposure [8]
Adult	Cardiac surgery (autologous transfusion)	Improved platelet function, minimized coagulopathy, reduced need for allogenic blood [9]
	Obstetric hemorrhage	Volume resuscitation, correction of coagulopathy [10]

World War II, it came to be agreed upon that donated whole blood could be used more efficiently if it was separated into packed red cells (PRBCs), fresh frozen plasma (FFP), platelet concentrates, and cryoprecipitate. This modern practice of blood banking makes it possible to correct hematologic deficiencies with specific components, so now a single donated unit of whole blood may serve many patients. Facing a potential shortage of donors in the years to come, this solution was much more desirable and economic. As a result, the use of whole blood therapy fell out of common practice in the civilian community. Over the 1970s and 1980s, the transition was made from whole blood therapy to component therapy [4]. The current-day indications for whole blood use are few and far between (Table 37.1). The current guideline for treatment of massive hemorrhage in civilian practice is replacement of components in a 1:1:1 ratio of PRBCs, FFP, and platelet concentrates, which has become accepted and promoted as a standard of care by the American College of Surgeons [5]. However, there is limited data to support this drastic shift in practice, the aim of which is to replicate whole blood.

Despite the advances in blood banking to come, fresh whole blood continued to be the military's treatment of choice for traumatic hemorrhage through World War II and Vietnam. It continues to saw widespread utilization, and has as recently as Operation Iraqi Freedom, where 13% of the patients who received blood transfusions received fresh whole blood. The continued use in the military was borne out of necessity. The earliest levels of care in the combat trauma chain are known as Forward Surgical Teams (FST). These teams focus on damage control, aiming to stabilize patients for transport to a higher level of care. Given the sometimes-remote locations of these teams, often the only available blood products are PRBCs. This is due to the level of resources required for the storage of FFP and platelets. Given the limited amount of blood products available, this supply can be rapidly depleted by one severe trauma. This necessitates the utilization of a "walking donor program" which allows the rapid integration of fresh whole blood (FWB) into the resuscitation algorithm during situations when RBC requirements have outpaced the available supplies. It is this recent utilization of whole blood that has piqued the interest of civilian trauma surgeons for possible utilization in the treatment of hemorrhage and coagulopathy.

Trauma and the Resultant Coagulopathy

Trauma is a major public health issue in the United States. Traumatic injuries remain the leading cause of death for Americans up to the age of 45, and it is the fourth leading cause of death overall for all ages in the United States [11]. Data from the US military shows that up to 80% of the preventable traumatic deaths are secondary to hemorrhage [12], and if this is applied to civilian data, it accounts for a substantial number of preventable deaths each year in the United States. Furthermore, data shows that deaths due to hemorrhage usually occur within the first 24 hours of presentation to a hospital [13], making early identification and control of hemorrhage, as well as correction of coagulopathy, a major priority in order to improve survival.

Coagulopathy has long been associated with trauma and recognized as a major contributor to trauma-related mortality [14]. Recent data shows that independent of all other variables, the initial prothrombin time (PT) and partial thromboplastin time (PTT) are independent predictors of all-cause mortalities in trauma patients. An initial PT elevated above 14.0 seconds is associated with a 35% increase in mortality, while an initial elevated PTT was associated with a 32% increase in all mortality [15]. With this in mind, it is important to understand the cause of the coagulopathy associated with trauma and the most efficient way to correct it in order to save future lives and resources [16].

In the setting of severe trauma coagulopathy is nearly universal is likely due to loss of coagulation factors and platelets to hemorrhage, as well as consumption of clotting component [17]. This will be further complicated and exacerbated by the triad known as the "vicious bloody cycle": hemodilution, hypothermia, and acidosis [18].

Hemodilution

First and foremost, coagulation factors and platelets will be lost directly in bleeding. This loss is exacerbated as blood pressure drops and interstitial fluid is mobilized into the vascular space to make up for the losses, further diluting the clotting elements that remain [17]. Lastly, the replacement of the lost blood volume during the resuscitation will further dilute the clotting elements in the blood. Recent studies show that in instances where larger volumes of crystalloid have been used for trauma resuscitation, a deleterious effect on outcomes, leading to an increased mortality and longer need for mechanical ventilation [19]. The repletion of lost blood volume with crystalloid will also lead to further hemodilution of clotting factors. While counterintuitive, this also holds true with blood components.

When a 500 mL unit of blood is processed into components, 180 mL of solutions containing a variety of preservatives (dextrose, mannitol, sodium phosphate, sodium bicarbonate, etc.) is added. The resulting 680 mL solution is one of components that is anemic (hematocrit < 30%), acidotic (pH < 7), and thrombocytopenic (80,000 platelets per microliter) and has a concentration of coagulation factors that is 60% that of whole blood [3]. If a patient were to receive 10 units of PRBCs, that patient will have lost around 70% of their plasma and coagulation factors, resulting in a prolongation of the PT and PTT.

Hypothermia

In the setting of trauma, hypothermia will usually begin at the time of the injury due to decreased motor activity resulting in decreased heat generation and increased loss of heat [17]. This will be continued upon arrival to a trauma center, as the patient is immobilized and exposed in the trauma bay for further examination. Resuscitation fluids are administered, which may not be warmed. If the patient undergoes surgery, conductive heat loss will occur as the patient lies on potentially blood saturated sheets, as heat is redistributed from the core to the periphery secondary to vasodilation from general anesthesia, and heat will be lost as moisture evaporated from the exposed visceral and serosal surfaces [20]. For each degree centigrade the body temperature lowers, the rate of the reactions of plasma coagulation is reduced by 10% [21]. Additionally, lower temperatures have adverse effects on the activation of platelets and von Willebrand factor, which will be completely inactivated at temperatures below 30 °C [22]. In conditions of hypothermia, platelets are unable to synthesize thromboxane, which is instrumental in the initiation of the vasoconstriction phase of the clotting cascade. This defect is completely reversible if the patient is rewarmed [23]. If core body temperature drops below 34 °C, coagulopathy rapidly progresses, and below 32 °C, the coagulopathy is so severe that bleeding often cannot be stopped and is fatal [17].

Acidosis

Acidosis will have a direct effect on both the intrinsic and extrinsic coagulation pathways, prolonging both the PT and PTT, as well as affecting platelet activation and aggregation. At a pH of 6.8, these tests will become abnormal. At a pH of 6.4, the function of coagulation factors is reduced by half, and platelet aggregation is decreased by more than half [24].

Component Therapy

As was previously mentioned, the current standard of practice in the resuscitation of severe hemorrhage is known as damage control resuscitation, where the patient receives equal parts RBCs, FFP, and platelets (i.e., 1:1:1 transfusion ratio) [25]. The aim of this resuscitation is to replicate whole blood in vivo. However, due to the addition of preservatives and anticoagulants to the stored blood components, it is not possible to duplicate whole blood in vivo.

One modern unit of packed, leukoreduced RBCs typically measures between 330 and 350 mL of volume. Around 195 mL of this will be RBCs and the rest in a suspending fluid. This unit will also subject the patient to a significant burden of acid and cold, as they are stored between 1 and 6 °C. After 2 weeks of storage, it will have a pH below 7. If not properly rewarmed during infusion, for example, during a massive transfusion situation when time is of the essence, 5 units of cold RBCs would be expected to lower the body temperature of a 70 kg man by 1 °C [17].

One unit of FFP contains 80% of the plasma from one unit of whole blood, usually in a volume of 220–250 mL. Of that total volume, 80% will be plasma and the rest additives. When transfused, one unit of FFP will deliver 500 mg of fibrinogen and 200 units of all of the other coagulation factors. This means that five units of FFP will contain close to one total liter of plasma, which is enough to replace only around 25% of the coagulation factors of a 70 kg man. Stored at 4 °C, thawed FFP will pose a thermal burden similar to that of RBCs [17].

Apheresis platelets contain at least 3.0 × 1011 platelets and are stored at 20–24 °C. Due to their higher storage temperature, they pose less of a thermal burden than RBCs and FFP [17]. However, stored platelets do demonstrate a decreased thrombotic function, secondary to a decrease in expression of high-affinity thrombin receptors during storage [26].

Bearing all of this in mind, it can seem irrational to approach massive transfusion situations with a clinical strategy that will deliver a mixture that is, under the best of conditions, anemic, thrombocytopenic, and acidotic with 60% the concentration of coagulation proteins [3]. This obligates providers to consider an alteration to the standard of care and to find a better solution for massive transfusion situations with a more physiologic profile. And providers need to look no further than whole blood.

The Re-emergence of Whole Blood

The original blood used for the first 250 years of transfusions, whole blood has worked its way back into the discussion for the treatment of massive hemorrhage. Its use in military settings has prompted discussion for implementation in civilian practice, including recent randomized controlled trials in the United States. One such pilot study was recently carried out at a level I trauma center in Texas [27]. When discussing transfusion options for whole blood, there are two to consider.

Warm Fresh Whole Blood

WFWB is defined as whole blood collected and transfused within a time span of 24 hours. In a combat situation, a transfusion may occur within minutes of donation. The "walking donor program" previously discussed relies on the utilization of WFWB to deliver large amounts of blood in a short amount of time. Due to the minimal amount of processing involved in the collection and the minimal amount of anticoagulant required upon procurement of the unit, this is the most optimal choice of resuscitation fluid in a massive transfusion situation. Due to the significant buffering capacity of whole blood, WFWB can be stored at room temperature for up to 24 hours and still remain usable with preservation of the function of platelets and plasma coagulation factors [28]. However, it is not approved for use in the civilian setting by the US Food and Drug Administration (FDA), as it does not undergo disease screening prior to use (this risk being mitigated in the military setting by the pre-screening of soldiers for blood-borne diseases).

Stored Whole Blood

Stored whole blood (SWB) is a unit of blood that is refrigerated to a temperature from 1 to 6 °C within 8 hours of donation and minimally processed. Although some preservatives are added, they are done so at smaller volumes, and the blood still undergoes leukoreduction. However, the final product does not undergo fractionation into the individual components [3]. This product can be refrigerated and stored for up to 21 days in citrate phosphate dextrose (CDP) or for up to 35 days in citrate phosphate dextrose adenine (CPDA-1) [29]. SWB is FDA approved for use in the civilian setting when stored in the appropriate anticoagulant solutions and tested for transfusion-related diseases [30].

The Argument for Stored Whole Blood

Recent studies show that in adhering to component therapy administered in a 1:1:1 ratio of PRBCs, FFP, and apheresis platelets, the product being delivered to the patient does not resemble blood in vivo as much as was initially believed. Due to the addition of preservative solutions and anticoagulants, the mixture of fluid delivered to the patient is diluted to a hematocrit of 29% and a platelet count of 90,000/μL (Table 37.2). In addition, the coagulation factors are only 62% as concentrated compared to those of SWB, and the endogenous thrombin potential is significantly reduced [31].

Historically, a concern with storage of blood products has been diminishing platelet and hemostatic function with storage. Current standards for storage of platelets mandate that they are maintained between 20 and 24 °C for no longer than 5 days from the date of collection [17]. This understandably poses a question about the viability of platelets during the storage of whole blood units. Despite these concerns, platelet function and the overall hemostatic function of a unit of cold whole blood stored for up 14–21 days remains comparable to that of a traditional unit of platelets stored at room temperature [32]. Furthermore, previous studies in cardiac surgery have also shown improved platelet function of SWB compared to the function of apheresis platelets delivered as a part of component therapy. In one such study, the data revealed that providing one unit of whole blood increased the patient's platelet count by a quantity comparable to providing six platelet units, with an increase in mean platelet volume to a level higher than that achieved by providing ten platelet units [33].

Current data shows that when transfused via a rapid rewarming infuser, SWB provides a superior product for resuscitation than component therapy. Whole blood provides a product that will most closely resemble what the patient is losing, and does so with a smaller overall volume of blood

Table 37.2 Comparison of blood components vs. stored whole blood [14, 17]

	PRBCs	FFP	Platelets	SWB
Volume (1 unit)	300–350 mL	220–250 mL	200–300 mL	500 mL
Contents	195 mL RBCs 155 mL suspending fluid (preservative solution, anticoagulant)	20% solution of citrate, sugar, and anticoagulant	50 mL anticoagulated plasma 10 mL citrate and sugar solution	70 mL anticoagulant and preservative solution
	Combination: Volume 720–900 mL Hematocrit 29% 90,000 platelets/μL 62% coagulation factor activity			Hematocrit 38–50% 150–400 k platelets/μL 100% coagulation factor activity

product required, and a smaller volume of preservative and anticoagulant solution exposed to the patient. An additional benefit to stored whole blood is decreased donor exposure.

Challenges for Implementation

While the benefits of whole blood transfusion have been reflected in recent data, there are still several obstacles to its widespread implementation in civilian practice. Due to the current prevalence of component therapy, most blood banks at this time will be unfamiliar with the storage and processing of whole blood. Another important logistical challenge will be the availability of whole blood for emergency medical services (EMS) on patient transport vehicles. In the prehospital setting, whole blood transfusion could have a tremendous impact on patient care and in preventing early coagulopathy of trauma. Given whole blood's relatively short shelf life compared to that of PRBCs, guidelines and protocols must be developed early to ensure proper storage and handling of cold whole blood.

These logistical challenges are best addressed by multidisciplinary teams involving every level of patient care under the direction of physicians from anesthesiology, surgery, and emergency medicine. Such teams will be crucial in the development of standardized protocols for the collection, testing, and storage of whole blood units, as well as the indications and contraindications for transfusion. These protocols will provide a firm foundation upon which to build a whole blood transfusion program and will help to overcome and adapt to any unforeseen obstacles with initiation of the program.

Conclusion

Once the only option for transfusion therapy, the use of whole blood for transfusion became less common with the emergence of modern blood banking and component therapy. However, continued successful use of whole blood transfusions in military theaters has prompted new investigations into its utilization in a civilian setting. The re-emergence of whole blood offers the most physiologic solution for treating coagulopathy and drastically simplifies transfusion protocols and therapy in guiding patient care. With current trials taking place at major trauma centers across the United States, whole blood transfusion offers a wealth of potential to have a profound impact anesthesia practices going forward.

References

1. Spinella PC. Warm fresh whole blood transfusion for severe hemorrhage: US Military and potential civilian applications. Crit Care Med. 2008;36(7):30–5.
2. Loong ED, Law PR, Healey JN. Fresh blood by direct transfusion for haemostatic failure in massive haemorrhage. Anaesth Intensive Care. 1975;9(4):371–5.
3. Zielinski MD, Jenkins DH, Hughes JD, Badjie KS, Stubbs JR. Back to the future: the renaissance of whole-blood transfusions for massively hemorrhaging patients. Surgery. 2004;155:883–6.
4. Repine TB, Perkins JG, Kauvar DS, Blackborne L. The use of whole fresh blood in massive transfusion. J Trauma. 2005;60(6):59–66.
5. American College of Surgeons Committee on Trauma. Advanced Trauma Life Support Student Manual; 1994:87–9.
6. Girelli G, Antoncecchi S, Casadei AM, et al. Recommendations for transfusion therapy in neonatology. Blood Transfus. 2015;13(3):484–97.
7. Jobes DR, Sesok-Pizzini D, Friedman D. Reduced transfusion requirement with use of fresh whole blood in pediatric cardiac surgical procedures. Ann Thorac Surg. 2015;99:1706–12.
8. Thottahil P, Sesok-Pizzini D, Taylor JA, Fiadjoe JE, Vincent A, Stricker PA. Whole blood in pediatric craniofacial reconstruction surgery. J Craniofac Surg. 2017;28(5):1175–8.
9. Martin K, Keller E, Gertler R, Tassani P, Wiesner G. Efficiency and safety of preoperative autologous blood donation in cardiac surgery: a matched-pair analysis in 432 patients. Eur J Cardiothorac Surg. 2010;37(6):1396–401.
10. Alexander JM, Sarode R, McIntire DD, Burner JD, Leveno KJ. Whole blood in the management of hypovolemia due to obstetric hemorrhage. Obstet Gynecol. 2009;113:1320–6.
11. American Association for the Surgery of Trauma [Internet]. Chicago; c2019. Trauma Facts. Available from http://www.aast.org/trauma-facts
12. Bellamy RF. The causes of death in conventional land warfare: implications for combat casualty care research. Mil Med. 1984;149:55–62.
13. Demetriades D, Murray J, Charalambides K, et al. Trauma fatalities: time and location of hospital deaths. J Am Coll Surg. 2004;198:20–6.
14. McNamara JJ, Burran EL, Stremple JF, Molot MD. Coagulopathy after major combat injury: occurrence, management, and pathophysiology. Ann Surg. 1972;176(2):243–6.
15. MacLeod JB, Lynn M, McKenny MG, Cohn SM, Murtha M. Early coagulopathy predicts mortality in trauma. J Trauma. 2003;55(1):39–44.
16. Kauvar DS, Holcomb JB, Norris GC, Hess JR. Fresh whole blood transfusion: a controversial military practice. J Trauma. 2006;61(1):181–4.
17. Armand R, Hess JR. Treating coagulopathy in trauma patients. Transfus Med Rev. 2003;17(3):223–31.
18. Johnson JL, Moore EE, Kashuk JL, et al. Effect of blood products transfusion on the development of postinjury multiple organ failure. Arch Surg. 2010;145(10):973–7.
19. Jones DG, Nantais J, Rezende-Neto JB, Yazdani S, Vegas P, Rizoli S. Crystalloid resuscitation in trauma patients: deleterious effect of 5L or more in the first 24h. BMC Surg. 2018;18:93.
20. Burch JM, Denton JR, Noble RD. Physiologic rationale for abbreviated laparotomy. Surg Clin N Am. 1997;4(1):779–82.
21. Watts DD, Trask A, Soeken K, et al. Hypothermic coagulopathy in trauma: effect of varying levels of hypothermia on enzyme speed, platelet function, and fibrinolytic activity. J Trauma. 1998;44:846–54.
22. Kermode JC, Zheng Q, Milner EP. Marked temperature dependence of the platelet calcium signal induced by human von Willebrand factor. Blood. 1999;94(1):199–207.
23. *Grosso SM, Keenan JO. Whole blood transfusion for exsanguinating coagulopathy in a US Field Surgical Hospital in Postwar Kosovo. J Trauma. 2000;49:145–8.
24. Green FW, Kaplan MM, Curtis LE, Levine PH. Effect of acid and pepsin on blood coagulation and platelet aggregation: a possible

contributor to prolonged gastroduodenal mucosal hemorrhage. Gastroenterology. 1978;74:38–43.

25. Holcomb JB, Jenkins D, Rhee P, et al. Damage control resuscitation: directly addressing the early coagulopathy of trauma. J Trauma. 2007;62(2):307–10.
26. Lozano ML, Rivera J, Gonzalez-Conejero R, Moraleda JM, Vicente V. Loss of high-affinity thrombin receptors during platelet concentrate storage impairs the reactivity of platelets to thrombin. Transfusion. 1997;37:368–75.
27. Cotton BA, Podbielski J, Camp E, Welch T, del Junco D, Bai Y, Hobbs RM, Scroggins JM, Hartwell B, Kozar RA, Wade CE, Holcomb J. A randomized controlled pilot trial of modified whole blood versus component therapy in severely injured patients requiring large volume transfusions. Ann Surg. 2013;258(4):527–33.
28. Hughes JD, Macdonald VW, Hess JR. Warm storage of whole blood for 72 hours. Transfusion. 2007;47:2050–6.
29. Kurup PA, Arun P, Gayathri NS, Dhanya CR, Indu AR. Modified formulation of CPDA for storage of whole bood, and of SAGM for storage of red blood cells, to maintain the concentration of 2,3-diphosphoglycerate. Vox Sang. 2003;85(4):253–61.
30. Administration FDA. Code of Federal Regulations Title 21. Chapter I – Food and Drug Administration Department of Health and Human Services 2018.
31. Ponschab M, Schöchl H, Gabriel C, Süssner S, Cadamuro J, Haschke-Becher E, Gratz J, Zipperle J, Redl H, Schlimp CJ. Haemostatic profile of reconstituted blood in a proposed 1:1:1 ratio of packed red blood cells, platelet concentrate and four different plasma preparations. Anaesthesia. 2015;70:528–36.
32. Pivalizza EG, Stephens CT, Sridhar S, Gumbert SD, Rossman S, Bertholf MF, Bai Y, Cotton BA. Whole blood for resuscitation in adult civilian trauma in 2017: a narrative review. Anesth Analg. 2018;127(1):157–.
33. Lavee J, Martinowitz U, Mohr R, Goor DA, Golan M, Langsam J, Malik Z, Savion N. The effect of transfusion of fresh whole blood versus platelet concentrates after cardiac operations. A scanning electron microscope study of platelet aggregation on extracellular matrix. J Thorac Cardiovasc Surg. 1989;97(2):204–12.

Normal Saline: Not So Normal at All in the Bleeding Patient

38

Brandan Kovacs, Hermandeep Dhami, and Erica Ash

Introduction

The discussion of blood products would be incomplete without mention of the role that non-blood fluids play in resuscitation. The infusion of crystalloid fluids is a clinical tool often used when blood products are limited or unavailable. Crystalloids serve as a means to rapidly volume resuscitate a patient that may be otherwise hypovolemic and hypotensive or, to a greater degree, in shock. The ultimate goal of intravenous fluid resuscitation is to maintain end-organ perfusion in situations where it is not feasible to rapidly infuse blood products.

While there are many crystalloid options, including plasmalyte, acetate buffered solutions, dextrose in water, normal saline, lactated Ringer's, and several more, the two most common crystalloids are lactated Ringer's and normal saline [1]. Normal saline is the focus of this chapter. The history and composition of normal saline, including its role and limitation in resuscitation, as well as current trends regarding crystalloid resuscitation are presented.

A Brief History of Normal Saline

What makes normal saline "normal?" The definitive origins for normal saline are not entirely clear. Historical references indicate that the first forays into the development of intravenous fluids occurred during the initial outbreak of the English cholera epidemic in 1831 [2]. Cholera-afflicted victims experienced severe diarrheal illness. The practitioners of the time sought a treatment that would improve survival in these patients who experienced dehydration secondary to significant gastrointestinal fluid loss. One of the potential treatments was to infuse a solution with a similar consistency to blood in the hopes of creating a net neutral fluid balance. These early fluid administration techniques are unrecognizable compared to common practices. With significant ongoing research into determining the composition of a physiologically neutral fluid, several fluids were investigated and proposed to fit this billing. It was during this period of research that the initial Ringer's solution was formulated, although even this formula is subtly different than the current design. W.S. Barlow cited the first reference to a study regarding 0.92% saline as nearly physiologic in the mid-1890s [2]. This cited study, performed by Dr. Hartog Jacob Hamburger, was an in vitro study of the effects of varying concentrations of saline on the hemolysis of blood. In his study, Hamburger discovered that saline concentrations of 0.9% had a similar freezing point to human serum and were the least likely to cause hemolysis. For physicians of this time, this discovery implied that 0.9% is the most physiological and therefore "normal." Hamburger subsequently referred to this fluid as "indifferent fluid" which was eventually altered to its current name, normal saline [3]. The exact trajectory from this single in vitro study to widespread in vivo use is unclear. One thought is that the simplicity of mixing salt and water was easy and inexpensive and therefore became ubiquitous [2]. While Hamburger's trial holds biological relevance as the lack of hemolysis being a particularly important quality of an infused fluid, he did not quite hit the mark. It is important to note that normal saline is neither "indifferent," "normal," nor physiologic to human serum.

B. Kovacs (✉) · H. Dhami
New York University Grossman School of Medicine, Department of Anesthesiology, Perioperative Care, and Pain Medicine, NYU Langone Medical Center, New York, NY, USA
e-mail: Brandan.Kovacs@nyulangone.org

E. Ash
NYU Langone Medical Center, Department of Anesthesiology, Perioperative Care, and Pain Medicine, New York, NY, USA

© Springer Nature Switzerland AG 2021
C. S. Scher et al. (eds.), *Essentials of Blood Product Management in Anesthesia Practice*,
https://doi.org/10.1007/978-3-030-59295-0_38

The Composition of Normal Saline

In the simplest terms, the composition of normal saline is merely sodium chloride, better known as salt water. Sodium and chloride dissociate when dissolved in water. One liter of normal saline contains 154 millimoles per liter (mmol/L) each of sodium and chloride. Normal saline has a pH of 5.0 and an osmolarity of 309 milliosmoles (mOsm) [3]. To compare these values to normal human physiology, blood sodium levels typically range between 135 and 145 mmol/L, and chloride is typically between 98 and 107 mmol/L. The normal physiologic pH of human blood is described as 7.4, and osmolarity ranges from 275 to 295 mOsm [3]. Thus, normal saline is hypernatremic, hyperchloremic, acidotic, and hyperosmolar when compared to human baseline, confirming that it is far from normal or physiologic. Infusion of normal saline has predictable side effects based on the obvious differences between the crystalloid fluid and human serum. Given the significant excess of chloride ions in normal saline compared to serum, hyperchloremic acidosis is perhaps the most notable. Rapid infusion of normal saline causes a rise in chloride ions which leads to a corresponding increase in the elimination of bicarbonate. This practice causes a predictable, dose-dependent hyperchloremic non-gap metabolic acidosis following normal saline administration [4]. While normal saline is clearly hypernatremic compared to human serum, studies demonstrate that the sodium burden is insufficient to cause clinical hypernatremia, provided preserved kidney function in the patient. It is important to note that critical patients with severe renal dysfunction are relatively incapable of regulating their intake and water-solute balance and may have subsequent sodium dysregulation. This notion, however, should be considered the exception rather than the rule [5].

Why Use Normal Saline?

Normal saline bears little resemblance to human serum, particularly in relation to sodium, chloride, and acidity levels. Why use normal saline at all? The exact historical reasons are nebulous; however, modern history offers context. Many soldiers in the Vietnam War who experienced severe blood loss had improved survival following rapid administration of blood products or crystalloid fluids. The observed ratio during this time of crystalloid infusion to blood loss was found to be roughly 2:1 or 3:1. This historical footnote was adopted into guidelines with little further study and became part of the Advanced Trauma Life Support (ATLS) protocol [6]. Perhaps the most significant reason for crystalloid administration as fluid resuscitation in the recent era relates to a study published in the early 2000s on fluid administration in sepsis. This 2001 *New England Journal of Medicine* published study demonstrated that the administration of a 30 milliliter per kilogram (ml/kg) bolus over the first 3 hours after identification of sepsis, known as early goal-directed therapy (EGDT), decreased mortality [7]. Sepsis is widely prevalent and has high rates of mortality. This study bore significant clinical promise and was quickly embodied in the guideline recommendations set by the following Surviving Sepsis Campaign. The significance of this finding has been challenged, however, as of late as three large multicenter trials demonstrated no survival benefit when employing EGDT. Furthermore, studies in resource-deprived environments support an increase in mortality when fluid bolus was used as early therapy [8]. With evidence of this contradiction emerging, the 2016 Surviving Sepsis Campaign guidelines issued a strong recommendation for continuation of the 30 ml/kg EGDT fluid resuscitation with crystalloids while simultaneously acknowledging that there was limited evidence to support the benefit of this intervention. The three large multicenter trials were specifically cited as giving evidence contrary to the initial position on EGDT, but the Surviving Sepsis authors also referenced that in the three multicenter trials, there was no clearly identified harm and as such the potential benefits of fluid resuscitation may outweigh any unidentified harms [9]. Other trials indicate that the known hyperchloremic metabolic acidosis from normal saline use is associated with increased mortality. Normal saline has been shown to preferentially decrease renal glomerular flow compared to plasmalyte. The combination of hyperchloremia, acidosis, and decreased renal perfusion is associated with an increased risk for acute kidney injury (AKI), particularly in critically ill patients. Use of alternative fluids avoided this increased risk in these trials [10].

Normal Saline Versus Balanced Crystalloids

While data demonstrates both support and opposition for normal saline use, several recent studies have compared the use of normal saline to balanced crystalloids in order to determine if the use of these fluids provides a greater physiological benefit than the theoretical harms of normal saline. Balanced crystalloids, such as plasmalyte and lactated Ringer's solution, have a content that better matches human serum parameters. Are the compositional differences between normal saline and balanced crystalloids distinctive enough to cause clinically significant differences in patient outcomes?

One meta-analysis looked at nine randomized controlled trials that compared the use of normal saline to balanced crystalloids in critically ill patients. The primary outcome was differences in mortality, and secondary outcomes included acute kidney injury and the risk of receiving renal replacement therapy related to previously established side effects of normal saline infusion. The findings ultimately determined no difference between the two groups, but the study listed a limitation of not further subcategorizing the critically ill patients. This limitation gives pause when considering whether normal saline differs from balanced crystalloids in a physiologically at-risk patient such as in decompensated heart failure or end-stage renal disease. This limitation highlights the importance of ongoing research [11].

Another recent study, a retrospective cohort, sought to compare the differences between normal saline and plasmalyte use in the treatment of diabetic ketoacidosis (DKA). This research was prompted by a prior study associating hyperchloremic metabolic acidosis related to normal saline use as a contributing factor in prolonging time to episode resolution in DKA patients [12]. Eighty-four patients with DKA were evaluated – 23 assigned to resuscitation with plasmalyte and 61 to normal saline. The primary outcome of mean time of resolution was similar between the two groups. However, there was a statistically significant rise in pH for the 4- to 6-hour and 6-to 12-hour period for those resuscitated with plasmalyte. The limitation of this study is that pH was only measured in a small portion of the study population [13]. Ultimately, both of these studies highlight the importance of further randomized controlled trials that explore the effects of normal saline's composition on resuscitation in various disease states, though they each failed to identify clinically significant differences between the administration of normal saline and balanced crystalloid.

Other studies have sought to determine which fluid is the best following initial resuscitation. One recent study in burn patients compared lactated Ringer's solution, a balanced crystalloid, to dextrose in normal saline in terms of maintenance for evaporative losses after burn injury. This study found that patients receiving exclusively lactated Ringer's solution were more likely to become hyponatremic over time, most likely due to the lower sodium concentration. Additionally, this study found that patients in the lactated ringer's solution only group were more likely to have lower blood glucose levels. Patients enrolled in the dextrose in normal saline group were more likely to have both a normal sodium level and higher blood glucose levels [14]. The authors refer to this study as evidence that even current balanced crystalloids are not physiologically similar enough to be used as maintenance fluids exclusively. There is no conclusive determination at this time whether normal saline or balanced crystalloids are superior. The decision of which fluid to use for resuscitation and maintenance will vary by situation until further research can show significant benefit toward a given fluid.

Emerging Trends in Crystalloid Administration: The Trauma Patient

The accepted protocol for administering crystalloid fluids to replace blood loss in trauma patients has existed since the Vietnam War [6]. With this recommendation ingrained in ATLS protocol for decades, change has been slow paced regarding this field. Recently, several studies challenged this dogma. These studies focus on the concept of damage control resuscitation (DCR), providing the least resuscitation possible to keep "the ship," in this case the human body, from sinking. The theory behind DCR is multifactorial, with hyperchloremic metabolic acidosis, mean arterial pressure, coagulopathy, and crystalloid volume infused as all factors. The final key component of DCR is damage control surgery to induce hemostasis prior to correcting any underlying abnormalities. Studies show that a focus on DCR leads to decreased mortality in severely injured trauma patients, yet is associated with other morbidity.

Comparatively low mean arterial pressure is a core concept of DCR. Studies demonstrate that goal mean arterial pressures (MAPs) of 50 mm of mercury (mmHg) are associated with decreased coagulopathy and bleeding when compared to the previously accepted standard of care of the MAPs of 65 mmHg goal. The prevailing theory as to the mechanism of this benefit is related to clot formation itself. In the actively bleeding trauma patient, hypovolemia leads to decreased blood pressure, and small, tenuous clots may be able to form at these sites of bleeding. While elevated MAPs may be advantageous for tissue perfusion, they may additionally be responsible for the rupture of these tenuous initial clots and lead to further bleeding. Maintenance of the lower goal MAPs of 50 mmHg has not been shown to be associated with increased 30-day mortality and is associated with increased incidence of lower blood loss volumes. The recommendation of DCR is to use fewer infused fluids and to infuse smaller volume boluses to maintain these low MAPs.

Coagulopathy is common in trauma patients. The underlying cause of this deregulation is unclear, but may be due to ongoing bleeding and consumption of coagulation factors. DCR proposes that the infusion of large volumes of clear fluids can cause further dilutional coagulopathy that will prolong bleeding. Instead, DCR focuses on goal-directed reversal of coagulopathy with blood products to minimize this dilutional coagulopathy. In resource-limited settings, or if blood products are not readily available, usage of limited clear fluids is an acceptable resuscitation strategy. Recent data shows that a more appropriate ratio of blood loss to crystalloid replacement may be closer to 1:1.6 rather than the traditional 1:3 espoused by ATLS.

Hyperchloremic metabolic acidosis is a concern addressed previously in this chapter but is again emphasized in

DCR. DCR recommends against using hyperchloremic fluids in non-cerebral trauma because of the risk of AKI. Instead, DCR favors balanced crystalloids for limited volume resuscitation. There is one notable exception to this recommendation in the case of cerebral trauma. Normal saline remains the recommended crystalloid fluid in cerebral trauma due to its association with reduced edema and swelling of brain tissue. Normal saline is slightly hypertonic compared to balanced crystalloid solutions. Overall, the advent of DCR may signal a significant paradigm shift in the usage of crystalloids in resuscitation [15–17].

Conclusion

Normal saline is a key crystalloid fluid that has been historically used for volume resuscitation. There are several known risks associated with normal saline, most notably hyperchloremic metabolic acidosis and kidney dysfunction. Despite these risks, studies have been largely unsuccessful in determining clinically significant differences between normal saline and balanced crystalloids, although emerging data may more clearly show an increased risk of AKI in specific populations. For decades, ATLS has delineated the accepted ratio of blood loss to crystalloid to be 1:3. This practice has been challenged of late, both by the suggestion of new blood loss to fluid ratios, 1:1.6, and new treatment algorithms such as DCR. These arguments both advocate for limited crystalloid resuscitation. While the growing body of data suggests that increased use of blood products may be beneficial compared to clear fluid administration, there will likely always be resource limitations that will drive providers to use crystalloid fluids. With many recent and ongoing trials providing new data, the future use of normal saline is ambiguous. For the time being, however, normal saline remains a valuable clinical tool.

References

1. Epstein EM, Waseem M. Crystalloid fluids. StatPearls [Internet]. Treasure Island: StatPearls Publishing; 2019.
2. Awad S, Allison SP, Lobo DN. The history of 0.9% saline. Clin Nutr. 2008;27(2):179–88.
3. Li H, Sun S-R, Yap JQ, Chen J-H, Qian Q. 0.9% saline is neither normal nor physiological. J Zhejiang Univ Sci B. 2016;17(3):181–7.
4. Eisenhut M. Adverse effects of rapid isotonic saline infusion. Arch Dis Child. 2006;91(9):797–.
5. Sam R, Feizi I. Understanding hypernatremia. Am J Nephrol. 2012;36(1):97–104.
6. Krausz MM. Initial resuscitation of hemorrhagic shock. World J Emerg Surg. 2006;1:14.
7. Rivers E, Nguyen B, Havstad S, Ressler J. Early goal-directed therapy in the treatment of severe sepsis and septic shock. N Engl J Med. 2001;345:1368–77.
8. Brown RM, Semler MW. Fluid management in sepsis. J Intensive Care Med. 2018;34(5):364–73.
9. Rhodes A, Evans LE, Alhazzani W, Levy MM, Antonellil M, Ferrer R. Surviving sepsis campaign: international guidelines for management of sepsis and septic shock: 2016. Critical Care Med. 2017;45(3):503–504.
10. Semler MW, Rice TW. Saline is not the first choice for crystalloid resuscitation fluids. Crit Care Med. 2016;44(8):1541–4.
11. Liu C, Lu G, Wang D, Lei Y, Mao Z, Hu P. Balanced crystalloids versus normal saline for fluid resuscitation in critically ill patients: a systematic review and meta-analysis with trial sequential analysis. Am J Emerg Med. 2019;37(11):2072–8.
12. Chua HR, Venkatesh B, Stachowski E, et al. Plasma-lyte 148 vs 0.9% saline for fluid resuscitation in diabetic ketoacidosis. J Crit Care. 2012;27:138–45.
13. Oliver WD, Willis GC, Hines MC, Hayes BD. Comparison of plasma-lyte a and sodium chloride 0.9% for fluid resuscitation of patients with diabetic ketoacidosis. Hosp Pharm. 2018;53(5):326–30.
14. Bedi MK, Sarabahi S, Agrawal K. New fluid therapy protocol in acute burn from a tertiary burn care centre. Burns. 2019;45(2):335–40.
15. Chatrath V, Khetarpal R, Ahuja J. Fluid management in patients with trauma: restrictive versus liberal approach. J Anaesthesiol Clin Pharmacol. 2015;31(3):308.
16. Chang R, Holcomb JB. Optimal fluid therapy for traumatic hemorrhagic shock. Crit Care Clin. 2017;33(1):15–36.
17. Wise R, Faurie M, Malbrain MLNG, Hodgson E. Strategies for intravenous fluid resuscitation in trauma patients. World J Surg. 2017;41(5):1170–83.

39 Blood Management for the Geriatric Patient

Arnaldo Vera-Arroyo and Richard A. Zack-Guasp

Longevity has been increasing, and there have been a rapidly growing number of elderly patients being treated in the medical ward and undergoing major surgical procedures. The elderly suffer from an aging physiology, chronic conditions, polypharmacy, and overall decreased physical performance. Overall, mortality for elderly patients undergoing major surgery has been low, but suffering from one or more complications while undergoing surgery is associated with a high 30-day mortality [1].

Anemia is commonly seen in the elderly. Studies have shown that 11% of men and 10.2% of women above age 65 are anemic, and these rates rose rapidly with increasing age and reached 20% above age 85 [2] with more recent literature placing it closer to 32% [3]. Anemia is defined since 1968 by the World Health Organization (WHO) with thresholds established as hemoglobin level (Hg) <13.0 g/dL in men and <12.0 g/dL in women [4]. The report places men and women >15 years of age into the adult category and does not differentiate ages further into subgroups. A recent publication from the WHO includes degrees of severity of anemia but yet groups adults above 15 years of age [5].

The aging patient suffers from anemia related to diseases like neoplasms; infections; inflammatory conditions; chronic kidney disease; malnutrition leading to iron, folate, or B12 deficiencies, and a wide array of acute bleeds, among others [3, 6]. These factors contribute to preoperative anemia. A multicenter survey revealed that the main reasons clinicians do not routinely treat preoperative anemia is the lack of organization and time, where results of blood test where near to the surgical date and postponement of the procedure was not accepted [7]. The preoperative period can allow for a comprehensive understanding of those patients that present with even mild degree of preoperative anemia have been associated with an increased risk of 30-day mortality and cardiac events in older, mostly male patients [8] and a wide array of comorbidities [9]. Identifying anemia and its causes will allow for providers to treat anemia which could impact outcomes. Perioperative surgical blood loss, coagulopathy, hemodilution and phlebotomies, and postoperative blunted erythropoiesis contribute to further degrees of anemia in surgical patients [10] (Table 39.1).

In the elderly population, we encounter that 6.9–50% of aging adults could be classified as frail, depending on the criteria used [11, 12]. Frailty is the state of vulnerability of a patient's physiologic reserve to stressors that could contribute to overall poor health outcomes [13]. It takes into account involuntary weight loss, exhaustion, muscle weakness, slow gait speed, and sedentary behavior [13]. Frailty has been associated with a higher hospital mortality in the general population [14] and 30-day mortality in octogenarians [15]. These patients are found to have lower levels of hemoglobin along with higher chances of congestive heart failure and lower mean Folstein's Mini Mental Status Examination (MMSE) scores when assessing cognitive impairment [12]. Anemia is an independent risk factor for decline in physical performance in the elderly [16] and affects activities of daily living (ADL). Anemia is a potential modifiable risk factor for frailty [11]. As the physiologic decline of adults progresses with aging and the importance of frailty and cognitive changes emerges, attempts are being made to focus on identification, management, and treatment in the elderly to decrease mortality, complication rates, adverse outcomes, and prolonged hospital stays.

The most efficient way to increase red blood cell (RBC) mass and hemoglobin (Hg) is by transfusion. Blood transfusions have been in practice for more than a century. During WWI, soldiers in the battlefield underwent arm-to-arm transfusions, and by the end of 1914, 44 cases were reported [17]. Other treatments have been identified to increase red blood cell mass and Hg. Recent studies have looked at the administration of intravenous and oral replacement of iron for iron deficiency anemia, folic acid, and B12 and erythropoietin administration.

A. Vera-Arroyo (✉) · R. A. Zack-Guasp
Department of Anesthesiology and Perioperative Medicine, University of Miami Miller School of Medicine, Miami, FL, USA

Division of Anesthesiology, Bruce W. Carter VA Medical Center, Miami, FL, USA
e-mail: averaarroyo@med.miami.edu

© Springer Nature Switzerland AG 2021
C. S. Scher et al. (eds.), *Essentials of Blood Product Management in Anesthesia Practice*,
https://doi.org/10.1007/978-3-030-59295-0_39

Table 39.1 Clinical relevance of low Hg levels [9]

Low hg levels are a risk factor for cardiovascular diseases	Cognitive impairment	Insomnia	Impaired mood	
Low Hg levels are associated with reduced executive function	Physical performance	Increased risk of falls and fractures	Frequent hospitalization	Longer hospital stays

Transfusion in the perioperative period has been identified among six other anesthesia intervention themes to have a significant impact on mortality [18]. Research has been done to establish safe transfusion thresholds for patients and, in our interest, the geriatric population. Thresholds are divided into liberal or restrictive, and most literature reports transfusion less than 8 g/dL and hematocrit < than 25% as restrictive [19]. A recent meta-analysis showed that older patients treated with a liberal transfusion strategy had a significant lower risk of 30-day mortality and better outcomes when it came to cardiac complications [20]. The concern regarding lower Hg levels in this population stems from the theoretical increased risk of myocardial ischemia or infarction, cerebro vascular, accidents and potential exacerbation of any underlying medical conditions. Interestingly, recent meta-analysis showed that transfusion strategies might differ for critically ill patients vs perioperative patients [21]. Others recommend that restrictive strategies in the perioperative period should be applied cautiously in high-risk patients undergoing major surgery as restrictive strategies seemed to increase the risk of adverse events from inadequate oxygen supply and mortality in cardiac/vascular surgery and similarly in orthopedic surgery but not in critically ill patients [22]. Guidelines for perioperative management of blood transfusions have been published and are applied to elderly patients as well.

Transfusions are not without complications with transfusion reactions occurring up to 1/100 transfusions. Degree of transfusion reactions are variable, and they could express mild to severe signs or symptoms. Signs and symptoms of adverse reactions to blood transfusion include hyperthermia, chills and rigors, rash and hives, urticaria, hemoglobinuria, microvascular bleeding, hypoxemia, respiratory distress, increased airway peak pressures, hypotension, and hypocalcemia [23]. Geriatric patients experiencing these could be detrimental in light of the current disease state in addition to a possible low reserve physiology (Table 39.2).

Table 39.2 Signs and symptoms of adverse reactions to blood transfusions [23]

Allergic and anaphylactic transfusion reactions	Hyper-hemolytic transfusion reactions	Septic transfusion reactions	Transfusion-related acute lung injury (TRALI)
Acute hemolytic transfusion reactions	Hypotensive transfusion reaction	Transfusion-associated circulatory overload (TACO)	
Delayed hemolytic or delayed serological transfusion reactions	Massive transfusion-associated reactions (citrate, potassium, and cold toxicity)	Transfusion-associated graft-versus-host disease	
Febrile non-hemolytic	Post-transfusion purpura	Transfusion-associated necrotizing enterocolitis	

Transfusion in Cardiac Surgery Patients

Patient undergoing cardiac surgery have a high likelihood of receiving blood transfusions. Historically, the Hg10/Hct 30 rule has been used for patients with coronary artery disease and acute myocardial ischemia. patients undergoing cardiac surgery, coronary artery bypass graft (CABG), and/or valve replacements carry a burden of disease, and anemia is common in this population. Their decision for surgery, could be elective or as an emergency which can contribute to morbidity. Age above 60 years has been a predictor of mortality in cardiac surgery but its impact has reduced throughout the years [24]. EURSCORE II is a modified version of the original score that includes age as one of its variables, and it is used as a tool to assess cardiac surgical risk [25]. Scoring systems have been developed to predict the need for blood transfusion in patients undergoing cardiac surgery. The Transfusion Risk Understanding Scoring Tool (TRUST) by Alghamdi et al. [24] and Transfusion Risk and Clinical Knowledge (TRACK) by Ranucci et al. [25] both take into account age as one of the variables: TRUST for age >65 and TRACK for age >67. These scoring systems can identify those patients at high risk for transfusion, and practices to optimize and avoid transfusion can be set in place [26]. Those patients might benefit from optimization prior to undergoing surgery and can be considered for interventions to reduce transfusion rates, including stopping platelet inhibitors and administration of folate, iron, and erythropoietin if feasible [26] (Table 39.3).

Early literature addressed hemodilution during cardiopulmonary bypass (CBP) which has an increased morbidity and mortality by causing ischemia and/or inflammatory or vital organ injury [27], especially renal injury [28], and stroke [29]. More recent RCTs, like the TRACS [30] (mean age ~ 69) and TRICS [31] (older population, mean age 72 years), have

Table 39.3 Scoring systems to predict the use of blood transfusions

TRACK [25]	Score	TRUST [24]	Score
Age >67 years of age	6	Age >65 years of age	1
Weight <60 kg for females and <85 kg for males	2	Preoperative hemoglobin level <13.5 g/dL	1
Female gender	4	Female gender	1
Complex surgery	7	Weight < 77 kg	1
Preoperative hematocrit	1 point per each % value below 40% (max 13 points)	Non-elective surgery	1
Transfusion risk in percentage is extrapolated to a TRACK score in the report		Serum creatinine level >1.36 mg/dL	1
		Non-isolated procedure	1
		Previous cardiac surgery	1
		Baseline risk = 0; probability of transfusion 0–19% Low risk = 1; probability of transfusion 20–39% Intermediate risk = 2; probability of transfusion 40–59% High risk = 3; probability of transfusion 60–79% Very high risk 4–8; probability of transfusion 80–100%	

placed restrictive strategies non-inferior to liberal ones, while TITRe2 [32] (median age 70 years) refers that restrictive strategies were not superior to liberal strategies with respect to morbidity which mortality. Others have associated intraoperative transfusion of red blood cells with increased mortality and was seen most commonly in patients of older age with higher EUROSCORE [33]. Meta-analysis refers that restrictive transfusion strategies with Hg 7–8 g/dL in patients undergoing cardiac surgery are safe [34, 35].

But patients who will require massive transfusions would benefit of less organ dysfunction and lower mortality with high-ratio transfusions [36]. For patients who are recognized to be anemic in the preoperative period, a RCT using an ultrashort-term combination treatment of intravenous iron, subcutaneous erythropoietin, alpha and vitamin B12, and oral folic acid will reduce blood product transfusions [37]. Further studies are required to explore benefits and adverse effects of this therapy.

Transfusion in Critical Care

Transfusion practices in the critical care unit are driven mostly by thresholds and influenced by patient factors such as age, severity of illness, reason for ICU admission, presence of gastrointestinal bleeding, comorbid heart disease, or acute myocardial infarction. One of the landmark studies done in the critical care setting is the TRICC (Transfusion Requirements in Critical Care) which showed that a restrictive transfusion strategy (Hg < 7.0 g/dL) was associated with a significant decrease in hospital mortality when compared to liberal transfusion strategies (Hg < 10 g/dL), but 30-day mortality was similar and significantly decreased among those less acutely ill and those younger than 55 years of age who received a restrictive strategy [38]. Patients in the critical care setting are sicker and have a wider range of comorbid medical conditions, and their admission diagnosis could be unique or multifactorial. The heterogeneity of the profile of the patients needs to be considered and could influence the threshold used to transfuse blood products. A mortality benefit has been observed when increasing the transfusion threshold for comorbid heart disease from 8 to 9 g/dL and 9 to 10 g/dL in patients admitted for acute myocardial infarction in a population with mean age of 66.1 ± 12.5 [39]. Anemia in this population could lead to myocardial ischemia and the inability to appropriately increase oxygen delivery by means of increasing the cardiac output.

Transfusion in Gastrointestinal Bleed

Gastrointestinal bleeding carries high morbidity and mortality, and it is common among elderly patients. Upper gastrointestinal bleeds (UGIB) is the most common due to PUD, and causes of lower gastrointestinal bleeds (LGIB) are diverticular bleeding, ischemic colitis, hemorrhoids, colorectal polyps/neoplasms, and angioectasia among others. There are various risk stratification scores used for patients who have gastrointestinal bleed. The Rockwall score is used to assess further bleeding and risk of death in patients with gastrointestinal bleeds. This is the only score to include age into its criteria: <60 (0 points), 60–79 (1 point), and >80 (2 points). Most of the studies include adults above 18 years of age, and information on the elderly is scant. In patients with acute upper gastrointestinal bleeding, patients randomized to restrictive transfusion practices had higher survival rates at 6 weeks when compared to a liberal strategy [39]. This meta-analysis included Villanueva et al.'s study that suggests that a restrictive transfusion strategy in adults with acute UGIB could have improved outcomes [40] but which excluded patients with recent ischemic events. Thus, the risk in myocardial infarction and other ischemic events is unknown. A post hoc analysis in patients with men age of LGIB found no difference between liberal and restrictive RBC transfusion strategies, but age was an independent risk factor for rebleeding and inpatient mortality [19].

Transfusion in Sepsis/Septic Shock

Another major cause of admission to the critical care unit is septic shock. The 2016 Surviving Sepsis Campaign guidelines recommend for blood transfusions in patients with septic shock to be reserved for Hg < 7.0 g/dL in the absence of myocardial ischemia, severe hypoxemia, acute hemorrhage, or other extenuating circumstances, fresh frozen plasma to correct clotting abnormalities in the presence of active bleeding and/or planned invasive procedures, and platelets at <10,000/mm^3 prophylactically, <20,000/mm^3 with significant risk of bleeding, and >50,000/mm^3 for active bleeding, surgery, or invasive procedures [41]. The recommendations come from two trials, the Transfusion Requirements in Septic Shock trial (TRISS) and the Protocol-Based Care for Early Septic Shock (ProCESS) trial which is less directed to transfusion therapy. TRISS concluded that the patients who received leukoreduced transfusions in a restrictive strategy, received less amount of transfusions and had similar mortality at 90 days, use of life support, and number of days alive when compared to those who were transfused liberally for hemoglobin levels less than 9 g/dL [24]. TRISS also showed no heterogeneity on mortality at 90 days for between patients with and without cardiovascular diseases and when patients were divided into younger than 70 and older than 70 years of age [25]. There was no difference at 60 in hospital mortality or 90-day mortality in the ProCESS trial where patients (mean age ~ 61 ± 16) were transfused at Hg < 10 g/dL when the ScVo2 was <70% vs the standard at Hg < 7.5 g/dL [25]. A recent trial observed a mortality benefit at 90 days in critically ill oncologic patients (mean age ~ 61 ± 13.5) who received a liberal transfusion strategy [24], but no subgroup analyses was done for elderly patients. Clinicians will base their decision-making following the Surviving Sepsis guidelines, but no specific transfusion guidelines have been published on elderly patients with sepsis/septic shock.

Transfusions in the Elderly Suffering Trauma

As the percentage of our population who suffer falls within the geriatric age increases, the number of geriatric patients presenting to the trauma setting is expected to increase accordingly. Statistically, trauma in the geriatric population has mostly been orthopedic secondary to falls, but every day more hemorrhagic blunt trauma is seen in this population. Most research in trauma has been done focusing on adults 18–45 years of age, which has left treatment of the elderly in this setting in the dark.

As is to be expected in the trauma setting, hemorrhagic complications secondary to primary trauma mechanism or extensive surgical interventions have made transfusion of blood products a mainstay of resuscitation efforts. Prevalence and adverse effects of baseline anemia are magnified in the setting of acute blood loss and trauma, which is associated with a proinflammatory state that leads to inhibition of bone marrow and iron metabolism, affecting, as a consequence, erythropoiesis. Elderly trauma patients were found to have lower hemoglobin levels on admission and discharge from trauma units, despite receiving more transfusions [42]. The hemoglobin levels at discharge were hypothesized to remain low due to an increased suppression of the bone marrow by trauma-induced hypercatecholaminemia, erythropoietin resistance, and overexpression of proinflammatory cytokines. Despite of this, anemia at discharge was not predictive of 60-day mortality or unplanned readmission in this population [43]. As for the increased rate of transfusions, it has been seen that despite the available guidelines, transfusion thresholds vary from clinician to clinician and historically have been higher in the elderly population in deference two their age-related cardiovascular physiologic alterations.

A retrospective study of patients >70 years old, which spanned 8 years and set restrictive thresholds below 7.0 g/dL and liberal thresholds below 10.0 g/dL, observed that liberal protocols in this population are not beneficial and receiving a transfusion was an independent risk factor for complications [44]. Survivors who had a liberal transfusion threshold were observed to have increased hospital length of stay and days in the ICU [44]. Transfusion strategies in the trauma geriatric population should adhere to a restrictive protocol, as this decreases the risk of developing adverse secondary effects.

Transfusions in the Elderly: Orthopedic Surgery

Orthopedic surgery is one of the most common surgical procedures performed in the geriatric population. These procedures could be performed electively but also could be as a result of a fall or trauma resulting in fractures and acute large amounts of blood loss. Many elderly adults are on anticoagulation medications depending on present comorbidities. These could impact ongoing bleeding, reversal of anticoagulants, timing on surgery, and requirement of blood transfusions. The FOCUS trial which included patients >65 of age (mean 81.6) with risks of cardiovascular disease suggests that liberal strategies did not reduce rate of death and withholding transfusion unless there are symptoms of anemia and Hg drops below 8 g/dL is reasonable [39]. This same group was followed for 3 years, and liberal transfusion strategies did not affect mortality when compared with restrictive strategies [40]. But an RCT of frail elderly patients from nursing homes or shelter suggests that implementation of a liberal transfusion strategy has a potential to increase survival among nursing home residents [19]. Retrospective studies suggest that in hip fracture surgeries, restrictive strategies show increased risk of cardiovascular events [41]. What has been seen though is that most patients undergoing hip fracture repair that required transfusions received them in the postoperative setting and in a more liberal manner. An increased number of infections and length of stay were observed, but without any changes in mortality in patients transfused liberally [24]. Either liberal or restrictive strategies showed no difference when observing for recovery from physical disabilities [25].

Transfusion in the Setting of Delirium

One of the major postoperative complications seen in the elderly is the development of delirium. This has been linked with prolonged length of hospitalization, poorer rehabilitation outcomes, increased institutionalization, and higher morbidity and mortality rates. Some studies have focused on examining the effect of blood transfusions in the postoperative development of delirium in hip fracture patients, and have found that more liberal strategies aiming for higher hemoglobin levels (above 10 g/dL) have not reduced the likelihood of postoperative delirium when compared to a more restrictive threshold of 8 g/dL [25]. These results have also been seen in studies focusing on elderly patients undergoing elective, unilateral, total hip replacement surgery. A post hoc analysis of data provided by the TRIFE study observed that liberal transfusion strategies aiming to a hemoglobin above 11.3 g/dL prevent delirium on postoperative day 10 [24]. Patients in this study were discharged back to their nursing facility within the first 2 postoperative days and followed by an orthogeriatric team. Having elderly patients in surroundings that are known to them has been a well-described factor that reduces incidence of delirium in this population. Although prevention of postoperative delirium is not currently an indication for transfusions, risks vs benefits should always be closely considered in elderly patients.

Although the literature mostly groups adults and the geriatric patients together, some studies have been done specifically on geriatric patients, but guidelines make no distinction on age but do take into account clinical condition. The American Society of Anesthesiologists guidelines of 2014 agree that a restrictive blood transfusion strategy will result in fewer transfusions and determine that red blood cell transfusion for Hg levels between 6 and 10 should be based on the risk of presence of bleeding, intravascular volume status, signs and symptoms of organ ischemia, and cardiopulmonary reserve [19].

An international consensus statement on anemia after major surgical procedures recommends testing, identification, treatment of anemia with iron and/or erythropoiesis-stimulating agents if required and feasible, and adoption of a restrictive transfusion threshold (Hg 7–8 d/d) in clinically stable patients [45]. The 2018 Frankfurt Consensus Conference published their clinical and research recommendations on blood management [39]. A strong recommendation is to detect and manage perioperative anemia and suggest conditional recommendations on the use of iron and erythropoiesis-stimulating agents in certain scenarios. They also strongly recommend a restrictive RBC transfusion threshold defined as Hg concentration <7 g/dL in critically ill but clinically stable intensive care patients and Hg concentration <7.5 g/dL in patients undergoing cardiac surgery. Conditional recommendations when the Hg concentration <8 g/dL in patients with hip fracture and cardiovascular disease or other risk factors and Hg concentration 7–8 g/dL in hemodynamically stable patients with acute GI bleeds. It is agreed upon that hospitals need perioperative blood management programs to improve appropriate RBC utilization.

Conclusion

More geriatric patients will be seen in the medical ward, will undergo elective procedures, and will be admitted for surgeries or intensive care units emergently, and there will be a high likelihood of these presenting with or developing with anemia. Not all anemias are made equally and should not be treated equally especially on the geriatric population. Transfusion decisions should be made taking into consideration comorbid disease, active symptomatology, initial hemoglobin levels, and the possibility of other forms of treatment of anemia, adequate control of source of disease, and adequate medical optimization. The lack of information of comprehensive data of the geriatric population renders us to fit them with the rest of the population according to the existing guidelines.

More data needs to be collected for evidence-based transfusion practices and medical decisions across the different medical and surgical specialties regarding transfusion and anemia in the geriatric population.

References

1. Hamel MB, Henderson WG, Khuri SF, Daley J. Surgical outcomes for patients aged 80 and older: morbidity and mortality from major noncardiac surgery. J Am Geriatr Soc. 2005;53(3):424–9.
2. Guralnik JM, Eisenstaedt RS, Ferrucci L, Klein HG, Woodman RC, Dc W. Prevalence of anemia in persons 65 years and older in

the United States: evidence for a high rate of unexplained anemia Prevalence of anemia in persons 65 years and older in the United States: evidence for a high rate of unexplained anemia. Blood. 2013;104(8).

3. Bach V, Schruckmayer G, Sam I, Kemmler G, Stauder R. Prevalence and possible causes of anemia in the elderly: a cross-sectional analysis of a large European university hospital cohort. Clin Interv Aging. 2014;9:1187–96.
4. WHO. Nutritional anaemias. Report of a WHO scientific group. [Internet]. Geneva: World Health Organization 1968. Available from: http://whqlibdoc.who.int/trs/WHO_TRS_405.pdf.
5. World Health Organisation, WHO. Haemoglobin concentrations for the diagnosis of anaemia and assessment of severity. Geneva, Switzerland: World Health Organization [Internet]. 2011;1–6. Available from: http://apps.who.int/iris/bitstream/handle/10665/85839/WHO_NMH_NHD_MNM_11.1_eng.pdf?ua=1%0Ahttp://scholar.google.com/scholar?hl=en&btnG=Search&q=intitle:Haemoglobin+concentrations+for+the+diagnosis+of+anaemia+and+assessment+of+severity#1.
6. Guralnik JM, Eisenstaedt RS, Ferrucci L, Klein HG, Woodman RC, Dc W. Prevalence of anemia in persons 65 years and older in the United States: evidence for a high rate of unexplained anemia prevalence of anemia in persons 65 years and older in the United States: evidence for a high rate of unexplained anemia. Blood [Internet]. 2004;104(8):2263–8. Available from: http://www.embase.com/search/results?subaction=viewrecord&from=export&id=L39331821%5Cn. https://doi.org/10.1182/blood-2004-05-1812.
7. Manzini PM, Dall'Omo AM, D'Antico S, Valfrè A, Pendry K, Wikman A, et al. Patient blood management knowledge and practice among clinicians from seven European university hospitals: a multicentre survey. Vox Sang. 2018;113(1):60–71.
8. Wu W-C, Schifftner TL, Henderson WG, Eaton CB, Poses RM, Uttley G, et al. Preoperative hematocrit levels and postoperative outcomes in older patients undergoing noncardiac surgery. JAMA. 2007;297(22):2481–8.
9. Stauder R, Valent P, Theurl I. Anemia at older age: etiologies, clinical implications, and management. Blood. 2018;131(5):505–14.
10. Muñoz M, Acheson AG, Auerbach M, Besser M, Habler O, Kehlet H, et al. International consensus statement on the peri-operative management of anaemia and iron deficiency. Anaesthesia. 2017;72(2):233–47.
11. Chaves PHM, Semba RD, Leng SX, Woodman RC, Ferrucci L, Guralnik JM, et al. Impact of anemia and cardiovascular disease on frailty status of community-dwelling older women: the Women's Health and Aging Studies I and II [Internet]. 2005 [cited 2019 Jul 8]. Available from: https://academic.oup.com/biomedgerontology/article-abstract/60/6/729/590335.
12. Khandelwal D, Goel A, Kumar U, Gulati V, Narang R, Dey AB. Frailty is associated with longer hospital stay and increased mortality in hospitalized older patients. J Nutr Health Aging [Internet]. 2012;16(8):1–4. Available from: http://www.embase.com/search/results?subaction=viewrecord&from=export&id=L52209305%0Ahttp://dx.doi.org/10.1007/s12603-012-0369-5%0Ahttp://findit.library.jhu.edu/resolve?sid=EMBASE&issn=12797707&id=doi:10.1007%2Fs12603-012-0369-5&atitle=Frailty+is+associat.
13. Cesari M, Calvani R, Marzetti E. Frailty in older persons. Clin Geriatr Med [Internet]. 2017;33(3):293–303. Available from: https://doi.org/10.1016/j.cger.2017.02.002.
14. Muscedere J, Waters B, Varambally A, Bagshaw SM, Boyd JG, Maslove D, et al. The impact of frailty on intensive care unit outcomes: a systematic review and meta-analysis. Intensive Care Med. 2017;43(8):1105–22.
15. Flaatten H, de Lange DW, Morandi A, Andersen FH, Artigas A, Bertolini G, et al. The impact of frailty on ICU and 30-day mortality and the level of care in very elderly patients (≥ 80 years). Intensive Care Med. 2017;43(12):1820–8.
16. Penninx BWJH, Guralnik JM, Onder G, Ferrucci L, Wallace RB, Pahor M. Anemia and decline in physical performance among older persons. Am J Med. 2003;115(2):104–10.
17. Garraud O, Tissot J-D. Transfusion, history and ethics: hundred years after WWI battlefield operations. Transfus Clin Biol [Internet]. 2019;26(1):1–2. Available from: https://doi.org/10.1016/j.tracli.2019.01.001.
18. Boet S, Etherington N, Nicola D, Beck A, Bragg S, Carrigan ID, et al. Anesthesia interventions that alter perioperative mortality: a scoping review. Syst Rev. 2018;7(1):1–15.
19. Practice guidelines for perioperative blood management: an updated report by the American Society of Anesthesiologists Task Force on Perioperative Blood Management*. Anesthesiology [Internet]. 2015;122(2):241–75. Available from: https://doi.org/10.1097/ALN.0000000000000463.
20. Simon GI, Craswell A, Thom O, Fung YL. Outcomes of restrictive versus liberal transfusion strategies in older adults from nine randomised controlled trials: a systematic review and meta-analysis. Lancet Haematol. 2017;4(10):e465–74.
21. Chong MA, Krishnan R, Cheng D, Martin J. Should transfusion trigger thresholds differ for critical care versus perioperative patients? A meta-analysis of randomized trials. Crit Care Med. 2018;46(2):252–63.
22. Hovaguimian F, Myles PS. Restrictive versus liberal transfusion strategy in the perioperative and acute care settings. Anesthesiology. 2016;125(1):46–61.
23. Delaney M, Wendel S, Bercovitz RS, Cid J, Cohn C, Dunbar NM, et al. Transfusion reactions: prevention, diagnosis, and treatment. Lancet [Internet]. 2016;388(10061):2825–36. Available from: https://doi.org/10.1016/S0140-6736(15)01313-6.
24. Alghamdi AA, Davis A, Brister S, Corey P, Logan A. Development and validation of Transfusion Risk Understanding Scoring Tool (TRUST) to stratify cardiac surgery patients according. Transfusion. 2006;46(7):1120–9.
25. Ranucci M, Castelvecchio S, Frigiola A, Scolletta S, Giomarelli P, Biagioli B. Predicting transfusions in cardiac surgery: the easier, the better: the Transfusion Risk and Clinical Knowledge score. Vox Sang. 2009;96:324–32.
26. Carson JL, Sieber F, Cook DR, Hoover DR, Noveck H, Chaitman BR, et al. Liberal versus restrictive blood transfusion strategy: 3-year survival and cause of death results from the FOCUS randomised controlled trial. Lancet. 2015;385(9974):1183–9.
27. Habib RH, Zacharias A, Schwann TA, Riordan CJ, Durham SJ, Shah A. Adverse effects of low hematocrit during cardiopulmonary bypass in the adult: Should current practice be changed? J Thoracic CArdiovasc Surg. 2003;125(6):1438–50.
28. Habib RH, Zacharias A, Schwann TA, Riordan CJ, Engoren M, Durham SJ, et al. Role of hemodilutional anemia and transfusion during cardiopulmonary bypass in renal injury after coronary revascularization: implications on operative outcome. Crit Care Med. 2005;33(8):1749–56.
29. Karkouti K, Djaiani G, Borger MA, Beattie WS, Fedorko L, Wijeysundera D, et al. Low hematocrit during cardiopulmonary bypass is associated with increased risk of perioperative stroke in cardiac surgery. Ann Thorac Surg. 2005;80(4):1381–7.
30. Hajjar LA, Vincent J-L, Galas FRBG, Nakamura RE, Silva CMP, Santos MH, et al. Transfusion requirements after cardiac surgery: The TRACS randomized controlled trial. JAMA. 2010;304(14):1559–67.
31. Mazer CD, Whitlock RP, Fergusson DA, Hall J, Belley-Cote E, Connolly K, et al. Restrictive or liberal red-cell transfusion for cardiac surgery. N Engl J Med. 2017;377(22):2133–44.

32. Murphy GJ, Pike K, Rogers CA, Wordsworth S, Stokes EA, Angelini GD, et al. Liberal or restrictive transfusion after cardiac surgery. N Engl J Med. 2015;372(11):997–1008.
33. Vlot EA, Verwijmeren L, van de Garde EMW, Kloppenburg GTL, van Dongen EPA, Noordzij PG. Intra-operative red blood cell transfusion and mortality after cardiac surgery. BMC Anesthesiol. 2019;19(1):1–7.
34. Carson JL, Stanworth SJ, Alexander JH, Roubinian N, Fergusson DA, Triulzi DJ, et al. Clinical trials evaluating red blood cell transfusion thresholds: an updated systematic review and with additional focus on patients with cardiovascular disease. Am Heart J [Internet]. 2018;200:96–101. Available from: https://doi.org/10.1016/j.ahj.2018.04.007.
35. Kheiri B, Abdalla A, Osman M, Haykal T, Chintalapati S, Cranford J, et al. Restrictive versus liberal red blood cell transfusion for cardiac surgery: a systematic review and meta-analysis of randomized controlled trials. J Thromb Thrombolysis [Internet]. 2019;47(2):179–85. Available from: https://doi.org/10.1007/s11239-018-1784-1.
36. Delaney M, Stark PC, Suh M, Triulzi DJ, Hess JR, Steiner ME, et al. Massive transfusion in cardiac surgery: the impact of blood component ratios on clinical outcomes and survival. Anesth Analg. 2017;124(6):1777–82.
37. Spahn DR, Schoenrath F, Spahn GH, Seifert B, Stein P, Theusinger OM, et al. Effect of ultra-short-term treatment of patients with iron deficiency or anaemia undergoing cardiac surgery: a prospective randomised trial. Lancet [Internet]. 2019;393(10187):2201–12. Available from: https://doi.org/10.1016/S0140-6736(18)32555-8.
38. Kherad O, Restellini S, Martel M, Sey M, Murphy MF, Oakland K, et al. Outcomes following restrictive or liberal red blood cell transfusion in patients with lower gastrointestinal bleeding. Aliment Pharmacol Ther. 2019;49(7):919–25.
39. Mueller MM, van Remoortel H, Meybohm P, Aranko K, Aubron C, Burger R, et al. Patient blood management: recommendations from the 2018 Frankfurt Consensus Conference. JAMA. 2019;321(10):983–97.
40. Cooper DJ, McQuilten ZK, Nichol A, Ady B, Aubron C, Bailey M, et al. Age of red cells for transfusion and outcomes in critically ill adults. N Engl J Med [Internet]. 2017;377(19):1858–67. Available from: http://www.nejm.org/doi/10.1056/NEJMoa1707572.
41. Ii E, Nashef SAM, Roques F, Sharples LD, Nilsson J, Smith C. EuroSCORE II †. Eur J Cardiothorac Surg. 2012;41:734–45.
42. Roubinian NH, Murphy EL, Mark DG, Triulzi DJ, Carson JL, Lee C, et al. Long-term outcomes among patients discharged from the hospital with moderate anemia a retrospective cohort study. Ann Intern Med. 2019;170(2):81–9.
43. Ong AW, Jaisingh NR, Butler S, Sigal A, Fernandez FB. Is it safe to discharge geriatric trauma patients with anemia? Am J Surg. 2018;215(3):419–22.
44. Deleon AN, Uecker JM, Stafford S v, Ali S, Clark A, Brown CVR. Restrictive transfusion in geriatric trauma patients. Am Surg. 2016;82(1):85–8.
45. Leff J, Romano CA, Gilbert S, Nair S. Validation study of the transfusion risk and clinical knowledge (TRACK) tool in cardiac surgery patients: a retrospective analysis. J Cardiothorac Vasc Anesth. 2019;33:2669–75.

Substance Abuse and Coagulopathy

40

Mitchell C. Fuller, George M. Jeha, Lu Sun, Ariunzaya Amgalan, Ivan Urits, Elyse M. Cornett, and Alan David Kaye

Introduction

Maintaining blood in a homeostatic liquid state is crucial for adequately supplying oxygen and nutrients to peripheral tissues. Conversely, when the body is exposed to vascular injury, it is a healthy physiologic adaptation for the blood to convert to a solid-state at the injury site. This mechanism is called *coagulation*. Coagulation is a highly dynamic process largely determined by a balance of pro-coagulation factors, anticoagulants, and fibrinolysis [1]. The set of diseases that alter this intricate balance of bleeding and vessel thrombosis is called *coagulopathies*.

Coagulopathies are a highly concerning cause of morbidity and mortality in hospitals that drive significant economic burden in our healthcare system. Common causes of coagulopathy are drug-related, drug-drug interactions, and nutraceutical agents. In this regard, nosebleeds, abnormal bruising, and GI bleeding are linked to oral anticoagulant use, while hemorrhoidal bleeding can be linked to drugs that cause constipation [2]. Additionally, several other factors contribute to drug-induced bleeding, including advancing age, polypharmacy, drug-drug interactions, and coexisting medical conditions. As the chronic disease burden continues to rise, multiple medical regimen therapies are more commonplace than ever and can be directly related to abnormal bleeding states.

More recent clinical literature has linked illicit and recreational drug use to coagulopathy with significant clinical consequences. Literature shows that recreational alcohol consumption is on the rise [3]. The role of alcohol on coagulopathy has been controversial, but it is currently hypothesized that alcohol has a bidirectional effect on coagulopathy and fibrinolysis [4].

In the setting of complex medication regimens and risk-adverse recreational drug use, patient education offers a rationale model for optimizing patient safety in both the hospital and outpatient settings. In particular, as an increasingly large number of drugs are introduced every year, it becomes no longer practical for the pharmacist to take sole responsibility of patient education or the physician to rely on memory to avoid drugs, which may induce bleeding [5].

Therefore, a *multidisciplinary approach* is necessary to develop pharmacotherapeutic regimens designed to minimize bleeding risk, downstream morbidity, and economic and clinical burden. Patients undergoing surgical operations and procedures require adequate anesthesia consultation to ascertain whether the drugs and medications they are taking can increase the risk of bleeding and consequently increase the risk of morbidity and/or mortality.

This chapter discusses the prevalence of substance abuse and coagulopathies and focuses on in-depth assessment of patients, anesthesia considerations, and treatment strategies.

M. C. Fuller
Froedtert Hospital, Medical College of Wisconsin, Milwaukee, WI, USA

G. M. Jeha
LSU School of Medicine, Department of Anesthesiology, New Orleans, LA, USA

L. Sun · E. M. Cornett (✉)
LSU Health Shreveport, Department of Anesthesiology, Shreveport, LA, USA
e-mail: ecorne@lsuhsc.edu

A. Amgalan
Georgetown University School of Medicine, Washington, DC, USA

I. Urits
LSU Health Shreveport, Department of Anesthesiology, Shreveport, LA, USA

Beth Israel Deaconess Medical Center Harvard Medical School, Boston, MA, USA

A. D. Kaye
Department of Anesthesiology and Pharmacology, Toxicology, and Neurosciences, Louisiana State University School of Medicine-Shreveport, Shreveport, LA, USA

LSU Health Shreveport School of Medicine, New Orleans, LA, USA

Tulane School of Medicine, New Orleans, LA, USA

© Springer Nature Switzerland AG 2021
C. S. Scher et al. (eds.), *Essentials of Blood Product Management in Anesthesia Practice*,
https://doi.org/10.1007/978-3-030-59295-0_40

States of Coagulopathy

Patients with liver disease may have complex alterations in procoagulant and anticoagulant profiles resulting in increased risk of bleeding and thrombosis [6]. This is further complicated by the etiology of liver disease, which may independently influence hemostasis. For example, in addition to its propensity to lead to chronic liver disease and cirrhosis, hepatitis C virus (HCV) infection causes changes in hemostasis by disrupting vascular endothelium, altering procoagulant and anticoagulant pathways, and influencing platelet function [7]. Furthermore, positivity for HCV is present in approximately 21% of HIV-infected adults [8, 9]. In patients such as these, the concomitant presence of liver cirrhosis, chronic HCV infection, HIV infection, and the potential presence of alcohol abuse, hepatitis B virus (HBV) infection, malnutrition, or other comorbid conditions further complicate the hematologic balance. This makes it difficult to fully elucidate the etiology of coagulopathy.

Chronic liver disease is a significant cause of morbidity and mortality in the United States and in the world, accounting for 44,000 deaths nationally and two million deaths worldwide each year [10–12]. Approximately 4.5 million people are living with diagnosed liver disease [13]. Infection with HBV and HCV is a known risk factor for the development of chronic liver cirrhosis and cancer. The prevalence of HBV in the United States is approximately 0.35%, and most HBV-related deaths are due to hepatocellular carcinoma and decompensated cirrhosis [12, 14, 15]. The prevalence of chronic HCV infection in the United States is 1% [12]. It is estimated that up to 68% of chronic hepatitis C infections remain undiagnosed [16].

HIV infection is associated with an increased risk for thromboembolic events. Although the precise mechanisms behind this effect are inadequately understood, it is thought that prolonged inflammatory states, chronic immune activation, and alterations in coagulation factors are contributing factors [17–19]. Thrombocytopenia is commonly associated with HIV, putting infected patients at increased risk for major bleeding events [20, 21]. The prevalence of HIV-related thrombocytopenia has decreased with the introduction of antiretroviral therapy (ART). In the pre-ART era, thrombocytopenia may have been present in up to 40% of patients with HIV [22]. In today's era of highly active antiretroviral therapy, this number is likely between 0.6% and 15% [21, 23, 24]. Comorbidities such as hepatitis C virus infection and cirrhosis are risk factors for thrombocytopenia in HIV-infected patients [20].

Drugs Associated with Coagulopathies

Synthetic Cannabinoids

The term "synthetic cannabinoids" describes a heterogeneous group of chemical compounds that functionally resemble Δ^9-tetrahydrocannabinol (THC) [25]. The development of synthetic analogs of THC has been an area of interest ever since its discovery as the active ingredient in marijuana [26]. Given their ease of synthesis, low cost, high potency, and inability to be detected on routine drug screenings, synthetic cannabinoids have become attractive to the illicit drug market and, in recent years, have emerged as a popular alternative to marijuana. They are listed as Schedule I substances under the Controlled Substances Act, and due to lack of regulation, the composition of these substances is highly variable [27]. They have become commercially available in products sold on the Internet and in convenience stores and gas stations, often under the name of herbal blends, incense, and air fresheners with labels such as "not for human consumption." [25, 28, 29]. Despite attempts to create legislation controlling the production and distribution of these compounds, manufacturers commonly manipulate chemical structures as necessary to evade legal ramifications [29–33].

The lifetime prevalence of synthetic cannabinoid use is between 0.2% and 4% and peaks in the late teen years and early 20s [34]. These drugs tend to be popular among recreational cannabis users [35]. Among US, high school seniors, the annual prevalence of synthetic cannabinoid use is second only to cannabis [36]. Between 6% and 17% of US college students have used synthetic cannabinoids at least once during their college years, and 1% of Europeans between the ages of 14 and 18 have used synthetic cannabinoids at least once in their lifetime [37–39].

In the United States, there have been hundreds of cases of contamination of synthetic cannabinoids with long-acting anticoagulant rodenticides (LAARs) resulting in coagulopathy and bleeding complications. Synthetic cannabinoids received national attention in March and April of 2018 when the Illinois Department of Public Health reported an outbreak of severe coagulopathies among patients with recent synthetic cannabinoid use [40]. Over 150 cases, including 5 deaths, were reported. Further investigation revealed that the coagulopathy was related not directly to the consumption of synthetic cannabinoids but rather to the contamination of the drugs with vitamin K antagonists such as brodifacoum, bromadiolone, and/or difenacoum, agents used in commercially available rodenticides [25, 40–42]. In July of 2018, the US. Food and Drug Administration issued a press release warning of significant health risks related to the use of synthetic cannabinoids contaminated with brodifacoum and other LAARs, stating that hundreds of patients have been hospitalized after consuming these products [29].

While the rationale for adulteration with LAARs is not clear, it is speculated that the compounds either prolong or enhance the psychoactive effect of the drug [27, 43]. Among reported cases of coagulopathy associated with the use of synthetic cannabinoids contaminated with vitamin K antagonists, brodifacoum seems to be the most common contaminant [25].

To date, state health departments in Illinois, Maryland, Florida, Indiana, Kentucky, Missouri, Pennsylvania, Virginia, and Wisconsin have reported at a total of 202 cases of accidental brodifacoum poisoning [40, 42]. The exact prevalence of synthetic cannabinoid-associated coagulopathy is unknown. However, given the relative lack of awareness and the illicit nature of the topic, it is not unquestionable that the total number of cases remains underrepresented [41].

Alcohol

Alcohol is a commonly used substance. According to the 2017 National Survey on Drug Use and Health, in the United States, 86.3% of people report that they have used alcohol at some point in their lifetime, and 70.1% report using it in the past year. An estimated 14.1 million people aged 18 and older have alcohol use disorder [44, 45]. Alcohol is responsible for as many as 88,000 deaths annually, making it the third leading cause of preventable death in the United States [46].

Alcohol is a known hepatotoxin that can cause hepatitis, steatosis, fibrosis, cirrhosis, and liver cancer [47, 48]. Additionally, alcohol consumption has been shown to affect the vascular endothelium, platelets, and the fibrinolytic system [49, 50]. Liver cirrhosis is associated with both increased bleeding risk due to abnormalities in procoagulant and anticoagulant protein synthesis and a prothrombotic state due to the systemic inflammation associated with liver dysfunction [51]. In a prospective study of over 48,000 men, alcohol consumption was associated with an increased risk of major gastrointestinal bleeding [52]. The number of annual deaths due to alcoholic liver disease is approximately 14,000 [53].

Patient Assessment

The first step in the clinical evaluation of a patient with suspected substance abuse is to perform an assessment – the next step is to treat, which will be covered later in this chapter. Depending on the clinical setting, there are two forms of initial substance abuse workup: assessment and screening. Screening is a process used in primary care to evaluate the possible presence of a substance abuse problem generating a simple "yes" or "no" answer (i.e., CAGE, AUDIT, and TCUDS II alcoholism questionnaires) [54]. Conversely, *assessment* is a process for defining the nature of the problem, determining the diagnosis, and developing treatment recommendations. An array of assessment tools are typically employed in anesthesia, intensive care, and emergent care settings to treat high-acuity patients and will be the subject of interest herein.

Normal Blood Homeostasis and Clinical Evaluation

A review of normal clot physiology will help make sense of the substance-induced disease states to follow in this review. There are two clotting pathways, the *extrinsic pathway* and the *intrinsic pathway*, that meet to form the *common pathway*. The extrinsic pathway is activated by endothelial secreted tissue factor (TF). In contrast, the intrinsic pathway is activated when vascular endothelium is damaged, exposing subendothelial type IV collagen, von Willebrand factor (vWF), and other negatively charged surfaces [55]. The extrinsic pathway involves a waterfall-type coagulation cascade of plasma factor VII and the common pathway. The intrinsic pathway is the long pathway made up of a similar coagulation cascade of plasma factors XII, XI, IX, and VIII, and the common pathway. The elaboration of both the intrinsic and extrinsic pathways is the common pathway summarized as a coagulation cascade of plasma factors X and V, thrombin (factor II), and insoluble fibrin clots (factor I) [56]. Alterations in fibrin clot homeostasis by exogenous substances (e.g., drugs) can induce clot formation and if left untreated, may progress to *disseminated intravascular coagulopathy* (DIC). DIC characterizes a group of systemic processes, not a single disease entity representing a pathologic balance between coagulation factor/platelet consumption and production leading to organ damage [56]. It is clinically imperative to understand the mechanisms of substance- induced coagulopathies to perform thorough clinical assessments.

Clinicians utilize a host of clinical tools to assess blood homeostasis and coagulopathies. Relevant labs include a complete blood count, clotting time assays (aPTT, PT, TT), individual clot-based assays (plasma fibrinogen, factor V), chromogenic assays (factor VIII), and cross-linked fibrin assays (D-dimer). Prothrombin time (PT) measures the time it takes plasma to clot post-exposure to TF, otherwise known as the extrinsic and common pathways, and is an easy first laboratory to measure, especially in patients who will be

Table 40.1 Parameter changers in setting of acute disseminated intravascular coagulopathy (e.g., substance-induced coagulopathy)

Parameter	Acute DIC
Platelet count	Reduced
Prothrombin time	Prolonged
Activated partial thromboplastin time (aPTT)	Prolonged
Thrombin time	Prolonged
Plasma fibrinogen	Reduced
Plasma factor V	Reduced
Plasma factor VIII	Reduced
Fibrin degradation products	Elevated
D-dimer	Elevated

undergoing surgical procedures or interventional pain procedures with appropriate histories or taking known medications that alter the coagulation cascade. INR is also a gold standard for monitoring warfarin and is simply the individual's PT/control subjects PT. A normal PT is 11–13 seconds. The activated partial thromboplastin time (aPTT) measures the time it takes plasma to clot when exposed to substances that activate contact factors known as the intrinsic and common pathways. A normal aPTT is 25–35 seconds. Thrombin time (TT) measures the final step of coagulation, conversion of fibrinogen to fibrin, and is usually 14–19 seconds. Clot-based assays assess a single clotting factor, like factor V or fibrinogen, by running a normal PT/aPTT assay with plasma deficient for a single factor. Slightly different, the chromogenic assay uses the cleavage activity of a colored/chromogenic substrate against a calibration curve to determine the percent activation of a particular clotting factor. Factor VIII chromogenic assays can be used to rule out haemophilia A (deficiency of factor VIII). Finally, fibrin degradation products assays – such as d-dimer – are ordered as non-specific markers to evaluate for the presence of thrombi.

If a drug inhibits the normal coagulation cascades clotting time will increase resulting in prolonged clotting times (aPTT, PT, TT). Table 40.1 displays the changes in blood homeostatic lab values when exposed to a drug that progress to a state of DIC characterized by a consumption of coagulation factors.

Clinical Management of Drugs Associated with Coagulopathies

Synthetic Cannabinoids

The clinical management of toxicities associated with synthetic cannabinoids is a challenge [57]. Current guidelines for reversal of LAAR-associated bleeding include administering blood products if necessary and vitamin K1 (phylloquinone/phytonadione) and adjusting doses based on close monitoring of coagulation assay values, clinical presentation, and serum LAAR concentrations [27, 57–65]. For acute severe bleeding with elevated INR, the recommendation is to give fresh frozen plasma or four-factor prothrombin complex plus intravenous vitamin K, check INR every couple hours, and repeat or adjust dose if INR remains elevated [58, 62–66]. Lowering vitamin K dose should be considered when INR returns to normal and serum levels of brodifacoum become non-detectable, keeping in mind that coagulopathy may persist even at this point [57, 62–64]. Most recently, in 2019, the Johns Hopkins Health System published a protocol for the acute treatment of LAAR toxicity; the protocol effectively reduced INR below two within 24 hours in 75% of patients in their study [27]. A few case reports indicated use of recombinant activated factor VII as an alternative for acute treatment of LAAR-associated coagulopathy, but it has a relatively short duration of action (around 3 hours), and there is limited data available on the effectiveness of this therapy [67, 68]. Given the long half-lives of LAARs and the possibility of persistent or recurrent coagulopathy, acute care needs to be followed with long-term maintenance therapy with vitamin K [62–64]. The management of LAAR coagulopathy is similar to management of warfarin overdose, but since LAARs are more potent than warfarin, patients with LAAR toxicity require higher doses of vitamin K [27]. Exogenous administration of vitamin K, with doses ranging from 20 to 600 mg/day, is required to treat LAAR-induced coagulopathy, but determining the exact dosing and duration of treatment is difficult due to the potency and long-half lives of LAARs [27, 62–64]. Depending on the degree of toxicity and LAAR serum levels, long-term daily administration of vitamin K may be required for weeks to over 1 year [57]. In addition to the typical treatment regimen for LAAR coagulopathy reversal, case reports have used phenobarbital, a cytochrome P450 inducer, to accelerate brodifacoum clearance, but the interactions of phenobarbital with vitamin K and safety data have not been established [69, 70]. For this reason, a 2019 review advises against the use of cytochrome P450 inducers for now until there is more research available to suggest otherwise [70]. An important complication to consider with cases of LAAR-induced hemorrhage is paradoxical thrombosis, which has been described in case reports [71–74]. Paradoxical thrombosis may be the result of early depletion of anticoagulant proteins C and S caused by LAAR or a complication of blood product transfusion therapy [71–74]. Effective management of patients with suspected LAAR toxicity requires careful examination of risk-benefit, factor levels, coagulation assays, and clinical presentation.

Nutraceuticals

There has been an explosion of over-the-counter products over the past two decades that are affordable and accessible and have not gone through the rigors required to achieve drug status. Many of these agents are marketed as wonder agents that can restore vitality and aid in complex medical conditions with limited therapies. In a study performed by Kaye et al. 70% of patients did not disclose that they were taking herbal products during routine anesthesia preoperative assessment. Furthermore, the prevalence of taking one or more of these herbal products was roughly one-third of the population scheduled to undergo surgery or a pain procedure [75]. In this regard, the kava plant, aloe vera, black cohosh, cascara, chaparral, comfrey, ephedra, and many other herbal products commonly sold worldwide over the counter have been linked to liver damage. Acetaminophen, aspirin, ibuprofen, and naproxen are examples of common over-the-counter analgesic that are linked to liver damage in a dose-dependent manner.

Alcohol

Alcohol use disorder is associated with trauma, liver cirrhosis, and end-stage liver damage (ESLD), which leads to massive reduction of pro- and anticoagulant factors. Additionally, previous studies showed a direct association between alcohol and coagulopathy in the trauma patients [76]. Therefore, proactive treatment of alcohol use disorder is a necessary prophylaxis to a subset of coagulopathies. Examples of prophylaxis include medication, psychosocial treatment, or both, depending on the severity of alcohol use disorder. For a mild disorder, the effectiveness of medication is unclear; thereby appropriate psychosocial treatments are recommended, including motivational interview, brief intervention, cognitive-behavioral therapy, residential treatment, mutual help group, and contingency management [77–79]. For moderate-to-severe disorders a combination of medication and proper psychosocial treatment are efficacious. Naltrexone and acamprosate are two commonly used medications to treat alcohol use disorder. Meta-analysis studies have shown no difference in efficacy between them [80, 81]. However, naltrexone may be a preferred choice for newly diagnosed patients because patients can initiate the administration while still drinking. Also, patients may be more compliant with naltrexone than acamprosate because they take one pill daily for naltrexone but two pills three times a day for acamprosate. On the other hand, in patients who are comorbid with liver damage (e.g., acute hepatitis and liver cirrhosis) due to chronic alcohol use disorder, acamprosate is the favored treatment because it is excreted mostly through the kidney rather than metabolized by the liver. In patients with liver cirrhosis, baclofen is considered safe and is associated with a higher abstinence rate. However, there is a lack of evidence regarding the efficacy of baclofen [82].

When surgical operations become necessary, patients with alcohol use disorder and cirrhosis are at higher risk in perioperative settings. Examples include aspiratory pneumonia, difficulty in the titration of oxygen, the special requirement of fluid and electrolytes, hypotension caused by dehydration, and wound infection due to immunosuppression [83]. A life-threatening postoperative complication is delirium tremens, which manifests as hallucinations, disorientations, tachycardia, hypertension, hyperthermia, agitation, and diaphoresis [84]. The first-line treatment is intravenous long-lasting benzodiazepines (e.g., diazepam and chlordiazepoxide) combined with supportive care. However, lorazepam and oxazepam are favored to treat patients with acute hepatitis or liver cirrhosis since their short-acting mechanism prevents oversedation.

When liver cirrhosis and the consequent liver failure develop due to chronic alcohol use disorder, balance between pro- and anticoagulant factors is disrupted, which may lead to coagulopathy and high bleeding risk. It is classically assessed by standard coagulation laboratory test in which prothrombin time (PT) is longer than 18 seconds, the activated partial thromboplastin time (aPTT) is longer than 60 seconds, the international normalized ratio (INR) is higher than 1.5, or any of these values is higher than 1.5 times of the laboratory reference value [85, 86]. Among them, the prolongation of the aPTT is more specific for diagnosis. Point-of-care techniques, including thromboelastography (TEG) and rotational thrombelastometry (RoTEM), measure the integrated viscoelastic properties of clot formation [76]. Vitamin K deficiency is often seen in decompensated liver cirrhosis. Injection of 10 mg vitamin K for three days is considered an adequate supplement to correct vitamin K deficiency-induced coagulopathy [87].

In trauma patients with massive hemorrhage, volume resuscitation with crystalloid and colloid is the first step to stabilize systemic circulation, although large-volume infusion may further dilute the concentrations of erythrocytes (RBC), coagulant factors, and platelets. Therefore, fresh frozen plasma (FFP) is often co-administered with packed RBC and platelet with a ratio of 1:1:1 [88, 89]. FFP contains pro- and anticoagulant factors, antifibrinolytic factors, albumin, and immunoglobin. FFP infusion offers fast compensation of coagulant factors, but associated risks such as acute lung injury, viral infection, exposure to immunoglobulin, and volume overload should be noted [90]; especially in patients with liver cirrhosis and ESLD, since potential volume overload may exacerbate the portal venous pressure [91].

Prothrombin complex concentrate (PCC) contains highly concentrated factors II, VII, IX, and X and small amounts of protein C and S, heparin, and antithrombin. It has been used to treat hereditary deficiency of coagulant factors mentioned above and rapidly reverse the effects of vitamin K antagonism (warfarin) [92]. PCC does not easily cause volume overload like FFP, and it has also been suggested to be superior to FFP in thrombin generation, which facilitates fibrin production [93]. Additionally, PCC is suggested to be not associated with the increased risk of thrombosis [94]. Therefore, PCC may be a good candidate in treating coagulopathy in patients with ESLD who are already at higher risk of venous thrombosis.

Recombinant FVII (rFVII) is commonly used, but its efficacy has become controversial. It is beneficial for obstetric hemorrhage and blunt trauma, where rFVII helped reduce massive transfusion without increased thromboembolic complications [90]. However, other studies suggested that rFVII may increase thromboembolic risk [54]. Given the inconsistent results from different studies, rFVII may be recommended only when other therapies fail.

The hyperfibrinolytic state that worsens bleeding has been discovered in patients with trauma and liver cirrhosis, probably due to the altered level of plasminogen activator inhibitor-1 [95]. Thus, antifibrinolytics are potentially beneficial in the situations of active bleeding and hemodilution. Currently available antifibrinolytics include lysine analogs, e-aminocaproic acid, and tranexamic acid. They strengthen the weak fibrin clots that are otherwise susceptible to plasmin. Lysine analogues have been reported to reduce blood loss and the need for RBC transfusion in cardiac, orthopedic, and hepatic surgery [96]. Randomized placebo-controlled trials have demonstrated the efficacy of tranexamic acid in the reduction of patient mortality [90].

Venous thrombosis is another primary concern in patients with liver cirrhosis and ESLD, due to the imbalance of the pro- and anticoagulation processes. Prevention of deep venous thrombosis and pulmonary embolism can be performed both mechanically and pharmacologically. Compression stockings and pneumatic compression exemplify the former. Commonly used pharmacological antithromboembolic prophylaxis includes enoxaparin, low-weight-molecular heparin, warfarin, and direct oral anticoagulants [54].

Summary and Conclusion

Coagulation is a dynamic process primarily determined by a balance of pro-coagulation factors, anticoagulants, and fibrinolysis. One particular cause of coagulopathy – drug induced bleeding – has gained attention because of increasing drug use, drug-drug interactions, and natural medicines. Drug-induced bleeding is commonly thought of as gastrointestinal bleeding after NSAID use. Still several other factors contribute to drug-induced bleeding including advancing age, nutraceuticals, polypharmacy, drug-drug interactions, and coexisting medical conditions. Recent clinical literature suggests that alcohol and synthetic cannabinoids are large contributors to drug-induced coagulopathies. There have been hundreds of cases of contamination of synthetic cannabinoids with long-acting anticoagulant rodenticides (LAARs), in the United States alone, resulting in coagulopathy and bleeding complications. Alcohol is a known hepatotoxin; however, alcohol consumption has been shown to affect the vascular endothelium, platelets, and the fibrinolytic system. Additionally, patients with liver disease may have complex alterations in procoagulant and anticoagulant profiles resulting in an increased risk of bleeding and thrombosis.

The first step in the clinical evaluation of a patient with suspected substance abuse is to perform an assessment. Screening is a process used in primary care to evaluate the possible presence of a substance abuse problem. Clinicians utilize a host of clinical tools to assess blood homeostasis and coagulopathies. Relevant labs include a complete blood count, clotting time assays (aPTT, PT, TT), individual clot-based assays (plasma fibrinogen, factor V), chromogenic assays (factor VIII), and cross-linked fibrin assays (D-dimer). Concerning treatment, proactive treatment of alcohol use disorder is a necessary prophylaxis to a subset of coagulopathy. This can be achieved by medication, psychosocial treatment, or a combination of both, depending on the severity of alcohol use disorder. When surgical operations become necessary, patients with alcohol use disorder and cirrhosis are at a higher risk for perioperative complications. The clinical management of toxicities associated with synthetic cannabinoids is a challenge. Current guidelines for reversal of LAAR-associated bleeding include administering blood products if necessary and vitamin K1 (phylloquinone/phytonadione) and adjusting doses based on close monitoring of coagulation assay values, clinical presentation, and serum LAAR concentrations. Ultimately, however, patient education about substance abuse and the potential for exacerbated existing coagulopathies or the development of coagulopathy is the most critical tool healthcare providers can utilize.

References

1. Othman M, Kaur H. Thromboelastography (TEG). In: Methods in molecular biology. Clifton: Humana Press Inc.; 2017. p. 533–43.
2. Hamrick J, Hykamp D. Drug-induced bleeding. 2015;40(12): 17–21.
3. Dawson DA, Goldstein RB, Saha TD, Grant BF. Changes in alcohol consumption: United States, 2001-2002 to 2012-2013. Drug Alcohol Depend. 2015;148:56–61.
4. Howard BM, Kornblith LZ, Redick BJ, Conroy AS, Nelson MF, Calfee CS, et al. Exposing the bidirectional effects of alcohol on coagulation in trauma: impaired clot formation and decreased fibrinolysis in rotational thromboelastometry. J Trauma Acute Care Surg. Lippincott Williams and Wilkins. 2018;84:97–103.
5. Hasnain H, Ali H, Zafar F, Sial AA, Hameed K, Shareef H, et al. Drug-drug interaction; facts and comparisons with national and international Bentch Marks. A threat more than a challenge for

patient safety in clinical and economic scenario. Prof Med J. 2017;24(03):357–65.

6. De Gottardi A. Coagulopathy of chronic liver disease. N Engl J Med. 2011;365(15):1452; author reply 1453–4.
7. González-Reimers E, Quintero-Platt G, Martín-González C, Pérez-Hernández O, Romero-Acevedo L, Santolaria-Fernández F. Thrombin activation and liver inflammation in advanced hepatitis C virus infection. World J Gastroenterol. 2016;22(18):4427–37.
8. Garg S, Brooks J, Luo Q, Skarbinski J. Prevalence of and factors associated with hepatitis C virus (HCV) testing and infection among HIV-infected adults receiving medical care in the United States. Infectious Disease Society of America (IDSA).
9. Yehia BR, Herati RS, Fleishman JA, Gallant JE, Agwu AL, Berry SA, et al. Hepatitis C virus testing in adults living with HIV: a need for improved screening efforts. PLoS One. 2014;9(7):e102766.
10. Kochanek KD, Murphy SL, Xu J, Arias E. National vital statistics reports. 2019;68(9). June 24, 2019 Deaths: Final Data for 2017.
11. Setiawan VW, Stram DO, Porcel J, Lu SC, Le Marchand L, Noureddin M. Prevalence of chronic liver disease and cirrhosis by underlying cause in understudied ethnic groups: the multiethnic cohort. Hepatology. 2016;64(6):1969–77.
12. Moon AM, Singal AG, Tapper EB. Contemporary epidemiology of chronic liver disease and cirrhosis. Clin Gastroenterol Hepatol. 2019.
13. Center for Health Statistics N. Table A-4. Selected diseases and conditions among adults aged 18 and over, by selected characteristics: United States, 2018. 2018.
14. Le MH, Yeo YH, Cheung R, Henry L, Lok AS, Nguyen MH. Chronic hepatitis B prevalence among foreign-born and U.S.-born adults in the United States, 1999-2016. Hepatology. 2020;71(2):431–43.
15. Szpakowski JL, Tucker LY. Causes of death in patients with hepatitis B: a natural history cohort study in the United States. Hepatology. 2013;58(1):21–30.
16. Cooke GS, Andrieux-Meyer I, Applegate TL, Atun R, Burry JR, Cheinquer H, et al. Accelerating the elimination of viral hepatitis: a Lancet Gastroenterology & Hepatology Commission. Lancet Gastroenterol Hepatol. Elsevier Ltd. 2019;4:135–84.
17. Funderburg NT, Lederman MM. Coagulation and morbidity in treated HIV infection. Thromb Res. 2014;133(Suppl 1):S21–4.
18. Hsue PY, Scherzer R, Grunfeld C, Nordstrom SM, Schnell A, Kohl LP, et al. HIV infection is associated with decreased thrombin generation. Clin Infect Dis. 2012;54(8):1196–203.
19. Baker JV, Hullsiek KH, Bradford RL, Prosser R, Tracy RP, Key NS. Circulating levels of tissue factor microparticle procoagulant activity are reduced with antiretroviral therapy and are associated with persistent inflammation and coagulation activation among HIV-positive patients. J Acquir Immune Defic Syndr. 2013;63(3):367–71.
20. Marks KM, Clarke RMA, Bussel JB, Talal AH, Glesby MJ. Risk factors for thrombocytopenia in hiv-infected persons in the era of potent antiretroviral therapy. J Acquir Immune Defic Syndr. 2009;52(5):595–9.
21. Nascimento FG, Tanaka PY. Thrombocytopenia in HIV-infected patients. Indian J Hematol Blood Transfus. 2012;28(2):109–11.
22. Morris L, Distenfeld A, Amorosi E, Karpatkin S. Autoimmune thrombocytopenic purpura in homosexual men. Ann Intern Med. 1982;96:714.
23. Vannappagari V, Nkhoma ET, Atashili J, Laurent SST, Zhao H. Prevalence, severity, and duration of thrombocytopenia among HIV patients in the era of highly active antiretroviral therapy. Platelets. 2011;22(8):611–8.
24. Ambler KLS, Vickars LM, Leger CS, Foltz LM, Montaner JSG, Harris M, et al. Clinical features, treatment, and outcome of HIV-associated immune thrombocytopenia in the HAART era. Adv Hematol. 2012;2012:910954.
25. Arepally GM, Ortel TL. Bad weed: synthetic cannabinoid-associated coagulopathy. Blood. 2019;133(9):902–5.
26. Gaoni Y, Mechoulam R. Isolation, structure, and partial synthesis of an active constituent of hashish. J Am Chem Soc. 1964;86(8):1646–7.
27. Bahouth MN, Kraus P, Dane K, Plazas Montana M, Tsao W, Tabaac B, et al. Synthetic cannabinoid-associated coagulopathy secondary to long-acting anticoagulant rodenticides. Medicine (Baltimore). 2019;98(36):e17015.
28. Seely K, Lapoint J, Moran J, Fattore L. Spice drugs are more than harmless herbal blends: a review of the pharmacology and toxicology of synthetic cannabinoids. Prog Neuropsychopharmacol Biol Psychiatry. 2012;39(2):234–243 7. 2014;39(0).
29. Gottlieb S, Marks P, Woodcock J. Press Announcements - Statement from FDA warning about significant health risks of contaminated illegal synthetic cannabinoid products that are being encountered by FDA. US Food and Drug Administration Home Page. Available.
30. Fattore L, Fratta W. Beyond THC: the new generation of cannabinoid designer drugs. Front Behav Neurosci. 2011;5(September):1–12.
31. Waugh J, Najafi J, Hawkins L, Hill SL, Eddleston M, Vale JA, et al. Epidemiology and clinical features of toxicity following recreational use of synthetic cannabinoid receptor agonists: a report from the United Kingdom National Poisons Information Service. Clin Toxicol (Phila). 2016;54(6):512–8.
32. Loeffler G, Hurst D, Penn A, Yung K. Spice, bath salts, and the US military: the emergence of synthetic cannabinoid receptor agonists and cathinones in the US Armed Forces. Mil Med. 2012;177:1041–8. https://doi.org/10.7205/MILMED-D-12-00180.
33. Brewer TL, Collins M. A review of clinical manifestations in adolescent and young adults after use of synthetic cannabinoids. J Spec Pediatr Nurs. 2014;19:119–26. https://doi.org/10.1111/jspn.12057.
34. Loeffler G, Delaney E, Hann M. International trends in spice use: prevalence, motivation for use, relationship to other substances, and perception of use and safety for synthetic cannabinoids. Brain Res Bull. 2016;126:8–28.
35. Winstock AR, Barratt MJ. Synthetic cannabis: a comparison of patterns of use and effect profile with natural cannabis in a large global sample. Drug Alcohol Depend. 2013;131(1–3):106–11.
36. Weaver MF, Hopper JA, Gunderson EW. Designer drugs 2015: assessment and management. 2015;1–9.
37. Egan KL, Suerken CK, Reboussin BA, Spangler J, Wagoner KG, Sutfin EL, et al. K2 and Spice use among a cohort of college students in southeast region of the USA. Am J Drug Alcohol Abuse. 2015;41(4):317–22.
38. Palamar JJ, Acosta P. Synthetic cannabinoid use in a nationally representative sample of US high school seniors. Drug Alcohol Depend. 2015;149:194–202.
39. Cottencin O, Rolland B, Karila L. New designer drugs (synthetic cannabinoids and synthetic cathinones): review of literature. Curr Pharm Des. 2014;20:4106–11.
40. Navon L, Moritz E, Austin C, Wahl M, Aks S, Layden J. The public health response to a large poisoning outbreak involving an illicit substance: synthetic cannabinoids contaminated with a long-acting anticoagulant rodenticide, Illinois, March–July, 2018. J Public Heal Manag Pract. 2019. 9000;Publish Ah.
41. Fasih A. Lethal coagulopathy resulting from the consumption of contaminated synthetic cannabinoids: the story of a public health crisis. J Public Health (Bangkok). 2019;(March 2018):1–6.
42. Center for Disease Control and Prevention. Outbreak of life-threatening coagulopathy associated with synthetic cannabinoid use. Available from https://emergency.cdc.gov/han/han00410.asp.
43. Waien S, Hayes DJ, Leonardo J. Severe coagulopathy as a consequence of smoking crack cocaine laced with rodenticide. N Engl J Med. 2001;345(9):700.
44. SAMHSA. 2017 National survey on drug use and health (NSDUH). Table 5.5A—alcohol use disorder in past year among persons aged

12 or older, by age group and demographic characteristics: numbers in thousands, 2016 and 2017.
45. Substance Abuse and Mental Health Services Administration. 2017 National Survey on Drug Use and Health. Table 2.19B—Alcohol use in lifetime, past year, and past month among persons aged 12 or older, by detailed age category: percentages, 2016 and 2017.
46. Mokdad AH, Marks JS, Stroup DF, Gerberding JL. Actual causes of death in the United States, 2000. JAMA. 2004;291: 1238–45.
47. Types of alcohol-induced liver damage. https://liverfoundation.org/for-patients/about-the-liver/diseases-of-the-liver/alcohol-related-liver-disease/.
48. Mellinger JL. Epidemiology of alcohol use and alcoholic liver disease. Clin Liver Dis. John Wiley and Sons Inc. 2019;13:136–9.
49. Tousoulis D, Ntarladimas I, Antoniades C, Vasiliadou C, Tentolouris C, Papageorgiou N, et al. Acute effects of different alcoholic beverages on vascular endothelium, inflammatory markers and thrombosis fibrinolysis system. Clin Nutr. 2008;27(4):594–600.
50. Shen CJ, Kao CH, Hsu TY, Chen CY, Lin CL, Shih HM. Effect of alcohol intoxication on the risk of venous thromboembolism. Med (United States). 2017;96(42):e8041.
51. Harrison MF. The misunderstood coagulopathy of liver disease: a review for the acute setting. West J Emerg Med. eScholarship. 2018;19:863–71.
52. Strate LL, Singh P, Boylan MR, Piawah S, Cao Y, Chan AT. A prospective study of alcohol consumption and smoking and the risk of major gastrointestinal bleeding in men. PLoS One. 2016;11(11):e0165278.
53. Stahre M, Roeber J, Kanny D, Brewer RD, Zhang X. Contribution of excessive alcohol consumption to deaths and years of potential life lost in the United States. Prev Chronic Dis. 2014;11:1–12.
54. Saner FH, Bezinover D. Assessment and management of coagulopathy in critically-ill patients with liver failure. Curr Opin Crit Care. 2019;25(2):179–86.
55. Grover SP, Mackman N. Intrinsic pathway of coagulation and thrombosis: insights from animal models. Arterioscler Thromb Vasc Biol. 2019;39(3):331–8.
56. Boral BM, Williams DJ, Boral LI. Disseminated intravascular coagulation. Am J Clin Pathol. 2016;146(6):670–80.
57. Rubinstein I, Weinberg G, van Breemen R, Hershow RC, Feinstein DL. Treatment for long acting anticoagulant rodenticide poisoning - beyond INR monitoring? Toxicol Commun. 2018;2(1): 59–61.
58. Watt BE, Proudfoot AT, Bradberry SMVJ. Anticoagulant rodenticides. Toxicol Rev. 2005;24(4):259–69.
59. Wang Y, Kotik V, Fahim G, Alagusundaramoorthy S, Eltawansy SA, Mathis S, et al. Treatment of brodifacoum overdose with prothrombin complex concentrate. Am J Health Syst Pharm. 2016;73(1):e14–7.
60. Bruno GR, Howland MA, McMeeking A, Hoffman RS. Long-acting anticoagulant overdose: brodifacoum kinetics and optimal vitamin K dosing. Ann Emerg Med. 2000;36(3):262–7.
61. Doyle RJ, Elfessi Z, Kolman K. Fixed dose 4-factor prothrombin complex concentrate for bleeding caused by long acting anticoagulant rodenticides. Am J Emerg Med. 2018;36(10):1922.e3–4.
62. Khan A. How to address bleeding reversal in synthetic cannabinoid users. Pharm Times. 2018.
63. King N, Tran MH. Long-acting anticoagulant rodenticide (Superwarfarin) poisoning: a review of its historical development, epidemiology, and clinical management. In: Transfusion medicine reviews, vol. 29: W.B. Saunders; 2015. p. 250–8. https://www.clintox.org/wp-content/uploads/2016/05/Anticoagulant-Rodenticide-Poisoning.pdf.
64. DeLoughery TG, Shatzel J. The superwarfarin chronicles. ASH Clinical News. 2018. p. 1.
65. Kelkar AH, Smith NA, Martial A, Moole H, Tarantino MD, Roberts JC. An outbreak of synthetic cannabinoid-associated coagulopathy in Illinois. N Engl J Med. 2018;379(13):1216–23.
66. Caravati EM, Erdman AR, Scharman EJ, Woolf AD, Chyka PA, Cobaugh DJ, Wax PM, Manoguerra AS, Christianson G, Nelson LS, Olson KR, Booze LLTW. Long-acting anticoagulant rodenticide poisoning: an evidence-based consensus guideline for out-of-hospital management. Clin Toxicol. 2007;45(1):1–22.
67. Zupančić-Šalek S, Kovačević-Metelko J, Radman I. Succesful reversal of anticoagulant effect of superwarfarin poisoning with recombinant activated factor VII. Blood Coagul Fibrinolysis. 2005;16(4):239–44.
68. Frontera JA, Lewin JJ, Rabinstein AA, Aisiku IP, Alexandrov AW, Cook AM, et al. Guideline for reversal of antithrombotics in intracranial hemorrhage: a statement for healthcare professionals from the Neurocritical Care Society and Society of Critical Care Medicine. Neurocrit Care. 2016;24(1):6–46.
69. Lipton RA, Klass EM. Human ingestion of a 'superwarfarin' rodenticide resulting in a prolonged anticoagulant effect. JAMA. 1984;252(21):3004–5.
70. Rubinstein I, van Breemen R, Nosal DG, Weinberg G, Hershow RC, Feinstein DL. Should cytochrome P450 inducers be used to accelerate clearance of brodifacoum from poisoned patients? Drugs R D. 2019;19(1):67–71.
71. Laposata M, Van Cott EM, Lev MH. Case records of the Massachusetts General Hospital. Case 1-2007. A 40-year-old woman with epistaxis, hematemesis, and altered mental status. N Engl J Med. 2007;356(2):174–82.
72. Papin F, Clarot F, Vicomte C, Gaulier JM, Daubin C, Chapon F, et al. Lethal paradoxical cerebral vein thrombosis due to suspicious anticoagulant rodenticide intoxication with chlorophacinone. Forensic Sci Int. 2007;166(2–3):85–90.
73. Franco D, Everett G, Manoucheri M. I smell a rat: a case report and literature review of paradoxical thrombosis and hemorrhage in a patient with brodifacoum toxicity. Blood Coagul Fibrinolysis. 2013;24(2):202–4.
74. De Paula EV, Montalvao SAL, Madureira PR, Jose Vieira R, Annichino-Bizzacchi JM, Ozelo MC. Simultaneous bleeding and thrombosis in superwarfarin poisoning. Thromb Res. 2009;123(4):637–9.
75. Kaye AD, Clarke RC, Sabar R, Vig S, Dhawan KP, Hofbauer R, et al. Herbal medicines: current trends in anesthesiology practice--a hospital survey. J Clin Anesth [Internet]. 2000 Sep [cited 2016 Dec 14];12(6):468–71. Available from: http://www.ncbi.nlm.nih.gov/pubmed/11090733.
76. Howard BM, Kornblith LZ, Redick BJ, Vilardi RF, Balhotra KS, Crane JM, et al. The effects of alcohol on coagulation in trauma patients: interpreting thrombelastography with caution. J Trauma Acute Care Surg. 2014;77(6):865–71; discussion 871-2.
77. Stecker T, McGovern MP, Herr B. An intervention to increase alcohol treatment engagement: a pilot trial. J Subst Abus Treat. 2012;43(2):161–7.
78. Tonigan JS, Toscova R, Miller WR. Meta-analysis of the literature on alcoholics anonymous: sample and study characteristics moderate findings. J Stud Alcohol. 1996;57(1):65–72.
79. Barnett NP, Celio MA, Tidey JW, Murphy JG, Colby SM, Swift RM. A preliminary randomized controlled trial of contingency management for alcohol use reduction using a transdermal alcohol sensor. Addiction. 2017;112(6):1025–35.
80. Jonas DE, Amick HR, Feltner C, Bobashev G, Thomas K, Wines R, et al. Pharmacotherapy for adults with alcohol use disorders in outpatient settings. JAMA. 2014;311(18):1889–1900. https://doi.org/10.1001/jama.2014.3628.

81. Rösner S, Leucht S, Lehert P, Soyka M. Acamprosate supports abstinence, naltrexone prevents excessive drinking: evidence from a meta-analysis with unreported outcomes. J Psychopharmacol. 2008;22(1):11–23.
82. Rose AK, Jones A. Baclofen: its effectiveness in reducing harmful drinking, craving, and negative mood. A meta-analysis. Addiction. 2018;113(8):1396–406.
83. Moran S, Isa J, Steinemann S. Perioperative management in the patient with substance abuse. Surg Clin North Am. 2015;95(2):417–28.
84. Abraham E, Shoemaker WC, Mccartney SF. Cardiorespiratory patterns in severe delirium tremens. Arch Intern Med. 1985;145(6):1057–9.
85. Brohi K, Cohen MJ, Davenport RA. Acute coagulopathy of trauma: mechanism, identification and effect. Curr Opin Crit Care. 2007;13(6):680–5.
86. Hoyt DB, Dutton RP, Hauser CJ, Hess JR, Holcomb JB, Kluger Y, et al. Management of coagulopathy in the patients with multiple injuries: results from an international survey of clinical practice. J Trauma - Inj Infect Crit Care. 2008;65(4):755–64; discussion 764–5.
87. Amarapurkar PD, Amarapurkar DN. Management of coagulopathy in patients with decompensated liver cirrhosis. Int J Hepatol. 2011;2011:695470.
88. Holcomb JB, Wade CE, Michalek JE, Chisholm GB, Zarzabal LA, Schreiber MA, et al. Increased plasma and platelet to red blood cell ratios improves outcome in 466 massively transfused civilian trauma patients. Ann Surg. 2008;248(3):447–58.
89. Johansson PI, Stensballe J. Hemostatic resuscitation for massive bleeding: the paradigm of plasma and platelets - a review of the current literature. Transfusion. 2010;50(3):701–10.
90. Bolliger D, Görlinger K, Tanaka KA. Pathophysiology and treatment of coagulopathy in massive hemorrhage and hemodilution. Anesthesiology. 2010;113(5):1205–19.
91. Giannini EG, Stravitz RT, Caldwell SH. Correction of hemostatic abnormalities and portal pressure variations in patients with cirrhosis. Hepatology. 2014;60(4):1442.
92. Ansell J, Hirsh J, Poller L, Bussey H, Jacobson A, Hijlek E. The pharmacology and management of the vitamin K antagonists: the Seventh ACCP Conference on Antithrombotic and Thrombolytic Therapy. Chest. 2004;126(3 Suppl):204S–33S.
93. Abuelkasem E, Hasan S, Mazzeffi MA, Planinsic RM, Sakai T, Tanaka KA. Reduced requirement for prothrombin complex concentrate for the restoration of thrombin generation in plasma from liver transplant recipients. Anesth Analg. 2017;125(2):609–15.
94. Sørensen B, Spahn DR, Innerhofer P, Spannagl M, Rossaint R. Clinical review: prothrombin complex concentrates - evaluation of safety and thrombogenicity. Crit Care. 2011;15(1):201.
95. Ferguson JW, Helmy A, Ludlam C, Webb DJ, Hayes PC, Newby DC. Hyperfibrinolysis in alcoholic cirrhosis: relative plasminogen activator inhibitor type 1 deficiency. Thromb Res. 2008;121(5):675–80.
96. Henry DA, Carless PA, Moxey AJ, O'Connell D, Stokes BJ, McClelland B, et al. Anti-fibrinolytic use for minimising perioperative allogeneic blood transfusion. Cochrane Database Syst Rev. 2007;(4):CD001886.

The Effects of Perioperative Transfusion of Allogenic Blood Products of Cancer Recurrence

41

Yang Jiang, Jay Karri, Kristen Mathias, and Alaa Abd-Elsayed

Background

Correction of anemias has traditionally been thought to improve outcomes in patients undergoing cancer resection [1, 2]. Consequently, allogeneic blood products are readily used in the perioperative setting to optimize this medically tenuous patient population. In recent years, however, there have been increasing studies suggesting that perioperative transfusion of blood products may paradoxically increase recurrence of cancer [3–5].

Cancer recurrence is a devastating clinical outcome as it often confers an increase in overall morbidity and mortality. Therefore, long-term outcomes must be considered even in early cancer management. Incorporating preemptive measures early in the treatment course may be consequential in preventing cancer recurrence and improving long-term patient outcomes. Conservative use of blood products has been proposed as a means of risk mitigation for cancer recurrence.

There has been increasing literature in cancer patients within the past decade that has associated blood transfusions with adverse perioperative morbidity, metastatic progression, and decreased disease-free and overall survival. These studies range in clinical context, cancer type, and surgical technique. The greatest evidence supporting this theory are in gastroesophageal, colorectal, pancreatic, and prostate cancers, with the most randomized control trials in colorectal cancer [3, 6, 7]. The association between perioperative blood transfusion (PBT) and adverse long-term outcomes remains controversial, however, because most studies to date have been retrospective and observational. Literature in other solid tumors are even more limited in quantity, quality, and consensus. Overall, despite PBT being a pervasive consideration in patients undergoing surgical management in malignancy, there exists a paucity of high-level evidence and recommendations for clinical practice.

While there have been multiple theories attempting to propose possible mechanisms for PBT contributing to cancer recurrence, the precise pathophysiology underlying this phenomenon remains poorly understood and has yet to be clearly delineated. Transfusion-related immunomodulation (TRIM) is considered the prevailing theory for contextualizing the molecular machinery responsible for post-PBT cancer recurrence [3, 8, 9]. This theory proposes that blood transfusions serve to downregulate the inflammatory response of the recipient, thereby producing a pro-tumor host environment. Pro-inflammatory cytokines, growth factors, and microparticles contained in the blood are all thought to change the immune milieu to favor oncogenesis [10, 11]. Secondary non-immune mechanisms proposed as to how blood transfusions lead to adverse patient outcomes include postoperative infectious complications, lung and cardiac injury, and disruption of the coagulation cascade [3]. There are also theories proposed that blood transfusion may lead to higher likelihood of leakage at the surgical anastomotic site and subsequent decrease in overall survival [12, 13]. However, the majority of the highest-level evidence exploring PBT and cancer recurrence has implicated dysregulated immunomodulation as responsible for the underlying pathophysiology.

Host immunity is suppressed in different degrees depending on the type of blood product used, features of the donor, quantity of blood transfused, and timing of transfusion. TRIM has been seen in the transfusion of all blood products, including whole blood, packed red blood cells, plasma, and

Y. Jiang
University of California Los Angeles School of Medicine, Department of Hematology and Oncology, Los Angeles, CA, USA

J. Karri
Baylor College of Medicine, Department of Physical Medicine and Rehabilitation, Houston, TX, USA

K. Mathias (✉)
University of Chicago, Department of Internal Medicine, Chicago, IL, USA

A. Abd-Elsayed
Department of Anesthesiology, University of Wisconsin School of Medicine and Public Health, Madison, WI, USA

© Springer Nature Switzerland AG 2021
C. S. Scher et al. (eds.), *Essentials of Blood Product Management in Anesthesia Practice*,
https://doi.org/10.1007/978-3-030-59295-0_41

platelets [14]. Autologous blood is less implicated in adverse outcomes than allogeneic [15]. Multiple studies have also suggested age of the blood donor affects patient outcome [16]. Dose of product transfused, leukoreduction status, and timing of the transfusion (whether pre-operative, intraoperative, or postoperative) also affect patient outcomes [3, 16–20]. Through these aforementioned parameters, host immunomodulation is disturbed in different capacities and leads to differences in tumor recurrence and patient outcome.

There are confounding factors unassociated with transfusion that oppose the view that PBT independently leads to adverse outcomes in cancer patients. Risks inherent to the patient population, cancer type, and surgical procedure must be considered. The patients and procedures that require more transfusions may also be the ones at higher risk for recurrent disease, separately from the transfusion itself. Baseline characteristics of patients who require perioperative transfusions typically include poor pre-operative nutrition, functional status, and anemia. Patients may also have advanced stage or poorly resectable cancers, requiring long procedures, high amounts of blood loss, and use of specific types of anesthesia. These surgeries may be more likely to increase malignant cells in circulation through tumor manipulation, and they may require more potent anesthetics and medications that can depress host immunity [21, 22]. Perioperative stress, inflammatory response, metabolic perturbation, and postoperative complications may also be higher in this patient subset. All of these confounding factors affect patient outcome and tumor recurrence separately from the transfusion itself. Some of the literature supporting TRIM account for these confounding factors through multivariable analysis, while others do not [23]. Additionally, most of our clinical evidence is retrospective, which creates difficulty separating confounding factors. This further necessitates quality randomized control trials to show transfusion can increase recurrence of the tumor independently of the factors associated with the surgical procedures and population at risk.

Although blood transfusions were long considered beneficial for perioperative management in persons undergoing cancer resection, increasing literature suggests that they may promote the risk of cancer recurrence. Unfortunately, this novel concept is substantiated by few well-designed and impactful studies and requires further exploration. Several existing studies are burdened with numerous clinical confounders and fail to clearly delineate PBT and long-term effects on recurrence-free and overall survival. Consequently, evidence-based data to dictate the judicious use of PBT for both optimizing perioperative risk and prevention cancer recurrence are largely lacking. Nonetheless, a thorough understanding of this phenomenon is instrumental for contextualizing forthcoming literature and transfusion guidelines. This chapter serves to present the proposed mechanisms of transfusion-related immunomodulation, risk factors for cancer recurrence, and clinical considerations for PBT.

Transfusion-Related Immunomodulation

The most investigated and cited mechanism suggested for perioperative blood transfusion and cancer recurrence is that of TRIM [3, 8, 9]. This theory suggests that the transfused blood changes the immune environment to suppress host immunity and allow tumor recurrence. Subsequently, metastatic progenitors may interact with immune modulators to survive and proliferate. By affecting the immune milieu, PBT theoretically adversely impacts postoperative complications, disease recurrence, metastasis, and overall mortality. Through immune dysregulation, PBT has been associated with patients having increased susceptibility to nosocomial infections in the short term and oncogenesis in the long term after surgery.

Host immune disruption has been suggested to occur through several mechanisms. These include transfusion-induced suppression of natural killer (NK) cell activity, depression of monocyte phagocytosis, increase in T-helper (Th) cell subtypes that favor host immunosuppression, upregulation in T-regulatory (Treg) cell activity with inhibition of interleukin-2 (IL-2) production, and augmented soluble microparticles such as human leukocyte antigen (HLA) Class I peptides and fibroblast-associated (FAS) ligand [3, 8, 9, 24]. Other mechanisms proposed include clonal deletion, induction of host anergy and tolerance, and alteration of B-cell antibodies in donor plasma that alter host response.

Cellular-based host interference primarily occurs through disturbance of normal Th cell subtype, Treg, NK, and monocyte activity [24–26]. Th1 cells are widely implicated in generating immune response against intracellular pathogens and tumorigenesis. Conversely, Th2 cells primarily target extracellular pathogens and permit tumor survival and invasiveness. PBT has been associated with gene expression profiles demonstrating decreased Th1 and increased Th2 activity, allowing for decreased host defense and recurrence of cancer. Tregs are similarly thought to suppress host immunity through decrease in IL-2 production. Additionally, NK cells and monocytes normally serve as immune regulators by decreasing the cytotoxic nature of tumor-infected cells and preventing tumor survival and metastasis. NK cell and monocyte reduction is also seen after transfusion, allowing for the cancer cells to not only recur in a debilitated host immune system but also survive and proliferate. Reduction of cytotoxic NK cells and phagocytic monocytes may also activate free tumor thrombus, causing postoperative recurrence and metastasis. Thus far, only decrease in Th1/Th2 ratio and suppression of NK cell activity have been studied, and these studies primarily exist in gastrointestinal cancers. The theory that PBT leads to host immune suppression and tumor recurrence needs to be further explored in other types of cancer and other cell types.

The details of the immune mechanisms responsible for oncogenesis are still being elucidated to prevent tumor recurrence. Leukodepletion is thought to decrease TRIM through limiting exposure to immune-stimulatory antigens. Decreased storage length is also hypothesized to minimize TRIM. Despite current standards of leukoreduction and blood storage, donor products are thought to still contain activated pro-inflammatory cytokines, chemokines, growth factors, prostaglandins and other biochemical microparticles (such as HLA Class I peptide and soluble FAS ligand) that shift the immune environment toward host immune suppression and tumor proliferation. These inflammatory biochemical substances are theorized to promote oncogenesis along every stage of tumor growth. They promote epithelial-mesenchymal transition and vascular permeability that facilitates cancer mobility and metastasis. Transfusion components may also include vascular endothelial growth factors, plasminogen activators, and other biochemical substances that subsequently allow metastasized cells to survive, invade, and proliferate. More laboratory research is necessary to further elucidate the exact molecules, pathways, and mechanisms of immune suppression and cancer survival. Nevertheless, TRIM remains the primary theory implicated in PBT and cancer recurrence.

Blood transfusions can also lead to poor patient outcomes through non-immune mechanisms. These non-immune sequelae of blood transfusion may independently cause increased perioperative and postoperative mortality. PBT confers increased risk of postoperative nosocomial infections (wound site, catheter-related) [5, 24, 27]. There have in fact been well-documented immunosuppressive patterns of gene expression associated with perioperative infective complications. Postoperative abdominal infection has also been shown to independently adversely affect overall outcome. PBT is also associated with pulmonary complications (thromboembolism, acute respiratory failure, and pneumonia), cardiac complications (myocardial infarction, angina, arrhythmia, and cardiac arrest), and non-immune transfusion-related complications (hemolytic reactions due to ABO mismatch, blood mismatch reactions, and concomitant hypoxia-induced factors that promote tumor angiogenesis).

Anastomotic leakage (AL) is a special category of complication that is frequent and well-established to be associated with blood transfusions in gastroesophageal junction and colorectal cancers [13]. PBT is intriguingly thought to compromise the microcirculation rheology and cause inflammation, especially at the anastomotic site. This phenomenon has mostly been seen to occur within 1 week of receiving perioperative blood products and may lead to the need for reoperation. Multivariate analysis data has shown AL to be an independent risk factor for decreased overall and cancer-specific survival. These non-immune mechanisms of PBT contributing to adverse patient outcome offer alterative explanations to the primary theory of TRIM leading to cancer recurrence. Whether through immune or non-immune mechanisms, PBT is implicated in adverse short-term and long-term outcomes following surgery.

Risk Factors for Cancer Recurrence

The risk factors associated with cancer recurrence significantly overlap with those of patients necessitating perioperative blood transfusion [1–6]. Patients who require PBTs are typically also ones with poor baseline functional status, advanced stage cancers, and need for lengthier surgical procedures. Cancer recurrence is thus more likely in these patients, separate from the effect of transfusions, and may confound the association of PBTs with overall outcome. While some of the literature account for these confounding factors and show PBT as an independent risk factor for cancer recurrence, others demonstrate a dependent association.

It is intuitive and supported by data that patients with poor ECOG and Karnofsky status generally have poor overall and cancer-specific survival after surgical intervention. Patients who are more malnourished and, anemic and have lower baseline functional reserve are more likely to have poor tolerance of the stressors introduced by surgery. This leads to more complications both intraoperatively and postoperatively that compromise outcome, separately from the effect of PBT [28–30].

Patients who have decreased survival also tend to have a higher proportion of tumor burdens that are high grade, advanced stage, and poorly resectable. Furthermore, these patients often require lengthier surgeries that are associated with more extensive blood losses. They may also necessitate stronger anesthetics and for protracted time periods that cause host immune suppression. There are also certain locations of tumors, such as intraabdominal or associated with the gastrointestinal tract, that are more likely to introduce malignant cells into circulation and have independently been associated with cancer recurrence. Thus, in a parallel way to PBT, immune and non-immune mechanisms contribute to adverse patient outcome. These high-risk patients, tumor types, and surgical procedures introduce perioperative stress, metabolic disturbances, and foreign products that confound the association of PBT with adverse patient outcome.

All of these confounding factors affect patient outcome and tumor recurrence separately from the transfusion itself. High-risk physiologic factors [e.g., older age, lower BMI, smoking status, worse performance status, pre-operative anemia, underlying comorbidities, neoadjuvant chemotherapy (NAC) requirements], or patient-specific surgical factors [pathologic stage, nodal metastases, tumor size, operative time, difficulty of the operation, estimated blood loss] affect not only the decision to transfuse but also cancer-specific outcomes. Significant postoperative complications that have been associated with worse patient outcomes after PBT that are separate from the effects of blood transfusion included thromboembolic events, delayed gastric emptying, uncontrolled hyperglycemia, and increased length of stay.

Some of the literature supporting PBT account for these confounding factors through multivariable analysis, while others do not. Still others do not perform multivariate analysis to adjust for confounding factors. Additionally, known data on PBT and adverse outcome association is primarily retrospective. Available clinical evidence creates difficulty separating confounding factors. This further necessitates quality randomized control trials to show transfusion can increase recurrence of the tumor independently of the factors associated with the surgical procedures and population at risk.

Certain cancer types are also more associated with poor outcomes after PBT. Specifically, gastroesophageal, colorectal, pancreatic, and prostate cancers have the most data supporting this theory [30–44].

PBT has also been implicated in bladder cancer and renal cancer; however studies available in current literature are more heterogeneous and poor in quality [45–52]. Unfortunately, evidence is even sparser in other tumor types. Conflicting or limited evidence exists in head and neck, lung, hepatic, biliary, peritoneal, ovarian, and cervical cancers [17, 18, 22, 53–55]. Available literature on PBT being unassociated with cancer recurrence includes spinal metastases of various primary tumors; however, this evidence is limited [56].

Overall, data is significantly lacking despite PBT comprising a universal problem surrounding surgical management of cancer. Most available evidence is retrospective and observational. Randomized control trials are limited, with the most associating PBT and cancer recurrence in colorectal cancer. More quality evidence is necessary to elucidate the association or lack of association of PBT with cancer recurrence. Public support is necessary to garner much needed high-level evidence to affect guidelines in clinical practice.

Clinical Practice Considerations for Perioperative Transfusions

Currently, as is reasonable and clinically appropriate, transfusion patterns are directed toward correcting the anemic statuses of cancer patients in anticipation of operative interventions [3]. These transfusion practice patterns themselves range from conservative to liberal, so as to prevent early transfusion-related adverse outcomes and effectively produce anemia correction. However, there exist very limited literature and no guidelines to direct transfusion practice patterns. Additionally, literature delineating the long-term adverse risks of cancer recurrence associated with various transfusion practices are also lacking. Regardless, the literature to date allows practitioners to consider several important parameters in their transfusion decision-making: conservative vs. liberal transfusion thresholds, low vs. high total transfusion dosages, and autologous vs. allogeneic donor sources. Of note, however, transfusion practices largely vary upon the particular clinical context, and parameters including cancer type, severity, and operative bleeding risk must always be considered.

Transfusion thresholds are highly dependent on the clinical context. Nonetheless, conservative transfusion parameters were thought to possibly be superior to more liberal parameters [17, 18, 41]. Xue et al. explored transfusion practices in a cohort of gastric adenocarcinoma patients undergoing surgical resection [34]. Firstly, they found that those patients who received transfusions had lower overall survival across a 150-month follow-up period. Most importantly, these trends were maintained when subgroup analyses exploring per-operative anemic status were considered, i.e., transfused patients had higher mortalities in the chronic phase irrespective of their pre-operative anemic status. While not overtly apparent in persons with 7–10 g/dl of pre-operative hemoglobin, those "non-anemic" persons with >10 g/dl of pre-operative hemoglobin that were transfused had much lower survival than their non-transfused counterparts. Additionally, they also found that transfusions were detrimental in "non-anemic" persons with stage 3 gastric adenocarcinoma. Following that, Liu et al. found that all stage 3 gastric cancer patients who received transfusions had lower cumulative survival regardless of anemic status [31]. Baumeister et al. also found similar patterns in a cohort of persons with head and neck cancers [22]. They conclude that restrictive transfusion thresholds should be utilized perioperatively in persons undergoing head and neck squamous cell cancer resection.

Past the decision toward transfusing patients, total transfusion loads are thought to carry a dose-dependent detriment in the perioperative phase [17, 18, 41]. This is particularly noteworthy as practitioners also utilize varied practices for total transfusion dosing after the decision to transfuse has been established. Thus, total transfusion loads are reflective of another point of possible intervention and investigation. Nizri et al. explored patient outcomes in persons with diffuse malignant peritoneal mesothelioma in the context of total transfusion dosages [17]. They found a direct dose-dependent relationship between total transfusion dosage inversely to both progression-free survival and overall survival.

Interestingly, similar explorations by Latif et al. in a cohort of persons with non-small cell lung cancer found that a single-unit packed red blood cell transfusion did not confer any increased risk of cancer recurrence [18]. However, they found that increased transfusions were inversely related to disease-free survival and overall survival. These findings support the utilization of judicious, conservative transfusion parameters.

In addition to the above factors, blood product donor source is vital to consider in the preparation of blood transfusions [3]. As expected, autologous transfusions are thought to be less detrimental compared to allogeneic products in regard to cancer recurrence [32, 33]. The superiority of autologous products has not been fully determined – largely because the vast majority of studies exploring this phenomenon involve allogeneic transfusions, as is standard in current clinical practice. Additionally, there exist safety concerns with autologous products given the theoretical risk that autologous blood may contain malignant cells that may be reintroduced following resection. However, the use of autologous products has been established as a safe practice across numerous cancer contexts. In fact, a few small, retrospective studies including cohorts with head and neck cancers have found that allogenic products confer greater cancer recurrence relative to autologous products [57]. More impactful evidence is largely lacking, however.

Conclusion

While PBTs are necessary in appropriate clinical contexts to correct pre-operative anemias, they have also been associated with increased risk of cancer recurrence in persons undergoing cancer resection interventions. Notably, it has been extensively shown that this increased risk was secondary to the PBT itself rather than the anemic status in this tenuous population. However, some studies have found that clinical parameters – ranging from cancer severity to performance status – ultimately drive cancer recurrence risk rather that PBT status. A clear understanding of PBT-induced cancer recurrence has yet to be clearly elucidated. The prevailing theory explaining this phenomenon suggests that TRIM downregulates immunogenic machinery in the transfusion recipient and facilitates the production of an oncogenic host environment. Regardless of the precise molecular mechanisms, judicious transfusion practices are necessary to optimize patient safety profiles and long-term disease-free survival. Unfortunately, this concern of PBT conferred cancer recurrence is still novel and further studies exploring underlying mechanisms and directing clinical practice patterns for PBT usage are necessary.

References

1. Dunne JR, Malone D, Tracy JK, Gannon C, Napolitano LM. Perioperative anemia: an independent risk factor for infection, mortality, and resource utilization in surgery. J Surg Res. 2002;102(2):237–44.
2. Schrijvers D. Management of anemia in cancer patients: transfusions. Oncologist. 2011;16(suppl 3):12–8.
3. Cata JP, Wang H, Gottumukkala V, Reuben J, Sessler DI. Inflammatory response, immunosuppression, and cancer recurrence after perioperative blood transfusions. Br J Anaesth. 2013;110(5):690–701.
4. Amato A, Pescatori M. Perioperative blood transfusions and recurrence of colorectal cancer. Cochrane Database Syst Rev. 2006;(1).
5. Vamvakas EC. Transfusion-associated cancer recurrence and postoperative infection: meta-analysis of randomized, controlled clinical trials. Transfusion. 1996;36(2):175–86.
6. Blumberg N, Agarwal MM, Chuang C. Relation between recurrence of cancer of the colon and blood transfusion. Br Med J (Clin Res Ed). 1985;290(6474):1037–9.
7. Foster RS Jr, Costanza MC, Foster JC, Wanner MC, Foster CB. Adverse relationship between blood transfusions and survival after colectomy for colon cancer. Cancer. 1985;55(6):1195–201.
8. Vamvakas EC, Blajchman MA. Transfusion-related immunomodulation (TRIM): an update. Blood Rev. 2007;21(6):327–48.
9. Blajchman MA. Transfusion immunomodulation or TRIM: what does it mean clinically? Hematology. 2005;10(sup1):208–14.
10. Qiu L, Wang DR, Zhang XY, et al. Impact of perioperative blood transfusion on immune function and prognosis in colorectal cancer patients. Transfus Apher Sci. 2016;54(2):235–41.
11. Zhu M, Zhu Z, Yang J, Hu K, Li Y. Impact of perioperative blood transfusion on gene expression biomarkers in patients with gastrointestinal cancer. Transfus Apher Sci. 2018;57(5):656–60.
12. Pang QY, An R, Liu HL. Perioperative transfusion and the prognosis of colorectal cancer surgery: a systematic review and meta-analysis. World J Surg Oncol. 2019;17(1):7.
13. Terp Fjederholt K, Svendsen LB, Mortensen FV. Perioperative blood transfusions increases the risk of anastomotic leakage after surgery for GEJ-cancer. Am J Surg. 2017;214(2):293–8.
14. Nakaseko Y, Haruki K, Shiba H, et al. Impact of fresh frozen plasma transfusion on postoperative inflammation and prognosis of colorectal liver metastases. J Surg Res. 2018;226:157–65.
15. Li SL, Ye Y, Yuan XH. Association between allogeneic or autologous blood transfusion and survival in patients after radical prostatectomy: a systematic review and meta-analysis. PLoS One. 2017;12(1):e0171081.
16. Loftus TJ, Lopez AN, Jenkins TK, et al. Packed red blood cell donor age affects overall survival in transfused patients undergoing hepatectomy for non-hepatocellular malignancy. Am J Surg. 2019;217(1):71–7.
17. Nizri E, Kusamura S, Fallabrino G, Guaglio M, Baratti D, Deraco M. Dose-dependent effect of red blood cells transfusion on perioperative and long-term outcomes in peritoneal surface malignancies treated with cytoreduction and HIPEC. Ann Surg Oncol. 2018;25(11):3264–70.
18. Latif MJ, Tan KS, Molena D, et al. Perioperative blood transfusion has a dose-dependent relationship with disease recurrence and survival in patients with non-small cell lung cancer. J Thorac Cardiovasc Surg. 2019;157:2469–77.
19. Wu HL, Tai YH, Lin SP, Chan MY, Chen HH, Chang KY. The impact of blood transfusion on recurrence and mortality following colorectal cancer resection: a propensity score analysis of 4,030 patients. Sci Rep. 2018;8(1):13345.
20. Moschini M, Soria F, Abufaraj M, et al. Impact of intra- and post-operative blood transfusion on the incidence, timing, and pattern

of disease recurrence after radical cystectomy. Clin Genitourin Cancer. 2017;15(4):e681–8.
21. Lopez-aguiar AG, Ethun CG, Mcinnis MR, et al. Association of perioperative transfusion with survival and recurrence after resection of gallbladder cancer: a 10-institution study from the US Extrahepatic Biliary Malignancy Consortium. J Surg Oncol. 2018;117(8):1638–47.
22. Baumeister P, Canis M, Reiter M. Preoperative anemia and perioperative blood transfusion in head and neck squamous cell carcinoma. PLoS One. 2018;13(10):e0205712.
23. Warschkow R, Güller U, Köberle D, et al. Perioperative blood transfusions do not impact overall and disease-free survival after curative rectal cancer resection: a propensity score analysis. Ann Surg. 2014;259(1):131–8.
24. Jensen LS, Andersen AJ, Christiansen PM, Hokland P, Juhl CO, Madsen G, Mortensen J, Meller-Nielsen C, Hanberg-Sørensen F, Hokland M. Postoperative infection and natural killer cell function following blood transfusion in patients undergoing elective colorectal surgery. Br J Surg. 1992;79(6):513–6.
25. Kaplan J, Sarnaik S, Gitlin J, Lusher J. Diminished helper/suppressor lymphocyte ratios and natural killer activity in recipients of repeated blood transfusions. Blood. 1984;64(1):308–10.
26. Tartter PI, Steinberg B, Barron DM, Martinelli G. Transfusion history, T cell subsets and natural killer cytotoxicity in patients with colorectal cancer 1. Vox Sang. 1989;56(2):80–4.
27. Manning-geist BL, Alimena S, Del Carmen MG, et al. Infection, thrombosis, and oncologic outcome after interval debulking surgery: does perioperative blood transfusion matter? Gynecol Oncol. 2019;153(1):63–7.
28. Zhou PY, Tang Z, Liu WR, et al. Perioperative blood transfusion does not affect recurrence-free and overall survivals after curative resection for intrahepatic cholangiocarcinoma: a propensity score matching analysis. BMC Cancer. 2017;17(1):762.
29. Liu J, Chen S, Chen Y, Wang N, Ye X. Perioperative blood transfusion has no effect on overall survival after esophageal resection for esophageal squamous cell carcinoma: a retrospective cohort study. Int J Surg. 2018;55:24–30.
30. Peng T, Zhao G, Wang L, et al. No impact of perioperative blood transfusion on prognosis after curative resection for hepatocellular carcinoma: a propensity score matching analysis. Clin Transl Oncol. 2018;20(6):719–28.
31. Liu X, Ma M, Huang H, Wang Y. Effect of perioperative blood transfusion on prognosis of patients with gastric cancer: a retrospective analysis of a single center database. BMC Cancer. 2018;18(1):649.
32. Motoyama S, Saito R, Kamata S, et al. Survival advantage of using autologous blood transfusion during surgery for esophageal cancer. Surg Today. 2002;32(11):951–8.
33. Li L, Zhu D, Chen X, Huang Y, Ouyang M, Zhang W. Perioperative allogeneic blood transfusion is associated with worse clinical outcome for patients undergoing gastric carcinoma surgery: a meta-analysis. Medicine (Baltimore). 2015;94(39):e1574.
34. Xue L, Chen XL, Wei-han Z, et al. Impact of perioperative blood transfusion on postoperative complications and prognosis of gastric adenocarcinoma patients with different preoperative hemoglobin value. Gastroenterol Res Pract. 2016;2016:6470857.
35. Xu D, Fang X, Li Y, Zhang Z, Li Q. Perioperative blood transfusion is one of the factors that affect the prognosis of gastric cancer. J BUON. 2018;23(3):672–7.
36. Kim JK, Kim HS, Park J, et al. Perioperative blood transfusion as a significant predictor of biochemical recurrence and survival after radical prostatectomy in patients with prostate cancer. PLoS One. 2016;11(5):e0154918.
37. Pushan Z, Manbiao C, Sulai L, Jun L, Ruidong Z, Hanshen Y. The impact of perioperative blood transfusion on survival and recurrence after radical prostatectomy for prostate cancer: a systematic review and meta-analysis. J Cancer Res Ther. 2018;14(Supplement):S701–7.
38. Amri R, Dinaux AM, Leijssen LGJ, Kunitake H, Bordeianou LG, Berger DL. Do packed red blood cell transfusions really worsen oncologic outcomes in colon cancer? Surgery. 2017;162(3):586–91.
39. Tokunaga R, Nakagawa S, Miyamoto Y, et al. The impact of preoperative anaemia and anaemic subtype on patient outcome in colorectal cancer. Colorectal Dis. 2019;21(1):100–9.
40. Mörner ME, Edgren G, Martling A, Gunnarsson U, Egenvall M. Preoperative anaemia and perioperative red blood cell transfusion as prognostic factors for recurrence and mortality in colorectal cancer-a Swedish cohort study. Int J Colorectal Dis. 2017;32(2):223–32.
41. Kneuertz PJ, Patel SH, Chu CK, et al. Effects of perioperative red blood cell transfusion on disease recurrence and survival after pancreaticoduodenectomy for ductal adenocarcinoma. Ann Surg Oncol. 2011;18(5):1327–34.
42. Mavros MN, Xu L, Maqsood H, et al. Perioperative blood transfusion and the prognosis of pancreatic cancer surgery: systematic review and meta-analysis. Ann Surg Oncol. 2015;22(13):4382–91.
43. Park HM, Park SJ, Shim JR, et al. Perioperative transfusion in pancreatoduodenectomy: the double-edged sword of pancreatic surgeons. Medicine (Baltimore). 2017;96(49):e9019.
44. Sutton JM, Kooby DA, Wilson GC, et al. Perioperative blood transfusion is associated with decreased survival in patients undergoing pancreaticoduodenectomy for pancreatic adenocarcinoma: a multi-institutional study. J Gastrointest Surg. 2014;18(9):1575–87.
45. Abu-ghanem Y, Zilberman DE, Dotan Z, Kaver I, Ramon J. Perioperative blood transfusion adversely affects prognosis after nephrectomy for renal cell carcinoma. Urol Oncol. 2018;36(1):12. e15–20.
46. Arcaniolo D, Manfredi C, Cindolo L, et al. Impact of perioperative blood transfusions on the outcomes of patients undergoing kidney cancer surgery: a systematic review and pooled analysis. Clin Genitourin Cancer. 2019;17(1):e72–9.
47. Iwata T, Kimura S, Foerster B, et al. Perioperative blood transfusion affects oncologic outcomes after nephrectomy for renal cell carcinoma: a systematic review and meta-analysis. Urol Oncol. 2019;37(4):273–81.
48. Tsivian M, Abern MR, Tsivian E, et al. Effect of blood transfusions on oncological outcomes of surgically treated localized renal cell carcinoma. Urol Oncol. 2018;36(8):362.e1–7.
49. Cata JP, Lasala J, Pratt G, Feng L, Shah JB. Association between perioperative blood transfusions and clinical outcomes in patients undergoing bladder cancer surgery: a systematic review and meta-analysis study. J Blood Transfus. 2016;2016:9876394.
50. Chalfin HJ, Liu JJ, Gandhi N, et al. Blood transfusion is associated with increased perioperative morbidity and adverse oncologic outcomes in bladder cancer patients receiving neoadjuvant chemotherapy and radical cystectomy. Ann Surg Oncol. 2016;23(8):2715–22.
51. Furrer MA, Fellmann A, Schneider MP, Thalmann GN, Burkhard FC, Wuethrich PY. Impact of packed red blood cells and fresh frozen plasma given during radical cystectomy and urinary diversion on cancer-related outcome and survival: an observational cohort study. Eur Urol Focus. 2018;4(6):916–23.
52. Wang YL, Jiang B, Yin FF, et al. Perioperative blood transfusion promotes worse outcomes of bladder cancer after radical cystectomy: a systematic review and meta-analysis. PLoS One. 2015;10(6):e0130122.
53. Xun Y, Tian H, Hu L, Yan P, Yang K, Guo T. The impact of perioperative allogeneic blood transfusion on prognosis of hepatocellular carcinoma after radical hepatectomy: a systematic review and meta-analysis of cohort studies. Medicine (Baltimore). 2018;97(43):e12911.
54. Bogani G, Ditto A, Martinelli F, et al. Impact of blood transfusions on survival of locally advanced cervical cancer patients undergo-

ing neoadjuvant chemotherapy plus radical surgery. Int J Gynecol Cancer. 2017;27(3):514–22.

55. Connor JP, O'shea A, Mccool K, Sampene E, Barroilhet LM. Perioperative allogeneic blood transfusion is associated with poor overall survival in advanced epithelial ovarian cancer; potential impact of patient blood management on cancer outcomes. Gynecol Oncol. 2018;151(2):294–8.
56. Paulino pereira NR, Beks RB, Janssen SJ, et al. Are allogeneic blood transfusions associated with decreased survival after surgical treatment for spinal metastases? Spine J. 2016;16(8):951–61.
57. Moir MS, Samy RN, Hanasono MM, Terris DJ. Autologous and heterologous blood transfusion in head and neck cancer surgery. Arch Otolaryngol Head Neck Surg. 1999;125(8):864–8.

Perioperative Management of Polycythemia

42

Jianli Zhao, Liang Huang, David Matson, Na Li, and Henry Liu

Introduction

Polycythemia refers to clinical scenarios in which there is an absolute increase in total red cell mass. This condition has also been termed as erythrocytosis. Polycythemia has three different forms being recognized: primary polycythemia, secondary polycythemia, and mixed (i.e., primary and secondary). Polycythemia vera (PV) is the most common form of the primary polycythemias, which is a clonal disorder of hematopoietic stem/progenitor cells [1]. While low-risk patients can be treated with aspirin and phlebotomy, high-risk patients will likely need cytoreductive therapy, which most commonly consists of hydroxyurea therapy in the United States. In perioperative settings, patients with PV may pose challenges because it may cause an increased incidence of thromboembolic and hemorrhagic complications [1, 2]. Contemporary medical management of PV consists of phlebotomy, anticoagulation, hemodilution, and cytoreductive therapy attempting to maintain the hematocrit (Hct) level at below 45% and prevent thromboembolic event. High-risk patients with PV often require cytoreductive therapy typically with hydroxyurea [3, 4].

J. Zhao
Thomas Jefferson University Hospital, Department of Pathology, Philadelphia, PA, USA

L. Huang
New York University Langone School of Medicine, Department of Anesthesiology, New York, NY, USA

D. Matson
Reading Hospital/Tower Health, Department of Anesthesiology, West Reading, PA, USA

N. Li
Hubei Women & Children's Hospital, Department of Anesthesiology, Wuhan, Hubei, China

H. Liu (✉)
Department of Anesthesiology and Perioperative Medicine, Milton S. Hershey Medical Center, Penn State College of Medicine, Hershey, PA, USA

Classification of Polycythemia

Primary Polycythemia

Primary polycythemia is caused by acquired (somatic) or inherited (germline) mutations expressed within the erythroid progenitors that increase their proliferation and cause an accumulation of erythrocytes in the blood circulation (i.e., polycythemia). Such mutations occur in PV and in dominantly inherited polycythemias caused by "gain-of-function" mutations of the erythropoietin receptor (EPOR) gene [3]. Primary polycythemias can usually be distinguished from secondary polycythemias by in vitro assays that reveal proliferation of erythroid progenitors with minimal or no added erythropoietin (EPO) [3].

Secondary Polycythemia

Secondary polycythemia refers to conditions in which there are circulating plasma factors (EPO, testosterone, etc.) that stimulate erythropoiesis. In rare instances, exposure to cobalt, dysregulated angiotensin/angiotensin receptor 1 erythroid signaling (e.g., in post-renal transplant erythrocytosis), or elevated plasma levels of insulin-like growth factor-1 can stimulate erythropoiesis [5].

Both primary and secondary categories of polycythemia can have acquired and congenital causes. Secondary polycythemia can be due to "appropriate" or "inappropriate" physiological responses. Typical examples of appropriate physiological response include physiological response to tissue hypoxia and hypoxemia which induce an increase in red blood cell (RBC) mass in the blood; this can also be seen in patients with pulmonary pathologies with low hemoglobin oxygen saturation level, and heavy smokers with high carboxy-hemoglobin level, or congenital diseases, such as mutant hemoglobin with increased oxygen affinity, inherited defect of 2,3-diphosphoglycerate [2,3-DPG] synthesis.

© Springer Nature Switzerland AG 2021
C. S. Scher et al. (eds.), *Essentials of Blood Product Management in Anesthesia Practice*, https://doi.org/10.1007/978-3-030-59295-0_42

Examples of inappropriate responses include EPO-secreting tumors or increased EPO due to congenital disorders of hypoxia sensing [6].

Mixed (primary and secondary) congenital disorders of hypoxia sensing: Some patients with polycythemia share features of both primary (i.e., increased sensitivity of erythroid progenitors to EPO) and secondary polycythemia (i.e., elevated EPO levels). Examples of mixed polycythemia include Chuvash polycythemia, congenital von Hippel-Lindau (VHL) gene mutations, and gain-of-function mutations of EPAS1 (encoding hypoxia-inducible factor (HIF)-2 alpha) [6, 7].

Pathogenesis

PV is the most common of the primary polycythemias. As with other Philadelphia chromosome-negative chronic myeloproliferative neoplasms (essential thrombocythemia and primary myelofibrosis), PV is often caused by more than one genetic, either acquired somatic or inherited germline, mutations in a single hematopoietic progenitor, leading to an increase in RBC production with simultaneous increase of platelets and myeloid cells at variable amount [8].

Clonality: PV arises from a single hematopoietic progenitor. Thus, the vast majority of the circulating myeloid cells are clonal in origin [8]. The mutational event leads to clonal myeloid expansion as in patient with PV with affected pluripotent stem cell. However, the majority of T lymphocytes and natural killer cells remain polyclonal [9]. The first in vitro abnormality in PV progenitor cells observed was these cells form erythroid colonies in the absence of exogenous EPO, a phenomenon not found in progenitor cells from normal subjects. This finding has been used as a diagnostic assay to help distinguish PV from other causes of polycythemia [9]. The unusual presence of erythroid colonies without exogenous EPO is called spontaneous, EPO-independent, or endogenous erythroid colonies. This atypical erythroid colony is the hallmark of PV.

JAK2 (JAK2V617F) mutation: Multiple studies have shown that JAK/STAT signaling plays a critical role in cellular proliferation and cell survival [10], particularly in EPO-EPOR signaling in erythropoiesis [11]. JAK2 deficiency in mice has shown embryonic lethality due to the absence of definitive erythropoiesis [12]. Additionally, JAK2-/- fetal liver myeloid progenitors failed to respond to several hematopoietic growth factors including EPO [13]. Abnormal signaling in PV through JAK2 was proposed first in 2004 [14], and then the finding of a single nucleotide JAK2 somatic mutation (JAK2 V617F) in the majority of PV patients [15], which was confirmed by four separate studies [16]. This single nucleotide change was shown to emulate many properties of native PV erythroid progenitors as EPO independence and hypersensitivity of PV erythroid colonies.

Several JAK2 inhibitors have been developed and tested in clinical trials, showing some clinical benefit in patients with PV, especially in primary and secondary myelofibrosis patients. Ruxolitinib is the first FDA approved of its kind for the use in primary myelofibrosis and also in patients with PV. While Ruxolitinib decreases symptoms and partially ameliorates splenomegaly, it does not seem to change the biology of the disease [16].

Additional genetic features: the vast majority of patients with PV will have a JAK2 mutation involving either exon 14 or 12. JAK2 mutations can also present in other myeloproliferative neoplasms with different clinical phenotypes, as essential thrombocythemia and primary myelofibrosis, and JAK2 mutations do not seem to explain the heterogeneity of prognosis among patients with PV. Potential mechanisms for these phenotypic variations may include mutations in additional genes, variabilities in the expression level of alternative genes, and epigenetic modifications.

Perioperative Complications

Thromboembolic complications are the main concerns for the perioperative care of patients with PV. The increased circulating RBCs in patients with PV are associated with blood hyperviscosity, which can lead to an increased risk of thrombotic/embolic complications such as cerebrovascular accidents, myocardial infarction, or peripheral vascular events. Almost half of the patients with PV may also have proliferation of other blood cell lines in addition to RBCs. Thus, these patients with PV may also suffer from thrombocytosis and leukocytosis [17, 18]. An increased risk of "hemorrhagic" (7.3%) as a complication of patients with PV has also been reported; this might be related to increased leukocyte burden during disease course [19]. A concurrently increased risk of bleeding has also been attributed to acquired von Willebrand disease, especially in PV patients with thrombocytosis, and possibly to other platelet function defects [9, 20].

Perioperative Management

Preoperative Evaluation

All patients with PV should have a complete history and physical examination preoperatively to document symptoms, signs, and laboratory studies that may potentially alter prognosis or management strategy. The preoperative evaluation should also include history of venous or arterial thrombosis; symptoms as pruritus, erythromelalgia, fever, sweating, weight loss, early satiety, fatigue, headache, lightheadedness, visual disturbances, atypical chest pain, and paresthesia; cardiovascular risk assessment; and assessment of spleen and liver size by physical examination. In addition to routine laboratory tests like a complete blood cell count with differential, peripheral blood smear, and chemistries with liver and renal function and electrolytes, tests for JAK2 V617F mutation and, if negative, for mutations of CALR exon 9 and MPL exon 10 should be done; testing for acquired von Willebrand disease in patients with clinical evidence of bleeding or platelet counts >1 million/mL also needs to be done. Some patients may need bone marrow biopsy. PV is a panmyelopathy. When it presents with erythrocytosis, leukocytosis, and thrombocytosis with or without splenomegaly, the diagnosis of PV is confirmed, regardless of the clonal marker. However, if it can present as isolated erythrocytosis, leukocytosis, or thrombocytosis, with splenomegaly and/or myelofibrosis, or any combination of these, JAK2 driver mutation expression eliminates the possibility of secondary or spurious erythrocytosis.

Perioperative Management

In general, treatment of PV has two goals: alleviating symptoms and prolonging survival by prevention of thrombosis, intractable splenomegaly, and leukemic transformation. Specifically, for perioperative care, the goal is simple, prevention and management of thromboembolic complications by phlebotomy therapy to reduce blood hyperviscosity and control of thrombocytosis [21]. A Dutch study showed that major clinical variations exist in treatment strategies for PV. Phlebotomy shortens the time to achieve hematocrit control, while hydroxyurea seems to better control platelet and leukocyte levels. The thrombotic vascular event rate remains clinically significant [22].

Phlebotomy

Thrombosis, without any doubt, is the most immediate threat to patient with PV. Phlebotomy is the cornerstone of management for these patients. Phlebotomy reduces the RBC mass and expanding the plasma volume [23]. Phlebotomy can be accomplished by daily or every-other-day procedures, or all at once by erythrocytapheresis [24]. Phlebotomy usually neither causes myelofibrosis nor stimulates hematopoiesis because PV hematopoiesis is autonomous [25].

Cytoreductive Therapy

PV patients at high risk of thrombosis is indicated to have cytoreductive therapy, typically with hydroxyurea, which is adopted by the PV Study Group. Hydroxyurea is a nonalkylating agent used to treat patients with PV [21, 26]. Hydroxyurea can decrease the production of deoxyribonucleotides via inhibition of the enzyme ribonucleotide reductase by scavenging tyrosyl free radicals as they are involved in the reduction of nucleoside diphosphates. It suppresses the bone marrow production of blood cells [25]. Hydroxyurea does impair DNA synthesis; it may cause therapy-related acute myeloid leukemia because they facilitate clonal expansion of hematopoietic stem cell bearing harmful mutations [27].

Prevention and Treatment of Thrombocytosis

Aspirin: Aspirin plays an important role in management of patient with PV [28]. A randomized, controlled study has demonstrated the efficacy of low-dose aspirin therapy in preventing thrombotic complications in PV patients [29].

Other Symptomatic Management

Aquagenic pruritus: Ruxolitinib, psoralen and ultraviolet A, PegFIN, and hydroxyurea are all therapeutic options depending on its severity. Thrombocytosis-induced von Willebrand syndrome usually does not cause spontaneous bleeding; for minor surgery or dental procedures, tranexamic acid or e-aminocaproic acid should be adequate treatment. For major surgery in patient with thrombocytosis-induced von Willebrand syndrome, platelet count reduction therapy to achieve normal ristocetin cofactor activity is necessary [21, 28]. Interferon: PegFIN is a good therapeutic option for the control of thrombocytosis for migraine relief or TIA [21].

For venous thromboembolism, anticoagulation should be immediately commenced. Low molecular weight heparin is still the first choice in the acute setting, followed by vitamin K antagonists as per guidelines [30]. Direct oral anticoagulants are also increasingly used in the non-myeloproliferative neoplasm population for prophylaxis and venous thromboembolism therapy [30].

Prognosis

Patients with PV require long-term management to prolong survival and improve quality of life. Nearly all patients should initially receive treatment with aspirin [29] and phlebotomy to achieve a target hematocrit <45% [28]; management should evolve with the natural course of the disease [8, 28]. Management decisions should be modified or updated by new conditions and new evidence (Fig. 42.1) based on

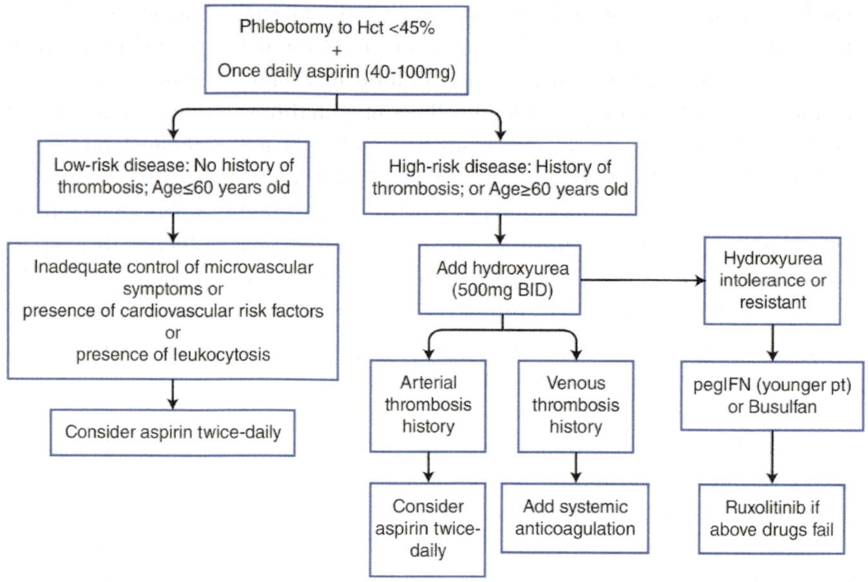

Fig. 42.1 Management of patient with polycythemia vera (Modified from [30])

both objective measures and subjective measures. Some patients will benefit from the addition or modification of therapeutic approaches [28, 31]. Early diagnosis and evidence-based patient management will improve long-term clinical outcomes and better quality of life.

Anesthetic Considerations

Patients with PV should have a thorough preoperative evaluation and risk stratification and control of hematocrit level to <45%. Intraoperatively hemodilution may be considered to avoid blood hyperviscosity by infusion of crystalloid fluids. Postoperative care should emphasize close monitoring of hematocrit level and occurrence of potential complications.

Summary

Perioperative patients more likely have anemic problem than polycythemia. Polycythemia means more total red blood cell mass than a normal human body needs. Polycythemia can be primary, secondary, and mixed types. PV is the most common type of primary polycythemias. PV is a neoplasm with overproduction of both morphologically and functionally normal blood cells. Polycythemia leads to high blood viscosity which predisposes patients to thrombotic/embolic complications as stroke, heart attack, and peripheral vascular events. Patients with PV may suffer from hemorrhagic complication as well. Patients with PV are usually treated with phlebotomy to Hct level < 45% and aspirin, which will suffice for low cardiovascular risk patients. High-risk patients will often warrant cytoreductive therapy with hydroxyurea. Sometimes interferon or Ruxolitinib will be needed. The anesthesia team should emphasize thorough preoperative evaluation and Hct control to <45%, and appropriate hemodilution intraoperatively, close monitoring of Hct level, and clinical indications of postoperative complications.

References

1. Campbell PJ, Green AR. The myeloproliferative disorders. N Engl J Med. 2006;355(23):2452–66. https://doi.org/10.1056/NEJMra063728. PMID: 17151367.
2. Tefferi A, Elliott M. Thrombosis in myeloproliferative disorders: prevalence, prognostic factors, and the role of leukocytes and JAK2V617F. Semin Thromb Hemost. 2007;33:313–20. https://doi.org/10.1055/s-2007-976165. PMID: 17525888.
3. Marchioli R, Finazzi G, Specchia G, Cacciola R, Cavazzina R, Cilloni D, et al. Cardiovascular events and intensity of treatment in polycythemia vera. N Engl J Med. 2013;368(1):22–33. https://doi.org/10.1056/NEJMoa1208500. PMID: 23216616.
4. Mesa R, Vannucchi AM, Yacoub A, Zachee P, Garg M, Lyons R, et al. The efficacy and safety of continued hydroxycarbamide therapy versus switching to ruxolitinib in patients with polycythaemia vera: a randomized, double-blind, double-dummy, symptom study (RELIEF). Br J Haematol. 2017;176(1):76–85. https://doi.org/10.1111/bjh.14382. PMID: 27858987.
5. Mehta J, Wang H, Iqbal SU, Mesa R. Epidemiology of myeloproliferative neoplasms in the United States. Leuk Lymphoma. 2014;55(3):595–600. https://doi.org/10.3109/10428194.2013.813500. PMID: 23768070.
6. Prchal JT, Sokol L. "Benign erythrocytosis" and other familial and congenital polycythemias. Eur J Haematol. 1996;57(4):263–8. PMID: 8982288.
7. Arber DA, Orazi A, Hasserjian R, Thiele J, Borowitz MJ, Le Beau MM, et al. The 2016 revision to the World Health Organization classification of myeloid neoplasms and acute leukemia. Blood. 2016;127(20):2391–405. https://doi.org/10.1182/blood-2016-03-643544. PMID: 27069254.
8. Barbui T, Thiele J, Carobbio A, et al. Disease characteristics and clinical outcome in young adults with essential thrombocythemia

versus early/prefibrotic primary myelofibrosis. Blood. 2012;120(3):569–71.
9. Passamonti F, Malabarba L, Orlandi E, Baratè C, Canevari A, Brusamolino E, et al. Polycythemia vera in young patients: a study on the long-term risk of thrombosis, myelofibrosis and leukemia. Haematologica. 2003;88(1):13–8. PMID: 12551821.
10. Randi ML, Putti MC, Scapin M, Pacquola E, Tucci F, Micalizzi C, et al. Pediatric patients with essential thrombocythemia are mostly polyclonal and V617FJAK2 negative. Blood. 2006;108(10):3600–2. https://doi.org/10.1182/blood-2006-04-014746. PMID: 16849644.
11. Sekiya Y, Okuno Y, Muramatsu H, Ismael O, Kawashima N, Narita A, et al. JAK2, MPL, and CALR mutations in children with essential thrombocythemia. Int J Hematol. 2016;104(2):266–7. PMID: 27209416.
12. Teofili L, Cenci T, Martini M, Capodimonti S, Torti L, Giona F, et al. The mutant JAK2 allele burden in children with essential thrombocythemia. Br J Haematol. 2009;145(3):430–2. PMID: 19208099.
13. Teofili L, Giona F, Martini M, Cenci T, Guidi F, Torti L, et al. The revised WHO diagnostic criteria for Ph-negative myeloproliferative diseases are not appropriate for the diagnostic screening of childhood polycythemia vera and essential thrombocythemia. Blood. 2007;110(9):3384–6. PMID: 17644735.
14. Jensen AW, Tefferi A, Arndt CA. Cerebral venous sinus thrombosis associated with essential thrombocytosis in a pediatric patient. J Pediatr Hematol Oncol. 2007;29(3):156–9. PMID: 17356393.
15. Khan AA, Kumar V, Anand I, Kumar M, Sharma P, Bhargava M. JAK2 mutation-negative essential thrombocythemia in a child presenting with cerebral venous thrombosis. Hematol Oncol Stem Cell Ther. 2012;5(1):66–8. PMID: 22446615.
16. Kurosawa H, Okuya M, Matsushita T, Kubota T, Endoh K, Kuwashima S, et al. JAK2V617F mutation-positive childhood essential thrombocythemia associated with cerebral venous sinus thrombosis. J Pediatr Hematol Oncol. 2009;31(9):678–80. PMID: 19707158.
17. Kearon C, Akl EA, Comerota AJ, Prandoni P, Bounameaux H, Goldhaber SZ, et al. Antithrombotic therapy for VTE disease: antithrombotic therapy and prevention of thrombosis, 9th ed: American College of Chest Physicians evidence- based clinical practice guidelines. Chest. 2012;141(2 Suppl):e419S–96S. https://doi.org/10.1378/chest.11-2301. PMID: 22315268.
18. Lim Y, Lee JO, Kim SH, Kim JW, Kim YJ, Lee KW, et al. Prediction of thrombotic and hemorrhagic events during polycythemia vera or essential thrombocythemia based on leukocyte burden. Thromb Res. 2015;135(5):846–51. https://doi.org/10.1016/j.thromres.2015.02.023. PMID: 25743883.
19. Guo L, Chughtai AR, Jiang H, Gao L, Yang Y, Yang Y, et al. Relationship between polycythemia and in-hospital mortality in chronic obstructive pulmonary disease patients with low-risk pulmonary embolism. J Thorac Dis. 2016;8(11):3119–31. https://doi.org/10.21037/jtd.2016.11.31. PMID: 28066591.
20. Giona F, Teofili L, Moleti ML, Martini M, Palumbo G, Amendola A, et al. Thrombocythemia and polycythemia in patients younger than 20 years at diagnosis: clinical and biologic features, treatment, and long-term outcome. Blood. 2012;119(10):2219–27. https://doi.org/10.1182/blood-2011-08-371328. PMID: 22262773.
21. Spivak JL. How I treat polycythemia vera. Blood. 2019;134(4):341–52. https://doi.org/10.1182/blood.2018834044. PMID: 31151982.
22. van de Ree-Pellikaan C, de Kreuk A, Schaar CG, Beeker A, Dompeling EC, Gerrits CJH, et al. Treatment strategies for polycythemia vera: observations in a Dutch 'real world' cohort study. Eur J Haematol. 2019. https://doi.org/10.1111/ejh.13291. PMID: 31298768.
23. Spivak JL. Polycythemia vera: myths, mechanisms, and management. Blood. 2002;100(13):4272–90. PMID: 12393615.
24. Teofili L, Valentini CG, Rossi E, De Stefano V. Indications and use of therapeutic phlebotomy in polycythemia vera: which role for erythrocytapheresis? Leukemia. 2019;33(1):279–81.
25. Messinezy M, Pearson TC. Incidence of myelofibrosis following treatment of primary polycythaemia by venesection [letter; comment]. Br J Haematol. 1995;89(1):228–30.
26. Randi ML, Bertozzi I, Cosi E, Santarossa C, Peroni E, Fabris F. Idiopathic erythrocytosis: a study of a large cohort with a long follow-up. Ann Hematol. 2016;95:233–7.
27. Wong TN, Miller CA, Jotte MRM, et al. Cellular stressors contribute to the expansion of hematopoietic clones of varying leukemic potential. Nat Commun. 2018;9(1):455.
28. Tefferi A, Barbui T. Polycythemia vera and essential thrombocythemia: 2019 update on diagnosis, risk-stratification and management. Am J Hematol. 2019;94(1):133–43. https://doi.org/10.1002/ajh.25303. PMID: 30281843.
29. Landolfi R, Marchioli R, Kutti J, European Collaboration on Low-Dose Aspirin in Polycythemia Vera Investigators, et al. Efficacy and safety of low-dose aspirin in polycythemia vera. N Engl J Med. 2004;350(2):114–24.
30. Tefferi A, Vannucchi AM, Barbui T. Essential thrombocythemia treatment algorithm 2018. Blood Cancer J. 2018;8(1):2. https://doi.org/10.1038/s41408-017-0041-8. PMID: 29321520.
31. Rumi E, Cazzola M. Diagnosis, risk stratification, and response evaluation in classical myeloproliferative neoplasms. Blood. 2017;129(6):680–92.

Blood Management in the Premature Neonate

43

Robert Jungerwirth, Hao Wu, and Hannah J. Hsieh

Introduction

Advances in neonatology over the past two decades have resulted in increased survival of preterm neonates. This has resulted in an increased number of procedures, anesthetics, and transfusions in this patient population [1]. Neonates (and particularly premature neonates) pose many unique perioperative challenges for the anesthesiologist (smaller size, increased airway complications, apneic and bradycardia episodes, developing cardiac and respiratory physiology, metabolic derangements due to immature renal and hepatic systems, and comorbidities of prematurity such as intracranial hemorrhage, necrotizing enterocolitis, sepsis). Anemia and thrombocytopenia are very common in neonates, especially preterm neonates [2–5]. Preterm infants are likely over-transfused in general as a population [6, 7]. Although rigorous regulations and screening of donor blood have decreased the incidence of infectious transmission, preterm infants are a vulnerable population and are at higher risk for complications given their comorbidities.

There is much debate regarding the effectiveness of transfusion and optimal transfusion thresholds, and there is no consensus among NICUs [8, 9] or pediatric anesthesiologists [10, 11]. Many of our current guidelines directing management are based on expert opinion. The research and evidence to guide transfusion practice in neonates is ongoing; research has come out attempting to define red blood cell transfusion triggers and thresholds in neonates and infants, and there are ongoing studies looking at platelet and plasma transfusions [12].

R. Jungerwirth · H. J. Hsieh (✉)
NYU Langone Health, Department of Anesthesiology, Perioperative Care, and Pain Medicine, New York, NY, USA
e-mail: Hannah.hsieh@nyulangone.org

H. Wu
NYU Medical Center, Department of Anesthesiology, New York, NY, USA

Causes and Risk Factors for Anemia

After birth, both term and preterm infants experience a progressive decline in hemoglobin (Hgb). For healthy term infants, Hgb concentrations range from 14.6 to 22.5 g/dL at birth and decline to a nadir of 10–12 g/dL by 8–10 weeks of age. This is often termed the "physiologic anemia of infancy" and is well tolerated in healthy term infants without need for treatment. Levels of Hgb gradually increase over time and reach adult levels by 2 years of age [13].

In contrast, preterm infants experience a more precipitous decline in Hgb concentration to a nadir of 7–8 g/dL at 4–6 weeks of age termed "anemia of prematurity" [14]. This is often accompanied by clinical signs of anemia such as pallor, poor weight gain, decreased activity, tachycardia, and tachypnea [15]. This anemia of prematurity occurs due to a combination of physiologic and nonphysiologic factors. Several of these physiologic processes are related to birth and the transition to extrauterine life, including shorter neonatal RBC survival time compared to adults, shift of the oxygen dissociation curve due to the change from high-oxygen-affinity hemoglobin F to low-oxygen-affinity hemoglobin A, and lower plasma concentrations of erythropoietin in response to anemia [13, 14].

Nonphysiologic factors that contribute to this anemia of prematurity include iatrogenic blood loss from phlebotomy, sepsis, inadequate nutrition, acute blood loss or hemorrhage, hemolytic disease of the newborn, and cardiorespiratory disease [13, 15, 16].

Surgery is a major cause of acute blood loss and anemia requiring transfusion in neonates. In an examination of all RBC transfusions over a period of 2 years at The Royal Children's Hospital in Melbourne, Australia, neonates were significantly more likely to receive an RBC transfusion than older children. Neonates were also more likely to undergo major surgery such as laparotomy and thoracic surgery, with laparotomy associated with a higher incidence of RBC transfusion in neonates than in older children [17].

© Springer Nature Switzerland AG 2021
C. S. Scher et al. (eds.), *Essentials of Blood Product Management in Anesthesia Practice*,
https://doi.org/10.1007/978-3-030-59295-0_43

Anemia has been shown to be significantly associated with mortality and increased incidence of red blood cell transfusion in premature neonates [18]. In a study by Goobie et al., preoperative anemia was an independent risk factor for postoperative mortality in neonates, with a preoperative Hct <40% as the optimal cutoff point to predict overall mortality [19].

Even though RBC transfusion can be a life-saving measure, especially in the setting of acute perioperative blood loss, transfusion of RBC has also been suggested to be associated with increased mortality in preterm infants [20–22]. There has been a concerted effort to find ways to prevent anemia and the need for unnecessary transfusion and their associated possible side effects.

Use of Hemoglobin and Hematocrit to Guide RBC Transfusion

In adults, guidelines for transfusion traditionally rely on maintaining a certain Hgb and Hct that we believe can adequately maintain oxygen delivery to tissues. However, in preterm neonates it is unclear what parameters best indicate an imbalance in oxygen delivery and demand and subsequently need for transfusion. Several countries have published national transfusion guidelines for neonates; however there are wide variability among them and no general consensus (Table 43.1).

Liberal Versus Restrictive RBC Transfusion Guidelines

As there is no consensus on what the threshold should be for transfusion in premature neonates, there have been several studies comparing restrictive and liberal Hgb thresholds to identify an optimal transfusion threshold. Adopting a restrictive transfusion threshold would not only significantly decrease the number of transfusions and exposure to blood products but will also result in financial savings. After implementing a program to improve guideline compliance, one center saw a financial savings of $780,074 over 12 months [27].

A randomized control trial by Bell et al. found that premature infants in the restrictive transfusion group had significantly higher rates of severe adverse brain events (defined as grade 4 intraparenchymal brain hemorrhage or periventricular leukomalacia, or both) and increased episodes and frequency of apnea compared to those in the liberal transfusion group. They postulated that those in the restrictive transfusion group likely had lower systemic oxygen transport to the brain, possibly leading to increased brain injury and apneic events. This decreased arterial oxygen content likely leads to increased cerebral blood and severe brain hemorrhage. It is unclear whether these short-term findings will result in long-term issues with brain development and function [28].

In comparison, there have been several studies that showed no significant difference in outcomes between patients transfused under liberal or restrictive guidelines [6, 7, 29, 30]. One study reported that after adopting a more restrictive transfusion strategy in ELBW infants, their transfusion rate decreased by 71% without a change in their primary outcomes of overall survival rate or acute complications. Of note, all of their study participants received concomitant weekly recombinant human erythropoietin treatment [7].

An observational study by Valieva et al. found that liberal transfusion had no significant effect on several clinical indices for anemia such as weight, heart rate, or apneic episodes. They did, however, see an increase in oxygen supplementation and use of diuretics after transfusion and found an association between transfusion and the development of necrotizing enterocolitis. Given these results, the center subsequently adopted a more restrictive transfusion strategy [29].

In the Premature Infants in Need of Transfusion (PINT) study, researchers found no difference in their primary outcome of death or major morbidity (defined as BPD, ROP, or ultrasound findings of brain injury) in premature ELBW

Table 43.1 Comparison of most recent international guidelines for RBC transfusion in neonates

	American Red Cross [23]		British Committee for Standards in Hematology [24]		Australian National Blood Authority [25]		Canadian Blood Services [26]	
Postnatal age	No respiratory support	With respiratory support[a]	No respiratory support	With respiratory support	No respiratory support	With respiratory support	No respiratory support	With respiratory support
0–7 days	Hct <20–30%	Hct <30–45%	Hgb <10 g/dL	Hgb <10–12 g/dL	Hgb 10–12 g/dL	Hgb 11–13 g/dL	Hgb 10 g/dL Hct 30%	Hgb 11.5 g/dL Hct 35%
8–14 days	Hct <20–30%	Hct <30–45%	Hgb <7.5–8.5 g/dL	Hgb <9.5–10 g/dL	Hgb 8.5–11 g/dL	Hgb 10–12.5 g/dL	Hgb 8.5 g/dL Hct 25%	Hgb 10 g/dL Hct 30%
≥14 days	Hct <20–30%	Hct <30–45%	Hgb <7.5–8.5 g/dL	Hgb <8.5–10 g/dL	Hgb 7–10 g/dL	Hgb 8.5–11 g/dL	Hgb 7.5 g/dL Hct 23%	Hgb 8.5 g/dL Hct 25%

[a]Respiratory support is defined as moderate to severe cardiopulmonary disease with need for supplemental oxygen, continuous positive airway pressure, or mechanical ventilation

infants randomized to restrictive versus liberal transfusion thresholds [6]. The same patients were subsequently followed up at 18 and 21 months of age, and researchers found no significant difference between groups in combined death or severe adverse neurodevelopmental impairment (cerebral palsy, cognitive delay, visual or hearing impairment) [31].

As of the date of publication, there are two ongoing trials looking at the neurocognitive development of premature infants who were transfused according to liberal or restrictive guidelines. The Effects of Transfusion Thresholds on Neurocognitive Outcome of Extremely Low Birth-Weight Infants (ETTNO) study included 920 ELBW neonates randomized into restrictive vs liberal blood transfusion groups. They followed the long-term development of these patients and will report on the incidence of death or major neurodevelopmental impairment at 24 months of age (ClinicalTrials.gov, NCT 01393496) [32]. The Transfusion of Prematures (TOP) trial included more than 1800 preterm ELBW neonates randomized to either a liberal or restrictive transfusion algorithm. Their primary outcome is death of neurodisability at 22–26 months of age. They will also follow up with these patients at 5–6 years of age to assess their neurological and functional outcomes (ClinicalTrials.gov, NCT 01702805). The results of these two upcoming studies are highly anticipated and will no doubt contribute to this field.

Other Transfusion Markers

In neonates, typical indications for transfusion include maintenance of specific Hgb or Hct level, replacement of phlebotomy losses, or clinical symptoms such as apnea, tachycardia, tachypnea, or growth failure [9]. More recent research has suggested that Hgb and Hct are not adequate measures of tissue oxygenation and need for transfusion [33–35]. In addition, evidence has shown that our conventional clinical and laboratory indices (such as hypotension, tachycardia, hematocrit, and metabolic acidosis) are poor predictors of measured blood volume and hypovolemia in sick preterm infants [36]. One study by Keyes et al. showed that transfusion in premature infants did not result in a predictable change in several traditional clinical indicators for transfusion (heart rate, respiratory rate, or incidence of apnea or bradycardias). There was also no correlation between these clinical variables and Hct [37]. More research needs to be done to find superior indicators of perfusion and oxygenation to possibly use as transfusion markers.

Red Cell Volume and Blood Volume

Red cell volume (RCV), the total amount of red cells in the circulation expressed as mL/kg body weight, has been purported to be superior to hematocrit as a surrogate for total blood volume [38]. Blood volume is important in anemia, as a reduction in total blood volume leads to redistribution of blood flow to essential organs such as the brain and heart. This results in hypoperfusion and hypoxia of low flow tissues in the early stages of anemia [39]. Additionally, very low RCV values have been associated with high mortality rate in high-risk newborns [40].

In healthy patients, Hct correlates with total body RCV. But in sick infants, there is a poor correlation between Hct and RCV [41], because plasma volume tends to fall and fluctuate due to impaired capillary integrity and subsequent extravasation of plasma components. In these patients, blood volume cannot be accurately predicted from Hgb or Hct concentration [36]. Some infants can maintain a relatively normal Hgb level while in fact they have a low RCV [42]. However, RCV is difficult to measure and likely has limited clinical utility in estimating total blood volume and need for transfusion [33].

Reticulocyte Count

Reticulocytes are immature red blood cells and a marker for the bone marrow response to anemia. In conjunction with Hgb and Hct, the reticulocyte count may be useful in determining whether a transfusion is indicated. Some guidelines have cited an absolute reticulocyte count of <100,000 cells/μL or reticulocyte count <5% along with Hgb and Hct as an indication for RBC transfusion [9, 43]. However, evidence for reticulocyte count as a reliable transfusion trigger is still lacking [44].

Serum Lactate

Lactate is an end product of anaerobic metabolism and can be an indication for hypoxia and hypoperfusion. It has been looked at as a possible biochemical trigger for transfusion in preterm neonates. Studies have shown that lactate significantly decreases after RBC transfusion. However, there has been no correlation between pretransfusion lactate and Hgb, Hct, or other clinical variables for anemia (heart rate, respiratory rate, number of apneas or bradycardias, or weight gain) [45–47]. Many clinical conditions such as sepsis, asphyxia, and congenital cardiac lesions and use of inotropes may also lead to increased serum lactate levels. While lactate is a marker for anemia, it is too nonspecific to serve as a transfusion trigger in preterm neonates [16, 44].

Near-Infrared Spectroscopy

Near-infrared spectroscopy (NIRS) is a noninvasive and continuous monitoring tool that measures regional tissue oxygen saturation (rSO2) by determining the ratio of oxygenated Hgb to total Hgb. NIRS has been advocated as an important clinical tool in conjunction with Hgb and Hct to determine an imbalance between oxygen delivery and demand and possible need for transfusion. Since 75–85% of the total cerebral blood volume is venous, NIRS measurement of cerebral regional tissue oxygen saturation (CrSO2) is therefore a surrogate for the cerebral venous saturation. Using pulse oximetry saturation (SaO2) as the measure for cerebral arterial saturation, the cerebral fractional tissue oxygen extraction (FTOE) can then be calculated. FTOE reflects the ratio of cerebral oxygen supply and demand and may serve as an indication of cerebral hypoxia and ischemia [48, 49].

Much of the research utilizing NIRS in neonates has looked specifically at cerebral saturation and perfusion, as it is thought that many of the neurological injuries in this patient population are due to imbalances in cerebral perfusion [50]. There is evidence showing that CrSO2 increases after RBC transfusion, consistent with the belief that CrSO2 is a marker for tissue oxygenation. This has not only been shown in adults after intraoperative RBC transfusion [51] but also in children and neonates [34, 35, 48, 52, 53]. While CrSO2 measurements in neonates were found to be reliable, several studies determined that NIRS is unreliable to measure absolute concentrations of oxygenated and deoxygenated Hgb [49, 54]. In fact, many studies have since shown a poor correlation between pre- and post-transfusion Hgb and CrSO2 [33–35, 48, 55], suggesting that Hgb is a poor marker for tissue oxygenation [34, 55].

A study by Wardle et al. found only a weak correlation between FTOE and Hgb, further supporting the idea that Hgb concentration is a relatively poor indicator of adequate tissue oxygenation. Interestingly they found a significant correlation btw RCV and FTOE. They also confirmed that preterm infants with symptomatic anemia had higher FTOE (increased tissue extraction of oxygen), while those with asymptomatic anemia had FTOE similar to controls [33]. Van Hoften et al. observed that FTOE decreased immediately after RBC transfusion along with a significant increase in CrSO2 [48].

NIRS has not only been utilized to measure cerebral saturation and perfusion in neonates, but also to measure the regional saturation of other peripheral tissues [34, 35, 53]. Bailey et al. saw a significant increase in regional splanchnic tissue oxygen saturation (SrSO2) after transfusion [34], and a study by Dani et al. showed that RBC transfusions resulted in increase in cerebral, splanchnic, and renal oxygenation in preterm infants with symptomatic anemia of prematurity. Of note, this study also observed an associated decrease in FTOE after transfusion [53].

A study conducted by Seidel et al. found that infants with very low initial NIRS values had the highest number of oxygen desaturations and after transfusion had the most reduction in the number of desaturations. This suggests that infants with low CrSO2 values (<55%), especially those with frequent desaturations, may benefit the most from RBC transfusions [35].

Bailey et al. looked at the usefulness of a metric called splanchnic-cerebral oxygenation ratio (SCOR) as a marker for need for transfusion in preterm infants. In the infants that clinically improved after transfusion, their pretransfusion SCOR was significantly lower than those who did not have a clinical improvement after transfusion. These patients also had a significant increase in SCOR during the transfusion. The authors hypothesized that symptomatic neonates had low SCOR because they maintained cerebral blood flow and oxygenation by shunting blood away from their splanchnic circulation. This evidence suggests that SCOR may be useful as a transfusion trigger in this patient population [55].

All of these findings suggest that NIRS may be a reliable marker for an imbalance between tissue oxygen delivery and demand and useful as a marker for the need for RBC transfusion.

Selection of RBC Products

Leukoreduced

Leukoreduction of RBCSrSO2 is the process of removing donor leukocytes from RBC units to decrease the risk of transfusion reactions such as febrile nonhemolytic transfusion reactions, allergic reactions, and alloimmunization [56]. Leukoreduction also filters out pre-inflammatory cytokines that have accumulated during the storage period such as tumor necrosis factor (TNF-alpha), interleukin-1 (IL-1), and interleukin-8 (IL-8). Leukoreduction may also decrease transmission of infectious agents commonly transmitted via leukocytes such as Epstein-Barr virus (EBV), cytomegalovirus (CMV), and human T-cell lymphocytic virus (HTLV)-I [57]. Leukoreduction of RBC however is not as effective at preventing transfusion-related graft-versus-host disease (GVHD).

Given their immature immune systems, donor leukocytes from red blood cell transfusions may depress the immune response, generate alloantibodies, and result in microvascular injury through the generation of free radicals in susceptible tissue beds such as the lungs and retina. After the institution of a nationwide Canadian universal pre-storage leukoreduction program in 1999, a study looking at premature infants showed that there were no significant reductions in NICU mortality or bacteremia. However, there was a reduction in clinical outcomes such as bronchopulmonary dysplasia, retinopathy of prematurity, necrotizing enterocolitis, and intraventricular hemorrhage. They also saw an average decrease of 11 days of NICU stay [58].

Irradiated

Exposing blood products to ionizing radiation damages nuclear DNA in order to inactivate donor T cells, thereby significantly decreasing the risk of transfusion-related GVHD in at-risk patients (including low birth weight neonates, neonates who have undergone intrauterine transfusions, newborns undergoing exchange transfusion, and those with congenital immunodeficiencies). For at-risk patients, all blood components with viable T cells should be irradiated, including RBCs, platelets, granulocytes, and fresh plasma. Cryoprecipitate is unlikely to contain viable T cells, and there is controversy whether irradiation of frozen plasma is necessary given the destructive effect of the freezing-thawing process on donor T cells. In comparison to leukoreduction, blood product irradiation does not produce a CMV-safe product.

Irradiation of RBC however can damage the cell membrane, reducing its shelf life to 28 days. This damage is also thought to cause increased concentrations of potassium in irradiated units. Reducing the time between irradiation and transfusion can minimize the potassium leak, and RBC washing is indicated prior to large-volume transfusions to reduce the risk of hyperkalemia. Platelet properties and storage, contrastingly, do not appear to be affected by irradiation.

Age of Blood

Refrigerated RBCs can be stored up to 42 days in the United States, with average shelf life between 2 and 3 weeks. There have been several studies investigating the effect of age of RBC on outcomes, without significant differences. The Age of Red Blood Cells in Premature Infants (ARIPI) trial was a double-blind, randomized controlled trial where 377 very low birth weight neonates were assigned to receive transfusions of RBCs stored less than 7 days (mean 5.1 days, SD 2.0 days) or standard blood bank practice (mean 14.6 days, SD 8.3 days). They found no significant difference in mortality or major neonatal morbidities (bronchopulmonary dysplasia, retinopathy of prematurity, necrotizing enterocolitis, intraventricular hemorrhage) [59]. These results may not be generalizable, however, given that transfusion thresholds were not standardized across patients, and average storage duration of refrigerated RBCs is around 18 days in the United States [12].

The Tissue Oxygenation by Transfusion in Severe Anemia with Lactic Acidosis (TOTAL) trial randomized 290 children aged 5 months to 5 years in Uganda with lactic acidosis from severe anemia (mostly secondary to malaria) to leukoreduced RBC transfusion of units stored 1–10 days (median 8 days) or 25–35 days (median 32 days). There were no significant differences in the groups in terms of clinical assessment, cerebral oxygen saturation, electrolyte abnormalities, adverse events, survival, or 30-day recovery [60]. There is also an ongoing study investigating outcomes after transfusion of RBC less than 7 days versus standard blood bank practice (oldest in inventory) called the Age of Blood in Children in Pediatric Intensive Care Units (ABC PICU) study [61].

Complications and Risks of Transfusion

Neonates pose some unique challenges with respect to anesthesia and blood products. Infants and neonates are disproportionately more likely to have adverse events from RBC transfusions – Stainsby et al. estimated the incidence of adverse events for infants less than 12 months to be 37:100,000, compared to 18:100,000 in children 1–18 years and 13:100,000 in adults [62]. Given the high probability of transfusion among preterm infants, there is a risk of exposure to multiple donors. Implementation of transfusion guidelines and transfusion reduction methods can reduce both the risk of blood transfusion and number of donors to whom infants are exposed. Some have suggested multipack collection or directed donation to minimize exposure to multiple donors.

Premature infants may be more susceptible to hyperkalemia (especially after transfusion of older or irradiated blood), hypocalcemia, hypoglycemia (possibly due to a reduction in glucose infusion during transfusion), and hypothermia with large-volume blood transfusions. Transfusion-related graft-versus-host disease occurs more often in sick neonates, so the use of directed donor products from close relatives and irradiated products is important [63]. Furthermore, an analysis of UK adverse outcomes of blood transfusion in children found a significant number of cases with errors at different stages in the transfusion chain including patients receiving a blood component that did not meet the required specification, and even was intended for a different patient [62].

Transfusion-Related Lung Injury

Although transfusion is relatively safe, neonates (particularly preterm neonates) are at increased risk for transfusion related lung injury (TRALI) [12, 62, 64, 65]. TRALI can be a difficult diagnosis, especially in neonates because they are often already critically ill. It is challenging to exclude a previous history of acute lung injury, as many are already intubated with abnormal chest radiographs. These patients are also very vulnerable to fluid overload, but it can be quite difficult to determine fluid status in these patients. They also have relatively immature immunosuppression and immature neutrophil physiology. This also contributes to the possible underreporting of TRALI in neonates and infants [65].

Infection

Blood transfusion carries the risk of transmitting bacteria, viruses, and other pathogens, the most common one being CMV. It is estimated that the prevalence of CMV is 30–70% in blood donors in the United States. As such, seronegative neonates should be transfused CMV-seronegative or leukoreduced units. Glanternik et al. also report three neonatal cases of transfusion-transmitted babesiosis, for which there is no FDA-approved test in donated blood nor is testing mandated. Susceptibility to babesiosis was correlated with lower birth weight and lower gestational age [66].

Bronchopulmonary Dysplasia

Bronchopulmonary dysplasia (BPD) is a chronic lung disease resulting from disrupted alveolar growth. It is the most common sequelae of preterm birth, characterized by supplemental oxygen requirement and severity assessment at 36 weeks, corrected gestational age. Many factors contribute to BPD, including oxidative and inflammatory injury to the immature lungs. RBC transfusion may increase oxidative stress, and neonates who developed BPD have been shown to have received more RBC transfusions than those who did not [67]. Valieva et al. however found that the incidence of BPD was significantly associated with number of transfusions at day of life 28, but not at 36 weeks corrected gestational age [29]. Similarly, Chen et al. did not find a significant difference in respiratory outcomes among 36 very low birth weight preterm babies randomized to liberal versus restrictive PRBC transfusion criteria. They did however find that development of chronic lung disease was associated with total transfused volume over 30 mL over 30 days in very low birth weight infants [30].

Necrotizing Enterocolitis

Necrotizing enterocolitis (NEC) is characterized by intestinal inflammation and ischemic necrosis. Incidence of NEC ranges from 2 to 15% among preterm infants and mortality rate of 15–30%, inversely related to gestational age and birth weight. Its pathogenesis is likely multifactorial, related to genetic predisposition, immaturity of neonatal GI tract vascular autoregulatory responses, anemia, changes in intestinal microbial colonization, intestinal and immunologic immaturity, and a highly immunoreactive intestinal mucosa [68].

There have been some studies reporting an association between RBC transfusion and increased risk of NEC [69, 70]. However, more recent studies have found no association between transfusion and NEC [71–73], and some have found transfusion to be protective against NEC [74]. Patel et al. conducted a prospective multicenter observational cohort study among 598 VLBW infants, adjusting for birth weight, center, breastfeeding, illness severity, and duration of initial antibiotic treatment. They found that severe anemia (within the week of developing NEC) was associated with increased risk of NEC (adjusted cause-specific HR 5.99, 95% CI 2–18). They however found no difference in the rate of NEC among patients who were transfused versus not transfused within a week of developing NEC (adjusted cause-specific HR 0.44, 95% CI 0.17–1.12) [75]. It is unclear that blood transfusion increases the risk of NEC, or rather that transfusion is a surrogate marker for severe anemia-related NEC. It has also been suggested that blood transfusion can blunt the prandial increase in mesenteric perfusion, and there is some evidence that withholding feeds during blood transfusion may reduce the risk of NEC [76].

Severe Intraventricular Hemorrhage

Intraventricular hemorrhage (IVH) is a significant cause of brain injury among premature infants, often due to germinal matrix fragility and changes in cerebral blood flow. A retrospective case-control study looking at VLBW with initial head US showing no hemorrhage found that those with subsequent grade 3 or 4 IVH were significantly more likely to have received a blood transfusion [77]. The same group looked at neonates with grade 1 IVH who subsequently extended to grade 3 or 4 hemorrhage and found that blood transfusion was associated with IVH extension. It is unclear however whether the extension of IVH is in part due to blood transfusion or rather the reason for transfusion itself [78]. In a multicenter prospective study of VLBW infants, Bednarek et al. (1998) suggest a higher risk of grade 3–4 IVH among patients in NICUs with liberal transfusion guidelines, though not clinically significant [8].

Retinopathy of Prematurity

Several studies have suggested that there is a correlation between both the number and volume of blood transfusions and retinopathy of prematurity (ROP); however, the pathophysiology is unclear. It is thought that transfusing premature infants with adult hemoglobin that has a greater affinity to offload oxygen causes increased oxygen delivery to the immature retina. Furthermore, increased free iron and free radical generation could contribute to retinal injury. Given their susceptibility to ROP risk factors as early as birth to 4 weeks of life, it is important to use methods to avoid unnecessary transfusions among preterm infants [79].

Several studies have found a correlation between blood transfusion and ROP. A prospective observational study of

45 preterm low birth weight infants found that transfusion volume during the first week (OR 1.16, 95% CI 1.03–1.3) and during the first 2 months of life (OR 2.93, 95% CI 1.52–5.62) were associated with the development of ROP. Inder et al. also found that among 56 VLBW infants, transfusion volume to 28 days was associated with risk of developing ROP (adjusted OR 2.03, CI 1.13–4.49). And among a cohort of 98 extremely low birth weight infants, the number of transfusions within 30 days was correlated with the development of ROP (OR 1.27, 95% CI 1.04–1.55) [22, 80, 81].

More recently, Lundgren et al. have conducted a prospective study of 78 and retrospective cohort of 227 extremely preterm infants, both of which found that anemia during the first week of life was an independent risk factor for ROP. In the cohort of 227 infants, both the duration of anemia and blood transfusion were associated with ROP warranting treatment; in the multivariate models however, only the number of anemic days during the first week of life was included in the best-fit model (as well as sepsis during the first 4 weeks of life and days of ventilation from birth to 35 weeks) [82, 83].

Alternatives to Transfusion

Prevention of anemia can significantly impact the number of blood transfusions among preterm infants, reducing its associated morbidity and mortality. A retrospective analysis of four western US NICUs with the same RBC transfusion guidelines found that despite no difference in compliance to their guidelines, blood transfusion rates varied widely between the units. The lower-transfusing NICUs had lower rates of NEC and IVH, as well as cost savings of $6970 per 1000 NICU days. Moreover, the units with lower rates of transfusion had written anemia-prevention guidelines which included measures like umbilical milking at VLBW delivery, use of cord blood for admission studies, and darbepoetin dosing for selected neonates [84].

Blood Conservation

Blood conservation methods can reduce the contribution of phlebotomy to neonatal anemia, especially among low birth weight infants. Such methods include microtechnique laboratory procedures, noninvasive monitoring, and the use of fetal blood from the placenta for baseline laboratory tests. Grouping lab draws can help reduce the amount of blood overdraw, and any blood waste can be re-administered.

Among 63 patients admitted to the PICU for greater than 48 hours, patients less than 10 kg had the greatest amount of phlebotomy-induced blood loss per kilogram, due to their small size and proportion of blood loss to body weight. They were also subjected to a greater number of blood draws with a longer length of stay and greater amount of blood loss per kilogram per PICU stay. Furthermore, blood drawn for single test had significantly more blood overdraw than for multiple tests [85].

Use of an in-line, ex vivo bedside monitor in the first 2 weeks of life of critically ill ELBW infants with UAC had significantly less laboratory blood loss (22%) and received significantly less RBC transfusion volumes (33%). The monitor drew 1.5 mL blood samples; analyzed them for blood gas, electrolytes, and hematocrit levels; and then reinfused all except 25 microL of blood. The study was terminated prematurely when one center's NICU changed its method of lab testing, however, and there were no differences in mortality, morbidity, and neurodevelopmental outcomes at 18–24 months [86]. Mahieu et al. also showed that the introduction of a point-of-care-testing analyzer (for bedside blood gases, hemoglobin, electrolytes, and bilirubin) significantly decreased transfusions among VLBW infants from 50% to 38.9%, with overall cost reduction of 8.51% per neonate [87].

Delayed Umbilical Cord Clamping and Cord Stripping

Delayed umbilical cord clamping (DCC) may provide a newborn more time for the transition from fetal to neonatal life, especially among premature infants. It also allows for placental transfusion which increases neonatal blood volume, ameliorates the hemodynamic changes associated with the transition, and may reduce the risk of IVH, blood transfusion, respiratory distress or support, and death.

A randomized controlled trial in which very preterm infants either had their cord clamped immediately or delayed showed that delayed cord clamping was significantly associated with decreased incidence of IVH and sepsis, with no difference in incidence of BPD and NEC [88]. Another study found that delayed cord clamping was associated with decreased hypothermia, neonatal respiratory interventions (surfactant therapy or intubation in the delivery room, in the first 24 hours of life, or during the NICU stay), and blood transfusions [89]. Strauss et al. however showed that although a 1-minute delay in cord clamping resulted in higher hematocrit and RBC volume and mass, there was no difference in number of blood transfusions [90].

In a retrospective cohort study of 4680 premature neonates, those who received DCC had reduced odds of severe neurologic injury (adjusted OR 0.80, 95% CI 0.64–0.99) and mortality (adjusted OR 0.74, 95% CI 0.59–0.93); there were no significant differences in the odds of BPD, ROP stage >3, NEC stage >2, late-onset sepsis, or receipt of >2 blood transfusions [91]. A case-control study of 45 infants monitored cerebral autoregulatory dampening using NIRS and mean arterial blood pressure among infants who had DCC versus early cord clamping. They found that the DCC group had a significantly more dynamic cerebral autoregulatory function and lower rate of IVH (OR 0.14, $p < 0.01$) compared to the early cord clamping group. They postulate that DCC is neuroprotective by stabilizing the cerebrovascular system and improving resistance to fluctuations in systemic blood pressure [92].

Umbilical cord milking (stripping) may enable blood to more quickly be transferred from the placenta to the infant, reducing the time away from neonatal care during DCC. Among 40 preterm infants randomized to early cord clamping or clamping after umbilical cord milking, the milked group was less likely to be transfused and had a lower number of transfusions, higher initial hemoglobin, and higher mean blood pressure. The milked group also had a shorter duration of ventilation or supplemental oxygen, with no significant difference in mortality [93].

A Cochrane review updated in 2019 of randomized controlled trials comparing early with delayed umbilical cord clamping for births before 37 weeks showed that delayed cord clamping may reduce the risk of death before discharge and any grade IVH for preterm infants, without sufficient evidence to show optimum timing of cord clamping or the effect of umbilical milking [94].

Erythropoietin

Erythropoietin (EPO) and darbepoetin have been suggested as methods to reduce neonatal transfusion, given that premature infants often have lower erythropoiesis and EPO levels. A randomized controlled trial of 157 preterm infants found that treating patients with recombinant human EPO versus placebo reduced the number (1.1 versus 1.6, $p = 0.046$) and volume (16.5 versus 23.9 mL, $p = 0.023$) of blood transfusions. Despite this reduction in transfusion, patients given EPO had higher reticulocyte counts ($p = 0.0001$) and hematocrit values ($p = 0.0001$); they found no difference in the incidence of major complications of prematurity [95]. Ohls and colleagues further compared EPO to darbepoetin and placebo in a randomized trial of 80 low birth weight infants. They found that EPO and darbepoetin recipients had higher cognitive scores and lower incidence of cerebral palsy when compared to placebo [96].

A Cochrane review of EPO or darbepoetin effect on blood transfusions among preterm or low birth weight infants found that early EPO reduced the risk of transfusion (risk ratio 0.79, 95% CI 0.73–0.85), volume of transfusion (mean difference 7 mL/kg, 95% CI 2–12), and number of donors to whom the infants were exposed (mean difference 0.54, 95% CI 0.20–0.89). There were no significant differences in outcomes such as mortality, IVH, and NEC, with varying neurodevelopmental outcomes. There was however an increased risk of ROP found in post-hoc analysis. Given the smaller reductions in transfusions and exposure with "likely...limited clinical importance," the authors did not recommend EPO (darbepoetin required further study) in light of the possible increased risk of ROP [15].

Studies have found increased levels of EPO in vitreous fluid when compared to serum. It has been proposed that EPO's effect in preventing vascular apoptosis and stimulating angiogenesis may be important in preventing ROP in its first phase (when low IGF-1 levels prevent angiogenesis) and worsening proliferative ROP [97]. A retrospective cohort study of 327 low birth weight preterm infants found that recombinant EPO exposure was associated with an increased risk of progression of retinopathy (OR 1.27, 95% CI 1.04–1.55) [98]. Suk and colleagues also found that the infants who received more than 20 doses of recombinant EPO were at higher risk of developing ROP (OR 3.53, 95% CI 1.59–7.85); of note, infants treated with EPO starting after 20 days of age (compared to starting EPO before 20 days) were similarly at higher risk (OR 3.57, 95% CI 1.59–8.03) [99].

Thrombocytopenia

Preterm infants are more likely to have thrombocytopenia compared to term infants [100]. Approximately 22–35% of neonates in NICU developed thrombocytopenia [101]. In addition to decreased platelet count, preterm neonates have platelet hyporeactivity for up to 3–4 days after birth. Thrombocytopenia is associated with bacterial and fungal infection, small for gestational age, low birth weight, pregnancy-induced hypertension, necrotizing enterocolitis, and DIC [102]. Thrombocytopenic babies also have significantly more skin, renal, pulmonary, or CNS hemorrhage, as well as higher mortality rate [100].

Causes/Risk Factors

Neonatal thrombocytopenia is defined as less than 150,000/mL [104]. Marked thrombocytopenia is defined as less than 100,000/mL, and severe thrombocytopenia is less than 50,000/mL. However, a study in 2009 suggested that the cutoff for neonatal thrombocytopenia may need to be revised, as normal platelet counts can fall below 150,000 and still be within the reference range of 5th–95th percentiles [100].

Thrombocytopenia can be divided into early onset (within 3 days of birth) and late onset (>3 days after birth) [5]. Causes of early onset thrombocytopenia are prenatal factors such as severe intrauterine growth restriction and maternal factors such as preeclampsia, HELLP syndrome, immune thrombocytopenia, pregnancy-induced hypertension, systematic lupus erythematosus, and cancer [103]. Late-onset thrombocytopenia can be caused by bacterial sepsis, necrotizing enterocolitis, or thrombotic events associated with the use of central lines [104].

The mechanisms of thrombocytopenia include decreased production, increased platelet consumption, increased extravascular loss, or a combination of these factors. Preterm infants with thrombocytopenia had fewer circulating megakaryocyte progenitors, compared to non-thrombocytopenic counterparts. Small for gestational age (SGA) neonates are also at risk for developing thrombocytopenia in the first week after birth [105]. A third of SGA infants have early thrombocytopenia. About 10% of these neonates have an obvious cause of thrombocytopenia, whereas 90% have thrombocytopenia that is hyporegenerative rather than platelet consumption or destruction [105]. Transplacental passage of maternal allo antibodies and auto-antibodies is responsible for 9–20% of all neonatal thrombocytopenias [106].

Very low birth rate infants have the highest rate of IVH, up to 25% [107]. Severe thrombocytopenia predisposes infants to intraventricular brain hemorrhage, but most preterm infants who develop a severe IVH do not have thrombocytopenia before their IVH, but rather develop thrombocytopenia and coagulopathy after the IVH [102]. IVH cause thrombocytopenia by increased consumption. Thrombocytopenia (platelet count below 150 × 109/L) is a risk factor for IVH among VLBW infants (hazard ratio of 2.17), but there was no relationship between severity of thrombocytopenia and risk of subsequent IVH.

Treatment (Platelet Transfusion)

Consider the condition of the neonate and the platelet count. Stable neonates have a much lower risk of ICH [102]. Among the different studies, there is no consensus in regard to the exact threshold to transfuse.

Thresholds

An observational study showed that of the neonates that had severe neonatal thrombocytopenia (platelet count <60 × 10^9 platelets/L), approximately 1/3 of them had platelet counts as low as <20 × 10^9. However, only 9% of these neonates developed major hemorrhage. There was no significant correlation between nadir of platelet count and risk of major hemorrhage. The majority of neonates that had major hemorrhage were gestational ages <28 weeks (85% of those with hemorrhage) and were within 14 days of birth. This suggests that gestational age and postnatal age were more of a risk factor. Majority (84%) of platelet transfusions were given to neonates with either no bleeding or only minor bleeding [5].

There was a randomized controlled trial that compared higher (<150 × 10^9/L) and lower (<50 × 10^9/L) platelet count thresholds for prophylactic transfusion. The incidence of ICH did not differ between the two groups. Early prophylactic platelet transfusion did not reduce the incidence or extent of intracranial hemorrhage [108].

A recent large randomized prospective multicenter trial of platelet transfusion thresholds in preterm infants showed that those transfused at a threshold of 50,000 cubic millimeter vs 25,000 cubic millimeter had a higher incidence of death or major bleeding up to day 28 of life. The odds ratio is 1.57 (95% confidence interval, 1.06–2.32; $P = 0.02$). Reasons for this difference is unknown. It could be 2/2 immunologic and inflammatory effects of platelets. This suggests that a restrictive platelet transfusion trigger may be preferable [109].

Platelet transfusion should not be given to patients with low risk of IVH for the sole purpose of maintaining platelet count above an arbitrary level. The mortality rate of infants who received transfusion is twice that of those who did not receive transfusions, although the mortality rate is likely secondary to underlying illness rather than negative effects of transfusion [3]. Furthermore, mortality is associated with number of platelet transfusions [103]. Severity of thrombocytopenia did not correlate with risk for IVH [110].

Transfusion Markers

Immature platelet fraction is a marker for megakaryopoietic activity in neonates and reflects the platelet production rate. The IPF can be useful in predicting the course of thrombocytopenia and can identify patients at risk of severe drop in platelet count. This information is helpful for identifying which neonates would benefit from platelet transfusions [111].

Complications

Platelet transfusion can worsen outcome in NEC [112]. Other risks of transfusion include bacterial contamination and CMV infection. Ways to decrease risk of platelet transfusion include photochemical inactivation by crosslinking DNA and RNA of viruses, bacteria, and host cells [107].

Treatment Alternatives

Alternative to transfusion includes recombinant human thrombopoietin (TPO). Thrombopoietin (Tpo) is the primary regulator of megakaryopoiesis and platelet production [100]. However, some patients developed anti-Tpo antibodies which can lead to aplastic anemia and severe hyporegenerative thrombocytopenia [113]. There are two thrombopoietin receptor agonists, eltrombopag and romiplostim, that have been approved by the FDA, but only few neonates have been treated with these agents [3]. Furthermore, Tpo receptor agonists require 7–10 days between commencement of dosing and a significant increase in platelet count [105].

References

1. Howarth C, Banerjee J, Aladangady N. Red blood cell transfusion in preterm infants: current evidence and controversies. Neonatology. 2018;114:7–16.
2. Keir AK, Yang J, Harrison A, et al. Temporal changes in blood product usage in preterm neonates born at less than 30 weeks' gestation in Canada. Transfusion. 2015;55(6):1340–6.
3. Christensen RD, Henry E, Wiedmeier SE, et al. Thrombocytopenia among extremely low birth weight neonates: data from a multihospital healthcare system. J Perinatol. 2006;26(6):348–53.
4. Roberts I, Stanworth S, Murray NA. Thrombocytopenia in the neonate. Blood Rev. 2008;22(4):173–86.
5. Stanworth SJ, Clarke P, Watts T, et al. Prospective, observational study of outcomes in neonates with severe thrombocytopenia. Pediatrics. 2009;124(5):e826–34.
6. Kirpalani H, Whyte RK, Andersen C, et al. The premature infants in need of transfusion (PINT) study: a randomized, controlled trial of a restrictive (low) versus liberal (high) transfusion threshold for extremely low birth weight infants. J Pediatr. 2006;149:301–7.
7. Maier RF, Sonntag J, Walkta MM, et al. Changing practices of red blood cell transfusions in infants with birth weights less than 1000g. J Pediatr. 2000;136(2):220–4.
8. Bednarek FJ, Weisberger S, Richardson DK, et al. Variations in blood transfusions among newborn intensive care units. SNAP II Study Group. J Pediatr. 1998;133:601–7.
9. Kasat K, Hendricks-Munoz KD, Mally PV. Neonatal red blood cell transfusions: searching for better guidelines. Blood Transfus. 2011;9(1):86–94.
10. Jouffroy R, Baugnon T, Carli P. A survey of blood transfusion practice in French-speaking pediatric anesthesiologists. Ped Anesthesia. 2011;21:385–93.
11. Wittenmeier E, Troeber C, Zier U, et al. Red blood cell transfusion in perioperative pediatric anesthesia: a survey of current practice in Germany. Transfusion. 2018;58(7):1597–605.
12. Goel R, Josephson CD. Recent advances in transfusions in neonates/infants. F1000 Research. 2018;7:609.
13. Widness JA. Pathophysiology of anemia during the neonatal period, including anemia of prematurity. Neoreviews. 2008;9(11):e520.
14. Strauss RG. Anaemia of prematurity: pathophysiology and treatment. Blood Rev. 2010;24(6):221–5.
15. Ohlsson A, Aher SM. Early erythropoietin for preventing red blood cell transfusion in preterm and/or low birth weight infants. Cochrane Database Syst Rev. 2014;4. Art No: CD004863.
16. Ree IMC, Lopriore E. Updates in neonatal hematology: causes, risk factors, and management of anemia and thrombocytopenia. Hematol Oncol Clin N Am. 2019;33:521–32.
17. Keung CY, Smith KR, Savoia HF, et al. An audit of transfusion of red blood cell units in pediatric anesthesia. Ped Anesthesia. 2009;19:320–8.
18. Banerjee J, Asamoah FK, Singhvi D, et al. Haemoglobin level at birth is associated with short term outcomes and mortality in preterm infants. BMC Med. 2015;13(16):1–7.
19. Goobie SM, Faraoni D, Zurakowski D, et al. Association of preoperative anemia with postoperative mortality in neonates. JAMA Pediatr. 2016;170(9):855–62.
20. Dos Santos AM, Guinsburg R, de Almeida MF, et al. Red blood cell transfusions are independently associated with intra-hospital mortality in very low birth weight preterm infants. J Pediatr. 2011;159(3):371–6.
21. Ghirardello S, Dusi E, Cortinovis I, et al. Effects of red blood cell transfusions on the risk of developing complications or death: an observational study of a cohort of very low birth weight infants. Am J Perinatol. 2017;34(1):88–95.
22. Wang YC, Chan OW, Chiang MC, et al. Red blood cell transfusion and clinical outcomes in extremely low birth weight preterm infants. Pediatr Neonatol. 2017;58(3):216–22.
23. Red blood cells: general information. In: A compendium of transfusion practice guidelines. 3rd ed. American Red Cross. 2017. Retrieved from: http://success.redcross.org/success/file.php/1/TransfusionPractices-Compendium_3rdEdition.pdf. Accessed on 25 Aug 2019.
24. New HV, Berryman J, Bolton-Maggs PHB, British Committee for Standards in Haematology, et al. Guidelines on transfusion for fetuses, neonates and older children. Br J Haematol. 2016;175:784–828.
25. National Blood Authority (NBA). Patient blood management guidelines: module 6 – neonatal and paediatrics. NBA, Canberra, Australia. 2016. Retrieved from: https://www.blood.gov.au/pubs/pbm/module6/#Table_F_1. Accessed on 25 Aug 2019.
26. Lau W. Chapter 13: Neonatal and pediatric transfusion. In: Canadian blood services, clinical guide to transfusion. 2017. Retrieved from https://professionaleducation.blood.ca/en/transfusion/guide-clinique/neonatal-and-pediatric-transfusion Accessed on 25 Aug 2019.
27. Baer VL, Henry E, Lambert DK, et al. Implementing a program to improve compliance with neonatal intensive care unit transfusion guidelines was accompanied by a reduction in transfusion rate: a pre-post analysis within a multihospital health care system. Transfusion. 2011;51:264–9.
28. Bell EF, Strauss RG, Widness JA, et al. Randomized trial of liberal versus restrictive guidelines for red blood cell transfusion in preterm infants. Pediatrics. 2005;115:1685–91.
29. Valieva OA, Strandjord TP, Mayock DE, Juul SE. Effects of transfusions in extremely low birth weight infants: a retrospective study. J Pediatr. 2009;155:331–7.
30. Chen HL, Tseng HI, Lu CC, et al. Effect of blood transfusions on the outcome of very low body weight preterm infants under two different transfusion criteria. Pediatr Neonatol. 2009;50:110–6.
31. Whyte RK, Kirpalani H, Asztalos EV, et al. Neurodevelopmental outcome of extremely low birth weight infants randomly assigned to restrictive or liberal hemoglobin thresholds for blood transfusion. Pediatrics. 2009;123(1):207–13.
32. ETTNO Investigators. The 'effects of transfusion thresholds on neurocognitive outcome of extremely low birth-weight infants (ETTNO)' study: background, aims, and study protocol. Neonatology. 2012;101:301–5.
33. Wardle SP, Yoxall WC, Crawley E, Weindling MA. Peripheral oxygenation and anemia in preterm babies. Pediatr Res. 1998;44:125–31.
34. Bailey SM, Hendricks-Munoz KD, Wells JT, Mally P. Packed red blood cell transfusion increases regional cerebral and splanchnic tissue oxygen saturation in anemic symptomatic preterm infants. Am J Perinatol. 2010;27:445–53.

35. Seidel D, Blaser A, Gebauer C, et al. Changes in regional tissue oxygenation saturation and desaturations after red blood cell transfusion in preterm infants. J Perinatol. 2013;33:282–7.
36. Aladangady N, Aitchison TC, Beckett C, et al. Is it possible to predict the blood volume of a sick preterm infant? Arch Dis Child Fetal Neonatal Ed. 2004;89:F344–7.
37. Keyes WG, Donohue PK, Spivak JL, et al. Assessing the need for transfusion of premature infants and role of hematocrit, clinical signs, and erythropoietin level. Pediatrics. 1989;84(3):412–7.
38. Jones JG, Holland BM, Hudson IRB, Wardrop CAJ. Total circulating red cells versus haematocrit as the primary descriptor of oxygen transport by the blood. Br J Haematol. 1990;76:288–94.
39. Wardrop CAJ, Jones JG, Holland BM. Detection, correction and ultimate prevention of anemias in the preterm infant. Transfus Sci. 1991;12:257–70.
40. Faxelius G, Raye J, Gutberlet R, et al. Red cell volume measurements and acute blood loss in high risk newborn infants. J Pediatr. 1977;90:273–81.
41. Phillips HM, Abdel-Moiz A, Jones JG, et al. Determination of red-cell mass in assessment and management of anaemia in babies needing blood transfusion. Lancet. 1986;327:882–4.
42. Hudson I, Cooke A, Holland B, et al. Red cell volume and cardiac output in anaemic preterm infants. Arch Dis Child. 1990;65:672–5.
43. Bishara N, Ohls RK. Current controversies in the management of the anemia of prematurity. Semin Perinatol. 2009;33(1):29–34.
44. Banerjee J, Aladangady N. Biomarkers to decide red blood cell transfusion in newborn infants. Transfusion. 2014;54(10):2574–82.
45. Moller JC, Schwarz U, Schaible TF, et al. Do cardiac output and serum lactate levels indicate blood transfusion requirements in anemia of prematurity? Intensive Care Med. 1996;22:472–6.
46. Frey B, Losa M. The value of capillary whole blood lactate for blood transfusion requirements in anaemia of prematurity. Intensive Care Med. 2001;27:222–7.
47. Takahashi D, Matsui M, Shigematsu R, et al. Effect of transfusion on the venous blood lactate level in very low-birthweight infants. Pediatr Int. 2009;51(3):321–5.
48. Van Hoften JC, Verhagen EA, Keating P, et al. Cerebral tissue oxygen saturation and extraction in preterm infants before and after blood transfusion. Arch Dis Child Fetal Neonatal Ed. 2010;95(5):F352–8.
49. Menke J, Voss U, Moller G, Jorch G. Reproducibility of cerebral near infrared spectroscopy in neonates. Biol Neonate. 2003;83:6–11.
50. Chakravarti S, Srivastava S, Mittnacht AJC. Near infrared spectroscopy (NIRS) in children. Semin Cardiothorac Vasc Anesth. 2008;12(1):70–9.
51. Torella F, Haynes SL, McCollum CN. Cerebral and peripheral oxygen saturation during red cell transfusion. J Surg Res. 2003;110:217–21.
52. Liem KD, Hopman JCW, Oeseburg B, et al. The effect of blood transfusion and haemodilution on cerebral oxygenation and haemodynamics in newborn infants investigated by near infrared spectrophotometry. Eur J Pediatr. 1997;156:305–10.
53. Dani C, Pratesi S, Fontanelli G, et al. Blood transfusions increase cerebral, splanchnic, and renal oxygenation in anemic preterm infants. Transfusion. 2010;50:1220–6.
54. Wolf M, Von Siebenthal K, Keel M, et al. Comparison of three methods to measure absolute cerebral hemoglobin concentration in neonates by near-infrared spectrophotometry. J Biomed Opt. 2002;7(2):221–7.
55. Bailey SM, Hendricks-Munoz KD, Mally P. Splanchnic-cerebral oxygenation ratio as a marker of preterm infant blood transfusion needs. Transfusion. 2012;52:252–60.
56. Hillyer CD, Silberstein LE, Ness PM, et al. Blood banking and transfusion medicine: basic principles and practice. 2. Philadelphia: Elsevier; 2007. p. 243.
57. Kim Y, Xia BT, Chang AL, Pritts TA. Role of leukoreduction of packed red blood cell units in trauma patients: a review. Int J Hematol Res. 2016;2(2):124–9.
58. Fergusson D, Hebert PC, Lee SK, et al. Clinical outcomes following institution of universal leukoreduction of blood transfusions for premature infants. JAMA. 2003;289:1950–6.
59. Fergusson DA, Hebert P, Hogan DL, et al. Effect of fresh red blood cell transfusions on clinical outcomes in premature, very low-birth-weight infants. JAMA. 2012;308(14):1443–51.
60. Dhabangi A, Ainomugisha B, Cserti-Gazdewich C, et al. Effect of transfusion of red blood cells with longer vs shorter storage duration on elevated blood lactate levels in children with severe anemia: the TOTAL randomized clinical trial. JAMA. 2015;314(23):2514–23.
61. Tucci M, Lacroix J, Fergusson D, et al. The age of blood in pediatric intensive care units (ABC PICU): study protocol for a randomized controlled trial. Trials. 2018;19(1):404.
62. Stainsby D, Jones H, Wells AW, et al. Adverse outcomes of blood transfusion in children: analysis of UK reports to the serious hazards of transfusion scheme 1996–2005. Br J Haematol. 2008;141:73–9.
63. Barcelona SL, Thompson AA, Cote CJ. Intraoperative pediatric blood transfusion therapy: a review of common issues. Part II: transfusion therapy, special considerations, and reduction of allogenic blood transfusions. Ped Anesthesia. 2005;15:814–30.
64. Gauvin F, Robillard P, Hume H, et al. Transfusion-related acute lung injury in the Canadian paediatric population. Paediatr Child Health. 2012;17(5):235–9.
65. Lieberman L, Petraszko T, Yi Q, et al. Transfusion-related lung injury in children: a case series and review of the literature. Transfusion. 2014;54:57–64.
66. Glanternik JR, Baine IL, Rychalsky MR, et al. A cluster of cases of Babesia microti among neonates traced to a single unit of donor blood. Pediatr Infect Dis J. 2018;37(3):269–71.
67. Cooke RW, Drury JA, Yoxall CW, James C. Blood transfusion and chronic lung disease in preterm infants. Eur J Pediatr. 1997;156:47–50.
68. Maheshwari A, Patel RM, Christensen RD. Anemia, red blood cell transfusions, and necrotizing enterocolitis. Semin Pediatr Surg. 2018;27(1):47–51.
69. Mally P, Golombek SG, Mishra R, et al. Association of necrotizing enterocolitis with elective packed red blood cell transfusions in stable, growing, premature neonates. AM Perinatol. 2006;23:451–8.
70. Blau J, Calo JM, Dozor D, et al. Transfusion-related acute gut injury: necrotizing enterocolitis in very low birth weight neonates after packed red blood cell transfusion. J Pediatr. 2011;158:403–9.
71. AlFaleh K, Al-Jebreen A, Baqays A, et al. Association of packed red blood cell transfusion and necrotizing enterocolitis in very low birth weight infants. J Neonatal Perinatal Med. 2014;7(3):193–8.
72. Sharma R, Kraemer DF, Toraazza RM, et al. Packed red blood cell transfusion is not associated with increased risk of necrotizing enterocolitis in premature infants. J Perinatol. 2014;34:858–62.
73. Wallenstein MB, Arain YH, Birnie KL, et al. Red blood cell transfusion is not associated with necrotizing enterocolitis: a review of consecutive transfusions in a tertiary neonatal intensive care unit. J Pediatr. 2014;165:678–82.
74. Sood BG, Rambhatla A, Thomas R, Chen X. Decreased hazard of necrotizing enterocolitis in preterm neonates receiving red cell transfusions. J Matern Fetal Neonatal Med. 2015;29(5):737–44.
75. Patel RM, Knezevic A, Shenvi N, et al. Association of red blood cell transfusion, anemia, and necrotizing enterocolitis in very low-birth-weight infants. JAMA. 2016;315(9):889–97.
76. Jasani B, Rao S, Patole S. Withholding feeds and transfusion-associated necrotizing enterocolitis in preterm infants: a systematic review. Adv Nutr. 2017;8(5):764–9.

77. Baer VL, Lambert DK, Henry E, et al. Among very-low-birth-weight neonates is red blood cell transfusion an independent risk factor for subsequently developing a severe intraventricular hemorrhage? Transfusion. 2011;51:1170–8.
78. Baer VL, Lambert DK, Henry E, et al. Red blood cell transfusion of preterm neonates with a grade 1 intraventricular hemorrhage is associated with extension to a grade 3 or 4 hemorrhage. Transfusion. 2011;51:1933–9.
79. Romagnoli C. Risk factors and growth factors in ROP. Early Hum Dev. 2009;85:S79–82.
80. Inder TE, Clemett RS, Austin NC, et al. High iron status in very low birth weight infants is associated with an increased risk of retinopathy of prematurity. J Pediatr. 1997;131:541–4.
81. Dani C, Reali MF, Bertini G, et al. The role of blood transfusions and iron intake on retinopathy of prematurity. Early Hum Dev. 2001;62:57–63.
82. Lundgren P, Athikarisamy SE, Patole S, et al. Duration of anaemia during the first week of life is an independent risk factor for retinopathy of prematurity. Acta Paediatr. 2018;107(5):759–66.
83. Lundgren P, Hellgren G, Pivodic A, et al. Erythropoietin serum levels, versus anaemia as risk factors for severe retinopathy of prematurity. Pediatr Res. 2019;86(2):276–82.
84. Henry E, Christensen RD, Sheffield MJ, et al. Why do four NICUs using identical RBC transfusion guidelines have different gestation age-adjusted RBC transfusion rates? J Perinatol. 2015;35:132–6.
85. Valentine SL, Bateman ST. Identifying factors to minimize phlebotomy-induced blood loss in the pediatric intensive care unit. Pediatr Crit Care Med. 2012;13(01):22–7.
86. Widness JA, Madan A, Grindeanu LA, et al. Reduction in red blood cell transfusions among preterm infants: results of a randomized trial with an in-line blood gas and chemistry monitor. Pediatrics. 2005;115(05):1299–306.
87. Mahieu L, Marien A, De Dooy J, et al. Implementation of a multi-parameter Point-of-Care-blood test analyzer reduces central laboratory testing and need for blood transfusions in very low birth weight infants. Clin Chim Acta. 2012;413:325–30.
88. Mercer JS, Vohr BR, McGrath MM, et al. Delayed cord clamping in very preterm infants reduces the incidence of intraventricular hemorrhage and late-onset sepsis: a randomized, controlled trial. Pediatrics. 2006;117(4):1235–42.
89. Song D, Jegatheesan P, DeSandre G, Govindaswami B. Duration of cord clamping and neonatal outcomes in very preterm infants. PLoS One. 2015;10(9):1–10.
90. Strauss RG, Mock DM, Johnson KJ, et al. A randomized clinical trial comparing immediate versus delayed clamping of the umbilical cord in preterm infants: short-term clinical and laboratory endpoints. Transfusion. 2008;48:658–65.
91. Lodha A, Shah PS, Soraisham AS, et al. Association of deferred vs immediate cord clamping with severe neurological injury and survival in extremely low-gestation-age neonates. JAMA Netw Open. 2019;2(3):e191286.
92. Vesoulis ZA, Liao SM, Mathur AM. Delayed cord clamping is associated with improved dynamic cerebral autoregulation and decreased incidence of intraventricular hemorrhage in preterm infants. J Appl Physiol. 2019;127:103–10.
93. Hosono S, Mugishima H, Fujita H, et al. Umbilical cord milking reduces the need for red cell transfusions and improves neonatal adaptation in infants born at less than 29 weeks' gestation: a randomized controlled trial. Arch Dis Child Fetal Neonatal Ed. 2008;93:F14–9.
94. Rabe H, Diaz-Rossello JL, Duly I, et al. Effect of timing of umbilical cord clamping and other strategies to influence placental transfusion at preterm birth on maternal and infant outcomes. Cochrane Database Syst Rev. 2012;8:CD003248.
95. Shannon KM, Keith JF, Mentzer WC, et al. Recombinant human erythropoietin stimulates erythropoiesis and reduces erythrocyte transfusions in very low birth weight preterm infants. Pediatrics. 1995;95(1):1–8.
96. Ohls RK, Kamath-Rayne BD, Christensen RD, et al. Cognitive outcomes of preterm infants randomized to darbepoetin, erythropoietin, or placebo. Pediatrics. 2014;133(6):1023–30.
97. Romagnoli C, Tesfagabir MG, Giannantonio C, Papacci P. Erythropoietin and retinopathy of prematurity. Early Hum Dev. 2011;87S:S39–42.
98. Brown MS, Baron AE, France EK, Hamman RF. Association between higher cumulative doses of recombinant erythropoietin and risk for retinopathy of prematurity. J AAPOS. 2006;10:143–9.
99. Suk KK, Dunbar JA, Liu A, et al. Human recombinant erythropoietin and the incidence of retinopathy of prematurity: a multiple regression model. J AAPOS. 2008;12:233–8.
100. Wiedmeier SE, Henry E, Sola-Visner MC, Christensen RD. Platelet reference ranges for neonates, defined using data from over 47,000 patients in a multihospital healthcare system. J Perinatol. 2009;29(2):130–6.
101. Mehta P, Vasa R, Neumann L, Karpatkin M. Thrombocytopenia in the high-risk infant. J Pediatr. 1980;97(5):791–4.
102. Christensen RD. Platelet transfusion in the neonatal intensive care unit: benefits, risks, alternatives. Neonatology. 2011;100:311–8.
103. Resch E, Hinkas O, Urlesberger B, Resch B. Neonatal thrombocytopenia-causes and outcomes following platelet transfusions. Eur J Pediatr. 2018;177(7):1045–52.
104. Lopriore E. Updates in red blood cell and platelet transfusions in preterm neonates. Am J Perinatol. 2019;36(suppl S2):S37–40.
105. Christensen RD, Baer VL, Henry E, Snow GL, Butler A, Sola-visner MC. Thrombocytopenia in small-for-gestational-age infants. Pediatrics. 2015;136(2):e361–70.
106. Beiner ME, Simchen MJ, Sivan E, Chetrit A, Kuint J, Schiff E. Risk factors for neonatal thrombocytopenia in preterm infants. Am J Perinatol. 2003;20(1):49–54.
107. Sola-Visner M, Saxonhouse MA, Brown RE. Neonatal thrombocytopenia: what we do and don't know. Early Hum Dev. 2008;84(8):499–506.
108. Andrew M, Vegh P, Caco C, et al. A randomized, controlled trial of platelet transfusions in thrombocytopenic premature infants. J Pediatr. 1993;123(2):285–91.
109. Curley A, Stanworth SJ, Willoughby K, et al. Randomized trial of platelet-transfusion thresholds in neonates. N Engl J Med. 2019;380(3):242–51.
110. Sparger KA, Assmann SF, Granger S. Platelet transfusion practices among very-low-birth-weight infants. JAMA Pediatr. 2016;170(7):687–94.
111. Cremer M, Paetzold J, Schmalisch G, et al. Immature platelet fraction as novel laboratory parameter predicting the course of neonatal thrombocytopenia. Br J Haematol. 2009;144(4):619–21.
112. Patel RM, Josephson CD, Shenvi N, et al. Platelet transfusions and mortality in necrotizing enterocolitis. Transfusion. 2019;59(3):981–8.
113. Li J, Yang C, Xia Y, et al. Thrombocytopenia caused by the development of antibodies to thrombopoietin. Blood. 2001;98(12):3241–8.

Coagulation and Regional Anesthesia

44

Chrissy Cherenfant and Uchenna Umeh

Overview of the Coagulation Cascade

Coagulation is the intricate process of clot formation that is fundamental in preventing bleeding and facilitating healing. This process is initiated by primary hemostasis, which entails platelet adhesion, aggregation, and plug formation. A platelet plug has the dual capability of activating the coagulation cascade while also being an unstable, temporary measure for bleeding cessation [3, 4]. The relationship between platelets and the coagulation cascade illustrates the importance of acknowledging the influence some antiplatelets may have on regional anesthesia.

Anticoagulants operate by inhibiting certain aspects of the coagulation cascade. The coagulation cascade is composed of calcium, phospholipids, and coagulation proteins. The proteins, also known as clotting factors, are sequentially activated into serine proteases to ultimately develop a fibrin clot. Clot formation is achieved through two collaborating pathways: extrinsic and intrinsic. Initiated by endothelial damage and exposure of blood to an artificial surface, the intrinsic pathway begins with the transformation of factor XII into its activated serine protease, factor XIIa [5]. Factor XIIa then serves as a stimulant of the downstream generation of activated factors XI and IX. Factor IXa forms a complex with factor VIII, as its cofactor, to activate factor X to factor Xa (Fig 44.1) [4, 5].

The extrinsic pathway is also initiated by vascular insult but through the release of tissue factor from endothelial cells. Tissue factor then activates factor VII to factor VIIa, and together they activate factor X to factor Xa, which is the converging point of both pathways [6, 7]. This convergence continues as the "common pathway" [3, 4, 8]. Thereafter, factor Xa is aided by factor Va as a cofactor to activate and cleave prothrombin (factor II) into thrombin (factor IIa). Thrombin then cleaves fibrinogen to fibrin (factor Ia). Thereafter, fibrin monomers aggregate with each other to form a fibrin mesh that stabilizes the platelet plug to facilitate the goal of the coagulation cascade and ultimately generate a fibrin clot [5–8].

Anticoagulants and Its Implications on Regional Anesthesia

Regional anesthesia encompasses spinal anesthesia, epidural anesthesia, and nerve blocks [9, 10]. Examples of surgeries that benefit from regional anesthesia include hip, knee, ankle, breast, thoracic, major abdominal, and cesarean sections [11–13]. As with most medical interventions, it is always important to weigh the benefits versus the risks of regional anesthesia. A major, yet rare, complication that may occur is a hematoma in the spinal or epidural space and its associated neurological complications [9, 14–16]. Thus, it is crucial to be cognizant of the risk factors that may make this occurrence more likely. Certainly, a patient's use of anticoagulants augments the possibility of bleeding and, similarly, spinal hematomas. To address this concern, guidelines have been developed to aid anesthesiologists in providing their patients with the benefits of regional anesthesia while diminishing the risks. The majority of guidelines mentioned in this chapter will be from the latest American Society of Regional Anesthesia and Pain Medicine (ASRA) guidelines from 2018. Fundamentally, these guidelines are evidence-based recommendations that assist anesthesiologists and other healthcare providers in executing safe peripheral and neuraxial regional anesthetic care [9, 17–20].

C. Cherenfant
Weill Cornell Medicine, Department of Anesthesiology, New York, NY, USA

U. Umeh (✉)
NYU Langone Health, NYU Langone Orthopedic Hospital, Department of Anesthesiology, Perioperative Care and Pain Medicine, New York, NY, USA
e-mail: Uchenna.umeh@nyulangone.org

© Springer Nature Switzerland AG 2021
C. S. Scher et al. (eds.), *Essentials of Blood Product Management in Anesthesia Practice*,
https://doi.org/10.1007/978-3-030-59295-0_44

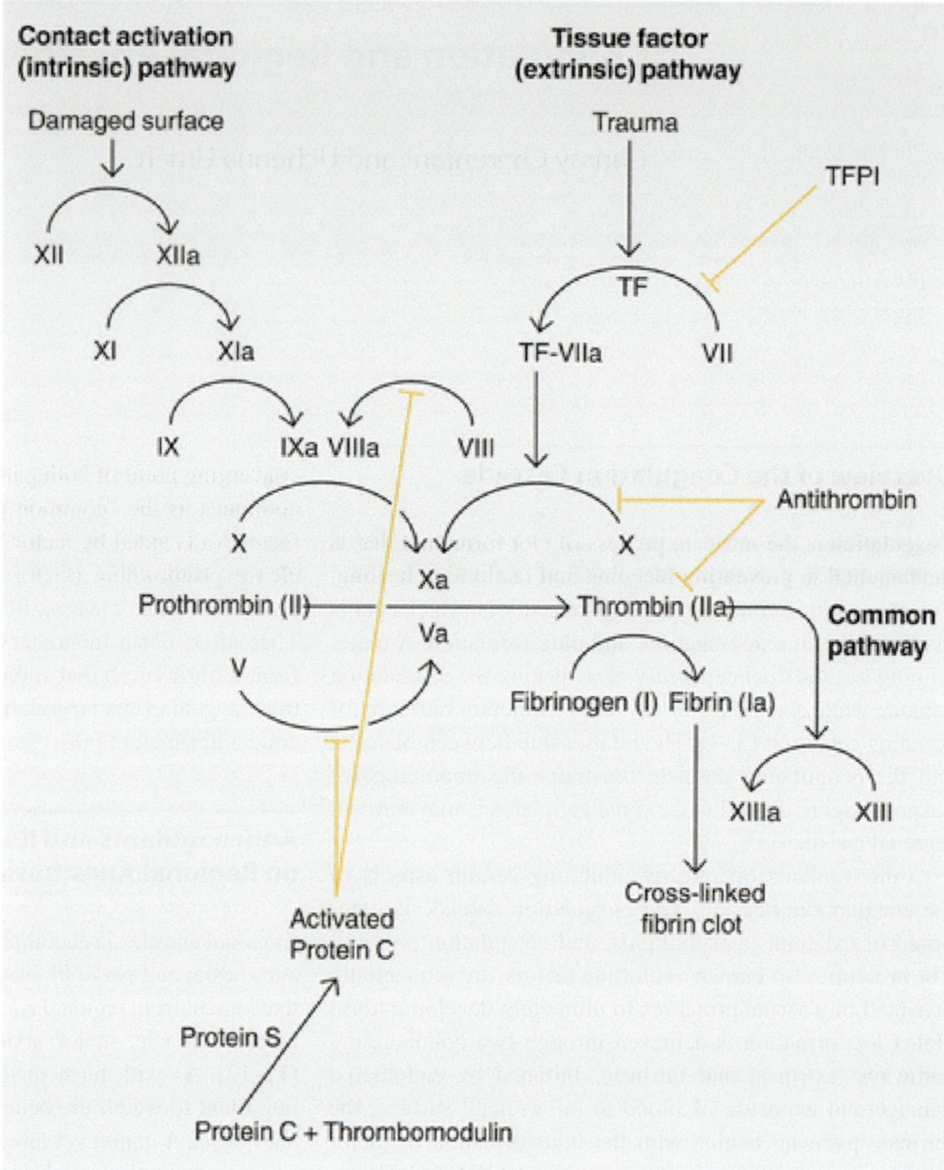

Fig. 44.1 Coagulation cascade

Heparin: Unfractionated and Low Molecular Weight

Heparin and its derivatives interfere with the coagulation cascade by binding to antithrombin, which inactivates thrombin (factor IIa), factor Xa, and factor IXa. Consequently, the fibrin clot is not formed [21, 22]. Heparin's anticoagulant effects can be reversed by protamine, with LMWH requiring more time for reversal due to reduced protamine binding. When given therapeutically, heparin can be monitored by partial thromboplastin time (PTT) and more accurately by anti-factor Xa. However, for neuraxial blocks, anti-factor Xa has not been found to be a predictor of the risk of bleeding. Since a specific level of anti-factor Xa has yet to be determined for optimal regional anesthesia, it is therefore not recommended as a mode of monitoring LMWH. During cardiopulmonary bypass, activated clotting time (ACT) is used to monitor the higher doses of heparin use.

Unfractionated heparin (UFH) and low molecular weight heparin (LMWH) have different biochemical and pharmacological properties, with LMWH often being preferred over UFH. LMWH has more favorable properties such as longer half-life, lower risk of hemorrhagic side effects, and more predictable pharmacokinetics [23, 24].

ASRA recommendations for spinal anesthesia with unfractionated heparin use include the following [9]:

- Discontinuing intravenous heparin 4–6 hours prior to neuraxial blockade.
- Verifying normal coagulation.
- Delaying heparin administration for at least 1 hour after needle placement.

- Removing neuraxial catheters 4–6 hours after the last heparin dose.
- Monitor the patient postoperatively to provide early detection of motor blockade, and consider the use of minimal concentration of local anesthetics to enhance the early detection of spinal hematoma.
- In the setting of more than a 4-day course of either UFH or LMWH, it is recommended to obtain a platelet count prior to neuraxial block or catheter removal, in light of the possibility of heparin-induced thrombocytopenia.

Of note, subcutaneous (SC) unfractionated heparin has different recommendations based on its dosing. For low-dose UFH with doses of 5000 units BID or TID, neuraxial block should occur 4–6 hours after last dose. There is no contraindication in maintaining catheters in the setting of low-dose UFH postoperatively. For higher doses such as 7500–1000 units BID or a daily dose greater than 20,000 units, it is suggested that neuraxial anesthesia occur 12 hours later. Postoperatively, these higher doses of UFH and their safety with indwelling neuraxial catheters have not been established. Thus, the management of these patients must be based on individual assessment of the risks and benefits [9].

The recommendations for spinal anesthesia among patients who use low molecular weight heparin are different from those regarding UFH. The difference in guidelines exist because of their distinct pharmacological profiles and knowledge acquired from case reports and clinical data. This data allowed the FDA to create a Drug and Safety Communication in 2013 that entailed updated information on LMWH, with the goal of decreasing the risk of neuraxial hematoma and paralysis. Interestingly, for LMWH, anesthetic and patient risk factors associated with spinal hematomas were ascertained such as female sex, age greater than 65, epidural technique, early postoperative administration (<12 hours), and greater than one dose daily [25]. Notable ASRA recommendations regarding low molecular weight heparin include the following [9]:

- Needle placement should occur at least 12 hours after a prophylactic LMWH dose.
- LMWH prophylactic dose should be administered no earlier than 12 hours after catheter/needle placement. If there is a second dose to be given, it should be administered at least 24 hours after the first dose. Remove the catheter 12 hours after the last dose of LMWH.
- If a dose of LMWH was given preoperatively within 2 hours, refraining from neuraxial technique is ideal, as needle placement would occur near peak anticoagulant activity.
- A delay of at least 24 hours prior to needle/catheter placement is recommended for higher (therapeutic) doses of LMWH (enoxaparin 1 mg/kg every 12 hours, enoxaparin 1.5 mg/kg daily, dalteparin 120 U/kg every 12 hours, dalteparin 200 U/kg daily, or tinzaparin 175 U/kg daily).
- After surgery with non-high bleeding risk, therapeutic dose of LMWH can be resumed in 24 hours. For high bleeding risk surgery, therapeutic dose LMWH can be reinstituted 48–72 hours after.

Warfarin

Warfarin is an oral anticoagulant that affects the clotting cascade by interfering with the synthesis of clotting factors II, VII, IX, and X. This is done by warfarin's ability to inhibit vitamin K epoxide reductase, which is necessary in the development of specific clotting factors from the liver [26]. Thus, warfarin's inhibition of vitamin K leads to decreased clotting factors and clot development by impeding both the intrinsic and extrinsic pathways. The anticoagulant effect of warfarin can be monitored by prothrombin time (PT) and international normalized ratio (INR). Warfarin can be reversed by fresh frozen plasma (FFP), prothrombin complex concentrate (PCC), and vitamin K [27]. PCC can be categorized as three-factor with factors II, IX, and X or four-factor consisting of factors II, VII, IX, and X. PCC may also be composed of protein C and S and heparin whose purpose is to balance the large clotting factor concentration that can be 25 times higher than that in normal plasma [28].

ASRA recommendations for regional anesthetic management for patients on warfarin are as follows [9]:

- Stop warfarin ideally up to 5 days prior to a neuraxial block and with INR normalization.
- Perform routine testing of sensory and motor function during epidural analgesia for patients on warfarin therapy, with the use of anesthesia that minimizes sensory and motor blockade.
- In the setting of reinitiating warfarin thromboprophylaxis, remove neuraxial catheters when INR is less than 1.5. Of note, although this recommendation was based on laboratory and clinical data, the risk of an INR greater than 1.5 but less than 3 is unknown.
- Hold or reduce warfarin in patients with indwelling catheters with an INR greater than 3.
- Continue neurologic assessment at least 24 hours after catheter removal.

Fondaparinux

Fondaparinux is an injectable synthetic pentasaccharide. Its benefits include rapid absorption, lack of platelet interaction, and a long half-life of 17–21 hours that allows for one-time dosing. However, a detriment of its use is that there is no reversal or antidote [29]. Fondaparinux's anticoagulant effect is that it inhibits factor Xa. During the initial clinical trials that helped determine the dose ranging of fondaparinux, no spinal hematomas were reported. This occurred because strict parameters were used such as patients being excluded from the study if needle placement was not accomplished on the first attempt or if there was traumatic bleeding. Therefore, the true risk of fondaparinux use on regional anesthesia is unknown, which provides more insight to the ASRA recommendations [9]:

- Until further clinical experience is available, performance of neuraxial technique should occur under the conditions used in clinical trials (single needle pass, avoidance of indwelling neuraxial catheters, atraumatic needle placement). If this is not feasible, an alternate method of prophylaxis should be considered.
- Neuraxial catheters should be removed 6 hours prior to the first postoperative dose.

Direct Parental Thrombin Inhibitors

Desirudin, bivalirudin, and argatroban are parenteral anticoagulants commonly used for treating heparin-induced thrombocytopenia. They all share the anticoagulant mechanism of inhibiting thrombin. Their effect can be monitored by activated PTT, and there is no pharmacological reversal. Due to the lack of information available to determine patient management and risk, ASRA recommends *against* the performance of neuraxial anesthesia in patients receiving these parenteral thrombin inhibitors [9].

Novel Oral Anticoagulants

Novel oral anticoagulants or non-vitamin K antagonist oral anticoagulants, also known as NOACs, are increasingly used due to many advantages. NOACs can be given without the need for monitoring. They are associated with less intracranial bleeding and more rapid onset and are often just as effective in preventing clots such as those seen in venous thromboembolism. NOACs include dabigatran, apixaban, betrixaban, edoxaban, and rivaroxaban [30–33].

Dabigatran is an oral direct thrombin inhibitor with a half-life of 12–17 hours. More than 80% of it is renally eliminated. The most reliable monitoring of dabigatran is by thrombin time (TT), ecarin clotting time (ECT), and diluted thrombin time (dTT) [34]. In 2015, the FDA approved idarucizumab as a rapid reversal of dabigatran. Idarucizumab is a monoclonal antibody that is a non-competitive irreversible inhibitor of the dabigatran-thrombin complex that works in minutes [35]. Initially, the manufacturer of dabigatran advised against placing epidural catheters due to limited experience, which consequently led to limited data on dabigatran and neuraxial anesthesia. However, with increased understanding of its pharmacokinetics and expert opinion, recommendations on neuraxial anesthesia amidst dabigatran use have been made. Of note, the suggestions are largely influenced by the renal excretion of dabigatran. The ASRA guidelines state [9]:

- We suggest that dabigatran be discontinued 120 hours prior to neuraxial block. However, if renal function has been reliably determined, and there are no additional risk factors for bleeding (e.g., age > 65 years, hypertension, concomitant antiplatelet medications), a more graded approach may be considered:
  - For all suggestions, consider checking ecarin clotting time and diluted thrombin time. However, an acceptable level of residual dabigatran activity to proceed with neuraxial block remains undetermined.
  - In patients with creatinine clearance (CrCl) 80 mL/min or greater, discontinue dabigatran 72 hours prior neuraxial block.
  - In CrCl of 50–79 mL/min, discontinue 96 hours prior.
  - In CrCl of 30–49 mL/min, discontinue 120 hours prior.
  - We suggest *against* the performance of neuraxial blocks in patients with a CrCl less than 30 mL/min.
- We suggest removing neuraxial catheters 6 hours before first postoperative dose.
- Before removing an indwelling catheter during administration, hold dabigatran for 34–36 hours or assess dTT or ECT.

Rivaroxaban, apixaban, edoxaban, and betrixaban are all NOACs that exhibit their anticoagulant effects by inhibiting factor Xa. Therefore, the best mechanism of monitoring their effect is by anti-factor Xa assays [9]. There are recently developed reversals for NOACs: idarucizumab, andexanet, and ciraparantag. Idarucizumab was previously discussed as a reversal agent for dabigatran. Andexanet binds to apixaban, edoxaban, rivaroxaban, and betrixaban as a decoy receptor, thereby inhibiting their mechanisms of action. It also reverses the antithrombotic effects of low molecular weight heparin, unfractionated heparin, and fondaparinux. Lastly, ciraparantag/aripazine uses its hydrogen bonding sites to bind to and reverse all NOACs and heparin [35, 36]. Since these reversals are fairly new and ciraparantag is still under investigation. Other antidotes are often used such as recombinant coagulation factor VIIa and PCC, which is a known reversal for warfarin [37]. Factor eight inhibitor bypassing activity (FEIBA) is another reversal agent that stops bleeding by generating thrombus due to its composition of factors II, IX, X, and VIIa, prothrombin, and prothrombin complex factors [38].

ASRA suggested management for patients on rivaroxaban as follows [9]:

- Discontinue rivaroxaban 72 hours prior to neuraxial block. Consider checking rivaroxaban or anti-factor Xa activity level if less than 72 hours. An acceptable level of residual rivaroxaban activity to proceed with neuraxial block remains undetermined.
- Remove neuraxial catheters 6 hours prior to the first postoperative dose.
- With unanticipated administration with indwelling catheter, hold rivaroxaban dosing 22–26 hours before catheter removal, or assess an anti-factor Xa assay calibrated to rivaroxaban until the catheter is removed.

ASRA suggested management for patients on apixaban as follows [9]:

- Discontinue apixaban 72 hours prior to neuraxial block. Consider checking apixaban or anti-factor Xa activity level if less than 72 hours. An acceptable level of residual apixaban activity to proceed with neuraxial block remains undetermined.
- Remove catheters 6 hours prior to the first postoperative dose.
- With unanticipated administration with indwelling catheter, hold apixaban dosing for 26–30 hours, or calibrate an anti-factor Xa assay to apixaban before catheter removal.

ASRA suggested management for patients on edoxaban as follows [9]:

- Discontinue 72 hours prior to neuraxial block. Consider checking edoxaban or anti-factor Xa activity level if less than 72 hours. An acceptable level of residual edoxaban activity to proceed with neuraxial block remains undetermined.
- Remove neuraxial catheters 6 hours prior to the first postoperative dose.
- Hold edoxaban for 20–28 hours, or perform an anti-factor Xa assay calibrated to edoxaban before catheter removal.

ASRA suggested management for patients on betrixaban as follows [9]:

- Discontinue a minimum of 72 hours prior to a neuraxial block. Consider checking betrixaban or anti-factor Xa level if less than 72 hours.
- There is a suggestion against the performance of neuraxial blocks in patients with CrCl less than 30 mL/min.
- Remove neuraxial catheters 5 hours prior to next dose.
- With indwelling catheter, hold betrixaban dose for 72 hours, and then remove the catheter.

Thrombolytic Therapy

Thrombolytics, also known as fibrinolytics, dissolve fibrin clots through the action of plasmin. Plasmin is derived from its inactive precursor plasminogen. Plasmin's mechanism of action is dissolving fibrin clots. This results in fibrin degradation products that inhibit platelet aggregation, furthering their role in anticoagulation. Examples of thrombolytics include exogenous plasminogen activators such as streptokinase and urokinase and formulations of tissue plasminogen activator (t-PA) like alteplase and tenecteplase. Plasminogen activators incite the reaction of plasminogen to plasmin and dissolve fibrin, thereby decreasing the amount of both fibrin and plasminogen. t-PA is more fibrin selective, where it binds to fibrin stimulating the dissolving of clots [9, 39, 40].

In patients taking fibrinolytics, ASRA recommends the following [9]:

- Against spinal or epidural anesthesia except in "highly unusual circumstances" [9].
- A 48-hour time interval and documentation of normalization of clotting studies, like fibrinogen, is suggested between discontinuation of these medications and the time of neuraxial puncture. This is because fibrinogen can be used to determine residual thrombolytic effect since it is one of the latter clotting factors to recover. It is also noted that puncture of "noncompressible vessels" was an original contraindication to thrombolytic therapy, with a now suggestion of 10 days following puncture for therapy.
- In patients who receive neuraxial anesthesia during or near the time of thrombolytic use, it is recommended for them to undergo neurological checks, no more than 2 hours apart. In this setting, if the anesthesia is an epidural catheter infusion, the anesthetic should have minimal sensory and motor block to allow for neurological monitoring.
- There is no recommendation for removal of neuraxial catheters in patients who receive thrombolytics unexpectedly, yet it is suggested to measure fibrinogen level.

Antiplatelets

Antiplatelet medications include nonsteroidal anti-inflammatory drugs (NSAIDs), aspirin, platelet receptor antagonists, and platelet phosphodiesterase IIIA inhibitors. NSAIDs and aspirin have not been found to increase risks for complications related to regional anesthesia, due to their minimal effect on platelet function. Therefore, there are no recommendations for timing of anesthesia administration or catheter techniques for patients on aspirin or NSAIDs [9, 41]. However, ASRA cautions performing regional anesthesia in the setting of NSAIDs or aspirin with simultaneous use of other medications such as antiplatelets and anticoagulants due to an increased risk of bleeding [9].

Ticlopidine, clopidogrel, and prasugrel are thienopyridine derivatives that irreversibly inhibit the P2Y12 component of ADP receptors on the platelet surface. This prevents the GPIIb/IIIa receptor complex from activating and consequently reduces platelet aggregation. Ticagrelor also has a similar mechanism of binding to the P2Y12 receptor; however, it is not a thienopyridine derivative, and its binding is reversible and noncompetitive. Cangrelor selectively and reversibly binds to the P2Y12 receptor, also preventing platelet activation and aggregation, but its administration is intravenous [42].

ASRA recommendations for patients taking these medications are as follows [9]:

- The recommended time interval between discontinuation of therapy and neuraxial blockade is 10 days for ticlopidine, 5–7 days for clopidogrel, 7–10 days for prasugrel, 5–7 days for ticagrelor, and 3 hours for cangrelor.
- Therapy may be reinstituted 24 hours postoperatively for ticlopidine, clopidogrel and prasugrel (thienopyridine therapy), and ticagrelor.
- Neuraxial catheters should *not* be maintained with prasugrel or ticagrelor due to their rapid onset.
- Neuraxial catheters may be maintained for 1–2 days with ticlopidine and clopidogrel, in the setting of no administration of a loading dose, since these antiplatelets do not have an immediate antiplatelet effect.
- Remove neuraxial catheter 8 hours prior to reinstitution of cangrelor therapy postoperatively.
- Thienopyridine and ticagrelor therapy may be resumed immediately after needle placement/catheter removal, if a loading drug is not given. If a loading dose is administered, a suggested time interval between catheter removal and administration is 6 hours.

GPIIb/IIIa receptor antagonists include abciximab, eptifibatide, and tirofiban. They greatly inhibit platelet aggregation, which impacts the recommendations made with their involvement in regional anesthesia. For context, after administration of abciximab, normal platelet aggregation reoccurs in 24–48 hours, while normalcy occurs 4–8 hours after eptifibatide and tirofiban [43]. In patients taking these medications, ASRA suggests avoiding neuraxial procedures until platelet function has recovered. If these therapies are given after neuraxial technique, it is recommended to use drugs that minimize sensory and motor blocking so patient can be monitored neurologically. No catheter removal time has been suggested; rather it is recommended to weigh the risk of spinal bleeding against the benefits of antiplatelet therapy [9].

Cilostazol reversibly inhibits platelet aggregation by inhibiting phosphodiesterase III. As its bleeding risk effect on neuraxial block is unknown, it is suggested that cilostazol be discontinued for 2 days prior to neuraxial anesthesia, which is based on its elimination half-life. ASRA also suggests neuraxial catheter removal prior to restarting therapy, with the first postoperative dose being administered 6 hours after catheter removal [9].

Dipyridamole's antiplatelet effect is also through inhibition of platelet aggregation. ASRA recommendations are as follows [9]:

- Discontinue the extended release form 24 hours prior to neuraxial block.
- Remove neuraxial catheters prior to reinstitution of therapy, with suggested administration 6 hours after removal.

Herbal Therapy

Examples of herbal remedies that are known to affect hemostasis are garlic, ginseng, and ginkgo. These therapies are all known to impact platelet aggregation and are therefore relevant to our discussion [44–46]. Although there are case reports of neuraxial bleeding following the consumption of garlic and ginkgo, larger studies have found no difference in bleeding after surgery among patients on herbal therapy [47–49]. This gives insight to the ASRA recommendation which states that herbal medications does *not* create a level of risk that will interfere with the performance of neuraxial block. Among patients on these herbal therapies, there is also a recommendation against the discontinuation of these medications or avoidance of regional anesthesia [9]. However, just as there are reservations against neuraxial anesthesia in patients using dual antiplatelet or antiplatelet and anticoagulant therapy simultaneously, there is a similar discretion regarding herbs with concurrent anticoagulation use [9].

Peripheral Nerve Blocks

Among patients who are on anticoagulants, the feared consequences of regional anesthesia via peripheral and plexus techniques are bleeding, hematoma formation, and subsequent neurological effects. There are limited case reports and studies that have evaluated and described the complications of peripheral nerve and plexus blocks in anticoagulated patients. Among the data available, profound bleeding has been found to be the critical complication, when compared to neurological deficits. This may be due to bleeding occurring into fixed, noncompressible, deep spaces, at which hemorrhage contributes to patient morbidity [9, 50]. For patients taking anticoagulants who undergo peripheral or more superficial plexus blocks, ASRA suggests that the similar guidelines for neuraxial techniques be used. However, for patients undergoing deep plexus or deep peripheral blocks, it is suggested that the anesthetic performance, catheter maintenance, and catheter removal be based on each site and its vascularity, bleeding consequences, and compressibility. Of note, the lack of more specific recommendations, like those pertaining to certain anatomical locations, serves as a reminder for the need of further studies and case reporting in this topic.

Anticoagulation in Obstetric Patients

Pregnancy is a state of hypercoagulability. Factors such as cesarean delivery, increased age, previous thromboembolism, and obesity all increase the preexisting prothrombotic state. The 6 weeks after pregnancy is also associated with higher rates of thrombosis [51]. These characteristics may contribute to certain patients benefiting from anticoagulation. Since neuraxial anesthesia is a common effective method of pain management during vaginal and cesarean delivery, it is important to acknowledge neuraxial anesthetic management in anticoagulated patients. Heparins are the main anticoagulant used in pregnancy because they do not affect fetal development [18, 51–53].

A systematic review of obstetric patients receiving thromboprophylactic dose of UFH or LMWH did not identify a single case of causally related spinal epidural hematoma (SEH) [54]. In contrast, a study involving direct oral anticoagulants during pregnancy resulted in miscarriages, fetal anomalies, and questionable efficacy with a lack of reported thrombotic or bleeding complication [55]. For parturients, ASRA suggests similar recommendations regarding anesthetic management amidst heparin use, which we previously discussed. However, in patients who are taking anticoagulants and require urgent intervention, these guidelines should be modified as found appropriate, and the risks of general anesthesia versus neuraxial anesthesia should be assessed [9]. Overall, the limited data on the implications of anticoagulant use during pregnancy on neuraxial anesthesia and epidural hematoma incidence serves as a reminder for the need of more studies [54].

Spinal Hematoma

Since bleeding is the major complication of anticoagulant therapy, neuraxial anesthesia in patients on anticoagulation poses a risk of hematoma formation. Hematomas can develop in the epidural, subdural, or subarachnoid space. However, bleeding occurs more commonly in the epidural space due to its venous plexus. Spinal hematomas are rare, and the true incidence in anticoagulated patients is unknown due to underreporting [9, 56].

Spinal hematomas are asymptomatic until they begin to compress the spinal cord, causing neurological symptoms and pain. These neurological consequences include bladder/bowel dysfunction and most commonly motor and sensory deficits [54, 57, 58]. MRI of the spine is the most sensitive and specific diagnostic method of spinal hematomas. If paralysis or significant deficits have not occurred, recovery can occur with conservative management that often includes close follow-up, frequent neurological exams, imaging, and coagulation. There have also been cases with spontaneous resolution of hematomas [57–62]. However, if paralysis occurs, the treatment is rapid surgical decompression of the spinal cord by laminectomy, evacuation of the hematoma, and coagulation of the bleeding [60–62].

Conclusion

The guidelines provided by the American Society of Regional Anesthesia and Pain Medicine are based on case reports, clinical studies, expert opinion, hematology, pharmacological data, and recommendations from other organizations like the European Society of Anaesthesiology. Although these guidelines are evidence-based reviews, it is crucial to note that they should not preclude weighing the risks and benefits for each individual patient. In performing regional anesthesia in patients on hemostasis-altering therapy, it is also important to determine their risk factors and enhance their coagulation status. Nevertheless, these recommendations are fundamental in aiding to provide safe, quality care to patients while simultaneously decreasing the risk of adverse events like spinal hematomas. The evidence-based guidelines discussed in this chapter are undoubtedly advantageous, but are not infallible. It is essential to remember that there is always a need for further studies, data, and case reporting to establish updated recommendations based on strengthened evidence.

References

1. Stults BM, Dere WH, Caine TH. Long-term anticoagulation. Indications and management. West J Med. 1989;151(4):414–29.
2. Barnes GD, Lucas E, Alexander GC, Goldberger ZD. National trends in ambulatory oral anticoagulant use. Am J Med. 2015;128(12):1300–5.e2.
3. Palta S, Saroa R, Palta A. Overview of the coagulation system. Indian J Anaesth. 2014;58(5):515–23.
4. Periayah MH, Halim AS, AZM S. Mechanism action of platelets and crucial blood coagulation pathways in hemostasis. Int J Hematol Oncol Stem Cell Res. 2017;11(4):319–27.

5. Smith SA, Travers RJ, Morrissey JH. How it all starts: initiation of the clotting cascade. Crit Rev Biochem Mol Biol. 2015;50(4):326–36.
6. Hall JE. Hemostasis and blood coagulation. In: Guyton and hall textbook of medical physiology: enhanced e-book. 11th ed. Philadelphia: Elsevier Health Sciences; 2010. p. 457–9.
7. Kumar V, Abbas AK, Fausto N, Aster JC. Hemodynamic disorders, thromboembolic disease and shock. In: Robbins and Cotran pathologic basis of disease. 8th ed. Philadelphia: Saunders Elsevier; 2010. p. 118–20.
8. Chaudhry R, Babiker HM. Physiology, coagulation pathways. [Updated 2019 Apr 17]. In: StatPearls [Internet]. Treasure Island (FL): StatPearls Publishing; 2019. Available from: https://www.ncbi.nlm.nih.gov/books/NBK482253/.
9. Horlocker TT, Vandermeuelen E, Kopp SL, Gogarten W, Leffert LR, Benzon HT. Regional anesthesia in the patient receiving antithrombotic or thrombolytic therapy: American Society of Regional Anesthesia and Pain Medicine Evidence-Based Guidelines (fourth edition). Reg Anesth Pain Med. 2018;43(3):263–309.
10. Torpy JM, Lynm C, Golub RM. JAMA patient page. Regional anesthesia. JAMA. 2011;306(7):781.
11. Smith LM, Cozowicz C, Uda Y, et al. Neuraxial and combined neuraxial/general anesthesia compared to general anesthesia for major truncal and lower limb surgery: a systematic review and meta-analysis. Anesth Analg. 2017;125:1931.
12. Johnson RL, Kopp SL, Burkle CM, et al. Neuraxial vs general anaesthesia for total hip and total knee arthroplasty: a systematic review of comparative-effectiveness research. Br J Anaesth. 2016;116(2):163–76.
13. Lirk P, Hollmann MW. Outcome after regional anesthesia: weighing risks and benefits. Minerva Anestesiol. 2014;80(5):610–8.
14. Ash EA. Chapter 119. Safety in regional anesthesia. In: Atchabahian A, Gupta R, editors. The anesthesia guide. New York: McGraw-Hill; 2013. p. 499–504.
15. Horlocker T, Kopp S. Epidural hematoma after epidural blockade in the United States: it's not just low molecular heparin following orthopedic surgery anymore. Anesth Analg. 2013;116(6):1195–7.
16. Benzon HT. Chapter 8. Regional anesthesia in the anticoagulated patient. In: Hadzic A, editor. Hadzic's peripheral nerve blocks and anatomy for ultrasound-guided regional anesthesia. 2nd ed. New York: McGraw-Hill; 2012. p. 107–13.
17. Enneking FK, Huntoon MA. Regional anesthesia in the patient receiving antithrombotic or thrombolytic therapy: if only the data were produced in a river not a pond! Reg Anesth Pain Med. 2018;43(3):223–4.
18. Regional anaesthesia and patients with abnormalities of coagulation: the Association of Anaesthetists of Great Britain & Ireland The Obstetric Anaesthetists' Association Regional Anaesthesia UK. Anaesthesia. 2013;68(9):966–72.
19. Gogarten W, Vandermeulen E, Van Aken H, et al. Regional anaesthesia and antithrombotic agents: recommendations of the European Society of Anaesthesiology. Eur J Anaesthesiol. 2010;27(12):999–1015.
20. Horlocker TT, Wedel DJ. Anticoagulation and neuraxial block: historical perspective, anesthetic implications, and risk management. Reg Anesth Pain Med. 1998;23(6 Suppl 2):129–34.
21. Hirsh J, Warkentin TE, Shaughnessy SG, et al. Heparin and low-molecular-weight heparin: mechanisms of action, pharmacokinetics, dosing, monitoring, efficacy, and safety. Chest. 2001;119(1 Suppl):64S–94S.
22. Gray E, Hogwood J, Mulloy B. The anticoagulant and antithrombotic mechanisms of heparin. Handb Exp Pharmacol. 2012;207:43–61.
23. Merli GJ, Groce JB. Pharmacological and clinical differences between low-molecular-weight heparins: implications for prescribing practice and therapeutic interchange. P T. 2010;35(2):95–105.
24. Hirsh J, Bauer KA, Donati MB, Gould M, Samama MM, Weitz JI. Parenteral anticoagulants: American College of Chest Physicians Evidence-Based Clinical Practice Guidelines (8th edition). Chest. 2008;133(6 Suppl):141S–59S.
25. Center for Drug Evaluation and Research. FDA drug safety communication: updated recommendations to decrease risk of spinal column bleeding and paralysis in patients on low molecular weight heparins. U.S. Food and Drug Administration. https://www.fda.gov/drugs/drug-safety-and-availability/fda-drug-safety-communication-updated-recommendations-decrease-risk-spinal-column-bleeding-and#tabs-3.
26. Crader MF, Johns T, Arnold JK. Warfarin drug interactions. [Updated 2019 Jul 5]. In: StatPearls [Internet]. Treasure Island (FL): StatPearls Publishing; 2019. Available from: https://www.ncbi.nlm.nih.gov/books/NBK441964/.
27. Hanley JP. Warfarin reversal. J Clin Pathol. 2004;57(11):1132–9.
28. Franchini M, Lippi G. Prothrombin complex concentrates: an update. Blood Transfus. 2010;8(3):149–54.
29. Reynolds NA, Perry CM, Scott LJ. Fondaparinux sodium: a review of its use in the prevention of venous thromboembolism following major orthopaedic surgery. Drugs. 2004;64(14):1575–96.
30. Cappelleri G, Fanelli A. Use of direct oral anticoagulants with regional anesthesia in orthopedic patients. J Clin Anesth. 2016;32:224–35.
31. Kaushal M, Rubin RE, Kaye AD, Gritsenko K. Anticoagulation and neuraxial/peripheral anesthesia. Anesthesiol Clin. 2017;35(2):e21–39.
32. Van den heuvel JM, Hövels AM, Büller HR, Mantel-teeuwisse AK, De boer A, Maitland-van der Zee AH. NOACs replace VKA as preferred oral anticoagulant among new patients: a drug utilization study in 560 pharmacies in The Netherlands. Thromb J. 2018;16:7.
33. De caterina R, Ageno W, Agnelli G, et al. The non-vitamin K antagonist oral anticoagulants in heart disease: section V-special situations. Thromb Haemost. 2019;119(1):14–38.
34. Demir M. Coagulation testing for new oral anticoagulants. J Atr Fibrillation. 2015;8(3):1089.
35. Abed HS, Kilborn MJ, Chen V, Sy RW. Reversal agents in the era of NOACs. J Atr Fibrillation. 2017;10(4):1634.
36. Levy JH, Douketis J, Weitz JI. Reversal agents for non-vitamin K antagonist oral anticoagulants. Nat Rev Cardiol. 2018;15(5):273–81. https://doi.org/10.1038/nrcardio.2017.223.
37. Rowe AS, Dietrich SK, Phillips JW, Foster KE, Canter JR. Activated prothrombin complex concentrate versus 4-factor prothrombin complex concentrate for vitamin K-antagonist reversal. Crit Care Med. 2018;46(6):943–8.
38. Turecek PL, Váradi K, Gritsch H, Schwarz HP. FEIBA: mode of action. Haemophilia. 2004;10(Suppl 2):3–9.
39. Baker WF. Thrombolytic therapy: current clinical practice. Hematol Oncol Clin North Am. 2005;19(1):147–81, vii.
40. Ali MR, Salim Hossain M, Islam MA, et al. Aspect of thrombolytic therapy: a review. Scientific World Journal. 2014;2014:586510.
41. Vela Vásquez RS, Peláez Romero R. Aspirin and spinal haematoma after neuraxial anaesthesia: myth or reality? Br J Anaesth. 2015;115(5):688–98.
42. Wijeyeratne YD, Heptinstall S. Anti-platelet therapy: ADP receptor antagonists. Br J Clin Pharmacol. 2011;72(4):647–57.
43. Schneider DJ. Anti-platelet therapy: glycoprotein IIb-IIIa antagonists. Br J Clin Pharmacol. 2011;72(4):672–82.
44. Wong WW, Gabriel A, Maxwell GP, Gupta SC. Bleeding risks of herbal, homeopathic, and dietary supplements: a hidden nightmare for plastic surgeons? Aesthet Surg J. 2012;32(3):332–46.

45. Hirsch GE, Viecili PRN, De almeida AS, et al. Natural products with antiplatelet action. Curr Pharm Des. 2017;23(8):1228–46.
46. Tsai TP. Chapter 12. Anticoagulation, antiplatelet medications. In: Atchabahian A, Gupta R, editors. The anesthesia guide. New York: McGraw-Hill; 2013. p. 50.
47. Gilbert GJ. Ginkgo biloba. Neurology. 1997;48:1137.
48. Lee A, Chui PT, Aun CS, Lau AS, Gin T. Incidence and risk of adverse perioperative events among surgical patients taking traditional Chinese herbal medicines. Anesthesiology. 2006;105:454–61.
49. Moss J, Yuan CS. Herbal medicines and perioperative care. Anesthesiology. 2006;105:441–2.
50. Doan L. Chapter 163. Management of continuous peripheral nerve blocks. In: Atchabahian A, Gupta R, Atchabahian A, Gupta R, editors. The anesthesia guide. New York: McGraw-Hill; 2013. p. 690–1.
51. James AH. Pregnancy and thrombotic risk. Crit Care Med. 2010;38(2 Suppl):S57–63.
52. Leffert L, Butwick A, Carvalho B, et al. The Society for Obstetric Anesthesia and Perinatology consensus statement on the anesthetic management of pregnant and postpartum women receiving thromboprophylaxis or higher dose anticoagulants. Anesth Analg. 2018;126(3):928–44.
53. ACOG Practice Bulletin No. 196: Thromboembolism in pregnancy. Obstet Gynecol. 2018;132(1):e1–e17.
54. Leffert LR, Dubois HM, Butwick AJ, Carvalho B, Houle TT, Landau R. Neuraxial anesthesia in obstetric patients receiving thromboprophylaxis with unfractionated or low-molecular-weight heparin: a systematic review of spinal epidural hematoma. Anesth Analg. 2017;125(1):223–31.
55. Lameijer H, Aalberts JJJ, Van Veldhuisen DJ, Meijer K, Pieper PG. Efficacy and safety of direct oral anticoagulants during pregnancy; a systematic literature review. Thromb Res. 2018;169:123–7.
56. Moen V, Dahlgren N, Irestedt L. Severe neurological complications after central neuraxial blockades in Sweden 1990–1999. Anesthesiology. 2004;101(4):950–9.
57. Lee LA, Posner KL, Domino KB, Caplan RA, Cheney FW. Injuries associated with regional anesthesia in the 1980s and 1990s: a closed claims analysis. Anesthesiology. 2004;101(1):143–52.
58. Nelson A, Benzon HT, Jabri RS. Diagnosis and management of spinal and peripheral nerve hematoma. In: Hadzic A, editor. Hadzic's textbook of regional anesthesia and acute pain management. 2nd ed. New York: McGraw-Hill; 2012.
59. Nam KH, Choi CH, Yang MS, Kang DW. Spinal epidural hematoma after pain control procedure. J Korean Neurosurg Soc. 2010;48(3):281–4.
60. Tailor J, Dunn IF, Smith E. Conservative treatment of spontaneous spinal epidural hematoma associated with oral anticoagulant therapy in a child. Childs Nerv Syst. 2006;22(12):1643–5.
61. Zhang S, Geng F, Wang J, Zhang Z, Du C. Rapid recovery of spontaneous spinal epidural hematoma without surgical treatment: case report and literature review. World Neurosurg. 2018;115:216–9.
62. Raasck K, Habis AA, Aoude A, et al. Spontaneous spinal epidural hematoma management: a case series and literature review. Spinal Cord Ser Cases. 2017;3:16043.

Iron Overload

45

Michael Godbold and Patrick D. McFarland

Anesthetic Implications of Iron Overload

Introduction

Iron overload is defined as excessive levels of circulating iron in the body. An estimated 16 million Americans have some form of iron overload with hereditary hemochromatosis being the most common form of iron overload [11]. It is estimated that 10–14% of the population are a genetic mutation carrier for some form of iron overload [14]. Iron overload affects a variety of organ systems including hepatic, cardiac, and endocrine. The symptoms of this condition range from changes in skin pigmentation to severe end-organ damage including cirrhosis and heart failure. Current treatment options are highly effective at controlling circulating iron levels. However, if left untreated, iron overload can progress to cirrhosis and increased morbidity and mortality associated with anesthesia.

Iron Metabolism

To understand iron overload and other disorders of iron balance, one must study how the body regulates iron metabolism. Iron metabolism is well regulated by specific proteins and homeostatic mechanisms including the balance between iron absorption and iron release from cells. Specific proteins involved in regulating this balance include transferrin, ferritin, ferroportin, and hepcidin, among others. Synthesized in the liver, transferrin is the primary protein responsible for iron transport in plasma. The transporter protein binds two ferric (Fe^{3+}) molecules at a time during iron trafficking [7]. Ferritin functions as a storage protein for iron in cells. A relatively large protein, ferritin has a molecular weight of 440 kDa and can store up to 4500 atoms of iron at a time [3]. Additionally, ferritin acts as an acute phase reactant and will experience elevated levels during times of stress and inflammation to protect against oxidative damage. Serum levels of ferritin are a good surrogate measure for total body iron storage. Roughly 1 ng/mL of ferritin equals 10 mg of total body iron [7]. Iron overload is characterized by an elevated ferritin level in the absence of any confounding infection or inflammation.

Iron exportation from cells into the circulation is accomplished by ferroportin. Ferroportin allows both enterocytes in the gut to export iron absorbed from diet and macrophages in circulation to export iron recovered from heme resorption. The protein hepcidin serves as the main regulator in the negative feedback mechanism ensuring normal iron balance. Hepcidin prevents iron overload by limiting iron absorption from diet and iron release from macrophages [13]. The protein's activity directly correlates with serum ferritin levels; in other words, when ferritin levels are high, hepcidin activity is also high, and vice versa. Mutations in hepcidin gene expression or protein dysfunction result in pathological primary iron overload states.

Normal total body iron levels are 3–4 grams with the majority found in heme [7]. The element is also found in iron-containing proteins, such as cytochromes and myoglobin, as well as transferrin-bound in plasma. Iron itself is insoluble in plasma and would result in toxicity from the generation of free radicals; however, transferrin acts to counter this effect, providing solubility to transferrin-bound iron. As such, virtually all iron circulating in plasma is bound to transferrin [7]. The remainder is mainly stored in the form of ferritin in organs such as the liver and spleen. Additionally, there are gender differences with regard to normal iron storage. Due to menstruation, adult women typically experience lower levels of iron storage as compared to adult men.

M. Godbold
University of Tennessee Medical Center – Knoxville, Department of Anesthesiology, Knoxville, TN, USA

P. D. McFarland (✉)
Department of Anesthesiology, University of Tennessee Graduate School of Medicine, Knoxville, TN, USA
e-mail: pmcfarland@utmck.edu

© Springer Nature Switzerland AG 2021
C. S. Scher et al. (eds.), *Essentials of Blood Product Management in Anesthesia Practice*,
https://doi.org/10.1007/978-3-030-59295-0_45

Absorption of iron occurs primarily through the gastrointestinal tract. The amount of iron absorbed varies by dietary intake and rate of gastrointestinal absorption. Gastrointestinal absorption is almost exclusively regulated by the protein, hepcidin. Produced by hepatocytes and expressed by the hepcidin antimicrobial peptide (HAMP) gene, hepcidin is the primary mechanism for control of iron absorption through the gastrointestinal tract. Hepcidin binds to the protein ferroportin and causes its internalization and degradation. As described above, ferroportin is the protein responsible for the transcellular movement of iron within the GI tract, macrophages, and hepatocytes. Inhibition of the function of ferroportin results in loss of iron through the GI tract and low iron states [13].

Homeostatic control of iron absorption through the gastrointestinal tract is primarily regulated through control of hepcidin production. The primary control of hepcidin production is through iron levels and erythropoietic activity. High levels of circulatory iron cause an increase in hepcidin synthesis and subsequently a decrease in iron absorption. Secondly, increased erythropoietic activity in the bone marrow will cause a decrease in production of hepcidin and increase circulatory levels of iron. In addition to these two primary mechanisms of control, hepcidin is also upregulated in states of inflammation, infection, and chronic kidney disease. Conversely, hepcidin is downregulated in states of hypoxia, hereditary hemochromatosis, and hepatitis C.

Hepcidin also controls iron release from macrophages. Through phagocytosis, macrophages will resorb heme from broken-down red blood cells. Depending on the local concentration of hepcidin, macrophages will utilize ferroportin to release the resorbed iron into the circulation or rely on ferritin to store iron for later release [9].

Iron loss is not regulated as strictly as iron absorption and release. Normal iron loss occurs at a rate of about 1–2 mg/day through processes such as sweating and gastrointestinal excretion [7]. Through diet alone, both adult men and women can compensate for these daily losses; however, adult women are more prone to deficiency given the additional iron losses experienced through menstruation. Regarding possible future pharmacological therapies, some studies have shown the kidney may contain possible excretory pathways that could be a drug target to combat iron overload states [2].

Signs and Symptoms of Iron Overload

Iron overload can cause a variety of clinical manifestations. Complications can be mild, such as in skin hyperpigmentation, or major, such as in advanced end-organ failure. In hemochromatosis, men are more likely than menstruating women to show symptoms of iron overload due to a lack of menses [11]. Ultimately, end-organ failure can be fatal if enough liver or cardiac damage occurs. The severity of damage is directly related to the degree of iron overload as toxicity results from free iron deposition in organ tissues [17]. Typical clinical findings are wide-ranging, depending on the extent of organ involvement, and include:

- Nonspecific abdominal pain and generalized malaise
- Bronze pigmentation of skin
- Joint pain
- Polyuria and polydipsia secondary to diabetes mellitus development
- Decreased libido and impotence due to hypogonadism from pituitary and gonadal involvement
- Abnormal liver function and inflammation that can progress to cirrhosis
- Palpitations, dyspnea on exertion, and peripheral edema secondary to dysrhythmias and cardiomyopathy from cardiac tissue deposition

In the past, iron overload had been referred to as "bronze diabetes" due to the bronzing of skin from hyperpigmentation and development of diabetes mellitus from free iron deposition in pancreatic tissue. The lack of specificity of early signs and symptoms often leads to a delay in diagnosis once advanced end-organ injury has already occurred [17].

Etiologies of Iron Overload

The etiology of iron overload can be divided into two main categories: increased iron intake and increased gastrointestinal absorption. Increased iron intake occurs primarily from either increased dietary intake or from a need for frequent blood transfusions. Iatrogenic increases in dietary intake include oral iron supplementation or intravenous iron administration. Iron overload resulting from chronic transfusion-related medical conditions is also called transfusion-associated iron overload. In this patient population, it is important to evaluate transfusion needs and requirements as each unit of transfused red blood cells contains roughly 200 mg of iron [17]. Transfusion-associated iron overload commonly results from the following medical conditions:

- Sickle cell disease and other hemolytic anemias
- Myelodysplastic syndromes
- Beta-thalassemia major
- Chemotherapy, bone marrow replacement, or stem cell transplantation
- Intrinsic RBC and hemoglobin abnormalities

Conditions resulting in increased GI absorption of iron include hemochromatosis, ineffective erythropoiesis, and chronic liver disease. Primary hereditary hemochromatosis is the most common form and results from a mutation in the HFE gene resulting in decreased production of hepcidin. Other forms of hemochromatosis include juvenile (which results from a mutation in the hemojuvelin gene) and neonatal hemochromatosis, which is normally not compatible with life. Anemias which result from ineffective erythropoiesis include thalassemias, sideroblastic anemias, and other inherited anemias. Ineffective erythropoiesis results in the destruction of RBC precursors, which subsequently increases overall erythropoietic activity, decreases hepcidin production, and increases circulatory iron.

Another way to classify iron overload is primary (genetic) versus secondary (acquired). Any intrinsic deficiency in the normal iron regulatory pathway resulting in excess iron burden is characterized as primary iron overload. Primary iron overload includes rare genetic disorders, such as hereditary hemochromatosis, hypotransferrinemia, and aceruloplasminemia. With low levels of transferrin available to transport iron, hypotransferrinemia results in excess iron storage in various organs. Ceruloplasmin is involved in the iron exportation and transportation pathway. Ceruloplasmin works with ferroportin and transferrin to process iron during exportation and transportation, respectively. Its absence results in inefficient iron recycling in the liver and excess iron accumulation. Hereditary hemochromatosis is described above.

Any extrinsic insult resulting in excess iron burden is characterized as secondary iron overload. Secondary iron overload includes chronic transfusion-related medical conditions as well as increased ingestion and excess intravenous administration of iron.

Laboratory Tests and Diagnostic Imaging

The diagnosis of iron overload is confirmed with two blood tests, ferritin level and transferrin saturation (TSAT). As previously described, ferritin correlates directly with the total amount of iron in the body. Elevated ferritin levels are 200–300 μg/L for men and 150–200 μg/L for women. Iron overload is defined as ferritin levels greater than 1000 μg/L [17]. Of note, ferritin is considered an acute phase reactant and can be elevated in non-iron overload states. Therefore, a transferrin saturation is also needed to confirm the diagnosis of iron overload. Transferrin saturation is calculated as serum iron divided by total iron-binding capacity. A normal TSAT ranges from 20% to 50%, and iron overload is confirmed with a TSAT greater than 50% [5].

In severe cases of iron overload, end-organ damage must also be considered when determining necessary diagnostic imaging. To evaluate iron content in the body, magnetic resonance imaging (MRI) is recommended over computed tomography (CT) as the latter has limited sensitivity [17]. Individuals with signs or symptoms of cirrhosis should have appropriate liver function testing. Cardiac evaluation with electrocardiogram (ECG), echocardiography (ECHO), or even cardiac MRI is also warranted in some circumstances. As always, clinical characteristics of the patient will dictate further cardiac and hepatic workup.

Iron Overload Complications

Complications due to iron overload are often encountered given the difficulty in recognizing the condition. Early signs and symptoms are nonspecific, and clinical manifestations can range from skin hyperpigmentation and joint pain to fatal end-organ disease. The liver is iron's primary storage site, and hepatocytes commonly experience cell death in iron overload states. Reactive oxygen species from toxic iron levels result in oxidative damage which can have cancer-causing effects [5]. Additionally, hepatoportal fibrosis can result from oxidative damage which can progress to cirrhosis and even hepatocellular carcinoma [4]. Some studies have shown patients dependent on blood transfusions can develop portal fibrosis and cirrhosis within 2–10 years if the disease is left untreated [8].

Excess iron burden can also significantly impact the myocardium. In fact, even small concentrations of free iron are toxic to cardiac cells [17]. Often, cardiac insult occurs only after the liver has experienced injury. The most frequent cardiac complication encountered with iron overload is congestive cardiomyopathy, although pericarditis and dysrhythmias can occur [10]. Furthermore, in advanced disease, sudden cardiac death has been reported [6]. Like other involved organs, the extent of cardiac injury directly correlates with the amount of free iron deposition in organ tissue. Studies have shown worsened outcomes with ferritin levels greater than 1000 μg/L [12]. Again, given the lack of specificity of early signs and symptoms, disease is often advanced once cardiac complications occur. When iron levels reach critical levels, systolic dysfunction eventually follows as well as the potential rapid deterioration of clinical status.

Other organ systems can be affected as well, including the endocrine system and the hypothalamic-pituitary-adrenal (HPA) axis. As previously mentioned, diabetes mellitus results from pancreatic dysfunction due to iron deposition and subsequent oxidative damage. Also, the development of hypocalcemia and its associated complications can occur due to parathyroid involvement. Free iron deposition in the pituitary gland can result in a wide array of symptoms, such as infertility and growth failure [5].

Perioperative Implications

In patients susceptible to chronic iron overload, one must carefully assess the degree of end-organ involvement prior to proceeding to the operating theatre. As always, preoperative cardiac risk stratification and optimization of medical co-morbidities should occur to guide intraoperative anesthetic management and to minimize risk of perioperative complications. As mentioned above, the nonspecific early manifestations of iron overload necessitate vigilance in screening at-risk patients who have yet to showcase advanced disease. Screening is accomplished with serum ferritin and transferrin saturation levels. A long-term study of hemochromatosis patients showed no change in survival if development of cirrhosis was avoided. Therefore, careful management of these patients includes early diagnosis of iron overload and continued attempts to reduce iron levels and prevent the life-shortening consequence of cirrhosis [1].

When advanced end-organ injury presents, one must assess the impact such injury will have on anesthetic management. Pharmacodynamic effects from advanced liver disease should be considered when selecting anesthetic agents as alterations in drug metabolism and protein binding may be observed. Additionally, altered hemostasis may result as platelets and coagulation factors become affected. In this patient population, a restrictive transfusion management strategy is prudent given the nature of chronic iron overload and the additional iron burden present in transfused blood units as well as to limit the other associated risks of a liberal transfusion strategy [15]. Cardiac involvement may warrant additional testing such as electrocardiogram to assess baseline rhythm and echocardiography to assess cardiac anatomy and systolic function. Decompensated heart failure and unstable dysrhythmias should be managed and optimized prior to proceeding with elective surgery.

Chronic iron overload is often treated with iron chelators or therapeutic phlebotomy. Iron chelation therapy has specifically been shown to benefit patients with transfusion-dependent anemia [16]. The anesthesia provider must consider the adverse effects of these medications during the perioperative period. Iron chelators, such as deferasirox and deferoxamine, can affect the cytochrome P450 drug-metabolism pathway, potentially affecting perioperative dosing of anesthetic medications [18]. Also, therapeutic phlebotomy schedules should be investigated, and appropriate cell counts assessed, to ensure adequate oxygen delivery to organ tissues.

Summary

Iron overload is an uncommon disease process that results in specific anesthesia-related implications. The homeostatic regulation of iron levels in the body is achieved through a complex process involving the liver, GI tract, and circulating hemoglobin. This chapter reviewed the roles that transferrin, ferritin, ferroportin, and hepcidin have in the metabolism and regulation of iron levels. Symptoms of iron overload vary greatly from mild abdominal pain to severe end-organ damage including liver and cardiac failure. Because of the wide range of symptoms, a high clinical suspicion is necessary to make the diagnosis of iron overload. This diagnosis is achieved through two blood tests, ferritin level and transferrin saturation (TSAT). Further testing is focused on identifying the primary cause of iron overload and assessing any end-organ damage if present. Hereditary etiologies of iron overload include hemochromatosis, hypotransferrinemia, and aceruloplasminemia. Secondary causes of iron overload include transfusion-associated iron overload and excessive supplemental administration.

The anesthetic management of a patient with iron overload should focus on addressing the degree of iron overload through laboratory testing as well as determining the cause of iron overload. Ultimately, assessing end-organ damage is the primary concern of the anesthesiologist. Thorough evaluations of the hepatic, cardiac, and hematologic systems are warranted and must be completed prior to conducting an anesthetic on a patient with iron overload syndrome.

References

1. Adams PC, Speechley M, Kertesz AE. Long-term survival analysis in hereditary hemochromatosis. Gastroenterology. 1991;101(2):368–72.
2. Andrews NC. Forging a field: the golden age of iron biology. Blood. 2008;112:219.
3. Arosio P, Levi S. Cytosolic and mitochondrial ferritins in the regulation of cellular iron homeostasis and oxidative damage. Biochim Biophys Acta. 2010;1800(8):783.
4. Asare GA, Massanda KS, Kew MC, Paterson AC, Kahler-Venter CP, Siziba K. Hepatocellular carcinoma caused by iron overload: a possible mechanism of direct hepatocarcinogenicity. Toxicology. 2006;219:41–52.
5. Bacon BR, Kwiatkowski JL. Approach to the patient with suspected iron overload. UpToDate. Topic 7157 version 70.0. 2019. Available: https://www-uptodate-com/contents/approach-to-the-patient-with-suspected-iron-overload. Accessed 05.09.2019.
6. Buja LM, Roberts WC. Iron in the heart. Etiology and clinical significance. Am J Med. 1971;51:209–21.
7. Camaschella C. Regulation of iron balance. UpToDate. Topic 7105 version 60.0. 2019. Available: https://www.uptodate.com/contents/regulation-of-iron-balance. Accessed 05.09.2019.
8. Hershko C, Peto TE. Non-transferrin plasma iron. Br J Haematol. 1987;66:149–51.
9. Korolnek T, Hamza I. Macrophages and iron trafficking at the birth and death of red cells. Blood. 2015;125:2893.
10. Liu P, Olivieri N. Iron overload cardiomyopathies: new insights into an old disease. Cadiovasc Drugs Ther. 1994;8:101–10.
11. McDowell L, Sticco K. Iron overload. StatPearls; Feb 2019.

12. Morrison ED, Brandhagen DJ, Phatak PD, et al. Serum ferritin level predicts advanced hepatic fibrosis among U.S. patients with phenotypic hemochromatosis. Ann Intern Med. 2003;138:627–33.
13. Nemeth E, et al. The role of hepcidin in iron metabolism. Acta Haematol. 2009;122:78–86.
14. Powell LW, George DK, McDonnell SM, Kowdley KV. Diagnosis of hemochromatosis. Ann Intern Med. 1998;129(11):925–31.
15. Schafer AI, Cheron RG, Dluhy R, et al. Clinical consequences of acquired transfusional iron overload in adults. N Engl J Med. 1981;304:319–24.
16. Shander A, Sazama K. Clinical consequences of iron overload from chronic red blood cell transfusions, its diagnosis, and its management by chelation therapy. Transfusion. 2010;50:1144–55.
17. Shander A, et al. Iron overload and toxicity: implications for anesthesiologists. J Clin Anesth. 2012;24:419–25.
18. Skerjanec A, Wang J, Maren K, Rojkjaer L. Investigation of the pharmacokinetic interactions of deferasirox, a once-daily oral iron chelator, with midazolam, rifampin, and repaglinide in healthy volunteers. J Clin Pharmacol. 2010;50:205–13.

46 Blood Product Management in Developing Countries

Kyle Gress, Karina Charipova, Mitchell C. Fuller, Ivan Urits, and Alan David Kaye

Introduction: Understanding the Problem

Transfusion of blood and blood products is not only critical in life-threatening emergencies but also facilitates management of acute and chronic conditions in routine patient care [1]. In developing countries (DGCs) such as those in sub-Saharan Africa, the greatest need for transfusions is in children with malaria-related anemia and women with obstetric hemorrhage [1, 2]. These clinical scenarios are associated with a mortality index of up to 25.5% [2]. Although the World Health Organization (WHO) included fresh frozen plasma, platelets, red blood cells, and whole blood on its Model List of Essential Medicines in 2019, many DGCs lack reliable access to these products [3].

Adequate blood product management requires a stable supply, a standardized procedure for processing and testing, and appropriate clinical and laboratory skills for use of products [1]. The problem faced by most DGCs can be broken down into three basic components: insufficient supply, excess demand, and inadequate quality of available supply. This problem is further complicated by the issue of cost. It has been shown that international organizations such as the Red Cross cannot permanently fund blood transfusion systems and that this responsibility belongs to national authorities [4]. In sub-Saharan Africa many countries have utilized external funding to establish national blood management services, but few have been able to convert to reliable self-sufficient systems [1].

Compared to developed countries, DGCs lack voluntary non-remunerated blood donors that are essential to maintaining adequate supply [5]. Due to a combination of infection-related apprehension and local and cultural beliefs, these countries rely heavily on replacement donations [5, 6]. Even so, proportions of repeat donors are low, resulting in an unstable supply of blood and a severe lack of plasma derivatives since very few DGCs have the fractionation plants required for their production [5]. The shortage of donors in DGCs is compounded by unindicated transfusion and a large volume of discarded blood [5]. Blood should be transfused only when clinically appropriate. Unfortunately, most clinical transfusion guidelines rely on formal assessments such as quality-assured hemoglobin measurements [1]. In places where these services are unavailable, clinicians rely solely on clinical judgment which, when faulty, can result in the transfusion of a unit of blood that costs 40 times more than an accurate hemoglobin test [1]. Despite the fact that the majority of transfusion-related research has focused heavily on preventing transfusion-transmitted infections rather than addressing blood shortage, the scope for increasing supply by reducing unnecessary transfusion is likely substantial [1].

Quality of available blood products in DGCs has benefited substantially from increased awareness of the human immunodeficiency virus (HIV), but efforts to improve testing for other transfusion-transmissible infectious agents are still warranted [5]. Recent data have shown that transfusion-associated infection rates in sub-Saharan Africa remain astronomically higher than those in high-income countries, with risk of HIV, hepatitis B (HBV), and hepatitis C (HCV)

K. Gress · K. Charipova
Georgetown Medical School, Department of Anesthesiology, Washington, DC, USA
e-mail: klg93@georgetown.edu

M. C. Fuller (✉)
Froedtert Hospital, Medical College of Wisconsin, Milwaukee, WI, USA
e-mail: mfuller@mcw.edu

I. Urits
Beth Israel Deaconess Medical Center Harvard Medical School, Boston, MA, USA

A. D. Kaye
Department of Anesthesiology and Pharmacology, Toxicology, and Neurosciences, Louisiana State University School of Medicine-Shreveport, Shreveport, LA, USA

LSU Health Shreveport School of Medicine, New Orleans, LA, USA

Tulane School of Medicine, New Orleans, LA, USA
e-mail: akaye@lsuhsc.edu

© Springer Nature Switzerland AG 2021
C. S. Scher et al. (eds.), *Essentials of Blood Product Management in Anesthesia Practice*,
https://doi.org/10.1007/978-3-030-59295-0_46

transmission reaching 1, 4.3, and 2.5 infections per 1000 units of blood, respectively [7]. In high-income countries, these rates are approximated to be 1 in 2 million, 1 in 100,000, and 1 in 2.5 million, respectively [7]. Unfortunately, these infection rates likely underestimate true transmission of disease since acquired viruses can be passed on via a wave of secondary infections [1]. As of 2016, antibody to HCV is not part of routine blood screening in many parts of Africa, and only a small proportion of blood banks use enzyme-linked immunosorbent assay (ELISA) kits for HBsAg because testing is not considered cost-effective given the endemic nature of the virus [1]. The delicate interplay between quantity and quality of supply is exemplified by malaria, a leading cause of anemia requiring transfusion in Africa that can also be transmitted by transfusion [1]. Despite the morbidity and mortality associated with malaria, excluding donors with low-grade parasitemia in endemic areas has the potential to significantly reduce supply of available blood [1]. Of note, it is equally important for DGCs to assure quality of blood products by pairing donors and recipients using appropriate blood groupings and crossmatching techniques [5]. Infection by bacterial components secondary to blood bank contamination and breakdown of the cold chain, often due to frequent power cuts during transport, are factors that are frequently overlooked yet have a significant capacity to decrease quality of available supply [1].

Looking Ahead: Solutions and Recommendations

The approaches that are typically used to secure an adequate supply of high-quality blood in high-income countries are not necessarily appropriate, validated, or practical for implementation in DGCs [8]. In DGCs, realistic solutions must encourage reliance on local resources, establish networks for research and education, and promote use of guidelines and audits for gradual improvement of clinical practice [1]. In many countries where inadequate supply and lack of funding are significant obstacles, progress can be made by reorganizing existing systems [4]. First, transfusion medicine should be integrated into the national health-care system [1, 4]. Second, a national blood policy must be created to define the organization(s) responsible for providing blood services, means of funding these services, acceptable forms of donation, and regulations for conducting procurement and transfusion [4]. Unfortunately, in 2016 while nearly all African states had established a national blood policy, more than half were unable to implement their policies [1]. In many cases, inability to carry out a national blood policy stems from a system of organization that relies on the ability of hospitals to run their own blood services without national control or coordination [4]. The International Foundation of Patient Blood Management (PBM) structures the development of a successful PBM program around the idea of "giving the right blood products in the right amount to the right patient at the right time" [9]. It provides formal recommendations for transfusion guidelines, appropriate education and training for clinical staff, and feedback mechanisms for evaluating appropriateness of transfusion [9]. Using this framework, countries like Uganda have been able to develop patient blood management (PBM) programs featuring national oversight committees and standard operating procedures within individual hospitals [9]. Currently, most sub-Saharan African countries, including Uganda, are in the early stages of developing PBM programs [9].

Bolstering Supply

It is important to keep in mind that at present, approximately 80% of the world has access to only 20% of the world's blood products [10]. Unfortunately, the best way to bolster supply is to encourage repeat donation by non-remunerated voluntary donors who, in a study of 2880 units of blood in Egypt, have been demonstrated to have significantly better health profiles than replacement or remunerated donors [11]. While it is difficult to motivate donors, entities like the Federal Ministry of Health in Nigeria have seen success by engaging the media and televising donations by public figures [1]. Nigeria has also implemented strategies such as Club 25 to recognize donors under the age of 25 years, while Zimbabwe created the Pledge 25 Club, a program that uses education incentives to attract students to give blood 25 times [1]. In India, issues in access resulting from a dispersed population were addressed by the institution of a system of "walking blood banks," which consists of a pool of pre-approved, healthy donors who can be recruited by rural hospitals to provide a reliable and timely supply of blood [12, 13]. Educational programs and materials created by the Red Cross and the WHO have proven helpful in dispelling apprehensions and false beliefs about the process of blood donation, especially in rural areas [1, 5]. It is likely that the most effective approaches for recruiting new donors and converting replacement donors to become repeat donors will involve the combined efforts of local and international organizations. Going hand in hand with augmentation of supply is reduction of waste. Some surgical procedures are associated with an inherent risk of blood loss and typically require preemptive crossmatching of blood, but this blood is often wasted at a cost of approximately $40 per unit [14]. Studies out of Britain recommend that crossmatching be performed only if audits suggest that there is a greater than 50% likelihood that the unit will be used. This practice, along with the general practice of auditing usage of blood supply, is likely to promote better stewardship of available products [14].

Decreasing Demand

A significant proportion of the blood requirement in DGCs is dedicated to the treatment of anemia, especially in children. In South Africa, the prevalence of anemia is estimated to be 31% in females and 17% in males [15]. While many of these cases of anemia require treatment, demand can be managed by considering alternative interventions such as use of hematinics for the treatment of nutritional anemia and stimulation of erythropoiesis prior to resorting to transfusion [5, 15]. Similarly, treatment with hydroxyurea can be used to decrease transfusion requirements in sickle cell anemia, and high-hematocrit placental blood can be useful for small-volume emergency transfusion in cases of neonatal anemia [1]. Novel strategies have also been developed to reduce excessive rates of exchange transfusions in infantile hyperbilirubinemia [16, 17]. It is proposed that formally assessing total serum bilirubin and clinical signs of encephalopathy allows for better prediction of kernicterus risk, reducing transfusion requirements and improving overall health outcomes [17]. In cases of trauma associated with significant blood loss, investigations like the Clinical Randomisation of an Antifibrinolytic in Significant Haemorrhage (CRASH-2) study demonstrated that tranexamic acid, an antifibrinolytic, reduces all-cause mortality by 10% when administrated within 3 hours of the initial trauma [1]. Per PBM recommendations, minimizing blood loss through anesthetic and surgical techniques as well as optimizing coagulation status before and during procedures is essential to reducing blood requirements in both emergency and scheduled operations [15]. Educating transfusion prescribers about appropriate protocols and available alternatives such as saline and colloids may also help decrease demand [5]. Given that strict enforcement of a transfusion protocol in a Malawian hospital reduced transfusion numbers by 75%, it is possible that implementation of these innovative interventions in conjunction with strict transfusion guidelines may help significantly decrease demand for blood and blood products in DGCs without negatively impacting mortality [1].

Improving Quality

There are two main strategies for improving quality of available blood and blood products: pre-donation testing and post-donation pathogen reduction. Recommendations for blood product monitoring include testing for direct antiglobulin and screening all donations for HIV, HBV, HCV, and syphilis, as well as regional pathogens such as arboviruses, *Trypanosoma cruzi*, and human T-lymphotropic virus [1, 5, 18]. Unfortunately, the specificity, sensitivity, ease of use, and costs associated with anti-HIV, anti-HCV, and HBsAg testing vary [1]. For instance, widespread use of nucleic acid testing (NAT) is limited in most DGCs by cost [1, 11]. Fortunately, more cost-effective substitutes for NAT such as the use of two anti-HIV ELISA tests performed in parallel are being investigated [1]. Similarly, there are data out of Egypt suggesting that core antigen testing is more effective than RNA testing for determining the presence of HCV without sacrificing specificity [18]. Rapid immunochemical tests, such as that developed for the HIV antibody, are under development for other infectious agents [1]. The development of these tests has the potential to cut costs by decreasing the need for highly skilled staff and advanced processing equipment [1]. Alternatively, researchers are considering the option of prophylactically treating recipients of red blood cells (RBCs) in endemic regions with antimalarial agents instead of excluding donors with low-grade parasitemia [1]. Pathogen reduction refers to a series of interventions that involve using heat or alcohol fractionation to eliminate viral components from plasma products. Pathogen reduction is promising but cannot be used for whole blood or packed RBCs and is associated with logistic concerns such as cost and requirements for complex equipment and skilled personnel [19]. It is important to note that as long as the prevalence of these viruses remains high, residual risk of transmission will not decrease even in the setting of adequate testing given the existence of the window period [1]. Thus, while it is important to channel efforts into developing adequate screening protocols, it is equally if not more vital to address availability of antiretroviral therapy.

References

1. Roberts DJ, Field S, Delaney M, Bates I. Problems and approaches for blood transfusion in the developing countries. Hematol Oncol Clin N Am. 2016;30:477–95.
2. Oladapo O, Adetoro O, Ekele B, Chama C, Etuk S, Aboyeji A, et al. When getting there is not enough: a nationwide cross-sectional study of 998 maternal deaths and 1451 near-misses in public tertiary hospitals in a low-income country. BJOG. 2016;124(6):928–38.
3. WHO. Model list of essential medicines. 21st ed. 2019.
4. Koistlnen J. Organization of blood transfusion services in developing countries. Vox Sang. 1994;67:247–9.
5. Gibbs WN, Corcoran P. Blood safety in developing countries. Vox Sang. 1994;67:377–81.
6. Abdel Jalil AA, Katzka DA, Castella DO. Approach to the patient with dysphagia. Am J Med. 2015;18(10):1138–42.
7. Jayaraman S, Chalabi Z, Perel P, Guerriero C, Roberts I. The risk of transfusion-transmitted infections in sub-Saharan Africa. Transfusion. 2010;50(2):433–42.
8. Custer B, Zou S, Glynn SA, Makani J, Tayou Tagny C, El Ekiaby M, et al. Addressing gaps in international blood availability and transfusion safety in low- and middle-income countries: a NHLBI workshop. Transfusion. NLM (Medline). 2018;58:1307–17.
9. Eichbaum Q, Murphy M, Liu Y, Kajja I, Hajjar LA, Sibinga CTS, et al. Patient blood management: an international perspective. Anesth Analg. 2016;123(6):1574–81.

10. Gani F, Cerullo M, Ejaz A, Gupta PB, Demario VM, Johnston FM, et al. Implementation of a blood management program at a tertiary care hospital. Ann Surg. 2019;269(6):1073–9.
11. Abdelrazik AM, Ezzat Ahmed GM. Priority needs and wisdom strategy for blood transfusion safety in developing low-resource countries. Transfus Apher Sci. 2016;54(1):147–9.
12. Sood R, Raykar N, Till B, Shah H, Roy N. Walking Blood Banks: An immediate solution to rural India's blood drought. Indian J Med Ethics. 2018;III(2):134–7.
13. Selvakumar S, Shahabudeen P, Paul RT. An analysis of re-configured blood transfusion network of urban India to improve the service level: a simulation approach. J Med Syst. 2019;43(2):28.
14. Faridi S, Ahmad A, Beg MA, Siddiqui F, Edhi MM, Khan M. Arranging blood for elective thyroid surgeries: dilemma continues in the developing world. BMC Res Notes. 2017;10(1):1–2.
15. Althoff FC, Neb H, Herrmann E, Trentino KM, Vernich L, Füllenbach C, et al. Multimodal patient blood management program based on a three-pillar strategy. Ann Surg. 2019;269(5):794–804.
16. Chhapola V, Sharma AG, Kanwal SK, Kumar V, Patra B. Neonatal exchange transfusions at a tertiary care centre in North India: an investigation of historical trends using change-point analysis and statistical process control. Int Health. 2018;10(6):451–6.
17. Olusanya BO, Iskander IF, Slusher TM, Wennberg RP. A decision-making tool for exchange transfusions in infants with severe hyperbilirubinemia in resource-limited settings. J Perinatol. 2016;36(5):338–41.
18. Abdelrazik AM, Abozaid HE, Montasser KA. Role of Hepatitis C Virus (HCV) core antigen in improving blood transfusion safety in high prevalence, resource limited countries, a step forward. Transfus Apher Sci. 2018;57(4):566–8.
19. Ware AD, Jacquot C, Tobian AAR, Gehrie EA, Ness PM, Bloch EM. Pathogen reduction and blood transfusion safety in Africa: strengths, limitations and challenges of implementation in low-resource settings. Vox Sang. 2018;113(1):3–12.

47 Considerations and Guidelines for Use of Anticoagulants and Antithrombotics in Patients Undergoing Interventional Pain Management

Jordan S. Renschler, Amanda L. Granier, George M. Jeha, John E. Scheinuk, Matthew E. Nungesser, Joshua M. Etienne, Abigail P. Erwin, Chrissy Cherenfant, Uchenna Umeh, Michael P. K. Webb, Erik M. Helander, and Alan David Kaye

Introduction

Chronic pain is increasingly treated via interventional pain management. This is an emerging specialty involving procedures used to both diagnose and to treat patients. In most interventional pain management cases, the procedures are performed percutaneously. Additionally, regional anesthesia and perioperative analgesia are percutaneously administered, all of which carry risks germane to bleeding [1]. Patients themselves may also have genetic risks of bleeding, and both inherent and the iatrogenic anticoagulated merit additional consideration for interventional techniques.

Procedures involving interventional pain management and regional anesthesia all can be significantly complicated by altered hemostasis. To address the risk of bleeding and hematomas following regional and neuraxial techniques, the American Society of Regional Anesthesia published guidelines, with the most recently updated guidelines from 2018 [2]. Importantly, several studies have offered conflicting recommendations that the guidelines seek to reconcile, especially in the setting of increasingly potent antithrombotic medications.

Interventional pain management is outpatient-oriented with a greater overall variety of procedures [3]. Although the ASRA guidelines address numerous important risks, they were not intended for interventional pain practitioners. In response, a summary of the literature and bleeding risk stratification was developed and updated for interventional pain physicians [1]. As in all procedures, the procedure's therapeutic benefit must outweigh the risk involved when assessing for the risk of bleeding in patients. Ultimately, the practitioner must make an informed decision about whether to continue the procedure after evaluating and analyzing the risks and benefits involved. To do so, the practitioner must understand coagulation physiology, pathophysiological mechanisms of bleeding disorders, anticoagulation pharmacology, and the technical risks associated with individual procedures.

J. S. Renschler · A. L. Granier · G. M. Jeha · J. E. Scheinuk
M. E. Nungesser · J. M. Etienne · A. P. Erwin · E. M. Helander
Department of Anesthesiology, LSUHSC New Orleans, New Orleans, LA, USA
e-mail: jrensc@lsuhsc.edu; gjeha@lsuhsc.edu; mnunge@lsuhsc.edu; ehelan@lsuhsc.edu

C. Cherenfant
NYU Langone Health, NYU Langone Orthopedic Hospital, Department of Anesthesiology, Perioperative Medicine, and Pain Medicine, New York, NY, USA

U. Umeh
NYU Langone Orthopedic, Department of Anesthesiology, Perioperative Care and Pain Medicine, New York, NY, USA
e-mail: Uchenna.umeh@nyulangone.org

M. P. K. Webb
Middlemore Hospital, Department of Anaesthesia and Pain Medicine, Auckland, New Zealand

A. D. Kaye (✉)
Department of Anesthesiology and Pharmacology, Toxicology, and Neurosciences, Louisiana State University School of Medicine-Shreveport, Shreveport, LA, USA

LSU Health Shreveport School of Medicine, New Orleans, LA, USA

Tulane School of Medicine, New Orleans, LA, USA
e-mail: akaye@lsuhsc.edu

© Springer Nature Switzerland AG 2021
A. D. Kaye, S. Leavitt (eds.), *Essentials of Blood Product Management in Anesthesia Practice*,
https://doi.org/10.1007/978-3-030-59295-0_47

Coagulation Physiology

Normally, a balance exists between hemostasis and bleeding, maintaining an equilibrium. To keep this equilibrium, there are complex interactions between activators, cofactors, and inhibitors. Three processes essentially comprise the overall process of hemostasis: (1) primary hemostasis, (2) secondary hemostasis, and (3) fibrinolysis.

Primary hemostasis results in a weak platelet plug, making platelets crucial to this step [4]. Needle trauma to the vascular endothelium induces the creation of a friable platelet plug to arrest bleeding. When the underlying extracellular matrix is exposed during endothelial injury, platelets change in a series of phases: adhesion, activation, and aggregation. This process resulting in platelet deposition is known as primary hemostasis.

Platelets are derived from fragments of bone marrow megakaryocytes and are surrounded by a coat of glycoproteins critical to the process of adhesion to the vascular endothelium. Upon endothelial injury, a subendothelial protein called von Willebrand factor (vWF) is exposed. Platelets express a glycoprotein Ib receptor that binds to the exposed vWF, which facilitates platelet adhesion to damaged endothelium. After glycoprotein Ib binds to vWF, the platelet activates, degranulating and changing shape. Upon activation, platelets express glycoprotein IIb/IIIa receptors, which initiate the platelet aggregation phase. Fibrinogen binds the glycoprotein IIb/IIIa receptors on the platelet surface, allowing other platelets to aggregate and form bridges between IIb/IIIa receptors via fibrinogen. This process is under tight regulation, with the surrounding intact endothelium, local anticoagulants, and humoral inhibiting factors preventing inappropriate platelet adhesion outside the area of vascular injury.

The coagulation cascade is the driving mechanism behind secondary hemostasis, which follows primary hemostasis to stabilize the weak platelet plug formed during primary hemostasis [4]. Inactive clotting factors constantly circulate until activation through exposure to tissue factor or damaged endothelium. All clotting factors are synthesized in the liver in zymogen form, except for von Willebrand factor (formed from platelet alpha granules and endothelial cells) and factor VIII (formed in endothelial cells). Activation of clotting factors involves proteolysis into the active enzyme. Cleavage of clotting factors occurs in a stepwise fashion with each clotting factor resulting in the cleavage and activation of a subsequent clotting factor. The final step is the activation of fibrinogen to fibrin by thrombin. Fibrin is water-insoluble, while fibrinogen is soluble before activation. Fibrin is the predominant factor that results in stabilization of the platelet plug formed in primary hemostasis. Cross-linking of fibrin then strengthens the already stabilized platelet plug, forming a clot.

Multiple theories exist about the precise mechanisms of secondary hemostasis. The leading theory for much of the time is founded on an intrinsic and an extrinsic coagulation pathway. More recent research suggests an alternate mechanism, that of a "cell-based" pathway.

The extrinsic and intrinsic pathways of secondary hemostasis merge into a common pathway leading to a stable hemostatic plug. The extrinsic pathway is activated only in the presence of endothelial trauma, exposing tissue factor. The exposure of tissue factor leads to factor VII activation to factor VIIa, initiating the clotting cascade pathway [5]. The intrinsic pathway does not require additional activation components, ki activating only with intrinsic components of blood upon contact with artificial surfaces [5]. Both intrinsic and extrinsic pathways lead to the common pathway with the activation of factor X to factor Xa with cofactor Va. Factor Xa then cleaves factor II (prothrombin) to factor IIa (thrombin), which cleaves factor I (fibrinogen) to factor Ia (fibrin).

The cell-based theory of coagulation espouses three distinct phases in clot formation: initiation, amplification, and the propagation phase. The central entity (i.e., the cell) in this pathway is the platelet, and it is thought to provide a substrate to and physical locale for the reaction. Tissue factor (TF) is the other key constituent. In initiation, TF-laden cells complex with factor VII and activate it. This complex then activates factors X and IX, which in turn activates factors V and II. In normal circulation this small amount of IIa is kept quiescent by local and humoral inhibitors, but in altered circulation, an amplification phase occurs. Platelets activated in primary hemostasis have an enlarged, procoagulant surface, and the small amount of thrombin (IIa) in turn activates IXa. IX and VIIIa form a stable complex. In the propagation phase, this IX + VIII complex readily activates X to Xa and is called the "Xase." The stable "Xase" then hydrolyzes multiple profactors into their active forms, primarily creating more Va and IIa. This is known as the thrombin burst [6].

Coagulation is under strict regulation as to only occur in areas of injury to prevent bleeding; dysregulation would have severe consequences manifest as arterial and venous thrombotic events. Three inhibitory pathways preside over-regulation: (1) antithrombin III, (2) thrombomodulin, and (3) tissue factor inhibitor. Antithrombin III inhibits factors IIa, IXa, XIa, and especially Xa. Thrombomodulin activates anticoagulant proteins C and S by binding thrombin, leading to proteolysis of factors Va and VIIIa. Tissue factor pathway inhibitor utilizes a negative feedback loop to prevent factor X activation. The fibrinolytic system also regulates coagulation through plasmin, the activated form of plasminogen. Plasminogen is cleaved to activated plasmin by tissue-type plasminogen activator (TPA). Plasmin is a proteolytic enzyme capable of degrading fibrin, fibrinogen, factor V, factor VIII, prothrombin, and factor XII.

Because TPA binds the clot to activate plasminogen, proteolysis is limited to a localized clot.

Coagulation Pathophysiology

Pathological disturbance of the coagulation cascade manifests as either a hemorrhagic or thrombotic disorder. Hemorrhagic disorders can be either acquired or inherited conditions. The three most common inherited disorders of hemostasis are von Willebrand disease, hemophilia A, and hemophilia B [7, 8].

von Willebrand disease affects approximately 1 in 1000 people, making it the most prevalent inherited bleeding disorder [8]. It is caused by either a quantitative or qualitative defect in von Willebrand factor (vWF) [7]. As mentioned above, vWF functions in primary hemostasis by binding subendothelial components and circulating platelets, causing platelet adhesion by forming a bridge between the platelet and subendothelial tissue. Additionally, vWF has a role in stabilizing factor VIII by acting as a carrier protein for factor VIII and increasing the half-life of factor VIII. In patients with von Willebrand disease, both of these functions of von Willebrand factor are impaired; platelet adhesion is degraded, and factor VIII levels are reduced. Hereditary von Willebrand disease is passed as an autosomal dominant disorder. Primary symptoms include bruising and mucosal bleeding, especially epistaxis and menorrhagia. In surgical procedures, prolonged oozing at the surgical site may also manifest. Bleeding time is not useful in diagnosing von Willebrand disease; instead, evaluation of closure time by platelet function analyzer (PFA-100) has better diagnostic value [7]. Treatment includes desmopressin and factor VIII replacement. Clarifying the specific type of vWD is important before treatment as "gain of function" mutations exist, whereby pharmacological treatment can result in disastrous thrombotic complications.

Hemophilia A is a bleeding disorder that results from a defect in factor VIII, preventing activation of factor X, therefore, interrupting the intrinsic coagulation cascade. The disease is X-linked and therefore primarily affects males. Plasma concentrations of vWF are unchanged in hemophilia A, but the risks associated with hemophilia A are high. Bleeding events can be life-threatening, particularly intracranial bleeding, which is associated with a 30% mortality rate. The activated partial thromboplastin time (aPTT), a measure of the intrinsic coagulation cascade, will be prolonged to diagnose hemophilia A. The prothrombin time as well as bleeding time will remain normal in hemophilia A. The severity of the disease depends on the plasma concentration of factor VIII; thus factor replacement is an essential component of therapy for hemophilia A [8]. While factor VIII replacement is an option, a more universal treatment in the setting of surgical or traumatic bleeding is recombinant activated factor VII, which is thought to ensure hemostasis by interacting with tissue factor and the platelet surface [8]. Hemophilia B is clinically indistinguishable from hemophilia A, but the deficiency is in factor IX. Treatment is similar to hemophilia A, except recombinant or plasma-derived factor IX is replaced, rather than factor VIII.

Vitamin K is crucial to the function of several coagulation factors; thus, a vitamin K deficiency can cause a defect of coagulation. Vitamin K deficiency can be caused by malnutrition, fat malabsorption, antibiotic use, and liver disease [4]. The liver enzyme microsomal carboxylase is necessary to convert factors II, VII, IX, and X into their gamma-carboxylated, active forms. Microsomal carboxylase is dependent on vitamin K; thus a vitamin K deficiency reduces functionality of all four coagulation factors. Vitamin K-deficient patients may develop melena, hematuria, ecchymosis, and hematomas as a result of the impaired coagulation [4]. In anticipation of a procedure, vitamin K can be supplemented to prevent bleeding complications.

Normal liver function is crucial to production of circulating coagulation factors. Grossly impaired hepatic synthetic function may impair coagulation in multiple ways. Liver dysfunction deranged hemostasis can occur via thrombocytopenia, platelet dysfunction, reduced production of clotting factors, increased clotting factor consumption, and increased fibrinolysis. Hemostatic dysfunction increases sequentially with the stage of liver disease, but at all stages, a risk of bleeding exists [8]. Screening for liver disease before a procedure may reduce the risks of unexpected bleeding events. By analyzing hemoglobin, PT, aPTT, platelet count, platelet function analysis, fibrinogen level, and bilirubin levels risk stratification can be performed. In patients identified with liver disease at risk of a bleeding complication, therapies include vitamin K supplementation, fresh frozen plasma, platelets, and cryoprecipitate. In patients with biliary tract disorders, vitamin K supplementation alone may suffice [9].

Impaired renal function may also lead to defective hemostasis [10]. Renal impairment may lead to qualitative defects in platelets, subendothelial metabolism, and platelet-vessel interactions. The effects of antiplatelet drugs and low molecular weight heparins are also enhanced by impaired renal function, primarily via reduced excretion of the drugs. In a renal failure patient, a complete coagulation study is critical to patient safety. Bleeding time may indicate platelet dysfunction due to renal disease, while elevated PT or aPTT may be indicative of coagulation factor deficiency. To restore homeostatic coagulation treatment of renally impaired patients may include dialysis, anemia correction, desmopressin, cryoprecipitate, estrogens, and avoiding antiplatelet drugs [10].

Hemostasis Pharmacology: Clinical Relevance to the Interventionalist

COX Inhibitors

Direct cyclooxygenase (COX) inhibitors work by directly inhibiting the COX-2 and/or COX-1 prostaglandin pathway, which results in numerous physiological changes ranging from deficits in homeostasis of coagulation to decreased bodily inflammatory responses [11]. Administration of nonspecific COX inhibitors results in reduced levels of thromboxane A2. This substance triggers platelet aggregation, vasospasm, and eventually serotonin release from the platelets themselves [12]. Aspirin is a COX-inhibiting drug that disrupts thromboxane A2 by irreversibly inhibiting the COX-1 pathway via enzyme acetylation. Related to this mechanism of action, it has been shown to be beneficial in decreasing thrombus formation and clotting by boosting the prostacyclin/thromboxane A2 ratio, which leads to reduced platelet aggregation [13]. This decrease in clot formation also puts patients at a theoretical risk for increased bleeding; however, this eventuality is uncommon. Aspirin at low doses can trigger an antiplatelet effect that lasts 7–10 days until the bone marrow can replace the current platelets [14]. In high doses ASA inhibits prostacyclin (PGI2) through COX-2, which can counteract the antiplatelet mechanism. NSAIDs also work in decreasing prostaglandin production to limit the inflammatory response that results in analgesic effects [15].

Warfarin

Vitamin K is needed for synthesis of the G1a protein family that includes four coagulation factors (II, VII, IX, X) needed for blood clotting in a normal individual [16]. These coagulation factors are important for homeostasis, and a deficiency can lead to life-threatening bleeding. Warfarin directly inhibits the gamma-carboxylation of glutamate residues in prothrombin and factors VII, IX, and X, preventing the vitamin K epoxide from adopting its active form. This inhibition is not immediate, but rather only becoming apparent when such time has passed that the active factors have been consumed or reabsorbed. The net effect on homeostasis caused by warfarin is reliant on the half-life of each coagulation factor it impacts, which ranges from 6–8 hours (VII) to 50+ hours (II) [17]. Warfarin, therefore, produces its maximal anticoagulant effect 3–5 days after administration. Paradoxically, owing to inhibition of proteins C and S, warfarin has a short procoagulant effect after initiation. Warfarin's efficacy is extremely dependent on the individual (age, gender, medical conditions, genetics, diet), and initiation of therapy requires close monitoring [18]. Warfarin effect is monitored by prothrombin time (PT) and international normalized ration (INR). PT measures the extrinsic and common pathways of coagulation to determine the amount of time a patient's plasma takes to clot via fibrinogen and factors V, VII, and X. INR helps to monitor PT and relate it to other patient labs to better control the dosage of anticoagulants [19].

Glycoprotein Receptor Antagonists

The platelet aggregation pathway has a final common receptor known as the glycoprotein IIb/IIIa receptor, which, if blocked or inhibited, will cause reversible blocking of aggregation [20]. This mechanism still allows for the early stages of the coagulation pathway and initial binding of platelets to damaged vascular surfaces to occur [21]. Inhibitors of the GPIIb/IIIa receptor include abciximab (ReoPro), eptifibatide (Integrilin), and tirofiban hydrochloride (Aggrastat). Abciximab is the Fab fragment of a humanized monoclonal antibody that works as an antagonist to the Glycoprotein IIb (GPIIb) receptor. It can inhibit close to 80% of platelet aggregation when administered intravenously. Eptifibatide blocks the fibrinogen binding site on GPIIb, causing a 50–80% drop in platelet aggregation. Tirofiban is a nonpeptide tyrosine derivative designed to mimic the natural ligand of the IIB/IIIa receptor [21].

Thienopyridine Inhibitors

These inhibitors work primarily by binding to P2Y12 receptor, which irreversibly modifies and significantly inhibits ADP-dependent platelet aggregation after 2 hours of administration with peak effect at 6 hours [22]. Platelets treated with this class are affected for their life (7–10 days); however, only 60–70% of the ADP receptors have been shown to be sensitive to thienopyridines. Due to their consideration as selective platelet-receptor inhibitors, thienopyridine inhibitors are considered relatively safe antiplatelet drugs. Drugs included in this category are clopidogrel (Plavix), prasugrel (Effient), and ticlopidine (Ticlid). Clopidogrel is used for the prevention of ischemic stroke, myocardial infarction, and vascular death in patients with a history of atherosclerosis or vascular disease [6].

Heparin

Heparin is one of the oldest biological medications used for the prevention and/or treatment of thrombosis [23]. Heparins work by increasing antithrombin III activity to inhibit clot-

Table 47.1 Comparison of commonly used anticoagulants

Drug class	Drugs	MOA	Effect	Monitored	Adverse effects
COX inhibitors (COX-1 and COX-2)	**NSAIDs** **Aspirin**	Block cyclooxygenase-1 and -2	Inhibit TXA2 (blood thinner) and inflammation (prostaglandins)		Increased bleeding (COX-1) Inhibited immune and inflammation response (COX-2)
Warfarin		Inhibits gamma-carboxylation of prothrombin, factors VII, IX, and X	Decreased coagulation	Prothrombin time (PT) + international normalized ratio (INR)	Increased probability of bleeding and/or hemorrhage Bruising Nausea and vomiting
Glycoprotein receptor antagonists	**Abciximab** (ReoPro) **Eptifibatide** (Integrilin) **Tirofiban Hydrochloride** (Aggrastat)	Antagonist to glycoprotein IIb receptor	Decreased platelet aggregation		Increased bleeding Thrombocytopenia
Thienopyridine inhibitors	**Clopidogrel** (Plavix) **Prasugrel** (Effient) **Ticlopidine** (Ticlid)	Binds P2Y12 leading to decreased ADP-dependent platelet aggregation	Decreased clotting ability		Increased bleeding Nausea and vomiting Thrombotic thrombocytopenic purpura
Heparin	**HMWH**	Increasing antithrombin III activity	Leads to inhibition of thrombin, IXa, and Xa, which decreases clotting	Partial thromboplastin time (PTT)	Increased bleeding Heparin-induced thrombocytopenia (HIT) Osteoporosis Injection site reactions
LWMH		Binding antithrombin	Increases inhibition of thrombin and factor Xa, leading to decreased clotting	Partial thromboplastin time (PTT)	Increased bleeding Injection site reactions HIT (less commonly than unfractionated heparin)

ting factors thrombin, IXa, and Xa. This activity is increased due to the conformational change that ATIII undergoes to reveal its active site. High molecular weight heparin (HMWH) is known for its higher molecular weight ranging anywhere from 5000 to 40,000 Da, making it unable to be absorbed from the GI tract. It is administered intravenously or subcutaneously and has limited utility in the outpatient setting due to its short 1-hour half-life. Heparin is commonly used in inpatient settings to prevent venous thrombosis. Heparin effectiveness is measured by partial thromboplastin time (PTT); however, close monitoring of heparin therapy is not required, unlike warfarin therapy.

Low Molecular Weight Heparin

Low molecular weight heparins (LMWH) are fractionated like their HMWH counterparts, but this process limits them to lower molecular weights (most molecules under 8000 Da). LMWH works by binding to antithrombin, causing a conformational change and increasing the propensity for inhibition of thrombin and factor Xa [24]. Compared to the high molecular weight fractions, LMWH have a higher bioavailability, longer half-life, and potential for once-daily dosing. The drug is given primarily subcutaneously [23] (Table 47.1).

Direct Thrombin Inhibitors

While heparins and vitamin K antagonists are the most commonly used agents in anticoagulation, direct thrombin inhibitors (DTIs) also play an expanding and key role in anticoagulation. DTIs work by inactivating free thrombin and thrombin already bound to fibrin. This inactivation is caused by binding the active site and/or the exosites of thrombin. The role of DTIs in the management of acute coronary syndromes was reviewed by the Direct Thrombin Inhibitor Trialists' Collaborative Group in a meta-analysis of data on individual patients. As compared with heparin, DTIs reduced the incidence of the composite outcome of death and myocardial infarction both at the end of treatment and at 30 days [25].

DTIs can be univalent or bivalent inhibitors. Univalent inhibitors, such as argatroban and dabigatran, work by binding to the active sites of thrombin. Bivalent inhibitors, such as hirudin derivatives desirudin, lepirudin, and bivalirudin, work by binding to the active site on thrombin with one of its exosites.

Argatroban reversibly binds to the active site on thrombin and inhibits thrombin's ability to activate several clotting factors. Importantly, argatroban has played a major role in heparin-induced thrombocytopenia (HIT), being used as an alternate form of anticoagulation when heparins are contraindicated. This can include systemic anticoagulation for cardiac bypass circuit initiation. Argatroban anticoagulation, compared with historical control subjects, improves clinical outcomes in patients who have HIT, without increasing bleeding risk [26]. Dabigatran is the other univalent DTI that is being used as a substitute for warfarin in acute venous thromboembolism and prevention of stroke in patients with atrial fibrillation. As with all anticoagulation, there is an increased risk of bleeding. Dabigatran's utility for atrial fibrillation had been questioned on these grounds, particularly before the advent of a widely available reversal agent (idarucizumab). Dabigatran administered at a dose of 150 mg, as compared with warfarin, was associated with lower rates of stroke and systemic embolism but similar rates of major hemorrhage [27]. Recombinant hirudin derivatives such as desirudin, lepirudin, and bivalirudin are all alternatives for heparin. Compared with historical controls, lepirudin treatment of HIT complicated by thrombosis was associated with reduced thrombotic events (relative risk reduction [RRR], 0.63–0.78) [28] (Table 47.2).

Factor Xa Inhibitors

Direct factor Xa drugs are a modern class of drugs that inhibit the clotting cascade. They have become popular in the treatment of patients with pulmonary embolism, deep vein thrombosis, and embolic stroke from atrial fibrillation. These drugs are used in clinical care because they can be administered in fixed doses without routine coagulation monitoring. Factor Xa inhibitor therapy is well tolerated, and the most common adverse event reported with the agents is bleeding. Factor Xa inhibitors have black box warnings for increased risk of stroke upon discontinuance of therapy and increased risk for developing epidural or spinal hematomas. There is no specific reversal agent for the factor Xa inhibitors, but a new drug, andexanet, is promising. Andexanet is biologically recombinant factor Xa, which acts as a decoy receptor, and reversed the anticoagulant activity of apixaban and rivaroxaban in older healthy participants within minutes after administration and for the duration of infusion, without evidence of clinical toxic effects [29].

Bleeding Complications and Risks in Regional Anesthesia

Neuraxial procedures carry risks that are rare but can be potentially devastating for patients, and bleeding complications are of particular concern [30]. This is especially true for patients who present with bleeding disorders and/or those taking antithrombic medication as this can increase the potential risk of bleeding. Physicians must weigh the risks and benefits for this subset of patients before the start of a procedure to reduce the chance of morbidity and mortality.

Some neuraxial procedure risk factors involve location of the target structure, size of needle, and the number of needle insertion attempts. A traumatic needle insertion can have minor consequences, such as post-dural puncture headache, or major consequences, such as spinal hematoma [31]. A traumatic needle insertion increases the likelihood of spinal hematoma by 11-fold [32]. The risk of needle insertion complications is influenced by age, gender, BMI, and spinal cord defects. For instance, patients without a spinal deformity have a 2.6 greater chance of first-pass success than those with spinal deformities [33]. Preoperative assessment of a patient's risk associated with a successful needle insertion can aid in reducing complications associated with multiple needle insertion attempts.

Spinal hematomas can result in permanent loss of neurologic function, and the incidence of hematomas is significantly greater for those on anticoagulant medications. For patients on anticoagulants, the approximated frequency of epidural hematoma is 33 in 100,000 patients for epidural anesthetics and 1 in 100,000 patients for spinal anesthetics. This is greater than the estimated number of 1 in 150,000 and 1 in 220,000 patients not on anticoagulation for epidural and spinal anesthetics, respectively [34].

Table 47.2 Direct thrombin inhibitors

Parameter	Lepirudin	Argatroban	Dabigatran
Class	Bivalent	Univalent	Univalent
Indication	Anticoagulation in HIT	Anticoagulation in HIT	Stroke prevention
Administration	Parenteral	Parenteral	Oral
Time to peak concentration	2.0 to 3.0 hours	2.0 to 4.0 hours	1.5 to 2 hours
Clearance	Kidneys	Liver	Kidneys

Anticoagulation medication such as heparin and warfarin must be timed appropriately for the administration of neuraxial anesthesia and removal of an epidural catheter. Analysis of drug-related factors in the development of spinal hematomas in neuraxial procedures showed that out of the 160 reported cases of spinal hematomas, 31% of the cases involved use of low molecular weight heparin, 24% involved unfractionated heparin, and 11% of the cases involved warfarin [35]. The FDA also highlighted 30 reports of patients who were on low molecular weight heparin and developed epidural or spinal hematomas [36]. There have been two cases reported through MedWatch system since 1998 that involved preoperative warfarin and the development of spinal hematomas when preforming a neuraxial block [37].

Physicians should also be aware of the increased risk of bleeding during neuraxial procedures in patients with medical disease. Hepatic failure may cause thrombocytopenia and other alterations in normal coagulation physiology [38]. In a report of 166 cases of spinal hematomas, 4 cases were associated with liver disease, and 10 cases were associated with renal insufficiency [35].

Antithrombic medications work to decrease thrombosis by interfering with the blood coagulation cascade. This results in increased bleeding, and as such, physicians may discontinue the use of this medication to decrease the risk of bleeding before performing pain management procedures. However, physicians must consider potential thrombosis complications posed by the removal of antithrombic medications, particularly for those with a history of coronary artery disease or cerebrovascular disease [35]. An online survey of interventional pain physicians reported withdrawal of antithrombic medication before pain management techniques in a substantial number of cases. According to the survey, "97% discontinued clopidogrel; 96% ticlopidine; 95% Aggrastat (tirofiban); 93% cilostazol, 85% dipyridamole, 60% aspirin 350 mg; 39% aspirin 81 mg; and 39% other non-steroidal anti-inflammatory drugs (NSAIDs) before performing interventional pain management techniques." An assessment performed indicated that complications due to thrombosis formation were more severe and three times more likely to occur than bleeding complications during pain management procedures [1]. This information should give practitioners pause for thought and the merits of ceasing medically indicated anticoagulation be carefully weighed. Knowing the reason why patients are on anticoagulants can help facilitate safe practices, and it may also be prudent to consult with the patient's prescribing physician regarding discontinuation of their anticoagulants.

Physicians must consider the risks associated with altering antithrombotic medication before, during, and after pain management procedures to ensure patient safety. For instance, NSAIDs, including aspirin, do not appear to pose risk of spinal hematomas during neuraxial procedures [32, 39]. Hence, discontinuing the use of low-dose aspirin may increase risk of thrombosis while having no impact on risk of bleeding. This is true only when aspirin is taken alone; aspirin taken with other antithrombic medications, SSRIs, and/or supplement such as fish oil increases the risk of hematomas [30]. For example, aspirin combined with the anticoagulation medication heparin increases risk of development of spinal hematoma during neuraxial procedures by a magnitude of 26 [32].

Recommendations and Safety

In patients undergoing interventional techniques, the management of antithrombotic therapy requires consideration of several factors, primarily the balance between the bleeding risk associated with continuation of antithrombotic therapy, the medical indication for anticoagulation, and the thromboembolic risk associated with its discontinuation or interruption [40–42]. While interruption is often required to minimize risk of bleeding after surgery, discontinuation, continuation, and recommencing of anti-clotting therapy in the perioperative setting come with associated risks [40–42]. In clinical practice, patients receiving antithrombotic therapy are routinely discontinued on their medication before undergoing interventional techniques despite a paucity of evidence of significant bleeding risk during these procedures and limited evidence to guide clinical practice [40, 43–46]. In fact, there is considerable risk with the traditional attitude of discontinuing medication 10 days before intervention and the indiscriminate use of bridging therapy [40, 46]. When managing anti-clotting medication in these patients, recent studies suggest that it is beneficial to stratify the anticipated surgical intervention into a low-risk (<4% per annum), moderate-risk (4–10%), and high-risk (>10%) category and adjust according to patient-specific risk factors [40, 46]. Additional considerations should include assessment for the need of bridging therapy, patient co morbidities, and the individual properties of the specific anti-clotting agent being utilized [41, 46, 47].

Estimation of Thromboembolic Risk

The three most common indications for anticoagulation therapy are atrial fibrillation, recent history of thromboembolism, and presence of prosthetic heart valves [41, 46–49]. The CHA2DS2-VASc score, a risk-stratification system used to predict future risk of stroke and thromboembolism in patients with nonvalvular atrial fibrillation (although not prospectively validated in the perioperative setting), may be useful in estimating relative thromboembolic risk in patients undergoing surgical procedures and assessing the need for bridging therapy. The CHA2DS2-VASc score calculator gives 1 point each for the presence of congestive heart failure, hypertension therapy, age 65–74 years, history of diabetes, history of vascular disease, and female sex. Two points are given for age greater or equal to 75 years and/or prior history of stroke, transient ischemic attack, or venous thromboembolism. Zero points are given for age less than 65 years and male sex. A score of 0–2 is considered low risk for thromboembolism; a score of 3–4 is considered intermediate risk; and a score of >4 is considered high risk [46, 47, 50]. With respect to thromboembolism, those in the first 6 months following an event are at the highest risk. Prosthetic heart valves are a non-native tissue within the body that may be non- or incompletely epithelialized. Replacement mitral valves and those of older generations (cage and ball/tilting disc) are the highest risk for an embolic phenomenon. Modern bi-leaflet prostheses at the aortic position confer moderate or even low risk dependent upon patient factors.

Risk Stratification for Severe Bleeding

Several factors influence the potential for severe bleeding complications, including the type of surgical/interventional technique performed, the anatomy of the region of interest, and individual factors such as patient age and obesity [40, 47]. There is good evidence for stratifying interventions into low risk for severe bleeding, intermediate risk for severe bleeding, and high risk for severe bleeding. This often relates to the compressibility of and access to the site to be operated upon. If performing a low-risk or intermediate-risk procedure on a patient with a high risk of bleeding, these patients should be regarded as intermediate-risk or high-risk, respectively. Examples of conditions that confer a high risk of bleeding include advanced age, history of bleeding tendency, concurrent treatment with other anticoagulant or antiplatelet agents, presence of advanced liver disease or cirrhosis, and presence of renal disease [40, 47]. Recommendations regarding when to discontinue antithrombotic and anticoagulant usage preoperatively and when to resume therapy post-operatively are influenced by the category of risk assigned to the intervention and patient and the type of anticoagulant used. In this regard, additionally it should be noted that many herbals and over-the-counter medications can interfere with the coagulation cascade and have additive and/or synergistic effects. Some of these agents have relatively short half-lives, and their effects last only a few days; however, the American Society of Anesthesiology recommends 2–3 weeks off these agents to ensure that there are not any significant effects since many of these products' half-lives are unknown and preparations vary considerably.

The risk stratification of several spinal procedures based on the potential risk for bleeding is outlined below [40]:

Low-risk procedures:

- Trigger point and muscular injections
- Peripheral joints
- Peripheral nerve blocks
- Sacroiliac joint and ligament injections and nerve blocks
- Caudal epidural injections
- Ganglion impar blocks

Intermediate-risk procedures:

- Facet joint interventions
- Lumbar transforaminal epidural injections at L4, L5, or S1
- Lumbar intradiscal procedures
- Hypogastric plexus blocks
- Lumbar sympathetic blocks
- Peripheral nerve stimulation trial and implant
- Pocket revision and implantable pulse regenerator/intrathecal pump replacement
- Caudal percutaneous adhesiolysis
- Lumbar percutaneous disc compression below L4
- Intervertebral spinous prosthesis
- Lumbar discography
- Lumbar interlaminar epidural injections at L5–S1

High-risk procedures:

- Cervical, thoracic, and high lumbar (above L4–L5) interlaminar epidurals
- Cervical, thoracic, and lumbar above L3 transforaminal epidural injections
- Spinal cord stimulator trial and implant
- Percutaneous adhesiolysis with interlaminar or transforaminal approach
- Percutaneous disc decompression above L4/L5
- Stellate ganglion, thoracic, splanchnic, or celiac plexus sympathetic blocks
- Thoracic and cervical intradiscal procedures
- Vertebral augmentation in the cervical, thoracic, and lumbar spine (above L4)
- Intrathecal catheter and pump implant
- Interspinous prosthesis

Abdominal hernia repair, axillary node dissection, and cholecystectomy may additionally be considered low risk for severe bleeding. Posterior chamber eye procedures, vascular surgery, general surgery, prostatic resection, and polypectomy are considered high risk for severe bleeding [47].

Bridging Therapy

The bridging of patients with heparin or other anticoagulation before or after procedural intervention is recommended only for patients with a significantly high thromboembolism risk. This may include patients with recent ischemic stroke or cerebrovascular accident, mitral position or older-generation mechanical heart valve, or CHA2DS2-VASc score of 5 or greater [46, 47]. In most patients, however, bridging therapy results in convoluted anticoagulation plans, excessive bleeding, longer hospital stays, and significant comorbidities while producing no significant difference in prevention of thromboembolism [40, 46, 48]. Multidisciplinary discussion with all stakeholders regarding the practicalities of bridging anticoagulation, the small risk of major complications off anticoagulation often leads to a plan that often does not include bridging.

Additional Considerations

Guidelines for the timing of anticoagulant interruption vary depending on the nature of the medication. For example, vitamin K antagonists must be discontinued sooner than factor Xa inhibitors due to the need for coagulation factors to be resynthesized. Patient age, weight, hepatic function, renal function, and other comorbidities must also be considered in the management of perioperative or periprocedural anticoagulant interruption [40, 46, 47].

If an interventional technique is deemed to have moderate to severe bleeding potential, most anticoagulant medications should be discontinued beforehand to minimize the risk of bleeding events. Of course, due to differences in pharmacologic properties, each specific agent or class of agents has different recommendations on the timing and method of discontinuation. ASRA and ASIPP have published recommendations for the handling of anticoagulant drugs based on extensive literature reviews [40]. Medication and class-specific management guidelines are summarized below based on low-, moderate-, and high-risk interventional pain management techniques.

Warfarin

Recommendations for the discontinuation of warfarin are based on the patient's INR. ASIPP and ASRA agree that pain interventions deemed low risk for adverse bleeding outcomes can safely be completed with an INR < 3. For moderate- to high-risk procedures, ASRA recommends a normal INR, while ASIPP considers an INR $\leq$ 1.5 adequate. In patients at high risk for thromboembolic events, consider a LMWH bridge [39, 50].

NSAIDs/Aspirin

For patients on daily aspirin, the decision to stop or continue the therapy should be based on the indication with bleeding and clotting risks weighed carefully. Patients taking aspirin for primary prophylaxis can stop therapy without hesitation. ASRA recommends stopping both high- and low-dose aspirin therapy 4 days before low- and moderate-risk interventional techniques and 6 days before high-risk interventional techniques. For low- to moderate-risk interventions, ASIPP recommends the physician's discretion to either continue aspirin therapy or discontinue for 3 days but recommends discontinuation of therapy 5 days prior to intervention techniques deemed high risk [39].

There is limited evidence for the stopping or continuation of NSAIDs around spinal procedures. The consensus between ASRA and ASIPP is that NSAIDs do not provide a protective effect; however, patients may complain of more uncontrolled pain with their discontinuation due to their use in analgesia. ASRA recommends discontinuing NSAIDs anywhere from 1 to 10 days before the procedure, suggesting drugs like piroxicam be stopped 10 days prior while drugs like ibuprofen and diclofenac be continued up until 1 day before. There is little evidence for significant bleeding risk with the use of NSAIDs, and clinicians may choose to continue these drugs perioperatively for their pain relief benefits to the patients. ASIPP suggests that regardless of risk stratification of the proposed intervention, NSAIDs can be continued or may be stopped 1–10 days before as stated in ASRA's guidelines [40].

ADP Receptor Inhibitors

ADP receptor inhibitors such as clopidogrel and ticagrelor block the aggregation of platelets. For spinal interventional techniques deemed low risk, both ASIPP and ASRA state that platelet aggregation inhibitors may be continued safely. For moderate-risk procedures, ASIPP leaves the decision to the discretion of the provider, stating that the agents may be continued or stopped for 3–7 days depending on the drugs's individual pharmacodynamic and pharmacokinetic properties. ASRA recommends stopping the platelet aggregation inhibitors for 7–10 days before moderate-risk interventions. Both ASRA and ASIPP recommend ceasing therapy with these agents before high-risk spinal pain interventions for 3–10 days, again depending on the properties of the individual agents [40, 51].

GPIIb/IIIa Inhibitors

Abciximab, eptifibatide, and tirofiban are GPIIb/IIIa inhibitors, which block platelet aggregation. Due to the little to no evidence of increased bleeding with continuation of these drugs in interventional pain procedures stratified as low risk, both ASIPP and ASRA state these drugs may be continued.

For moderate- to high-risk interventional spinal procedures, ASIPP recommends stopping abciximab for 1–2 days and eptifibatide and tirofiban for 8 hours, while ASRA recommends stopping abciximab 2–5 days and eptifibatide and tirofiban 8–24 hours before the interventional techniques are performed [40].

Phosphodiesterase Inhibitors

Cilostazol and dipyridamole reversibly inhibit platelet aggregation through inhibition of phosphodiesterase. Aggrenox is also a phosphodiesterase inhibitor that combines dipyridamole with aspirin. For interventional pain procedures classified as low or moderate risk, both ASRA and ASIPP state these agents may be continued except for Aggrenox. Due to the aspirin component, ASRA recommends discontinuation of this drug for 4 days, consistent with their aspirin recommendations. Aggrenox should be stopped 5 days before a high-risk intervention according to ASIPP. According to ASRA, Aggrenox should be stopped 6 days before a high-risk intervention. For patients undergoing high-risk intervention taking cilostazol or dipyridamole alone, ASIPP states that therapy may be continued or stopped for 2 days, while ASRA recommends stopping therapy for 2 days [40].

Heparin/LMWH

Heparin and low molecular weight heparin are frequently used for bridging other anticoagulants up until the time of the procedure. Both ASRA and ASIPP share recommendations for the use of these drugs around spinal pain procedures. For IV heparin treatment, regardless of the procedure's risk stratification level, discontinue therapy for 4 hours before. For subcutaneous heparin treatment, discontinue 8–10 hours before the intervention. For low molecular weight heparin, ASRA and ASIPP recommend discontinuation of therapy for 24 hours before any interventional spinal procedure [40, 52].

Direct Thrombin Inhibitors (Dabigatran)

Direct thrombin inhibitors, such as dabigatran, directly block thrombin's ability to convert fibrinogen to fibrin. Careful consideration of a patient's renal function must be considered with decisions to cease therapy before spinal procedures for pain intervention [52, 53]. For procedures classified as low risk, both ASRA and ASIPP state that dabigatran can be continued or stopped for 2 days. For both moderate- and high-risk interventions, ASRA and ASIPP recommend stopping therapy for 4–5 days in patients with normal renal function and 6 days for patients with impaired renal function [40].

Conclusion

The **pharmacopeia of agents that impact coagulation is extensive. This is a vast and expanding medical field, and knowledge of the pharmacodynamics and pharmacokinetics is essential for any proceduralist.** The physician's responsibility is to carefully weigh the risk of bleeding and the risk of developing thrombosis when performing neuraxial procedures. A bleeding risk score can enable physicians to quickly and effectively decide whether to perform the neuraxial procedure. Evaluating the risk involves understanding the technical risks of a procedure, and the complications that can arise with patients who have a higher risk of bleeding [30]. Absolute risk of neuraxial procedures cannot be eliminated but can be reduced with adherence to guidelines. Like the one proposed by the American Society of Regional Anesthesia, a risk score enables the physician to evaluate the risk effectively and efficiently to ensure patients receive adequate interventions with minimal risks of adverse sequelae [30]. Finally, herbals, over-the-counter products, fish oils, and many other agents can interfere with the coagulation cascade and provide additive and/or synergistic anticoagulant effects. These effects can increase the risk of bleeding and catastrophic complications.

References

1. Manchikanti L, Falco FJE, Benyamin RM, Caraway DL, Kaye AD, Helm S, et al. Assessment of bleeding risk of interventional techniques: a best evidence synthesis of practice patterns and perioperative management of anticoagulant and antithrombotic therapy. Pain Physician. 2013;16:SE261–318.
2. Horlocker TT, Wedel DJ, Rowlingson JC, Enneking FK. Executive summary: regional anesthesia in the patient receiving antithrombotic or thrombolytic therapy. Reg Anesth Pain Med. 2010;35(1):102–5.
3. Manchikanti L, Abdi S, Atluri S, Benyamin RM, Boswell MV, Buenaventura RM, et al. An update of comprehensive evidence-based guidelines for interventional techniques in chronic spinal pain. Part II: guidance and recommendations. Pain Phys. United States. 2013;16:S49–283.
4. Meisenberg G, Simmons W. Hemostasis and Thrombosis. Principles of medical biochemistry. Saunders. 29th April 2011:p.608.
5. Smith SA, Travers RJ, Morrissey JH. How it all starts: Initiation of the clotting cascade. Crit Rev Biochem Mol Biol. 2015;50:326–36.
6. Bahuleyan B. Hemostasis: a cell based model journal of physiology and pharmacology advances. J Phys Pharm Adv [Internet]. 2019;2015:638–42. Available from: www.grjournals.com.
7. Sadler JE, Budde U, Eikenboom JCJ, Favaloro EJ, Hill FGH, Holmberg L, et al. Update on the pathophysiology and classification of von Willebrand disease: a report of the Subcommittee on von Willebrand Factor. J Thromb Haemost. John Wiley & Sons, Ltd (10.1111). 2006;4:2103–14.

8. Mannucci PM, Tuddenham EGD. The Hemophilias — from royal genes to gene therapy. N Engl J Med. Massachusetts Medical Society. 2001;344:1773–9.
9. Sallah S, Bobzien W. Bleeding problems in patients with liver disease. Postgrad Med. Taylor & Francis. 1999;106:187–95.
10. Weigert AL, Schafer AI. Uremic bleeding: pathogenesis and therapy. Am J Med Sci. 1998;316:94–104.
11. Hawkey CJ. COX-1 and COX-2 inhibitors. Best Pract Res Clin Gastroenterol. 2001;15:801.
12. Hamberg M, Svensson J, Samuelsson B. Thromboxanes: a new group of biologically active compounds derived from prostaglandin endoperoxides. Nutr Rev. 2009;44:208.
13. Bates SM, Greer A, Middeldorp S, Veenstra DL, Prabulos AM, Vandvik PO. VTE, thrombophilia, antithrombotic therapy, and pregnancy – antithrombotic therapy and prevention of thrombosis, 9th ed: American College of Chest Physicians evidence-based clinical practice guidelines. Chest. 2012;141(2 Suppl):e691S–736S.
14. Patrono C, García Rodríguez LA, Landolfi R, Baigent C. Low-dose aspirin for the prevention of Atherothrombosis. N Engl J Med. 2005;353:2373.
15. Vane JR, Botting RM. Anti-inflammatory drugs and their mechanism of action. Inflamm Res. 1998;47:78.
16. Vermeer C, Vitamin K. The effect on health beyond coagulation – an overview. Food Nutr Res. 2012;56:5329.
17. Appadu B, Barber K. Drugs affecting coagulation. Anaesth Intensive Care Med. 2018;19:656.
18. DeLoughery TG. Warfarin. Hemostasis and Thrombosis. 3rd ed. Springer International Publishing. 2015:3. https://doi.org/10.1007/978-3-319-09312-3
19. Hirsh J, Dalen JE, Anderson DR, Poller L, Bussey H, Ansell J, et al. Oral anticoagulants: mechanism of action, clinical effectiveness, and optimal therapeutic range. Chest. 2001;119:8S.
20. Cook NS, Kottirsch G, Zerwes HG. Platelet glycoprotein IIb/IIIa antagonists. Drugs Future. 1994.
21. Stangl PA, Lewis S. Review of currently available GP IIb/IIIa inhibitors and their role in peripheral vascular interventions. Semin Intervent Radiol. 2010;27:412.
22. Ibanez B, Vilahur G, Badimon JJ. Pharmacology of thienopyridines: rationale for dual pathway inhibition. Eur Hear J Suppl. 2006;8:G3–9.
23. Gray E, Mulloy B, Barrowcliffe TW. Heparin and low-molecular-weight heparin. Thromb Haemost. 2008;99(5):807–18. https://doi.org/10.1160/TH08-01-0032.
24. Bussey H, Francis JL. Heparin overview and issues. Pharmacotherapy. 2004;24:103S.
25. Di Nisio M, Middeldorp S, Büller HR. Direct thrombin inhibitors. N Engl J Med. 2005;353(10):1028–40.
26. Lewis BE, Wallis DE, Berkowitz SD, Matthai WH, Fareed J, Walenga JM, et al. Argatroban anticoagulant therapy in patients with heparin-induced thrombocytopenia. Circulation. 2001;103:1838.
27. Larsen TB, Rasmussen LH, Skjøth F, Due KM, Callréus T, Rosenzweig M, et al. Efficacy and safety of dabigatran etexilate and warfarin in "real-world" patients with atrial fibrillation: A prospective nationwide cohort study. J Am Coll Cardiol. 2013;61:2264.
28. Schulman S, Beyth RJ, Kearon C, Levine MN. Hemorrhagic complications of anticoagulant and thrombolytic treatment: American College of Chest Physicians evidence-based clinical practice guidelines (8th edition). Chest. American College of Chest Physicians. 2008;133:257S–98S.
29. Siegal DM, Curnutte JT, Connolly SJ, Lu G, Conley PB, Wiens BL, et al. Andexanet Alfa for the reversal of factor Xa inhibitor activity. N Engl J Med. 2015;373:2413–24.
30. Shah R, Kaye AD, Kaye A, Tsai JY. Anticoagulation and regional anesthesia concerns. Essentials Reg Anesth. 2012;
31. Allen DJ, Chae-Kim SH, Trousdale DM. Risks and complications of Neuraxial Anesthesia and the use of anticoagulation in the surgical patient. Baylor Univ Med Cent Proc. 2002;15:369.
32. Stafford-Smith M. Impaired haemostasis and regional anaesthesia. Can J Anaesth. 1996;43:R129–41.
33. Ružman T, Gulam D, Drenjančević IH, Venžera-Azenić D, Ružman N, Burazin J. Factors associated with difficult neuraxial blockade. Local Reg Anesth. 2014;7:47–52.
34. Claerhout AJ, Johnson M, Radtke JD, Zaglaniczny KL. AANA journal course: update for nurse anesthetists. Anticoagulation and spinal and epidural anesthesia. AANA J. 2004;72(3):225–31.
35. Kaye AD, Manchikanti L, Novitch MB, Mungrue IN, Anwar M, Jones MR, et al. Responsible, safe, and effective use of antithrombotics and anticoagulants in patients undergoing interventional techniques: American Society of Interventional Pain Physicians (ASIPP) guidelines. Pain Physician. 2019;22:S1–74.
36. Lumpkin MM. FDA public health advisory. Anesthesiology. 1998;88:27A–8A.
37. Horlocker TT, Wedel DJ, Rowlingson JC, Enneking FK, Kopp SL, Benzon HT, et al. Regional anesthesia in the patient receiving antithrombotic or thrombolytic therapy: American Society of Regional Anesthesia and Pain Medicine Evidence-Based Guidelines (Third Edition). Reg Anesth Pain Med. 2010;35:64–101.
38. Harrop-Griffiths W, Cook T, Gill H, Hill D, Ingram M, Makris M, et al. Regional anaesthesia and patients with abnormalities of coagulation: the Association of Anaesthetists of Great Britain & Ireland the Obstetric Anaesthetists' Association Regional Anaesthesia UK. Anaesthesia. 2013;68(9):966–72.
39. Vela Vásquez RS, Peláez Romero R. Aspirin and spinal haematoma after neuraxial anaesthesia: Myth or reality? Br J Anaesth. 2015;115:688.
40. Kaye AD, Manchikanti L, Novitch MB, Mungrue IN, Anwar M, Jones MR, et al. Responsible, safe, and effective use of antithrombotics and anticoagulants in patients undergoing interventional techniques: American Society of Interventional Pain Physicians (ASIPP) Guidelines. Pain Physician. 2019;22(1S):S75–S128.
41. Moesker MJ, De Groot JF, Damen NL, Huisman MV, De Bruijne MC, Wagner C. How reliable is perioperative anticoagulant management ? Determining guideline compliance and practice variation by a retrospective patient record review. BMJ Open. 2019;9(7):e029879. https://doi.org/10.1136/bmjopen-2019-029879 PMID: 31320357 PMCID: PMC6661608.
42. Arthroplasty A, Barlow BT, Hannon MT, Waldron JE. Preoperative management of abstract. 2019;00:1–9.
43. Horlocker TT, Wedel DJ, Rowlingson JC, Enneking FK, Kopp SL, Benzon HT, Brown DL, Heit JA, Mulroy MF, Rosen- quist RW, Tryba M, Yuan CS. Regional anesthesia in the patient receiving antithrombotic or thrombolytic therapy: American Society of Regional Anesthesia and Pain Medicine Evidence-Based Guidelines (Fourth Edition). Reg Anesth Pain Med. 2018;43(3):263–309.
44. Horlocker TT, Bajwa ZH, Ashraf Z, Khan S, Wilson JL, Sami N, Peeters-Asdourian C, Powers CA, Schroeder DR, Decker PA, Warfield CA. Risk assessment of hemorrhagic complications associated with nonsteroidal antiinflammatory medications in ambulatory pain clinic patients undergoing epidural steroid injection. Anesth Analg. 2002;95(6):1691–7.
45. Horlocker TT, Wedel DJ, Schroeder DR, Rose SH, Elliott BA, McGregor DG, Wong GY. Preoperative antiplatelet therapy does not increase the risk of spinal hematoma associated with regional anesthesia. Anesth Analg. 1995;80:303–9.
46. Rechenmacher SJ, Fang JC. Bridging anticoagulation. J Am Coll Cardiol. Elsevier Inc. 2015;66:1392–403.
47. Patel RB, Tassiopoulos AK. Anticoagulants and surgery: so many agents, so many taking them. Adv Surg. Elsevier Inc. 2019;53:235–51.
48. Shaw JR, Woodfine JD, Douketis J, Schulman S, Carrier M. Perioperative interruption of direct oral anticoagulants in patients with atrial fibrillation: a systematic review and meta-analysis. Res Pract Thromb Haemost. 2018;2(2):282–90.

49. Haas E, Onel E, Miller H, Ragupathi M, White PF. A double-blind, randomized, active-controlled study for post-hemorrhoidectomy pain management with liposome bupivacaine, a novel local analgesic formulation. Am Surg. 2012;78(5):574–81.
50. Coppens M, Eikelboom JW, Hart RG, Yusuf S, Lip GYH, Dorian P, et al. The CHA2DS2 -VASc score identifies those patients with atrial fibrillation and a CHADS 2 score of 1 who are unlikely to benefit from oral anticoagulant therapy. Eur Heart J. 2013;34:170–6.
51. Douketis JD, Spyropoulos AC, Spencer FA, Mayr M, Jaffer AK, Eckman MH, et al. Perioperative management of antithrombotic therapy. Antithrombotic therapy and prevention of thrombosis, 9th ed: American College of Chest Physicians evidence-based clinical practice guidelines. Chest. 2012;141(2 Suppl):e326S–50S.
52. Spyropoulos AC, Douketis JD. How I treat anticoagulated patients undergoing an elective procedure or surgery. Blood. 2012;120(15):2954–62.
53. Stangier J, Rathgen K, Sthle H, Mazur D. Influence of renal impairment on the pharmacokinetics and pharmacodynamics of oral dabigatran etexilate: an open-label, parallel-group, single-centre study. Clin Pharmacokinet. 2010;49(4):259–68.

The Red Blood Cell Storage Lesion: A Controversy of Biology Versus Randomized Controlled Trials

48

Lauren Smajdor and Bruce D. Spiess

Introduction

Blood transfusion (Tx) has been a mainstay of modern medicine since the early 1900s, when ABO histocompatibility antigens were discovered [1, 2]. Today, Tx of banked blood is the leading hospital therapy in the United States and in most developed countries. Blood banking evolved (never having undergone safety/efficacy testing) prior to and during World Wars I and II as refrigeration improved in parallel with methods to anti-coagulate blood [2]. Focus in the blood banking field upon infrastructure has assured supply for ever growing demands. Transfusion safety has focused on the elimination of transmissible viral, parasitic, and bacterial contamination with wonderful success [1–4]. The HIV crisis of the 1980s spurred action to assure that the blood supply was the "safest" possible, with a laser focus only upon viral diseases [1–4]. Progress in safety should not be underappreciated. Reduction of viral transmission risk by advanced testing and self-reporting by donors has made risk of HIV and hepatitis C so small as to be only calculable by computer modeling (as opposed to actual measurements) [1–6].

Blood may be kept up to 42 days in the United States and 49 days in some European countries. More recently, transfusion risk research has shifted to outcomes: immunomodulation (infection in hospital and cancer recurrence), transfusion-related acute lung injury (TRALI), organ dysfunction (renal and lung), as well as some oxygen (O_2) delivery data [6]. Retrospective work sparked anxiety regarding relationships between age of red blood cells (RBCs) and negative outcomes [7]. Because of a sentinel paper [7] and others that preceded, RCTs have been sponsored to investigate the link between age of blood and outcome (mortality) [8–13]. This review will first examine what is known today regarding the biology of RBC storage lesions and second look at retrospective data and third the RCTs. Does a dichotomy between biologic storage changes and the majority of RCTs exist? Doctors examining this data without understanding the implications and limitations of such studies should be rightly confused. Retrospective comparisons triggered RCTs, not the biologic data alone [14]. Few criticisms and considerable praise exist regarding the negative outcomes of the RCTs [15]. Blood bankers do not completely agree with their own conclusions that have been drawn from the RCTs. A survey of blood bankers (97% agreement) demonstrated that the utilization of fresher blood at their hospitals could produce clinical benefits though 80% believed the RCTs [16]. Sixty-six percent stated they feel length of storage is a major concern, but 81% said their institutions are doing nothing to improve usage of fresher blood [16]. Confusion exists, therefore, not only due to the conflicting biologic and outcome data but also due to messages from "experts," i.e., blood bankers. This manuscript is meant to help health-care workers understand the conflicting/confusing data.

Storage Lesions

Stored RBCs (up to 42 days) demonstrate biochemical, metabolic, structural, inflammatory, and physiologic changes that occur over time as well as worsen with time. These changes are collectively known as the storage lesion [17]. With time, RBCs undergo deterioration, shape changes, loss of cell membrane material, leakage of intracellular ions, changes in membrane protein expression, and hemolysis. These complex changes have relations to oxidative stress (inflammation/heme release and reactive oxygen species) overload combined with consumption of antioxidants during storage [18–

L. Smajdor (✉)
University of Florida, Department of Anesthesiology, Gainesville, FL, USA
e-mail: lsmajdor@anest.ufl.edu

B. D. Spiess
University of Florida Health, Gainesville, FL, USA
e-mail: bspiess@anest.ufl.edu

© Springer Nature Switzerland AG 2021
C. S. Scher et al. (eds.), *Essentials of Blood Product Management in Anesthesia Practice*,
https://doi.org/10.1007/978-3-030-59295-0_48

21]. Survival of transfused RBCs is measured by radioactively labeling infused RBCs with sodium chromate and then sampling periodically to determine the clearance and kinetics of RBCs after transfusion [19]. Regulatory standards are that there should be no more than 1% hemolysis in the stored blood bag prior to infusion and that 75% of RBCs infused should survive in vivo for 24 hours (US FDA). Tests for storage were done on a small number of units, and then it was assumed that all other units treated in the same manner will comply with the initial findings from those original units that led to regulations. For the in vivo breakdown, healthy volunteers were given blood stored, and then hemolysis was calculated at 24 hours. A substantial portion of transfused RBCs is cleared from the patient's circulation within the first 24 hours, and the percentage of these non-viable RBCs increases with duration of storage. Currently, the FDA requires that stored RBC experience less than 1% hemolysis and that at least 75% of stored RBC survive in the recipient 24 hours after transfusion [20]. Conversely, it is deemed acceptable by regulators that 25% of infused cells are cleared within the body as cellular debris. There are no regulatory requirements that any of the transfused cells function normally, and in vivo testing for hemolysis has not been done in patients with abnormal vasculatures, or who are inflamed with disease processes.

Oxygen (O_2) Carrying/Delivery

RBCs have no aerobic respiration. They lack mitochondria. RBCs rely on anaerobic glycolysis for adenosine triphosphate (ATP) production, which produces 2,3-diphosphoglycerate (2,3-DPG) as a byproduct. Stored blood may contain dextrose, phosphate, citrate, and adenine to aid in energy production for membrane integrity. As storage time increases, lactate accumulates, and pH decreases, as does ATP and 2,3-diphosphoglycerate (2,3-DPG) [22–32] (Fig. 48.1).

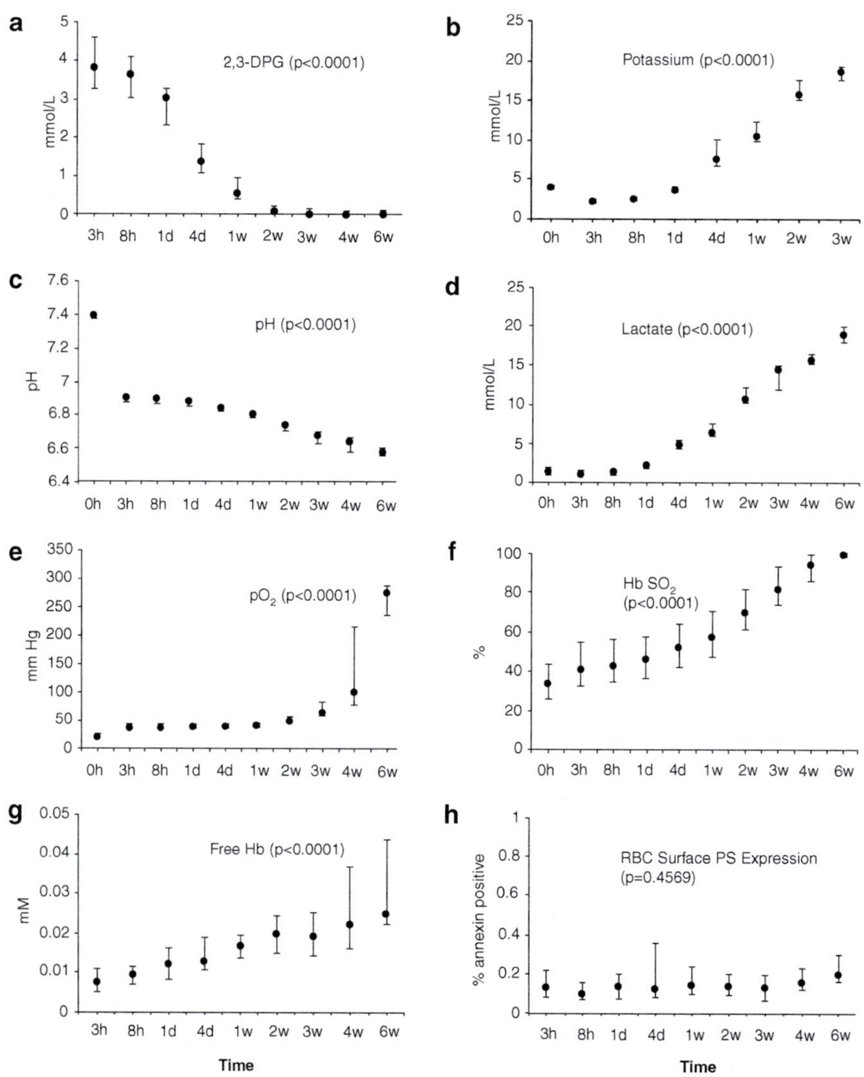

Fig. 48.1 Values for plasma levels of key cellular indicators of red cell storage lesions are noted from the time period of 3 hours to 6 weeks of storage. Note that 2,3-DPG is depleted by 1 week and other levels begin to change within 1 day of storage (Adapted and reprinted with permission from Bennett-Guerrero E, Veldman TH, Doctor A, et al. Evolution of adverse changes in stored RBCs. Proc Nat Acad Sci 2007; 104: 17063–17,068)

Decreased 2,3-DPG results in increased affinity of hemoglobin (Hgb) for O_2, a lowered P_{50}, with decreased O_2 delivery. The decrease in 2,3-DPG acts much as would sickle cell or fetal Hgb [31]. Aged blood (from transfusion) passing through the lungs is oxygenated but does not unload its O_2 well in the peripheral tissues [28–33]. Transfusion results in a left P_{50} shift persisting for up to 3 days [32]. Human gastric mucosal O_2 levels after transfusion show a decrease, exacerbated when older blood was infused [33]. Transfusion has not always demonstrated an increase in tissue O_2 delivery [30–35]. In contrast, one of the recent RCTs (to be discussed later) demonstrated improved cerebral oxygenation after transfusion [36].

In a rodent model of hemorrhagic shock with species-specific blood for resuscitation, the blood pressure, central venous pressure, and mixed venous O_2 tension all improved equally upon infusion of either fresh or aged stored blood [31]. However, if aged blood was infused, sensitive intracellular monitors of O_2 tension found a 400% decrease in cellular O_2 tension. Only fresh whole blood restored cellular O_2 delivery [31]. Healthy humans do not hit critical O_2 delivery until the Hgb level is below 5gm/dl, as seen in the African study of old vs. newer blood in children with sickle cell disease and malaria [36, 37]. A study of healthy volunteers who donated their own blood and were electively hemodiluted to 5.5 gm/dl began having neurologic changes which was relieved by getting their own blood back. The investigator used this as indirect proof of critical O_2 delivery in humans [38].

Efforts to slow the storage decay of 2,3-DPG are ongoing. Additives to banked blood can enhance 2,3-DPG levels up to 8 days before all 2, 3-DPG is exhausted. On average, blood is approximately 21 days old when transfused [16]. Efforts to use additives to preserve 2,3-DPG thus far are functionally ineffective if average blood utilized is 21 days old. Rejuvenation additives to boost both erythrocyte ATP and 2,3-DPG exist [37]. These agents are not often used because they require a minimum of an hour to rejuvenate the blood followed by another hour in cell washing [37]. Rejuvenation technologies have not been studied in RCTs. 2,3-DPG changes are an area of controversy when discussing old vs. fresh blood.

Cell Rigidity/Fracture and Inflammation

Increased membrane rigidity from storage causes RBCs to aggregate, adhere to endothelial cells, become inflexible, and inhibit movement through capillaries. RBC rigidity leads to increased microvascular resistance [39–41]. Models of red cell shear stress involving older erythrocytes interacting with live single layer endothelial cells demonstrated that the increased shear-related cellular injury of endothelial cells mimics what has been described in the pulmonary microvasculature after transfusion [39].

In 21 patients receiving chronic frequent transfusion, standard blood transfusion (mean age 24.5 days) was compared within each subject at different transfusion events to blood less than 5 days old [40]. Endothelial function was measured using a previously validated hyperemia tonometry index. Hyperemic response was decreased by the infusion of older blood, signaling endothelial cell dysfunction and inflammation [40].

Other data regarding older blood and endothelial cell functions was implicated in a novel metabolomics study [42]. Over 280,000 patients from Denmark had profiles of their blood studied with and without transfusion [42]. The metabolomics changes are far more detailed than pH, or free Hgb. RBC flexibility indices from metabolomics were associated with outcome in the 280,000 transfused patients as markers of cellular RBC quality [42].

In healthy volunteers given their own autologous blood aged 5 days or 30–42 days, there was no difference in pulmonary artery pressures depending upon the age of blood infused [43]. The lack of pulmonary artery vasoconstriction after older blood was interpreted to be an indication of no difference in aged nitric oxide binding activity [43]. Perhaps it could be that young healthy volunteers given 1 unit of their own blood (roughly 5% volume) have a great capability to adapt and do not have reactive pulmonary vasculature. This same group of researchers demonstrated that aged blood did indeed worsen endothelial dysfunction by measuring pulmonary artery pressures in either obese or those with underlying endothelial dysfunction [39–43]. We rarely transfuse perfectly healthy patients [43].

Functional capillary density (the number of open capillaries per unit of tissue) decreases with age, in many diseases, and with the transfusion of older blood [28, 29]. Older and more ill patients with a lower functional capillary density at baseline are exactly the patients who are most likely to be transfused. No animal research has focused upon transfusion in such diseases.

Data from a cardiac RCT has demonstrated differences in delirium outcome – perhaps related to microvascular impairment [44].

Dysfunctional shape along with reduced RBC flexibility leads to endothelial cell dysfunction with a tendency toward more inflammation as the age of RBCs increases [45–47]. Endothelial cells are sensitive to vascular shear forces from flowing blood. Older blood increases endothelial shear stress and upregulates these cells' reactivity to platelets, white cells, and other cellular insults [45, 47]. This data is in contradistinction to the previously noted findings with healthy volunteers instrumented with PA catheters. Herein we see the contrast between some basic science animal model research and RCTs.

Hemolysis, Potassium, and Free Hgb

As storage time increases, RBCs release free Hgb, a nitric oxide scavenger. In the RBC, Hgb is surrounded by large amounts of glutathione, an antioxidant. Hgb is toxic to neurological tissues, endothelial cells, and renal cells, if it is free and unbound. The release of free Hgb results in vasoconstriction, endothelial dysfunction, and the potential for more platelet and neutrophil adhesion to the microcirculation. With longer storage RBCs may have reduced nitric oxide arteriole vasodilatation in response to hypoxia [47]. Again this nitric oxide response is in contrast to what was found with healthy volunteers but fits with research on functional capillary density.

Free Hgb is toxic to tissues and is scavenged by haptoglobin. Iron metabolism is central to multiple metalloproteins (Hgb, cytochromes, catalase, tryptophan pyrolase); hence free iron is tightly scavenged. Free iron as well as unbound heme are profound oxidizers [48–51]. High levels of free Hgb are associated with renal dysfunction/kidney failure. In a guinea pig model of massive transfusion, older blood (2-days-old vs. 21–28-days-old blood) demonstrated an increase in hypertension, vascular injury, and renal insufficiency [48–51]. The amount of post-transfusion hemolysis and free Hgb was correlated with the severity of the organ injuries as well as the age of the units transfused. Furthermore, when haptoglobin was infused along with transfusion, the levels of free Hgb dropped as did adverse outcomes [48–50]. Other work regarding transfusion release of free Hgb discussed ektacytometry or shear stress analysis of aged versus younger erythrocytes [51]. In a small sub-group analysis of a randomized trial in 20 septic patients who received fresh blood, <10 days vs. > 15 days old, sublingual microcirculation function was measured by sidestream dark field imaging. Dark field imaging in humans can be utilized to assess functional capillary density as well with newer techniques to assess the thickness of the endothelial glycocalyx. Furthermore in this study, the assessment of the glycocalyx was performed in conjunction with near-infrared spectroscopy to find tissue O_2 levels [51]. Functional capillary density decreased (worsened) in conjunction with increased free Hgb, and tissue Hgb index (a measure of red cell transit per gram of tissue) was worse with aged blood [51]. What might be especially interesting about this study is that the rise in free Hgb occurred after the aged red cells were transfused, meaning they were broken apart in the circulation with lysis in vivo [51]. This finding fits with what has been described earlier regarding the biology of increased cellular fragility with storage [51, 52]. As stated, extravascular hemolysis seems to be the prevalent destruction of transfused erythrocytes, not destruction in the stored bag. When comparing blood aged up to 6 weeks in healthy volunteers, more red cell destruction and free Hgb was found in older blood samples [53]. That is an important piece of biology because it signals that the red cell membranes after storage are indeed fragile.

As erythrocytes are stored, extracellular potassium rises [29, 54, 55]. Hyperkalemic arrest in pediatric patients has occurred [54, 55]. This mortality risk is increased when patients have underlying acidosis, low cardiac output, hypocalcemia, hyperglycemia, and hypothermia [38]. Critically ill infants are susceptible to Tx-related incidents with case reports of sudden death in young children being transfused [47, 54, 55]. A recommendation exists in pediatric cardiac surgery; if 4 or more units may be transfused, they should receive the freshest blood [56].

In 2014, the Society for Pediatric Anesthesia (SPA) and its patient safety organization, "Wake up Safe," released an advisory in response to concern about transfusion-related hyperkalemic cardiac arrest. SPA advocated for "anticipating and replacing blood loss before significant hemodynamic compromise occurs" [55]. Baseline electrolyte abnormalities, impaired renal function, using larger-bore peripheral IVs which allow for longer infusion times (faster infusion rates pose a greater hyperkalemic burden to the body), and less RBC hemolysis were advocated [54]. It is unclear how RCTs might affect these recommendations.

Unique Proteins/Micro-particles

Band 3 ion exchanger protein is an anchor for many glycolytic enzymes. Its destruction has detrimental effects on the erythrocyte. Longer storage stimulates RBCs to release submicron-sized fragments of the cell's plasma membranes into the supernatant – micro-particles [57–65]. It is thought that the oxidization of cell membrane lipids in stored erythrocytes as well as oxidization of many proteins leads to destabilization of the membrane. Band 3 ion exchange protein is involved in this process with increased oxidative dysfunction during blood bank storage [66].

When band 3 ion exchanger is destroyed, its aggregates move within the cell membrane for vesiculation serving as a signal for the body to remove the senescent or damaged (oxidized) cell [66]. The movement of damaged parts of band 3 ion exchanger protein to the cell surface creates neo-antigens, which in turn stimulates macrophages to clear these cells. The breakup of band 3 ion exchange protein may be related to a series of pro-inflammatory events and is implicated in TRALI. Other cell markers associated with apoptosis, such as phosphatidylserine (cell membrane structures), along with the number of vesicles that express them, increase proportionally due to the duration of storage. The release erythrocyte micro-particles in normal physiology serves a protective role, allowing the older/damaged RBCs to be cleared away when these detrimental oxidized proteins are present. However, micro-particle formation and band 3 expression could also have the opposite effect when we transfuse large numbers of dysfunctional cells into the circulation [66].

The term "eryptosis" was coined by Lang and colleagues in 2006 to describe the suicidal death of erythrocytes [65]. Micro-vesicles/ micro-particles, expressing oxidized phosphatidylserine (dysfunctional cell membrane components), actually create a surface for pro-coagulant reactions [60]. These surface oxidized lipids are capable of facilitating thrombin generation, and platelet activation which is a process detrimental to the vasculature and an amplifier of inflammation [60].

Solomon and Klein studied the effects of transfusing older blood to septic dogs, using a canine model of *Staphylococcus aureus* pneumonia to represent critically ill patients in an ICU setting [67]. Just as in human patients, the dogs were treated with mechanical ventilation, fluid infusions, vasopressors, sedation, and antibiotics. The animals were randomized into groups that received 7-day-old canine blood, or 42-day-old blood. Mortality in the older blood group significantly increased. Notably the dogs receiving older blood also had worsening of lung injury and degree of shock. Pertinent to this discussion, the older blood had increased free Hgb, which can scavenge NO. This canine study was the first blinded randomized trial that used standard blood banking techniques to show that older transfused blood increased mortality in a large animal model [67]. It is important to note how much different canine model is than what will be described in the human RCTs. The canine study examined blood at the far ends of the aging spectrum, something avoided in RCTs. Also, it examined animals in extremes of clinical stress, not done in RCTs.

Micro-particles are budded pieces of cell membrane, and with storage they are found from both red cells and platelets [60–63, 68]. They are particularly pro-inflammatory as well as stimulate thrombin generation and fibrinolysis [69]. 42-day-old blood has been shown to have more micro-particles than does fresh blood [61]. The older the blood, the more micro-particles. In animal studies red blood cell micro-particles from stored blood scavenge nitric oxide and contribute to pneumocyte dysfunction as well as pulmonary artery dysfunction [62, 67]. Micro-particles are present in fresh frozen plasma (FFP) both of which have been implicated in TRALI [62]. Oxidized micro-particles are immunomodulatory, upregulating macrophages initially. With enough micro-particle loading, the effect can overwhelm, leading to immunosuppression [57]. The literature regarding micro-particles in transfusion should be a review paper unto itself [57].

Retrospective Outcome Data

Observational/retrospective studies have not always shown increased morbidity and mortality in patients who have undergone cardiac surgery or trauma or are critically ill after receiving older blood. As early as 1997, in a 37-patient retrospective study in critically ill patients, the age of the blood transfused was shown to be associated with increased mortality [64]. Shortly thereafter, in trauma patients with large blood transfusion loads, the age of blood using multi-variable logistic regression was found to have relation to multi-system organ failure [68]. In contrast, in cardiac surgery when confounders were loaded into models, age of blood transfused did not influence outcomes [69].

Colorectal cancer recurrence was associated with age of blood during resection [70]. Of 740 patients analyzed in this national database study with follow-up for a mean of 6.8 years, age of blood infused was traced. Those who received older blood had more cancer and worse outcomes [70]. In trauma, relationships between more and older blood, immunomodulation was manifested by increased infection rates in those that survived when older or more blood was utilized [71]. In two cardiac surgery databases, associations between age of blood and adverse outcomes were not forthcoming [72, 73]. However, the one big study that changed focus was the one by Koch and of course was in cardiac patients [7].

In 2008, Koch et al. did a retrospective (1998–2006) single-center study at the Cleveland Clinic, comparing CABG or valve surgery patients who received "newer blood" (≤14 days) versus "older blood" (>14 days) [7]. In order to reduce confounding factors, data from patients who received a mixture of older and newer blood were excluded. The study found that older blood increased in-hospital mortality (2.8% vs. 1.7%, $P = 0.004$), with more prolonged ventilation (9.7% vs. 5.6%, $P < 0.001$), increased renal failure (2.7% vs. 1.6%, $P = 0.003$), sepsis (4.0% vs. 2.8%, $P = 0.01$), and/or multi-system organ failure (0.7% vs. 0.2%, $P = 0.007$). Older blood was associated with multiple serious adverse events (25.9% vs. 22.4%, $P = 0.001$). A 1-year survival of 92.6% was found in the group receiving newer blood and 89.0% for the group receiving older blood ($P < 0.001$) [7].

Koch's study was both praised and criticized [14]. It was praised since she analyzed the age of transfused blood as a continuous variable. That has been done also in the delirium in cardiac surgery study noted above [36]. The major criticisms were that ABO grouping was different in the two groups and other potentially important confounders were not evenly distributed. The editorial criticism pointed out that over the time of the study, 8 years, perhaps the utilization of leukoreduced blood may have changed as did severity of disease of the patients studied [14]. Together the criticisms further strengthened the calls for RCTs.

In 2012, a retrospective/prospective meta-analysis of 21 studies (18 observational studies with an n = 409,966 and three randomized, controlled trials with n = 126) of cardiac and trauma patients did indicate that each unit of older blood was associated with a 16% increase in the risk of death (OR 1.16) [74–77]. Clearly the RCTs in this meta-analysis were overwhelmed with the data driven by the large retrospective studies.

Randomized Controlled Trials

Most RCT findings stand in contrast to the biologic as well as the retrospective data. A meta-analysis from 2016 evaluated 12 RCTs that had enrolled 5229 participants [77]. No effect of fresher versus older RBCs on mortality was found (relative risk [RR], 1.04; 95% confidence interval [CI], 0.94–1.14; P = 0.45; $I^2 = 0\%$, moderate certainty evidence) or on adverse events (RR, 1.02; 95% CI, 0.91–1.14; P = 0.74; $I^2 = 0\%$, low certainty evidence) [78]. This analysis had limitations. The trials analyzed had a priori variable cut-points to define fresher versus older RBCs. The profiled trials also used different values, such as the mean or median, to report the blood transfusion utilization range. None looked at age of blood as a continuous variable, which is important. Also the trials had transfusion for a number of different disease states, and some were not limited to only one age of blood versus another. Some studies had leukoreduced or irradiated blood, while others did not. Manipulating RBCs through irradiation or washing can change the impact of a storage lesion. The methods of blood processing and storage solutions varied throughout the studies. This was a sample size of greater than 5000 patients, and while such a sample size might appear adequate, no power analysis can be done to judge the power when searching for a negative outcome.

The ARIPI (Age of Red Blood Cells in Premature Infants) study examined 377 neonates (potentially at risk for transfusion adverse outcomes with potassium as well as necrotizing bowel) across Canada who were randomized to receive either extremely fresh blood (≤7 days old) versus standard blood banked blood of many different ages (mean of 14.6 days) [79]. There were no differences in outcome. ARIPI was one of the first RCTs. They looked at super fresh versus fresh blood. One can criticize it in that the "standard age" blood had a wide range of ages of units transfused but in the end it was what would be otherwise considered fresh. There was no defining power analysis based upon the necrotizing bowel complication which in this age group is the feared complication associated with blood transfusion [79]. Also, the centers doing this study were very focused upon the adverse events of blood transfusion, so perhaps a bias existed in the study for selection toward "best practices."

In 2015, the "ABLE" (Age of Blood Evaluation) study enrolled 2510 patients from tertiary care intensive care units at 64 centers in 5 countries across Canada and Europe [80]. ABLE compared patients who received "fresh" blood (mean age 6.1 days) to those who received standard Tx (mean 22 days) [80]. Patients were assigned in a 1:1 ratio to one of the two study groups with permuted blocks of 6, 8, or 10. Using an "intention to treat" analysis, they found that at 90 days into the study, 37% of the patients who received fresh blood had died, compared to 35% of patients in the standard group. While there was no benefit to fresher blood, the groups did note that they used a "restrictive transfusion strategy," with their patients having a mean pre-transfusion level of 7.7 g/dl. This is significant because many institutions transfuse at higher or more liberal levels, which could affect outcomes as these patients are exposed to higher levels of blood products. In addition, the overall adherence rate to protocol was said to be >95%; however 16% of patients randomized to the "fresh" group received at least 1 RBC unit that had been stored for >7 days, so clearly adherence was not 95% [80]. Does 1 unit of old blood invalidate the data when intention to treat analysis is done?

The INFORM (Informing Fresh versus Old Red Cell Management) trial was prospective/randomized from 2012 to 2015 at multiple centers with all types of surgery, in over 31,000 patients who were recruited, but 29,000 had usable data (outwardly a large number) focused on mortality [81]. The study had a 1:2 randomization (more received old blood) for fresh blood – ≤ 7 days old vs. 8–35 days old and a very few who received older than 35-day-old blood. Mean age of blood in the old grouping was 23.6 days, whereas the mean age in the fresh blood group was 13.0 days. Extremes of aged blood were not studied, nor was blood age evaluated as a continuous variable although they drew the conclusion that blood over 35 days old was just fine. Many patients had overlap of aged vs. fresh blood. Furthermore, many patients received platelets, FFP, and cryo, yet these blood products were disregarded as having any influence upon outcome. Because it was such a large study, INFORM could be construed as being the final answer. It complimented itself for a "pragmatic" design, investigating relatively small amounts of transfusion, in other words a study that could be done.

The design did not compare oldest versus freshest blood as was done in the canine septic shock study. Even though INFORM had as its strength that multiple types of surgery were recruited, enrollment bias may have crept in. For one example, it was considered a strength that cardiovascular surgery was included, as a subset. There were over 9000 patients with cardiovascular surgery. The outcome found was alarmingly high in hospital mortality rate for heart surgery which was 12.3% in short-term storage and 11.2% in long-term storage. Most cardiovascular surgery programs accept in-hospital mortality rates at or below 5%. Such an alarming high mortality rate in cardiac surgery begs the question – who were these patients?

A strength to INFORM could be argued that if in routine surgery there is no difference in 29,000 patients. The outcome examined was death. What is the expected mortality rate in those particular 29,000 surgeries? Is mortality the correct outcome for RCTs in transfusion to begin with? If mortality is the end point, then one needs to know the risk of mortality due to blood transfusion before we can dichotomize or segregate transfusion age as a variable (segmented or continuous). Mortality due to transfusion is not known because nobody has ever done the study comparing transfusion to patient blood management (PBM) (non-transfusion).

The largest cause of mortality due to transfusion is TRALI. The incidence of TRALI is quoted at 1/6000–20,000 cases. With such an infrequent incidence, the power analysis for an RCT based upon this one side effect is astronomical. It begs the question once again that perhaps RCTs cannot be performed with old vs. fresh blood where mortality is the end point unless we go to immense numbers of patients (perhaps millions with very clear separation of groups). That realization supports the contention that if it takes that many for power to be accumulated, then age of blood really makes little difference. But, perhaps, the question should not be examined for "all comers" but for high-risk groups who have a considerably higher mortality related to TRALI. Researchers are loath to design such studies. In contrast TRALI in ICU critically ill patients may be higher than 1/200 units transfused with 50% mortality [82]. Would not the power needed to understand that randomization be considerably less?

Within INFORM there were over 10,000 patients who spent time in the ICU. But that does not mean that ICU care was their primary site for transfusion intervention. An editorial published along with the INFORM study took the RCTs at the time and stated that now we know the answer that older blood is of no consequence.

A non-randomized, but prospective observational, study was conducted focusing upon the extremes of blood age. Extremely aged blood, 35–42 days old, was associated with an increased death rate. Just as in canine septic shock, this study was focused upon highest-risk patients. Observational studies have been deemed less "weighty" than RCTs [83].

The Red-Cell Storage Duration Study (RECESS) was designed to compare clinical outcomes after complex cardiac surgery in 1481 patients, 12 years or older, who received a transfusion [84]. Patients were selected to receive blood that was stored for ≤10 days or ≥ 21 days, perhaps trying to mimic the timing of blood Tx that Koch utilized. It should be pointed out that all patients were already undergoing hemolysis by virtue of having cardiopulmonary bypass. The effect of on-going hemolysis might be a confounder. Investigators measured the change in Multiple Organ Dysfunction Score (MODS) from before and after surgery on a scale of 0 to 24, with 24 being death of the patient. The scores were obtained 7 days after surgery or until the patient's time of death, whichever came first [84]. The primary outcome of the study showed the mean 7-day change was 8.5 points in the short group compared to 8.7 in the long group, a difference of 0.2 points in favor of shorter-term storage but of no significance (95% confidence interval for difference, −0.6 to 0.3; P = 0.44). Their conclusions were that all-cause mortality was similar. Fifteen patients in the shorter-term group and 11 in the longer-term group died by post-operative day 7 (p = 0.43). There were no differences in hospital or ICU stays. One limitation was that the expiration dates of each transfused unit were not concealed due to hospital policies, which could have introduced bias into the study. The researchers also noted that they were unable to design the study to differentiate differences in mortality or other uncommon clinical events. Once again, another limitation of the study is that while the effects of fresh and moderately old blood were examined, they did not study the effects of oldest blood (35–42 days) [84].

The study from Africa wherein severely anemic critically ill children who had elevated serum lactate levels along with very low Hgb levels were randomized to get newer vs. older blood had been mentioned before [36]. This study deserves special mention because it looked both at mortality but also in depth at key physiologic events: lactate production/ clearance, pulmonary dysfunction, coma and electrolyte disturbances. This study found no differences between newer and older blood for these physiologic measurements. In other words, older blood corrected the lactate production/acidosis and cerebral oxygen deficit as quickly as did fresher blood [36]. The median age of units used in the fresher blood group was approximately 8 days old, while the older units had a mean age of 32 days, a considerable difference to be sure. Does this single RCT then settle the question or negate all the biologic research to date? That is hard to say, but it certainly is worthy of note for all those interested in this complex quandary. This study was well designed in terms of separation of age of blood, and it looked at complex physiologic events that have previously been implicated in aging of stored blood. Indeed, it is very hard to reconcile this single RCT with the animal- and biochemical-based data.

One RCT did find differences in outcome and was performed in cardiac surgery. That RCT demonstrated differences in delirium with older versus fresh blood when the blood age was analyzed as a continuous variable [44]. The analysis was complicated, but blood beyond 21 days increased delirium (odds ratio of 1.02–1.23 per day of increased storage) [44]. They found no difference with a lumped comparison of fresh (<14 days) versus older (21 days) blood. Examination of blood age as a continuous variable, as Koch did, may be extremely important [44].

As noted above a major problem completing RCTs is that patients might receive blood with different ages, and unless all blood used is tightly controlled, such variations in age of blood may invalidate some findings. How does the research team deal with transfusions that involve units of many different ages of banked blood, perhaps being used outside of the "study period"? Relatively few patients who are critically ill get only 1 unit of blood. Some RCTs controlled the age of blood only during certain parts of the hospitalization, leaving other time periods to get a transfusion of any age of blood.

By limiting RCTs such that they cannot compare the farthest ends of the blood age spectrum and being "pragmatic" (meaning most patients got multiple different ages of blood – INFORM study), bias has been created. All units of blood do not age the same. Wide ranges of lactate levels, micro-particle production, potassium level, and free Hgb are found in aged blood. Therefore each 14-day-old or 35-day-old unit is not alike.

In Koch's analysis age of blood was analyzed both as a lumped (averaged age) and as a continuous variable. The RCTs mostly examine data by only comparing mean or median unit ages. If groups overlap, like they did in INFORM, then continuous variable analysis makes the most sense.

Conclusions/Going Forward

No research to date has studied really fresh warm whole blood which is what was given during the World Wars and then shown (non-randomized) to be most effective in the Iraq conflict. Also, no research has been done to compare standard practice (21–25-day-old) to the best practices of patient blood management limiting all blood transfusions. It is fundamental that we do not know the mortality risk of transfusion. Therefore, a power analysis of all the RCT studies attempting to find no difference is impossible. To show no difference in outcome, one has to rigorously design a non-inferiority trial with proper controls [85]. Such design should be based upon the known biology from prior work, as well as the known risk of the adverse outcome being tested (mortality – an unknown in this case). For blood transfusion, TRALI is the largest cause of mortality. INFORM and all the other RCTs did not consider the FDA guidelines for non-inferiority trials [86]. Without proper design, RCTs cannot claim the question has been answered. This review was not focused upon study design for each RCT.

The current practice at some blood centers is to give tertiary centers old blood to avoid outdating. Sicker patients as well as complex trauma patients tend to be in tertiary care centers. These patients in particular could be more sensitive to older blood products, as they are often in more critical condition. Few of the randomized prospective trials, with the exception of the African study in severely anemic children and the cardiac study of delirium, have been built upon hypotheses generated from biologic changes that are known in the storage lesion. In other words, we have not translated the physiology-based research to hypotheses-based human trials. Rather we have created trials that seemingly (just because they seem big), but not really, answer the question about age of blood and outcomes.

So, what should the anesthesiologist conclude? There is a paucity of data to show that Tx improves outcome in subgroups of high-risk patients. There is a tremendous amount of association data implicating transfusion in immunosuppression, TRALI, prolonged length of hospital stay, increased renal dysfunction/failure, and many other adverse outcomes. There are extensive biological reasons for the potentially increased danger of infusing stored and aged blood. Yet, RCTs to date have given medicine some conflicting evidence that older blood does not create worse outcome. Perhaps it is more accurate to say that the biologic individual mechanistic studies, retrospective studies, meta-analyses, and RCTS are rather contradictory. The RCTs were not designed as hypothesis testing or non-inferiority testing of oldest blood versus youngest blood.

The opinion poll of blood bankers is very instructional in that most (97%) still believe that minimizing the RBC storage lesion would provide clinical benefit [16]. Most (81%) know that their centers are not changing practice to fresher blood [16].

Medicine is not completely practiced based upon RCTs, and transfusion is the prime example. RCTs never proved a link between smoking and cancer, heart disease, and vascular disease. Biology in that case made sense.

It seems for the time being there will be few if any new RCTs since the American Association of Blood Bankers has said the question is answered [87]. One has to ask the rhetorical question: if the RCTs were not designed to reflect and test the biologic questions, and the RCTs had inherent flaws/bias (not designed for non-inferiority testing according to FDA guidelines), are we indeed done?

New technologies to improve storage are being developed. If age of stored blood makes no difference and the blood banking industry truly believes that (which they appear not to), then how can industrial money be put forward to reducing the storage lesions? Indeed, the question is far from settled. The reader should remember that when blood transfusion was first utilized in war zones, it was practiced with warm, fresh, whole blood from soldiers in the theatre of operation. We know the efficacy of allogeneic blood itself has not yet been appropriately tested to give us best practice answers, as well as to provide mortality risk from which non-inferiority testing should have been designed.

References

1. World Health Organization global database on blood safety: report 2004–2005. Geneva: World Health Organization; 2008.
2. Starr D. Blood: an epic history of medicine and commerce. New York: Harper Collins; 2002. p. 53–146.

3. Seghatchian J. Multilayer-strategy to enhance optimal safety of the blood supply: the role of pathogen inactivation for optimizing recipient safety and helping health care cost containment. Transfus Apher Sci. 2015;52:233–6.
4. Blood Connects Us All. World Health Organization. N.p., n.d. Web. 13 June 2016.
5. Leparc GF. Safety of the blood supply. Cancer Control. 2015;22:7–15.
6. Bolton-Maggs PH, Cohen H. Serious Hazards of Transfusion (SHOT) haemovigilance and progress in improving transfusion safety. Br J Haematol. 2013;163:303–14.
7. Koch CG, Li L, Sessler DI, et al. Duration of red-cell storage and complications after cardiac surgery. N Engl J Med. 2008;358:1229–39.
8. Weinberg JA, McGwin G Jr, Griffin RL, et al. Age of transfused blood: an independent predictor of mortality despite universal leukoreduction. J Trauma. 2008;65:279–82; discussion 282–284.
9. Robinson SD, Janssen C, Fretz EB, et al. Red blood cell storage duration and mortality in patients undergoing percutaneous coronary intervention. Am Heart J. 2010;159:876–81.
10. Eikelboom JW, Cook RJ, Liu Y, Heddle NM. Duration of red cell storage before transfusion and in-hospital mortality. Am Heart J. 2010;159:737–743.e1.
11. Edgren G, Kamper-Jørgensen M, Eloranta S, et al. Duration of red blood cell storage and survival of transfused patients. Transfusion. 2010;50:1185–95.
12. Leal-Noval SR, Muñoz-Gómez M, Arellano-Orden V, et al. Impact of age of transfused blood on cerebral oxygenation in male patients with severe traumatic brain injury. Crit Care Med. 2008;36:1290–6.
13. Gauvin F, Spinella PC, Lacroix J, et al. Association between length of storage of transfused red cells and multiple organ dysfunction syndrome in pediatric intensive care patients. Transfusion. 2010;50:1902–13.
14. Dzik W. Fresh blood for everyone? Balancing availability and quality of stored RBCs. Transf Med. 2008;18:260–5.
15. Belpulsi D, Spitalnik SL, Hod EA. The controversy over age of blood: what do clinical trials really teach us? Blood Transf. 2017;15:112–5.
16. Roback JD. Perspectives on the impact of storage duration on blood quality and transfusion outcomes. Vox Sang. 2016;111:357–64. https://doi.org/10.1111/vox.12441.
17. Qu L, Triulzi DJ. Clinical effects of red blood cell storage. Cancer Control. 2015;22:26–37.
18. Carl H, Soumya R, Srinivas P, Vani R. Oxidative stress in erythrocytes of banked ABO blood. Hematology. 2016;21:630–24.
19. Nagababu E, Scott AV, Johnson DJ, et al. Oxidative stress and rheologic properties of stored red blood cells before and after transfusion to surgical patients. Transfusion. 2016;56:1101–11.
20. The International Committee for Standardization in Hematology. Recommended methods for radioisotope red cell survival studies. Blood. 1971;38:378–86.
21. Yoshida T, Shevkoplyas SS. Anaerobic storage of red blood cells. Blood Transfus. 2010;8:220–36.
22. Paglia G, D'Alessandro A, Rolfsson Ó, et al. Biomarkers defining the metabolic age of red blood cells during cold storage. Blood. 2016;128:e43–50.
23. Rinalducci S, Zolla L. Biochemistry of storage lesions of red cells and platelet concentrates: a continuous fight implying oxidative/nitrosative/phosphorylative stress and signaling. Trans Apher Sci. 2015;52:262–9.
24. Pallotta V, Rinalducci S, Zolla L. Red blood cell storage affects the stability of cytosolic native protein complexes. Transfusion. 2015;55:1927–36.
25. Tarasev M, Chakraborty S, Alfano K. RBC mechanical fragility as a direct blood quality metric to supplement the storage time. Mil Med. 2015;180:150–7.
26. Grau M, Freiderichs P, Krehan S, et al. Decrease in red cell blood cell deformability is associated with a reduction in RBC-NOS activation during storage. Clin Hemorrheol Microcirc. 2015;16:215–29.
27. Hu X, Patel RP, Weinberg JA, et al. Membrane attack complex generation increases as a function of time in stored blood. Transfus Med. 2014;24:114–6.
28. Hess JR. Measures of stored red blood cell quality. Vox Sang. 2014;107:1–9.
29. Bennett-Guerrero E, Veldman TH, Doctor A, et al. Evolution of adverse changes in stored RBCs. Proc Natl Acad Sci U S A. 2007;104:17063–8.
30. Tsai AG, Hofmann A, Cabrales P, Intaglietta M. Perfusion vs. oxygen delivery in transfusion with "fresh" and "old" red blood cells: the experimental evidence. Transf Apher Sci. 2010;43:69–78.
31. Tsai AG, Cabrales P, Intaglietta M. Microvascular perfusion upon exchange transfusion with stored red blood cells in normovolemic anemic conditions. Transfusion. 2004;44:1626–34.
32. Scott AV, Nagababu E, Johnson DJ, et al. 2,3-diphosphoglycerate concentrations in autologous salvaged versus stored red blood cells in surgical patients after transfusion. Anesth Analg. 2016;122:616–23.
33. Marik PE, Sibbald WJ. Effect of stored-blood transfusion on oxygen-delivery in patients with sepsis. JAMA. 1993;269:3024–9.
34. Walsh TS, McArdle F, Mclellan SA, et al. Does storage time of transfused red blood cells influence regional or global indexes of tissue oxygenation in anemic critically ill patients? Crit Care Med. 2004;32:364–71.
35. Fitzgerald RD, Martin CM, Dietz GE, Doig GS, Potter RF, Sibbald WJ. Transfusing red blood cells stored in citrate phosphate dextrose adenine-1 for 28 days fails to improve tissue oxygenation in rats. Crit Care Med. 1997;25:726–32.
36. Dhabangi A, Ainomugisha B, Cserti-Gazdewich C, et al. Effect of transfusion of red blood cells with longer vs shorter storage duration on elevated blood lactate levels in children with severe anemia. JAMA. 2015;314:2514–23. https://doi.org/10.1001/jama.2015.13977.
37. Koshkaryev A, Zelig O, Manny N, Yedgar S, Barshtein G. Rejuvenation treatment of stored red blood cells reverses-storage-induced adhesion to vascular endothelial cells. Transfusion. 2009;49:2163–43.
38. Weiskopf RB, Feiner J, Hopf H, et al. Fresh blood and aged stored blood are equally efficacious in immediately reversing anemia-induced brain oxygenation deficits in humans. Anesthesiology. 2006;104:911–20.
39. Seo J, Conegliano D, Farrell M, et al. A microengineered model of RBC transfusion-induced pulmonary vascular injury. Sci Rep. 2017;7:3413.
40. Parviz Y, Hsia C, Alemayehu M, et al. The effect of fresh versus standard blood transfusion on microvascular endothelial function. Am Heart J. 2016;181:156–61.
41. Bordbar A, Johansson PI, Paglia G, et al. Identified metabolic signature for assessing red blood cell unit quality is associated with endothelial damage markers and clinical outcomes. Transfusion. 2016;56:852–62.
42. Nemkov T, Hansen KC, Dumont LJ, D'Alessandro A. Metabolomics in transfusion medicine. Transfusion. 2016;56:980–93.
43. Hayek SS, Neuman R, Ashraf K, et al. Effect of storage-aged red blood cell transfusions on endothelial function in healthy subjects. Transfusion. 2015;55:2768–9.
44. Brown CH 4th, Grega M, Seines OA, et al. Length of red cell unit storage and risk for delirium after cardiac surgery. Anesth Analg. 2014;119:242–50. https://doi.org/10.1213/ANE.0000000000000134.
45. Berra L, Pinciroli R, Stowell CP, et al. Autologous transfusion of stored red blood cells increases pulmonary artery pressure. Am J Resp Crit Care Med. 2014;190:800–7.

46. Karger R, Lukow C, Kretschmer V. Deformability of red blood cells and correlation with ATP content during storage as leukocyte-depleted whole blood. Transfus Med Hemother. 2012;39:277–82.
47. Callan MB, Patel RT, Rux AH, et al. Transfusion of 28 day-old leukoreduced or non-leukoreduced stored red blood cells induces an inflammatory response in healthy dogs. Vox Sang. 2013;105:319–27.
48. Manlhiot C, McCrindle BW, Menjak IB, et al. Longer blood storage is associated with suboptimal outcomes in high-risk pediatric cardiac surgery. Ann Thorac Surg. 2012;93:1563–9.
49. Schaer DJ, Buehler PW, Alayash AI, Belcher JD, Vercellotti GM. Hemolysis and free hemoglobin revisited: exploring hemoglobin and hemin scavengers as a novel class of therapeutic proteins. Blood. 2013;121:1276–84.
50. Baek JH, et al. Hemoglobin-driven pathophysiology is an in vivo consequence of the red blood cell storage lesion that can be attenuated in guinea pigs by haptoglobin therapy. J Clin Invest. 2012;122:1444–58.
51. Gladwin MT, Kanias T, Kim-Shapiro DB. Hemolysis and cell-free hemoglobin drive an intrinsic mechanism for human disease. J Clin Invest. 2012;122:1205–9.
52. Damiani E, Adario E, Luchetti MM, et al. Plasma free hemoglobin and microcirculatory response to fresh or old blood transfusions in sepsis. PLoS One. 2015; https://doi.org/10.1371/jopurnal.pone.0122655.
53. Rapido F, Brittenham GM, Bandyopadhyay S, et al. Prolonged red cell storage before transfusion increases extravascular hemolysis. J Clin Invest. 2017;127(1):375–82.
54. Dietrich HH, Ellsworth ML, Sprague RS, Dacey RG Jr. Red blood cell regulation of microvascular tone through adenosine triphosphate. Am J Physiol Heart Circ Physiol. 2000;278:H1294–8.
55. Raza S, Ali Baig M, Chang C, et al. A prospective study on red blood cell transfusion related hyperkalemia in critically ill patients. J Clin Med Res. 2015;7:417–21.
56. Lee AC, Heitmiller ES. Preventing pediatric transfusion-associated incidents of hyperkalemic cardiac arrest: Anesthesia Patient Safety Foundation; 2014. https://www.apsf.org/newsletters/html/2014/June/01_pedhyper.htm. Accessed October 31, 2016.
57. Weed RI, LaCelle PL, Merrill EW. Metabolic dependence of red cell deformability. J Clin Invest. 1969;48:795–809.
58. Cognasse F, Hamzeh-Cognasse H, Laradi S, et al. The role of microparticles in inflammation and transfusion: a concise review. Transfus Apher Sci. 2015;53:159–67.
59. Fischer D, Büssow J, Meybohm P, et al. Microparticles from stored red blood cells enhance procoagulant and proinflammatory activity. Transf. 2017; https://doi.org/10.1111/trf.14268.
60. Levin G, Sukhareva E, Lavrentieva A. Impact of microparticles derived from erythrocytes on fibrinolysis. J Thromb Thrombolysis. 2016;41:452–8.
61. Rubin O, Deloble J, Prudent M, et al. Red blood cell-derived microparticles isolated from blood units initiate and propagate thrombin generation. Transfusion. 2013;53:1744–54.
62. Gamonet C, Mourey G, Aupet S, et al. How to quantify microparticles in RBCs? A validated cytometry method allows the detection of an increase in microparticles during storage. Transfusion. 2017;57:504–16.
63. Said AS, Doctor A. Influence of red blood cell-derived microparticles upon vasoregulation. Blood Transfus. 2017;15:522–34.
64. Jy W, Ricci M, Shariatmadar S, et al. Microparticles in stored red blood cells as potential mediators of transfusion complications. Transfusion. 2011;51:886–93.
65. Rubin O, Canellini G, Delobel J, Lion N, Tissot JD. Red blood cell microparticles: clinical relevance. Transfus Med Hemother. 2012;39:342–7.
66. Lang F, Lang KS, Lang PA, Huber SM, Wieder T. Mechanisms and significance of eryptosis. Antioxid Redox Signal. 2006;8:1183–92.
67. Rinalducci S, Ferru E, Blasi B, Turrini F, Zolla L. Oxidative stress caspase-mediated fragmentation of cytoplasmic domain of erythrocyte band 3 during blood storage. Blood Transfus. 2012;10(Suppl 2):s55–62.
68. Solomon SB, Wang D, Sun J, et al. Mortality increases after massive exchange transfusion with older stored blood in canines with experimental pneumonia. Blood. 2013;121:1663–72.
69. D'Alessandro A, Liumbruno G, Grazzini G, Zolla L. Red blood cell storage: the story so far. Blood Transfus. 2010;8:82–8.
70. Sweeney J, Kouttab N, Kurtis J. Stored red blood cell supernatant facilitates thrombin generation. Transfusion. 2009;49:1569–79.
71. Purdy FR, Tweeddale MG, Merrick PM. Association of mortality with age of blood transfused in septic ICU patients. Can J Anaesth. 1997;44:1256–61.
72. Zallen G, Offner PJ, Moore EE, et al. Age of transfused blood is an independent risk factor for post injury multiple organ failure. Am J Surg. 1999;178:570–2.
73. Vamvakas EC, Carven JH. Length of storage of transfused red blood cells and postoperative morbidity in patients undergoing coronary artery bypass graft surgery. Transfusion. 2000;40:101–9.
74. Mynster T, Nielsen HJ, Danish RANXO5 Colorectal Cancer Study Group. Storage time of transfused blood and disease recurrence after colorectal cancer surgery. Dis Colon Rect. 2001;44:955–64.
75. Offner PJ, Moore EE, Biffl WL, Johnson JL, Silliman CC. Increased rate of infection associated with transfusion of old blood after severe injury. Arch Surg. 2002;137:711–6.
76. Leal-Noval SR, Jara-Löpez I, Garcia-Garmendia JL, et al. Influence of erythrocyte concentrate storage time on postsurgical morbidity in cardiac surgery patients. Anesthesiology. 2003;98:815–22.
77. Van de Watering L, Lorinser J, Versteegh M, Westendord R, Brand A. Effects of storage time of red blood cell transfusions on the prognosis of coronary artery bypass graft patients. Transfusion. 2006;46:1712–8.
78. Wang D, Sun J, Solomon SB, Klein HG, Natanson C. Transfusion of older stored blood and risk of death: a meta-analysis. Transfusion. 2012;52:1184–95.
79. Alexander PE, Barty R, Fei Y, et al. Transfusion of fresher vs older red blood cells in hospitalized patients: a systematic review and meta-analysis. Blood. 2016;127:400–10.
80. Da F, Hébert P, Hogan DL, et al. Effect of fresh red blood cell transfusions on clinical outcomes in premature, very low birth-weight infants: the ARIPI randomized trial. JAMA. 2012;308:1443–51.
81. Lacroix J, Hébert PC, Fergusson D, et al. The ABLE study: a randomized controlled trial on the efficacy of fresh red cell units to improve the outcome of transfused critically ill adults. Transfus Clin Biol. 2015;22:107–11.
82. Heddle NM, Cook RJ, Arnold DM, et al. Effect of short-term vs. long-term blood storage on mortality after transfusion. N Engl J Med. 2016;375:1937–45.
83. Rana R, Fernández-Pérez ER, Khan SA, et al. Transfusion-related acute lung injury and pulmonary edema in critically ill patients: a retrospective study. Transfusion. 2006;46:1478–83.
84. Goel R, Johnsons DJ, Scott AV, et al. Red blood cells stored 35 days or more are associated with adverse outcomes in high-risk patients. Transfusion. 2016;56:1690–8.
85. Non-Inferiority Clinical Trials to Establish Effectiveness-Guidelines for Industry, United States Department of Health and Human Services Food and Drug Administration, Center for Drug Evaluation and Research (CDER) Centers for Biologics Evaluation and Research (CBER), November 2016, pages 1–56.
86. Steiner ME, Ness PM, Assmann SF, et al. Effects of red-cell storage duration on patients undergoing cardiac surgery. N Engl J Med. 2015;372:1419–29.
87. AABB. Press Release: October 24, 2016: International trial shows no survival advantage with fresh red blood cells. http://www.aabb.org/press?Pages?pr161024.aspx.

Index

© Springer Nature Switzerland AG 2021
C. S. Scher et al. (eds.), *Essentials of Blood Product Management in Anesthesia Practice*,
https://doi.org/10.1007/978-3-030-59295-0

I

Printed in Singapore by Markono Print Media Pte Ltd